Lecture Notes in Medical Informatics

Edited by D. A. B. Lindberg and P. L. Reichertz

11

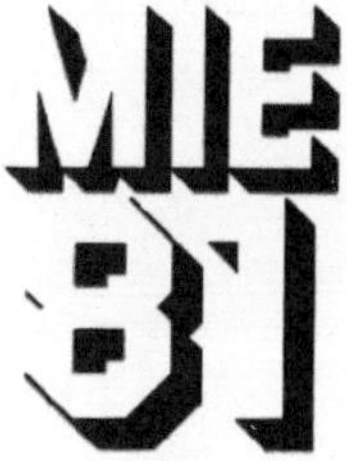

Medical Informatics Europe 81

Third Congress of the European Federation of Medical Informatics

Proceedings, Toulouse, France

March 9–13, 1981

Edited by

F. Grémy, P. Degoulet, B. Barber, and R. Salamon

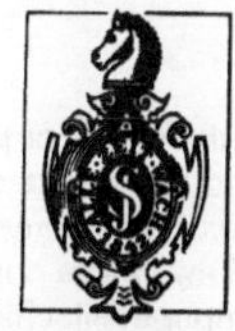

Springer-Verlag

Berlin Heidelberg New York 1981

Editors

F. Grémy
P. Degoulet
Départment de Biophysique et de Biomathématiques
Faculté de Médecine PITIE-SALPETRIERE
91, boulevard de l'Hôpital, Paris 13ème, France

B. Barber
North East Thames Regional Health Authority
40, Eastbourne Terrace, London, W2 3QR, Great Britain

R. Salamon
Département Informatique, Université BORDEAUX II
146, rue Léo Saignat, 33076 BORDEAUX CEDEX

Program Committee

F. Grémy
B. Barber
P. Degoulet
P. Dragsted
W. van Eimeren
A. Fernandes Perez de Talens
M. Laudet
J. Martin
A. Michel
F. Roger
O. Wigertz

Organizational Committee

T. Brichteau
B. Doyon
P. Fernet
F. Grémy
A. Remond
M. Valerguic

ISBN-13:978-3-540-10568-8 e-ISBN-13:978-3-642-93169-7
DOI: 10.1007/978-3-642-93169-7

2145/3140-543210

INTRODUCTION

The European Federation for Medical Informatics has established itself as a regional body coordinating activity in medical informatics. The Congress in Toulouse, MIE-81, from 9 - 13 March 1981, is the third congress in the series following MIE-78 in Cambridge, and MIB-79 in Berlin with a gap during 1980 for the world congress MEDINFO-80 in Tokyo. The rationale behind all these congresses is the scientific need to share results and ideas and the educational need to train a wide variety of professional staff in the potential of health care and medical informatics. All the caring professions are involved, doctors, scientists, nurses, para-medical staff, administrators, health care planners, community physicians, epidemiologists, statisticians, operations analysts together with specialists from the computing profession dealing with system analysis, hardware, software, languages, data-bases and the marketing of systems.

Medical Informatics is a very wide subject with ramifications throughout the health care and preventive services; it offers a key to the monitoring and improvement of patient care and to the provision of a healthier environment. The collection and evaluation of relevant data improves our understanding of the ways in which health care is provided while the availability of cheaper computer hardware and more versatile software enables us to design and implement more revealing and intelligent medical systems.

Even though typical systems take a substantial amount of time to design, implement and evaluate, there is the continuing need for informaticians to assess the current state of development across the whole field with their colleagues and for new-comers to the profession to be exposed to the variety of systems in current use and the extent of the role that medical informatics can play in health care. The rapid publication of conference papers from a multi-stream congress enables participants to follow work presented to sessions that they could not attend but more importantly this approach provides a published record with a relevant bibliography for research workers to assess which groups are active in which areas of medical informatics. In this sense such collections help to define the field and they are particularly valuable in a rapidly expanding multi-disciplinary environment. The keynote of the approach is rapid publication using camera-ready copy provided by the author. This precludes more than a minimal amount of editing; only a few of the most obscure papers can be retyped in the time scale that such an approach makes possible. Also, it does not attempt to include the actual papers as presented at the congress, which often depart from the published text, or to include any assessment of the papers and any consequential discussion. These are valuable but different areas of interest and the lack of them does not diminish the value of the papers from the point of view of a detailed examination of a topic as it would be normal to establish direct contact with professionals working in an area of interest in order to obtain their latest papers, internal reports and suggestions.

The papers for MIE-81, Toulouse, are well up to standard in presenting a variety of topics in medical informatics from a wide variety of countries in Europe and beyond.

The main focus of the congress is on three specific areas:-

1. Analysis, Evaluation & Improvement of Health Systems
2. Chronic Diseases
3. Informatics, Robotics and the Handicapped

rather than the whole range of medical and health care informatics. These are areas where the potential for growth is considerable and it is expected that they will attract considerable interest. It is hoped that this congress will have helped to foster and encourage this interest.

During the next decade medical and health care informatics will provide essential tools for the clinical care of patients, for the evaluation of patient care and for the administration and planning of health services. Computer systems will proliferate in more and more interesting medical and nursing applications providing specialised facilities to more and more practitioners. These papers represent another milestone in the growth of the subject and offer some further insight into its current development and future potential.

FRANCOIS GREMY
PATRICE DEGOULET
BARRY BARBER
ROGER SALAMON

PARIS
NOVEMBER 1980

TABLE OF CONTENTS

* Paper could not be included

Session E3: Evaluation of institutions: Out-patients care

Chairperson: Peterson, H. (Sweden)
Vice Chairperson: Fokkens, O. (Netherlands)

Session E4: Patient care: Special application to intensive care

Chairperson: Rateau, O. (IBI, Rome)
Vice chairperson: Le Gall, J.R. (France)

Session E5: Evaluation of institutions: In-patients care

Chairperson: Roger, F.H. (Belgium)
Vice chairperson: de Heaulme, M. (France)

Session E6: Evaluation of diagnostic and therapeutical procedures

Chairperson: Salamon, R. (France)
Vice chairperson: Dragsted, P. (Denmark)

* Paper could not be included

Session C2: Data Handling

Chairperson: Reichertz, P.L. (F.R.G.)
Vice chairperson: Degoulet, P. (France)

Session C4: Statistical methods, therapeutical trials

Chairperson: Überla, K. (F.R.G.)
Vice chairperson: Chastang, C. (France)

* Paper could not be included.

Session C5: Chronic diseases

Chairperson: Bernard, J. (France)
Vice chairperson: Peto, J. (U.K.)

Session C6: Methodology and epidemiological studies

Chairperson: Lechat, M. (Belgium)
Vice chairperson: Boisvieux, J.F. (France)

* Paper could not be included

Session H1: Handicapped and society

Chairperson: Woolf, H. (U.K.)
Vice chairperson: Henrard, J.C. (France)

Session H2: Informatics and handicapped

Chairperson: Rabischong, P. (France)
Vice chairperson: Tomović, R. (Yugoslavia)

* Paper could not be included

Session H3: Informatiques and handicapped

Chairperson: Townsend, H. (U.K.)
Vice chairperson: O'Moore, R. (Ireland)

Session G: General topics

Chairperson: Roux, M. (France)
Vice chairperson: Anderson, J. (U.K.)

* Paper could not be included

THE COMPUTER IN THE DOCTOR'S OFFICE

- Report on an IMIA working Conference -

by

J.R. Möhr
Universität Heidelberg
Im Neuenheimer Feld 325

Contents:

The proceedings of the conference are summarized and a personal view of the conference's results is given. Throughout references refer to the speaker of a given contribution instead of a complete list of authors.

1. Introduction

Computer applications in practicing physicians' office have become a reality by now. There are a substantial number of applications operational in different sites and the suppliers have become alerted on a broad scale of this growing market with great potential.
Therefore the IMIA working conference dealing with "The Computer in the Doctor's Office" came extremely timely with its intention to summarize the available experience and to outline directions for further developement.
The conference was organized by P.L. REICHERTZ in Hannover and took place immediatly subsequent to the Hannover Industrial Fair where a number of relevant products had been displayed. During several years of preparation, an international programme committee had shaped the conference by defining the main topics as

1 System Analysis of Ambulatory Care with Regard to EDP Support
2 Ambulatory Care Information Needs
3 Examples of Computer Applications
4 Examples of Administrative Functions
5 Evaluation of Computer Applications
6 New Technologies.

A selection of internationally renowned specialists was invited to contribute to the working sessions with these titles. In addition, the conference was opened to the interested public upon application. The discussion evolving among the scientists, physicians and industrial representatives who formed the roughly hundred attendants, were summarized by rapporteurs and included in the Proceedings, which the editors O. RIENHOFF and M.E. ABRAMS achieved to published within four month after the conference (1).

In the following, I will attempt to give an overview of the contents and the results of the conference. For this purpose, I will first give a chronologic overview of the contents and emphasize some prominent aspects of the subjects that were brought to our attention as a result of the conference.

2. Contents

2.1 Opening Leture

The Opening Lecture by H. VUORI of WHO summarized the current policy of the Regional Office for Europe in the light of the Alma Ata Conference on Primary Care and drew some conclusions concerning information requirements. VUORI stressed that the Alma Ata declaration is relevant not only for developping countries but also for affluent industrialized nations in that goals like "universal accessability and social acceptance, utilization of practical and scientifically sound methods, affordability and self determination" are equally as relevant for health care systems of industrialized nations as of developing countries. On the basis of a schematic overview of different organisational patterns of health care systems, the current trends in the development of primary care were characterized as concerning the relations of

1 institutionalized versus ambulatory care
2 secondary and tertiary care versus primary care
3 more versus less specialized services
4 health services versus social services.

Whereas currently the view prevails that secondary and tertiary care rely on a basis of primary care, and control and direct it, it was stressed that in the spirit of the Alma Ata conference this view should be reversed so that secondary and tertiary care should support primary care were it is insufficient. This means that instead of looking at the conditions of the patient that require specialized services one should look for services that are required to help the patient care for himself or to make primary care sufficient.

Therefore the beginning of the conference was marked by a very distinct and comprehensive contrast programm to the rest of the conference. It is clear that the WHO goals outlined by VUORI constitute a marked contrast to the contents of most current health care information systems in ambulatory care or elsewhere and that this view should be kept in mind by all those active in the developement of

such information systems, but even more by those determining general health care policies.
It is also clear that these views provide some clues to the questions on health care information needs,which were addressed later but were much more characterized by an acceptance of the current practice of health care. On the other hand, there was no question that the proposed changes in attitude will be difficult and slow to attain, that they will require a lot of painstaking research and development, particularly in the area of data procurement and information processing. But by outlining the way and encouraging the initiative to proceed in its direction, an appropriate frame for the conference had been defined.

2.2 Systems Analysis of Ambulatory Care with Regard to EDP Support.

This session comprized academic outlines (Cl. DIETRICH, J.R. MÖHR) as well as practical suggestions (J. ZIMMERMAN) for analyzing the requirement for EDP support of an ambulantory health care system as a whole as well as of an individual office. Ilustrative examples were given for the basic approach as well as for its results.
There was an unanimous agreement on the requirement of such analysis if one wants to come up with workable solutions that have resonably broad applicability and are not only geared to the personal and subjective requirements of an individual physician. The scope of such analysis was briefly outline by REICHERTZ in his introduction. During the discussion, it became absolutely clear that environmental factors do profoundly influence medical practice and hence information systems designed to support it. For this reason, the transfer of solutions that succeeded in one environment - the limits of which frequently coicide with the limits of a nation and its health care system - may not prove success full in another. Simple transfer is therefore risky and systems analysis is a very basic requirement. Systems and analysis is moreover feasible and not too costly compared to the costs of a failure of an entire project. The amount of systems analysis is of course relative to the project. A minimal amount is necessary if a selection among turnkey systems for given office has to be made. For the purpose of the development of such a turn

key system, analysis may well accompany the entire life cycle of the system and consume a substantial fraction of the development effort.

2.3 Ambulatory Care Information Needs.

This session was intended as a continuation of the previous one in that it attempted to define the information needs arising in physicians' offices, which should represent the focus of impact for information systems. Even though the session was affected by the inability of several speakers to attend, it served to give an overview of the means to identify information needs and their results. Again a highly pragmatic view of the fundamental needs indentified as a consequence of several years' experience as a vendor (M. BARRETT-MOORE) from the United States contrasted with a subtle and detailed analysis of subjective needs elaborated in several years of research in the Federal Republic of Germany (B. SCHWARZ). Both reports contain lists of identified requirements that should be usefull to all those active in the field. An additional report (B. SHIRES) emphasized the benefits for patient care as well as office management that may be derived from unconventional and thorough use of the data available to such information systems. An additional paper that could not be presented orally summarized the data processing requirements and related functions of an information system in a dispensary from the German Democratic Republic (W. GRIMM).

The discussion, besides emphasizing again the need to relate to the basic health care system in which needs are perceived and defined, pointed out that it may be worth while to take several steps back and to question whether it is not advisable to may be alter the operation of doctor's offices extensively in order to improve the overall systems approach and to arrive at a definition of information needs rather than data processing needs.

This requirement was illustrated by an account of the background of the approach that was taken by the group around TEMMERMAN and PEUMANS from Belgium. (See also subsequent session). The relevance of the introduction became apparent.

2.4 Examples of Computer Applications.

After the question of what should be done had been addressed in the previous session, the emphasis shifted towards the question of what had actually been done and how this was achieved. The real value of an international assembly as the one gathered during this conference became appparent during this session. Not only were different approaches to hardware (H. PETERSON, P. SJÖBERG) and software solutions (B. WAXMAN) outlined, but again the fundamental differences between perceived needs and their impact on solutions became apparent, this despite the fact that all contributors disposed of several years of solid experience. The contrasts could hardly be greater and served well to illustrate the amount of possible variation between approaches.

One type of experience is the one gained during development and application of COSTAR (B.WAXMAN). The system was developped as a highly modular adaptive system on the basis of the requirements of a community health center. It prooved transportable to a number of group practices with overwhelming success. The system was presented in a manner illustrating operational characteristics, as a supplement rather than a repeat of the published version of the paper. It became evident that a highly useful system has been made available, that supports the administrative and medical functions of larger group practices comprehensively. Its efficacy was well illustrated.

Perhaps the greatest contrast to this approach was contribution from the Netherlands (H.LAMBERTS). In his environment, the medical care process requires very little administrative processing, and the competitive situation of family physicans is secure. The result is a computer project aimed at analysis of the care process rather than support of the care processess as currently perceived. This is done effectively in a cooperative project of several physicians with minimal EDP support.

A different approach had been taken for nearly a decade by physicians in Belgium. On the basis of support generated by a successful central laboratory for private physicians, G. TEMMERMAN and W. PEUMANS were able to concetrate on support of medical functions, the gathering of medical data, its processing to insure better and more comprehensive care for patients. Unconventional and stimulating examples for useful data processing approaches for family physicians in solo practice are given in their report.

A contribution from Great Britain by J. PERRY outlined the design considerations for a primary care information system in the Oxford Community Health Project. Different types of records and a compact codification scheme that allows entry of patient data and their analysis for monitoring individual patients, or entire practice populations for various purposes was outlined in principle on the basis of ten years' experience.

A contribution from Sweden by H.PETERSON described the design characteristics and features of a specialized function key terminal used for patient registration in a comprehensive outpatient system.

2.5 Examples of Administrative Functions

Administrative functions are an important sector of the overall spectrum of doctor's office systems. There was little disagreement on this statement among conference participants although the contribution by LAMBERTS in the previous session indicated that health care systems may be organized in such a way as to make administrative chores much less bulky and dominant than in the environments from which the contributions to this session came. M.E. ABRAMS as reporteur to this session noted that there was a notable consensus on what the functions are that deserve our attention, and that it is essential that the systems should be as general as possible while appearing to the individual user as though designed specially for him.

On the basis of the experience with an extencive goverment supported development programme, an account on what should be done and what obstacles one is likely to encounter was given by E. GEISS. An extensive description of systems functions used in outpatient clinics in the U.S. was given by D.H. WILSON. Among his evaluation of failing and successful approaches, the account that the system made it possible not only to smoothe the patient management, but by interface with algortihmic management of disease, to delegate medical management functions to "physician extenders", i.e. nurses, and in doing so, to achieve a control of hypertensive patients in the order of 90% with a drop out rate of less thats 10% is likely to be remembered by the attendants.

Specific attention was given to the require ment and benefits of scheduling systems - again on the basis of experince with the COSTAR System (Mc INTOSH). These three cited constributions were the ones primarily concerned with administrative functions.

A different topic was addressed by J. ROUKENS who decribed an integrated regional system developped in the Netherlands and designed to provide data processing services to hospitals as well as practicing physicians on the basis of a multilevel computer network.

Finally the session contained a compact contribution of the experience gained by a vendor in marketing systems for solo- or small group practices. This paper has very little overlap with other papers and may be particularly appreciated by other vendors, but certainly not only by those, since all developpers in this field are in some way required to market their product.

In a very compact and comprehensive manner M. BARRETT - MOORE gave answers to the crucial questions

- Why do these companies (doctors' office computer vendors) fail?
- Why are marketing costs so great?
- Why are support requirements so large - much larger than with any previous computer system market?
- Why are there so many companies venturing in to the business of supplying turnkey computer systems to medical offices?

and

- what is the formula for successfully introducing a product in today's marketplace?

The answers shall not be repeated here but the referral to this account and the internalization of the outlined principles is highly recommended to anyone venturing into the business.

2.6 Evaluation of Computer Applications

Even if based on a thorough systems analysis, the design principles of a given system remain to some extent hypothetical. Evaluation therefore, is a must. This the more so, since the developments tend to be oriented towards realization of preexisting procedures and schemes, the efficacy of which is frequently ill understood. The contributions of this session were of two types

1. Concerning the objectives of and means and techniques for evaluation.
2. Concerning the results of evaluation.

J.P. BARRETT ho also chaired the session, introduced the topic by identifying shortcomings of current computer applications with respect to ambulatory care needs on the basis of previous evaluations. D. SIMBORG and C. VALLBONA outlined the issues that an evaluation should cover. According to the latter they may be classified according to the views of different groups of persons having contact with such systems.

- health care planners
- care providers
- consumers

On the basis of a specification of the goals relevant for these groups, he addressed the different conceivable frameworks for evaluation. With this respect a computerized information system may be evaluated as

1 a component of the health care system
2 a technological development
3 a special purpose health information system.

All these diffrent frames require different approaches to evaluation. These were outlined and finally a list of indicators of short term effects is given.

SIMBORG, differenteated between

- patient outcome measures
- process measures
  - generic process methodology
  - information theoretic methods.

The advantages and disadvantages of these methods are discussed with respect to their

- bias
- sensitively and specificety
- practicality
- validity.

These theoretical constributions were complemented by an account of an actual field test of computers which was given by P.L. REICHERTZ. In this comprehensive evaluation, subjective and objective characteristics of attitudes, processes and financial aspects were analyzed in several offices before, during and after introduction of a computer in these offices. The results were compared to several hypotheses formulated before the experiment. The relevant results are that the system, even though suboptimal, experimental, supporting only a small spectrum of essentially administrative functions, proved marginally costeffective. The subjective acceptance however was not entirely predictable by efficiency or by indicators thought to identify suitable practices.

2.7 New Technologies

The question dominating this session was formulated by G. WIEDERHOLD, its chairman, as "which novel technologies should be included in the next system".
He pointed out that the decision in answer to this question has to weigh the benefits of the new technology against its cost, recommending that the amount of change should be kept to a minimum, focussing on the satisfaction of needs rather than the attainment of an absolute optimum.

The session then emphasized mainly hardware advances -

without attempting comprehensiveness. The priciple and potential of optical discs as mass storage medium were described (J. DINKLO) and the application of voice output systems, using recorded as well as synthetic voice segments in the medical context was demonstrated (R.B. FRIEDMAN). Two contributions concerned compact systems for dedicated use in the analysis of ECG's (S. PÖPPL and J. DUDECK).

A comprehensive assessment of the impact of new VLSI technology on the interface of systems with users and their consequences for software development was given by P. LE BEUX. Finally, an account of a complex development comprising hardware and software components of a computer network for use in hospitals and doctor's offices was given by H. KUMA.

Based on the spectrum from purchasable systems over components and systems in various developmental stages to theoretical considerations, the session therefore conveyed a sense of the direction in which system development will proceed:

- networks will become available consisting of quite independent components
- at limited cost several functions will become available, which do not yet form part of current systems
- the potential for improvement of interaction with the user is considerable

3. Consequences of the Conference.

Looking back at the conference from half a year's distance, it seems like the major objectives were accomplished. The field has been covered and a starting point for future coordinated efforts has been achiened. The highlights from the point of view of someone active in the field for some years as well as invclved i designing the conference, are the following:

- At a time, when the activity of vendors in the field is drastically increasing and the consumers have become alerted of the services that may become available to them, a summary of the international experience has become available.

- Even though health care systems are vastly different, the development effort is common to all industrialized countries. It is dominantly triggered by a demand from care providers trying to improve aspects of their practice.
- The principle is usefull and practical, not only in large group practices but also solo practices.
- The functions and detailed characteristics of a given system, however are profoundly influenced by their environment.
- The requirements of the environment and of a given health care installation are amenable to analysis. The methodology for this is available. The benefits of the process exceed costs.
- Functional integration and adaptive global solutions are required and may be the key to dramatic improvement of the outcome of medical care.
- A high degree of transportability is attainable for well designed systems.
- Even if all prior requirements are met, systems evaluation is still required. The methodology of evaluation is still under development, and is not meeting all conceivable objectives. The insights that can be be gained with the available methodology do nevertheless represent a wealth of knowledge as compared to what is available without them.
- The impact of new technologies will render the systems more usable and extend the scope of applicability
- No one at the conference reported on any serious disadvantageous side effects of the use of computers in doctors' offices, appart loss of money due to unsuccessfull development.

As a direct consequence of the conference, an IMIA work study group on

Ambulatory Care Information Needs

was founded. It has meanwhile been approved by the IMIA general assembly. P.L. REICHERTZ, Hannover, is chairing the group who will address itself to the systematic comparison of different ambulatory care systems and their respective information needs. This, I am sure, will provide for the coordination demanded by several speakers at the conference as well as from the audience for further improvement of the necessary work in this field.

Reference:

1 O. RIENHOFF, M.E. ABRAMS
The Computer in the Doctor's Office
(Amsterdam, New York, Oxford: North Holland, 1980)

MESURE DE LA SANTE INDIVIDUELLE ET MESURE DE LA SANTE D'UNE POPULATION

M. GOLDBERG, W. DAB, F. GREMY

INSERM U 88 - GERSS
91, bd de l'Hôpital, F-75634 Paris Cedex 13

The classical concepts of mortality and morbidity, upon which the major health indexes are based are revisited regarding their main limitations. This paper investigates the recent attempts to improve these aspects : extension of the concept of morbidity by the introduction of disability measurements and the development of a "positive health" concept. Indexes based on these concepts are described.

"La santé est un état temporaire, et qui ne présage rien de bon"
J. Romains (Knock)

I. POURQUOI "MESURER" LA SANTE

La médecine (qui a affaire à des individus), la santé publique (qui s'occupe de populations) sont des disciplines de décision et d'action ; or toute décision dans le domaine de la santé suppose une évaluation plus ou moins explicite de l'état de santé des individus ou de la population concernés.

Choisir une thérapeutique, décider d'une intervention chirurgicale, prescrire des activités de réhabilitation sont des décisions pour lesquelles la connaissance d'un diagnostic médical, si précis soit-il, n'est pas suffisante : il faut savoir tenir compte également de l'état général du patient, de ses capacités de récupération, de son environnement économique et social. Bref, évaluer son "état de santé". Cela sera nécessaire également pour porter un jugement sur l'efficacité du traitement, car on sait bien qu'il ne suffit pas toujours de faire disparaître un symptome ou une maladie pour considérer le patient "guéri".

Pour le spécialiste de santé publique, il faut pouvoir apprécier le niveau de santé de la population dont il a la charge; identifier et évaluer l'ampleur de problèmes sanitaires spécifiques, choisir et optimiser l'allocation des ressources à mettre en oeuvre pour améliorer l'état de santé général ou pour résoudre un problème particulier et évaluer les résultats des actions entreprises : mesurer l'état de santé d'une population, c'est se donner un instrument pour définir une politique de santé au niveau de la collectivité et en apprécier les résultats.

Toutes ces raisons sont suffisantes pour justifier des recherches dans le domaine de la mesure de la santé. Il faut cependant en rajouter deux autres, à notre avis, qui sont d'un intérêt plus actuel et qui expliquent sans doute la multiplication des travaux dans ce domaine durant la dernière décennie : (i) la remise en cause de l'idéologie du triomphalisme médicale : l'idée d'un progrès continu de la science médicale s'accompagnant d'une efficacité toujours accrue des techniques en découlant est contestée par beaucoup. Le cancer n'est pas toujours vaincu, les maladies cardio-vasculaires déciment la population des pays industrialisés, les enfants des pays pauvres sont toujours au moins aussi nombreux à mourir (quand on se donne la peine de les compter), l'espérance de vie stagne depuis plusieurs années ... alors que les dépenses de santé croissent partout à un rythme que nul ne parvient à contrôler ; (ii) le public de plus en plus, ne se contente pas de s'intéresser à sa santé, mais veut participer à la gestion du système. Beaucoup d'observateurs ont décelé une crise de confiance envers les professionnels et une volonté d'être impliqué dans les changements profonds qui s'opèrent aujourd'hui un peu partout dans les systèmes de santé. Le retentissement considérable du livre d'ILLICH (1), la multiplication des ouvrages consacrés par des économistes, des sociologues, des philosophes... au domaine de la santé en sont des signes évidents.

Face à ces attentes, à ces critiques plus ou moins radicales, le monde des professionnels de la santé ressent la nécessité de relever le défi et de prouver son efficacité : nous verrons que la voie obligée d'une telle démarche passe par une amélioration des outils de mesure de la santé.

II. PEUT-ON MESURER LA SANTE ?

Selon le Petit Robert, mesurer est "l'action de déterminer la valeur de certaines grandeurs par comparaison avec une grandeur constante de même espèce prise comme terme de référence (étalon, unité)". On voit immédiatement que la possibilité d'une mesure de la sante implique le choix d'un terme de référence, d'une norme, qui semble difficilement compatible avec la définition de l'OMS : "la santé n'est pas la simple absence de maladie ou d'infirmité, c'est un état de complet bien-être physique, mental et social" (2). Que peut-être le terme de référence d'un état de complet bien-être ?

Nous verrons dans les pages qui suivent comment on a pendant longtemps esquivé ce problème, et comment on a, depuis peu, tenté de le résoudre.

III. LES OUTILS TRADITIONNELS DE LA MESURE DE LA SANTE +

Jusqu'à une période très récente, nul ne s'est avisé de mesurer l'état de

+ Cette communication, pour l'essentiel, résume les travaux publiés par les auteurs dans un article récent (5) et un rapport (6). Nous ne reprendrons notamment pas ici la bibliographie complète de ces publications, auxquelles nous renvoyons le lecteur intéressé.

santé d'un individu : il y avait bien trop à faire à tenter de lutter contre les maladies et la mort. C'est donc au niveau des populations que les premières tentatives d'une mesure quantitative ont vu le jour. On peut dater de 1693 l'établissement de la première table de mortalité pour la ville de Breslau par l'astronome HALEY (3).Le principe d'une mesure de l'état de santé en termes de morbidité semble pouvoir être attribué à CHADWICK, qui proposa de comparer en 1842, l'état de santé de deux groupes de population londonnienne (4). Depuis cette époque, l'appréciation de l'état de santé d'une population a entièrement reposé sur les concepts de mortalité et de morbidité (c'est-à-dire de dénombrement de cas de maladies codifiées par la science médicale du moment). Aujourd'hui encore, les statistiques sanitaires établies pour les ministères de la santé à travers le monde se contentent, dans les meilleurs des cas (hormis quelques tentatives que nous verrons plus loin), de compter les malades et les morts et de résumer par quelques indicateurs les chiffres obtenus. Pour la mortalité, les indicateurs reposent soit sur la fréquence des décès (il s'agit alors de nombres absolus, de taux,de ratios, bruts ou standardisés, souvent éclatés par causes spécifiques ou par classe d'âge) soit sur la durée de vie (permettant de calculer notamment des espérances de vie). Pour la morbidité aussi, les indicateurs sont construits à partir de la fréquence et de la durée des maladies : on calcule ainsi des incidences et des prévalences de maladies, qu'on ajuste souvent selon des critères simples (âge, sexe, catégorie sociale notamment).

Il ne faut certainement pas sous-estimer l'intérêt de tels indicateurs, et ce qu'ils ont pu apporter dans un contexte où les décès prématurés et les épidémies de maladies transmissibles ont dominé le tableau sanitaire de tous les pays - et continuent de le dominer dans les pays en voie de développement. Aujourd'hui encore, ils gardent leur actualité et pouvoir établir de façon fiable de tels indicateurs reste la préoccupation majeure des responsables des statistiques sanitaires dans bien des pays, même dit "développés".

On peut cependant sentir, notamment à la lumière des besoins et des critiques exposés dans l'introduction, les limites des indicateurs reposant uniquement sur la mortalité et la morbidité, spécialement dans les pays industrialisés.

Ils ne permettent pas de mesurer la répercussion (individuelle ou socio-économique) des atteintes pathologiques, ni l'efficacité des actions médicales destinées à à les combattre. Prenons l'exemple d'un malade atteint de polyarthrite chronique évolutive : dans l'état des connaissances actuelles, on ne sait pas guérir la maladie, mais on peut atténuer ses effets ; ni l'incidence ni la prévalence ne permettent d'apprécier la répercussion de la maladie (douleur, gêne fonctionnelle se traduisent par des limitations physiques ... pour l'individu, journées de travail perdues pour l'économie, etc ...). Ces indices ne permettent pas non plus d'évaluer l'amélioration éventuelle apportée par un traitement. En effet, l'incidence ne montrera que les cas nouveaux ; la prévalence est sans intérêt puisqu'il s'agit d'une maladie chronique ; la mortalité non plus, car il s'agit d'une affection réputée non mortelle.

Un autre problème que l'on rencontre avec les indicateurs classiques est qu'ils ne reflètent qu'une tendance négative de la santé, mais ne disent rien de ce que pourrait être la santé au sens extensif donné par l'OMS, ou par de nombreux autres auteurs.

La reconnaissance de ces limites ne remet pas en cause la nécessité de poursuivre dans la même voie, d'améliorer constamment les classifications utilisées et les procédures de recueil et de validation de l'information correspondante, de chercher de nouveaux indicateurs plus précis ou plus pertinents.

Il n'en reste pas moins que ces limites existent, et qu'on voit depuis quelques années de nombreux travaux tentent de proposer des solutions diverses.

IV. LES INDICATEURS DE SANTE RECENTS

Aux notions classiques de mortalité et de morbidité, deux nouveaux concepts se sont ajoutés pour former la base du développement des indicateurs de santé récemment proposés : celui de "morbidité étendue" et celui de "santé positive".

4.1. Le concept de morbidité étendue s'inscrit toujours dans le domaine d'une santé évaluée de façon négative, mais ici il ne s'agit plus de dénombrer simplement des cas de maladie, mais de prendre en compte leurs répercussions défavorables. Récemment, WOOD (7), dans le cadre de la 9ème révision de la Classification Internationale des Maladies de l'OMS, a proposé une classification des Déficiences, Incapacités et Handicaps. La déficience est considérée comme un trouble de fonctionnement, qui peut entraîner une limitation fonctionnelle, laquelle peut à son tour provoquer une restriction d'activité (ces deux derniers éléments constituant l'incapacité) ; le handicap est l'inconvénient en résultant, inconvénient de nature physique, sociale, financière, etc ... Cette catégorisation proposée par WOOD représente certainement l'état le plus achevé des tentatives de classification dans le domaine de la répercussion des problèmes de santé. Mais depuis longtemps déjà, certains auteurs ont imaginé des indicateurs applicables, soit à l'échelle individuelle, soit à celui d'une population, pour quantifier le degré d'incapacité ou de handicap (sans toujours faire une distinction claire entre ces notions complémentaires).

Ainsi, toute une famille d'indicateurs basés sur des limitations des activités de la vie quotidienne, dont le principe a été fondé par KATZ (8) sous le non "d' ADL Indexes" 'Activities of Daily Life) a été développée notamment en gériatrie. Il s'agit d'indicateurs individuels, qui prennent en compte le degré d'indépendance des personnes pour ce qui concerne des actes quotidiens comme s'habiller, se nourrir, etc. L'objectif d'une mesure quantitative ici, car les indices ADL attribuent une note globale à l'état du patient, est l'optimisation de l'allocation des ressources infirmières dans le cadre de la gestion d'institutions de soins pour malades chroniques.

Bien d'autres indicateurs individuels reposant sur la limitation des capacités fonctionnelles ont été proposés. Citons encore le classique indicateur de GROGONO et WOODGATE (9), développé pour évaluer l'amélioration de l'état de santé de patients hospitalisés : dix activités ou aspects de la vie quotidienne sont pris en compte, et une note (0 si l'activité est impossible, 0.5 si elle est gênée et 1 si elle est possible sans difficulté) comprise entre 0 et 10 est obtenue par sommation des notes partielles.

A l'échelle d'une population, plusieurs indices reflètant l'incapacité ont également été proposés. On peut par exemple classer dans cette catégorie le taux d'Années Potentielles de Vie Perdue (APVP) imaginé par ROMEDER et Mc WHINNIE (10).Il ne s'agit ici que mettre en évidence l'impact socio-économique des principales causes de décès en soustrayant l'âge de survenue des décès de 70 ans, âge choisi arbitrairement. On obtient ainsi un tableau de la mortalité par causes, classées par ordre d'importance, bien différent de celui basé sur la fréquence simple des décès. Les statistiques sanitaires publiées par le ministère de santé fédéral du Canada sont organisées de cette façon (11) et ceci n'est pas sans conséquence sur le planification des priorités sanitaires.

Mais il ne s'agit dans cet exemple que de pondérer la mortalité par l'âge de survenue des décès. On a également proposé des indicateurs qui intègrent la notion de morbidité étendue, isolément ou en association avec la mortalité. Ainsi, à partir de l'enquête nationale de santé des Etats Unis, établit-on trois indicateurs d'incapacité calculés pour des populations : nombre de jours de restriction d'activité, nombre de jours de perte d'activité majeure, et nombre de jours passés au lit (12). L'OCDE a également proposé une série d'indicateurs d'incapacité au niveau d'une population : ces indicateurs doivent refléter la perte fonctionnelle causée de facon permanente par des problèmes de santé (trois niveaux fonctionnels sont distingués : niveau organique, de la vie courante et niveau social), ainsi que la perte fonctionnelle temporaire reflètant un problème passager (13).

C'est SULLIVAN (14) qui, le premier, a proposé un indicateur composite reflétant simultanément mortalité et morbidité étendue : l'Espérance de Vie Sans Incapacité (complété par l'Espérance d'Incapacité) : il s'agit de l'espérance de vie de laquelle on retranche le temps perdu pour incapacité. Le même groupe d'experts de l'OCDE (13) a également suggéré un indicateur similaire : l'Espérance de Vie en Bonne Santé.

4.2. Le concept de santé positive est plus ambitieux, puisqu'il ne s'agit plus d'évaluer la mauvaise santé, mais d'identifier des niveaux quantifiables dans un domaine commençant à partir de l'absence de toute morbidité apparente.

Nous renvoyons le lecteur aux publications déjà citées (5, 6) pour une revue des différentes conceptualisations de la santé proposés dans la littérature.

On peut schématiquement indiquer ici qu'une mesure opérationnelle de la santé positive comporte deux étapes successives : conceptualisation de la notion de santé, avec introduction de niveaux positifs , classification des états de santé négatifs et positifs.

Pour ce qui concerne le premier point, on peut constater, à travers la littérature que la notion de santé s'apparente tantôt à des aspects <u>perceptuels</u> (se sentir en bonne santé), tantôt à des aspects <u>fonctionnels</u> (peut-on réaliser ce qu'on veut faire) ou enfin à des aspects <u>adaptatifs</u> (peut-on s'adapter à des situations de changement ou d'agression).

Quel que soit l'aspect que l'on choisit ou privilégie, il est nécessaire ensuite d'introduire des niveaux différents.Ceci peut se faire de deux façons : (i) on établit une liste d'items décrivant différents aspects de la santé ; chaque patient est alors confronté à cette liste. Finalement une méthode d'agrégation plus ou moins sophistiquée est utilisée pour composer une note globale quantifiant le niveau de santé de l'individu (ou d'une population si ont fait la somme des scores individuels). On peut citer dans cette catégorie l'indice de BRESLOW et al.,(15) qui explore les trois dimensions préconisées par l'OMS : santé physique, mentale et sociale, ou le Sickness Impact Profile (16) , orienté également vers un abord perceptuel de la santé ; (ii) on établit d'emblée une liste d'états de santé globale ; sous-jacente à cette approche apparaît l'idée introduite par REED (17) qu'il existe un continuum des états de santé, allant du meilleur au plus mauvais et permettant d'établir des listes ordonnées d'états de santé. Les auteurs qui opèrent de cette façon proposent donc une telle liste, chaque état étant caractérisé par un ensemble d'activités, de situations et/ou de jugements : le patient est confronté à la liste et affecté à un des états qui la composent. Il faut ensuite attribuer un score à chaque état pour quantifier l'état de santé individuel (ou d'une population, par sommation).

Plusieurs indicateurs de ce type existent. Nous ne citerons que celui de FANSHEL et BUSH (18) qui en est le prototype et qui a été très bien validé. Schématiquement, il s'agit d'un indicateur reposant sur une liste de onze états fonctionnels distincts (depuis cette première publication, l'indicateur a été développé d'une façon plus sophistiquée : voir (5) pour une description plus détaillée, ainsi que pour la présentation d'autres indicateurs de ce type) auxquels chaque patient est affecté selon ses réponses à des questions concernant des actes de la vie quotidienne ainsi que des symptomes et problèmes de santé. Une "utilité" (au sens de la théorie de la décision) est attribuée à chaque état afin de refléter la "préférence sociale" accordée à celui-ci. On a donc ainsi une mesure du "niveau de bien être" individuel, qu'il est possible d'agréger dans un indicateur de population qui n'est autre qu'une "espérance de vie ajustée par valeur".

5. DISCUSSION - CONCLUSION

Cette très rapide présentation des tendances actuelles des recherches dans le domaine de la mesure de la santé débouche sur plusieurs problèmes de fond. Nous n'en aborderons que deux,qui nous semblent essentiels ici.

5.1. Les limites de l'utilisation d'une expression quantifiée de la santé doivent être envisagées. Dans un article en cours de publication (19), les auteurs proposent une grille d'analyse des indicateurs de santé destinée notamment à préciser leur utilisation possible. Ils distinguent les indicateurs adaptés pour l'identification de priorités sanitaires, l'estimation de l'importance des problèmes, l'allocation des ressources et l'évaluation des actions de santé. Mais il faut clairement voir que pour aucun de ces objectifs, il n'existe d'indicateurs "parfait". Notamment, il ne faut pas oublier que beaucoup de facteurs spécifiques de l'individu et du contexte socio-culturel ont une importance souvent majeure qui ne peut être reflétée par un indicateur, si sophistiqué soit-il.

5.2. L'aspect normatif de toute mesure de la santé ne doit pas être négligé. On le retrouve à tous les niveaux de l'élaboration d'un indicateur : choix d'une conceptualisation de la santé, choix des phénomènes mesurés, introduction de pondérations diverses. Certes, une telle normativité est déjà présente dans les indicateurs traditionnels de mortalité et de morbidité, mais elle prend un caractère plus systématique encore pour les indicateurs reposant sur les concepts de morbidité étendue et de santé positive.

Malgré ces limites, il ne fait pas de doute que les travaux actuels concernant la mise au point d'indicateurs permettant d'améliorer la connaissance de l'état de santé ont permis des progrès notables par rapport aux critiques formulées au début de cet exposé. Jusqu'à présent, les spécialistes des sciences du traitement de l'information en santé se sont peu occupé de ce domaine. Ils se doivent cependant de participer à la définition, au recueil, à la validation et à la gestion des informations destinées à mesurer l'état de santé des individus et des populations.

REFERENCES

1 Illich I. Nemesis médicale. L'expropriation de la santé. Ed. du Seuil, Paris, 1975.

2 Organisation Mondiale de la Santé : Constitution de l'OMS. Annexe 1. OMS, Genève, 1958.

3. Susser M. Causal thinking. in the Health sciences (Citations des travaux de Halley,p. 17) Oxford University Press, New York London, Toronto, 1973.

4 Chadwick E. Report on the sanitary condition of the labouring population in Great Britain, 280, Edinburgh University Press, Edinburgh, 1842, Réimpression 1965.

5 Goldberg M, Dab W, Chaperon J, Fuhrer R, Grémy F : Indicateurs de santé et "Sanométrie" : les aspects conceptuels des recherches récentes sur la mesure de l'état de santé d'une population. Rev Epidem Santé Publ, 1979, 27, 1ère partie:

51-68 ; 2ème partie : 133-152.

6 Dab W. La mesure de la santé d'une population : étude critique à partir d'une typologie desindicateurs de santé. Paris, Pitié-Salpétrière, GERSS, 1980.

7 Wood PHN. Edition française du projet de Classification des déficiences, incapacités et handicaps. WHO/ICD, 9/Rev Con 7/15.15. Centre OMS pour la classication des malades. INSERM, Paris, 1975.

8 Katz S, Ford AB, Moskovitz RW, Jackson BA, Jaffe MW. The index of ADL : a standardized measure of biological and psychological function. J Am Med Assoc, 1963, 184, 914, 21.

9 Grogono AW. Woodgate DJ. Index for measuring health. Lancet II, 1971, 1024-1026.

10 Romeder JM, Mc Whinnie JR. Potential years of life lost between ages 1 and 70 : an indicator of premature mortality for health planning. Int J Epidemiol. 1977, 6, 2, 143-151.

11 Ministère de la santé nationale et du bien être social. Indicateurs du domaine de la santé, 21-24, Ottawa, 1976.

12 National center for health statistics : Disability days. United States, July 1965, June 1966, Vital and Health Statistics PHS Publication, 1000, Series 10, 47, 1968.

13 Organisation de coopération et de développement économiques : Mesure du bien-être social. Progrès accomplis dans l'élaboration des indicateurs sociaux. OCDE, Paris, 1976.

14 Sullivan DF. A single index of mortality and morbidity. HSMHA, Health reports, 1971, 86, 4, 348-354.

15 Breslow L. A quantitative approach to the World Health Organisation definition of health : physical, mental and social well-being. Int J Epidemiol. 1972, 1, 4, 347-355.

16 Bergner M, Bobbitt RA, KRESSEL S, Pollard WE, Gilson BS, Morris JR. The Sickness Impact Profile : conceptual formulation and methodology for the development of a health status measure. Int J Health Serv. 1976, 6, 417.

17 Reed LJ. Principles applying to the collection of information on health as related to socioenvironmental factors. In : Backgrounds of social medicine, 24-32, Milbank Memorial Fund, New York, 1949.

18 Fanshel S, Bush JW. A health status index and its application to health services outcome. Operations Research, 1970, 18, 6, 1021-1066.

19 Dab W, Goldberg M. Un outil multicritère d'analyse des indicateurs d'état de santé d'une population. Application à l'élaboration d'une typologie de l'utilisation des indicateurs de santé. Soumis pour publication à Rev Epidém et Santé Publ.

MEDICAL INFORMATION SYSTEMS IN THE U.S.A., 1980*

A Selected Review of Current and Future Trends in Medical Information Systems

Marion J. Ball, Ed.D.
Temple University Health Sciences Center
Philadelphia, PA 19140

The author has addressed the current state-of-the-art of Medical Information Systems in the United States as we enter the decade of the 80's. Special emphasis has been placed upon the various classes of information systems with examples in each category. An attempt has also been made to address the experiences in medical data processing over the past fifteen years with the view towards where we have failed and what we have learned from these early attempts.

I. THE PRESENT STATUS OF MEDICAL INFORMATION SYSTEMS IN THE U.S.A.

In this paper the term Medical Information Systems (MIS) is defined as "a computer-based system that receives data normally recorded about patients, creates and maintains from these data a computerized medical record for every patient, and makes the data available for the following use: patient care, administrative and business management, monitoring and evaluating medical care services, epidemiological and clinical research and planning of care resources."[1]

In the present (1980), however, it is clear that no MIS incorporating all of the above mentioned components currently exists. A future ultimate, though formable, objective could be to develop an integrated "Total Medical Information System."

Seeing the all encompassing definition of MIS, the following subdivisions of Medical Information Systems will be defined and discussed separately with an emphasis in this paper on Hospital Information Systems (HIS):

Class A Individual stand-alone Medical Systems which address the specific requirements of single departments, research users or specialities (e.g., laboratory system, drug information system, family practice system).

Class B Defines a Medical Information System specifically for hospital use called a Hospital Information System (HIS). Such a system crosses interdepartmental and specialty boundaries. Its base is institutionally and administratively oriented and has a communications network superimposed on this administrative base. The network may extend to the transmission of orders between patient floors and departments. It also may include integrated ancillary applications as well. (A further refinement into levels of distinction are defined below.)

Class C Defines another type of Hospital Information System. This type of system is oriented to the patient medical record and computer linkage of historical patient information as the foundation. When communication networks are superimposed on Class C systems they have many similarities with Class B systems. The major difference lies in structure. Class B systems use administrative or fiscal systems for a base, while Class C systems use the patient medical record as a base. The Class C system by design includes fully integrated ancillary subsystems or applications.

A further refinement of Class B Hospital Information Systems is defined as follows:

---

*Portions of this material has been submitted for publication in the Journal of Hospital Financial Management.

Class B-Level 1 Hospital Information System: A system which includes an ADT* subsystem and a data collection message switching subsystem. On-line terminals are in place throughout the hospital for order entry, communication of the orders, and for charge capture. Periodically, once or twice a day, the system must be cleared of captured charges. The only permanent data base for the duration of the patient stay is the demographic data maintained by the ADT subsystem.

Class B-Level 2 Hospital Information Systems (HIS): Includes all the capabilities of a Level 1 HIS but in addition it maintains some archival structure for retaining the patient medical record of orders, results, progress notes, etc. It also maintains data bases for ancillaries. As such it can generate medication schedules, nursing care plans, cumulative lab test results, etc. It can also provide a wealth of information upon inquiry, such as all active orders, medication profiles, incompleted laboratory tests, etc.

1.1 Class A Systems

The current proliferation of Class A Systems has been escalated as a result of major technological breakthroughs with mini-micro data processing technology, particularly during the past three years.

The vast number of specialty areas that could not have dreamed of extensive processing capabilities are now utilizing computers from the extremes of office management to esoteric individual research projects. Many physicians are supporting their own micro systems in their home.

Taking a brief look at Class A Systems used for medical consultation purposes, not necessarily mini-computer based, but addressing a specific requirement are as follows:

Duke University Cardiovascular Information System. The system provides physicians with a large data base regarding clinical experiences with coronary artery disease. The physician's management decision can be based on far more accurate and unbiased information then could be possible without the computer.[2]

Electrolyte and Acid-Base Consultation System. Beth Israel Hospital in Boston, Massachusetts has constructed a computer consultation program to help physicians manage patients with electrolyte and acid-base disorders.[3]

HELP. The HELP system is the core of a complex group of computerized subsystems developed at the Latter Day Saints Hospital in Salt Lake City, Utah. A variety of findings on symptoms data and patient status information is incorporated into the system after being acquired through laboratory tests, blood gas analysis, intensive care monitoring units, multiphasic health testing stations, and medical record abstracts. The rapidly growing data base and the decision logic are also being used in evaluation and research.[4]

INTERNIST. The INTERNIST was developed at the University of Pittsburgh as a computer-based diagnostic consultation system for problems in internal medicine.[5] It is based on assigning rough estimates of the likelihood of the association of a disease, given a finding, and a similar estimate of the likelihood of the finding, given a disease.[6]

Indiana University Medical Center Computing Reminders System. The Computer Reminders System is based on the assumption that the physician must apply a few simple rules to a few items of information many times.[7] The system provides reminders for a large percentage of the simple clinical decisions.[8]

---

*(Admissions, Discharge and Transfer)

A Class A module addressing ambulatory medical and administrative needs is incorporated into a system called COSTAR. COSTAR (Computer-Stored Ambulatory Record) is a computer-based ambulatory information system with prime emphasis on the patient record. COSTAR is also an information and communication system designed to meet both the medical care and financial-administrative needs of group practices.[9] The system also demonstrates educational and quality assurance links with Medical Information Systems.

2.1 Class B Systems

The typical Class B Hospital Information System consists of: (1) the communications network, (2) the clinical, and (3) the financial/administrative applications, among which communication occurs. The overall communications component integrates these parts into a coordinated information system. A typical Hospital Information System may have terminals of some type on each of the nursing stations, and in, or accessable to, each of the ancillary areas in the hospital. The terminals are tied together through one or more computers, which may be off-site. There are basically two levels of Class B information systems which are described below:

Class B-Level 1

To state the difference between Level 1 and Level 2 systems, reference is made to an earlier paper by Shannon and Ball.[10]

Level 1 systems emphasize communications and administration oriented applications. In general, they transmit orders, capture a day's charges, prepare census, often provide some report functions such as laboratory or pharmacy, and they frequently allow inquiry to patient financial records on the accounting computer which may be off site.

Class B-Level 2

Level 2 systems include the functions of Level 1 systems, but also provide significantly more support for various aspects of the clinical record. They not only offer expanded reporting features from such areas as laboratory, radiology, dietary and the like, but also maintain record files of these areas during the patient's hospital stay. In addition, these systems commonly support the nursing service as well.

It cannot be overemphasized that the difference between these two levels is not primary in their communications, but rather in the complexity of their integrated application functions. It is true that some systems can handle a larger variety of messages than others. Some systems have more sophisticated provisions for validating, checking, editing and formating than others. Some respond faster and offer a better variety of displays. These variations are differences in the communication portion of the system. They are important, but criteria based on these factors are not those used to distinguish between Level 1 and Level 2. <u>It is the integrated application structure and data retention that makes the difference.</u> As the evolution of Hospital Information Systems continue, Level 1 and Level 2 will most likely merge.

3.1 Class C - Medical Information Systems

A somewhat different example of a comprehensive computerized Hospital Information System defined as Class C type of Medical Information System is that which is described as still being in the process of development in the 450 bed teaching hospital at the University of Vermont in Burlington. PROMIS (the name given this system) is described as unique in two respects. It not only radically restructures the medical record, but also directs the process of clinical care "in order to address problems hindering the provision of medical care dependence on the physician's memory, ineffective organization for massive amounts of medical data, and lack of meaningful feedback about the appropriateness of care."[11] Priorities are stated to be: implementing the system throughout a hospital; continued development; validation; maintenance of the medical content display frame library; and incorporation of medical audits to ensure quality of care.[12]

The configuration of such a Hospital Information System may appear similar to Class B Hospital Information Systems, but the content is primarily oriented to the patient record. Purely administrative functions tend to be secondary. Much more patient information such as history, physical and progress data is contained in these systems because their emphasis is on reorganization and integration of direct clinical information. It is on the basis of this approach that the eventual integration of medical education and self-assessment will be based.

Looking at the marketplace of Hospital Information Systems and their currently developmental status, reference is made to a recent survey by Ball and Jacobs from which can be concluded that at present the action is in Class B-Level 1 HIS's using mini computers.[13] Four tables are presented for review from the study. This survey showed the following with regard to the current status of a Hospital Information System.

1. A least 18 vendors in the U.S. are marketing and selling Level 1 systems.
2. At present approximately 500 Level HIS systems have been installed in U.S. hospitals since 1974.
3. Hospitals over 100 beds, primarily, are opting for Level 1 Hospital Information Systems with a few in the larger hospitals planning to blend into a Level 2 Hospital Information System.
4. Mini-computers have successfully met the Level 1 Hospital Information Systems market needs.
5. CRT's have, to date, proven to be utilized by most vendors. This is to solve the man-machine interface, particularly true in the admitting area.
6. About one-half of the Level 1 vendors surveyed also provide a shared business and financial system.
7. Five out of 18 vendors marketing Level 1 systems also are presently marketing a Level 2 system.

The seven points above address only Class B-Level 1 systems. In the Class B-Level 2 system marketplace Stanley Jacobs, in a soon to be published report, identifies seven major Level 2 vendors with a total of 50 installations in the USA.

In summary, the action in U.S. Hospitals as we enter the decade of the 80's is in Class B-Level 1 Hospital Information Systems.

TABLE I

PRESENT VENDORS OF LEVEL 1 HIS

Vendor	No. Installed or in Process - April 1980	No. of Beds Least	No. of Beds Most	Order Entry Terminal
HBO & Company (HBO)	237	100	829	CRT[1]
Shared Medical Systems Corporation (SMS)	100	154	1,725	CRT
McDonnell Douglas Automation Co. (MCAUTO)	53	103	650	CRT
IBM Corporation (IBM)[3]	50 (est)			CRT
NCR Corporation (NCR)	25	284	641	BCWR or OCR
Burroughs Corporation[3]	20	191	737	CRT
DATX Corporation (DATX)	10	176	534	CARD READER
Pentamation Enterprises	9	280	800	CRT & OCR
Tymshare Medical Systems	5	80	436	CRT
Compucare, Inc.	4	250	440	CRT
Space Age Computer Systems, Inc.	4	349	845	CRT
Hospital Data Center of Virginia (HDC)	4	256	800	BCWR[2]
Spectra Medical Systems, Inc.	2	140	600	CRT
Technicon Medical Information Systems Corporation	3	446	719	CRT
Interpretive Data Systems, Inc. (IDS)	1	250	250	CRT
National Data Communications, Inc. (NADACOM)				CRT
Genitron, Inc.				BCWR
Informational Resource Electronics Corp. (IREC)				CRT (Intelligent)

NOTES: [1] CRT = Cathode Ray Tube
BCWR = Bar Code Wand Reader
OCR = Optical Character Reader

[2]HDC also utilized CRT's for inquiry purposes.

TABLE II

VENDORS OF SHARED BUSINESS AND FINANICAL SYSTEMS WHICH OFFER LEVEL 1 HIS

Vendor	1979 Data No. of Hospitals in Shared System	1980 Data No. of Level 1 HIS Installations
MCAUTO	561	53
SMS	490	100
Tymshare	150	5
Technicon	45	3
Pentamation	31	9
Space Age	26	4
HDC	24	4
HBO (IFAS)[1]	14	237

[1]HBO introduced a new real-time, terminal/network based financial system in 1979. Their new IFAS System directly interfaces in-house to HBO's Hospital Information System (MEDPRO System).

TABLE III

VENDORS OF LEVEL 1 HIS WHICH ALSO OFFER LEVEL 2 HIS

Vendor	No. of Hospitals with Level 2 HIS	No. of Hospitals with Level 1 HIS
Spectra	18	2
Technicon	17	3
NDC (NADACOM)	10	0
Burroughs	8	20
MCAUTO	6	53
IREC[1]	4	0
IBM	Not available from IBM (estimate 50)	50 est.

[1]IREC is a relatively new vendor of HIS. Its development site was The Sisters of St. Mary Hospital Group, St. Louis. Its system is modular, and IREC claims that its complete system is a genuine Level 2 HIS. This system together with facilities management therefore is also being marketed by Electronic Data Systems, Dallas, Texas.

TABLE IV

VENDOR RESERACH & DEMONSTRATION BUDGETS FOR HOSPITAL INFORMATION SYSTEMS
(SURVEY: M.J. BALL, 1980)*

Firm	R & D $ Invested to Date	R & D $ to be Invested Next 2 years
Compucare (HIS)	3,500,000	2,000,000
Datacare (PCIS)	4,000,000	1,000,000 (vary by client needs)
HBO and Company	6,000,000 (approx.)	6,000,000 (approx.)
Hospital Data Center of Virginia (HDC)	Not available	250,000
Interpretive Data Systems (IDS)	1,000,000 (approx.)	300,000
McDonnell-Douglas Automation Co.	20,000,000	4,000,000 plus
Meditech	300,00/yr. since 1969 (3,300,000)	600,000
NADACOM	15,000,000 on full line of patient data systems	will continue to make a significant investment in new development
NCR Corporation	6,000,000	3,000,000
Shared Medical Systems	6,200,000 during 1979	no specific data, but in keeping with past efforts
Spectra (Medicus)	25,000,000	"proprietary information"
Technicon Medical Information Systems	24,000,000 (incl. Lockheed)	4,000,000
Tymshare Medical Systems	"well over the million dollar mark"	not available
Burroughs	"does not report R & D expenditure specifically for the health care industry"	"does not report R&D expenditure specifically for the health care industry"
IBM (PCS)	"not available for public disclosure"	"not available for public disclosure"

*The data listed are intended to convey the scope of the aggregate funds currently spent on development activities. This data in no way should be used to compare individual vendors to each other since each of the vendors budgeting and reporting conventions differ. The main point is that HIS development is not a minor expense.

II. WHAT HAVE OUR EXPERIENCES DURING THE PAST 15 YEARS WITH MEDICAL INFORMATION SYSTEMS (MIS) TAUGHT US?

The initial expectation associated with general purpose computers for Medical Information Systems did not occur in the timeframe anticipated. The following are some of the reasons hospital information systems have not developed as rapidly as expected.[14]

1. The complex information and communication structure which takes place to deliver patient care in hospitals was grossly under-estimated. As new procedures and technology continued to be implemented, health care delivery grows more complex with or without computers.
2. The hardware and software of the 60's was grossly inadequate, rigid, unreliable and very expensive. Many hospitals are still suffering from this early failure.
3. The staffing requirements in terms of systems and data processing professionals who could manage, define, communicate and implement systems in hospitals was grossly underestimated.
4. The vendor world and mass media over sold the capabilities of computer systems which lead to unrealistic expectations and "programmed" disappointments.

What we have learned from the above experiences is as follows. To avoid future failures:

1. Top administration must be involved in the design and implementation of complex information and communication systems related to patient care and management.
2. The total commitment to long range planning integrated into all aspects of management decisions must be undertaken by the leaders in a health care facility if computerization is to have long range benefits. This function is currently in the hands of middle management in most health care institutions.
3. Staffing of hospital and/or medical computer facilities with competent individuals continues to be a major problem. However, with the evolution of successful vendors who provide services, the need is less acute because vendors perform staff functions. More emphasis will be placed on good consultants, facilities managers and vendor user relationships.

Ten years ago, at a symposium by the American Medical Association, G. Octo Barnett, M.D. gave a paper entitled "The Use of Computers in Clinical Data Management: The Ten Commandments". The same ten commandments are as valid today as they were then. Maybe in this decade of the 80's, more heed will be given to these caviots listed below:[15]

1. "Thou shall know what you want to do."
2. "Thou shall construct modular systems."
3. "Thou shall build a system that can evolve in a graceful fashion."
4. "Thou shall build a system that allows easy and rapid programming development and programming modification."
5. "Thou shall build a system that has a consistently rapid time response and is easy for the non-computernik to use."
6. "Thou shall have duplicate hardware systems."
7. "Thou shall build and implement your system as a joint effort with real users in a real situation with real problems."
8. "Thou shall be concerned with realities of the cost and projected benefit of the computer system."

9. "Innovation in computer technology is not enough; there must be an equal commitment to the potentials of radical change in other aspects of health care delivery, particularly those having to do with organization and manpower utilization."
10. "Be optimistic about the future, supportive of good work that is being done, passionate in your commitment, but always be guided by a fundamental skipticism."

III. WHAT FUTURE IMPLICATIONS INFLUENCING ADOPTION AND USE OF MEDICAL INFORMATION SYSTEMS ARE INDICATED DURING THE DECADE OF THE 80'S?

The question has been addressed by Don Lindberg as follows:

> "...as to the future of MIS (Medical Information Systems) development is that it will be strongly influenced by certain internal technical changes as well as by new concepts. The strongest internal effects will be: microprocessors, optical disk memories, artificial intelligence techniques, and computer communications technology. The first three will have a generally centrifugal effect, supporting even further decentralization of the health care system. Communications technology could also potentially support direct computer access in remote areas, but will more likely serve to centralize control over health care because of its potentiation of central file structures."[16]

From this statement, it is clear that the introduction of mini-computers and microprocessors in the area of medical computing will revolutionize the older concepts of centralized data processing. More decentralization and distributed networking is inevitable in the years ahead.

Real-time distributed computer use, in conjunction with data processing, is a rapidly growing trend. Furthermore, the cost of hardware has decreased with new options for the user becoming increasingly feasible. Indeed, major technological changes, as stated by Lindberg above, will influence the entire medical and health sciences profession.

It is hoped that government policy statements will lead to further growth and support of computers in both clinical and educational uses of health related computing. This has further implications for quality assurance, data security and communication accesses to health related data for rural medicine.

In a 1977 publication by the Office of Technology Assessment entitled, Policy Implications of Medical Information Systems," the following statements were made that are relevant to future trends in MIS:

1. Pertaining to Acceptability of Medical Care Providers. "Experience with the three computer systems discussed in this report (Technicon's MIS, COSTAR, Larry Weed's PROMIS system, also addressed as a Class C system) indicates that familiarity with a system encourages medical personnel to accept it. Providers who regularly use a system support it more strongly than those who are only occasional users."[17]
2. Technical Transferability. "Medical Information Systems will have a major impact on the provision of medical care only if they can be successfully transferred to many medical institutions. Prototype systems have been made adaptable to the various conditions of different institutions."[18]
3. Cost. "Medical Information Systems are an expensive technology. However, a majority of institutions using medical information systems have reported considerable cost savings, particularly in labor expenses. Moreover, costs of computing hardware and thus the cost of medical information systems are expected to decrease."[19]

4. General Factors. "Rate of use of medical information systems will depend on multiple factors applicable to any new technology. New developments in computing hardware and software, federal policies, and economic incentives and constraints could facilitate or impede adoption. The effect of these factors on medical information systems is now predictable."[20]

A final prediction can be made and that is that in the next decade the physician will have his own mini or micro computer in his office with access to many of the systems discussed in this paper. He will use it for his continuing medical education and self-assessment as well as a link to libraries and other national data banks not yet developed.

The next major step in HIS development, in the opinion of the author, will be in linking HIS or MIS systems with the actual practice of medicine and to the continuum of medical education. The current leader of continuing medical education in the USA, Dr. Phil R. Manning, has stated this point as follows:

> "The next big step in continuing education will come through the linking of education to real events in practice, at the time and place when the physician is developing his diagnostic and therapeutic plans for his patients."[21]

(1) Computer Technology in Medical Education and Assessment (Congress of the US, Office of Technology Assessment, Washington, D.C.) 3.

(2) Ibid., 64.

(3) Cleich HI. The Computer as a Consultant. New Engl J Med. ; 284 : 141-146.

(4) Computer Technology in Medical Education and Assessment (Congress of the US, Office of Technology Assessment, Washington, DC) 64.

(5) Lawrence SB. Internist. Forum on Med. 1 ; 4 : 44-47.

(6) Computer Technology in Medical Education and Assessment (Congress of the US, Office of Technology Assessment, Washington, DC) 3.

(7) McDonald CJ. Protocol Based Computer Reminders: The Quality of Care and the Nonperfectability of Man. New Engl J Med. ; 295 : 1351-1355

(8) Computer Technology in Medical Education and Assessment (Congress of the US, Office of Technology Assessment, Washington DC) 3.

(9) Barnett GO. A Computer-Based Medical Information System for Ambulatory Patient. Publication pending.

(10) Ball MJ and Shannon RH. Introduction to Medical Information Systems. Manual of Computers in Medical Practice (1977) : 143-149.

(11) Weed LI. A New Paradigm for Medical Education (ed.) in Recent Trends in Medical Education (The Josiah Macy, Jr. Fdn., New York, 1976).

(12) Weed LI. Medical Records, Medical Education and Patient Care (Case Western Univ., Cleveland, Ohio, 1969).

(13) Ball MJ and Jacobs SE. Information Systems: The Status of Level 1. Hospitals ; June 16, 1980 : 179-186.

(14) Ball MJ and Boyle TM. Hospital Information Systems: Past, Present and Future. Hospital Financial Management Journal ; February 1980 : 12-24.

(15) Barnett OG. The Use of Computers in Clinical Data Management: The Ten Commandments ; Comp Med. Forum : 6-8.

(16) Lindberg DAB. The Status of Medical Information Systems Technology, Hospital Information Systems--An International Perspective on Problems & Prospects (Elsevier North-Holland, Inc., New York, 1979) 19-28.

(17) Policy Implications of Medical Systems (Congress of the US, Office of Technology Assessment, Washington, DC, 1977) 55.

(18) Ibid., 56.

(19) Ibid., 58.

(20) Ibid., 62.

(21) Manning PR. The Computer and Continuing Medical Education, Hospital Information Systems--An International Perspective on Problems and Prospects (Elsevier North-Holland, Inc. New York, 1979) 49.

INTEGRATED COMPUTING & TELECOMMUNICATIONS IN BIOMEDICAL RESEARCH AND MEDICINE

A Perspective for the Eighties

Jacques J. Vidal

Computer Science Department & Brain Research Institute

University of California, Los Angeles, USA

SUMMARY

This paper reflects on the development of computer assisted medical decision making and biomedical research, and concludes that, despite long standing difficulties in these areas, routine reliance on computers will become firmly established within the current decade.

1. INTRODUCTION

In an all too familiar pattern, the real computer revolution in medicine, loudly announced in the sixties has not yet fully materialized. High hopes for computer automated patient care have been consistently frustrated during the following two decades. Hospital computers, not counting administration, are mainly found hiding in advanced instrumentation, for such functions as patient monitoring, evaluation of electrocardiograms and medical imaging.

These applications will continue to expand dramatically as low cost microprocessors will find their way into virtually every medical device. By contrast, the more challenging applications to diagnosis or treatment decisions where the physician directly interacts with the system are still in their infancy. From that angle, the impact on actual physician care has in fact remained minuscule. This situation has persisted despite a number of successful experiments in the university environment, some of which will be mentioned later.

Computer assisted decision making properly belongs to the still emerging discipline of artificial intelligence. This is the area with the highest potential impact for all tertiary activities of the human race. It is also the most difficult for the computer scientists as the field still lacks an adequate theoretical foundation and must use the digital machines of the day with the realization that they are only marginally suitable for the job.

In more than one way medicine is the worst conceivable candidate for interactive computing: the intrinsic disarray of its structures is a formidable obstacle. It has been said that the inputs of the medical record, consisting as they do of unstructured handwritten notes from the physician, numbers from test results, graphs from ECG and EEG recordings and pictorial data in the form of X-rays or scanner output, violate all rules of data organization.

There are other complex causes for the slow progress that cannot simply be traced to physician conservatism or unwillingness to change. There was initially a widespread misapprehension of what the machines could really do, both by computer professionals and by those physicians who genuinely wanted to get involved with the technology.

These caveats notwithstanding, we can safely predict that irreversible changes are in the cards for this decade although the psychological resistances and the limits imposed by cost and the lack of qualified professionals and support staff, will not disappear. On the other side, at least in the United States, many graduating physicians entering the ranks have been acquainted with computers during their school years. What their elders may have seen as a threat or, at best, a frivolous nuisance, they are more likely to perceive as an opportunity for improved practice and to understand that computer potential will have to be brought up over the years by a gigantic collaborative effort involving practitioners from both sides.

Powerful and inexpensive hardware is a necessary, if not sufficient, condition for a successful implantation into ordinary hospitals and clinics. In that respect certainly, the state of the art is quite different from that of ten years ago. explosion, the personal computer will progressively but dramatically revolutionize the work habits of everyone involved with manipulating information. There is little doubt that personalized computer environments will become as much a necessity to the physicians as to most other professionals, a projection I can draw from personal experience with integrated computing and the use of networks in biomedical research. With flexible graphics, speech output and, in the most advanced systems, speech input, the human interface will become also progressively friendlier. This in turn will induce increased participation of the medical end user rather than reliance on staff.

The second technological agent of change is the tremendous development of computer networks, public or private, accessed through common carriers. For the price of a telephone connection, networks open new doors for an integrated computerized environment with unprecedented opportunities for interpersonal communication and for gaining access to remote resources in the form of hardware, software or data.

In medical terms, access to complex information in medical data bases will yield benefits that will become impossible to ignore in anything more complex than completely routine care.

2. MANAGING THE MEDICAL RECORD

As mentioned before, the fuzzy structure of the medical record offers special challenges. A successful medical data acquisition program demands an interaction between a reference depository of medical knowledge maintained separately, and the patient data entered on line, the latter a conglomerate of inputs that include informal comments as well as a host of other data types and must allow for change over time.

A survey of the recent literature reveals a few advanced systems in active service at major universities, that tackle with the medical record in its generality.

These include PROMIS (University of Vermont)[1,2], a pioneer system initiated in 1968. PROMIS was designed with a menu oriented user interface intended for direct use by medical personnel. To each patient record in the system is associated a problem list, which in turn serves as the base for a plan of medical intervention, with the help of a shared pool of stored knowledge.

Another large system, ARAMIS, developed at Stanford, provides similar features with added facilities from monitoring patient evolution over time and identifying causal relationships[3,4]. These systems and others such as HELP[5,6] combine the generation of a computer based patient record (including in the latter case explicit entries for medical history data), with the treatment planning discussed in the next section. Others like MEDUS at Harvard [7] or the tumor registry maintained at the University of Illinois[8], are more exclusively focussed on data management and retrieval rather than interpretation.

It may be pointed out that these systems do more than simply provide a computer based record for patient management. They generate data banks for the benefit of researchers.

While this is obviously a desirable goal for the academic designers of the systems, one should realize that in clinical practice the medical record never had such lofty purpose and thus could accomodate omissions that would invalidate it as research data.

This ambivalence has not always been recognized; that aspect of the task requires a large machine. Furthermore, under the still primitive systems presently in operation, it places added demands on the acting physician which can become major stumbling blocks to eventual acceptance in the field.

By contrast, small, microprocessor based stand-alone medical data systems very similar in cost and complexity to many other clinical instruments, are now realizable[9]. It is more than likely that systems of this type will proliferate in the future.

3. DIAGNOSIS AND THERAPEUTICS: THE DECISION TOOLS

Once the problems associated with the computer formatting of patient data have been overcome, the stage is set for the decision making aspects and the management of the medical intervention. The decision tools are programs for diagnosis, consultation and the planning of treatment including prescription of tests as well as drug selection and dosages.

Medical Diagnosis has been a tempting problem for researchers in pattern recognition and decision theory, a broad field at the juncture of system theory and artificial intelligence. Serious work in that area has been underway for some time: a 1974 survey of pattern recognition in medical diagnosis[10] already shows more than 120 references.

Some of the systems mentioned in the previous section are in fact integrated diagnostic and treatment systems that exploit the computerized medical record. Typically they are confined to a specialized area of expertise such as arthritis[3], or abdominal pain[11].

While the pattern recognition methodology varies among authors, the basic problem remains the assignement of likelihoods to a given illness on the basis of the recorded "symptoms" and history data. This is a difficult problem, not all elements of which are quantifiable. Straightforward Bayesian classification has been often used although it is clear that more sophisticated methods are advisable. Isolated symptoms are seldom additive in their contribution to the disease probabilities. To form primitives for the decision process symptoms should be grouped for interdependence or causality. The Bayesian approach is also a one step decision. A more sensible alternative uses sequential decision trees and adjusts likelihood values at each step[9,12].

Regardless of the algorithm chosen for decision however, the reference data translates into symptom probabilities conditional to each disease. It must be acquired either by expert consultation or from statistical analyses of large number of medical records for which positive diagnosis have been procured.

One promising approach is to organize knowledge in the form of production rules[13]. consisting of premises and conclusions, each bound to a "certainty" factor or "strength" reflecting the relative power of the premises in their support of the conclusion. The general purpose MEDICO program[14] is a clinical system of this type.

It is clear that computer-aided diagnosis is still very limited in scope and power and will be so for some time to come. Human experts actually perform well in diagnosis and some of the factual and procedural knowledge they use cannot be specified a priori[15]. As a result, to acquire and internally structure a proper knowledge base into the system (a process sometimes called "priming") is a major undertaking. Ideally, it requires systems capable of natural language understanding and concept identification.

Work on such capabilities and on the underlying theories of fuzzy logic and inexact reasoning are contemporary topics in artificial intelligence and are progressing rapidly. It is however doubtful that full scale applications will reach the medical environment before the end of the eighties or well into the next decade.

Computer assistance in the areas of drug therapeutics, specifically drug selection and dosages fall in somewhat different categories. One may first observe that drug selection could greatly benefit from access through computer networks to large pharmaceutical data bases, independently maintained and containing cross-indexed information about drug indications, contraindications, toxicity, side-effects, cost etc... Pharmaceutical information is accumulating fast and few physician can claim to be completely informed. For functions of this type, computerized data bases have enormous advantages over printed compendiums, in terms of retrieval, association and updating. There are however thorny problems associated with financing of such facilities and with garanties of integrity and completeness of content.

By contrast, the determination of drug dosage does not require a large infrastructure and for which some very successful prototypes have been implemented. This application has great social and economic significance because of the high incidence of adverse reactions in hospitalized patients especially to digitalis based, anti-arrythmia and antimicrobial drugs[16]. Drug effects are quantifiable. Precise prescriptions depends on characteristics such as weight age and sex, some physiological variables with different values for each patient, and on pharmacokinetic variables which can be assessed empirically from population studies. Theoretical models of action for a given drug can relate these quantities to the target blood level and can be used to obtain optimal dosagés and time distribution of drug delivery[16,17,18,19].

References

1. Schultz, J. R., "PROMIS, Problem-oriented medical information system," in Proc. Third Illinois Conf. on Medical Information (1976).

2. Weed, L.L., in Computer Application in Medical Care: Proc. 2nd. Annual Symposium, ed. Orthner, F.H., Washington D.C. (November 1978).

3. Fries, J., "Time-oriented patient records and a computer databank," JAMA Vol. 222(12), pp.1536-1542 (1972).

4. Wiederhold, G., Fries, J., and Weyl, S., "Structured organization of clinical data bases," AFIPS Conference Proc., pp.49-485 (1978).

5. Warner, H. R., Olmsted, C., and Rutherford, B., "HELP - A program for medical decision-making," Comput. and Biomed. Research Vol. 5, pp.65-74 (172).

6. Warner, H.R., Rutherford, B., and Houtchens, E., "A sequential approach to history taking and diagnosis," Computers and Biomedical Research Vol. 5, pp.256-262 (1972).

7. Miller, P. and Strong, R., "Clinical care and research using MEDUS/A, A medically oriented data base management system," pp. 288-297 in IEEE Second Annual Conference on Medical Applications.

8. An integrated database system for managing medical information:, IEEE Second Annual Conference on Medical Applications.

9. Fisher, P.R. and Kurlander, D.J., "Microcomputers in medical diagnosis," pp. 75-79 in ACM Proc. Ann. Conf. (1980).

10. Patrick, E., Stelmock, F., and Shen, L., "Review of pattern recognition in medical diagnosis and consulting relative to a new system model," pp. 1-16 in IEEE Trans on Systems, Man, and Cybernetics (1974).

11. deDombal, P. T., Leaper, D., Horrocks, J., Staniland, J., and McCann, A, "Human and computer-aided diagnosis of abdominal pain," Brit. Med. J., Vol. 1, pp.376-380 (174).

12. Kulikowski, C. A., "Pattern recognition approach to medical diagnosis," pp. 173-178 in IEEE Trans. on Systems Science and Cybernetics, (1970).

13. Davis, R., Buchanan, B., and Shortliffe, E., "Production rules as a representation for a knowledge-based consultation program," Artificial Intelligence Vol. 8, pp.15-45 (1977).

14. Walser, R. and McCormick, B., "Organization of clinical knowledge in MEDICO," Proc. Third Annual Conference on Medical Information Systems (1976).

15. Gorry, G. A. , "Computer-assisted clinical decision-making," Method. Inform. Med. Vol. 12, pp.45-51 (1973).

16. Sheiner, L. B., Rosenberg, B., and Melmon, K., "Computer-aided drug dosage," Proc. AFIPS Spring Joint Computer Conference, pp.1093-1099 (1972).

17. Peck, C. C., Sheiner, L., Carrol, M., Martin, M., Combs, D., and Melmon, K., "Computer-assisted digoxin therapy," N. Engl. J. Med., pp.289-441 (1973).

18. Bleich, H. L., "Computer-based Consultation: Acid-base disorders," American Journal of Medicine Vol. 53, pp.285-291 (1972).

19. Shortliffe, E. H., Computer-Based Medical Consultations, MYCIN, Elsevier/North Holland, New York (1976).

CENTRALIZATION AND DECENTRALIZATION ASPECTS IN HOSPITAL INFORMATION SYSTEMS

A.R. Bakker
BAZIS, University Hospital Leyden,
The Netherlands

ABSTRACT

Initially because of restrictions in the computer technology hospital information systems (HIS) were set up as centralized systems. Nowadays the usefulness of centralization for these systems is questioned a lot.
In this paper various aspects of a HIS are considered with regard to centralization. It is concluded that centralization is essential for datadefinition and coordination of software development while decentralization is essential for the i/o functions. Attention is further given to: long-term storage, short-term storage processing and operating. It is concluded that a centralized structure of a HIS is still attractive in general. Limitations for centralization are indicated.

1. INTRODUCTION

Initial attempts to realize an integrated hospital information system were based on a centralized structure of these systems (1), (2), (3), (4), (5).
These centralized structure was at that time hardly questioned because the state of the art in computer technology and the price of hardware forced the designers towards that structure. Most attempt to realize a HIS lead to disappointments with a lot of critics as to user-friendliness, performance, reliability and flexibility. The problems are at least partly caused by reasons like lack of experience with complex information systems, restrictions in hardware and system software facilities, experience in introduction of systems with such an intensive user interface. Nevertheless the centralized structure itself was often blamed for the lack of success.
Modern developments in computer technology like decreasing price/performance ratio, storage facilities, micro processors and network software, stimulate discussion on the question centralized versus decentralized (6).
Users often have the feeling that 'buying their own computer' might solve a lot of problems.
This paper deals with considerations on aspects of centralization and decentralization in integrated hospital information systems. It will be tried to answer the question whether decentralization is attractive as an answer to the existing disadvantages of integrated information systems.
Also limitations of the centralized approach will be discussed.

2. OBJECTIVES OF HOSPITAL INFORMATION SYSTEM

Before discussing the various aspects of centralization and decentralization the main objectives of integrated hospital information systems will be summarized first. An integrated hospital information system can be described as an information system for a hospital where data are stored in their mutual relationship within a computer system. The data are gathered near the source and supplied to authorized users at the moment and at the place where they need those.
The information system is also charged with tasks in the area of coordination of activities within the hospital.

With the introduction of a hospital information system one is aiming at:

- improvement of the quality op patient care; up-to-date information on the patient will be available quicker, more accurate and more complete,
- more efficient utilization of the available resources; activities can better be coordinated, a part of human activities can be taken over by equipment and processes can be accelerated,
- support of research and management; from the data stored in the computer system well-ordered selections and overviews can be made according to various points of view,
- support of educational activities; from the data stored relevant cases or illustrations can be selected.

3. THREE DIFFERENT STRUCTURES OF HOSPITAL INFORMATION SYSTEMS

It is considered to be essential that various users have access to the data that become available for a specific patient at various places in the organizations that use the information system concerned. For that reason organizations using a number of stand-alone computer systems, which is as a matter of fact a very decentralized approach, are not considered here because the fast access to data is not realized and according to the description given in chapter 2 such a way of information processing is not called a HIS.
Although the primary way of use of the hospital information system is of a conversational character a number of batch type functions have to be carried out, mainly to support administration, statistical analysis and archives.
Although there are a lot of appearances of hospital information systems three basically different structures can be distinguished.

A. The centralized structure

In this structure there is a central computer system with a central database. For reasons of availability the system is often duplicated. To this system various types of remote terminals are connected that may even be dedicated computer systems. It is considered to be essential in this structure A that all data that are of common interest to users of the system are stored in the central database. If satellite computers are connected these may hold their own files, but only as far as these files are only of local importance to the unit where the satellite is installed.

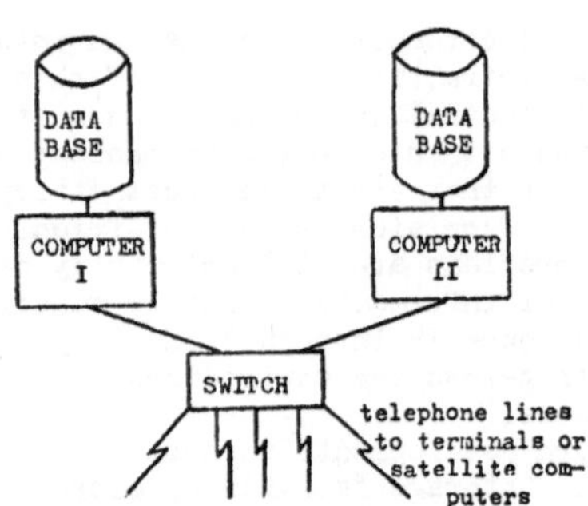

Fig. 1. Centralized system, one computer system for production purposes, the other for back-up.

Most of the well-known operational systems like El Camino, London Hospital, Stockholm county, Leyden University Hospital, Hannover, Geneva, Kiel etc. (1), (2), (4), (9) are of the structure A. Examples of terminal-type satellites are: 1. computers for ECG analysis, where reporting of results and archiving is carried out by the central system. 2. Satellite computers for process control of measurement equipment in laboratories.
The scope of the information systems may be quite different and vary from a medium size hospital to a region where several hospitals and other health care organizations are serviced by the system.

B. The star-type network

In this structure a number of computer systems (nodes) is organized around a central system and connected to it by means of data communication facilities. Terminals in general are connected to the remote computer systems that hold their own (part of the) database. The central computer system also has its database

that is mainly applied for long-term storage of data and as a back-up for the remote computer systems. The filosophy behind this structure is that users mainly will need access to data in their local database and only for a restricted percentage of the use need access either to the central database for historical data or to other remote computers for data gathered at another place in the organization.
Batch processing is carried out mainly by means of the central computer system. In this structure at remote computer systems only a limited attendance of computer professionals is supposed.
This type of structure may even consist of more layers where e.g. in a hospital there is in itself a star-type network where the central systems from this hospital-level are hooked up to a central regional computer system.

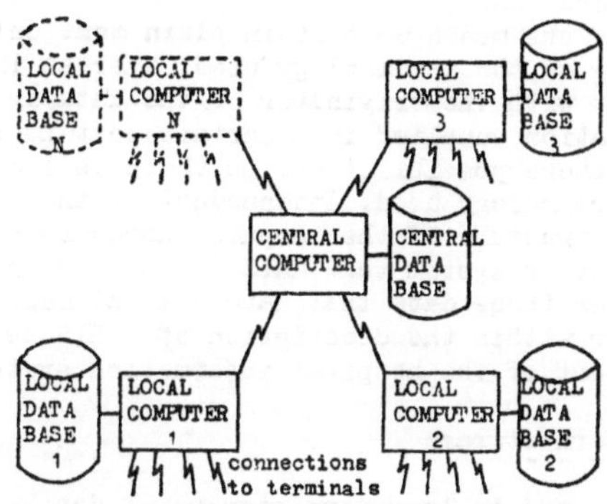

Fig. 2. The star network.

C. Mesh-type network

In this type of network there is in principle no hierarchy between the composing computers. For each computer system there is a database facility where both short-term and long-term storage is realized for the organization where this computer belongs to.
Back-up facilities can either be realized by means of duplication at each node in the network or by duplication of storage at one of the other nodes together with data communication switching facilities for the terminal equipment. Batch-processing is carried out at each node for the own organization. The nodes in itself may be of star-type structure including satellite computers.

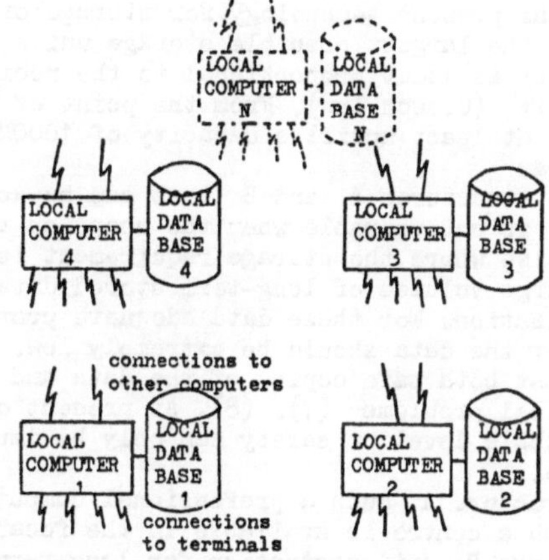

Fig. 3. The mesh network.

4. ASPECTS TO BE CONSIDERED

In this chapter various aspects will be considered that are of importance in the discussion as to (de-)centralization. For some of these aspects firm conclusions can be drawn as to the desirability of either decentralization or centralization. For other aspects only a number of remarks can be made about advantages and disadvantages at the present time and expectations for the forseeable future.

Data definition and database management

Since hospital information systems are meant amongst others to improve the exchange of information both within and between the participating organizations an environment should be created where this exchange of information is feasible. This implies that there should be agreement as to shape and meaning of messages to be exchanged.
It makes no sense to set up an information system with as one of the objectives a more up-to-date overview of the data that has been collected at various places for the same patient if no rules exist about the shape and meaning of the

registered data.
Even if the messages contain plain text only agreement should exist as to the meaning of the terminology used. Whereas in manual information systems the direct contact with the originator of the data or his way of handwriting may put the information supplied in a certain context the automatic exchange of information lacks these possibilities. So there is a clear need for a unique definition of the terminology used. Independent of the choice of a centralized or a decentralized structure of the computer hardware system it is essential for a hospital information system that data definition and maintenance be centralized.
Only for those data that have a local meaning only some freedom can be allowed. However within the description of a HIS as given in chapter 2 these data hardly make part of the hospital information systems database.

Long-term storage

With regard to long-term storage of data we not only have to think of data on patient history and utilization of available resources, but also of medical knowledge, the description of the organization and the procedures applied.
For the long-term storage of data we'll have to deal with a considerable volume. For the present state of the art of hospital information systems several hundreds of millions of bytes is a typical storage requirement. It can be expected that with the increase of application of a HIS within 10 years this size will increase with at least a factor ten.
With the present technology for storage of large volumes of data it is attractive to use the largest possible storage units since the price per megabyte storage-capacity is about proportional to the reciprocal of the squareroot of the capacity per unit (Grosch law). From the point of view of cost it is attractive at the moment at least uptill a capacity of 1000Mbytes to centralize long-term storage of data.
In the structures A and B this can be achieved while in structure C this cost aspect is unfavourable when the scope on the nodes in this structure is limited at a size where the storage requirement is considerably below 1000Mbytes.
The large volumes of long-term stored data are of great value to the using organization. For these data adequate protection is very important. The risk of loss of the data should be extremely low. Data protection measures should include at least both safe copies of the data and procedures for reconstruction after technical problems (7), (8). At present data protection measures that give an acceptable level of safety can only be implemented within a professional computercentre.
In structure A such a professional computercentre is implicit while in structure B such a centre is available in the focal point of the system. If within structure B data protection for long-term storage is realized in the focal computer system an acceptable level of protection can be reached. In structure C such measures only can be implemented when the node computercentres are above a critical size. Again we find restrictions as to the level of decentralization in structure C.
As long as the data stored are text type data or comparable quantities, data transmission sets no restrictions as to the location where the data are stored.
When complete images are stored however (e.g. x-ray images) transmission over large distances of images with about one million pixels gives serious timingproblems with technology available at present. Because of these timing problems and the cost involved in their solution it may be necessary to store those imagedata at the location close to the main users (in this case probably the x-ray department itself). Since storage of those imgaes on a large scale within a HIS is no common practice yet and new technologies for transmission are developing it is unclear at this moment whether this problem will set serious restrictions on the centralization of storage capacity.

Short-term data

For short-term storage of data the required volume of storage capacity is much smaller than that for the long-term storage. The cost advantage of centralized storage because of Grosch law is here less attractive than in the former case.

A considerable percentage of the short-term storage of data is made up of working files. These working files often are mainly of importance for one department or group of users.. In the case these working files are only necessary for the preparation of data that only finally are of interest to other users (e.g. data of a sample plate in a laboratory before the data are authorized) there is no functional disadvantage in decentralization.
In the case other users are interested in the contents of the working files, decentralization, if applied, should not restrict the accessability by other users. This implies that good communication facilities should be realized and as far as data definition is concerned also those working files should be controlled by a central database management.
When the working files for a certain application are implemented on a dedicated computer system the measures for availability and data protection may be geared to the special requirements of this application. In some cases the requirement of duplication of equipment may be avoided in this way. For instance if a good manual emergency procedure can be developed.
For some batch type activities temporary files of considerable size may be necessary. This need for additional storage capacity should be taken into account and can best be realized in a central facility.

Input-Output facilities

It is essential within the concept of a HIS that input and output of data can be realized at the place where users are active. This implies that these facilities should be heavyly decentralized. Nowadays the number of terminals installed in hospitals with an advanced information system amounts to 15 to 25% of the number of beds. It should be realized that these terminals are not only installed in wards and outpatient departments but also in central supporting facilities, laboratories and administration. With the decreasing price of computer terminals it can be expected that these decentralization will proceed even further. As a long-term trend we can expect the number of terminals in a hospital to become of the same order of magnitude as the number of telephones.
There will be hardly a difference in cost for the various structures A,B and C. The message switching facilities and data communication equipment show a large range of variation. There is no evidence for an essential difference in cost level. With an increasing number of terminals installed the requirement for availability of terminal hardware may decrease because it will be easier to use a near-by other terminal in case of problems. On the other hand when emphasis on conversational use increases the need for a high availability of the systems functions increases. Decentralized i/o puts heavy requirements on the data protection (8); hardware, software and organizational measures should be implemented to regulate the users access rights. Since each of the structures A,B and C is meant to yield users access to the data in essence the data protection requirements are the same. Because of the decreasing price and increasing performance of printing terminals the need for central lineprinters will be decreasing in the coming years.

Software development and maintenance

The costs for development and maintenance of application software for a HIS are very high (at least in the order of magnitude of hundred manyears). Because of the decreasing price/performance ratio of computer hardware the implementation of more functions within a HIS will become attractive.
This effect will lead to an even further increase of the software effort. Although some improvement in efficiency of software development can be expected, as a total the software effort for a hospital information system can be expected to increase in the future.
The level of cost for software development and maintenance leads to the need to share this increasing cost between various using organizations. This may lead to a centralization of development. It should be realized that transportation of application software from one approach (to an integrated hospital) to another approach is in general not possible. Transportation of application software is

only possible when a strong coordination of development is achieved.
The centralization of software development can be achieved when integrated hospital information systems are marketed on a commercial base. Another way may be cooperation of various organizations that use a similar information system (9). The cost of software development and maintenance will depend heavily on the scope of application of the resulting system. Quality of software can be expected to be better for products with a broad scope than for those with only one or two using organizations. Also for dataprotection a broad scope of the product gives a better chance that sufficient attention can be paid to problems in the field of availability, data and program integrity and usage integrity.

Processing

We should distinguish between the processing of data that is directly related to a certain process e.g. analysis of ECG's, computation of a measurement result, formatting of screen lay-outs and output messages on one hand and the processing of data from the databank when more than one data type is involved on the other hand. In the former case decentralization may be a means to unload the central computer system. There are no principal disadvantages of such a decentralization. For the latter case we should realize that the integration aspect is essential here, restricting the possibility to decentralize the processing from the location of the integrated database.
In laboratory information processing for instance, the medication of the patient, his diet, his location in the hospital together with his demographic data will be taken into account when reporting the result of a certain test. With a further evolution of the information handling concepts dealing with the integrated character of the HIS the attractivity of department related computer systems will diminish. The task of department related systems will more and more be restricted to the local housekeeping of the department and the basic processing of the data (e.g. ECG analysis).
Since the cost of processing capacity has reduced dramatically because of the introduction of new technologies there is no strong cost evidence for centralization at the moment as far as CPU consumption is concerned.
However the processing will need access to the integrated database which will set limits to the decentralization. Modern data communication facilities on the other hand make communication of complete medical and administrative history of patients between various nodes in a HIS system feasible. Handling of display screens and the formatting of messages might be distributed quite a lot,even to the terminal devices itself,by means of the application of micro-processors that might hold both menu systems and department related data. Although at this moment from a cost point of view simple terminals are still attractive unloading of the central CPU capacity when necessary can be expected to become feasible within a few years.
Decentralization of CPU capacity as e.g. indicated in structure B and C leads to increased intensity of use of data communication facilities which might lead to need for additional measures in the data protection area.
Where the measures to be taken to achieve a high availability of processing capacity are rather obvious in structure A (duplication of equipment) the choice of these measures in structure B and C is less simple, since full duplication probably is not the best solution here and back-up by means of remote equipment should be organized.

Operating

Although hospital information systems are meant for automatic processing of data in the hospital, the system itself needs operating assistance.
Operator activities comprise:
- handling and supervision of equipment (support of malfunctioning terminals is a large percentage of the effort in this area)
- supervision of batch type jobs and handling of the resulting output
- production of safecopies of files and handling of these,
- effectuation of data protection measures.

The costs of operating form a considerable percentage of the total running cost of a operational HIS. In literature figures of 30 to 40% are reported (9).
Although it would be very interesting to know the effect of the choice between the structures A,B and C on the operating cost no figures are available in this area till now. The situation is complicated by the fact that in a highly distributed environment certain operator tasks will be carried out by employees of the using departments. About the effects on operating effort to be expected when decentralization is applied the following remarks can be made:

- supervision of computer equipment itself will be simpler when this equipment is concentrated in one centre like in structure A.
- supervision of terminals might be easier when this is carried out by a local responsible person, as long as he has access to suffiecient spare equipment.
- supervision of batch jobs probably will be more efficient when these are concentrated in one centre as in structures A and B. The output of batch jobs might be distributed (at least partly) via the terminal network.
- Since performance of storage devices increases with increasing capacity, the time needed for back-up copies of files will be least in the centralized approach for the database as in structure A and (more or less) in structure B.
- data protection measures can best be maintained in a professional computercentre of a certain size as realized in structure A. Especially in structure C considerable effort will be necessary to realize an acceptable level of dataprotection.

5. COSTS, AVAILABILITY AND DATA PROTECTION ONCE MORE

In the previous chapter various aspects have been considered, attention has been given amongst others to cost, availability and data protection. In this chapter these three aspects are considered in itself.

Costs

The cost aspect is important as far as development effort is concerned, sharing of cost is essential to arrive at an acceptable costlevel. This sharing of costs is only possible for a centralized set-up of the development effort or at least with a strong central coordination. Centralization of long-term storage has advantages as long as Grosch law applies (at present up to a capacity of about 1000Mbytes).

Availability

Measures to arrive at a high availability of the services of the system are easier in structure A (duplication of equipment) and become gradually more difficult when structure B or C is chosen.
Although there is some progress in the development of software for distributed databases, technical problems in this area, especially in case of hardware failures, are still considerable. In case of malfunction of the system, the effect on the organization is highest in structure A because the problems are synchronized for all participating organizations.

Data protection

It is rather popular misunderstanding that data protection can easier be realized in a decentralized approach as e.g. structure C. Since also in that approach users can get access to data stored in other systems, regulations of access rights should be of the same order of sophistication as the other structures. Protections measures in hardware, software and procedures require a certain level of professional climate around the computer system. This level can only be realized if the composing computer systems in the structure are not too small. Necessary measures for dataprotection comprise amongst others safecopies of files, user authentication, access to computer facilities, fire protection, etc. (8)

6.LIMITATIONS OF CENTRALIZATION

In the preceeding chapters no significant advantages of structure B and C as compared to A have been found. On the contrary centralization still has attractive advantages. In additioning the overwhelming majority of succesful hospital information systems is of structure A, so it might be concluded that this structure A should be preferred anyhow. On the other hand nobody suggests to build one worldwide or even nationwide HIS according to structure A. In such a gigantic system the problems of the volume of work to be processed would be practically unsolvable. Moreover the datacommunication problems would become considerable. As indicated earlier in this paper (scale effect on cost, size of operation that makes professional quality attainable easy exchange of information) appear already at a much smaller size of system. In practice the biggest systems operational are at most aiming at the region of about 10,000 hospital beds or consist of local hospital information systems that share a common batch processing facility and file back-up.
Limits to centralization are on the upper side set by:
- capacity of computer systems,
- the unit size of the largest mass-storage units,
- data communication cost if participating organizations are spread over a wide area,

Limits at the lower end are set by:
- relative increase of operating costs for smaller centres,
- relative increase of equipment cost for smaller units (Grosch law),
- cost of data protection.

Of course several separate systems can be more or less loosely connected to allow for some exchange of information between these systems.
The optimum working area for a system according to the centralized approach seems to be somewhere around 3000 beds at the moment.
It is not expected that this figure will change dramatically in the coming years.

7. CONCLUSION

When considering three types of structures of an integrated hospital information system (fully centralized system A, star-type network B, mesh-type network C) according to a number of aspects it is found that:
- data definition should be centralized anyhow,
- development effort should be shared between different organizations and need a strong central coordination,
- cost for long-term storage are least when organized at the central location (structure A or B),
- professional operating (that's especially important for batch type activity and data protection measures) is best realized in a computercentre of considerable size as present in structure A and to some extent in structure B
- structure A gives the best opportunities for realization of adequate data protection measures,
- over-all availability of services of the system can best be realized in structure A. However the scope of the problems arising in case of system fâilure is also largest for structure A.

It is concluded that the centralized approach is most attractive for a HIS, with a limit of scope of around 3000 beds.

References

1. Shannon, R.H.(ed); Hospital Information Systems; IFIP working conference. North-Holland Amsterdam 1979.
2. van Egmond, J., de Vries Robbé, P.F., Levy, A.H.; Information systems for patient care.
North-Holland Amsterdam 1976.

3. Abrahamsson, S.,et al; Danderyd hospital computer system 11, total regional system for medical care.
Computers in biomedical research 3 1970.

4. Lindberg, D.A.B.; Growth of medical information systems in the United States.
Lexington Books Boston, Mass. 1979.

5. Collen, M.F. (ed); Hospital computer systems.
Wiley New York 1975

6. Bakker, A.R.; centralized versus decentralized hospital information systems.
Proc Medinfo 77 pp 895-899. North-Holland Amsterdam 1977.

7. Griesser, G.G.(ed); Realization of dataprotection in health information systems.
North-Holland Amsterdam 1977.

8. Griesser, G.G.,et al; Dataprotection in health information systems.
North-Holland Amsterdam 1980.

9. Bakker, A.R.; Scope and limitations of a mini-based centralized hospital information system.
Proc Medinfo 1980 pp 505-509. North-Holland Amsterdam 1980.

HEALTH INFORMATION SYSTEMS FOR REMOTE AREAS.

b/ Jan-Ivar Kvamme, Alta, Norway.

SUMMARY.

Information systems may turn out to be an important means in the solution of some of the main problems in remote areas:

(1) absence of general medical survey,

(2) shortage of doctors

(3) lack of continuity

(4) absence of a system of evaluation.

Some projects in Northern Norway aimed at solving this problems are discribed:

(1) Before - after investigations

(2) Cardiovascular diesease prevention programme

(3) The hypertension programme and

(4) A computer record keeping system for general practice.

Some of the main problems in primary health care in remote areas are

- the absence of a general medical survey of the area
- the shortage of doctors and health personell
- the lack of continuity
- the absence of a system of evaluation

Information systems may turn out to be an important means in solution of these problems. I shall discuss some projects in Northern Norway aimed at solving them.

First some introductory remarks about the area:
During the last 17 years I have been working as a medical doctor in the primary health care in Finmark, the northernmost and the most sparsely populated county in Norway. The population is about 79 000 scattered over an area of about 48 600 km2. The main sources of insome are fishing, agriculture, mining and service trades. A sizeable part of the population are of Lappish origin. Another ethnic minority are the Fins descendants of those who left Finland during the famine in the 19th century. Most of them are by now naturalized, and have lived in the area for generations. Skilled hands and professionals are recruited from southern part of Norway. They move back to more attractive positions after up to 5 years in Finmark. This is perticularly the case with medical doctors, which the following figure indicate:

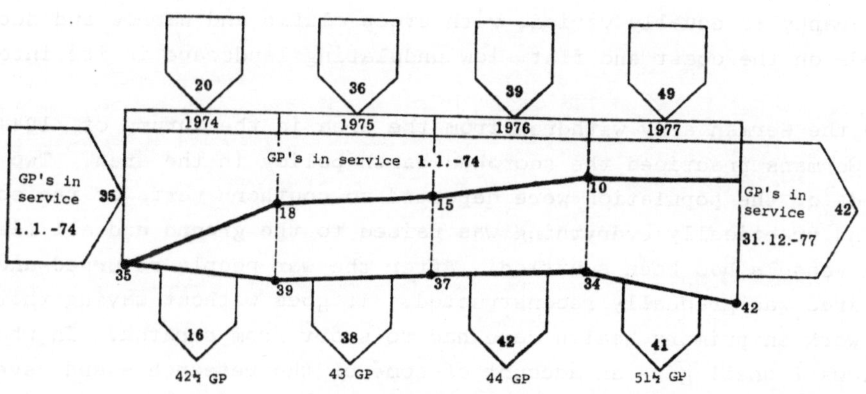

Figure 1: General practioners (GP) in the primary care in Finmark, Norway, 1974-1977. SUM: 179 GP.

In january 1974 were 35 doctors working in primary health care in Finmark. After a year 18 of them were left, the year after again there were 15, then 10 and at the end of the year 1977 10 out of the 35 were working as doctors in the area. Of course new doctors moved in, but the point is that they only stayed for a short time, as the figure illustrates:

In 1974 20 doctors were appointed and 16 left
In 1975 the figures were 36 and 38
In 1976 the figures were 39 and 42
And in 1977 the figures were 49 and 41

In short during a periode of 4 years 179 doctors had been in and out of 35 to 42 positions. These figures speaks for themselves. The need of an information system which ensures efficiency and continuity has been the prime force behind the research work done up to now.

There are extreme seasonal climatic variations in Finmark, ranging from 24 hours sunshine in summer to polarnights in midwinter. Its topography is equally varied, with steep cliffs and narrow and deep fjords on the coast and flat, low undulating landscape in its interior.

When the German army withdrew from the area in the autumn of 1944, the Germans practiced the scorched earth policy in the area. Two thirds of the population were deported to southern parts of the county and practically everything was raised to the ground and all fishing vessels had been scuttled. After the war people returned and the area was gradually reconstructed. It goes without saying that the work in primary health care had to start from scratsh. In what follows I shall give an account of some of the research - and developmental projects carried out under the reconstruction scheme.

1. BEFORE - AFTER INVESTIGATIONS

In 1968 the planning of a new primary health care started based on health centers spread over the entire county. A collaboration was established very early with the University of Tromsø to develop an information system for primary health care in the area.

The objective was to develop a system which was designed to meet local needs within each individual area - in other words: a decentralized system wich was simple and hence easy to operate

The first stage of this developmental work was the SDS-system - a registering and statistics program. It is based on micro-computer which requires the following equipment:

- micro-computer
- storebox for magnetic discs
- a writer
- a data screen with a key board

The SDS-system is easy to operate and it requires little space. It is comparatively inexpensive and reliable, and no previous training is necessary. All registering is done on an ordinary typewriter keyboard in Norwegian. It takes 30 minutes training to master it. This system is developed primarily for registering and statistical treatment of data in each individual area.

I have made use of it myself in a large scale before - after investigation at the Alta healthcenter of which I am in charge myself. The Alta healthcenter is one of the major ones providing health and social services. It cost about 30 million Norwegian kroners and it covers an area with about 13 000 inhabitans. We have some where between 80 000 and 90 000 consultations a year.

The problem was how such a healthcenter affected primary health care in the area. Specified records were made before and after the healthcenter was opened. The material was analysed locally by means of the SDS-system.

The findings was as follows:

1. Increased efficiency.
   The number of consultations increased from 2,7 per head before the center was opened to 3,0 per head after it was opened.
2. A more even geografical dispersion was achieved. The increase was notably significant for the remotest areas.
3. The elderly were rendered poor service.
4. The number of home visits decreased.
5. The number of those admitted to hospitals was reduced.
6. Hospital costs per head were reduced.

The findings forced us to concentrate our work on the elderly and on home visits. It would have been difficult to carry out this project without the SDS-system. Our future plans are to develope a continious evaluation and product control system.

2. CARDIOVASCLAR DISEASE PREVENTION PROGRAMME

For cardiovascular disease and ischemic heart disease, Finmark has the highest male mortality rates in Norway. Therefore during the years 1974 to 1977 an extensive cardiovascular screening programme was carried out with special attention attached to risk - factors as

- hypercholesterolaemia
- cigarette smoking
- hypertension
- lack of physical activity during leasure time

In the days of tuberculosis Finmark used to be the county with the highest mortality rate. In the fight against tuberculosis. The National Mass Radiography Service was an important collabotator together with the primary health care. Mobile teams of buses and boats covered every small place in the sparsely populated area. A computer at the organisation's headquaters in Oslo was used to help analyse the data.

The same service-system was used in the cardiovascular screening examinations recently. During the years 1974/75 17 517 persons were examined. Exactly 3 years later (1977/78) the same persons were reexamined. The data were analyzed by the large computer at the headquaters. In addition it carried out a series of routine tasks such as

- wrighting of calling - in letters
- analysing answers to tests and questionnaires
- finding of persons at risk
- reporting the findings to the local medical offcer in each rural district
- analysing the findings of follow-up examinations of persons at risk.

Technically the entire system worked smoothly. Vast amounts of data were gathered for prospective epidemiologic analyses of cardiovascular disease. Without the help of the centrally located service institution, we simply would not have been able to carry out the project. The work was centered on persons at high risk. The follow-up examinations 3 years later offered an opportunity of further analysis of previous findings. The intervening treatment of persons at risk revealed that

- serum cholesterol had been significantly reduced
- cigarette smoking had been significantly reduced
- Persons at risk had increased their physical activities only minimally
- No reduction of average blood pressure ($p > 0,05$)

In other words we carried out an evaluation of our own work. This would have been impossible without our computer service.

3. THE HYPERTENSJON PROGRAMME

The negative result of the hypertension treatment resulted in change and increased efforts in the hypertension treatment in my district. The findings of the screening examinations were transfered from the large central computer to the microcomputer at the local health-center in Alta. New data were registered as the new hypertension programme was carried out.

After two more years (that is 5 years after the first examination), the material was reanalysed. Now the reduction of both systolic and diastolic blood pressure was significant ($p < 0,001$).

The combined use of the two information systems revealed weak points in our hypertension treatment. By improving the system we could successfully improve the results.

4. A COMPUTER RECORD KEEPING SYSTEM FOR GENERAL PRACTICE

One of the most serious problems in the primary health care in remote and sparsely populated areas is the constant change of doctors as I suggested introductorily. The lack of continuity in health care is the result. The patient records are one of the most importans tools in individual treatment. They are also the most important sources when necessary administrative data are needed and when there is a need of a qualitative assessment of the work that is beeing carried out.

We have developed a manual record system which is now used all over the country. It works very well, but is unfortunately not capable of more systematic analyses. The University of Tromsø has therefore in collaboration with the primary health care developed a computer record keeping system for general practice. This is now beeing tested out.

Like the SDS-system it aims at meeting local needs and is easy to operate. It consists of a combination of a minicomputer and several micro-computers connected with each terminal at the healthcenter.

Each individual doctor has his own terminal where he can obtain:

1. Information picture: Personal data, family, occupation.
2. Over-all picture: Previous diagnosis, symptoms, episodes of immediate concern.
3. Repeat medication: A survey of previous and present medicines are automatically prescribed on the basis of this medication.
4. All previous laboratory findings.
5. A survey of all persons on the sick-list.
   On the basis of these data sick reports are automatically made.

The system offers:

1. More systematized records which are easily available.
2. Better survey of social and occupational status of the patients.
3. A safer and easier way of prescribing medicines.
4. A better survey of the status of those reported sick.
5. Administrative evaluations.
6. Qualitative evaluations.
7. Qualitative analysis of treatment.
8. Reduction of administrative routines concerning patients.
9. Establishment of at - risk register.

By means of this system we hope to neutralize the constant change of doctors, to have a better survey of the work done and, most important of all, raise the quality of medical practice in primary health care.

5. PERSPECTIVES.

Only 10 years back the picture in remote areas in Northern Norway was quite different from the point of view of primary health care. I each district there were up to two doctors. They were responsible for all the health care of the population for 24 hours a day. They knew almost every patient. They knew their health status and had a survey of the most important groups of diagnosis. Every individual doctor stayed for a lengthy periode in his district.

In recent years the working hours of doctors have been reduced to 38 hours a week. But there are 168 hours in a week. This means that each doctor only covers 23 % of the week's hours. The old doctors' memory was a way of databank and the doctors received information through 24 hours a day the week on end. If we are to keep of the most important chronical diseases in the future, the old race of doctors must be replaced by information systems.

MEDICAL DATABASES - CONCEPTUAL AND TECHNICAL ASPECTS

Karl SAUTER
Abt. Medizinische Statistik und Dokumentation
Klinikum der Universität
Kiel, Fed. Rep. of Germany

SUMMARY

Within the last decade much conceptual and technical work has been done to support the management of structured medical and medico-administrative information by computer systems resulting in a large number of database and medical record applications. In focusing primarily on a few major aspects, this paper mainly comprises a conceptual part, stressing the role of the database within a medical information system, and a database-oriented technological part. Important problem areas and current trends are discussed as well.

1. INTRODUCTION

One basic issue in applying computers in the medical field is that of management of information in order to support health care delivery systems, coping with the inflation of information (01,02). A key concept used from computer science is that of the database. From a system-analytical view-point a database is an integral part of an information system overlaying a real or object system such as a health care delivery system and supporting the various information processes within it. Most medical information systems (MIS) are dealing with patient information, representing various forms and/or subsets of medical records (MR).

Due to the complexity and dynamics of the whole field, the scope of this contribution cannot comprise all relevant topics. A number of aspects, e.g. the current trends in hardware technology or cost-effectiveness considerations, had to be omitted, others could only be mentioned.

2. DATABASES IN MEDICAL INFORMATION SYSTEMS

2.1. The Medical Record

Within the last years a variety of computer-supported patient record systems emerged. They greatly differ with regard to structure and contents, according to the functions of the underlying MIS. The most comprehensive one is the hospital (inpatient) MR (03, 04), possibly comprising major parts of the traditional MR and recently including data of medical images as well. The availability of an extensive MR may be of particular importance for the rather small percentage of 'problem-cases'. It is recognized, however, that merely collecting all available data within a computer database is not useful and that the degree of integration has to be defined carefully. Of increasing importance is the class of ambulatory MR's (05).

2.2 Basic Concepts of MIS

A computer-supported information system consists of a database, comprising the data of an organization, all programs and the technical equipment to support the various information processes related to operation, control and planning of the real or object system. Major objectives for MIS are the support of patient care, management, research and education.

Computerized MIS may be roughly classified in:

a) Institution/organization - oriented MIS, comprising nation-wide or regional systems, hospital information systems (HIS) and ambulatory care systems, as well as

b) function-oriented MIS, consisting mainly of systems for specific medical care, dedicated systems, medical information service systems and systems supporting clinical and epidemiological research.

3. DATABASE TECHNOLOGY

3.1 Definitions and Objectives

One of the major tasks of an information system is that of information integration and the vehicle generally used is the database. A database is a structured and organized (possibly large) collection of logically related data in which it is possible to define and manipulate application-specific data substructures ('views') according to specific information needs. The database management system (DBMS) is the software supporting the description, creation and maintenance of the database. A database system consists of the database software (DBMS) and the database (06, 07). However, in the literature on MIS the term 'database' is sometimes used in a less rigorous sense, fulfilling only partially this definition.

An overall objective for supporting an IS by a database is that of centralized control of data. The following are generally considered to be the major advantages:

- The (operational) information of an organization, e.g. a health care delivery system, can be integrated according to one or more aspects
- A multitude of users with different functions and resulting information needs can be supported by appropriate sharing of stored data
- Data integrity can be maintained and the amount of data redundancy can be reduced
- Data independence can be provided which means that the description of data and access techniques is not built into the application programs
- Standardization can be accomplished
- Flexibility for the users in developing and maintaining application systems can be achieved
- Data security restrictions can be met by applying centralized built-in security functions channelling and controlling selectively the access to the database (07).

3.2. Data Modelling

A data model describes the information contents of a database in terms of objects and relationships between these objects. Objects are elementary things in the user's view of reality which are characterized by attributes (properties). For a HIS, these logically related objects may be: PATIENT, ADMISSION, DIAGNOSIS, THERAPY etc. (fig. 1 and 2). Within the computer system data models are represented by data structures.

In medical database applications various data models are used, according to the MIS objectives and to technological and economical boundary conditions. Well-known are (06):

3.2.1. The hierarchical model, supported by many existing DBMS, is implemented in several application areas such as HIS, diagnostic centers or research - oriented systems. A basically hierarchical structure, too, has been defined for a regional health information system (08). The hierarchical or tree-structured approach, representing one-to-many relationships, appears to be appropriate for modelling MR data in quite a natural way (fig. 2).

3.2.2. The network model is a more general approach than a hierarchy allowing for the representation of many-to-many relationships between objects (09). In the medical field the network approach has been mainly applied to HIS as well (fig. 1).

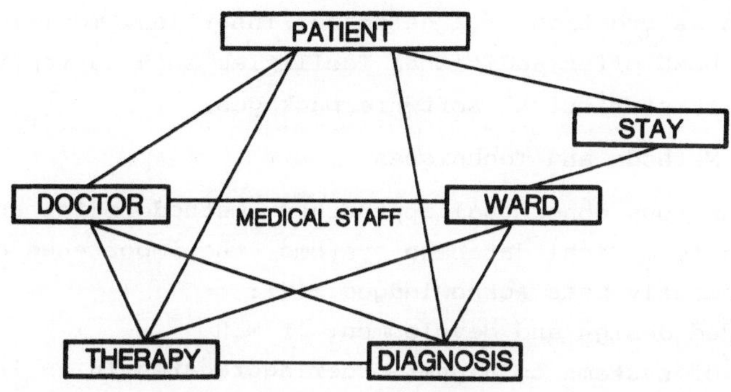

Figure 1: Logically related objects of a computer-supported medical record system (07)

3.2.3. The relational model (10) is based on the mathematical theory of relations. Relations are used to represent data about objects and (many-to-many) relationships between these objects. Since relations may be represented by tables, this data-view is considered to be especially user-friendly. Relational DBMS are still an object of research however (11). There exist a number of implementations in the medical field, offering the major functions or, at least, retrieval facilities of a relational DBMS.

3.3 Database Description

A DBMS must be provided with a formal description of the data which have to be handled and stored. The same is true for any generalized software tool to access and update data (12). This description of the database is formulated in a so-called data description language (DDL). The principle of data independence implies the separate description of logical and physical data views, resulting in a multi-level system architecture. Recently, a 3-schema model has been proposed (13) which comprises the internal, external and conceptual schemas representing the machine, the 'users' and the global data views respectively.

3.4 Database Access

For the maintanance and retrieval of data so-called data manipulation languages (DML) are used which enable a user to formulate data access functions such as creation of a database, insertion, modification etc. of data. Many DBMS offer additional facilities such as report generators or links to statistical software packages.

3.5 Concepts, Methods and Techniques

Amongst the numerous conceptual approaches, methodologies and technologies applied to medical database systems, the importance of the following have recently been acknowledged (14):

- Computer-aided design and development of MIS
- Integration of systems to higher-order aggregates in an integrated, modular systems approach
- Representation of medical knowledge as data in so-called knowledge bases comprising information on relationships between events or variables, interpretation rules for medical data etc.
- Concepts and techniques to improve the <u>software</u> <u>quality</u> with regard to reliability, portability and flexibility, stressing particularly the formalization of the software design process
- Database design: The conceptual schema, as introducted in chapt.3.3 and describing the information <u>contents</u> of a database in a global view, has proved to be a valuable tool - not only for central control and communication - but also for database design and redesign (15) (fig. 2).

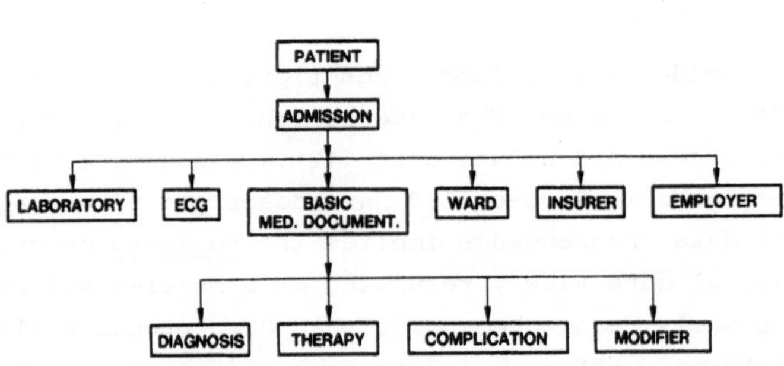

Figure 2: Conceptual Schema of the Medical System Hannover Patient Database (12)

4. USER INTERFACES

The interface between the database system and the user is established by the data model, the data description language(s) and the data manipulation language(s). Effectiveness and acceptability of database-supported MIS greatly depend on the availability of powerful, yet easy-to-handle interfaces of users. In recent years considerable progress has been achieved in this area:

a) The use of complex data structures (chapt. 3) may greatly reduce the complexity of the high-level language application programs

b) Specific classes of interactive user languages emerged, e.g. query and command languages, promoting the man-computer communication through various dialogue interaction concepts. Own experiences with the use of relational query languages indicate - however - limitations in their suitability as a direct user interface.

5. PROBLEM AREAS

Due to the conceptual as well as the technological complexity of database-supported MIS and their relationships to the 'real-world', there exist a number of problems areas. The following two deserve particular consideration:

a) Maintenance of data and program integrity should be considered as part of a comprehensive quality concept for data including the validation of data and the correctness and reliability of all programs used. Syntactic data integrity constraints may be described centrally as part of the conceptual schema (chapt. 3.3, (16)). Experience shows that data integrity problems increase rapidly with the degree of information integration.

b) Guarantee of data security: The problems encountered increased in line with the development of modern computer systems possibly serving a large number of users simultaneously: stored data as well as programs may be shared and users may interact with the information system via remotely located terminals. Security concepts comprise hardware precautions, software facilities and organizational measures (07, 17) with a trend from software to more efficient hardware solutions.

6. CONCLUSION

There is an important impact of computer technology on the management of information in health care. The following trends may be recognized:

a) Due to decreasing hardware costs and the development of advanced modular and 'packaged' software, the application systems will be:
   - provided with more and more functions
   - usable with less qualification and knowledge.
b) MIS will be provided with knowledge bases supporting the interpretation of database information, decision making and education.
c) 'Cautious' integration of systems to higher-order structural aggregates or networks with a global logic will, due to progress in 'distributed informatics', improve:
   - the integration of patient information
   - the sharing of medical resources
   - the insight and control in the health sector in general.

REFERENCES

(01) Barber, B., Grémy, F., Überla, K., Wagner, G. (eds.): Medical Informatics Berlin 1979, Proceedings. Lecture Notes in Medical Informatics 5 (Springer, Berlin, 1979).

(02) Grémy, F.: The Future of Information Processing in Medicine and Public Health. Comput. Progr. Biomed. (1980) 71-80.

(03) Schneider, W., Bengtsson, S.: The Application of Computer Techniques in Health Care with Special Regard to Hospitals. Comput. Progr. Biomed. 5 (1976) 169-249.

(04) Shannon, R.H. (ed.): Hospital Information Systems. IFIP Working Conference, Cape Town, 1979 (North-Holland, Amsterdam, 1979).

(05) Reichertz, P.L. et al.: Results of a Field Test of Computers for the Private Practice. In: (01) 283-294.

(06) Date, C.J.: An Introduction to Database Systems (Reading, Massachusetts: Addison - Wesley Publ. Co., 1975).

(07) Sauter, K.: Data Security in Health Information Systems by Applying Software Techniques. Meth. Inform. Med. 18 (1979) 214-222.

(08) Sauter, K. (ed.), Griesser, G., Jainz, M., Schneider, W.: A Data Structure Model for a Health Information System. Comput. Progr. Biomed. 6 (1976) 171-177.

(09) CODASYL Programming Language Committee: Data Base Task Group Report. Association for Computing Machinery, New York, 1971.

(10) Codd, E.F.: A Relational Model of Data for Large Shared Data Banks. Comm. ACM 13 (1970) 377-387.

(11) Kim, W.: Relational Database Systems. Comput. Surv. 11 (1979) 185-211.

(12) Sauter, K., Reichertz, P.L., Weingarten, W., Schwarz, B.: A System to support High Level Data Description and Manipulation. Medical Informatics 1 (1976) 15-26.

(13) ANSI/X3/SPARC. Study Group on Data Base Management Systems. Interim Report, Amer. Nat. Stand. Inst., CBMA, Washington DC, 1975.

(14) Lindberg, D.A.B., Kaihara, S.: MEDINFO 80, Proceedings of the Third World Conference an Medical Informatics, Tokyo, 1980 (North-Holland, Amsterdam, 1980).

(15) Klonk, J., Sauter, K.: Steps Towards a Methodology for Data Base Design. In: (14) 470-474.

(16) Sauter, K., Klonk, J., Rienhoff, O.: Integrity Problems within a Database-Supported Patient Information System. In: (01) 570-579.

(17) Griesser, G. et al. (eds.): Data Protection in Health Information Systems, Considerations and Guidelines (North-Holland, Amsterdam, 1980).

EXPERIENCES FROM A REGIONAL MEDICAL DATA BASE

Matti KATAJA[=] and Matti AHO[+]

Central Public Health Laboratory, Helsinki[=]

Tampere Central Hospital, Tampere[+]

Finland

SUMMARY

A computer application for data retrieval from a regional medical data base is described. The data covers nearly all discharge summaries during the past ten years in the Tampere region. The region has about 410 000 inhabitants and it is served by a central hospital (1200 beds), two municipal hospitals (900 beds), three district hospitals (400 beds), two mental hospitals (850 places) and many health centres (400 beds). Each discharge summary includes the exact patient identification, date, place, duration of the stay and the diagnosis. The retrieval system consists of a parameter driven universal searcher and of seceral report programmes. Physicians use the system through a form, usually without a programmer's activity. The response time is short enough for all practical purposes.

1. BACKGROUND

Hospital discharge records are collected in Finland since 1961 by a uniform national system. This was planned by Dr Sakari Härö of the National Board of Health (1) and it operates still nearly in its original form. The attending physician completes a discharge form for every inpatient irrespective of the type of the hospital. Thus the discharge file is virtual medical data base on the hospital care of all Finns since 1961. The national system is discussed also elsewhere in this Congress by Eero Linnakko & al.

The data set of the discharge form has about the same structure as in all other systems (2) serving a similar purpose. The most important items are:

- personal ID, called previously the social security code, which is unique for every individual in the country
- the code of the place of residence, by commune (ca 470 communes in Finland)
- hospital code including the hospital type
- code for medical speciality
- type of admission (emergency or regular)
- date of admission
- date of discharge
- where remitted
- main diagnosis according to ICD-7 (3)
- additional diagnoses or causes of treatment.

Patient's name, sex and age are not included, because the name is not needed for the purpose,and the sex as well as the age are derived from the personal ID and from the dates.

During the recent years the National Board of Health has keypunched this data of about 800 000 cards yearly and has compiled out national and regional summaries. During the past 2-3 years the central hospitals in Finland have taken the duty to write discharge data from their region into a machine readable form. Thus, regional data bases are built in many places as a byproduct of this nation-wide effort.

2. TAMPERE REGION

Tampere is the second biggest city in Finland with about 165 000 inhabitants. Tampere region (4) is a roundly area (Figure 1) having about 8 % of the population of Finland (410 000 out of 4.8 million). The Central Hospital has about 1200 beds, while the two big municipal hospitals and the three district hospitals have together about 1300 beds. The number of acute care beds in the region totals about 1800. There are 4300 beds or places for other care.

2.1. Data processing facilities

The Central Hospital has a close co-operation with Tampere University, but they both have data processing facilities of their own. The university concentrates in research and teaching whilst all data processing concerning the patient care is carried out by the computers in the Central Hospital. The data processing unit was established in 1967 and, since then, its main duty has been in assistance of patient examination and care. However, the medical data flown through has been stored, and it is used mainly for regional planning and to some extent for research. The DP-staff consists of 27 people, 7 of which are capable of programming.

2.2. Discharge data collection in Tampere region

Most hospitals of the region use a standard form for discharge data. Some hospitals have planned their own forms by integrating more administrative data on the sheet. All hospitals and health centres of the region send their discharge forms to the Central Hospital for keying to magnetic tapes, which is the form used in sending that data to the National Board of Health.

Tampere Central Hospital itself uses a combined data transmission and collection set, which is used in keying medical data to the collection files after the discharge of the patient. The discharge record is then generated by the computer from this file.

The data processing unit runs a comprehensive set of reports on the basis of the discharges (about 70 000) collected during a year. In the main report for each commune the local health board may learn what care, how much and where, has been delivered for the inhabitants of the commune. For regional planning purposes the separate reports of each medical speciality have the widest use.

3. TAMPERE REGION MEDICAL DATA BASE

3.1. Purpose

The discharge data collected on magnetic tapes had been used already for many years as the main source of information for administrative and research purposes concerning hospital utilization in the region. This activity always required a programmer's intervention and a lot of time. To shorten the computer time and the waiting period in the user's unit a disc resident data base was drafted and actually realized as a prototype within one month. The original purpose was to save time but now the main purpose may be said to be in a better service to medical and administrative experts in the region.

3.2. Environment and the file structure

The data base resides on a 90 megabyte removable disc pack continuously spinning in a Data General Eclipse C/300 computer. This computer is in one type of real time use, having continuously updated file of the inpatients of the Central Hospital. The running mode of the computer allows a simultaneous batch processing, which makes it possible to respond quickly enough to enquiries. The data base occupies about 18 % of the disc pack. A summary of 12 words, equivalent with 24 bytes, is stored from every discharge in a contiguous file. The data base thus consists of about 670 000 summaries.

Because of the rather high speed of the above computer and because of the common need to use the data on a yearly basis, no indexing or other tricks are applied. The data is kept in 24 subfiles, one for each year and hospital group. Thanks to this structure and to the use of big reading buffers, the search procedure normally runs very quickly, i.e. 20..30 seconds per year both groups processed. This is at least 30 times faster than the competition.

3.3. Content

The discharge record is processed to 12 words of information of which all parts can be used as searching keys. Thus the file is practically a key-file to the medical record archives on paper. The main use for data from years earlier than 1979 is in fact the search of the personal ID's for finding medical records from the archives. The content of a record in the files is as follows: (The number of the word in the first column.)

1 Hospital code and the code for medical speciality
2 Personal ID, the day of birth
3 Personal ID, the latter part with sex
4 Age on admission, sex decoded for a key
5 The code of home minucipality
6 Date of discharge
7 Duration of stay
8 Dichotomous variables for admission type, payment class and death
9 Main diagnosis by ICD-7 code, integer part
10 Main diagnosis, decimal part
11 Second diagnosis, integer part
12 Second diagnosis, decimal part.

4. THE USE OF THE DATA BASE

From the administrative viewpoint this data is a part of the medical record archives in the region. Thus the data base is treated according to the rules for medical records. A physician or a researcher needing some support from the data base must fill in a form and he must provide a signature of the chief physician of the hospital. If the problem is restricted to one speciality the signature of the head of the department in question is enough. The data processing unit then runs, in most cases within one hour the desired results. In complicated cases, when a programmer's intervention is needed, 1 to 2 days delivery time is expected.

The program system consists of a general searcher which collects records fulfilling the given requirements. Virtually all cases within the past two years were run without a programmer in this phase. The searcher uses AND function with different key items and OR function within a key. Thus with the notion: "age = 40-60", "sex = male", "dgn = 250.xx" all male diabetics in the age range from 40 to 60 years are put to the intermediate file for further processing.

AND function within a key is realized by using the searcher once more, the output data from the first phase as the input. For example, if diabetes as a complication of some hearth disease is under study, the diagnosis of this hearth disease is used in the first phase and "dgn = 250.xx" in the second phase. The next operation is then the report writing for which we have developed a series of programmes fulfilling the needs of most users. Normal listing is provided if nothing else is required. The diagnose summaries are the most popular other output forms.

The system has a very powerful feature to search by the personal ID but this is hidden so that there is in the inquiry form no hint of this. Only the searches to the chief physicians are allowed to be produced by the DP-staff.

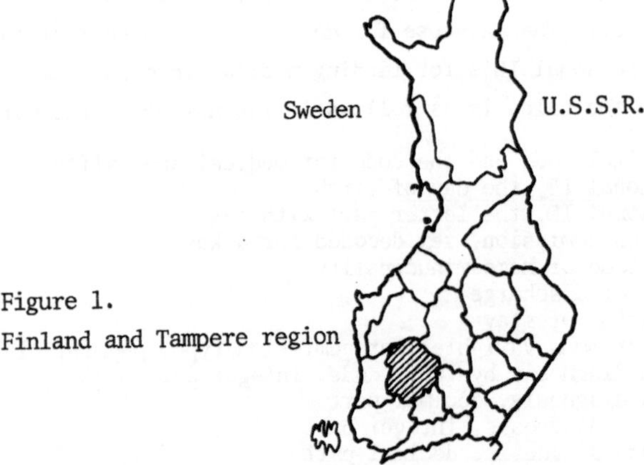

Figure 1.
Finland and Tampere region

5. AN EXAMPLE OF THE APPLICATION OF THE REGIONAL DATA BASE

5.1. The task

The senior author had a request to produce data on the treatment of tuberculosis in the Tampere region. The main questions were:

1. Are there differences which can be explained on the basis of some local foci of the disease.
2. Are there areas free of tuberculosis.
3. What are the trends of tuberculosis treatment in the past ten years.
4. How many patients were treated for tuberculosis at the hospitals of the region during the past ten years. Note: Not how many hospital stays but how many individuals.

5.2. The Solution

The calling sequence of the searcher includes all possible files, since all the hospitals in the region are searched. For the diagnosis range 010-019 is given and switch for both diagnoses is set on. It took some 15 seconds to write the calling sequence, some 4 minutes to run the first phase and some half an hour to do all necessary processing to answer the four questions stated above.

The report program for output by communes gives the hospital stays in absolute and in proportional form. The latter is counted per 1000 inhabitants. The trends were studied by dividing the total time period into three intervals and by calculating the rate of stays for each of them. One routine program counts the number of patients, counts on patients treated twice, three times and so on. It also counts the cumulative number of treatment days in each group. Thus the question 4 was answered, moreover with additional data about the mean stay per patient and per treatment period. An other program reports separately all the stays if a patient is treated "n" times or more. With n = 3 some interesting information was obtained about the treatment system.

5.3. Results

The definitive answer for the question one was yes. In the region there are some corners where 2 to 3 times more patients are treated for tuberculosis as compared to the mean. The newly grown areas in the neighbourhood of the region capital are not quite free of tuberculosis (as reflected by hospital treatment) but the incidence of the disease is lower than that in the capital itself or in the peripheral communes. Thus the question 2 was answered properly.

The figures for the years 1970-1972 concerning the treatment rates and numbers are more than twice as high as those for years 1976-1978. The number of hospital stays during the past ten years was about 3400 corresponding to 2400 treated individuals. This means that about 0.5 % of the population had been treated in a hospital for tuberculosis during past ten years.

6. DISCUSSION

6.1. Validity of the data

Since many years the discharge system is an integral element of the hospital information collection in Finland, and it has gained an unquestioned acceptance throughout the country. Thus the data is very reliable as compared to all other data collection except that of deaths. Coding and transmission errors destroy 0.01 % to 2 % of the records depending on the hospital and its tradition. Concerning the Tampere region the data from the years 1975 to 1977 from some heath centres is still incomplete since the collection sheets were sent directly to the National Board of Health, in spite of the orders from the Central Hospital. The correction of this defect is under process at the moment (December 1980).

The validity of the data has been checked nationwide in several studies during the past two three years but the reports are for internal use and in Finnish. The biggest source of error is the lack of data from certain health centres from the late seventies. In the system described the mental care was not included before the year 1977. In the data base discussed here there is no data of the outpatient visits. In Tampere Central Hospital the outpatient visits have been registered during the past 7 years and there are similar but slower programmes to process them by feeding the data from magnetic tapes.

6.2. Costs and benefits

It took about one month for a programmer to write the prototype version of the system and to collect the primary data. After the verification that the system works well the program was rewritten to meet the quality and documentation standards,and further report programmes were added. The total effort now used for the development and tuning of the system corresponds to about half a year programmer's time. The recent system is the third version, and it is realized by using DGC's FORTRAN 5 compiler which speeds up the execution of the search phase by 50 % as compared to normal FORTRAN IV compiler.

The benefits are remarkable because the computer time needed for data query and report generation was reduced to a small fraction of the time needed earlier. Also the time of the computer staff used for queries was reduced, especially since in normal cases no programming is needed and every operator is able to run the queries just from the form.

So far, no drawbacks have been identified. There is a potential danger of the abuse of certain personal data because the system is capable to search and combine data by personal ID. To avoid misuse a security system is used so that only written questions are accepted, every form must be signed by an authorized chief physician and searching by personal ID's is carried out ounly personally to the physicians in charge of the hospitals who are responsible of the medical record archives.

6.3. Other implementations

The rumours of a well functioning system will spread to the neighbouring regions although the penetration of such knowledge is in the medical world rather slow. However, the system is just under implementation in another region south-east of Tampere. The implementation takes three weeks' time and is realized by the second author of this paper.

6.4. Effects

There are two main effects gained by a data retrieval system from the medical data base. First, the summary data for various acute needs can be obtained so easily and so quickly that the effort is worthwhile and the work is really done. In most other regions in the country this is not done because it simply would cost too much, and in most cases would take too much time. Secondly, the medical staff receives feedback to their work, which results in better information handling in the hospital.

REFERENCES

(1) Härö AS. Hospital Discharge Reporting System. Hospital Statistics and a Minimum Basic Data Set, Edinburgh, 1976.

(2) The status of hospital discharge data in six countries. Hyattsville, Md. National Center for Health Statistics, U.S. Department of Health, Education, and Welfare, 1980.

(3) The National Board of Health, Classificatio Morborum et Causarum Mortis, Helsinki, 1969.

(4) Bridgman RF. Hospital Utilization, Oxford University Press, 1979.

CONSTRUCTION OF A POPULATION INDEX TO IMPROVE COMMUNITY HEALTH: A SCOTTISH APPROACH TO HEALTH COMPUTING

BRYDEN J.S., DAVIDSON D., MARR A.C., McQUEEN I., MELVILLE A.G. and RANKIN J.
Argyll and Clyde Health Board, Gilmour House, Paisley SCOTLAND.

It seems to be natural instinct to grudge money spent on health services. As a result only limited resources are allocated to health care. If money is tight then health resource allocators must ensure that health value is obtained from every expenditure.

As Scots we have an international reputation of being careful about money. Our team here describe how we are trying to use health computing to promote health. We belong to a non-academic department and have to argue our monies for health computing out of the same budget that pays for nurses or drugs. We have to justify this expenditure under the public eye and especially under the ever prying eyes of the local newspapers.

Medicine continues to be practised as art more than science. There is a danger that when sophistocated technology, such as medical informatics is grafted onto such an art that the resultant growth can be uncontrolled and might (continuing the analogy of grafting) ultimately kill off the host.

Health computing often emulates mountaineering. Peaks of effort are sometimes scaled solely because they are there. Such efforts may be laudable because they expand the scientific base of medical information processing. However, like any other form of medical research there has to be a discard pile, as well as adopted new therapies. Many antibiotics have been researched and tested - only a few are actually used. We were perhaps fortunate in arriving late on the computer scene. Although some of us had been involved with informatics for several years, the actual group was only brought together following the first re-organisation of the U.K. Health Service in 1974. We were thus able to look at some of the approaches that had been evolved in Europe and compare them with our objectives.

Management by objectives has been one of the many techniques tried to unravel the complexities of multifacetted organisations. Health is a nebulous entity about which it is difficult to be objective. All of us depending on our background and our own personal and family health have differing concepts of health. Even the WHO's definition of health is so all embracing as to make the objectivity more diffuse. However, we feel strongly that one must be objective about health services - their management is unusual and cannot be by directive but must be by persuasion and facilitation. We feel health targets should be met and medical informatics projects should only be adopted if they wll move the complex system towards one or many of these targets.

We have looked carefully at the computing of the medical record, especially the hospital medical record, typified by major often "all singing - all dancing" systems. These can now work well but that do they do for health? Can they emulate the pictographic quality of the good tectural medical record - "This cheery old lady sitting comfortably in bed ?" Can that picture be retained by each hospital computer system?

So in the first instance we rejected hospital medical record systems as producing major health value for money. We did see, however, good low cost schemes using the computer as an index to the total medical record and more of this anon.

We see greatest value for money in using the computer where it differs most from the humans that control it. The ability of the computer not to forget, not to be tired and to be constantly accurate.

Health promotion, prevention of illness or hardship frequently fall because of human lethargy, apathy or inaccuracy. At a busy diabetic clinic if a patient does not attend - the natural reaction of the doctor and nurses is relief. One less to see on a busy day, and yet perhaps the missing patient had most need to be seen - surely a need for automatic recall. As described in some of our subsequent papers there have already been recall systems well tried in the U.K. In Scotland we have a national thyroid treatment follow-up scheme which, If I remember, was described here before in Toulouse in one of the Journees d'Informatique Medicale. This recall scheme promotes better thyroid care by recalling patients to their family doctors. As a result more treated patients continue to be euthyroid and less iatrogenic disease results.

Parents may have well meaning motives towards their babies being immunised but often they forget, treatment courses are not completed, and many children are left unprotected. Computer recall for immunisation has produced higher immunisation rates, often at lower cost. Yet such recall is dependant on non-mobile families. As you will hear later, yet community data base is needed to ensure inclusion of mobile children. Well meaning recall systems have been tried and failed. The need for exfoliative cervical cytology, although originally somewhat unproven, is now accepted yet most "At Risk" recall systems have failed over the problems of continuing to identify the women at risk over several years - a further case for community data base.

How do you find the target groups needing better health promotion or better care?

Often these can be simply identified by age, sex and even by geography. Here in France you have given much thought to the problems of perinatal mortality. In Scotland sadly we have even worse figures. Baird, Brotherston et al over many years have demonstrated the relationship of socio-economic status with perinatal mortality. Marr, from our team, has highlighted that within the low income socio-economic groups there are further increases in perinatal mortality related to living in urban ghettoes. Again a case for recall through a community index.

Measuring health or hardship is never easy. Most indicators really measure illness or even provision of service. Any measurements that can be made need a meaningful denominator. The national census in most countries is only carried out every ten years. Population movement in the intercensus period can be so marked as to invalidate calculations using the census figures. For accurate rates a more up-to-date meaningful denominator is required. Moreover, it is important to link events to individual persons. Care may be given by family doctors, local hospitals, health visitors, dentists, community nurses, family planning clinics, regional hospital centres and so forth but only by centralised identification can these episodes of care or health promotion be brought together and measured. The main body of this paper and the paper tomorrow describe our efforts over the last few years of how we created a community health index as the base for our health promotion approach to medical informatics.

Many aspects of what we are tackling are controversial. Society has to be reassured that with "1984" approaching rapidly we are not a subtle form of "Big Brother". We control confidentiality and security by making personal appointments of named and identifiable medical holders of all the health data.In negotiations with individual medical practitioners, area medical advisory committees and local health consumer councils this concept of personal responsibility for confidentiality has done much to reassure natural misgivings. We are now supporting these data holders with a watchdog data privacy committee.

This paper is an introduction to our work. We have a long history of interest and responsible attitude to the public health in Scotland. We have exported medical officers of health throughout the world.

We hope you find our approaches to community health computing effective and, coming from a Scottish stable, low cost.

We belong to the West of Scotland and all health services are provided through four Health Boards serving 1.1 million of Scotland's 5 million population. It includes on the one hand problems of urban deprivation and on the other rural and island isolation.

In our health services like many others we keep many indexes to our patients.

DESCRIPTION	SIZE
National Health Service:	
Family Doctor Payment Index	Whole population
Hospital Registration Indexes	2-3 times population
Health Centres/GP Individual Family Practices	Whole population
Local Public Health Indexes	Approximately ½ of population

Each index will contain the following common information, name age, address and sex together with other information relevant to the particular use of the index. In general, information on one index will not be linked or easily linkable to any other, and amendments to one will not create a similar amendment to the others. In this situation the accuracy of each index may be quite low. The decreasing cost of computer hardware and the increasing cost of clerical staff are leading towards the computerisation of many previously manually administrative procedures. If systems are computerised in isolation this creates duplication of common data. Rather than merely computerise the existing files it is of value to consider the possibility of using a Central Index which is linked or replaces other indexes. In Scotland the most comprehensive index is that used by the administration which funds family doctors because it contains the details of all patients registered with general practitioners. In a national Health Service this is very close to the whole community, whole health is being cared for - The Community Health Index (CHI). This caters not only for those currently receiving care but potential users or hopefully non-users if preventive medicine is successful.

The CHI was originally created in batch and is subsequently maintained and updated on-line. We used a similar optical character reading technique to that described here in Toulouse. Almost all people are registered with family doctors. Each central administration hold its details on file cards. These cards were typed up on golf-ball typewriters using an OCR font and OCR read. This was followed by a validation update cycle until the computer "ledger" figures matched the former manual system - to each family doctor very important because this is how they are paid.

Once the information has been captured the index is run on-line using conventional video terminals. The index was originally established for the biggest of the four Boards in whose office is housed the centralised computer and the on-line service is provided to the family doctor administration sited in that office.

It took some considerable time to carry out the input cycle for the first half-million people - almost 18 months. The funding for this exercise was provided, however by a non-health service source - that is the British Manpower Services Commission who fund work experience programmes as part of the effort to combat our unemployment problems. We used temporary typists and clerkesses funded thereby. Now the system is running on-line for routine updating no extra staff are used - former clerkesses, who ran the previous filing system have been retrained as VDU operators and in fact that department has now taken on new work without staff increase.

The four Boards had already conbined to provide a computing and information services consortium, and had been funded nationally for this. These systems/programming staff, as well as the computer, did not have to be increased for this exercise and we have made use of modified, already existing software.

You can see that apart from the capital costs involved that this almost no cost approach has been very appealing to us as "canny Scots". Once happy with the first Board and its half million population, work began creating the index for the other Boards. This uses a combination of distributed processing and remote job entry. However, in the two other Board offices are mini computer systems linked on-line to the central computer. The data capture exercise is being repeated using type-writers and OCR and the daily running is carried out by the local minis linked to the mainframe some 30 to 250 kilometres away. We have thus with hard effort created a community index and we now see this as the base for all our health promotion activities.

For the community index to be of maximum use to the Health Board it should meet three major requirements, i.e. it should be (1) accurate, (2) up-to-date and (3) complete. To achieve these objectives it is necessary to check the data against other sources or patient data and feed data into the index from all possible Health Board sources. The Community Health Index serves as the nerve centre of the Primary Care Division, e.g., when a patient arrives in the area and registers with a GP the patient's name is added to the index. When a patient moves out of the area and registers with another GP the index is up-dated. When a patient submits a claim for a prescription excemption the index is checked. When a patient dies, notification is made to the Primary Care Division by the Registrar General. As the index is an integral part of the work of the Primary Care Division the staff continuously work with and modify the index.

Where are the points of contact between patient and Health Services from which data can be fed into the index? Four main sources are:-

(a) Primary Care Division (already covered)
(b) General practitioners, either in the health centre or surgery premises or on a home visit.
(c) Hospitals, as inpatients, elective or emergency and as

outpatients - consultative, accident/emergency or paramedical attendance.

(d) Community Health Departments - clinics, schools or home visits.

The general practitioner is normally the most frequent point of contact between the patient and the Health Service and the most likely source to provide up-to-date information on change of name (in marriage), change of address etc. Temporary residents also make use of this branch of the service.

The hospital has certain contacts which can be regular and long-term - the patient with a slow growing cataract who attends a consultative eye clinic every six months or annually, or the boy with a hearing aid who calls at the hospital to have the aid adjusted or repaired, or even to collect batteries. There is one type of hospital contact which can be the only health service contact with certain patients i.e., the patient who does not register with a general practitioner but who calls at the Accident/Emergency Department for advice and treatment when ill. These patients are mainly the "drop-outs," the patient with no fixed abode who may lodge in one of the hostelries which provides overnight accommodation for people with no home.

Community doctors and health visitors keep surveillance on young children and the elderly. In the School Health Service routine examinations are carried out in the school. Specific groups, for example, handicapped, are kept under regular review.

If one is to look to these three sections to provide a feed-in of up-to-date information following patient contact, one should consider what incentive there can be for the staff to encourage their participation. The obvious answer is the use that these people can make of the index in their own particular situation. Can the community health index become the "local" index? As an index at local level the CHI has the following advantages:-

1. It is maintained centrally
2. It can be provided in different forms (i) microfiche (ii) computer printout (iii) individual patient cards (iv) individual patient self-adhesive labels.
3. It can be produced singly, in duplicate, triplicate etc.
4. It is not subject to the "human" error misfiling of manually kept index.

Can the Community Health Number become the local medical record identifier? Although the CHI number consists of ten digits and for identification purposes requires the complete ten digits for filing purposes, one can reduce the filing requirement to the first six digits, i.e., date of birth. What are the advantages of date of birth filing? The date of birth is a permanent six digit number which remains constant throughout life and is known by the patient, and used by the patient for many purposes. It is a standard character length, i.e. six digits, and a record can be located if date of birth is known without reference to an index.

In general practice, whether a single-handed practice or group practice, the medical records have been filed in alphabetical order in the past. What could we offer? With regard to the actual general practitioner medical record, which has remained virtually unchanged for many years , it consists of small, awkwardly sized envelopes - in Scotland the personal details are horizontal and in England the details are vertical. Reports from laboratories, radiology departments, correspondence from hospital consultants, community health doctors, are folded and placed in the envelope and it is therefore difficult to locate any particular document. The Ministry of Health in England and the Scottish Home and Health Department have recently produced a standard record folder, which can accommodate unfolded international size A4 inserts. In addition, certain inserts have been provided for:-

> Clinical notes, summary of important illnesses and investigations, immunisations and screening investigations, antenatal/maternity recording, paediatric development, x-ray and pathology investigations (mount sheet) and nurses and health visitors notes.

General practitioners were keen to adopt these new records but the conversion of existing records was most time-consuming and disruptive to the day-to-day work of a busy practice. The opportunity was there to consider how the CHI could be used to assist in the conversion. It was realised that if clerical support could be made available, it was possible to convert the existing records and set up an improved records system. The procedures to effect such a conversion were devised. Two main obstacles had to be overcome. (1) The agreement of a single general practitioner to allow his records to be used for a trial scheme, and when such agreement was reached, (2) The preparation and submission of a case to the Manpower Services Commission to provide the necessary manpower. The first hurdle was rapidly overcome by the agreement of one partnership of the Port Glasgow Health Centre, who allowed their records to be used in the trial. The submission to MSC was then approved.

The change over programme follows the pattern set out below:-

(1) A computer printout is provided listing all patients registered with the practice in alphabetical order, male and female listings together or separated according to the existing practice filing arrangements.

(2) Listing is checked against the medical records envelopes (MREs) and matched on name, date of birth and address, or name and date of birth or name and address. Partial matches are checked with the practice secretaries or receptionists or with the patients.

(3) Listing is returned to Primary Care where CHI is up-dated.

(4) Corrected listing is provided, also a self-adhesive printed label for each patient.

(5) Label is affixed to the front of each folder, number boldly printed above.

(6) Folder is colour coded (a) Practice code (b) Sex code (3) Filing number code. (By day and month or year and month).

(7) Standard inserts as agreed by each practice are inserted.

(8) Folders are married with MREs i.e., the MRE is inserted into the back pocket of the folder.

(9) Comfiche of practice index - alphabetic, and numeric is provided.

(10) Folders are re-filed according to date of birth.

(11) Contents of MREs are removed re-arranged in agreed order and filed within the folder.

From the initial success of the 3-doctor practice, a single-handed GP followed by a 4-doctor practice was later converted in the same health centre. Secretaries and receptionist, initially apprehensive of the change-over and new filing sequence became rapid converts. The most obvious improvement was the disappearance of mis-filed and lost records. In moving on to the next health centre in Gourock a modification was made to the Port Glasgow procedures. In this health centre there is a three-doctor practice and a single-doctor practice. Here, there was agreement to have total integration of the records of both practices. The third health centre now being converted is the Greenock Health Centre, where currently nine practices, from 6-doctor to single-handed practice having a total of approximately seventy-thousand records is underway.

Practice records have been checked, many for the first time against the Primary Care Index. A more acceptable clinical record, the contents of which follow a particular pattern, has been introduced. Confidentiality is better protected as access is more difficult. A patient index on Comfiche is easily kept under lock and key outwith office hours. Records cannot be easily located unless the filing system is known. Most records can be located by staff without reference to the index as the date of birth can be easily quoted by the patient. The system has been accepted quickly by both the professional and administrative staff and already the CHI number is quoted in all correspondence relating to a patient.

Plans are in progress to convert the hospital records system to a date of birth filing system using the CHI as the hospital index. Unlike general practice the change-over would start from a particular date and would be actioned on contact by the patient to any part of the hospital i.e., either outpatient or inpatient. Only records of patients making contact with the hospital after the starting date would be brought forward to the "date of birth" system. As the CHI would become the patient record number in the hospital (i.e. the number quoted by consultants on patient correspondence) the patient would be identified by the same number in both hospital and general practice. This has great benefits to laboratories, radiology departments etc.

Once the same system is extended to the Community Health records, medical, nursing and school health service, the Inverclyde District will be the first District in Scotland to use a common patient identifier in all three branches of the National Health Service.

A DISTRICT HOSPITAL WITH RESTRICTED ACUTE BEDS: A Mini Computer System Linked to the Community Health Index for Optimising Empty Beds for Acute Admissions

There is now a tendency for hospitals to operate with fewer beds than in the past. To achieve this without a decline in service to patients greater use must be made of the beds which are available. This is not unique to the United Kingdom - Canada at the moment is taking steps to reduce its hospital acute beds. Inverclyde Royal Hospital (IRH) is a case in point having 366 beds to provide acute services to 140,000 population. The IRH is a new hospital replacing 7 old hospitals with 482 beds. In order to provide the information necessary to plan and monitor the use of the beds in IRH a computer based system has totally replaced certain tasks previously done manually. The system produces up-to-date details of the location of individual patients and summary statistics of the number of patients in each ward (vital since convalescent patients may be moved to allow new admissions to be accommodated in wards best staffed to give the intensity of nursing care required - making it difficult to ascertain the whereabouts of both patients and empty beds for new admissions).

THE SYSTEM: The mini computer system consists of a number of interlinked files which contain details of each patient and of the hospital itself, lists of consultants, size of wards etc. A 'database' approach is taken. An outline of the structure is shown in Figure 1. A piece of information on a patient is held on only one file but may be accessed from another file, using the unique patient number as a pointer. Each item is assigned a name in a 'dictionary' for the file. This dictionary automatically assigns column headings when items are listed. The standard software on the computer includes a powerful enquiry language which in conjunction with the dictionary enables detailed lists and summary statistics to be produced. New items may be defined (as combinations or as arithmetic functions of one or more items from one or more files) which in turn may be used as the basis of a report. In reports all items on a record are automatically reported but an option which is almost always used is to list only specified items in each report.

OPERATION OF THE SYSTEM: A typical patient record would be processed by an operator working interactively at a VDU as follows:-

1. When the admission is planned the details of the patient and the planned details of the admission are keyed into the computer. This creates an entry in the personal file - name, date of birth, address and patient number - and in the pre-registration (planned admission) file - date and time of admission, ward, consultant etc.
   The mini computer is linked to the mainframe (which holds the CHI) and the VDUs may control both computers simultaneously passing information from the CHI as necessary (personal identification details and identification details only).

2. When the patient arrives to be admitted any details which have previously been placed on file are checked and any missing information which is now available is supplied. Data may be transferred from the CHI if required. Multi-part admission documents are automatically printed. One copy is retained by the records department, one stays with the patient while one serves as a notification of movement or discharge document.

3. Any patient movement (notified by the nurses using a copy of the admission document) is keyed into the computer and the inpatient record is amended. Corrections may be made at any time.

4. On discharge, the inpatient information is transferred to the discharge file along with certain personal details which need to be retained as at the time of discharge. The personal file remains unchanged and may be used to identify the patient on subsequent contacts.

5. The discharge information is expanded to show various items required for local and national research and for statistical purposes. Coded information on diagnosis, operations and place of residence are added and the information transferred from the inpatient file is checked against the case notes. A summary of the discharge information is copied on to tape to be processed for Scottish national morbidity analysis.

CHECKING THE SYSTEM: A list of named patients is produced at a set time each day (midnight) for each ward and this is taken to the wards for the nurses to check.

REPORTS: As previously indicated the reporting is very flexible. Some standard reports are -

1. Alphabetic list of inpatients giving location - produced twice daily.
2. Summary of occupancy by ward and/or specialty - produced thrice daily. These summaries are circulated to the main receiving wards for each specialty and to the Community Medicine Specialist who is responsible for the overall monitoring of the availability of beds. The system may be interrogated at any time to produce the current status of bed occupancy. The response time is generally under a minute.
3. List of patient movements - daily.
4. Midnight status by ward/specialty/sex. This is produced weekly and maintained on line so that any specified summary over any time period may be produced as required.
5. List of deaths in hospital - weekly.
6. List of discharges - as required (monthly).
7. Special reports - easily produced to user specifications.

These examples and tomorrow's paper show how we have used an interlinked philosophy to promote total health.

S U M M A R Y

Four Health Boards in the West of Scotland have combined to produce a Community Health Index of their populations.

The paper describes this exercise and its use as the basis for a wide series of health promotion activities.

ETABLISSEMENT D' UN SYSTEME D' INFORMATION SUR L' ACTIVITE MEDICALE DE BASE: UNE APPROCHE.

F.L. Ricci, Municipalité de Rome, Italie.

A. Rossi Mori, F. de Rosis, Groupe de Recherche sur les Systèmes d' Information, Istituto Tecnologie Biomediche, CNR, Rome, Italie

SUMMARY

This paper outlines the objectives followed in establishing an information system for the evaluation of the activity performed by general practitioners in the Municipality of Rome. The general approach is described (to bring together and to integrate the information already collected by the administration), with some preliminary results obtained by applying this approach to the analysis of the distribution of general practitioners and of the administration of drugs.

1. INTRODUCTION

Au début de 1980, la mise en place d'un Service de Santé Publique (SSP) a ouvert dans notre pays une phase de transformation du système de soins. Jusqu'à ce moment-là, un ensemble d'institutions (Sociétés d'Assurance Mutuelle, Organismes de Gestion des Hôpitaux, etc.) gérait, d'une façon séparée et avec des logiques différentes, des sous-secteurs de la santé publique pour des sous-groupes particuliers de la population. Le SSP se propose de construire un système intégré qui garantit à tous les citoyens les services qui s'avèrent nécessaires, sur la base d'une évaluation des besoins de la population. Le Premier Plan National de Santé, 1980-82, met en évidence l'exigence de programmer les activités et d'évaluer et redéfinir de façon continue les programmes développés.

La gestion coordonnée du système de soins est assurée, au niveau local, par l' USL (Unità Sanitaria Locale), qui est la cellule politico-administrative du Service, avec autonomie de programmation, financement, évaluation et gestion des activités, pour une population de 200.000 individus au maximum.

L'administration des soins diagnostiques et thérapéutiques est réglée, dans le SSP, par le système suivant:

- l'activité de médecine générale est effectuée par des médecins en pratique libérale, qui sont liés au SSP par une convention à payement "pro capite": chaque citoyen doit choisir son "médecin de confiance" (médecin personnel) parmi une liste de médecins disponibles et acceptés par l'USI. L' USI verse périodiquement à chaque médecin inscrit dans ses listes un montant proportionnel au nombre de ses patients, à leur distribution par classes d' âge, et aux caractéristiques d'ancienneté et qualification professionnelle du médecin lui-même.

- l'activité de médecine spécialisée est effectuée dans les cabinets de consultation de l' USI et dans un réseau de cabinets privés conventionnés, auxquels l' USI rembourse les soins fournis aux citoyens sur demande du médecin de confiance.

- les médicaments prescrits au moyen d'ordonnances dressées par le médecin de confiance sur des formulaires standardisés sont fournis gratuitement par les pharmacies, qui sont ensuite remboursées tous les mois par l'USI, après contrôle des listes présentées.

D'après les évaluations disponibles, l'ensemble de ces activités correspond à 25 % environ du budget global du SSP (16.000 milliards de lires par an, ce qui correspond à peu près à 300.000 lires pro capite): la seule consommation de médicaments dépassant 50 % de ces frais.

De ce tableau ressort la position centrale du médecin de confiance, qui garantit les soins de première ligne, et qui est en même temps le canal-filtre indispensable pour les soins spécialisés et pharmacéutiques, et pour les admissions hospitalières.

La réqualification de l'activité médicale de base, indiquée parmi les objectifs prioritaires du Plan 80-82, demande donc que l' USI dispose d'un système d'information qui lui permet l'évaluation et le contrôle continu de cette activité, et la mise au point de programmes d'information et de formation adaptés aux exigences des médecins et des usagers, plutôt que de contrôle bureaucratique et policier.

Au niveau du système national de statistiques, il n'existe toutefois actuellement aucune information sur la plupart des secteurs de soins, et de l'activité médicale de base en particulier: l' Institut Central de Statistique ne publie que des données comptables et administratives sur l'activité des hôpitaux; les Sociétés d'Assurance Mutuelle publiaient, jusqu'à 1976, des informations sur leur activité dans le domaine de la médecine générale et spécialisée et de la consommation de médicaments: ces informations étaient toutefois recueillies, présentées et élaborées suivant des critères non unifiés.

De ces informations, si sévèrement limitées, on faisait d'autre part une utilisation très faible, en raison du fait que l'activité de programmation et d'évaluation, effectuée par le seul Organisme Gouvernemental existant (le Ministère de la Santé) était bien limitée elle-même.

2. OBJECTIF DE CETTE RECHERCHE

Dans le cadre des initiatives organisées par l' "Observatoire Epidémiologique" de la Région Lazio, et sur demande de l' Autorité Municipale responsable de la Santé, nous avons abordé le problème du système d'information sur la médecine de base dans la ville de Rome. Suivant la Loi Régionale, le Service de soins est assuré, dans cette ville, par 20 USI, placées dans les différents quartiers: dans la phase actuelle de construction du SSP, l' Autorité Municipale a le rôle d'entamer l'étude et l'expérimentation du nouveau système d'information, qui, à terme, sera géré d'une façon autonome par les différentes USI.

L'approche que nous avons choisi est la suivante:

a. au lieu de s'engager dans un travail lourd de recueil d'information ad hoc, évaluer dans quelle mesure les informations déjà disponibles, recueillies à des fins administratives, pouvaient être utilisées à fin d'évaluation (par des petites modifications adéquates). Cela correspond à l'exigence, souvent affirmée chez nous (1), que le système d'information sur la santé ne soit pas subdivisé en différentes sections (administration, épidémiologie, clinique et gestion) gérées par différentes institutions et insuffisamment reliées entre elles, mais resulte du travail intégré des différents services;

b. à partir du cadre ainsi esquissé, définir la méthodologie pour la mise en place d'un étude plus approfondie (par échantillons, et orientée vers les problèmes principaux qui seraient mis en évidence) des modalités suivant lesquelles est effectuée l'activité médicale de base, des facteurs qui l' influencent, de son adéquation aux besoins réels de la population.

c. utiliser l'ensemble des informations obtenues pour établir un procèssus de discussion et de collaboration entre l'institution de santé et les opérateurs de base et les usagers. De ce processus, l'institution va tirer des indications précises sur les exigences de transformation du système de soins, les opérateurs une habitude et une méthode pour l'évaluation de leur activité, et les usagers une orientation pour une utilisation correcte du système lui-même.

la <u>phase préliminaire du travail</u> a demandé la reconstruction des différents flux d'information qui relient le médecin généraliste aux structures de soins et administratives qui sont dans le territoire. Cette analyse nous a confirmé l'existence d'un ensemble de flux et de supports, temporaires ou permanents, gérés de façon totalement séparée par différentes institutions, ce qui est le reflêt de l'intrication des compétences qui existe encore, dans cette phase de réorganisation du SSP.

Il en résulte, de toute façon, la possibilité d'évaluer, dès maintenant ou bien par des modifications opportunes, les <u>quatre connexions principales du médecin généraliste</u> avec l'extérieur (figure 1):

- les patients soignés par chaque médecin, déjà mémorisés pour le payement des médecins mêmes;
- les ordonnances de médicaments, actuellement mémorisées pour le remboursement des pharmacies;

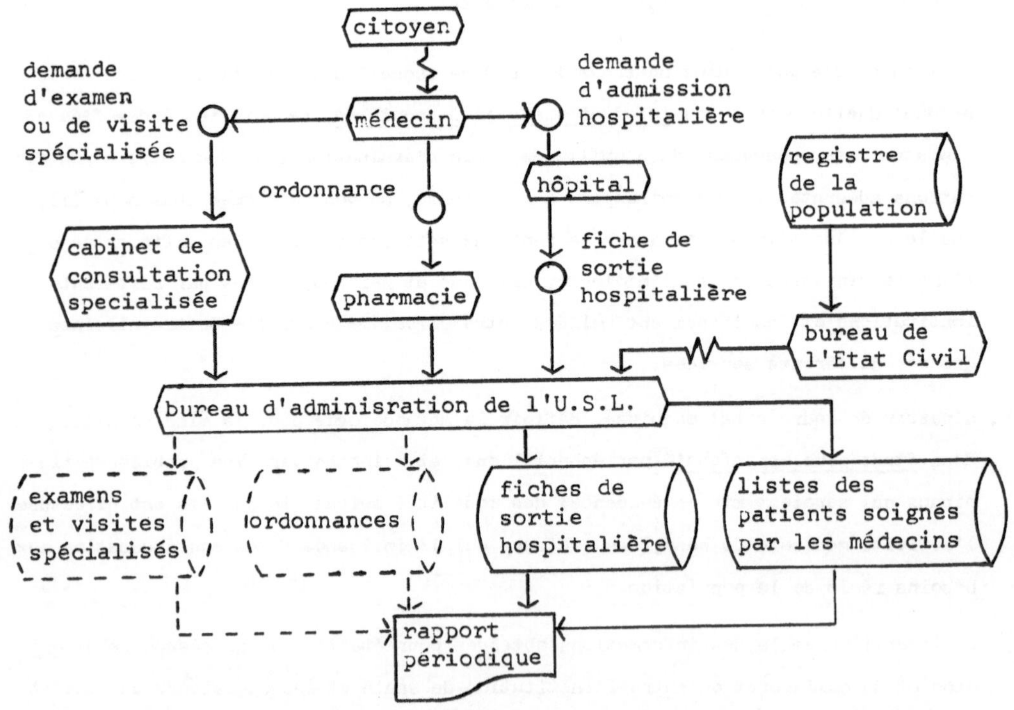

fig.1 Sujets (▭), flux, supports temporaires (o) et permanents (▭) d'information, actuels (———) et prévus (- - -).

- les examens et les visites spécialisés effectués, qui seront mémorisés pour le remboursement des cabinets conventionnés;
- les fiches de sortie hospitalière, qui seront mémorisées pour l'évaluation de l'activité des hôpitaux et de la morbidité qu'ils prennent en charge.

3. LE CONTEXTE INTERNATIONAL

Les éléments qui nous semblent caractériser le système d'information adopté, dans les expériences d'autres pays, sont les suivants:

- la nature de l'institution qui utilise le système, et donc les buts auxquels le système même se propose de répondre: en géneral (2,3,4) il s'agit d'institutions scientifiques, qui utilisent des données recueillies par l'administration, pour effectuer des analyses détaillées mais épisodiques de problèmes spécifiques. Les expériences de gestion - utilisation du SI par l'Autorité de Santé Publique se sont déroulées en Islande et aux Etats Unis (5), dans le cadre du Medicaid Management Information System (6): en ce cas, les objectifs rentrent dans le programme général de rationalisation des aspects financiers et d'organisation du système de soins, qui semble caractériser la phase actuelle au niveau international: contrôle des fraudes et des abus majeurs, évaluation de la qualité des soins fournis, et formation des différents opérateurs impliqués;
- les formes de contrôle exercées, et donc le niveau d'organisation et d'élaboration de l'information: le recueil et l'élaboration sont fait, en général, au niveau central (l' Etat) et les essais pour établir un contrôle local effectué par des représentants des opérateurs mêmes ont produit des résultats douteux;
- les niveaux d'integration entre les différents sous-systèmes d'information relatifs à des secteurs spécifiques de l'activité de diagnostic et de soins.

L'approche que nous avons adopté est d'établir un système d'information étendu à la population entière, qui intègre les sous-systèmes actuellement séparés,pour reconstruire une image globale de l'activité médicale de base, et soit confié à la gestion de l' USI à des fins de programmation: dans cette optique, la dimension de la population desservie et des services impliqués, et la nature non seulement technique, mais aussi politique et administrative de l'organisme chargé de l'utilisation de l'information, offrent à notre avis quelque garantie de reduire certains des insuccès de l'expérience américaine.

4. MATERIEL ET METHODES

Dans la phase actuelle du travail, nous avons analysé le sous-système: choix du médecin - ordonnance de médicaments, dont le schéma "entités - relations", representé suivant une modification du modèle de Chen (7), est indiquée en figure 2.

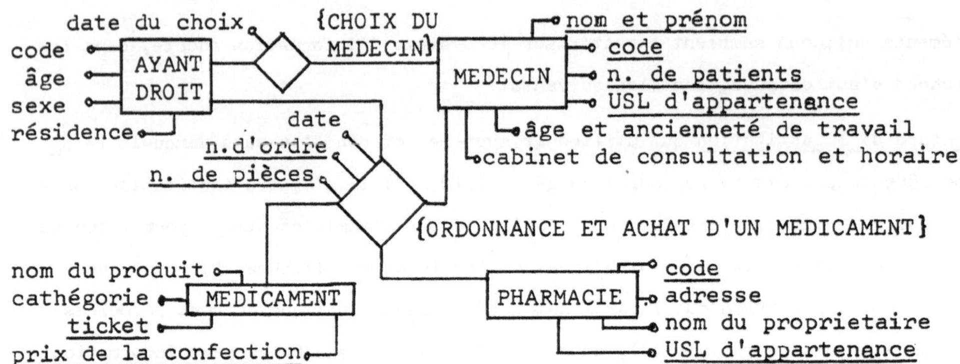

fig.2 Modèle Entités-Relations du sous-système "choix du médecin/ordonnance de médicaments":
▭ entité (cathégorie d'objects qui font partie du S.S.P.)
◇ association (relation logique entre entités)
—o attribut (propriété d'une entité ou d'une relation).
Les attributs soulignés correspondent à des informations enregistrées dans les fichiers sub a et b; les attributs non soulignés correspondent à des informations recueillies, mais actuelment non enregistrées dans les fichiers sub a et b.

Les fichiers utilisés sont les suivants:

a. Registre des médecins conventionnés,

b. Fichiers mensuels des ordonnances (environs 2 millions par mois, qui correspondent à une dépense de 2 milliards de lires par an).

Le lien entre les informations contenues dans ces deux fichiers, effectué au moyen du code du médecin, a donné un couplage correct pour le 91.5 % des médecins. Ce lien nous a permis de mesurer les distributions et les relations qui existent dans un ensemble très simple d'<u>indicateurs d'offre et d'activité</u>:

- le nombre de citoyens inscrits dans la liste de chaque médecin;
- le nombre et le coût moyen des médicaments ordonnés par chaque médecin, par rapport au nombre de patients inscrits dans ses listes.

Nous avons abordé, de cette façon, une évaluation:

- de la collectivité desservie par chaque généraliste, avec une analyse des phénomènes d'hyper et d'hypo activité, du respect de la norme (1500 patients/médecin), des critères suivant lesquels est effectué le choix du médecin de la part de la population;
- du rôle exercé par les médecins mêmes dans la prescription des médicaments, et des facteurs qui l'influencent.

5. PREMIERS RESULTATS

Bien que l'objectif immediat de notre travail soit plutôt la mise au point d'une méthodologie que l'évaluation de l'activité médicale de base dans la ville de Rome, nous allons indiquer ici quelques resultats descriptifs obtenus, qui nous semblent prouver la validité de la méthode et indiquer les démarches ulterieures à poursuivre.

a. Du point de vue de la disponibilité globale des médecins, il semble y avoir une situation très favorable (valeur moyen de l'index "patients soignés par médecin" = 496), ce qui correspond au fait que, en Italie aussi, les médecins ont tendance à se concentrer dans les grandes villes: la distribution par USI n'est toutefois pas homogène, et les zones péripheriques et à composition sociale moins élevée sont plus défavorisées, par rapport aux zones du centre historique.
Face à cette situation générale, il y a toutefois un nombre très élevé (43.6 %) de médecins pratiquement "inactifs" (ayant moins de 50 patients dans leur liste), et un nombre assez important (10.0 %) de médecins "hyperactifs", qui dépassent la norme de 1500 patients.
Plus le nombre moyen de patients par médecin est élevé, plus la population "se presse" progressivement vers les groupes de médecins ayant un nombre de patients plus élevé, plutôt que s'adresser de façon privilégiée aux médecins dont le nombre de patients est inférieur: cela nous semble prouver la nécessité d'établir un système d'information qui oriente le médecin au moment du choix de l'USI dans laquelle il veut établir son cabinet, et la population au moment du choix du médecin.

b. Le taux moyen de médicaments administrés par patient ne semble pas être lié au nombre de patients du médecin: il y a en fait une légère diminution de ce taux (mineure, toutefois, de la variation entre deux mois successifs) qui serait en accord avec les résultats d'autres études, suivant lesquels le niveau d'ordonnance diminuerait proportionnellement au nombre de patients, puisque ainsi la fréquence des visites effectuées diminuerait. Il est toutefois possible que d'autres facteurs inter viennent pour "masquer" le phénomène réel. P.e., les médecins signent les ordonnances aussi pour des individus non inscrits dans leur listes: ce phénomène décroit en importance proportionnellement à la dimension des listes mêmes, en introduisant dans le taux d'ordonnance un biais de poids décroissant.

6. DEVELOPPEMENTS IMMEDIATS

Dans les mois prochains, nous allons expérimenter:

a. le lien des deux fichiers cités en 4 a. et b. avec le fichier des "ayant droit", au moyen du code d'identification du citoyen, pour vérifier quel est le poid exercé sur la consommation de médicaments par des variables telles que l'âge et le sexe du patient, déjà remarquées comme très importantes dans les études conduites en d'autres pays (8).

b. Pour un échantillon des USI, l'enrichissement de l'information actuellement recueillie dans le fichier des ordonnances avec d'autres informations nécessaires pour avoir une image plus détaillée de la consommation de médicaments; p.e., la catégorie du médicament, qui permet d'effectuer des analyses spécifiques sur les produits et les associations de produits.

c. Dans le même échantillon des USI, la réalisation du système d'information complet indiqué en figure 1, par le lien des trois fichiers susnommés avec les données relatives aux examens et aux visites effectués dans les cabinets conventionnés, et aux fiches de sortie hospitalière.

Il faudra aussi étudier des formes convenables pour les rapports périodiques qui seront utilisés par les administrations des USI; ils devront, en tout cas, réduire autant que possible l'information contenue, et adopter des modalités de présentation opportunes, afin de permettre une lecture simple et rapide. A terme, il s'agira donc de rapports pour les cas exceptionnels, dans lesquels seront indiqués seulement les médecins, les groupes de patients, les médicaments, les zones, etc., qui sortent de une situation "de référence", definie sur la base des tendances passées et des objectifs du plan.

REMERCIEMENTS

Les aspects operationnels de ce travail n'auraient pas été possibles sans la collaboration de A.M. Bocchi, à laquelle vont nos remerciements.

REFERENCES

(1) De Rosis F, Pizzutilo S. Health care reorganisation and information system building in Italy. Methods of Information in Medicine. 1980 ;

(2) Contandriopoulos AP, Rivard JY. Development of a master file for the professional corporation of physicians of Quebec for use in planning and analysis. Proceedings of Medinfo 77. North Holland Publishing Company

(3) Wade OL, Hood HE. An analysis of prescribing of an hypnotic in the community. Brit. J. Prev. Soc. Med. 1972; 26: 121 - 128

(4) Wade OL, Hadden DR, Hood H. The prescribing of drugs used in the treatment of diabetes. Brit. J. Prev Soc. Med. 1973; 27 : 44 - 88

(5) Grimsson A., Olafson O. Drug prescription in Iceland. Brit.J.Prev.Soc.Med. 1977; 31 : 65 - 66

(6) Knoben JE, Mc Ghan WF. Surveillance of drugs use utilizing the Medicaid Information System. Medical Informatics in Europe. Paris, 1979

(7) Batini C, Santucci G. Top-down design in the Entity-Relationship model. Int.Conf. on the E-R approach to system analysis and design. Los Angeles, dec. 1979

(8) Johnes DA, Sweetnam A, Elwood PC. Drug prescribing by GPs in Wales and in England. Journal of Epidemiology and Community Health. 1980; 34 : 119 - 123

EVALUATION DE LA MORBIDITE HOSPITALIERE PUBLIQUE ET PRIVEE DES BOUCHES-DU-RHONE APPROCHE DE L'ADEQUATION DES MOYENS DEFINIS PAR LA CARTE SANITAIRE

[x]BENECH J-M, [x]BRUNEL M., [xx]SAMBUC R., [xx]FIESCHI M.

x Service Médical de l'Assurance Maladie des Travailleurs Salariés : Médecins Conseils - Echelon Régional du Contrôle Médical de la Région de Marseille 195, boulevard Chave - 13005 MARSEILLE

xx Service Universitaire de Biomathématique, Statistiques Médicales et Epidémiologiques, Informatique. Pr M. ROUX - Faculté de Médecine de Marseille 13385 MARSEILLE CEDEX 4.

SUMMARY :

The study related in this paper can be considered as an attempt to evaluate the "Bouches-du-Rhône" (BDR) morbidity in hospitals, and the suitability of the resources offered by sanitary charts. This work has been achieved by the BDR control service from data collected a given day over all the patients who were in the hospitals. (January 1, 1978)

Here are shown results applied only to medical, surgical, gynoecological and obstetrical fields. They put into relief the differences of the patient's origins among public, private and non profit-making private sectors. High occupation rates may be then explained, but not entirely justified, by different flows of patients coming from their residence places to hospitals.

The interest of such a study is the instantaneous photography it provides of the entire set of BDR patients in hospitals.

INTRODUCTION :

Cette communication présente une double tentative d'évaluation de la morbidité hospitalière des BDR et l'adéquation des moyens définis par la carte sanitaire. Elle est réalisée à partir de données recueillies dans le cadre d'une enquête de type transversal portant sur l'ensemble des malades présents, un jour donné, dans les établissements d'hospitalisation privés (PR), privés à but non lucratif (PNL) et publics (PU) pour les disciplines médecine, chirurgie, gynéco-obstétrique.

Le traitement statistique a été effectué par le Service Médical de l'Assurance Maladie, en collaboration avec le Service Universitaire d'Informatique Médicale (Pr M. ROUX).

L'enquête porte sur 17.374 malades ; les données recueillies comportent l'identification de l'établissement et du service, et pour le malade : l'adresse, le motif de l'hospitalisation (code OMS Liste D 300 rubriques 1968), le régime, le risque, la situation, le sexe, l'âge, la date d'entrée et le mode d'entrée.

I/ - EVALUATION DE LA MORBIDITE HOSPITALIERE

Les lits d'hospitalisation ont une vocation dont la réalité doit être appréciée au travers des caractéristiques socio-démographiques et épidémiologiques de la population hospitalisée.

Les variables *sexe et âge* sont inter-dépendantes. La majorité des malades a plus de 65 ans et on constate, par rapport à la population générale, dans les lits de médecine PR, PNL et de chirurgie PR, une sur-représentation féminine, alors qu'elle est masculine dans les lits de médecine PU (non retrouvée à l'AP de Paris [3] et [4]). On trouve en médecine PU et PNL ainsi qu'en chirurgie PU des sujets de moins de 16 ans, de sexe masculin, en proportion comparable à celle de la population. Les lits d'obstétrique PU se singularisent par la présence de femmes âgées de plus de 45 ans atteintes d'affections génito-urinaires.

L'étude du *régime* d'assurance met en évidence une proportion importante de malades non salariés non agricoles dans les établissements PNL, cette caractéristique paraît liée à l'implantation de ces établissements dans le secteur de Marseille et de malades du régime agricole dans les établissements PU, qui semble expliquée par la part importante des lits PU dans les secteurs de résidence de ces malades.

La répartition des malades entre *assurés et ayants-droit, conjoints et enfants* présente certaines particularités : les 12,5% d'enfants hospitalisés en médecine et en chirurgie ne se trouvent que dans les lits PU et PNL, ce qui traduit l'absence de lit de pédiatrie dans le PR.

Le *mode d'entrée* caractérise le type d'hospitalisation : 60 à 70% des malades du PR dans les trois disciplines, sont adressés par le médecin traitant, l'autre mode caractéristique en médecine PR étant le transfert d'un autre établissement, PU le plus souvent, faisant jouer ainsi un rôle de moyen séjour à certains établissements PR. Les malades du PNL sont adressés : en médecine, en majorité par le médecin traitant ou recrutés dans une proportion trois fois moindre par consultation externe, en obstétrique la grande majorité entre en urgence, et en chirurgie les malades sont à égalité (40%) adressés par le médecin traitant ou recrutés par consultation externe. Dans le PU les malades sont admis en urgence ou après consultation externe, en chirurgie et en obstétrique ; en médecine aux deux modes précédents s'ajoutent les malades adressés par le médecin traitant.

Du fait du caractère transversal de l'enquête, il est impossible de calculer une durée moyenne de séjour, seule est connue la *durée de présence* réelle au jour de l'enquête, elle permet de mettre en évidence le rôle de moyen séjour joué par certains lits de médecine PR : 37% des malades sont présents depuis plus de 30 jours et moins de 365 jours. En chirurgie ce sont les établissements PNL qui présentent le plus grand étalement dans la distribution des durées de présence. En obstétrique retenons que 68% des malades sont présents depuis moins de 6 jours. En général les durées de présence les plus longues sont le fait des classes les plus âgées.

L'étude de la *morbidité* doit permettre de justifier l'utilisation des lits. Elle a été réalisée de deux manières : la première en prenant en compte les grandes classes nosologiques et en mettant en évidence les diagnostics les plus fréquents, ainsi en médecine prédominent les affections de l'appareil circulatoire avec les cardiopathies et les maladies cérébro-vasculaires et celles de l'appareil respiratoire avec les bronchites chroniques et l'asthme ; la deuxième en classant les diagnostics par ordre de fréquence jusqu'à caractériser 60% de la population hospitalisée, au-delà la dispersion des diagnostics étant trop grande. Cette répartition a été affinée par rapport au type d'hospitalisation, au sexe, à l'âge et aux durées de présence, ainsi, par exemple, viennent en tête en médecine PU les états morbides mal définis, ce qui paraît être en rapport avec une vocation particulière à résoudre les problèmes diagnostiques, leur disparition dans les durées de présence longues le confirme. De même viennent en tête les bronchites chroniques et l'asthme dans le PR et le PNL. Certaines affections sont caractéristiques du type d'hospitalisation : pour le PU les états morbides mal définis, les leucémies, les thalassémies, l'alcoolisme ; dans le PR le cancer du sein, les névroses, les fractures du col du fémur ; dans le PNL le cancer du poumon, du larynx, de l'oesophage et la pathologie du disque inter-vertébral chez l'homme, le cancer du sein, l'obésité et une part non négligeable des névroses chez la femme. Si l'on prend en compte l'âge et le sexe on trouve en exergue dans la classe 31-40 ans les névroses chez la femme et les discopathies chez l'homme. L'étude des durées de présence les plus longues fait ressortir que ces malades sont des femmes de plus de 70 ans, atteintes de troubles cérébro-vasculaires et de fractures du fémur hospitalisées dans un établissement jouant le rôle de long séjour ; de même les hommes atteints de troubles mentaux hospitalisés dans une clinique médicale "psycho-somatique" jouant en fait le rôle de clinique psychiatrique. En obstétrique le motif de l'hospitalisation oppose les établissements PR, 69% des hospitalisées le sont pour des accouchements simples, aux établissements PU et PNL où l'on retrouve les avortements et les accouchements compliqués ainsi que les affections génito-urinaires déjà citées.

L'étude de l'ensemble des résultats permet de caractériser les établissements PU, PR et PNL suivant la pathologie motivant les hospitalisations et suivant les caractéristiques socio-démographiques des hospitalisés. On note une relative identité entre les populations des établissements PU et PNL, mais ces derniers ne sont-ils pas dénommés hôpitaux privés ?

II/ - APPROCHE DE L'ADEQUATION DES MOYENS DEFINIS PAR LA CARTE SANITAIRE

La carte sanitaire définit, pour chaque discipline, un indice théorique lits-population. Les lits existants correspondent à ceux recensés le jour de l'enquête. L'évaluation de l'adéquation des moyens définis par la carte sanitaire consiste certes à analyser les différences constatées entre besoins théoriques et lits existants mais aussi les taux d'occupation. Ces deux indicateurs sont cependant insuffisants puisqu'on constate des flux de population entre les divers secteurs. Cette enquête essaie d'en rendre compte en considérant la pathologie et la spécialisation de certains établissements présentant une attraction particulière.

1°/ Médecine

Dans cette discipline, les besoins théoriques s'élèvent à 4025 lits, 6898 lits ont été recensés le jour de l'enquête ; on constate donc un excédent de 2873 lits (71%). Cet excédent, ainsi que le taux d'occupation instantané, globalement de 89%, varient par secteur et suivant le type d'hospitalisation.

SECTEURS	MARSEILLE			AIX		ARLES		AUBAGNE		MARTIGUES		SALON	
Indice lits-pop.	2,3°/₀₀			2,1°/₀₀		1,9°/₀₀		1,9°/₀₀		1,9°/₀₀		1,9°/₀₀	
Besoins th. lits	2.710			487		188		216		220		204	
Lits réels	4.811			684		508		411		275		209	
Variations %	+ 77			+ 40		+ 170		+ 90		+ 25		+ 2,5	
ETABLISSEMENTS	PNL	PR	PU	PR	PU	PR	PU	PR	PU	PR	PU	PR	PU
Taux d'occup.inst.%	83	97	87	94	72	83	90	94	78	74	85	110	85
Provenance % :													
BDR (même secteur	85	85	70	58	77	92	82	8	78	92	86	27	74
BDR (secteur ≠	6	6	8	33	9	4	10	39	17	5	13	64	24
Hors BDR	9	9	22	9	14	4	8	53	5	3	1	9	2

Le recrutement des établissements se fait dans leur propre secteur, sauf pour les établissements PR des secteurs d'Aix et d'Aubagne, dont nous étudierons les flux propres par la suite. L'étude du secteur de Marseille (4341 malades présents le jour de l'enquête, taux d'occupation instantané 89%) semble révéler une sous-évaluation du nombre de lits théoriques ; mais si l'on admet, d'une part, qu'en moyenne le double de la durée de présence au jour de l'enquête constitue un bon estimateur de la durée réelle de séjour, sous certaines hypothèses, d'autre part, qu'au-delà de 40 jours de séjour on est manifestement dans le cadre du moyen séjour, on peut retrancher les malades dans ce cas, soit 1.646. On obtient 2695 lits utiles, alors que l'estimation théorique est de 2710. En ce qui concerne le secteur d'Aix, les établissements PR, occupés en quasi totalité (94%), recrutent leurs malades dans d'autres secteurs des BDR (33%), essentiellement pour une pathologie cancéreuse, en provenance en général des établissements PU. De même, dans le secteur d'Aubagne, les établissements PR, et notamment deux d'entre eux, recrutent des malades provenant soit d'autres secteurs, soit de l'extérieur des BDR ; il s'agit d'établissements spécialisés en pathologie respiratoire et circulatoire. L'excédent de lits est bien réel, ces établissements jouant le rôle de moyen séjour.

2°/ Chirurgie

Dans cette discipline, les besoins théoriques s'élèvent à 4226 lits, 6030 ont été recensés le jour de l'enquête ; on constate donc un excédent de 1084 lits (42,6%). Cet excédent, ainsi que le taux d'occupation instantané, globalement de 85% varient là encore en fonction des secteurs et du type d'hospitalisation.

SECTEURS	MARSEILLE			AIX		ARLES		AUBAGNE		MARTIGUES		SALON	
Indice lits/pop.	2,5°/°°			1,9°/°°		2°/°°		2°/°°		2°/°°		2°/°°	
Besoins th. lits	2.913			441		198		228		231		215	
Lits réels	4.366			412		367		316		299		259	
Variations %	+ 49,8			- 6,6		+ 85,4		+ 38,6		+ 29,4		+ 20,5	
ETABLISSEMENTS	PNL	PR	PU	PR	PU	PR	PU	PR	PU	PR	PU	PR	PU
Taux d'occup.inst.%	88	95	76	101	78	94	74	88	76	100	68	107	42
Provenance % :													
BDR (même secteur	76	81	65	84	77	82	77	80	79	90	93	90	72
BDR (secteur ≠	7	10	10	5	5	9	9	11	13	8	7	8	22
Hors BDR	17	9	25	11	18	9	14	9	8	2	-	2	6

Si l'on considère que les séjours d'une durée supérieure à 30 jours ne correspondent pas à la vocation de lits de chirurgie aiguë, le nombre de malades qui auraient dû être hospitalisés le jour de l'enquête est de 3734, ce qui par rapport aux besoins théoriques ou à l'excédent que représentent les 6030 lits recensés, n'a rien de comparable, même si un certain nombre de malades sont recrutés à l'extérieur du département, du fait de la renommée du chirurgien, de la spécialisation ou du plateau technique de certains établissements. Ainsi, dans le cadre de la pathologie ostéo-musculaire, et dans le secteur de Marseille, les établissements PU recrutent à l'extérieur du département, le PNL dans le secteur de Marseille et le PR dans les autres secteurs des BDR et les départements adjacents. Autre exemple, dans le secteur de Salon, l'hôpital recrute une proportion non négligeable de ses malades en urgence et pour des traumatismes (antenne chirurgicale réputée).

3°/ Gynéco-obstétrique

Dans cette discipline, les besoins théoriques s'élèvent à 821 lits, 1033 ont été recensés le jour de l'enquête ; on constate donc un excédent de 212 lits (26%).

SECTEURS	MARSEILLE			AIX		ARLES		AUBAGNE		MARTIGUES		SALON	
Indice lits/pop.	0,5°/..			0,5°/..		0,5°/..		0,4°/..		0,5°/..		0,4°/..	
Besoins th. lits	509			116		49		46		58		43	
Lits réels	579			140		107		56		89		50	
Variations %	+ 14			+ 21		+ 118		+ 22		+ 53		+ 16	
ETABLISSEMENTS	PNL	PR	PU	PR	PU	PR	PU	PR	PU	PR	PU	PR	PU
Taux d'occup.inst.%	88	89	95	72	47	70	55	69	15	61	102	150	57
Provenance % :													
BDR (même secteur	77	90	78	72	84	96	90	64	67	96	90	80	91
BDR (secteur ≠	7	8	11	14	8	-	5	18	-	4	10	20	9
Hors BDR	16	2	11	14	8	4	5	18	33	-	-	-	-

Le taux global instantané est de 78%. On constate que 83% des malades proviennent du même secteur et 10% d'autres secteurs. Il est difficile de ne prendre en compte, que les séjours inférieurs à 12 jours, ces établissements, notamment PU et PNL, recrutant des malades atteints de tumeurs malignes ou d'affections génito-urinaires qui nécessitent une hospitalisation plus longue. Toutefois, il faut noter que 93% des malades restent moins de 30 jours et 66% d'entre eux moins de 12 jours. Les établissements PR du secteur de Salon présentent un taux d'occupation instantané de 150% alors qu'ils recrutent 20% de leur clientèle dans le secteur adjacent d'Arles, où on note pourtant un excédent de lits de 118%, et où les taux d'occupation sont de 70% pour le PU et 55% pour le PR.

L'appréciation de l'adéquation de la carte sanitaire ne peut être réalisée uniquement à partir de l'indice lits-population et du taux d'occupation. Il est nécessaire aussi de tenir compte des flux de population, des pathologies les motivant, qu'elles réclament des compétences ou des équipements techniques appropriés ou qu'elles relèvent de causes sociales ou du libre choix. Vouloir apprécier tous ces éléments de façon continue est illusoire en raison du volume des données. Il est donc souhaitable de réaliser de telles enquêtes transversales, dont le coût est moindre. On peut proposer l'estimation de la durée réelle du séjour comme étant, en moyenne, le double de la durée de présence au jour de l'enquête, sous certaines hypothèses, en particulier l'indépendance statistique entre la durée de séjour et la date d'entrée. Le fait de constater, un jour donné, un taux d'utilisation des lits voisin de l'estimation annuelle, n'implique pas obligatoirement la justification de tous les séjours, d'où l'intérêt d'exclure ceux dont la durée ne correspond pas à des lits de court séjour.

En conclusion, ce type d'enquête, au terme de l'analyse succincte présentée, recèle un grand nombre de possibilités d'appréciation du fonctionnement du système hospitalier de soins, mais à cette photographie panoramique, dont le champ couvre la quasi totalité de la structure médico-chirurgico-obstétricale du département, devraient succéder d'autres enquêtes, dont le champ restreint permettra de préciser les différents profils hospitaliers et d'apprécier médicalement l'adéquation du malade à la structure hospitalière.

BIBLIOGRAPHIE

1 - EICHER C, HATCHUEL A : Les admissions en urgence à l'Assistance Publique. Ecole des Mines. Assistance Publique (Juillet 1978)

2 - EICHER C, HATCHUEL A. - SIMON JM, LE GAIL JR. Des facteurs qui influencent la décision d'admission en urgence à l'Assistance Publique de Paris, la nouvelle presse médicale 9/2/80 9 n°7 ; p. 449, 450, 451.

3 - BELLEVILLE -SEJOURNE AM, BIENTZ M, CHEVALIER J, DAGON L et JOLLY. Morbidité et mortalité dans les hôpitaux de Paris de 1978. Association des amis de l'Assistance Publique de Paris 1980.

4 - LIESS M, BEAUVAIS N. Essai d'analyse de l'hospitalisation publique sous trois aspects : Admission - Séjour - Remboursement effectué par le Régime Général de la Sécurité Sociale, au moyen d'une enquête par sondage, Revue Médicale de l'Assurance Maladie CNAMTS n° 2 (1973) p. 43 à 66.

5 - AURRAN Y, GOUVERNET J, SAMBUC R, SIVIRINE F. "Système de gestion de dossiers médicaux en mode conversationnel : Système SYCVAR".
Symposium on medical informatics 14 - 17 mars 1978 TOULOUSE.

o

o o

REGIONAL PATIENT DATABANK

K. Schuurman

SAZZOG Foundation
6835 GN ARNHEM
The Netherlands

This paper explains the aims of SAZZOG in relation to the aims and scope of the preferred regional patient databank. In addition, some characteristics of the SAZZOG Foundation are presented.

It is explained how the preferred structure of the information services organisation in healthcare in the Netherlands will be.

A quantitative discription of the use of all kinds of healthcare facilities in a region of 1 million people is given followed by a discussion of the need for regionally acquired and available patient-oriented data.

This discription is based on a study directly related to the relevance of regional patient databanks in the Netherlands.

Within this context the architecture of the planned informationsystem in the SAZZOG-region will be given.

SAZZOG IN A NUTSHELL

The SAZZOG Foundation was established in 1974, with the aim to develop the automatic information services for the hospitals in the southern and eastern parts of the province of Gelderland in the Netherlands (see fig. 1).

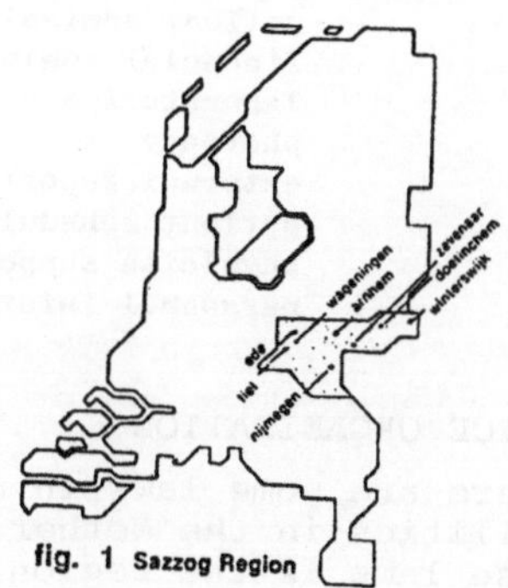

fig. 1 Sazzog Region

The number of inhabitants in the region is about 1 million.
The health care facilities in this area or region were considered relatively well-connected from the managerial as well as the patient mobility points of view, and all together large enough to develop the services foreseen on an economical basis. Although at the moment of its inception the rendering of services to other health care facilities than hospitals was not excluded, such aim had no priority.
For a better understanding by readers from outside the Netherlands, it is necessary to know that health care in this country is largely based on "private initiative", only indirectly and globally controlled by the government. The influence of the government is mainly oriented towards the direction of development of the different sectors of the care system, much less to the organizational and operational aspects. New laws will be passed through parliament in the near future, which will give more power to government and which will restrict the autonomy of the individual institutions, but that will not challenge the private character of the health care system.
Within this context, the SAZZOG has gradually developed the concept of the comprehensive Regional Health Information Service, comprising hospitals and the other health care facilities. Whether this idea can be realized in its full consequence is doubtful, because there is no accepted policy in this country to promote and support the cohesiveness of the health care facilities in a region (and not on the local or national level either). Because of this uncertainty, the aims and scope of the organization are double-tongued: the idealistic approach is concerned with the development of the comprehensive regional health information services as mentioned. The other one, maybe more realistic, is to support the health care institutions and practices with information services according to their own needs. It is a main task to maintain the compatibility between these two aims.

To give an impression of the SAZZOG-organization the number and kind of users, the machines and the applications that are operational are given (see fig. 2).

USERS	MACHINES	APPLICATIONS
8 hospitals	1 medium size computer	patient registration
3 nursing homes	20 mini-computers	patient admission
4000 beds	125 terminals	financial administration
6 G.P.'s	20 printers	laboratories
		pharmacy
		external reporting
		patient scheduling
		physician support
		personnel information

fig. 2

STRUCTURE OF INFORMATION SERVICE ORGANISATION

As already mentioned above there are some laws in development which concerned all health care facilities in the Netherlands.
One of the main topics of these laws is the regionalization of health care.
Regionalization is defined as follows:
The devision of the country into (geografical) area's, in which a

transparant and coherent system of health care facilities functions. In addition it is thought necessary to develop a structure for the information services organization in health care to serve the performance, evaluation and adjust of health care management.
It is stressed that in health care informationstreams can be distinguished, namely
- informationstream of data of health care facilities
- informationstream of data per patient.

Until now there are some general accepted starting points, namely
- It is not necessary for the enforcement of the law that the government has data at his disposal about individual patients.
- The creation of a rigorous separation between data, needed for health care management and data, needed for treatment of individual patients is in practice not possible.
- It can be necesary in relation to enforcement of the law to make links between different databanks for example to gather information about patientstreams.
- Acumulated or aggregated data on the national level should be dirived from existing databanks.

The most logical structure of information service organization can be shown as follows (see fig. 3).

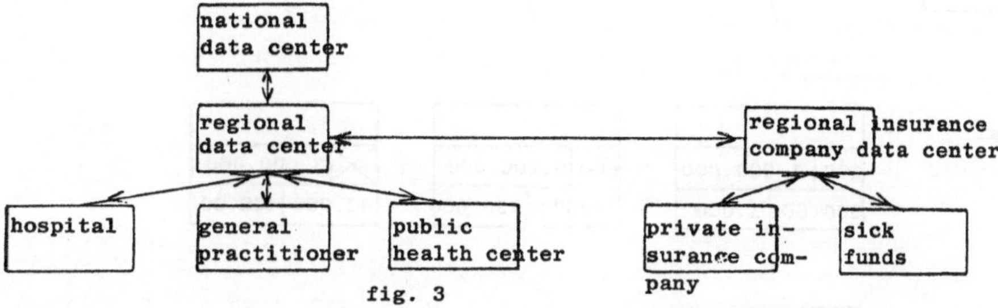

fig. 3

In this filosofy it is essential that the health care facilities on the local level are in principle responsible for their own methodology of information service.
In what extent and in what time this structure becomes reality in the Netherlands depends on many factors.

NEEDS FOR A REGIONAL PATIENT DATABANK

First of all it is relevant to know what is realy happening every day in a region of for instance 1 million inhabitants.
Fig. 4 gives an impression of the use of all kinds of health care facilities in a region.
The numbers are very roughly estimated and depend on the definitions used; so be careful in interpretation.

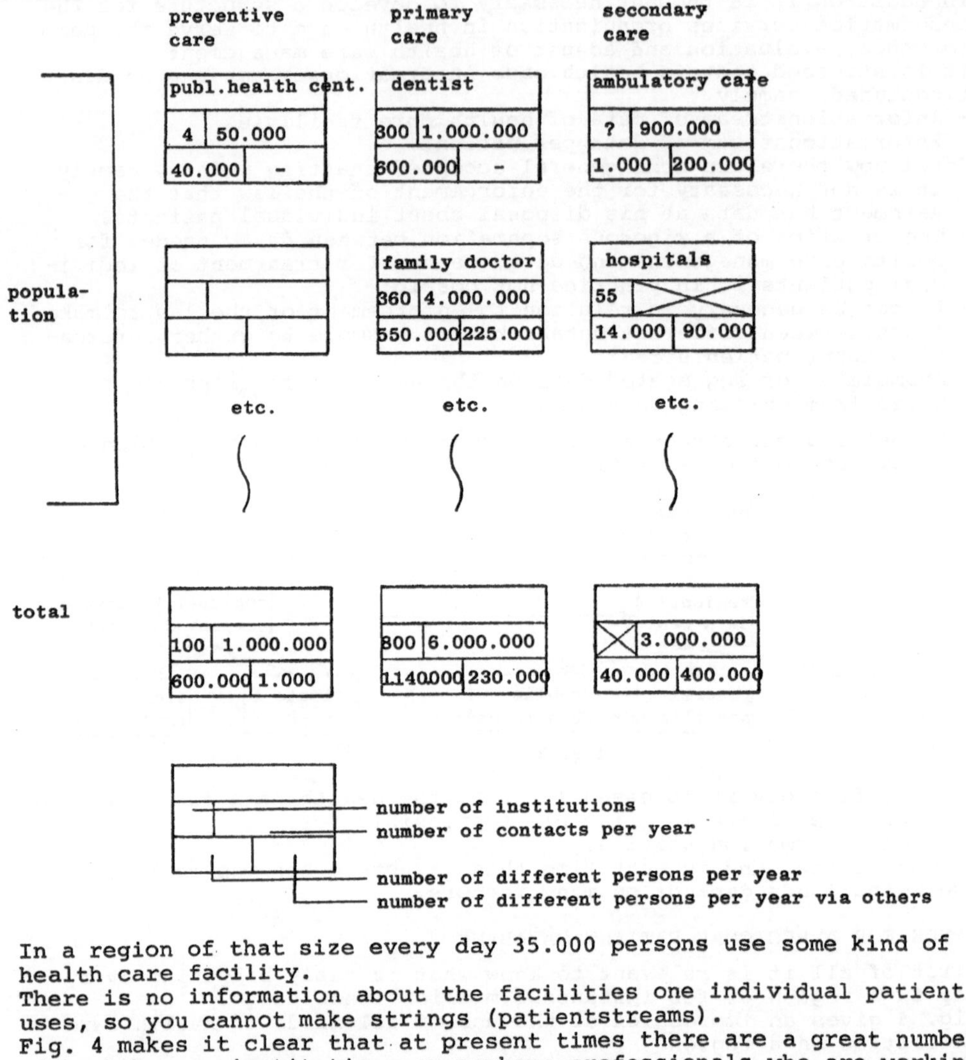

In a region of that size every day 35.000 persons use some kind of health care facility.
There is no information about the facilities one individual patient uses, so you cannot make strings (patientstreams).
Fig. 4 makes it clear that at present times there are a great number of health care institutions or perhaps professionals who are working on the medical care of individual persons; this in contradistinction to the past.
In the past for many people the family doctor was the only physician they met.
The above and the increased mobility of the people results in the fact that a patient at present times will be treated by much more physicians during his life.
Every physician gives his own contribution to the recording of the case history of the patient.

The patient has good reasons to hope that:

- the data on the different pages who are spread over a number of health care institutions are not in contradiction with each other;
- the access to the data is fast when necessary and the data is readable, so that for instance known allergies etc. will not be established in an empirial way by every next doctor, who treats the patient.

In short: Medical care has become team-work, but the recording of the history remained in many cases one-man work.

In many hospitals in the Netherlands this problem is solved in such a way that the medical record is recorded and controled on the institutional level.

This solves only a part of the problem given above, because the case-history is only known in the health care institutes where the patient has been treated.

The next step should be the development of communication facilities between the different health care units.

A well known example of an operational system is Sweden where a network functions in the region Stockholm and a regional patient databank is the central part of that system.

At this moment there are some examples of a regional patient databank in the Netherlands too. The contents of the databank exist only of administrative data and the number of participating institutions is very limited (a few hospitals, some nursery homes etc.).

The benefits are of a pragmatic kind such as:

data collection, data processing and datastorage is once-only, the reliability of data is improved and uniformity is stimulated.

A recent investigation in the Netherlands shows a real need of information that can only become available when data is stored per patient This data is needed for patient treatment, health care management, research and epidemiology.

Besides the more administrative oriented data like person-related data, family relation, insurance data etc. there is also a real need for contact data, data on essential medications, allergies, patient's condition etc.

As important benefits are mentioned:

- the use of on different places stored information of one patient is stimulated;
- better and more information will become available to serve a combination of aims like health care management, research and epidemiology;
- the availability of statistics describing the performance of the health care system and the health status of the population;
- a lot of administrative work becomes easier;
- uniformity is stimulated.

Important problems and conditions are:

- there have to be good rules for data management;
- the privacy, accescibility and data exchange requires special attention;
- what data-elements are needed on departmental, institutional, regional or national level?

Whether a regional patient databank in an expanded shape (all kinds of health care facilities, many data elements) will be quickly implemented or not is not known at this moment.

However one aspect is clear anyway namely:
there is a real need of information that can only be derived when data is stored and is accessible per patient. As for we know now the idea of the regional patient databank fits into the ideas about the structure of the information services organisation in the Netherlands.
As far as concerned the SAZZOG organization the first step will be the implementation of a regional patient databank to replace the separate patient databanks of all health care institutions who are member of the SAZZOG foundation.
In the beginning the record length will be very limited (only administrative data).

ARCHITECTURE OF THE PLANNED INFORMATION SYSTEM

Distribution of computer processing and storage facilities has been the SAZZOG hardware policy from the very beginning. More important however is the policy that the input and output facilities should be in the hands of the health personnel, and their operation an integral part of the daily work of these people.
Centralized processing power can in principle provide for such decentralized input/output machines, of course. The policy to distribute processors is mainly based on economical and psychological arguments.
The inter-user communication that is required in a comprehensive regional information system is provided for by networks to which the processors are connected. The regional network will be composed of a hierarchy of rings and brooms (fig. 5). The ring allows the processors attached to the ring to communicate with each other directly. Processors connected to a broom cannot communicate with each other, but only through the intermediary of the broom processor.

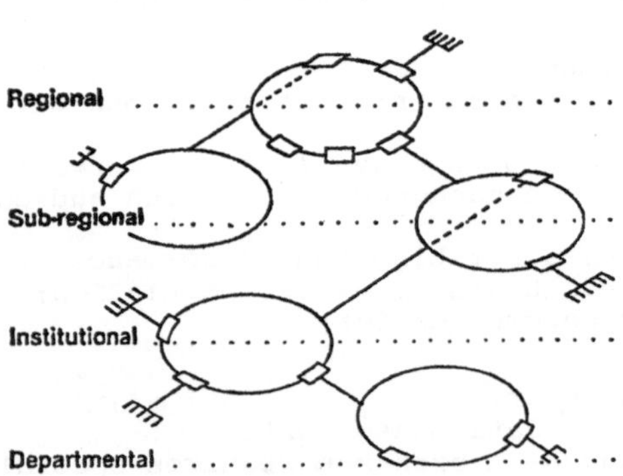

fig. 5

A connector processor attaches a ring to the next higher ring. At this moment, six rings are operational at the institutional (hospital) level, each with a considerable number of combs connected to them.

At the regional level there is a broom which connects terminals located in nursing homes throughout the region, as well as terminals located in G.P. offices throughout the region. The latter will be taken over by brooms at the sub-regional level as soon as this level is implemented. In the near future, the terminals in nursing homes and G.P. offices will be exchanged for processors with storage facilities, but this will not essentially change the system, as they will be broomed in the same way. They may, of course, constitute brooms or rings themselves.

It should be stressed that to a very large extent identical programs are used for basically identical functions, even if they are implemented for quite dissimilar institutions. E.g., the programs that identify and register patients for G.P.'s and for hospitals are identical. This makes it even possible for both to access the same program copies that may operate on different patient files.

In the next two years, the network as drawn in fig. 5 will be operational completely. Then, and only then, will it be possible to have only one master copy of a patient identification for the whole region. These patient identification data will be distributed among the processors at the regional level, with relevant copies at each lower level. For the more distant furure this suggests a problem of great importance which we have not solved yet. It is the question whether the basic patient data that may comprise significantly more than identification data, will be stored at the "highest", or rather at the "lowest" level. The latter would mean that, for all practical purposes, the data would be stored in the patient's G.P. office (in the Netherlands the great majority of the people have one and only one so-called family doctor).

CONCLUDING REMARKS

In this paper only some aspects of the development of a regional patient databank related to regional informationsystem are discussed. There are some aspects who concerns the way in which the health care in the Netherlands is organized, but also a number of aspects who have an international character.

Exchange of knowledge on this particular field seams very useful.

REFERENCES

1. Wills, A.R. (1978): Replicable, multi-purpose patient index systems - an analysis of some necessary features. Proceeding MIE 78.
2. Peterson, H.E., e.a. (1978): The Stockholm County Medical Information System, Springer-Verlag, Berlin-Heidelberg-New York, 1978.
3. Verhoef, E. (1979): Gebruik van gezondheidszorgvoorzieningen in Nederland (Use of health care facilities in the Netherlands).
4. Roukens, J. (1980): Information system for general practitioners in the context of a regional information service. Proceeding "The computer in the doctor's office", april 1980.

Prévision régionale de la main d'oeuvre dentaire: le cas du Québec

Alain Saucier, Jean-Marc Brodeur, André-Pierre Contandriopoulos,
Gilles Dussault
Département d'administration de la santé
Université de Montréal

Quebec dentists are poorly distributed over the territory of Quebec as a whole. They tend to establish themselves in the large centres - a feature that has become accentuated over the last few decades. This inadequate distribution hinders the progress of existing free dental-care programs.

A study of the population of Quebec according to certain socio-demographic characteristics permitted the authors to divide the province into light homogenous regions based on a regrouping of census areas.

On the basis of these eight regions, it was possible to illustrate the future evolution of dental care supply, by using two multiregional projection models - firstly a projection of the number of dentists, and secondly a projection of the studied population.

Prévision régionale de la main d'oeuvre dentaire: le cas du Québec[1]

La problématique: l'accessibilité géographique

Les professionnels de la santé en général et les dentistes en particulier constituent des sous-populations spécifiques dont la mauvaise répartition risque de faire obstacle aux interventions de l'Etat au niveau de la couverture des soins. Les objectifs d'accessibilité aux soins et d'égalisation des ressources préoccupent de plus en plus le planificateur. Au cours de cette communication, nous verrons comment l'établissement de régions homogènes et l'utilisation de modèles simples de projections permettent d'illustrer l'accessibilité régionale aux soins et son évolution. En ce qui concerne les services dentaires au Québec, le problème d'effectifs se situe à deux niveaux: manque d'effectifs provincialement et disparités interrégionales.

En 1977, on dénombrait au Québec 3.5 dentistes pour 10 000 habitants tandis que le rapport souhaitable est environ 4.5 pour 10 000; le nombre de dentistes était donc insuffisant à l'époque pour assurer une offre de services adéquate à l'ensemble de la population. Une projection au niveau provincial pour déterminer le moment où l'objectif de 4.5 dentistes pour 10 000 habitants sera atteint constitue une partie de ce travail. Cette projection tente aussi d'illust er les disparités importantes qui existent entre les régions. En 1977, la région du Montréal métropolitain comptait en effet 5.38 dentistes pour 10 000 habitants tandis que les régions du Bas St-Laurent/Gaspésie et de la Côte Nord se classaient aux derniers rangs avec respectivement 1.55 et 1.57 dentistes pour 10 000 habitants.[2]

Nous nous interrogerons donc sur l'évolution provinciale de l'offre de soins dentaires et sur les changements au niveau des différences entre les régions.

La méthode de regroupement des comtés de recensement en régions homogènes. Quel type d'unité régionale choisir pour une telle analyse.

Les régions recherchées doivent répondre à deux critères: elles doivent être en nombre assez restreint et être homogènes par rapport au phénomène à étudier. Si on décide de travailler à partir des divisions de recensement[3] relativement homogènes, on se retrouve avec 76 régions; si par contre le choix se porte sur les 12 régions socio-sanitaires existantes[4], on néglige le critère d'homogénéité.

Afin de constituer les régions homogènes, nous privilégierons donc la notion d'uniformité en fonction de l'objet d'étude plutôt que la notion de régions géographiques continues. Ainsi, deux unités de base faisant partie du même regroupement pourront ne pas être géographiquement voisines.

Plus une unité est petite, plus elle est homogène et c'est à partir de telles unités que nous devons construire les groupes homogènes. Il faut donc une unité géographique de base qui puisse être considérée comme homogène et pour laquelle les données statistiques soient facilement disponibles; les 76 divisions de recensement constitueront les unités de base utilisées.

Il s'agit de regrouper les 76 divisions de recensement en un nombre restreint de régions constituées d'un ensemble de divisions aussi semblables que possible entre elles et aussi différentes que possible des autres régions.

Pour ce faire, il a fallu caractériser chacune des divisions de recensement à l'aide des 29 variables suivantes:

1) Variables démographiques

Pourcentage de la population âgée de moins de 15 ans; population âgée de 65 ans et plus; population habitant dans des municipalités de 2,500 habitants et plus; population dans les municipalités de 10 000 habitants et plus; degré d'urbanisation du comté; écart relatif de la population (1966-1976); densité de la population; taux de migration (1966-1971); taux de natalité (1976).

2) Variables socio-économiques

Revenu disponible per capita (1977); écart relatif du revenu (1971-1977); population de 15 ans et plus selon le niveau de scolarité (moins de 9 ans et post-secondaires); population de langue maternelle française.

3) Variables concernant les dentistes et les services de santé

Rapport dentistes-population; dentistes selon le nombre d'années de pratique (2 ans et moins, 31 ans et plus); rapport dentistes-population en fonction des comtés avoisinants; présence de dentistes spécialistes; variation de la densité relative (1966-1976); écart relatif du rapport dentistes-population (1966-1976); population consommant de l'eau fluorée; dentistes de sexe féminin; classification du comté; rapport denturologistes, hygiénistes dentaires, médecins généralistes et médecins spécialistes par

10 000 habitants; nombre d'hôpitaux de plus de 50 lits.

Note: Toutes les variables concernant les populations sont exprimées en pourcentage.

Il s'agissait ensuite de comparer les 76 divisions ou régions deux à deux pour identifier celles dont l'indice de ressemblance était le plus significatif[5]. On fusionne alors ces deux divisions et l'on se retrouve avec 75 régions qui sont soumises au même processus jusqu'à ce que l'on atteigne un nombre de régions acceptable. Le choix du nombre de régions est déterminé par un indice de ressemblance incorporé dans une fonction-objectif qui mesure la perte d'information du regroupement lui-même. C'est à partir de l'écart des valeurs prises par la fonction-objectif que nous avons déterminé le nombre de régions car au-dessous de ce nombre la perte d'information devenait trop importante.

La figure I illustre ce processus qui débute par la fusion des comtés de Lotbinière et de Dorchester, puis vient celle des comtés regroupés Montmorency 1 et 2 avec celui de Napierville, etc. On doit ici préciser que quelques divisions ont été réunies avant même d'être soumises au regroupement vu la très grande importance du voisinage géographique de ces régions. On retrouve donc, au départ, 69 régions. La description détaillée de la méthode de regroupement a déjà été publiée par l'un des auteurs (Contandriopoulos, 1974).

Résultats du regroupement

La figure II représente les huit régions homogènes obtenues. C'est à partir de ces régions que nous avons mené l'analyse. Nous avons comparé les régions homogènes obtenues et les régions socio-sanitaires afin d'estimer les avantages de notre regroupement. Pour ce faire nous avons mis en relation le pouvoir explicatif des deux regroupements face aux 29 variables choisies. La fonction-objectif qui mesure la perte d'information des regroupements n'est que 28.8 pour les régions homogènes comparativement à 45.7 pour les régions socio-sanitaires. Même si le nombre de régions socio-sanitaires (douze) est plus grand que le nombre de régions homogènes (huit) ce qui devrait favoriser les régions socio-sanitaires, la perte d'information est de beaucoup supérieure avec les régions socio-sanitaires. Nous avons aussi comparé pour chacune des variables les valeurs du R^2 obtenues pour les deux regroupements en rapportant la valeur du R^2 des régions homogènes sur celle des régions socio-sanitaires. Des 29 variables étudiées, 23 voient leur variance totale mieux expliquée par le regroupement en régions homogènes.

Méthode de projection du nombre de dentistes

Globalement, il s'agit de déterminer, à chaque année, pour chacune des régions, le nombre de départs et d'arrivées. Etant donné l'absence de renseignements précis concernant la retraite et la migration des dentistes, nous avons calculé un taux brut de sorties par région en nous basant sur la période 1971-1976. Nous pouvons ainsi dédui-

Figure 1: Regroupement des divisions de recensement

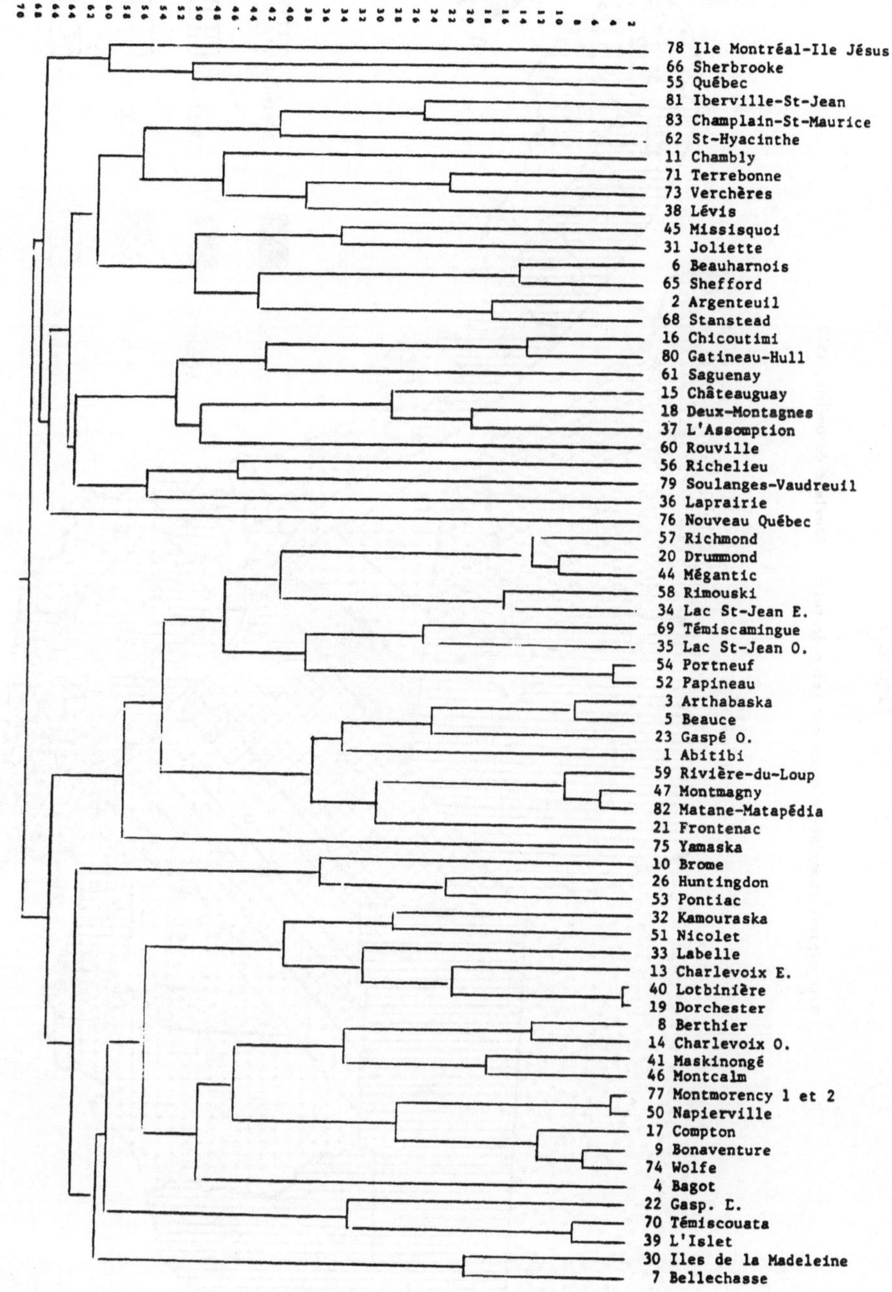
78 Ile Montréal-Ile Jésus
66 Sherbrooke
55 Québec
81 Iberville-St-Jean
83 Champlain-St-Maurice
62 St-Hyacinthe
11 Chambly
71 Terrebonne
73 Verchères
38 Lévis
45 Missisquoi
31 Joliette
6 Beauharnois
65 Shefford
2 Argenteuil
68 Stanstead
16 Chicoutimi
80 Gatineau-Hull
61 Saguenay
15 Châteauguay
18 Deux-Montagnes
37 L'Assomption
60 Rouville
56 Richelieu
79 Soulanges-Vaudreuil
36 Laprairie
76 Nouveau Québec
57 Richmond
20 Drummond
44 Mégantic
58 Rimouski
34 Lac St-Jean E.
69 Témiscamingue
35 Lac St-Jean O.
54 Portneuf
52 Papineau
3 Arthabaska
5 Beauce
23 Gaspé O.
1 Abitibi
59 Rivière-du-Loup
47 Montmagny
82 Matane-Matapédia
21 Frontenac
75 Yamaska
10 Brome
26 Huntingdon
53 Pontiac
32 Kamouraska
51 Nicolet
33 Labelle
13 Charlevoix E.
40 Lotbinière
19 Dorchester
8 Berthier
14 Charlevoix O.
41 Maskinongé
46 Montcalm
77 Montmorency 1 et 2
50 Napierville
17 Compton
9 Bonaventure
74 Wolfe
4 Bagot
22 Gasp. E.
70 Témiscouata
39 L'Islet
30 Iles de la Madeleine
7 Bellechasse

Figure 2

Huit régions homogènes d'accès aux soins dentaires, Province de Québec, 1977.

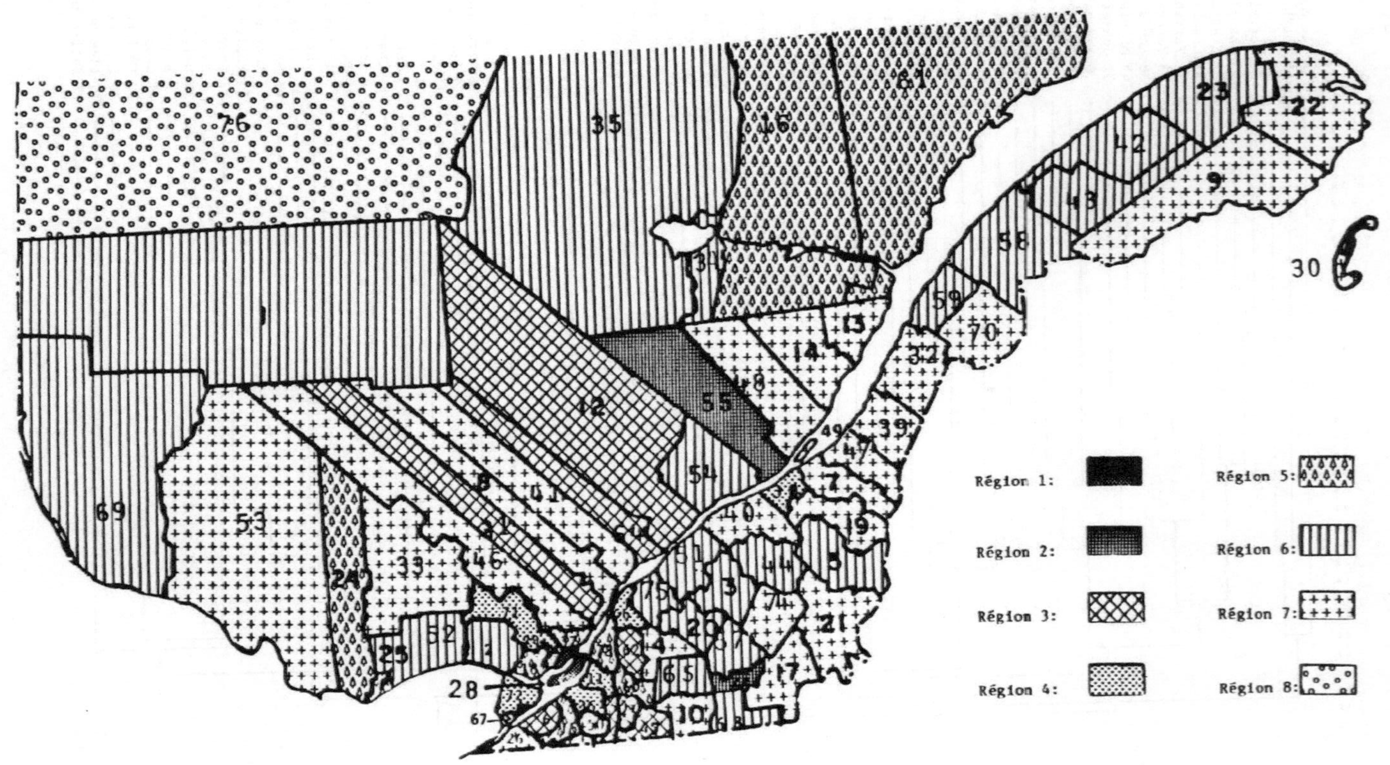

re le nombre de dentistes qui demeuraient dans une région i donnée et additionner ce nombre à celui des nouveaux diplômés venus s'installer dans cette région.

L'estimation de ces nouveaux dentistes s'effectue en trois étapes:

- estimation du nombre futur d'inscriptions dans les facultés de médecine dentaire pour les années à venir;
- multiplication de ce nombre par un taux de passage correspondant à la probabilité d'obtenir un diplôme quatre ans plus tard et de s'installer au Québec;
- répartition de ce produit parmi les huit régions homogènes.

La plupart des taux utilisés dans cette projection ont été estimés en considérant le lustre 1971-1976 et nous les avons laissés constants de sorte que le terme "projection" est utilisé non seulement parce qu'elle couvre une longue période mais aussi à cause des limites des hypothèses.

Méthode de projection de la population

Nous avons choisi de projeter la population à l'aide d'une méthode dite agrégée à cause de sa très grande flexibilité. Il nous fallait, en effet, une méthode assez souple pour effectuer une projection multirégionale (Rogers, A. 1974) à partir de n'importe lequel des regroupements des 76 divisions de recensement. De plus, comme le personnel de l'équipe était limité, on ne pouvait songer à des méthodes plus élaborées comme celle des composantes par exemple.

Pour illustrer facilement la complexité d'une projection de type régional, il suffit de penser aux 64 transferts possibles qu'engendre la migration entre huit régions; heureusement, le calcul matriciel permet de tenir compte de l'ensemble de ces mouvements. On peut ainsi mieux saisir l'importance de la migration interne quant au calcul du rapport dentistes-population. Prenons par exemple la région 4, en ne considérant que le taux d'accroissement de la population totale pour la période 1971-1976, on aurait passé de 718 220 personnes en 1976 à 1 898 979 en 2001. Ceci suppose que l'émigration de la région de Montréal vers ses banlieues continue au même rythme pendant 30 ans. Comme cette hypothèse est difficilement soutenable, nous avons opté pour le modèle multirégional qui permet une projection tenant compte à la fois de la population soumise au risque de migrer ainsi que des diverses composantes de la migration.

Les probabilités de migrer d'une région à l'autre ont été calculées à partir des données sur la migration de la période 1971-1976 contenues dans les statistiques du recensement de 1976 (Statistiques Canada, 1978). Quant à l'évolution de la fécondité, de la mortalité et de la migration externe, nous avons utilisé les taux projetés par Statistiques Canada (1979).

En ce qui concerne la mortalité nous avons supposé qu'elle était identique pour toutes les régions de la province contrairement à la fécondité où nous avons considéré le rapport entre le taux de natalité de la région et celui de la province en 1976. Il s'agit ensuite de calculer le taux d'accroissement naturel de chacune des régions puis d'intégrer les résultats des migrations.

Résultats des projections

Ces calculs ont permis d'illustrer l'évolution du rapport dentistes-population (graphique I). En général, toutes les régions verraient leur situation s'améliorer mais à des rythmes bien différents. En effet, même si provincialement, le rapport de 4.5 dentistes pour 10 000 habitants est atteint en 1989, seules trois régions se retrouvent au-dessus de cet objectif et ce jusqu'à l'an 2000. Exception faite des deux premières régions déjà favorisées, seule la région 4, actuellement en pleine expansion atteindrait cette valeur.

Nous avons également explorer ce que serait la situation future si l'on pouvait agir sur la répartition des nouveaux dentistes pour la période 1981-1990. Pour ce faire, nous avons divisé la province en trois zones: la région homogène 1, la région homogène 2 et le reste de la province; puis, nous avons posé comme contrainte qu'entre 1981 et 1991, on empêche tous les nouveaux diplômés de s'établir dans les régions 1 et 2. On s'aperçoit qu'à l'aide de telle mesure, en moins de dix ans, on corrigerait le problème d'accessibilité des régions éloignées (graphique II, courbes en trait plein).

GRAPHIQUE I: RAPPORT DENTISTES-POPULATION POUR LES HUIT REGIONS HOMOGENES, QUEBEC 1977-2001.

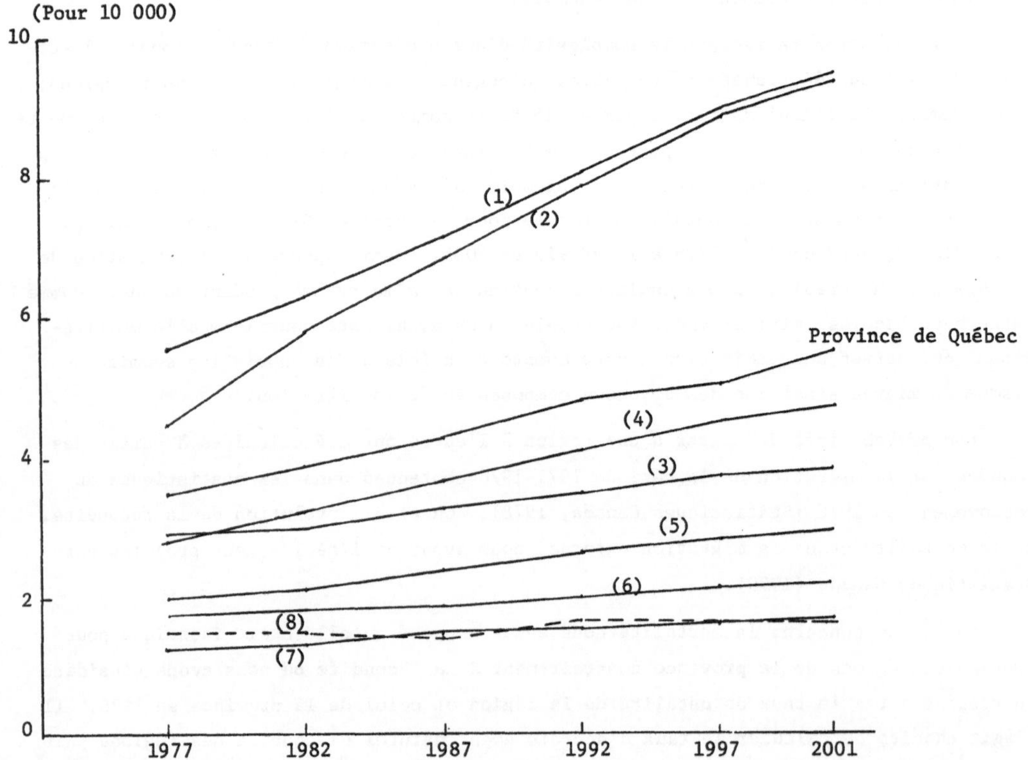

Une autre hypothèse exploratoire intéressante consiste à supposer que certaines mesures incitatives soient si efficaces que 50% des nouveaux gradués, qui se seraient normalement installés dans les régions 1 ou 2, s'établiraient dans le reste de la province. Ces mesures permettent aux régions 1 et 2 de maintenir un rapport à peu près constant tandis que le reste de la province voit sa situation s'améliorer progressivement (graphique 2, courbes en tiret)

Conclusion

Ces projections effectuées à partir de modèles simples ont permis d'illustrer la nécessité d'agir sur la répartition des futurs gradués; elles ont également démontré l'importance des migrations internes dans l'analyse de la variable population. La méthode de regroupement et les modèles présentés constituent deux instruments facilement applicables avec les données habituelles des recensements et les fichiers des corporations professionnelles. Il est entendu que le rapport dentistes-population constitue un indice incomplet de l'offre de soins (Cole, 1971). Dans la poursuite de nos travaux, nous avons pondéré cet indice par la production différentielle des dentistes selon la région en tenant compte des variables sexe, expérience, heures de travail, organisation de la pratique. Nous comptons aussi raffiner notre modèle à partir des changements dans le choix de lieu de pratique des futurs gradués et des différences de besoins entre les régions.

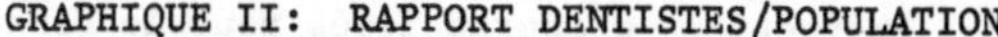
GRAPHIQUE II: RAPPORT DENTISTES/POPULATION

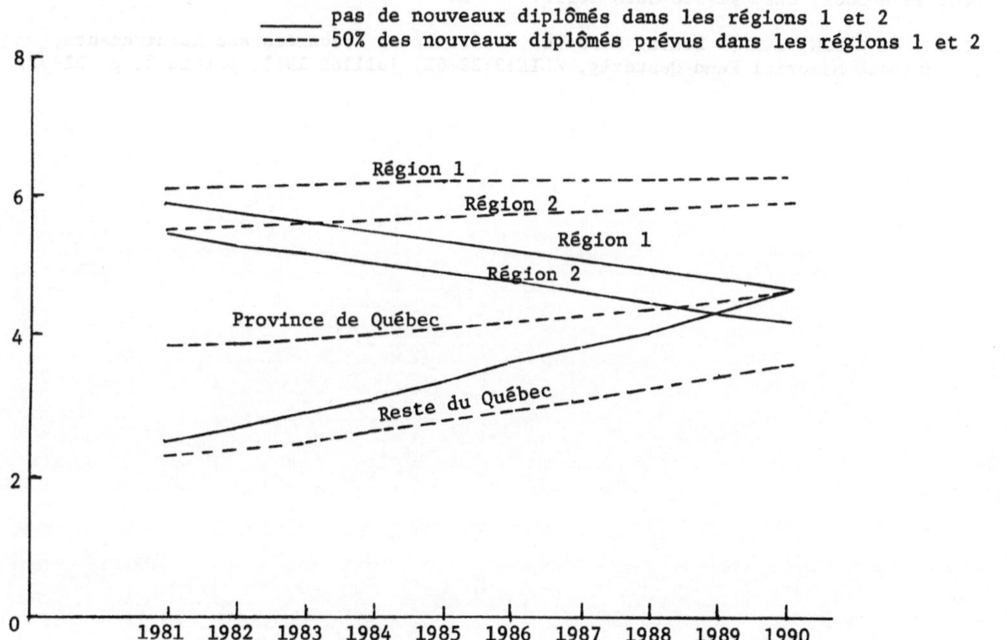

Références

(1) Projet de recherche financé par le Conseil de la Recherche Socio-Economique du Québec et le Conseil de la Recherche en Santé du Québec.

(2) Le système des honoraires modulés. Rapport du Comité sur la rémunération des professionnels de la santé du Québec. Ministère des Affaires sociales, Québec, mars 1980.

(3) Une division de recensement est une division administrative pour laquelle les données de recensement les plus détaillées et les plus complètes sont disponibles.

(4) Les régions socio-sanitaires ont été établies par le ministère de l'Industrie et du Commerce. Elles ont chacune un pôle de développement et se caractérisent par un certain degré d'autonomie.

(5) Cet indice, la distance euclidienne au carré, mesure l'écart existant entre deux régions à partir des 29 variables retenues.

Bibliographie

CONTANDRIOPOULOS, A.P.; LANCE, J.M.; MEUNIER, C., Un regroupement des comtés de la province de Québec en régions homogènes. L'Actualité économique, Oct. 1974: 572-586

ROGERS, A., Introduction to Multiregional Mathematical Demography, John Wiley & Sons, New York, 1974, 203 p.

CANADA, Statistique Canada, Migrants de 5 ans et plus selon le lieu de résidence en 1971, l'âge et le sexe, Microfiche SDDEMB30.

CANADA, Statistique Canada, Projections démographiques pour le Canada et les provinces, 1976-2001, Cat. 91-520 hors série.

COLE, R.B., et COHEN, L.K., Dental Manpower - Estimating Resources and Requirements, The Milbank Memorial Fund Quaterly, KLIX:3:29-62, juillet 1971, partie 2, p. 31-32.

ORGANISATION, TECHNICAL SOLUTIONS AND UTILISATION OF PATIENT DISCHARGE REGISTERS IN FINLAND

Eero Linnakko, Hilkka Seppälä[x] and Esko Hillebrand[xx]
Finnish Hospital League, Helsinki, Finland
[x]National Board of Health, Helsinki, Finland
[xx] State Computer Centre, Jyväskylä, Finland

The National Board of Health has since 1967 collected information from all patients discharged from all hospital wards into the centralised computer register. Because of the difficulties in using the register at the regional and hospital level the system was reorganised on the regional base in 1976. In the co-operation project between the National Board of Health, the Finnish Hospital League and hospitals agreements were made on uniform registration principles. Also a common software for input and output was created. Due to the reorganisation, the discharge information is more up to date and also more accurate. The utilisation of data is increased both at the national and regional level.

1. BACKGROUND

The main responsibility for organising and producing healthcare services in Finland lies on the local authority, i e a commune. They or groups of them own the hospitals and health centres. The central government subsidises and controls these activities through the National Board of Health (NBH). To manage this it has traditionally collected information concerning the structure and the process of the healthcare system. To get more accurate data on hospital use for the purpose of management, evaluation and research, the NBH started in 1960 to gather the discharge summaries from general hospitals. The collecting of discharge summaries in tuberculosis sanatoria and in mental hospitals started already in 1956. Because of the technical restrictions the collection was disrupted until 1967. Since then the summaries concerning all ward patients in all hospitals - private hospitals included - have been collected into the centralised data base. Today the NBH's computerised data base contains approximately 12 million records, and about 800,000 new ones are added to this data base each year. Every record includes 19 data items concerning the producer (hospital, speciality), the patient (ID-number, from which also age and sex can be derived, occupation, education etc) and the cause and duration of hospitalisation.

At first the summaries were coded and key punched by the NBH. Because of limited resources file maintenance was slow and caused a delay of two to three years. Even when the data were accurate for administrative purposes at the national level, the use of central data for regional and hospital level was very restricted due to the delay and the high price of retrieving the data. Also the validity of the data was not always very reliable. For example in 1972 over 10 per cent of the expected summaries were missing and 15 per cent of the ID-numbers were incorrect. However, other variables have been found to be very accurate (1). Some other countries, where centralised discharge registers are kept, seem to experience the same difficulties (2).

In the middle of the 1970s the need for a computerised patient data base increased also at the regional and hospital level because of the new planning system. Realising the difficulty to utilise the national data base, many hospitals decided to start to collect similar data into their own files. Some of the central hospitals also started to gather discharge information from other hospitals within the region thus creating a regional data base. However, the co-operation between regions was lacking and the registration practice was developing without any common standards. This caused twice as much work and reduced the possibilities of comparing information between regions.

2. REORGANISATION OF THE DISCHARGE REGISTERS

2.1 Development project

From the beginning of 1976 the NBH slightly decreased the data items collected into the central register. The aim was to reduce the coding work and errors. Now there was also a good opportunity to get a more uniform registration practice for regional registers. The NBH and the Finnish Hospital League together with some hospitals established a co-ordination and development process. Because the regional summaries in many cases include more data items than the central register it was decided that the regional registers adopt a 200 character long record for a patient discharged. The record was divided into three logical parts.

- The first part is uniform with the national discharge summary record (96 characters),

- the second part is common for all regional registers and
- the rest of the record is for the special purposes of a region if needed.

A software for input and checking of discharge data was also developed. Thus all regions were using the same checking principles for the same variables. Also a general tabulation program especially for discharge information was created.

In principle hospitals can still send their discharge summaries to the NBH on the data collection sheets but only very few do so. Over 90 per cent of the summaries is sent into the central register directly on magnetic tapes. Smaller hospitals within the region send their summaries to the central hospital once a month. They create a regional patient history data base from which the necessary data are sent to the central register at the end of each year. The statistics needed in hospitals concerning different time periods are produced from regional registers. (Figure 1.) The central register is used now mainly for administrative and research purposes at the national level.

Figure 1. Possibilities to organise the data processing of discharge summary system.

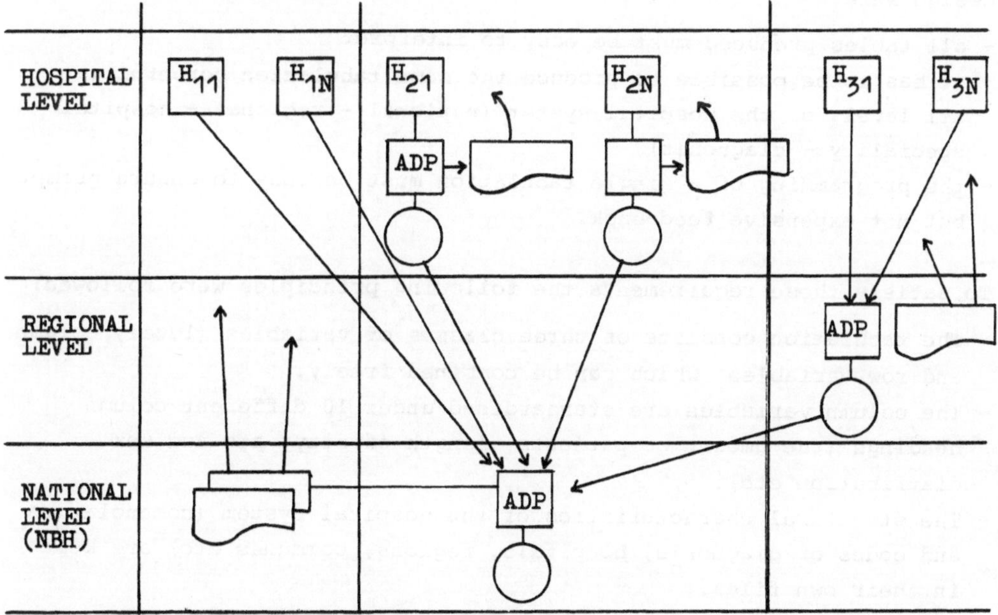

After the close of the project the maintenance of the created system was transferred to the permanent steering committee for hospital edp-systems (such as patient administration, personnel management, fiscal management etc). In the meetings of the committee agreements are made on how to develop the systems further and how to share the cost of developing.

The developed discharge summary edp-system is now employed in every region (21) except two. Because of longer tradition and greater edp-capacity these two have developed their own regional discharge information systems. However, also these regions were included in the project and they use the results of it when they are applicable.

2.2 Software for discharge summary statistics

The main shortcomings of the discharge registers both at the national and the regional level were the limited utilisation of the collected data. To increase the use of data a tailored software for output, Discharge Summary Statistics (DSS)were developed for better data handling, manipulation and presentation. It is a report-generation program to obtain listing and tabulations from discharge registers mainly for administrative purposes. The objectives of the system design were:

- all tables produced must be easy to interpret
- it has to be possible to produce the same tabulation concerning all levels of the hospital system (national - regional - hospital - speciality - diagnosis)
- the programming of a single tabulation must be easy to ensure prompt but not expensive feed-back.

To satisfy these requirements the following principles were followed:

- The tabulation consists of three classes of variables (level, column and row variables) which can be combined freely.
- The column variables are standardised under 10 different column headings (the amount of patients, length of stay, age and sex distribution etc).
- The structural characteristics of the hospital system (nomenclature and codes of diagnosis, hospitals, regions, communes etc) are kept in their own files.
- The structure variables can be both of row and level variables. There can be nine level variables in the same table.

- For each table there are certain default rules kept on the file.
- The whole name of each level and row variable is printed on the table.
- It is possible to produce the table sorted according to one of the column variables (for example average length of stay).
- Every table has a name, which is derived from the column and row variables. (e g "age and sex distribution"/by diagnosis or by speciality).
- The time period covered by data is printed out (e g 01.01.-31.03. 80.
- The size of the table is A4-standard form.

The layout of the table is standardised as presented below.

Level variables	Name of the table Time period
Code name	Column heading
Row variables	Data
Total	

The simple non-procedural language was developed especially for discharge registers. It is possible to determine

- which file is used (national or one of the regional ones) (compulsory)
- which one of the standard "headings" is chosen (compulsory) and how the variables are classified if needed
- what is the row variable (compulsory) and how it is classified
- what is (are) the level variable(s) (optional)
- what is the time period (optional)
- how the name of the table is changed (optional).

The structure of the edp-application is divided into three parts:

1. The main program, which
   - reads and interprets the parameters of the language
   - retrieves the records which are needed for each table

2. The table modules where all necessary calculations, classifying and tabulations are executed.

3. The data base where all standard specifications and classifications concerning files, records, tables and nomenclatures are kept.

The DSS system was programmed by using the computer independent FAS (FORTRAN-ASSEMBLER-SYSTEM) language for administrative purposes developed by the State Computer Centre. Thus it was possible to apply the same programs to all computers where discharge data were handled without a conversion. FAS-language is widely used also in other edp-applications in Finnish hospitals which have for their use different computer equipment.

The DSS system has fulfilled the objectives mentioned above. It is used also for other tabulation task systems like outpatient statistics and hospital management reporting system.

3. UTILISATION OF DISCHARGE INFORMATION

3.1 Administrative use

Until the mid-1970s the use of collected information was restricted mainly for administrative purposes at the national level. Certain standard output was produced annually for the NBH from the data base. The listings were producer,hospital oriented (the amount of patients and patient days, age and sex distribution by hospital, by region or by diagnosis etc). Especially the information concerning diagnosis (case mix of hospitals) was difficult to obtain from other sources. Although the handling time was long the information obtained was useful for the NBH when collecting yearly data for official healthcare statistics.

The hospitals had an opportunity to order the same standard outputs concerning their own data from the national register, but because of the reasons mentioned earlier very few hospitals in fact used the central register. Only mental hospitals had a regular and prompt feed-back for their yearly statistics. But when the registration practice was regionalised the administrative use of information was made easier for hospitals. The utilisation of regional registers in

Finland is discussed also elsewhere in this Congress[1)].

3.2 Central discharge register as a source of information for research

At the end of the 1970s the data bases both at the national and the regional level have been increasingly used for utilisation studies, for epidemiological research and even for clinical research. However, the first utilisation studies were made using the data collected in 1960. Because the information concerning the area of residence of the patient is included in the record, it is also possible to obtain and utilise patient oriented information and not only producer oriented one. In these studies attention was paid to the amount of the use of hospital services by various population and sickness groups and by the population in different communes within special need groups (3). The same material was used to clarify the influence of social factors on the use of hospital services among men of working age. The results of these and some other unpublished research were adapted in the planning of the national and regional hospital bed requirements.

Because of the long history of the national discharge system one important research approach has been the time-series analysis. The most recent and most comprehensive study concerning the use of the general hospital services is being made in the NBH by Doctor O. Nikiforow. All patients discharged from 1967 to 1977 are included. In this study the trends of the use of services according to age, sex, disease group, region and type of hospital etc have been established. The results are, however, still unpublished. In order to make the discharge data more accurate for this study a special analysis of the possibilities of correction was carried out and relevant correction coefficients were used. It was found that the proportion of erroneous data is very low (0.2 - 0.4 %). This suggests that the register gives feasible information for epidemiological and operational research.

Also two other time-series analysis were made recently. In the first one the current provision and use of resources for respiratory

---

1) Kataja M. Experiences from a regional medical data base.

hospital patients in Finland were examined and an estimate of the requirements for hospital beds and personnel in 1985 was derived. In the study the discharge records concerning all hospital visits from 1969 to 1975 were used together with resource information derived from other sources. (4) The second study describes the admission and the discharge processes in psychiatric hospitals and the patient population which is determined by these two processes. Also theoretical models were used in estimating future patient populations until 1985. The main source of information was the mental hospital patient census data from 1958 to 1977. (5)

As an example of recent cross-sectional utilisation analyses partly based upon the discharge information we can take two ones concerning the year 1975. In these studies the discharge information was linked to resource data and to the information concerning the use of other types of services, such as social welfare or out-patient visits, visits to private physicians etc. The unit of studies was a commune and a health centre area. The first of them analyses the division of services for elderly and how the services substitute each other. (6) In the second one the health service resource variables and the use variables were analysed by multiple regression model. (7)

The national discharge register has been a source of several epidemiological studies of different problems, such as alcoholism, traumas etc. Most recent ones are the studies made by the Institute of Public Health at the University of Helsinki. The discharge register in combination with death certificate records has been used in studying the incidence and survival from coronary heart disease (8) and also to study prospectively the coronary heart disease experiences of a large number of disease-specific cohorts (9).

In the case of clinical research the use of the registers is mainly limited to seek out the relevant research population. By using the patient ID-number it is possible to find the basic documents - i e medical records whereever they are located. When the patient ID-number is printed out from the register there is the problem of confidentiality. However, there are strict rules governing the retrieval of information about a single patient. The permission must be obtained from the Ministry of Social Affairs and Health. For the use in statistical information only, clearance may be given by a medical officer of central hospital in the case of the regional register and by the NBH concerning the central one.

4. FUTURE DEVELOPMENT

It has been considered that in the future some data items now generally kept in the regional registers would be useful also to maintain in the national one (e g the treatment). However, the amount of data must be restricted in this kind of a large and comprehensive system. The data needed for special purposes are more economical and accurate to collect using samples. Some regions have enlarged their systems to cover also out-patient visits. However, because of the large amount of out-patients (15 million/year) it seems not possible to collect patient oriented out-patient information at the national level.

REFERENCES

(1) Kaprio J, Pulkkinen P. Accuracy of the national hospital discharge register. The Institute of Public Health, University of Helsinki. 1978 (in Finnish)

(2) The status of hospital discharge data in six countries. Hyattsville, Md. National Center for Health Statistics, U.S. Department of Health, Education, and Welfare, 1980

(3) Vauhkonen, O. A Study of Regional Differences in the Utilisation of General Hospital Services, Helsinki, the National Board of Health, 1967 (in Finnish)

(4) Kokkola K. Hospital Services for Respiratory Patients. Department of Community Medicine, London School of Hygiene and Tropical Medicine, 1978

(5) Hakkarainen A. Estimating Future Mental Hospital Population. Second International Conference of System Science in Health Care, Montreal, 1980

(6) Vauhkonen O, Kataja M, Linnakko E, Vauramo E. The Elderly Population as a User of Health Care Services. The Finnish Hospital League, Helsinki, 1979 (in Finnish)

(7) Kekki P. Analysis of the Relationship between Resources and the Use of Health Service in Finland. Social Insurance Institution, Helsinki, 1979

(8) Koskenvuo M, Kaprio J, Kesäniemi A. Diseases predisposing to IHD. Abstract Book, VII European Congress of Cardiology, Paris, 1980; 87

(9) Koskenvuo M, Kaprio J. Survival from attacks of IHD by marital status, social class and book, VII European Congress of Cardiology, Paris, 1980; 65

THE FINNISH HOSPITAL LEAGUE
THE FINNISH SOCIETY FOR HEALTH INFORMATICS

Paul Grönroos, Head of Laboratory Tampere Central Hospital

Raija Tervo-Pellikka, chief of Section for Informatics The Finnish Hospital League

THE LIFE-LONG OR UNIT MEDICAL RECORD SYSTEM AND ITS CONNECTION TO THE REGIONAL DATA-BASE

The Finnish Hospital League set up in 1971 a committee with the following three tasks:

1 to present a proposal for an unit medical record system for all the general hospitals in the country;

2 to establish to which extent it would be possible to use this system for introducing a so-called problem-orientated approach in the care of the patient;

3 to make a proposal about how the medical record system could be expanded to cover the different medical institutions, i.e. to find out whether it would be possible to have one medical record per patient in one medical district.

The committee submitted its proposal for a unit medical record system to the National Board of Health in 1973 and it was adopted by most of the general hospitals by 1977. The system has become compulsory and should be in general use by 1981.

It was, however, found out that the unit medical record system could not be used in all the regional hospitals without being connected to the regional medical data-base. For this reason a committee was set up by the Finnish Hospital League to outline and make a proposal for the connections. Meanwhile, the committee was given also other tasks and all the different items proposed by the committee have not yet been accepted by the authorities. It seems, however, that any attempt to produce a unit medical record system requires its connection to the persons "health record". The National Board of Health has, accordingly, set up a committee with the tasks to propose a structure for a health record and to outline its connection with the unit medical record system.

A complete unit medical record system should naturally also include the records of psychiatric patients. Because the psychiatric care is given by a separate organization in our country the newly developed psychiatric medical record is kept in a separate file and connected through the computer system to the unit medical record.

As to the principles of the new psychiatric medical record it is quite similar to the unit medical record and thus it may, later on, make a real part of the unit medical record system.

The unit medical history system

The different levels of information can be seen in Fig. 1. Each patient is supplied with a cardboard or plastic file, red for women and blue for men. On the file is indicated with black tape the subject's date of birth, i.e., the first digits of the Finnish personal identification number. The National Board of Health requires that the patient's personal identification number is controlled at the various contacts.

The first real information level (Fig. 1) is represented by the blank form called SUMMARY. The summary is a collected review of all the medical consultations of the patient at both the outpatient department and in the ward.

On the following level there are the forms for the use of the clinics. All the clinics of the hospital are spread out on this level. The forms are blank and may be printed according to the needs of the clinic. However, a problem-orientated approach has been suggested. The forms of the different clinics are identified by colour e.g. brown is for surgical forms throughout the country and green for x-ray, each service department has a form of own colour etc. The 3-letter abbreviations of the specialities have also become standards.

A feature common to all level B forms is that they are bundled together after each visit to the hospital. B forms contain in principle basic data. They are evaluated by the physician who makes the summary which for its part is recorded on the level A forms.

For the registration of every medical event there is a set of special forms marked XYZ:

X Data needed for accounting the patient.

Y Data needed to produce the necessary statistics for planning, etc.

Z Minimum data needed for the acute treatment of a patient while waiting for the complete unit medical record to be transported from the previous hospitals or health center.

X and Z contain entirely patient-bound data, while Y data are relevant without identification of the patient.

The data on the form Z are collected to make a minimum database for the ADP. Thus it must contain information that is important for the patient's later treatment as well as a statement, where the patient's paper-bound unit medical record is filed. The data on this form are the basis for a later expansion of the system to the whole region (one medical record per patient and region). Furthermore, a similarly constructed public health record that is connected to the unit medical record, will be necessary. Accordingly, if the patient has permanently settled down in a new district his health record has to be sent to his new health center.

A MINIMUM DATA-BASE

The Finnish Hospital League set a committee in 1978 aiming to specify the main implementation alternatives of a so-called minimum data-base, to calculate their costs and to estimate the benefits of the various alternatives.

The proposal for the minimum data-base was given already in 1976 (see fig. 3) and the committee work was finished in 1979. The main proposals put forward by the committee are, shortly following:

A regional patient data base is the central part of the regional patient information system. The data base is separate for each central hospital region and is maintained centrally by the central hospital. The base holds data on the population and its health status, and the use of health care services within the central hospital region. At the first stage, health centres and hospitals providing general medical services should be included within the system.

Regional health care causes certain needs and problems related to data processing concerning the population and the treated patients.

The medical records of a patient are stored at the health care unit where he/she has been treated. Therefore, as a result from the implementation of the multi-level principle, there may be medical records of one patient at several health care units within a central hospital region. The inefficient use of medical records is a big problem, especially in the smaller, remote health care units within a central hospital region.

Regional health care organisation and efficient implementation of the multi-level principle require well functioning follow-up and reporting systems.

The information contents of the data base can be divided in six main groups:

1 Personal data. These data form the fixed, permanent part of the data base. They include the personal identification number, name, address, occupational code etc.

2 Data regarding the care episode. These data are the central, active part of the data base. They contain medical and patient administrative information of the local people who have received outpatient or inpatient medical services at the health care units within the central hospital region.

3 Reference data. These data indicate where the patients paper-bound medical records are kept, and also if the patients are entered in some treatment scheduling of problem-oriented registers within the region.

4 Treatment scheduling data. These data briefly indicate the situation of patients who are waiting for a place at various health care units within the region.

5 Cumulative treatment data. These data include brief summaries of those episodes in the treatment that have been transferred to the passive part of the regional patient data base.

6 The critical medical data.

The regional patient data-base system improves the unilisation of the regionally scattered medical records by the aid of the reference data. Thus, by using the vital parts of the episodic data arising from treatment, it is possible to produce a minimum data-base for the patient, and use it in combination with the paper-bound unit medical record.

It can produce statistics that describe the performance of the health care system and the health status of the population. The system is necessary for controlling health care on the institutional, regional and national level.

A MODEL OF EVALUATION OF HEALTH SERVICES "BY OBJECTIVES"

P.M.MANACORDA,P.PIETROBONI

SOGESS-Sistemi Organizzazione e Gestione Servizi

Sociali e Sanitari

Via Turati, 29 20121 MILANO -ITALY-

A model for the evaluation of health services is proposed. It allowy to assess the degree of obtainment of quality and organization objectives in every service of an area. From the objectives one can derive exactly the necessary conditions for their obtainment an express these in form of questions gathered in a questionary. The answers are compared with standards (when possible) or measured by a three degrees scale.

Introduction: la réforme du système sanitaire italien.

La loi n° 833 ("La réforme sanitaire") a été approuvée en décembre 1978, après un débat culturel et politique qui a duré presque 10 ans. Elle réorganise le système sanitaire italien sur la base des éléments suivants:

- la prévention-traitement-réhabilitation comme objectif;
- la planification et la programmation comme méthode;
- la décentralisation comme principe d'organisation;
- la participation des citoyens, (d'une façon opportune), à l'organisation et à l'evaluation des interventions;
- l'assistance sanitaire gratuite étendue à tous les citoyens.

Du point de vue de l'organisation, la structure s'articule sur quatre niveaux:

- l'Etat (coordination et contrôle);
- la Région (législation régionale et planification stratégique);
- les U.S.L. (50-250.000 hab.) (érogation de l'assistance).

Le premier Plan Sanitaire National a été promulgué au cours de l'année 1979. Ce plan est valable pour les années 1980-81-82, et il se donne des objectifs stratégiques ainsi que les moyens pour les atteindre. Dans ce plan on a souligné trois projets-objectifs, concernant respectivement:

- la tutelle de la santé de la mère et de l'enfant;
- la tutelle de la santé des travailleurs et la prévention de la nocivité des lieux de travail;
- la tutelle de la santé des personnes âgées.

Insuffisance des évaluations traditionnelles

La situation qui existait avant la Réforme était caractérisée par le manque de programmation et d'évaluation des structures sanitaires, qui dépendaient de plusieurs organismes et institutions. La réussion de tous les services (y compris les hôpitaux) au sein des unités sanitaires locales (U.S.L.) devrait permettre d'activer ces mécanismes de programmation-contrôle-évaluation des interventions que l'on considère aujourd'hui comme necessaires à l'efficacité et à l'efficience du système sanitaire. Pour atteindre cet objectif, les U.S.L. ont besoin d'instruments d'information gouvernementaux instruments qui doivent permettre de vérifier non seulement le fonctionnement régulier et coulant des services (efficience), mais aussi la capacité effective de ces services d'agir d'une façon positive sur la santé de la population (efficacité). Traditionnellement, l'organisme responsable ne contrôlait les services sanitaires que du point de vue quantitatif: le nombre d'interventions effectuées permettait de contrôler l'activité des services, et le rapport entre le nombre des interventions et le nombre des opérateurs (indice de charge) donnait une évaluation de la productivité. Mais aucun des deux éléments ne contribuait à donner une image de la qualité du service, et encore moins de son efficacité. Cette optique a engendré des systèmes d'information souvent très riches du point de vue de la "quantité des données" mais très pauvres du point de vue de la qualité des informations. En définitive, le manque d'un modèle d'évaluation de la qualité des services a fait en sorte que les données recueillies, même si elles étaient abondantes,complètes et fiables,ne puissent pas être utilisées pour le but principal,c'est à dire la programmation et la vérification des interventions. Comme tout le monde sait, la véritable évaluation d'efficacité doit être réalisée à travers la "lecture épidémiologique" de l'état de santé de la population, et donc à travers la lecture des statistiques de mortalité et de morbidité et les recherches épidémiologiques spécifiques. L'évaluation que l'on peut faire de l'intérieur des services se rapporte surtout à la qualité et au caractère é conomique de ce service. Ces deux caractéristiques sont à leur tour deux éléments importants du concept plus global d'efficacité.

Méthode: le modèle d'évaluation "pour objectifs"

L'optique de laquelle nous sommes partis en proposant un "modèle d'évaluation de la qualité et de l'efficience des services" ainsi que du système d'information relatif est totalement différente. La méthodologie adoptée consiste en:

a) détermination d'une série d'objectifs que les services doivent atteindre pour tendre à l'efficacité;

b) détermination d'une série de conditions auxquelles les services doivent répondre afin d'atteindre les objectifs cités au point a);

c) détermination de certains éléments cognitifs (informations) nécessaires pour vérifier l'existence des condiitons b) et la réalisation des objectifs a).

Nous estimons que séul une méthodologie qui tire les informations des objectifs, et non pas le contraire, comme il arrive souvent, permet de tenter, avec toutes les attentions nécessaires, une évaluation de qualité et d'efficacité. Les objectifs que nous avons pris en considération sont les suivants:

1) capacité de connaître la demande; 2) efficience technique; 3) efficience économique; 4) intégration des interventions sectorielles; 5) flexibilité; 6) accessibilité; 7) caractère essentiel des procédures bureaucratiques; 8) capacité de produire des informations; 9) transparence et possibilité d'être soumis à un contrôle. On a défini chaque objectif dans des termes plus précis, par exemple intégration des interventions sectorielles signifie "la capacité et/ou la possibilité d'exercer des activités qui sont propres à plusieurs secteurs (sanitaire, social, culturel, récréatif)"; transparence et possibilité d'être soumis à un contrôle signifient "la capacité de favoriser la consultation, l'évaluation et le contrôle de la part de la population et des organismes gouvernementaux".

Aprés avoir déterminé et défini les objectifs, ces derniers ont été concrétisés dans les conditions ou les caractéristiques du service nécessaires à évaluer la possibilité d'atteindre ces objectifs.

Par exemple l'obiectif du "caractère essentiel des procédures bureaucratiques" dépend des conditions suivantes:

- qu'on ne demande pas à l'usager de démontrer son droit à l'assistance, sauf en cas exceptionnels;

- que le passage des informations bureaucratiques entre les différents services, et entre ces derniers et d'autres bureaux de l'Organisme local, ne soit pas effectué par l'usager;
- que les procédures bureaucratiques éventuellement nécessaires soient effectuées dans le lieu de résidence (district) afin d'éviter le déplacement de l'usager.

Après avoir déterminé les conditions nécessaires pour atteindre chaque objectif, il faut préciser ces mêmes conditions par une série d'élements d'information qui sont l'objet réèl d'un questionnaire. Sur la base des exemples précédents, afin de vérifier l'objectif du caractère essentiel des procédures bureaucratiques concrétisé de la façon déjà citée, il s'impose de poser les questions suivantes:

- combien de passages bureaucratiques se révèlent-ils nécessaire pour avoir accès au service?
- l'usager doit-il démontrer, en général, son droit à l'assistance?
- si votre service exige l'intervention d'un autre service, qui doit la demander: l'usager ou le service même?
- s'il faut une autorisation pour avoir accès au service, où est elle donnée: dans le district ou au siège central de l'U.S.L.?

Chaque "condition" donne donc lieu à une liste de questions, recueillies dans un questionnaire, qui est soumis aux services.

Discussion: les problèmes de l'évaluation

Le problème le plus difficile quand on établit un modèle d'évaluation de ce genre est de définir les termes de confrontation, c'est à dire ceux qui permettent une évaluation réelle. Ils peuvent être représentés par:

- des réponses de type binaire (oui/non, présent/absent)
- des standards qualitatifs
- des échelles métriques.

Ainsi que dans tous les cas d'évaluation complexe, les trois types de confrontation se révèlent nécessaires; mais ces confrontations trouvent encore plus de difficultés à cause du manque de standards pour beaucoup de variables importantes, comme par exemple le nombre d'interventions par heure/opérateur, le nombre de mètres carrés ou d'installations par service, le rapport numérique entre les differentes catégories de personnel (médical, paramédical, technique) dans les différents services.
En Italie, seul l'hôpital est réglé par des standards d'espace, d'équipements et de

personnel définis par la loi; au cours des dernières années, de nouveaux services ont été crées parallèlement à des indications sur les dimensions des bassins d'utilisation et les typologies du personnel à employer.

Ces indications doivent être complétées par celles qui dérivent des conventions que l'Etat Italien a stipulé avec les généralistes et les pédiatres. Ces indications établissent le nombre maximum de personnes qui peuvent être assistées par chaque médecin. Dans cette situation, l'utilisation de standards de référence pose des problèmes. Certains standards ont été intégrés au modèle d'évaluation. Ils ont été tirés de source supranationales comme l'Organisation Mondiale de la Santé, nationales comme celles du Service Sanitaire anglais, sourtout pour ce qui concerne le service médical de base) et de certaines Régions Italiennes.

Les problèmes concernant les échelles métriques sont venus s'ajouter à celui, bien connu, de la définition des valeurs "normales" d'un certain paramètre. Si par exemple le rapport entre personnel sanitaire et personnel administratif est trop bas, cela indique un niveau élevé de bureaucratisation, mais au-dessus d'un certain seuil cela révèle un manque d'efficience et de fonctionnalité. Loursqu'on a établi ces échelles métriques on a également tenu compte du différent degré de complexité des services du premier et du second niveau. Il faut aussi souligner que plusieurs informations qu'il faut acquérir revêtent un caractère qualitatif, comme par exemple la qualitè des appareils et le niveau professionnel des opérateurs. Dans plusieurs cas l'échelle métrique ne peut donc être exprimée que par la forme haut-moyen-bas. En général, on a essayé de ramener toutes les réponses, y compris celles de type qualitatif, à une échelle à trois niveaux: haut-moyen-bas, que l'on exprime respectivement par trois-deux-un. Une phase de précodification qui trasforme toutes les réponses en réponses à trois niveaux se révèle nécessaire quand les réponses sont du type descriptif-qualitatif. Par exemple, lorsqu'on étudie la connaissance du service de la population, les questions visent à sonder cette connaissance de façon directe ou indirecte; à la fin, le codificateur, qui doit être une personne ayant reçu une formation spécialisée, doit tirer un jugement de: "connaissance haute-moyenne-basse", sur la base des réponses aux questions spécifiques.

Dans certains cas, les questions, ou même chaque modalité de réponse, peuvent être caractérisées par un "poids" qui en indique l'influence différente sur la détermination de la réalisation de l'objectif; il y aura des poids différents d'après les services. Ainsi par exemple, il est important que tous les services d'une U.S.L. puissent connaître les statistiques de mortalité de la population de l'U.S.L.; cette ré ponse bénéficiera d'un poids important. Les autres statistiques changent suivant les services: le centre de consultation familiale doit connaître les statistiques de la santé de la mère et de l'enfant, le service de médecine du travail celles des accidents du travail, et ainsi de suite.

Pour cette raison le niveau de réalisation d'un objectif peut être tiré d'un algorithme adéquat qui doit être rendu explicite dans le modéle d'évaluation et qui est suffisamment flexible pour s'adapter aux différentes impostations locales de politique sanitaire. Le niveau de réalisation de l'objectif, ou plutôt des différents objectifs indiqués dans le modèle s'exprime également sur une échelle ternaire du type: haut- moyen-bas. Le résultat du modèle est donc constitué par la connaissance du niveau auquel les neuf objectifs différents ont été atteints dans chaque service.

Résultats: l'utilisation du modèle d'évaluation

Le modèle peut être utilisé à quatre niveaux différents:

- celui de chaque service
- celui du réseau de services homogènes
- celui du domaine problématique
- celui du domaine territorial

Par réseau de services homogènes on entend l'ensemble constitué, dans une zone déterminée (Région ou Unité Sanitaire Locale), par tous les services du même type, par exemple tous les généralistes ou tous les centres de consultation pour les problèmes de la mère et de l'enfant.

Par "domaine problématique" on entend une partie de la population caractérisée par une homogénéité des problèmes; normalement, en ce qui concerne la situation italienne, le secteur de la mère et de l'enfant, celui des travailleurs, celui de l'âge évolutif, celui des personnes âgées et des inadaptés sont considérés des "domaines problématiques". Les différents types de services peuvent être groupés en un domaine problématique qui du point de vue institutionnel est représenté par un "Département" de l'U.S.L..

Le domaine territorial enfin, correspond généralement à un territoire administratif (U.S.L.) ou bien à une partie de celui-ci (Mairie ou District). Les quatre niveaux sont compatibles entre eux, et peuvent tous être tirés du modèle-base développé dans les neuf objectifs déjà cités. En particulier, on peut les définir en déduisant quelques questions spécifiques du modèle général, et/ou en donnant à ces questions des poids différents. Par exemple, on évalue l'objectif "accessibilité et jouissance" pour chaque secteur à travers une série de questions qui visent à connaître les conditions de localisation, la facilité d'accès, les barrières architecturales et les horaires d'ouverture. Pour évaluer l'accessibilité et la jouissance d'un réseau de service, il faut introduire des questions qui visent à vérifier les conditions de localisation de l'ensemble du réseau et surtout le niveau d'homogénéité dans la distribution des services dans les différentes zones.

On peut atteindre un niveau ultérieur de synthèse essayant d'exprimer un seul jugement, toujours à trois niveaux, sur un seul service. Dans ce but il faut encore attribuer des poids aux différents objectifs spécifiques et au niveau auquel ils ont été atteints. Au début on a pensé d'attribuer plus de poids aux deux premiers objectifs, c'est à dire respectivement l'efficacité et l'efficience technique, en donnant moins de poids aux autres. Ainsi un service qui aura atteint le premier objectif de façon insuffisante, sera considéré comme étant " inefficace" et s'il a atteint également le second objectif de façon insuffisante, il sera donc considéré comme étant "inefficient".

Il s'agit évidemment de jugements approximatifs qui facilitent toutefois leur interprétation et les décisions, surtout si l'on doit utiliser ce modèle pour des réseaux de service et pour des zones entières.

L' output du modèle sera donc constitué par une série de tableaux avec des niveaux différents d'agrégation. Des tableaux seront dressés pour chaque service, chaque objectif ainsi que le niveau relatif de réalisation au sein du service. Comme nous avons déjà dit, on peut utiliser ces tableaux pour un nombre limité de services (jusqu'à 20/30). Quand le nombre de services à analyser augmentera on utilisera des tableaux de fréquence relatifs à une série de services, à un domaine problématique ou à un domaine territorial.

Elaboration automatique du modèle

D'après la description précédente, il résulte que le modèle ne contient pas d'algorithmes particulièrement complexes; pour des quantités limitées de questionnaires (quelques dizaines), l'élaboration à la main de ce modèle se révèle probablement plus avantageuse que l'élaboration automatique. L' avantage de l'élaboration manuelle, dans ce cas, est constitué par le fait que la lecture des questionnaires permet de connaître d'autres éléments d' information, comme par exemple les observations des opérateurs et certaines réponses qui doivent être obligatoirement en texte li -

bre, et, ne peuvent entrer dans le modèle automatisé.

Au-dessus de ces dimensions, au contraire, la quantité des variables examinées rend nécessaire le recours à l'élaboration automatique. Comme dans plusieurs cas d'élaboration automatique, la partie la plus consistante du travail est constituée par l'input des données, alors que les programmes qu'il faut utiliser ne sont que des programmes statistiques banals.

Le questionnaire et le modèle relatif, en version simplifiée, ont été expérimentés à l' occasion du recensement des services dans une grande ville italienne, Milan. On estime qu'à l'état actuel d'évolution du système sanitaire italien, le questionnaire complet et le modèle relatif ne sont utilisables que dans certaines réalités suffisamment évoluées. Dans les autres situations, au contraire, la capacité actuelle de reflexion et d'auto-évaluation des services ne permet pas d'obtenir des réponses satisfaisantes et complètes. On retient toutefois que c'est justement un modèle de ce type, qui laisse beaucoup de place au relèvement des conditions et des modalités de travail, et non seulement à la "quantité", qui peut représenter un istrument utile pour faire évoluer dans le temps l'attitude à l'évaluation des opérateurs et donc indirectement, la qualité du service offert.

THE ROLE OF ECONOMICS IN HEALTH CARE EVALUATION

Alastair M. Gray

Health Economics Research Unit
University of Aberdeen
Scotland

Summary

As pressure increases in many Western countries to contain health service costs and restrict growth of health care expenditure, so policy and decision-makers need to make use of the techniques of economics in analysis, evaluation, and planning. This paper outlines some of the more important methods of economic evaluation, and illustrates how their use may assist the process of improving resource allocation and resource use in the health care sector. In particular, the techniques of cost-effectiveness analysis and cost-benefit analysis are considered. The paper concludes with some comments on the problems of applying these techniques, and notes that their routine application will depend upon changes in the way relevant information is collected and presented.

Introduction

Whatever we may think of the aggregate provision of resources to the health care sector, it is clear that the resources available will always be finite, and therefore that choices must be made. Given that economics may be defined - at least in part - as "the study of how men and society end up choosing .... to employ scarce productive resources that could have alternative uses ...."(1), we might expect the discipline to have something to offer health service planners, and hope in turn that planners might draw upon economics in the processes of policy-formulation and evaluation.

Two techniques which economists are endeavouring to promote in the health sector are cost-effectiveness analysis and cost-benefit analysis. Each has specific applications, but both can aid the rational appraisal of alternative uses of scarce health care resources, if used correctly. But in order to be used correctly, both techniques are crucially dependent upon the information they make use of. In discussing these techniques, therefore, this paper stresses the importance of ensuring that a more widespread adoption of economic methods in the health care sector is not handicapped by lack of appropriate information.

Cost-Effectiveness Analysis

The uses of cost-effectiveness analysis are perhaps the least far-reaching of the techniques discussed here. Cost-effectiveness analysis is constrained to considering <u>how</u>, at least cost or with a fixed budget, to attain a particular objective. Such studies have four broad requirements: defining the objective; listing the options available to meet the objective; quantifying the effect of the different options; and measuring the costs associated with each option.

To illustrate these requirements, consider a screening programme for breast cancer. The objective might be any of the following:

(i) the lowest screening cost per woman screened;

(ii) the lowest cost, including treatment and screening costs, per true positive case detected;

(iii) the lowest cost, including treatment and screening costs and allowing for savings in treatment costs for cases which would have presented symptomatically, per year of life extended.

Clearly the selection of objective ultimately rests not with economists but rather with policy-makers. What the economist may request is that the objective is stated in terms of 'final' outputs where possible: 'lives saved' rather than 'women screened'.

Once the objective has been defined, it is important to try to assemble as many feasible options as possible to meet the objective. Unless this has been done it will be largely a matter of luck whether or not the most 'cost-effective' option is actually selected.

The third requirement, that of quantifying the effects of different options, hinges upon good data. Previous cost-effectiveness studies (for example Piachaud and Weddell's study[(2)] of varicose vein treatments) have often been obliged to generate this information specifically for the evaluation, and the general lament about clinical procedures being undertaken without a proper awareness of their effectiveness is thus strongly supported by economists.

Finally, the costs associated with each option must be measured. By costs is meant not only those costs incurred by the health service, but also costs falling on patients themselves, other social services, etc. The problems of obtaining relevant health service costs will be returned to in this paper; the measurement of other costs such as waiting-time or stress and anxiety present problems which are no less difficult, but in this context are principally the concern of economists rather than information scientists.

If all these requirements are met, then options can be ranked in terms of their relative cost-effectiveness. If a level of output is specified, then each option will be ranked by total cost in meeting the objective. If the objective specifies the type of output but not the total quantity, then the ranking from cost-effectiveness analysis will be by cost per unit of output for each option. Again if the objective is stated in terms of a fixed budget to obtain some type of output, then the ranking will be by number of units of output obtainable within this budget for each of the options.

Cost-Benefit Analysis

For all that cost-effectiveness analysis can be a valuable technique, it cannot say anything about whether or not something is worth doing, or how much to do. In order to address these issues it is necessary to weigh costs against benefits, and it is here that cost-benefit analysis takes its place.

The technique is neatly propounded by Williams as follows: "Cost-benefit studies stress the simple truth that the decision whether or not to pursue a particular course of action depends on both costs and benefits." He continues: "we see far too many recommendations based on assertions that x is cheaper than y (without adequate consideration of relative benefits) or that x is more effective than y (without adequate consideration of relative costs)".[3]

Thus by assessing the costs and benefits of different policies, judgments can be formed about the relative worthwhileness of committing scarce resources in different ways. Cost-benefit analysis thus has all the virtues and requirements of cost-effectiveness analysis plus the capacity to assist in decisions about 'worthwhileness'.

As with cost-effectiveness analysis, the costs to be considered should include the pecuniary and non-pecuniary costs falling on society as a whole, and not only on the health service.

The same principle applies on the benefit side i.e. that the relevant benefits are those accruing to society at large. But the problems of benefit measurement are considerable. While accepting that this issue cannot be handled adequately in a paper of this length, let us consider one particular facet of it.

Every decision in health care which involves the commitment of resources to a particular policy implies measurement of benefit as does any decision not to pursue a particular policy. If policy A is implemented at a cost of £10,000 this implies that the decision-makers have formed the judgment that the benefits of the policy are at least £10,000. Failure to implement policy A would imply a value of less than £10,000 for the benefits.

While it is certainly true that the theory underlying cost-benefit analysis suggests that the consumer knows best what is good for him (i.e. the principle of consumer sovereignty), in health care it can be argued that the consumer does not know best what is good for him. Without wishing to pursue here the debate on the nature of the commodities health and health care, what is clear is that decisions are being made daily by politicians, planners, administrators, clinicians and indeed patients which imply values for the benefits provided in the health care sector.

Two very simplified examples will serve to illustrate this. In 1971 the UK government decided on grounds of cost not to proceed at that time with the child-proofing of drug containers. Allowing for the cost of drug proofing and savings to the NHS from reduced hospital admissions, it was calculated by Gould[4] that the cost per child's life saved would have been of the order of £1000. Since the child-proofing was not pursued at that time, the implied value of a child's life was less than £1000.

The second example of implied values arises from the changes in building regulations following the partial collapse of a high rise block of flats in London (Ronan

Point), which resulted in the deaths of some of the residents. Calculations made by the Science Policy Research Unit at the University of Sussex suggested that, given estimates of the expected numbers of lives saved by, and the costs involved in the changes in the regulations, the implied value of life was at least £20 million.(5)

Three important points are illustrated by these examples. First, the valuation of benefits cannot be avoided or ignored, for values are continually being applied - even if only by implication - to apparently intangible benefits, including life itself. Secondly, these implied valuations of, for example, lives saved, show little measure of agreement in magnitude. Thirdly, by placing these valuations on an explicit basis, better - because more consistent - decisions might be reached.

Cost-benefit analysis cannot act as a decision-making tool in health care; but its potential as a decision-aiding tool remains underexploited. There are perhaps some who would argue that it can only be of assistance in planning health care once the problems of measurement of costs and benefits are overcome. If this were so we would have a long wait indeed before looking to it to assist planning. Fortunately, even without the ability to measure all costs and benefits, cost-benefit analysis as an approach to and philosophy of planning can make an important contribution to health care decision-making.

Economic Techniques in Practice

Cost-effectiveness and cost-benefit analysis are not without methodological problems, and these have been touched upon, albeit briefly. A far more important set of obstacles to their widespread use, however, lies in the way in which information is currently generated within the health service. Most obvious to the economist is the inappropriateness of much of the cost data the health service produces. Costing information is still largely geared to the needs of accountants, whose principal preoccupation is the maintenence of itemised expenditure accounts, rather than the pattern of expenditure on health care objectives. Despite the increasing adoption of 'programme budgeting', that is, relating expenditure to programmes such as care of the elderly or mentally handicapped, it remains the case that health service accounts far more readily yield information on the cost of inputs - electricity, drugs, linen and bedding, etc. Thus evaluative studies face a considerable task in reorientating costing data from inputs towards inputs. The implementation of data-gathering systems more geared to the requirements of planning and evaluation than of book-keeping would represent a significant step towards the planning of health care systems which maximise patient welfare within their budget constraints.

In addition to this need to improve the basis on which costing information is assembled, the evaluative techniques discussed here require accurate information on the other side of the equation: that is, on outputs and effectiveness. It was noted that the definition of output in cost-effectiveness analysis is preferably to be stated in terms of final outputs, such as lives saved, additional years of life expectancy produced, sick-days avoided, and so on, rather than in terms of intermediate outputs such as bed-days, discharges or cases treated. It remains the case, however, that the great bulk of routine health care statistics is concerned with these intermediate outputs. No doubt this is in part due to the relative ease with which such statistics can be generated, and the difficulty of stating output in more final measurements. The lack of any clear operational definition of health itself, and the problems encountered by researchers in trying to devise health status indexes underline this difficulty. Nevertheless, if decision-makers can be persuaded to acknowledge explicitly the deficiencies of intermediate output measures, this in itself would impart valuable momentum to the search for more appropriate alternatives.

Measuring final output is not strictly separable from the issue of measuring the effectiveness of medical procedures. That medical practitioners have frequently resisted attempts to scrutinize the effectiveness of their methods can hardly be questioned, although the reasons for this resistance are not always clear. To finish on a debating point, it might be suggested that one factor which has influenced the attitude of clinicians is a lack of confidence (hitherto frequently justified) in the techniques used to measure effectiveness, and that if interdisciplinary efforts by economists, information scientists, epidemiologists and others could win this confidence the consequences could be beneficial not only to their own disciplines but to the health care system at large.

References

(1) Samuelson, P.A., Economics, Tenth ed, McGraw Hill, 1976

(2) Piachaud, D. and Weddell, J.M., The Economics of Treating Varicose Veins, Int.J. Epidem. 1972; 1, 3: 287-294

(3) Williams, A., The Cost-Benefit Approach, Brit. Med. Bull. 1974; 30, 3: 252-256

(4) Gould, D., A Groundling's Notebook, New Scientist 1979; 51: p 217

(5) Science Policy Research Unit, Human Life and Safety in Relation to Technical Change 1972, University of Sussex

RENAL REPLACEMENT SERVICES PLANNING - A MATHEMATICAL APPROACH

A.R. Shah, S.J. Foot and J. Hollowell
North East Thames Regional Health Authority
Management Services Division
St. Faith's Hospital
Brentwood, Essex.
ENGLAND

1. INTRODUCTION

The provision of renal replacement therapy (R.R.T.) is an expensive commitment on the part of the National Health Service in the United Kingdom. The revenue cost for renal replacement services has been estimated to be over £4,000 per patient per annum. The resources available for this specialty are very limited - even by the most conservative estimate of need for renal replacement therapy, only a third of the total need is currently being met by the renal units in the United Kingdom. Moreover, it is an area of medical care that has seen relatively rapid technical developments and where future changes are likely. These factors, costliness and scarcity of resources and the technical developments, make renal replacement services an obvious area for planning.

This paper presents an analysis of the quantitative dimension of the problem and highlights the use of mathematical models in forecasting the expected number of patients on the renal replacement therapy programme for varying levels of intake of new patients. The study was carried out in one of the health Regions - The North East Thames Region.

2. INCIDENCE OF CHRONIC RENAL FAILURE

The 'potential demand' for the renal replacement service is a function of the incidence of chronic renal failure and the size of the population being served.

Several studies have been carried out to measure the incidence of chronic renal failure, (5,7,8,9,10). The estimates obtained from these studies very between 20 and 75 new patients per million population per year. The main reason for such a wide range of estimates is that the studies differ in their definition of need for renal replacement therapy and also in the criteria used for acceptability of patients. However, in all these studies the age limit of the patients was found to be a crucial factor in determining the number of patients who would be accepted for treatment. If the limitations on age and fitness criteria are completely relaxed, it is estimated that 150 new patients per million population per year could benefit from renal replacement therapy (7). In the United Kingdom, it is generally accepted that about 40 new patients per million population develop potentially treatable chronic renal failure.

3. TREATMENT OF CHRONIC RENAL FAILURE

Chronic renal failure is a disease process which involves 'a slowly progressive loss of nephrons, frequently accompanied by vascular narrowing, with clinically irreversible impairment of function'. (8)

More than twenty years ago a patient with such an impairment of kidney function would have died within a few weeks. However, as a result of the development of medical technology in this specialty over the last twenty years, a patient who has reached the terminal stage of this disease can now undergo one of two available treatment procedures: dialysis or transplantation.

The basic principle of dialysis exchanging substances from the blood to a dialysis fluid by means of a special membrane - is applied in two different ways. The predominant method, used in more than 95% of the cases receiving dialysis in Europe, is haemodialysis in which the dialysis is performed by a kidney machine. In the remaining few cases, peritoneal dialysis is used. This form of treatment is relatively recent and uses a natural membrane (the peritoneum) instead of an artificial membrane outside the patient's body.

The alternative form of treatment is for a patient to undergo a kidney transplant operation. In this case, a patient receives a kidney from a living donor or a cadaver kidney. Although the graft survival rate for living donor transplants is slightly higher than that of cadaver grafts, such operations tend to be few because of the difficulty in obtaining satisfactory donors. Thus, the total number of transplant operations is mainly governed by the number of cadaver kidneys available for such operations.

In the U.K., most patients start treatment with dialysis in hospital, and at the same time are trained to use the kidney machine usually with the help of a relative. Most of the patients are put on a waiting list for a transplant. For some patients, home haemodialysis may not be a suitable form of treatment; the patient will then be given priority for a transplant, but in the meantime will remain on hospital haemodialysis, which is relatively expensive due to staff costs. Conversely a patient may return to dialysis if a transplant fails. Thus patients may change their form of treatment several times. In such circumstances, it is difficult to make comparisons between the different treatments and their survival rates. (See figure 3)

4. PATIENT DATA

In health problems it is usually difficult to obtain adequate data for model construction. The data for this study, however, were readily available.

All the four renal units within the North East Thames Region submit data to the European Dialysis and Transplant Association (E.D.T.A.). This is an organisation which was set up on the initiative of the clinicians themselves and it collects patient data from over a thousand renal units in Europe. The data includes treatment profiles of all the patients.

Table 1 gives the numbers of new patients accepted for treatment within the North East Thames Region over the past ten years. In recent years an average of 76 new patients have been accepted annually. However, less than 60% (45 patients) of these patients came from within the North East Thames Region.

5. NEGATIVE EXPONENTIAL MODEL

An incidence rate for chronic renal failure of 40 new patients per year per million population gives a 'potential demand' of 150 new patients per year for the North East Thames Region. If the 'flows' of patients across the boundaries of the region were to continue to be taken into consideration, a crude estimate for the 'potential demand' for renal replacement services in the Region would be about 200 new patients per year. The present rate of intake of about 76 new patients per year is thus meeting less than half the need for the Region.

The relatively high cost of treatment severaly limits the provision of services in this specialty. Moreover, a patient once accepted on the renal replacement programme, continues to receive treatment until his death. The total number of patients on the programme is therefore sensitive to the level of intake of new patients. Thus, a model which examines the implications of increasing the level of intake is an important and useful planning tool.

The E.D.T.A. data was initially used to determine the total length of stay of each patient on the programme, irrespective of any changes in treatment. These were then used to plot the survival probabilities. Figure 1 shows that the overall survival data for this region fit a negative exponential distribution with a mean of 15 years.

The results obtained using the model show (Figure 2) that the total number of patients on the programme will increase each year even if the present rate of intake remains constant. Considerable additional resources will therefore be required to meet the demands of the renal replacement services in the coming years.

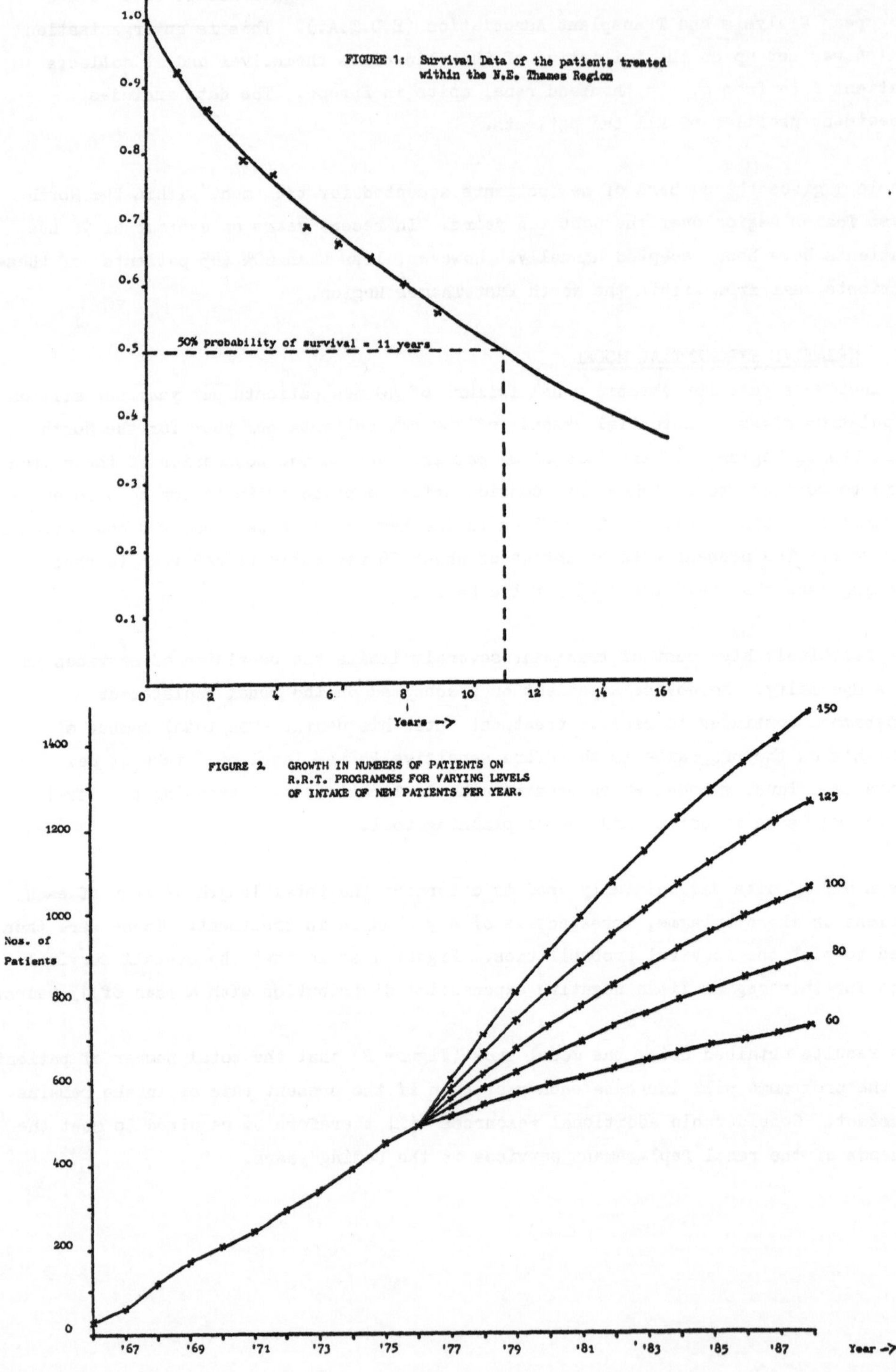

FIGURE 1: Survival Data of the patients treated within the N.E. Thames Region

FIGURE 2. GROWTH IN NUMBERS OF PATIENTS ON R.R.T. PROGRAMMES FOR VARYING LEVELS OF INTAKE OF NEW PATIENTS PER YEAR.

6. MATHEMATICAL MODEL

The different forms of treatment show wide variations both in cost and survival rates. The following estimates of costs (at 1976/77 prices) per patient per year for the treatments have been obtained (7, 10).

Hospital (unit haemodialysis)	£8,000 - £11,000
Home Haemodialysis	£4,500 - £6,000
Transplant patients	£1,000 - £2,500

Given such wide variations in cost, it was necessary therefore in this planning exercise to obtain not only forecasts of the total numbers of patients on R.R.T. programmes, but also to sub-divide these into the numbers on each individual form of treatment.

Furthermore the region was very interested in establishing whether increasing the facilities for transplant operations would significantly affect the additional number of new patients that could be treated each year. Thus a more complex model (for the technically minded a semi-markov model) was developed to enable forecasts to be made for patients on each form of treatment. The model framework is shown in Figure 3, where a distinction has to be made between first and subsequent periods of treatment as the survival rates are different.

7. RESULTS

Patients enter the programme via unit haemodialysis, hospital peritoneal dialysis or receive a transplant. Various inputs of numbers of patients were considered to examine the effect of different intakes on future forecasts. The results obtained are given in Table 2. These results show that if current treatment policies are continued and the present intake of new patients is maintained, the total number of patients will be more than doubled in 12 years.

The results also show that the greatest increase will be in the number of patients on unit dialysis. The detailed results for patients on unit haemodialysis are given in Table 3. This shows that the proportion of patients on first time of treatment compared to those on subsequent periods of treatment will change from 52% to 29%. The main conclusion which emerges from these figures is that even if the number of transplant operations and home dialysis machines are substantially increased, this shift towards a greater proportion of patients on second and subsequent periods of unit haemodialysis treatment will severely limit the number of new patients who can be accepted for renal replacement therapy. The present capacity of the renal units will thus need to be increased physically or through reduction in dialysing time with improved dialysis techniques.

TABLE 1. Intake of New Patients 1967–1976.

Year	Patient Intake	Year	Patient Intake
Bef. '67	31	1972	73
1967	33	1973	67
1968	70	1974	75
1969	64	1975	91
1970	48	1976	73
1971	50		

TABLE 2: 1988 FORECASTS FOR THE REGION

	Unit Haemo-Dialysis	Home Haemo-Dialysis	Hospital Peritoneal Dialysis	Home Peritoneal Dialysis	Transplant	Total
Position in Dec'76	110	209	5	14	161	499
72 New Pats./Yr	291	389	10	15	297	1002
84 New Pats./Yr	321	444	10	16	324	1115
96 New Pats./Yr	346	521	13	20	324	1224
76 New Pats./Yr	301	438	10	15	281	1045
100 New Pats./Yr	361	526	12	18	343	1260

TABLE 3: NO. OF PATIENTS ON UNIT HAEMODIALYSIS (76 pats./yr)

	UNIT HAEMODIALYSIS	
	First Treatment	Second & Subsequent Treatment
Dec. 1976	57 (52%)	53 (48%)
Dec. 1988	86 (29%)	215 (71%)

8. IMPLEMENTATION

The treatment of patients with chronic renal failure has been modelled before (1,2,6). Contrary to the conclusions reached in previous studies (3,4), the results obtained here suggest that a steady state will not be reached for many years.

In the planning study the output from the model was used to determine the maximum number of patients who could be treated within a given budget allocation. Specifically it was possible to show that:

(1) The development of minimal care hospital facilities which allow more than one patient to be dialysed on a machine with minimal support of trained staff.

(2) An increase in transplant operations

would greatly improve patient intake levels. These additional facilities are now being provided by the region.

Finally, a feature of the planning work has been the general recognition that there is uncertainty about long term survival rates in this new specialty and the possible effects of technological development, therefore further work is now being planned and undertaken to provide the basic patient data on a routine basis and to update the forecasts regularly.

9. REFERENCES

1. Davies Ruth, Johnson D. and Farrow S., Planning Patient Care with a Markov Model, Operational Research Quarterly, Vol. 26 3 ii (1975) 599-607.
2. Davies Ruth, A Model of the treatment of patients with Chronic Renal Failure in Oxford and its implication for Policy, Report, Operational Research Health and Social Services Unit, University of Reading.
3. Farrow S.C., Fisher D.J.H. and Johnson D.B., Statistical Approach to Planning an Integrated Haemodialysis/Transplantation Programme, British MedicalaJournal (1971) 671-676.
4. Fisher D.J.H., Farrow S.C. and Johnson D.B., Renal Transplantation trends and prospects, British Journal of Hospital Medicine, (1975) 451-454.
5. Fisher D.J.H., An enquiry into some of the Medical, Social and Economic Implications of Renal Failure amongst the Adult Population in the North East Metropolitan Region, M.D. Thesis, London University (1976).

6. Trent R.H.A., Correspondence: A simulation model of a Renal Dialysis and Transplantation Services.
7. Laing W., Renal Failure - a priority in health?, Report No. 62, Office of Health Economics, 162 Regent Street, London, W.1 (1978).
8. McCormick M.C. and Navarro V., Epid miological bases for planning kidney dialysis units, Uses of Epidemiology in Planning Health Services - Proceedings of the 6th International Scientific meeting, (1971) 114-138.
9. Pendreigh D.M. et al, Survey of Chronic Renal Failure in Scotland, The Lancet (1972) 304-307.
10. Pincherle G., Kidney Transplants and Dialysis, D.H.S.S. Report 2 in series Topics of our Time, H.M.S.O., London, (1979).

FIGURE 3 : A FLOW DIAGRAM SHOWING THE STATES SPECIFIED IN THE MODEL AND THE MAIN TRANSITIONS BETWEEN THEM

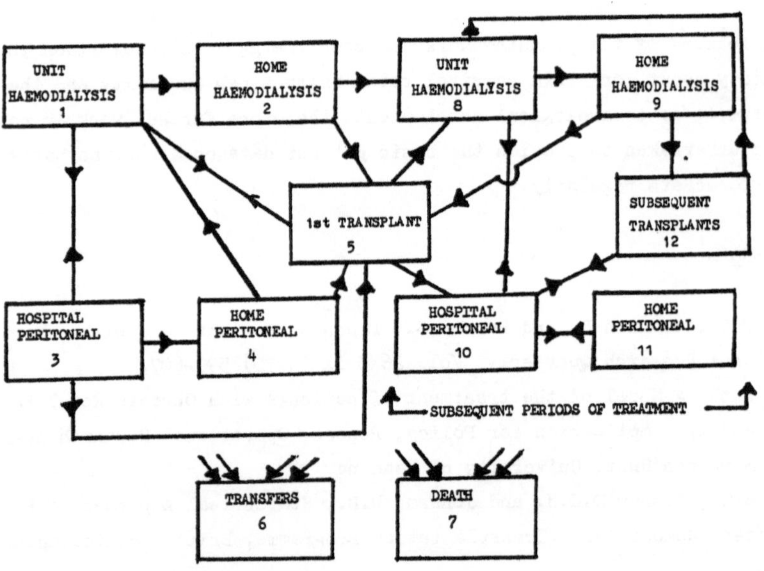

SELECTION IN RECRUITING PATIENTS VIA A RANDOM SAMPLE OF GYNECOLOGISTS

Ursula KELLHAMMER

ISB-Institut für medizinische Informationsverarbeitung, Statistik und Biomathematik
Ludwig-Maximilians-Universität
München, Federal Republic of Germany

SUMMARY

In 1977, a field study was started, in which randomly selected gynecologists should recruit five pairs of patients each, a pair consisting of a pilltaker and an age-matched control between 16 and 35 years. 51.9% of the physician sample contributed a total of 373 patient pairs. Each patient should get a medical examination and complete a questionnaire at the start and after one year. Complete information was received in 59.2% of all pairs. Adherence to the recruitment criteria was fairly close at the beginning. After one year 27.5% of the pairs were split up by a change of contraception. Two major features of the study design should therefore be newly assessed in the future: If possible, one should recruit individuals rather than pairs. Social data should be collected through a separate organization.

1 INTRODUCTION

1.1 The project 'Side-effects of oral contraceptives - pilot stage'

Since 1975, a Study group at the ISB-Institut (Director Prof. Dr. K. Überla) conducted pilot studies to find out the best way of longitudinally investigating side effects of oral contraceptives in the German population. The project is financed by the 'Bundesministerium für Forschung und Technologie' under No. MT 281. The data used here stem from the Pilot III Field survey, which started in autumn 1977.

1.2 Study Design

A stratified random sample of gynecologists practising ambulatory care in Bavaria was drawn. The 20 strata were defined by community size and age of the doctor's office (i.e., time period, the physician had been working there). We approached eight gynecologists per stratum. Each of them was asked to recruit five pairs of patients, a pair consisting of a pilltaker (= case) and a nontaker (= control). The inclusion criteria were: oral contraception during six months prior to the Study; the patient's intention to remain in the oral contraception status of the recruitment phase for one year; age between 16 and 35 years. Exclusion criteria were: absolute contraindications to the pill; no need for contra ception. The maximum age difference allowed in a pair was one year. The women underwent a gynecological examination (documented on the Study group's standardized forms) and they received a self-administered questionnaire from the physician. After one year the data collection was to be repeated in all cases, where the documentation of the first medical examination existed. Details of the Study layout are described in (1).

2 THE DATA

2.1 The physicians' cooperation

105 gynecologists (i.e. 65.6% of the gross physician sample) stated their intention to participate in the study. From these 90 physicians contributed at least one patient document, thus building up the gross patient sample of 809 cases. Since questionnaires and medical examination forms were returned independently, the patient pairs could only be established after termination of the fieldwork. Out of the 809 cases 373 pairs were considered eligible for the evaluation. These cases were recruited by 83 gynecologists. 63 patients (= 809 minus 746) had to be excluded for the following reasons: 46 cases returned a questionnaire only. In seven cases the study group received the medical documentation of a single patient. Three pairs of patients had to be eliminated, because one partner did not even roughly correspond to the admission criteria. Two further pairs were excluded, because both partners were wrongly defined.

The 83 gynecologists who recruited the 373 pairs admitted to the evaluation represent 51.9% of the gross physician sample. The distribution of these initially cooperative physicians over the sample strata is given in Table I. The distribution does not statistically significant deviate from a constant distribution.

TABLE I: COOPERATING PHYSICIANS

	Age of doctor's office					
Community Size	-1960	1961-65	1966-70	1971-77	total	
under 20,000	3	4	4	3	14	χ^2= 13.6
20,000-u. 50,000	3	4	7	5	19	D.F.= 19
50,000-u. 100,000	1	2	5	6	14	
100,000-u.1000,000	2	3	4	7	16	
1000,000 or more	5	3	5	7	20	
total	14	16	25	28	83	

The initial intensity of cooperation appears to be independent from the sample strata. In Table II the average number of recruited pairs per stratum is shown.

TABLE II: AVERAGE NUMBER OF RECRUITED PAIRS PER PHYSICIAN IN THE STRATA

Community Size	Age of doctor's office -1960	1961-65	1966-70	1971-77	total
under 20,000	5.0	5.5	3.8	4.3	4.6
20,000-u. 50,000	4.7	5.0	4.0	4.4	4.4
50,000-u. 100,000	5.0	4.0	5.0	3.5	4.2
100,000-u.1000,000	4.5	5.0	4.0	5.0	4.7
1000,000 or more	5.2	3.7	4.8	4.1	4.5
total	4.9	4.8	4.3	4.3	4.5

We had asked the physicians to recruit five pairs each. The 373 pairs represent therefore a return rate of 89.9%.

The physicians' 'longitudinal' cooperation has to be judged by the return of documents in the repeat phase. Since a noticable part of the physicians refused to disclose their patients' addresses, the return of questionnaires was not independent from the return of the examination forms. Therefore it is not always easy to discern between the physician's and the patient's cooperation. The returns of the second data collection phase are given in Table III.

TABLE III; RETUREND FORMS OF THE REPEAT PHASE

Returns, 2nd phase, from the case	Returns, 2nd phase, from the control: none	questionn. only	medical form only	both forms	total
none	35	2	2	24	63
questionnaire only	3	-	-	4	7
medical form only	2	-	3	16	21
both forms	36	4	12	230	282
total	76	6	17	274	373

The longitudinal dropouts of pairs attributable to a deficiency in physician's cooperation lie between 9.4 and 10.7% (depending on the definition). Between the returns of the second phase and the sample strata no contingency was apparent. But on account of the small numbers this result has to be interpreted with some reservation.

2.2 The patients' cooperation

The structure of information received from the pairs is given in Table IV.

TABLE IV: OVERALL INFORMATION STRUCTURE OF THE STUDY

Information of the case*	Information of the control*: EX1	EX1,Q2	EX1,EX2	EX1,Q2 EX2	EX1,Q1	EX1,Q1 Q2	EX1,Q1 EX2	EX1,Q1 EX2,Q2	total
EX1	-	-	-	-	4	1	1	3	9
EX1,Q2	-	-	-	-	-	-	-	-	-
EX1,EX2	-	-	-	-	1	-	-	4	5
EX1,Q2,EX2	-	-	-	-	-	-	-	4	4
EX1,Q1	2	-	-	-	29	1	1	21	54
EX1,Q1,Q2	-	-	-	-	3	-	-	4	7
EX1,Q1,EX2	-	-	-	-	1	-	3	12	16
EX1,Q1,EX2,Q2	5	-	2	5	31	4	10	221	278
total	7	-	2	5	69	6	15	269	373

*EX = medical examination form
Q = questionnaire (example: Q1 = questionnaire of the first phase)

Again it is not absolutely unequivocal, what is to be considered as patients' cooperation. If one defines a pair as cooperative by the completion of both questionnaires, then the Study achieved patient cooperation in 61.4%. This result compares rather unfavourably with that of the Pilot I Study, where patients were approached directly by the Study group (2).

3 METHOD OF ANALYSIS

The results are analyzed under two aspects: First, how closely were the patient recruitment criteria followed? Secondly, are there major differences between the characteristics of the cases and of the controls? The latter comparison is drawn in three subgroups: (1) 341 pairs, where both partners completed the first questionnaire. (2) the 221 pairs with complete information. (3) the 291 pairs, where the partners are not more than one year apart in age.

Throughout the evaluation classified variables are analyzed in two-dimensional contingency tables, one dimension representing the cases' values, the other the controls' values. For each of the continuous variables the mean in the case group and the control group is given.

4 RESULTS

4.1 Adherence to the recruitment criteria

Contraception: The definition of cases and controls regarding the current pill status at the beginning appears to be nearly always correct. According to the contraceptive history taken by the physician four cases are open to doubt.
The information of the first questionnaire mostly bears out the physician's classification. It should be noticed, that 75.7% of the controls classify themselves as ex-takers. This fact appears to justify the rather broad definition of the control, which came under discussion in comparison to the Oral Contraception Study (3) (for the discussion see (1), p. 183).
It was not possible exactly to control for the condition of the contraceptive status during the six months prior to the Study on account of the very poor documentation of the contraceptive history in the medical documentation forms. However, the questionnaire data seem to indicate, that the case group has been on the pill for about five years on the average, whereas the ex-takers of the control group claim an average consumption period of 4.5 years.
The adherence to the initial contraceptive status is measured by the status of the second questionnaire. This is to be done with some reservation, since only 229 pairs have completed this form.

TABLE V: ORAL CONTRACEPTIVE STATUS IN THE SECOND QUESTIONNAIRE

OC-status of the case	OC-status of the control: current taker	ex-taker	never taker	no answer	total
current taker	17	124	34	8	183
ex-taker	5	36	5	-	46
never taker	-	-	-	-	-
no answer	-	-	-	-	-
total	22	160	39	8	229

The change of plans is more frequent in the cases (20.1%) than in the controls (9.6%). The consequences for the matched- pair-comparison are grave: After one year 27.5% of the pairs are disrupted in the central criterion of oral contraception.
Age: The 373 pairs were all born between 1940 and 1960. As the Study started in 1977, the age condition can be considered as more or less

fulfilled. But the age-matching condition was not quite so carefully observed. The age difference between case and control varies between -4 yrs and +13.8 yrs. The birthday differences (case minus control) have the following distribution: In 36 pairs the control is too young, in 291 pairs the difference is to be tolerated, in 46 pairs the case is too young. There appears to exist some association between 'age of the doctor's office' and correct matching. The 'younger' physicians adhere closer to the matching condition, the association is significant at the 1%-level.

4.2 Structural comparison of cases and controls

Reproductive history: In the variable 'nullipara yes/no' the pairs are remarkably similar. In all the analyzed subgroups 71 to 72% of the pairs are alike in this respect despite the fact, that the marginal distributions show about 50% in each class. In number of children and birth-year of the first child there are no differences to speak of.
Miscarriages are slightly more frequent in the control group. More controls state to have had an abortion (22 controls vs 8 cases).

Use of IUDs: More controls have IUD-experience (46.6% controls of all pairs with second questionnaire vs 7.8% cases) and the controls were on the average twice as long exposed compared to the cases.

Contact to the health care system: The physicians recruited the patients mainly from their longterm clientele. Only 9.5% of the pairs consist of last year's patients. The cases have markedly shorter intervals between gynecological check-ups than the controls (58.4% at least twice/yr vs 45.2%). The data allow no causal interpretation of this fact. Regarding the family doctor there is no difference between the two groups and no pairwise association either.

Sociodemographic critera: 67.3% of the pairs have the same marital status. This might be an unconscious matching, but more probably this likeness is caused by the age matching. 70.3% of the catholic cases have a catholic control, but only 37.9% of the protestant cases have a partner of the same religion. This effect is to be considered as an artefact produced by the sample stratification.
There is no apparent association between 'education' and the pair-building. The cases appear to have as a group slightly more fulltime jobs, but there is no pair-effect. 41.9% of the cases do smoke vs 37.0% of the controls, but there is no difference in the number of cigarettes/day or in the age they started smoking.

5 DISCUSSION

5.1 Physicians' cooperation

(1) Enlisting physicians for such a study and monitoring the data collection is a time-consuming task. In most cases telephone contacts with the physician proved to be necessary to enlarge the physician's awareness of the Study or to clear up misunderstandings. At the study center a person has to be available, who is able to point out the underlying ideas and to discuss the recruitment criteria. In addition to that the monitoring of data returns occupies one person fulltime during the fieldwork phases.

(2) Physicians tend to underestimate the difficulties in adhering to recruitment criteria. Only 79.0% of the physicians willing to cooperate actually contributed to the data under evaluation. The 373 patient pairs represent 89.9% of the aspired total (i.e. 415 pairs from 83 physicians).

(3) Once the cooperation has been established, it continues fairly well. Pairwise patient losses after one year are attributable to the physician in about 10% (of the initial pairs).

5.2 Adherence to the recruitment criteria

(1) The criterion of current contraceptive status was strictly observed by the physicians. The age rules were followed less closely. The matching condition (age ± one year) was exactly fulfilled in only 78.0%. Younger physicians were significantly more cooperative than older ones in this respect.

(2) It appears to be unrealistic to incorporate the patients' future plans into the recruitment criteria, as it was done here ('oral contraceptive status constant during the Study'). After one year 27.5% of the pairs were split up, because one or both partners had changed their contraception.

(3) Recruitment by using variables out of the patient's medical history appears to be rather unreliable. Despite the fact, that the oral contraception during the six months prior to the Study constituted one of the recruitment conditions, this variable was documented so poorly (both by doctors and by patients), that no strict control of the adherence to this criterion could be undertaken.

(4) There appears to exist quite a noticable amount of unconscious matching in medical or medically relevant variables (e.g. number of children, use of IUDs). Social variables like the patient's education or occupation were of no importance for the construction of pairs in this Study.

5.3 The patient's cooperation

Patients who undergo a gynecological examination, are usually highly motivated for a cooperation (see 2)). But the return of questionnaires in this Study fell short of our expectations. Return rates were markedly lower than 80%, whatever combination of questionnaire returns is termed 'patient cooperation'.

5.4 Sociodemographic description of pairs

(1) In the marginal distributions of the more 'basic' sociodemographic variables (e.g. marital status, education, number of children, occupation) there exist no obvious deviations from the population average. In this respect no marked selection effect could be detected.

(2) Social variables seem to be of no importance for the physician in constructing the pairs. Therefore the pairs were rather heterogeneous when considered by the sociodemographic description alone. This could turn out as a problem in studies, where the hypotheses involve sociodemographic variables.

6 CONCLUSIONS

- The patient recruitment by randomly selected gynecologists in ambulatory care is feasible.
- The handing out of self-administered questionnaires (SAQs) to the patients via the physicians is not advisable. The study center should receive the patients full addresses and then mail and monitor the SAQs independent from the medical forms.
- The pairwise recruitment on changable conditions (e.g. contraception) for longitudinal studies is too costly in terms of dropouts. Possibilities of individual sampling and posterior matching should be discussed for that type of problem.

REFERENCES

(1) Kellhammer U. A field survey of oral contraceptives with patient pairs out of gynecological practices (Pilot III). In: Kellhammer U, Überla K (Eds). Long-term studies on side effects of contraception - state and planning. Lecture Notes in Medical Informatics, vol 3, Springer, Berlin-Heidelberg-New York, 1978; 175-183

(2) Kellhammer U. The Pilot-I Study: Analysis of drop-outs and some results of a pilltaking typology. In: Kellhamer U, Überla K (Eds). Long-term studies on side-effects of contraception - state and planning. Lecture Notes in Medical Informatics, vol 3, Springer, Berlin-Heidelberg-New York, 1978; 93-114

(3) Kay CR. Oral Contraceptives and Health. An Interim Report from the Oral Contraception Study of the Royal College of General Practitioners, Pitman Medical Publishing, London, 1974

EFFICACITE DU SYSTEME DE SOINS ET PAIEMENT A L'ACTE[1]

A.P. Contandriopoulos
Département d'administration de la santé
Université de Montréal
Montréal, P.Q., Canada

The presentation comprises three sections: the analysis framework, the evaluation of the Quebec medical care system, and a proposal for a new form of reimbursement.

__Analysis Framework__: The objective of the medical care system is to render the highest quality of care possible to the entire population by making the best use of resources available. The proposed evaluation model for the medical care system establiches the existing links between the prevalent organizational structure and degrees of attaining the objectives of the medical care system.

__Evaluation of the Quebec Medical Care System__: The proposed analysis model is used to evalue the Quebec medical care system. The conclusions of the evaluation are that the two main factors limiting the effectiveness of the Quebec medical care system are the fee-for-service method within a third party system of reimbursement and the lack of physicians' integration in the organization and functioning of the medical care system.

__Proposal for a New System of Reimbursement__: In order to correct the imperfections identified in the present system, a new method of payment is proposed, dissociating physicians' income from the volume of services offered, and encouraging physician - patient contacts. For better physician integration, this method or reimbursement should be an integral part of the restructuration of the present medical care system based on the following principles: decentralized management entrusted to physicians, financing of physicians in each region within a global envelope proportional to that region's population, peer group control of professional activity, and instituting of a permanent mechanism for evaluation and planning.

Nous commencerons par proposer un cadre d'analyse permettant d'évaluer de façon générale un système de soins, puis nous utiliserons ce cadre pour apprécier l'efficacité du système de soins du Québec de façon à porter un jugement sur une de ses caractéristiques: le paiement à l'acte des médecins. Dans la dernière partie de la présentation, nous donnerons les grands principes autour desquels un nouveau mode de rémunération pourrait être envisagé.

I. Cadre d'analyse

Idéalement, l'évaluation du système de soins devrait se faire en appréciant son efficacité à améliorer l'état de santé de la population. Malheureusement, d'une part il n'existe pas d'indicateur global permettant de mesurer l'état de santé d'une population et d'autre part il est à toute fin pratique impossible de connaître l'influence relative des différents déterminants de la santé (facteurs biologiques, environnement, habitudes de vie et système de soins) sur l'état de santé.[2]

Les différents facteurs qui déterminent l'état de santé constituent le système de santé. Le système de soins qui peut se définir comme un ensemble de ressources (professionnels, établissements, équipements, etc.) structuré en vue de fournir des services de santé (services hospitaliers, médicaux, dentaires, etc.) à la population dans le but de contribuer à améliorer son état de santé, ne constitue qu'un des éléments du système de santé.[3]

Pour pouvoir évaluer dans quelle mesure le système de soins contribue à améliorer l'état de santé d'une population, il faudrait non seulement résoudre plusieurs problèmes méthodologiques difficiles mais aussi pouvoir postuler que tous les autres déterminants de l'état de santé sont restés inchangés pendant toute la durée de l'évaluation. L'irréalisme de ce postulat conduit à centrer l'évaluation du système de soins, non plus sur des indicateurs de résultats, mais sur des indicateurs de processus.[4] Pour ce faire, il faut définir de façon normative quelles devraient être les caractéristiques des services de santé puis comparer ces caractéristiques théoriques avec celles des services réellement utilisés par la population. Les caractéristiques théoriques des services découlent des objectifs spécifiques du système de soins.

Au Québec, les objectifs du système de soins ont été énoncés par la commission Castonguay-Nepveu.[5] Ils peuvent être résumés de la façon suivante:

Le système de soins doit: fournir à toute la population quelles que soient les caractéristiques sociales, économiques et géographiques tous les services qu'elle requiert (accessibilité); s'assurer que ces services sont de la meilleure qualité possible, c'est-à-dire qu'ils sont globaux, continus et conformes aux normes de la bonne pratique (qualité); être organisé de façon à utiliser au mieux les ressources disponibles (productivité); satisfaire les aspirations de la population ainsi que celles des professionnels (satisfaction); et être administrable d'une façon efficace.

L'évaluation du système de soins consistera à transformer chacun de ces objectifs en indicateurs opérationnels puis à définir la norme qui permettra d'apprécier dans quelle mesure les objectifs ont été atteints. Les jugements que l'on portera à la suite de cette évaluation devront considérer non par chaque objectif indépendamment mais tous les objectifs simultanément.[6] C'est en effet seulement dans la mesure où tous les objectifs seront atteints que le postulat implicite au type d'évaluation qui est entrepris, c'est-à-dire que mieux le système de soins atteind ses objectifs, meilleur est son efficacité à améliorer la santé de la population, est acceptable.

Après avoir porté un jugement sur l'atteinte des objectifs, il faudra identifier les éléments de l'organisation du système de soins qui peuvent expliquer les résultats obtenus. Cette démarche se fera en considérant que le fondement du système de soins peut être schématisé ainsi:[7] l'utilisation des services de santé résulte d'une interaction entre d'une part le comportement du consommateur qui décide de faire appel au système de soins et d'autre part le comportement du professionnel qui après avoir établi un diagnostic, propose un plan de traitement à son patient. C'est lors de l'établissement du diagnostic et de la mise en oeuvre du traitement prescrit que les différentes ressources du système de soins sont utilisées. Les comportements qui à l'origine de l'utilisation des services de santé sont influencés d'une part par l'importance du problème de santé qui a été à l'origine de la démarche entreprise et par toutes les caractéristiques personnelles des individus en cause (éducation, niveau socio-économique, croyance, etc) mais aussi par la façon dont est organisé le système de soins. C'est sur ce dernier facteur que nous nous attarderons de façon à apprécier d'abord dans quelle mesure la façon dont est organisé le système de soins peut, en créant toutes sortes de stimulants, influencer le comportement des professionnels et celui de la population et ensuite si ces stimulants sont cohérents ou non avec les objectifs du système de soins.

II. Evaluation du système de soins

Avant de présenter les résultats de l'évaluation du système de soins, il convient de rappeler les principales caractéristiques de l'organisation du système de soins québécois, surtout celle qui portent sur les services médicaux puisque l'évaluation portera surtout sur eux.

Ces caractéristiques sont les suivantes: (a) existence d'un régime général d'assurance pour tous les services hospitaliers et médicaux; (b) le principal mode de rémunération des médecins est le paiement à l'acte avec tiers payant; (c) les tarifs de remboursement des actes ainsi que les conditions de pratique sont définies par des ententes négociées entre le gouvernement et les associations de médecins; (d) la quasi totalité des médecins participent au régime d'assurance-maladie; (e) les dépassements d'honoraires sont interdits; (f) les libertés professionnelles (liberté thérapeutique, liberté du choix des patients, liberté du choix du lieu et du mode de pratique, liberté du choix de la spécialité, liberté de ne pas participer au programme d'assurance-maladie) sont garanties; (g) tous les hôpitaux sont financés par des fonds publics; (h) les médecins peuvent utiliser gratuitement les ressources hospitalières; (i) les coûts de fonctionnement des cabinets privés sont à la charge des médecins.

Les résultats de l'évaluation qui est présentée ci-dessous a été faite essentiellement en utilisant les études disponibles et les statistiques existantes.[8]

1. Accessibilité

Le degré d'accessibilité au système de soins a été évalué en analysant successivement l'accessibilité provinciale, l'accessibilité régionale, l'accessibilité sociale et l'accessibilité organisationnelle.

L'accessibilité provinciale concerne la relation entre les effectifs existants, leur évolution récente et leur prévision, et les effectifs requis pour offrir des services de qualité à toute la population de la province.

Elle est bonne, il y a déjà au Québec un médecin pour 540 personnes. La croissance prévue des effectifs est rapide. Elle l'accompagne d'une augmentation de la proportion des femmes (37% des nouveaux médecins sont des femmes) et la proportion des omnipraticiens qui se stabilisera à environ 60% du corps médical.

L'accessibilité régionale concerne la répartition géographique des effectifs et l'évolution de cette répartition en fonction des besoins des populations.

Le nombre des médecins par rapport à la population a augmenté dans toutes les régions; toutefois, cette amélioration de la répartition géographique découle plus de l'abondance des effectifs dans les régions métropolitaines que de la prise en considération des besoins des populations. La répartition des médecins spécialistes reste problématique.

L'accessibilité sociale concerne l'existence et l'importance des divers obstacles (psychologiques, sociaux, économiques, culturels) que la population peut rencontrer dans l'utilisation des services de santé.

D'une façon générale, l'introduction du régime d'assurance-maladie a permis une amélioration de l'accessibilité sociale en réduisant les barrières financières à l'accès aux services. Toutefois, les disparités régionales dans la distribution des effectifs font en sorte que tous les québécois n'ont pas accès de la même manière aux services. Il semble ainsi subsister des différences dans les types de services médicaux utilisés en fonction des niveaux socio-économiques.

L'accessibilité organisationnelle concerne la disponibilité des ressources existantes.

Globalement, l'accès aux ressources existantes est apparu acceptable. Toutefois, le niveau d'accessibilité à certains services est trop dépendant des tarifs en vigueur (consultations téléphoniques, visites à domicile, etc...).

2. Qualité

La qualité des services est une notion difficile à cerner qui a été appréciée sous trois aspects: la globalité, la continuité, la qualité technique.

Pour évaluer la globalité, il faut voir si le système de soins favorise la dispensation de la gamme complète des services (prévention, cure, réadaptation) à l'endroit le plus approprié (cabinet, domicile, établissement). Il faut examiner aussi dans quelle mesure il existe une intégration entre les différents types de services (médicaux, sociaux, hospitaliers, etc.) et une orientation des services vers les besoins des populations considérés dans leur environnement économique et social.

Dans le système actuel, la globalité apparaît particulièrement insuffisante. De façon générale, les activités qui ne sont pas reliées directement aux soins aux patients, tels la prévention, les tâches administratives, l'enseignement, ne sont pas favorisées. Dans plusieurs cas, elles ne sont pas rémunérées, ou si elles le sont, c'est selon des modes de rémunération différents ce qui limite l'intégration de ces services aux autres dimensions de l'activité médicale.

Dans le cas des services médicaux, la prévention auprès des populations particulières est peu encouragée. Le temps consacré aux contacts humains est souvent déprécié par rapport aux dimensions techniques de l'exercice de la médecine.

L'objectif de continuité est atteint lorsqu'il y a une interaction cohérente entre les différents professionnels pour que la prise en charge de l'individu (prévention, cure, réadaptation) soit assurée à tout moment et quel que soit le lieu de l'intervention.

Dans le système actuel, cet objectif n'est pas atteint. En effet, la pratique individualiste qui caractérise la rémunération à l'acte ne favorise pas la constitution d'équipes pluridisciplinaires, ni l'intégration des activités dans un système cohérent où les différentes catégories de services seraient harmonisées. On observe un manque important de communication entre les différents professionnels.

La qualité technique des services mesure le degré de concordance entre les services fournis et les normes de la bonne pratique.

Bien qu'il existe au Québec un certain contrôle de l'activité professionnelle, de nombreuses interrogations subsistent. Le maintien des compétences n'est pas favorisé. L'encadrement de l'activité professionnelle existe surtout dans le milieu hospitalier, et de nombreux omnipraticiens sont absents de ce milieu. De plus, la qualité des services n'est pas valorisée, l'acte est payé de la même façon quelle qu'en soit la qualité.

3. Productivité

La productivité est la relation entre les ressources existantes et le volume des services offerts.

L'utilisation accrue des examens complets plus rémunérateurs que les examens sommaires, la facturation d'actes mineurs (exérèse de cérumen, funduscopie, pansements de plus de vingt centimètres carrés, etc.) et l'élargissement des indications de certains actes diagnostiques ou thérapeutiques (électrocardiogrammes, scopies digestives, radiographies dentaires, étude simple de la vision des couleurs, etc.) entraînent un accroissement du nombre des actes et du coût des services souvent indépendants des besoins de la population c'est-à-dire une pseudo-productivité.

Cette pseudo-productivité est possible à cause du double rôle que joue le médecin à la fois conseiller et fournisseur de services. Ce conflit d'intérêt va aussi parfois à l'encontre d'une utilisation rationelle des ressources en retardant l'introduction de technologies automatisées ou en restreignant le regroupement de certains services très spécialisés.

La faible utilisation du personnel auxiliaire diminue la productivité des médecins et des dentistes, mais elle représente un comportement économique cohérent avec les plafonnements des revenus bruts, les restrictions au paiement d'actes qui n'ont pas été posés par le dispensateur lui-même, et le fait que le tarif des actes est fixe et qu'il ne peut donc être ajusté selon les coûts de fonctionnement des cabinets.

4. La satisfaction des professionnels

Les professionnels sont généralement satisfaits du régime d'assurance-maladie et ils jouissent d'une liberté étendue dans leur pratique.

Leur rémunération place les médecins québécois aux premiers rangs parmi les provinces canadiennes, et les situe favorablement par rapport aux professionnels à leur compte. Leurs heures de travail diminuent et la durée de leurs vacances augmente.

5. Administrabilité

L'administrabilité concerne le niveau de complexité de la gestion du système de santé, et la capacité du système à évaluer ses performances, à planifier son développement et à contrôler la croissance de ses coûts.

La gestion du système de soins est très lourde. La Régie de l'assurance-maladie doit multiplier les vérifications pour tenter d'empêcher des abus mais l'application de mécanismes de contrôle de la pratique individuelle payée à l'acte par une organisation centrale reste relativement inefficace parce qu'il est souvent difficile de distinguer si les différences dans le nombre et le type de services dispensés sont reliées à des variations du jugement clinique ou au conflit d'intérêt inhérent à la rémunération à l'acte.

Le système de rémunération à l'acte ne fonctionne pas de façon intégrée avec l'ensemble du système de soins. La négociation s'est substituée au processus de planification et de gestion; et il n'existe pas de mécanisme systématique d'évaluation.

Le contrôle de la croissance des coûts est plus tributaire du rationnement budgétaire global appliqué aux établissements que d'une réallocation sélective et rationnelle des ressources selon des objectifs d'ensemble qui tiendraient compte des populations à desservir.

6. La satisfaction de la population

Elle est en général bonne, mais il faut être conscient que le consommateur est peu amené à se servir de son jugement critique lorsqu'il doit utiliser les services de santé, et que de plus, l'insatisfaction générée par cette utilisation n'est pas toujours canalisée vers les organismes ayant pour fonction de recevoir les critiques et les plaintes et susceptibles de fournir des statistiques à ce sujet.

Au terme de cette évaluation, il faut conclure que les objectifs du système de soins sont loin d'être atteints et qu'il n'y a aucune raison pour que dans le système actuel, ils puissent l'être sans des changements importants.

III. Influences du paiement à l'acte sur les faiblesses observées

Les faiblesses observées sont en bonne partie reliées aux modes de rémunération en vigueur, c'est-à-dire principalement au paiement à l'acte avec tiers payant dans un régime public d'assurance-maladie. Ce mode de rémunération a en effet trois caractéristiques qui le rendent incompatible avec les objectifs du système de soins.[9]

Ce mode de rémunération ne permet pas de rémunérer la totalité de l'activité professionnelle. Cette dernière est un ensemble complexe d'interactions entre le professionnel, les patients et l'environnement dans lequel elle s'exerce. Cette activité ne peut être entièrement définie par des actes aussi nombreux et précis soient-ils; ainsi la prévention auprès de populations, l'administration, le suivi des patients, la psychiatrie dans une large mesure, et d'une façon générale, toutes les activités qui dépendent plus de l'interaction entre le professionnel et son patient que de la nature de l'acte posé, sont difficiles ou impossibles à rémunérer à l'acte.

C'est pour pallier ces faiblesses que le paiement à l'acte a été complété par du paiement au temps (salaire, vacations, actes avec une référence explicite au temps). Cette juxtaposition de modes de rémunération de nature différente qui complique l'administration du système et engendre de nombreux abus, ne résoud que de façon très imparfaite les lacunes du paiement à l'acte; certaines activités continuent à ne pas être rémunérées (les consultations téléphoniques, l'éducation continue, etc.) et dans les autres, le passage d'une rémunération à l'acte à une rémunération au temps nuit à la continuité et à la globalité des services.

Enfin, le paiement à l'acte est, le plus souvent, sans relation avec la qualité de l'acte ou les compétences particulières des professionnels.

Avec le paiement à l'acte, la pratique individualiste est valorisée. Le professionnel est rémunéré pour un service spécifique fourni à un patient particulier. Cette situation décourage l'interaction entre les professionnel (la pluridisciplinarité est difficilement compatible avec un paiement à l'acte tout comme le recours optimal à la consultation), et surtout elle empêche l'intégration des professionnels à l'organisation et au fonctionnement du système de soins, ce qui a des effets négatifs sur la qualité des services et surtout sur l'administrabilité du système.

Avec le mode de rémunération actuel, le professionnel est orienté vers le traitement des maladies et non vers la santé de la population.

Il existe une relation entre le revenu et la quantité des actes. Cette relation, associée à la capacité des professionnels d'influencer le volume et l'éventail des services qu'ils dispensent, les place dans une situation de non-neutralité dans leurs décisions. Les actes clairement identifiables, ceux qui font appel à la technologie plus qu'à la relation humaine, se multiplient. Les populations particulières qui demandent beaucoup de temps ne reçoivent pas toujours tous les services que leur état requiert. Certains actes sont posés sans qu'il y ait un besoin véritable (pseudo-productivité); la quantité prend le pas sur la qualité, et il est impossible d'appliquer des mécanismes efficaces de contrôle.

IV. Vers un nouveau système de rémunération

S'il y a incompatibilité entre les objectifs du système de soins et les façons actuelles de payer les médecins, seul un changement radical du mode de rémunération et de l'organisation dans lequel il s'inscrit permettra au système de soins de mieux atteindre ses objectifs.

Ces changements reposent sur le postulat qu'il y a fondamentalement un accord de principe entre les différents intervenants (population, professionnels, gouvernement, etc.) sur les objectifs du système de soins. De plus, pour être réalisables, les modifications envisagées devront rester compatibles avec les valeurs socio-culturelles de la société québécoise. Parmi les valeurs à préserver mentionnons la liberté de la population de choisir son professionnel et le maintien des principales libertés professionnelles des médecins.

Le système de rémunération qui a été conçu pour corriger les faiblesses du système de soins actuel est appelé système des honoraires modulés. Il est constitué par un mode de rémunération et par un réaménagement de l'organisation du système de soins.

Le mode de rémunération

1. Le mode de rémunération doit être unique, c'est-à-dire s'appliquer à tous les professionnels.

2. Le même mode de rémunération doit s'appliquer à toutes les activités des médecins, c'est-à-dire couvrir aussi bien les activités cliniques que la prévention, l'administration, l'enseignement, la recherche, la formation continue. Ce mode de rémunération s'appliquerait ainsi à tous les services rendus par les professionnels qu'ils soient assurés dans le cadre des programmes d'assurance-maladie ou non. L'accessibilité de la population aux services serait ainsi indépendante de considérations économiques. Ce principe implique que des mécanismes de recouvrement du coût des services non assurés auprès de la population devraient être instaurés.

Les caractères unique et complet du mode de rémunération veulent dire que les médecins auraient à choisir entre une complète participation au système ou une non participation intégrale. Dans ce cas, le coût des services serait entièrement à la charge du patient.

3. La rémunération devrait être fonction du temps consacré par le médecin à ses différentes activités professionnelles. Les honoraires devraient être modulés pour tenir compte d'une part de certaines caractéristiques du professionnel (expérience, durée de la formation, etc.) et d'autre part du caractère particulier de certaines ac-

tivités (soir, week-end, intervention chirurgicale particulièrement stressante, etc.).

4. Le paiement des honoraires serait effectué selon le principe du tiers payant par la régie de l'assurance-maladie sur réception d'une formule de déclaration du temps consacré par le médecin à différentes activités, des patients vus et d'informations succintes sur les services rendus.

5. Ce mode de rémunération ne s'applique qu'aux activités professionnelles. Le financement des cabinets devrait faire l'objet d'un financement particulier et être clairement distingué des honoraires.

Organisation du système de soins

L'autonomie et les libertés professionnelles que le mode de rémunération permet doivent être encadrées, pour éviter des abus, par une organisation dans laquelle les médecins collectivement prennent des responsabilités face aux objectifs du système de soins. Cette responsabilité collective des médecins sera favorisée par les modalités suivantes:

1. La décentralisation des responsabilités de planification, de gestion et de contrôle de la distribution des services professionnels.

2. Dans chaque district (120 000 personnes, 200 médecins, au moins un hôpital), tous les médecins constituent l'assemblée de district. Les médecins élisent aussi des représentants qui forment l'assemblée régionale des médecins.

3. Tous les services professionnels sont payés aux médecins de chaque district à même un budget global de district établi en fonction de la population desservie par les médecins du district.

4. Les médecins, dans leur assemblée de district acceptent la responsabilité de fournir à leur population les services requis en respectant leur budget global. Ceci implique qu'ils sont responsables de la gestion de leur budget global, du contrôle de leurs effectifs ainsi que de l'encadrement de leurs activités professionnelles.

5. Les assemblées de district et de région sont intégrés au système de soins. La cohérance et la coordination du système est assuré par des organismes comme les Conseils régionaux de la santé et des services sociaux.

6. L'information nécessaire, pour permettre aux différents organismes d'évaluer leurs activités, et de planifier leurs développements, est compilée et fournie régulièrement et systématiquement par la Régie de l'assurance-maladie.

V. Conclusion

Il faut noter que le système des honoraires modulés ne peut être assimilé ni au paiement à l'acte, ni au salariat. Il apparaît comme un système nouveau de rémunération qui devrait contribuer à améliorer l'état de santé de la population en favorisant la dispensation de services plus globaux, plus humains, où les relations médecins-patients sont plus valorisées que le volume des services; en améliorant l'accessibilité aux services; en permettant aux professionnels d'assurer leurs responsabilités dans l'organisation et le fonctionnement du système de soins; en stimulant la pluridisciplinarité, et en offrant à toute la population un accès équitable aux soins.

Notes de références

(1) Cet article est en quelque sorte un résumé du rapport du Comité sur la rémunération des professionnels de la santé du Québec (Le système des honoraires modulés, ministère des Affaires sociales, Québec, mars 1980). Son contenu est fortement inspiré de la réflexion de tous les membres du comité bien que l'auteur reste seul responsable de la formulation proposée ici.

(2) Voir entre autres Goldberg, M. et al. Indicateurs de santé et "Sanométrie": Les aspects conceptuels des recherches récentes sur la mesure de l'état de santé d'une population. Rev. Epid. et Santé Publ., 27, 1979, et Lalonde M. Nouvelle perspective de la santé des canadiens, Ministère de la santé et du bien-être social, Ottawa, 1974. McKeown, T. The role of Medicine, Nuffield Provincial Hospitals Trust, London, 1976.

(3) Ces définitions sont inspirées par celles de Dab, W. et al. Glossaire des principaux termes utilisés en épidémiologie informatique et statistique, G.E.R.S.S., Paris, Juin 1979.

(4) Pineault, R. Rationnalisation de l'évaluation et du contrôle dans les organisations de santé, Admin. Hospitalière et Sociale, Mars-Avril 1977 et Grémy, F. Evaluation de l'action médicale et de l'action en santé publique, INSERM, Paris, 1979.

(5) Rapport de la Commission d'enquête sur la santé et le bien-être social, Gouvernement du Québec, Québec, 1970.

(6) Donabedian, A. Issues in National Health Insurance, Am. J. of Public Health, 66:4, 1978, et Greenlick, M.R. A framework for assessing the impact of health policy alternatives on Medical Care efficiency and effectivness. U.S. Dept. of Commerce, Feb. 1976.

(7) Donabedian, A. Aspects of Medical Care Administration, Harvard Univ. Press, 1973.

(8) En particulier les statistiques de la Régie de l'assurance-maladie du Québec et celles de la Corporation professionnelle des médecins du Québec.

(9) Rivard, J.Y. et Boudreau, T. "Les effets de la rémunération et de l'organisation de l'exercice de la médecine sur les objectifs du système de santé, P.N.R.D.S. Santé et Bien-être, Ottawa, 1975, et Gobel, J.R., Redisch, M.A. Alternative Physician Payment Methods: Incentives, Efficiency, and National Health Insurance, Health and Society 57:1, 1979.

BABY IMMUNISATION AN AID TO ILLNESS AND HANDICAP PREVENTION.

MARR, A.C., MELVILLE, A.C., RANKIN, J., BRYDEN, J.S., DAVIDSON, D. and McQUEEN, I.
Argyll and Clyde Health Board, Gilmour House, Paisley, SCOTLAND.

A standard register and recall system for child health purposes is being developed by the Welsh Health Technical Services Organisation, providing child register, immunisation, pre-school health and school health modules. The first of these has been running in Glasgow since January 1978.

Argyll and Clyde Health Board also opted to use the Standard Scottish System but have related it to the Community Health Index by using the CHI number for registering the children. The aims of the Argyll and Clyde system are not only to record accurately the immunisation history of the children in the Area, but to give the facility to identify the non-attenders for immunisation of those refusing consent, in order that those who are most at risk may be encouraged to attend, thus helping prevent morbidity and handicap. A further benefit is more accurate and therefore more useful statistics as well as improved feedback of information for the General Practitioners, clinical doctors and health visitors of the state of immunity of these patients.

Because of problems and criticism surrounding the confidentiality of data in the pre-school and school health modules these have not been accepted at the present time for use in Scotland, and so the Argyll and Clyde System consists of an immunisation module linked to the Child Register module, with the register using the CHI number, but not so far physically linked to the Index. It is hoped that this will be a future development.

CHILD REGISTER MODULE

Since 1st April 1980 all Argyll and Clyde births have been registered on to the system. This includes all children born within the Area, as well as those born outside but resident in Argyll and Clyde. The record is generated on receipt of the Statutory Notification of Birth form, or by use of a Transfer-in document for children moving into the area. From this register a periodic print-out is produced for each district for use by the districts as a check list - to compare with their own registers which are kept and for comparison with the Registrar General's print-out. Quarterly and annual statistics for districts and area will be produced from the register.

As each new Child Register is created, pressure-sensitive adhesive labels are produced. These are used for Health Visitor Cards, the Immunisation Consent form and the Low Birth Weight Baby Report. The information available on the labels includes name, address, date of birth, general practitioner and health visitor reference, and the child's reference number in Argyll and Clyde: this being the CHI number - a ten digit number made up of date of birth (dd mm yy) and a three digit personal number plus a check digit.

It is the responsibility of the health visitor to ensure completion of the consent form, in consultation with and signed by the child's parent or guardian. This form is then returned to the Health Board where the relevant information including the child's forenames, family doctor and either the surgery or the Child Health Clinic information is coded. The general practitioners' surgery or the Child Health Clinic where the immunisations are carried out are referred to as treatment centres.

The father's occupation is also ascertained and is used for statistical purposes. The Low Birth Weight Report is completed only for those children who weighed 2,500 grammes or less at birth, and is required in order to produce the annual statistics for ISD (S) 7. The label for this contains information on name, address, date of birth, place of birth, birth weight, sex and reference number.

IMMUNISATION MODULE

This system is linked to the child register module and maintains a separate record for each child, showing consent details, treatment centre and immunisation history. The record is created either on receipt of a completed and signed consent form or, for children subsequently moving into the area, on receipt of the Notification of a Child Moving into Area Form.

The computer scans all the immunisation records of those children whose parents have consented and for immunisations that are due at treatment centres holding a session in that period a postcard is produced to notify the patients of the time and place of the appointment. An appointment list is also produced for use by the treatment centre. Treatment Centres are able to choose their method of appointment from six options - varying from timed appointments on specified days through untimed appointments within specified weeks, to receipt by the treatment centre of postcards and clinic lists in order that they might arrange their own timings. The latter option is for use mainly by rural practices. It is possible by temporary variation to alter sessions due to holidays or sickness or if extra sessions are required. Permanent variations are also possible. A further postcard is sent out if a child defaults a clinic attendance and a listing produced for the treatment centre of those children who have missed two appointments without reason.

The treatment centre marks the results of each session on to the appointments list before returning it to the Health Board. This allows the child's immunisation record to be updated. No further appointments are made while a result is outstanding. Unscheduled attendance at a treatment centre is notified to the Health Board on a separate form in order that these details can be entered on to the child's record. The information required on the appointments list includes batch numbers of the vaccine used, whether or not the child attended, and whether or not the scheduled immunisation was given (in the case of the latter a reason is given for this). It is also possible at this stage to input to the child's record any significant medical information relevant to immunisation. Family doctors are entitled to payment for immunisations and the system allows for a quarterly schedule of these payments to be produced, as well as a list of children to whom treatments have been given. Quarterly and annual statistics are produced from the results.

IMMUNISATION SCHEDULE

The system allows for two schedules to be in operation but in practice only the revised schedule which was recommended in 1978 is used, with the possibility of an extra or different schedule being brought into operation as and when required. The determining time for minimum age for certain immunisations is the minimum time interval between doses. At the present time only the basic course of immunisations is scheduled but the facility for recording information on BCG vaccinations is available, as this Health Board has continued to recommend this vaccination in infancy.

GP73 FORMS

If a general practitioner does not participate in the computer scheme a separate form is available for the recordings of immunisation and for claiming the relevant fee. This form is also used for those children (or adults) who attend a participating general practitioner for immunisation but were born before 1st April 1980 and were not on the computer system previously used by the Health Board.

TREATMENT CENTRE NOTIFICATION

Apart from the appointments list which is sent to the treatment centre, a results analysis of the previous session is also sent giving totals of scheduled and unscheduled courses registered during the update run, and payments to general practitioners are based on this information. Computer runs are carried out twice monthly.

When immunisations are carried out at a child health clinic, each general practitioner is sent a list of those children registered as his patients, who have received treatments. Quarterly payment lists are produced for each GP treatment Centre to enable primary care to make the appropriate payments. This gives the total of each course given, the rate of payment for that course and the payment due. Along with this list primary care receives a detailed listing of the children included in the payment summary and a listing of any results input at a date prior to the period for which the contemporary payment rates apply.

ROUTINE DEFAULTERS LIST

Missed two appointments reports are produced for each treatment centre where children have failed to attend on two consecutive appointments without reason. No further appointments are sent until the Health Board is notified, so this gives the opportunity for the GP or Health Visitor to investigate the reason for non-attendance.

CHANGE OF ADDRESS

A major problem in any recall system is population movement and the difficulty in maintaining up-to-date addresses. It is particularly essential that children do not miss their appointment for immunisation and therefore information regarding change of address must be notified promptly by as wide a group as possible to the various groups who need to update their records.

The problems also arise in the Community Health Index system but perhaps less urgently. However, general practitioners do have a system of notifying changes of address of their patients to primary care and because of the interaction of the two systems, CHI and Immunisation, which have been set up by the primary care department, this information can be used to update both registers. Child Health sources such as health visitors can also be used to update the system and a two-part change of address form giving information on other members of the child's family as well as the child is sent into primary care, the botton copy being sent to the child's doctor for his information.

ADDITIONAL FACILITIES

A treatment centre may be given a list of patients with immunisation status and an analysis of the state of protection of the live children in the practice or attending the clinic. This is accompanied by a list of children requiring follow-up. If there is any doubt of the immunisation state of that child, or of the details held on the computer files for that child a printout is available giving full information. This may also be used when a child transfers to another area and the information is to be passed on.

Immunisation is an important factor in public health both by protection of the individual and prevention of spread of disease. An effective administration system can help to bring about an improvement in immunisation statistics. A computer system releases trained medical and nursing staff from the repetitive clerical duties involved in manual systems and releases them for the work for which they are trained.

Argyll and Clyde Health Board in common with many others had a mixture of schemes both manual and computer based - the computer being owned and operated by the local authority. It is of course, preferable for any health care scheme to be run on a health service computer and it was to this end that changes had to be made in the area. It was not possible for technical reasons to transfer the existing computer system to the Health Board computer, and so the Scottish Standard System was adopted and modified for use by the West Coast Consortium Health Boards. Because Argyll and Clyde Health Board was operating a computer system as well as a manual system before registering of all births from 1st April 1980, the children on the existing computer register who were being scheduled for that system were transferred to the new one. This was in order to have the minimum possible time for treatment centres to cope with two concurrently running systems.

The Scottish Standard System is so organised that most of the routine work is done by the computer with data preparation by a small team of clerical staff. Great reliance is placed on the district offices who process the information for transmission to area.

The computer system takes the initiative of inviting the parent or guardian to bring the child for immunisation so increasing the penetration of the service to reach those children most in need and most at risk in the community. It does not of course guarantee success in encouraging all children to attend but goes far along these lines and gives us the means of identifying those not protected and so enabling more concentrated follow-up and discussion.

SUMMARY

Parents no matter how well motivated often fail to take up the benefits of immunisation. Computer systems have been used before with effect to improve the take up by effective recall.

This system is linked to a Community Health Index described elsewhere in these proceedings and is a more effective way of reaching the missing child.

INTERET DE L'ORDINATEUR DANS LE CONTROLE DES VACCINATIONS

Gilbert MARTIN-BOUYER (1),
Gilbert ESTAVOYER (2) and Gérard FOULON (1)

(1) INSERM Unité 165
Maladies Transmissibles et Accidents Toxiques
Le Vésinet, France

(2) Compagnie internationale de Services
en informatique
Paris

SUMMARY

It is essential, for health authorities, to know the actual immunization status in the population. This should be expressed in terms enabling one to appraise the programs, to study the time course of events and to compare various population types.
Although these data are simple in nature, it is not always easy to bring them together by manual recording.
In this field, therefore, computers can provide irreplaceable contributions.
This has been confirmed by GALLOWAY, in CHICHESTER, since 1962.
We, in France, have taken over this method since 1972, and have extended it to about twelve cities from this year onwards. We have studied its cost and results.

1. INTRODUCTION

La situation vaccinale de la population française est connue par l'exploitation des rapports annuels établis par les Directions Départementales de la Santé sur la pratique vaccinale dans chacun des 95 départements français.

L'analyse de ces données, en 1978 (1), a pu montrer, par exemple, que pour les enfants nés en 1971, au moment de leur 5ème anniversaire,

- 55% n'étaient pas vaccinés contre la variole
- 44% n'étaient pas vaccinés contre la diphtérie et le tétanos
- 43% n'étaient pas vaccinés contre la poliomyélite.

Pour les enfants nés en 1968, ces pourcentages étaient respectivement de 49%, 41% et 38%.

L'étude de cette situation a mis en évidence une double défaillance :

Défaillance des circuits d'informations

L'acte vaccinal doit être consigné au niveau des communes dans un fichier vaccinal géré par les municipalités, décret 52.247 du 28/2/1952, ces fichiers servant de base à l'information adressée aux Directions Départementales de l'Action Sanitaire et Sociale pour établir leur rapport annuel. Une étude préliminaire a montré qu'à chacun de ces niveaux, des défaillances étaient sensibles et donnaient une information incomplète sur l'activité vaccinale réelle.

...

Défaillance vaccinale réelle

Par enquête dans la population (2), on a pu mettre en évidence une défaillance vaccinale réelle essentiellement due au manque d'information des familles sur les dates optimales à observer pour la vaccination de leurs enfants.

Tenant compte de cette double observation, un travail a été réalisé par l'Unité 165 de l'I.N.S.E.R.M. consistant à utiliser l'ordinateur comme incitateur de la réalisation des programmes vaccinaux. Cette étude a repris des travaux anglais réalisés par GALLOWAY depuis 1962 à CHICHESTER (3,4 et 5).

En France, elle s'est appuyée sur trois villes pilotes : MONTPELLIER, VITRY, SAINT-MAUR et est opérationnelle depuis Janvier 1972 (6).

2. DEVELOPPEMENT

Ce système informatique (PASTEUR) est actuellement implanté dans 12 villes françaises généralement de taille importante. Un des objectifs consiste à impulser l'adhésion à cette réalisation du plus grand nombre possible d'agglomérations, en s'adaptant à la fois aux configurations informatiques et aux structures démographiques, quelle que soit la taille de la ville.

Parallèlement, est étudié un nouveau système plus sophistiqué, capable de travailler en temps réel et d'intégrer, non seulement les données relatives aux vaccinations, mais celles relatives aux maladies transmissibles à déclaration obligatoire. De plus, ce nouveau programme permettrait d'envisager des stratégies vaccinales originales, correspondant aux possibilités actuelles des nouveaux vaccins.

Enfin, certaines collectivités ont souhaité l'adaptation de ce programme à leurs problèmes particuliers, et c'est le cas de certaines entreprises souhaitant améliorer la surveillance de la vaccination de leur personnel. Un cas particulier est à mentionner, celui de la demande formulée par les hôpitaux.

3. RESULTATS

Dans chacune de ces trois villes, l'information vaccinale est maintenant connue d'une manière parfaitement exhaustive, elle montre, par rapport à des populations témoins, des progrès importants dans la pratique vaccinale, c'est ainsi qu'à l'âge d'un an, 75% des enfants ont reçu leur vaccination par le B.C.G. lorsqu'ils sont suivis par l'ordinateur, contre 10% dans les villes témoins. Pour diphtérie-tétanos, 60% d'enfants ont été vaccinés dans les villes informatisées, contre 35% dans les villes non informatisées (7).

La couverture vaccinale est également excellente, puisqu'elle dépasse 80% pour l'ensemble des vaccinations dans les populations informatisées. Figures I, II, III, IV.

4. COUT

Une première étude a été réalisée par l'équipe de SAUNDERS et GALLOWAY, elle montre que l'informatisation entraîne une baisse du coût de l'acte vaccinal (tableau I) (5).

...

TABLEAU I

DEPENSES REELLES POUR UNE IMMUNISATION

(1968-1969)

	ANGLETERRE et PAYS de GALLES (Non Informatisé)	SUSSEX OUEST (Informatisé)
Acte vaccinal	4 s	2 s 11 d
Secrétariat Général	1 s 6	7 d
Dépense totale	5 s 6 d	3 s 6 d

s = shilling

d = pence

D'après J. SAUNDERS Brit. J. Prev. Soc. Med. 1970, 24, 187-191.

Le coût global de l'opération a été estimé pour une ville de 100.000 habitants.

Mise en place du système

. 40.000 F

Entretien et fonctionnement

a. Maintenance annuelle du programme

. 4.000 F

b. Fonctionnement

. 25.000 F/an
pour les frais de timbres, d'imprimés, du service informatique (perforation - vérification, temps d'ordinateur).

Soit en calculant l'étalement de l'investissement sur 10 ans : une dépense annuelle de l'ordre de 43 000 F/an avec un nombre d'actes vaccinaux réalisés, datés et enregistrés de l'ordre de 11 000 F/an en vitesse de croisière, soit un chiffre de l'ordre de 4 F par acte vaccinal.

5. CONCLUSION

Ces résultats sont en accord avec ceux obtenus dans le West Sussex (7) où l'utilisation de l'outil informatique semble avoir été un élément déterminant dans le maintien à un haut niveau de la pratique vaccinale entre 1970 et 1976.

Le développement du système,en une version temps réel, a pour but essentiel de procéder aux adaptations rendues nécessaires par l'évolution technologique.

Références

(1) Radenac H, Pichet C, Martin-Bouyer G. Vaccination contre la variole, le tétanos, la diphtérie et le poliomyélite antérieure aiguë. Santé Sec. Soc. stat. et com. 1980, 3 : 101-119.

(2) Martin-Bouyer G, Veiga-Pires H, Pavillon G, Brandimiller P A. Modification du comportement vaccinal de la population par la mise en place dans 3 villes françaises d'un fichier vaccinal géré par ordinateur. Colloques IRIA : informatique médicale, Toulouse 5-7 Mars 1975, 335-346.

(3) Galloway T McL : management of vaccination and immunization procedures by electronic computer. Med. Off. 1963, 109 : 232-233.

(4) Galloway T McL : l'emploi des ordinateurs pour les programmes de vaccination. La santé publique en Europe : maladies transmissibles, OMS, 1974, 3 : 71-78.

(5) Saunders J : results and costs of a computer-assisted immunization schema Br. J. Prev. Med. 1970, 24 : 187-191.

(6) Martin-Bouyer G, Veiga-Pires H, Brandimiller P A : utilisation d'un ordinateur pour la gestion d'un programme vaccinal. Arch. frc. péd., 1977, 34 : 121-132.

(7) Bussey A L, Holmes B S : immunization levels they all decline ? Lancet : 1977 : 970-971.

Figure I

ENQUETE DANS UNE DES VILLES PILOTES : TAUX DE COUVERTURE VACCINALE POUR L'ENSEMBL

DU FICHIER AU 5 FEVRIER 1980

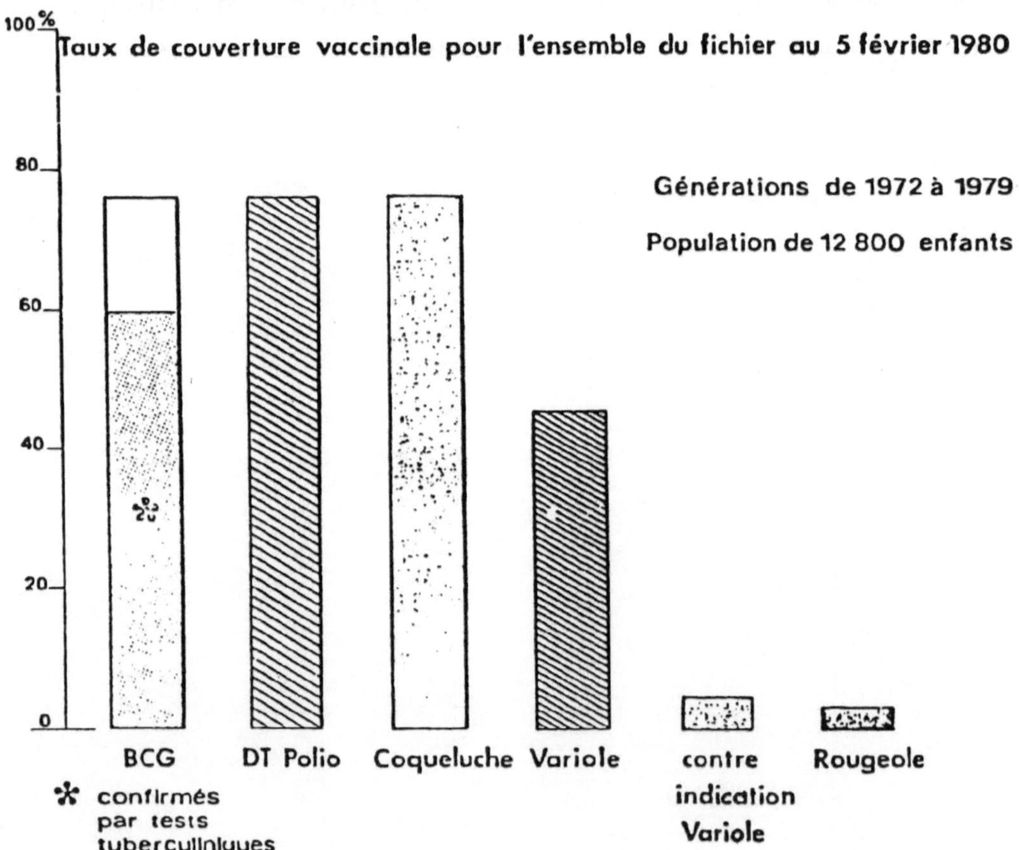

Figure II

SCHEMA COMPARATIF DES TAUX DE COUVERTURE VACCINALE PAR GENERATION (72 à 78)

DT COQ POLIO (PRIMO)

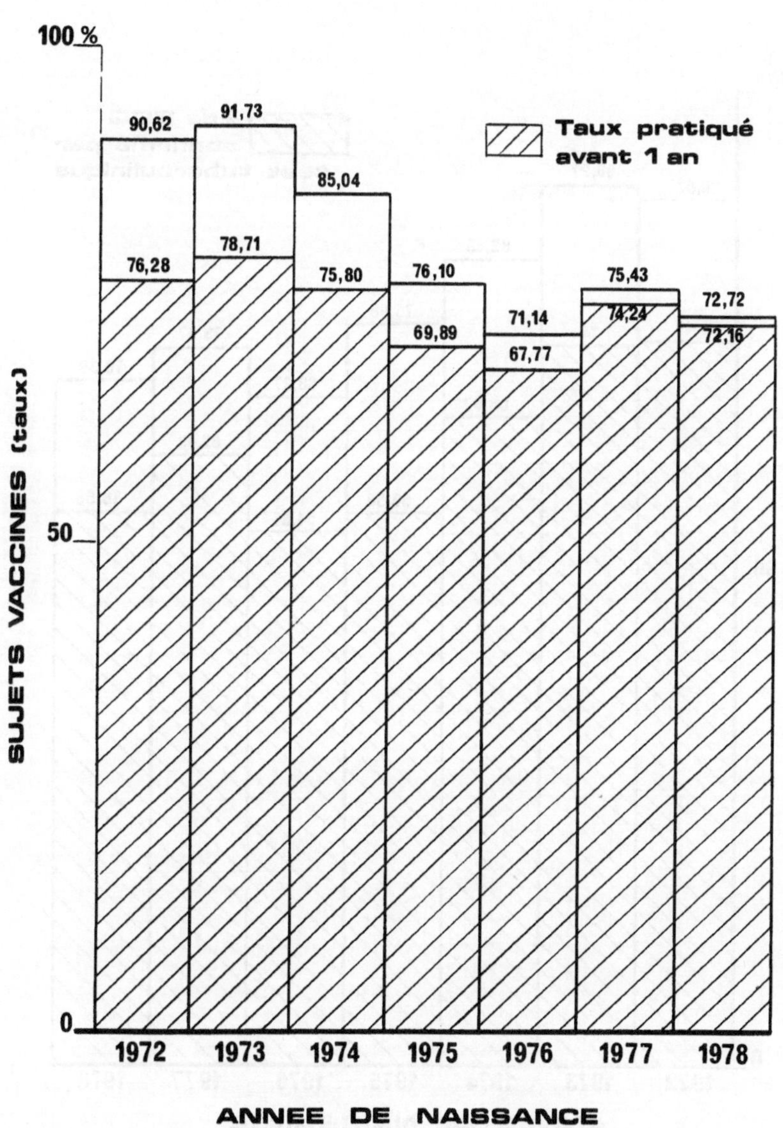

Figure III

SCHEMA COMPARATIF DES TAUX DE COUVERTURE VACCINALE PAR GENERATION (72 à 78)

BCG - TEST TUBERCULINIQUE

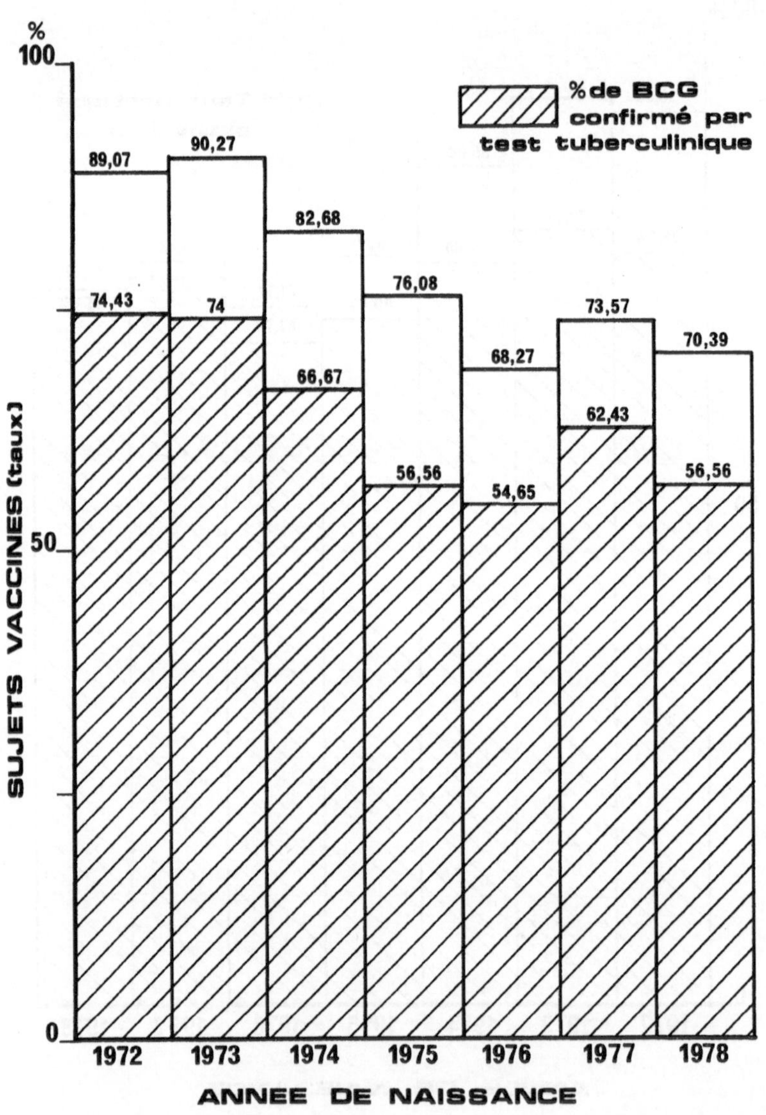

Figure IV

SCHEMA COMPARATIF DES TAUX DE COUVERTURE VACCINALE PAR GENERATION (72 à 78)

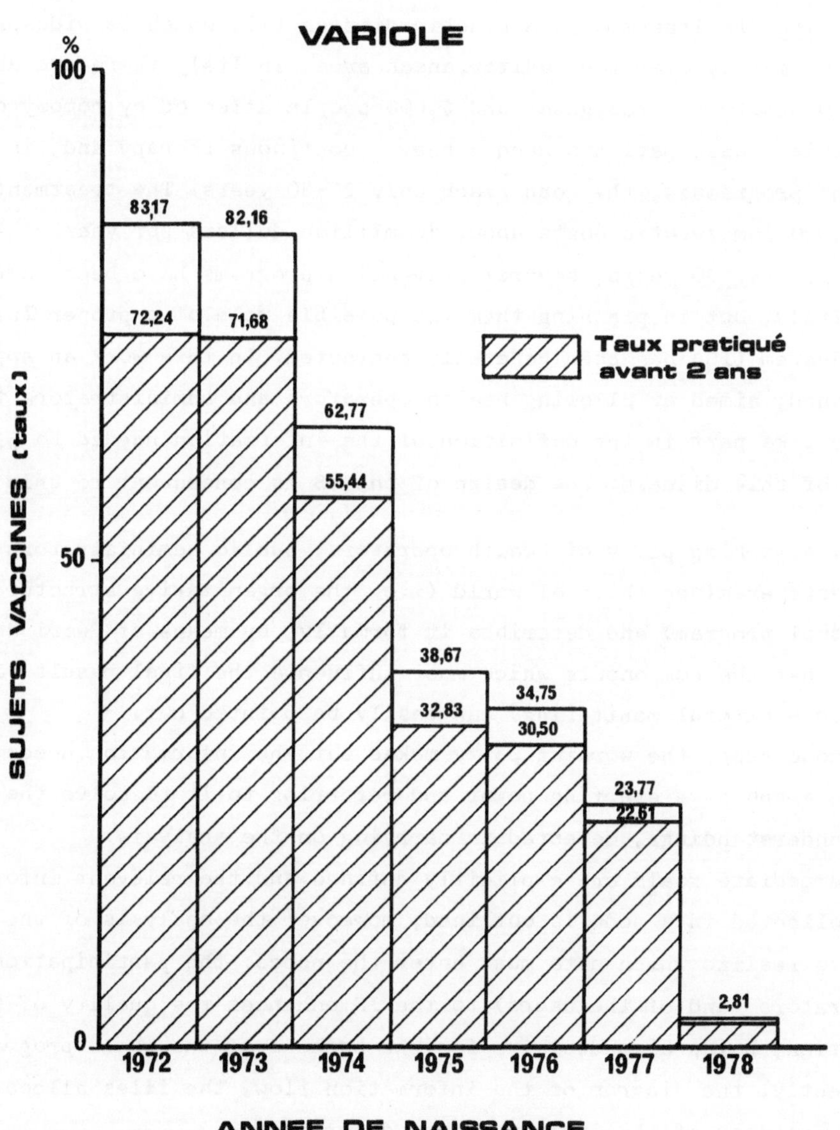

The role of the information system in planning the control of a genetic disease

F.L.Ricci, B.Rossi, A.Rossi-Mori
Group on Information Systems, Institute for Biomedical Technologies
National Research Council, Rome, Italy

Introduction. Thalassemia is a genetic disease (1), which is widespread, in Europe, mainly over the Mediterranean area. In Italy there are about 2,000,000 healty heterozygotes and 6,000 people affected by homozygous thalassemia. These patients need a heavy, continous therapy and, in spite of recent progresses, they can reach only 20-30 years. The treatment of these 6,000 homozygotes costs about 40 million dollars per year.
During the past 30 years, several prevention programs have been carried out in Italy, but in planning them the possible role of a proper Information System (IS) has been generally neglected. In this work an approach is examined, aimed at allowing health operators and administrators to actively take part in the definition of the information needed to plan the control of this disease. The design of the IS is consequent to this phase.

Methods. A working party of health operators, public administrators and IS analysts examines the real world (i.e. the organizative structure of the control program) and describes it formally, by means of Petri Nets (2), so that the components which most influence the final result (and thus need a careful monitoring) can easily be pointed out.
In a second step, the working party makes out the information needs, taking the graph as a starting point and referring to it to solve the possible misunderstandings, detected in carrying on the analysis.
The intermediate goals are explicitly defined and the relevant information to be collected in a node is outlined; moreover the analysis of the net allows to realize which data must enter the nodes: the participation of the operators (and of the users) to the IS enhances the quality of input information, being also decisive for the success of the whole program.
Consequently, the diagram of the information flow, the files allocation and the features of the indicators are determined.
The IS analyst carries out the description of the conceptual scheme, by means of current methods (3), and leads to implement the most appropriate

information structures (not necessarily computerized).

Results. The evaluation of a therapeutic action in this field is (theoretically) relatively easy; the same thing can not be said for prevention. This intervention is in fact made of several components (such as Health Education, Heterozygote Screening, Genetic Counselling, Prenatal Diagnosis), whose final goal is unique: namely the reduction of homozygote births. A feedback, for this part of the program, may be obtained by comparing the observed number of born homozygotes with the estimated incidence in the population, in absence of prevention. However, this feedback is slow in comparison with operational times; moreover, since it gives a global evaluation of the results, it can not be used for the optimization of each single component of the program. Two new indicators have therefore been proposed, to be used together with more simple or already known ones, in the evaluation of the Heterozygote Screening: the estimate of the potentially avoided homozygotes, as future possible offsprings of identified "at-risk" couples, and the estimate of the mean elapsed time, from the identification of an "at-risk" status to the potentially avoided birth. A National Register, specific for thalassemia, has been outlined. The register is made up of two complementary sections: homozygotes and "at-risk" couples. It is regionally operated, but nationally coordinated, so that duplicate records are avoided and selected data are analysed homogeneously at regular intervals. In order to experiment such a register, a sample of Regions has been selected.

Discussion. The achievement of prenatal diagnosis for different genetic diseases is boosting voluntary heterozygote screenings worldwide (4). Such interventions are no longer limited experiences, but represent by now a service (undoubtely at a very high level) for the community. It is therefore necessary to set up precise planning methods, namely to fix evaluation criteria based on efficacy, rather than on volumes of activity as those now in use (5). The design of such indicators can originate only from the detailed analysis of the program features, carried out by a working party, where public administrators and health operators collaborate with IS analysts. It must therefore be avalaible a method for the modelling of the real world, which is at the same time powerful for the subsequent analysis of information flows and easy to be understood and used by not experienced people. The Petri Nets approach was chosen, rather than the classical methods (Gantt, PERT), to fulfill this purpose. The first shows up the casual connections existing between the various entities, identified throught the modeling of the real world, and then allow to study time links and parallelisms; whereas the seconds appeared devoted to the description of time relationships.

Conclusions. A suitable approach was described, for the definition of information needs in planning the control of a genetic disease. With a top-down process, it is possible to carry out the modeling of every part of the therapeutic and preventive interventions and of their relationshi This description easily leads to build up a first set of indicators, whi could result in high descriptive power and simple meaning. This method appears consistent with its main purpose, to get not experienced people to take part in outlining the role of the information system inside a global project, and namely to express well formalized specifications for the design of the appropriate files.

Acknowledgements. The autors are grateful to many health operators, and mainly to I.Bianco, A.Cao, R.Galanello, L.Tentori, C.Vullo.
This work was partially supported by a grant to the unit coordinated by I.Barrai of the P.F.Medicina Preventiva, SP Malattie Ereditarie dell'Eritrocita, contract CNR 79.01010.83.

References.

(1) Weatherall, D.J., Clegg, J.B.: The thalassaemia sindromes. Blackwell Publications, Oxford 1972.

(2) Peterson, J.L.: Petri Nets. Computing Surveys, vol.9, n.3, 1977.

(3) Chen, P.P.S.: The Entity-Relationship model. Toward a unified view of data. ACM Trans. on Database Systems 1, n.1, 1976, pag.9-36.

(4) - : Population Screening for Carriers of Recessively Inherited Disorders. Lancet, 1980, ii, pag.679-680.

(5) A.Rossi-Mori: Criteri per la valutazione dei programmi di screening. 3rd Congress of the Italian Soc. of Medical Genetics, Ferrara 1980.

Progress and Prospects for Patient-Controlled Medical Information Systems

by

Richard J. Giglio
University of Massachusetts
Amherst, MA 01003

Summary

Medical information systems are predominately controlled and used by professionals such as physicians and administrators. Patients' use of information systems could help personalize the medical system, could help educate patients, give them a greater feeling of control of their lives and could reduce the demand on medical personnel. Some of the experience reported in this paper demonstrates that many patients would benefit from the use of health records, that such a process is logistically and economically feasible and that patient training should start in the schools and be reinforced by the medical establishment. Furthermore, it is conjectured that direct patient interaction with decision-making algorithms could relieve physicians of much routine screening and referral work while providing them with imporved instantaneous data bases. The technology is available; a series of pilot studies is needed to work out the details.

Introduction

Since medicine is information-based and information-intensive, information systems, in particular the medical record, are central to an effective system for delivering and promoting health care. Historically, information systems have been controlled by professionals; physicians have responsibility for medical records, epidimiologists deal with aggregate data on disease and accountants and administrators are concerned with cost-monitoring and control systems. The increasing use of digital computers has probably reinforced this pattern because a new breed of specialists has been introduced.

Although current practices have much to offer, it is the thesis of this paper that professional use and control of information systems must be balanced by an increase in the control and use of health information by the individual patient. Following arguments supporting this position, we will summarize experience, primarily the author's, with patient-controlled information systems and speculate on future prospects.

The argument for patient-controlled systems

In the industrialized countries, most causes of mortality and morbidity are diseases which are greatly affected by "life style" (eg. heart disease, lung cancer, auto accidents,) or conditions which are often best diagnosed by the patient (eg. breast cancer). Thus, the greatest improvements to the current health care system may arise from involving individuals to a greater extent in their own health care.

Health education, a primary phase of preventive medicine, seeks to change the actions of individuals as a means of preventing disease or injury. However, traditional health education programs have not been especially successful and means must be sought to expand and augment them.

Figure 1, depicting the disposition of 100 "typical" patients who visit a primary care physician, graphically illustrates the limitations of the medical system. Since only about 15% of the patients who visit physicians can be helped by them, some efficient method of patient-initiated screening would greatly decrease the burden on the medical system and insure that each individual was seen by the most appropriate party. A properly designed information system or screening algorithm could serve that purpose.

Figure 1
Disposition of 100 Typical Encounters with a primary care Physician
(From Carmichael, (1))

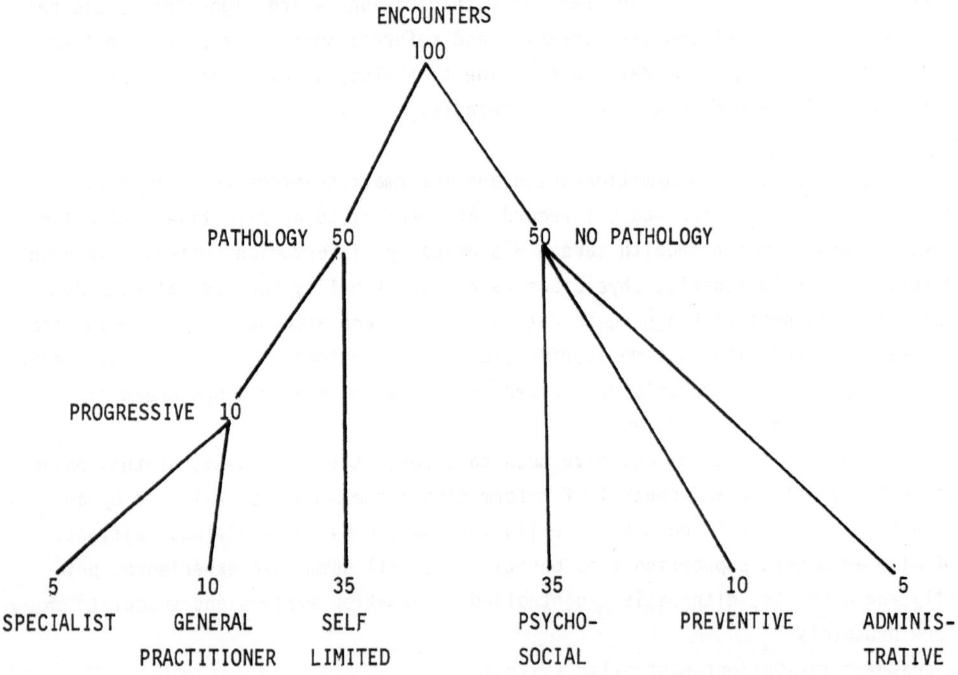

still more comprehensive form of record. (Giglio,(5)). That record contains most of what is in a medical chart, plus a number of sections which deal with health maintenance, behavior changes and the use of the health care system. The contents of the record are listed in Table 1. Participatory records are designed to be maintained by the patient with initial instruction and reinforcement by physicians and nurses.

Table 1

Contents of the participatory record (Giglio, (5))

Past Health	Future Health
Family tree	Current activities and future health
Birth certificate	Health Hazards
Historical problem list	Health maintenance plans
Immunization record	Periodic health assessments
Current health	**Data**
Health strengths	Summary of important data
Goals/Challenges	Urinalysis
Health habits	Blood count
Typical day	Medication record
Life stress	Physical exam
Current health problems	Hospital discharge summaries
Summary of current problems	Dental Health
	Vision screening
	Hearing tests
	X-ray exposures
	Allergies

A study currently underway with a population from U.S. Public Health Service shows that individuals like receiving a record but need follow-up to use anything but the simplest records. Physicians feel the records have value but by and large believe it is peripheral to their role. More will be known upon completion of this study but it is anticipated that simple records can be introduced easily and with little cost and that they will help provide continuity of care and spark patient interest.

Using a more complex record such as the PLHP requires greater care. Of key importance is the process by which the record is introduced and reinforced. This process must be designed to strike a balance between providing too little structure and providing so much that the goal of encouraging self responsibility is counteracted. The PLHP has been tried in several settings including a University Health Service employing 14 physicians and a group practice/HMO which had 6 physicians and two nurse practitioners.

A patient was introduced to the PLHP by a nurse or aide who explained its concept in general terms and helped fill out some specific items (measurements of height, weight, pulse, and blood pressure). Present evidence indicates this should take approximately 20 minutes/person if done singly. Clients were also asked to fill out

Perhaps the most important reason for patient involvement is psychological. The increasing expense and complexity of medicine and apparent mechanization of procedures tends to isolate patients and contribute to feelings of anomie and helpnesses which are claimed to permeate modern societies. There have been many studies (see Strickland, 1973, for a review) which show significant correlations between those conditions and the onset of diseases such as cancer in addition to obvious ones such as suicide and accidents.

It is our contention that education, self screening and a feeling of control over ones life can be enhanced by involving the patient in the operation of the medical information system. A mechanism for expanding the clients role should have several characteristics if it is to be successful:

1. It should be integrated with the professional care an individual receives. In that way clients' belief in their role is reinforced and not diminished by the health system, and medical professionals can monitor progress.
2. It should be consistent with the principles of behavior modification; individuals should help set objectives, concentrate on specific behaviors, and receive feedback and selective reinforcement.
3. It should be applicable to a broad segment of the population and have the flexibility to enable different individuals to tailor it to their own needs and interests.
4. It must be cost effective from both an overall social perspective and from the perspective of a significant number of individual health care organizations.
5. The process should be simple to initiate with the clients' involvement increasing throughout their lives as their knowledge expands.

A number of models for patient-centered information systems are described below.

Patient Use of Medical Records

The medical records has been selected as a foundation on which to build an information system for increasing client participation by Bouchard,(2), Hertz,(3), Shenkin, (4). Giglio, et al, have extended the work of others and studied patient use of various forms of records (Giglio,(5) Eddy,(6)). Two general types of records have been outlined below.

1. A small, compact record, the size of a passport or even small enough to be folded to wallet size can contain a brief problem list and lists of allergies and innoculations. This record can help maintain continuity of care when visiting a different facility and increase patients' understanding of their medical problems.
2. A record in which the patient participates in the preparation and up-dating such as the Personal Life Health Plan (PLHP), is a

"Life Stress" in the various sections of "Past Health," and, if they wished, "Health Strengths" when they return home. The introduction included a brief meeting with a physician who sanctioned the PLHP concept. Patients were next invited to come in for a physical and to discuss the "Health Hazzards" section. A health maintenance program was discussed at the meeting. If the client wished to change behavior, a contract was suggested and programs or personnel were suggested to help in that difficult task. (Miller, (7).

For most clients the next major interaction with the PLHP process occurred when the individual scheduled a visit with the professional for an acute problem. The health professional reinforced the concept of the PLHP during the course of that visit in the following way:

1. The client was encouraged to fill out the "Current Problems" section with the professional's diagnosis and plan. This only took a minute or two, but it stressed the fact that the professional believed that the PLHP is important and the process of providing care was demystified as the individual was made a party to it. The physician/nurse also used the record to ascertain if the individual understood the instructions and to monitor past compliance.
2. The physician suggested that the individual record illnesses in the "Current Problems" section when no visit to a professional is made (eg.,a cold or fatigue or depression) and reviewed past entries.
3. Time permitting, the physician asked a leading question about the individual's "Health Hazards" section. If the person were interested, the physician emphasized the importance of health maintenance and discussed a contract for health maintenance.

After its initial introduction the use of the PLHP was integrated into the professional-client relationships and little extra time required of physicians and nurses. The physician or nurse continued to reinforce the use of the PLHP by the simple actions mentioned above. Group instructional courses were offered to satisfy interests stimulated in clients. The topics were chosen by the participants, and seminars on the physical examination and prescription and over-the-counter drugs were held.

The detailed results of the study are given elsewhere (Giglio et al,(5). They indicated that twenty to sixty percent of the population will volunteer to use the PLHP and that the start-up time for the process was modest. (5-20 minutes per person) Patients showed a high rate of continued participation during the several months of activities and they exhibited a high use of all sections of the record. Over 50% of the participants throughout the process was worthwhile and would recommend it to a friend. The small sample and short span of the study made it difficult to assess the effectiveness of the PLHP in changing behaviors. However, some positive health-related attitude changes were noted.

Health Record as the Basis for a Health Education Course

Because the use of health records involves long term changes in the attitudes and perceptions of patients, it was thought that the use of patient information systems might best be taught in schools as the basis of a health education course. Then, the use of a client-held medical record can be the thread which continues through life allowing individuals to gain both knowledge and control of their health.

An inter-disciplinary team which included a system analyst, a physician, a physician's assistant, an undergraduate engineering student and a graduate student in public health, designed a 12-week course and presented it at two high schools (Eddy, et al, (6)). The schools were chosen to span the middle class as defined by the income and education of parents. Twenty-seven juniors and seniors from each school were enrolled in the course which was offered one day a week after normal school hours. The purpose of the course was to teach and motivate students to construct, maintain and use health records. At regular intervals throughout the course, students' use the health record was monitored and four indicators were taken to measure the effects of the course:

1. the interest of students in the client-held health record,
2. students' performance in learning how to use the record.
3. the extent of usage of the record, and
4. the effect usage had on health habits and attitudes.

Also three questionnaires measuring health habits, attitudes and "locus of control" were administered to the students at the beginning and end of the course. (See Strickland, (8) for a description of locus of control)

Seventy-four percent of the students in both high schools completed the course, and 65-75% of the students attended eight or more of the 11 sessions at which attendance was recorded. In disucssing topics with the students, it was surprising to see how open they became with problems and worries which were quite personal in nature. Small group discussions and actual participation in class exercises (eg. taking blood pressure, looking in ears) was the most favored class format.

Remarks on the anonymous evaluation questionnaire shed light on the way students viewed the course. For example:

> "Personal health, as I have discovered through this course, is very important to me. When I first heard of this course, I thought, 'Boring!' I have since learned that this was not so....keeping a record is quite useful and necessary."

In the final evaluation questionnaire, one of the questions asked whether participants planned to continue using the PLHP. 78% answered "positively yes" or "probably," while 7% (two individuals) answered "probably not" or "no". Table 2 gives a breakdown of the results comparing the two high schools. There is a substantial difference between the two schools for reasons which we are unable to verify. Students in High School A were considerably more assertive and apparently more highly motivated throughout the course and we suspect this was related to family background.

Table 2
Plans to Continue Use of Record

	Positively #	Positively %	Probably #	Probably %	Uncertain #	Uncertain %	Probably Not #	Probably Not %	No #	No %
High School A -	5	27.8	11	61.1	1	5.5	1	5.5	0	
High School B -	1	11.1	4	44.4	3	33.3	0		1	11.1

Three months after completion of the course, an attempt was made to reach all participants by telephone. Although vacations and leaving for college lowered the rate of response, a total of 18 participants were contacted and asked if they had used the PLHP since the end of the class or whether they intended to use it. 83% said they had either used the document or intended to use it.

Another interesting use of patient-controlled information systems was reported by Dr. Schade, a physician, who has his patients carry their own chart (Schade,(9). He keeps only a 5 x 7 file card for each patient containing a major problem list, allergy list and information useful in emergencies. The patient is requested to bring the full record in at each visit.

Dr. Schade has found that his system works well. People seldom forget or lose their charts and when they do the summary information is sufficient for treatment. He has encountered no legal problems and, of course, his record-keeping has been simplified. Also, he believes that his patients gain a great deal by having the responsibility for their charts because they can learn from them and the process emphasizes that they, ultimately, are responsible for their own health.

Patient Interaction with Computer Medical Systems

"Hands-on" experience with health and medical records has many advantages. However, patient involvement need not stop there. They can, and we believe, should be able to take advantage of compter technology.

One obvious way to do this is by using medical decision-making algorithms. Patients, using their phones and their TV's could interact with a question-asking decision program housed at their medical facility to replace telephone screening and diagnosis which is common in the United States, especially at night or on weekends. The decision algorithms would be conservative; if the symptoms could possibly be serious the patient would be instructed to call and speak to a nurse or physician or to make an appointment which could be automatically scheduled.

Other outcomes of an interaction would be diagnosis and advice (common cold; take aspirin, fluids, etc.), instructions to call again if there is no improvement in a specified period of time, or a referral to another provider as Figure 1 suggests should often be done. The central program could maintain a running count (daily and weekly) on the types of complaints which were coming in. Thus, physicians would know almost immediately when "something was going around", information which would be useful in treatment. The algorithms could be modified on a spot basis to handle special contingencies or emergencies. Finally, the system could automatically contact patients with advice and appointment remainders.

The electronic technology for the above already exists. So do the diagnostic algorithms - see, for example the book by Vickery (Vickery, (10) . Undoubtedly, programs will be sold for home computers as they become popular and it would be far preferable to have patients use one which was approved and maintained by a medical facility.

REFERENCES

(1) Carmichael, Lynn, Carmichael, Joan: The relational model in family practice. J. of Health & Social Behavior, May, 1976.

(2) Bouchard, R., et al. The patient and his problem-oriented record. In: Implementing the Problem Oriented System. J.W. Hurst and H.K. Walker, Eds. New York, Medcom Press, 1973.

(3) Hertz, C.G, Bernheim, J.W., Perloff, T.N. Patient participation in the problem oriented system: A health care plan. Medical Care, 14:77,1976.

(4) Shenkin, B. Warner, D. Giving the patient his medical record: A proposal to improve the system. New England J. Med. 289:688,1973.

(5) Giglio, R,et al Encouraging behavior changes by use of client-held health records. Medical Care, September,1978.

(6) Eddy, N, et al A client-held health record in a health education curriculum. J. of School Health, October,1979.

(7) Miller, P.M. The use of behavioral contracting in the treatment of alcholism: A case report. Behavi. Ther. 3:593,1972.

(8) Strickland, B.R. Locus of control: Where have we been and where are we going?

(9) Schade, H.I. My patients take their medical records with them. Medical Economics, 1976.

(10) Vickery, Donald, Fries, James Take care of yourself. Addison-Wesley Publishing Co. Reading, Mass., 1976.

A METHOD TO MEASURE THE DEGREE OF HEALTH CARE COVERAGE IN PRIMARY CARE

Birgit SCHWARZ and Peter L. REICHERTZ
Dept. of Biometrics and Medical Informatics
Medical School Hannover, Hannover/FRG

A simulation model was developed to describe the degree of primary care coverage focussing on the aspect of supply (providers) and demand (consumers) of a health care delivery system. It describes variables influencing supply and demand and reflects the relationships between these parts. The model determines the degree of primary care coverage for a region and prognosticates trends within a region. The model was tested on four different regions: a metropolitan area, a suburban area, a small city and a rural area.

1. Introduction

Health care delivery systems imply both to be able to provide people with medical care if they enter the health care system and demand medical services and health resources and to foresee and predict to a certain degree the needs in order to cover them in time. In this context, the factors equity, equality, availability and health care coverage play an essential role among other factors on each level of a health care system: primary, secondary and tertiary care.
Considering primary care in the Federal Republic of Germany (FRG), the mandatory physicians organizations are obliged by legislature to guarantee primary medical coverage. The aim is to guarantee the insured persons and their families equity and equality of medical care which also comprise a sufficient emergency service and stand-by service within a reasonable distance as well as to guarantee the actual status of medical science and technology and the possibility of optimization and modernization. In order to ensure primary medical care the physicians organizations are obliged to develop a health need plan for each defined catchment area of a region. This health need plan is essentially oriented on the method of the population-per-physician ratio comprising additional informations about supply, demand and socio-economic structure of the catchment area. The purpose of these annually health need plans is to detect health surplus and health scarcity areas and to determine and evaluate primary medical coverage. The main goal of our approach was to develop a dynamic model which describes in a more adequate way than the statistical population-per-physician ratio the degree of health care coverage in primary care,

especially focussing on the aspect of supply and demand. Besides quantitative aspects, the model includes qualitative aspects of medical coverage, e.g. the physicians' intensity of care, their spectrum of activities, social structure of the population, industrial structure, migration etc.
The model determines the degree of coverage for a region and prognosticates trends within a region when changing parameters of the model. Such parameters comprise e.g. number and age structure of physicians in primary care, number and age structure of inhabitants, social structure, health resources factors etc.
Predictive values should be obtained for actual comparison and planning purposes.

2. Model

The principal concept of this model was to determine and subdivide the determinants of the degree of primary medical coverage into two parts representing supply (i.e. providers, e.g. physicians) and demand (i.e. consumers, e.g. patients). The term demand is understood as the actual use of medical services by the consumer. In the health care market demand is also determined by physicians. Thus, physicians play a dual role in this area: they act as providers and partly as consumers resp. demand regulators. In the model no consideration is made concerning health status, morbidity, incidence, prevalence or actual needs.
On the basis of these determinants, the model calculates the 'effective' number of physicians participating in primary medical care (providers) and the 'effective' number of inhabitants (probably) demanding medical care. The model basically adjusts the number of providers according to the regional situation and structure of the providers and relates this effective number of providers to the adjusted ('effective') number of inhabitants. The term effective number of providers describes with which factor a physician of a region is computed for the determination of the degree of primary medical coverage. The term effective number of inhabitants describes with which factor an inhabitant participates in the demand. The degree of primary care coverage is determined by the ratio of effective number of providers and effective number of inhabitants.
The dynamic aspects of the model are presented by feedback loops and performed by simulation runs. The model is written in CSMP (Continuous System Modeling Program). It was tested on four different regions in Lower Saxony, a state ('Land') of the FRG: a metropolitan area, a

suburban area bordering this metropolitan area, a small city and its environment and a rural area. The model was mainly based on empirical data of the regional physicians organization (2) as well as on the results of a structural analysis of about 2,000 general practices in Lower Saxony (5).

2.1 Determinants of the model

2.1.1 Supply

The variables used (1-17) to determine the adjustment of the providers are:

1) age structure of the physicians of the region,
2) sex structure of the physicians of the region,
3) number of treatment cases in the region,
4) percentage of partnership practices in the region,
5) physician's time in general practice,
6) working hours of the physician,
7) average waiting time per contact,
8) location of practice (rural, small city, large city),
9) number of auxiliary personnel,
10) number of house calls,
11) size of laboratory,
12) degree of organization of practice,
13) postgraduate training of the physician,
14) spectrum of diagnostic assessment,
15) spectrum of procedures recorded,
16) time spent per patient,
17) participation in emergency services,
18) estimate of primary care provided by specialists in the region (SPECE)
19) accessibility of practices.

In order to calculate the adjustments of these variables some assumptions had been made in the model because of the lack of empirical, actual data for the 4 analyzed regions. Actual data could be obtained only for the variables: age and sex structure of the physicians, number of treatment cases, percentage of partnership practices and estimate of primary care provided by specialists. For the other variables mean values were taken from the data of the structural analysis in Lower Saxony (5) or adjustments were made based on previous analyses in Lower Saxony (2). Some correlations between variables were taken into account and adjusted to the variables, e.g. number of treatment cases and annual turnover etc. (5). Adjustments for the percentage of primary care provided by specialists were made according to the mix of specialties in the regions. In the health care system of the FRG, specialists participate to a varying degree in primary care. Thus, pediatricians were adjusted with a factor of 0.9 (compared to GP's with 1.0), internists with 0.8, gynecologists with 0.5, ophthalmologists with 0.2 etc. Adjustments for age structure were made concerning case load resp. work time provided by female versus male physicians. Data for work time were obtained from a demographic analysis which showed that 84% of the female physicians worked more than 40 hrs/week compared to 95% of male colleagues (4). Adjustments for waiting time were based on a previous analysis taking into account the type of the region, i.e. urban, suburban, small city, rural. Similarly, adjustments were calculated for the other variables, e.g. home visits in the region, number of paramedical personnel etc. Another important indicator of the supply of medical services in health care is the accessibility of the practice. An overall ideal or operational measure to determine the reasonable distance for a patient to a practice is unknown and depends on various factors, e.g. time, distance, population density, traffic network in the region, availability of other institutions, e.g. schools, shopping centers etc. Several attempts have been made to determine the reasonable distance either by assumption (e.g. half an hour) or by methods. In our approach accessibility was based on an algorithm which determines the average distance of an inhabitant to a primary care physician in a region (1):

$$DS = \frac{\sum_{i=1}^{n} e_i E_i}{TE} \cdot D$$

E_i: number of inhabitants/region
DS: distance to the next physician
n: number of agglomeration in the region
e_i: distance of the i-th agglomeration to the next settlement of a primary care physician
TE: total number of inhabitants of the region
D: density of population of the region

However, this score DS did not enter the model as such but it was calculated separately. The score was between 100 and 170 for the tested regions; values greater 200 may indicate an undercoverage.

The effective number of physicians in primary care (GP) was computed by the formula:

$$GPE = NGP \cdot \frac{\sum_{i=1}^{17} V_i}{17} + SPECE$$

GPE: effective rate of GPs
NGP: normal rate of GPs
SPECE: specialists participating in primary care
V_i: variables of the i-th agglomeration

Some variables, e.g. age and sex structure of the physicians, work time, organization of practice, number of treatment cases were assumed to have a greater importance than other. In another equation, they were weighted.

2.1.2 Demand

The variables (v_i) determining adjustments of the inhabitants (consumers) were considered to be:

1) age structure of population,
2) sex distribution of population,
3) educational structure of population,
4) mix of professions,
5) population density,
6) economic structure of the region,
7) percentage of commuters (MIG),
8) employment rate,
9) accessibility to information,
10) style of living,
11) family situation,
12) financial situation,
13) standard of living,
14) nationality,
15) degree of urbanization.

The first 6 socio-demographic variables entered the simulation run for each of the 4 tested regions. For calculation of adjustments some variables, e.g. age, sex and educational structure of the population and population density were set into relation with the number of inhabitants. The effective number of inhabitants actually demanding medical services in primary care was computed by determining the mean value of the variables multiplied by the total number of inhabitants of a region plus or minus the number of people commuting into or out of the region:

$$INH = T_i \cdot \frac{\sum_{i=1}^{6} V_i}{6} + MIG$$

INH: inhabitants of the region
MIG: migration of the region
T_i: total number of inhabitants of the region of the i-th agglomeration
V_i: variables of the i-th agglomeration

2.2 Feedback loops

According to the suggestions of KLIMKE (3), 4 feedback loops were implemented in the model to reflect the feedback mechanism between supply and demand:

- feedback between the number of patients and overload of primary care physicians: it is assumed that general practitioners (GPs) are demand regulators, e.g. generating demand by more attractiveness, less referrals (vice versa), number of treatment cases (e.g. recalling patients for encounter etc.).

- feedback between the number of physicians in primary care and their workload: this is the relation between demand and number of physicians. Increase (decrease) of number of cases treated increases (decreases) the demand for new physicians in the region.

- feedback between the number of providers and demand resp. number of treatment cases: it is assumed that the number of GPs in a region has an influence on demand of the population for primary care.
- feedback between the number of hospital physicians going into primary care and the attractiveness of work in primary care: it describes the migration of hospital physicians into private practice and considers workload and resulting attractiveness as factors of the degree of migration (figure 1).

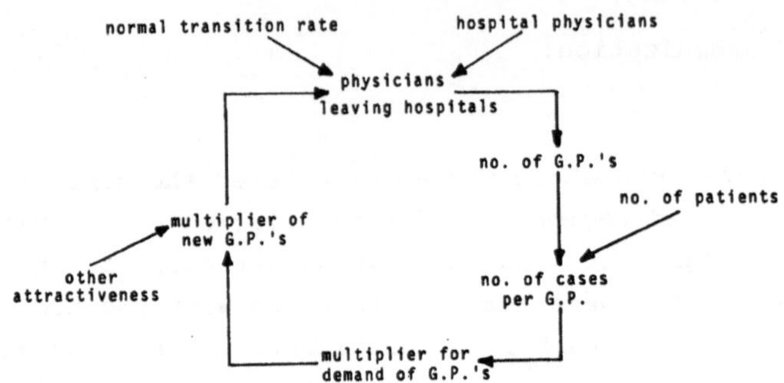

Figure 1: Migration of physicians from hospital positions into private practice (3)

The two subsystems 'supply' and 'demand' of the model are constructed using these feedback loops (figures 2, 3).

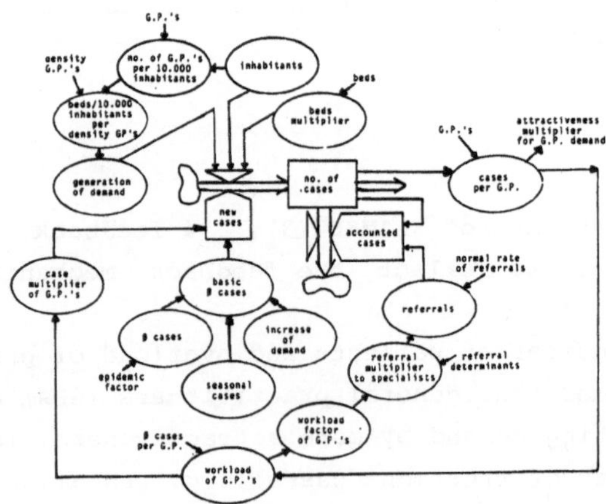

Figure 2: Model of the subsystem 'demand' (3)

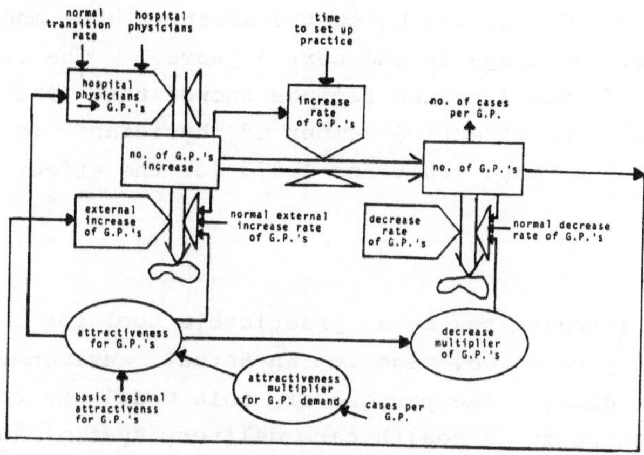

Figure 3: Model of the subsystem 'supply' (3)

3. Results

The time interval for the simulation runs of the 4 analyzed regions was chosen to be one week over a period of five years. A population growth rate of 1% was assumed based on population changes in previous years (2). The ideal population-per-physician ratio is unknown and most frequently handled by assumption or arbitrary definition. In the FRG, the critical value for beginning undercoverage is assumed to be 1 GP per 2,400 inhabitants or 4.2 GPs equivalents per 10,000 inhabitants. The model prognosticated a decrease of coverage of 2% over the next 5 years for the metropolitan area. This will be a result of the growing tendency of specialization as well as of the age structure of the primary care physicians which will have a greater declineation rate than population (in 1977, 53% of the physicians were over 60 years old). The suburban area can be described as a health scarcity area considering the critical value for beginning undercoverage of 4.2 GP equivalents per 10,000 inhabitants. The model predicted a further decrease of 19% in the next 5 years resulting by population declineation of 15%. The degree of coverage in the small city is similarly as to the metropolitan area due to a great number of specialists with their respective GP equivalents. The prognosticated decrease of coverage of 9% will be a result of population increase versus a relatively constant effective number of GPs. The rural area showed the best actual degree of primary care coverage compared to the other three regions due to a low population density and a relatively high number of primary care physicians. Despite of this, the number of treatment cases per GP was not below the average. The model predicted a 23% decrease of coverage in the next 5 years. The results of the simulation runs of the 4 tested regions showed that the overall factors to calculate the effective number of physicians in primary care varied between 0.996 resp. 1.015 and 1.073 for the effective number of inhabitants.

4. Conclusions

This model was intended to be a practicable tool for measuring the degree of primary care coverage in an actual environment based on actual available data. The purpose of this model was to reflect the causal relationships in a health care delivery system and to provide help in decision making under consideration of the requirements of health need plans. The primary concern for further refinement of the model is to include e.g. changes in the physicians population due to increasing student numbers.

REFERENCES

1) Beske F. Kassenärztliche Bedarfsplanung. Gutachten zum Entwurf eines Planungsansatzes für die Bedarfsplanung der kassenärztlichen Versorgung in der Bundesrepublik Deutschland. Zentralinstitut für die kassenärztliche Versorgung in der Bundesrepublik Deutschland, Heftreihe Bd. 9, Deutscher Ärzteverlag, Köln 1977.
2) Bossmann A. Praxis 72, Praxisanalyse der Kassenärztlichen Vereinigung Niedersachsen. Kassenärztliche Vereinigung Niedersachsen, Hannover 1972.
3) Klimke WA. Dynamische Systemanalyse der ambulanten und stationären Krankenversorgung einer Region. Eine System-Dynamics Studie. In Wahl (Ed.): Wissenschaftliche Reihe Karlsruhe, Karlsruhe 1976.
4) Koller S. Ärzteanalyse - Zahl, Struktur und Nachwuchsbedarf der Ärzte. Bundesministerium für Jugend, Familie und Gesundheit (Ed.), Bonn 1970.
5) Reichertz PL, Schwarz B, Meldau HJ. The structure of physicians' activities in general practice and modelling their degree of coverage. In Wagner G, Reichertz PL, Mase E. (Eds.): Technology and Health. Man and his World, Springer Verlag, Heidelberg, 1980; 208-228.
(see further literature)

PROBLEMS OF EVALUATING OUTPATIENT CARE WITH ROUTINE DATA

Detlef SCHWEFEL[1], Elisabeth REDLER[1], Wilhelm van EIMEREN[1], Stefan SCHEWE[2]
[1]Institute for Medical Informatics and Health Services Research, GSF
[2]Institute for Medical Informatics, Statistics and Biomathematics, LMU
Munich, Federal Republic of Germany

SUMMARY

Routine data from a 5% sample of medical records involving 8 873 ambulatory patients in 3 Bavarian districts for the second quarter of 1976 are analyzed according to their suitability for the evaluation of ambulatory care. The sources of error in the original data, in data transfer, coding and analysis that are subsequently discussed reveal that basic descriptions based on physician and patient variables are expedient, although they have the usual weaknesses of secondary analyses. It is also apparent that any interpretation of data on diagnoses and physicians' services must take into account substantial sources of error. A comprehensive evaluation of ambulatory care by means of routine data is hardly practicable, since interfering variables required for interpretation are not contained in the data made available. Supplementary investigations are essential.

1. INTRODUCTION

In the Federal Republic of Germany 59 036 private physicians (1.1.79) are active in ambulatory care. Due to a highly differentiated fee-for-service system comprising 1 580 individual services, virtually all these physicians document their services and diagnoses on special forms for the 58.1 million subscribers of the GKV (German public health insurance scheme). It is believed that these data may be used for evaluative purposes as (i) they pertain to all patients in 94.7 % of the population, (ii) virtually all private physicians record them, (iii) they are comparable for all insurance schemes under the GKV, (iv) they are recorded on a regular basis and (v) they are readily available at the end of each quarter.
Taking as an example the analysis of routine data made available by the Kassenärztliche Vereinigung Bayerns (Bavarian association of physicians subscribing to the public health insurance) we shall use selected findings to discuss problems related to the evaluation of ambulatory care.

2. DATA

The following discussion will be based on considerations of experts (1), observa-

tions in physicians' offices (2) and a 5 % random sample of records covering patients in three Bavarian districts for the second quarter of 1976 (3).
The 10 436 records involving 8 873 patients contain the following information:
Physician: name and identification number with medical discipline and district.
Patient: name, age, insurance status, insurance scheme, place of residence.
Treatment: diagnoses, services, date of treatment, if applicable reason for transfer, type of accident, etc.
In order to maintain confidentiality of personal data the subjects were made anonymous. The transfer and processing of data were subjected to several error checks.

3. PROBLEMS OF THE DATA ON PHYSICIANS AND PATIENTS

FINDINGS: Initial contact according to physician group and social class: For first contact only 78% of the patients choose a general practitioner. Patients covered by a so-called Substitute Fund (Ersatzkasse), virtually all white-collar employees, i.e. members of a higher social class, are more inclined to take up initial contact with a specialist than patients of other insurance schemes, where mostly blue-collar workers are eligible. These findings remain valid after adjustment for influences of age and sex.
Patterns of contacts: 27.3 % of the patients call upon a physician only once in the quarter. 8 % of the patients see more than one physician. Substitute Fund patients have more initial contacts with different physicians, i.e. they call upon more than one physician, than patients of other insurance schemes. 2 patients use 6 original vouchers for 6 different physicians, although insurance regulations allow only one original voucher per quarter. This regulation is followed by 92,2 % of the patients.
Age structure of the patients: Eye and lung specialists, internists and urologists have a more elderly clientel than other specialists.
PROBLEMS: Findings of this nature should not be employed for evaluative purposes without taking into due consideration problems that arise in the original material and in the transfer and analysis of the data.
Sources of error in the original records can only be determined by means of auxiliary surveys and occur, for example, in the following areas:

- Misidentification of the patient, that is, processing with the wrong insurance form, e.g. in the case of insured patients and close relatives.
- Lack of documentation interest: Some entries, e.g. the area code, seem to be negligable to the physician and patient alike, as it is missing on 31,7% of the forms.
- Lack of documentation checks: Certain entries, e.g. age and address, are never checked if previously being entered by the insurance company.
- Uncertainty about documentary procedure: It is unclear who makes certain entries and when.

- No relation to disease episodes: Only formal statements can be made on the initial contact, as the data have no relation to disease episodes, but rather to the quarters of the calendar year.

Transfer errors generate the following problems:

- Information losses through anonymization: The obligation to maintain confidentiality of data - in our case realized by alphanumerical coding of name and sex on the original forms and blacking out of the original data - gives rise to identification problems and confusions in sex for 5.5 % of the patients. When there are several different records belonging to one patient, this rate rises to at least 21 %.
- Other transfer errors: In a random sample of 172 original records 38.4 % of the records reveal at least one erroneous entry. The average formal error amounts to 4.7 % of all entries, the variation ranging from 0.9 % to 21.7 % depending on the variable in question. The average error in content amounts to 3.4 %.

CONCLUSIONS: The problems mentioned are not singular to this project but arise rather in all primary and secondary analyses handling data restricted in time, space or number of variables, but certainly to a more limited extent in well-controlled primary surveys. If due consideration is given to the error sources and sufficient care is exercised in interpreting the findings, routine data would seem to provide meaningful evaluations in questions of supply and use of ambulatory care.

4. PROBLEMS OF THE DATA ON DIAGNOSES AND SERVICES

We shall now discuss the suitability of routine data for the evaluation of physicians' activities, analyzing the relationship between diagnoses and services. We concentrate on two diagnoses known in the literature as tracers, namely hypertension and infection of the urinary tract (4).

FINDINGS:

Prevalence: At least 8.6 % of the patients have the diagnostic entry "hypertension", 0.8 % "labile hypertension", 1.8 %" "infection of the urinary tract".

Prevalence according to sex: Hypertension and urinary tract infection occur in 72 % and 69 % respectively of women, although they make up 56 % of the patients.

Prevalence according to age: Hypertension is more common in higher age groups than urinary tract infection.

Multiple diagnoses: For 96.7 % of patients suffering from hypertension and 91.2 % of those afflicted with urinary tract infection further diagnoses were given.

Multimorbidity: There exist between various diagnoses highly significant, plausible correlations and low contingencies in accordance with Pearson.

Medical services related to diagnoses: Of those services that according to experts should be rendered at least once a year to hypertensive patients, in the case of 56 hypertensive patients, for whom no further diagnosis was stated, the service "complete examination" was calculated a total of 55 times, "urinary sedimentation" 5 times, "ECG" twice, "funduscopic examination" once, yet "complete blood analysis" not a single time.

Fees related to diagnoses: The fee was DM 64 per patient suffering from hypertension and DM 99 per patient with urinary tract infection.

PROBLEMS: For the s e r v i c e s one highly differentiated fee-schedule exists (at the time of the study two largely comparable schedules) that entails the following problems:

Excessive scope: Many service categories are irrelevant or unknown to most physicians. Of the 1 580 services only 595 were cited by physicians, and 150 of those only once.

Differentiation.: The differentiation between many services is not very sharp. This ambiguity leads to intersubsitution of categories.

Imbalanced aggregation: The aggregation levels vary widely with no differentiation being made for the most common medical services such as consultations and physical examinations. These two service categories account for roughly 32% of the physicians' fees.

Variability: The fees listed in the schedules are subject to frequent changes as a result of fee negotiations. Furthermore, unofficial abridged versions are offered for various situations in practice.

Unclear documentation practice: Uncertainty exists as to who documents when. In part assistants record the services rendered by the physician or the physician the services of the assistants - sometimes concurrently with the services, sometimes at the end of the quarter.

Modification: In checking the calculations of the physicians the Kassenärztliche Vereinigung makes corrections in the service entries.

Validity: There is a lack of agreement between services specified in the fee-schedules and treatment criteria cited in the literature. In the case of hypertension only 12 of the 29 diagnostic criteria of the "German League Against High Blood Pressure" and 7 of the 43 criteria listed by Kessner can be accounted for with services in the fee-schedules (5). The latter provide no information on details of the case history or on the determination of pathological blood pressure and the method of measurement.

Informal entries: The entries in the forms are made in free format. Often texts by the physicians are added.

Computerization: The storage of 1 580 service categories with the available program packages SAVOD, SPSS and BMDP poses processing problems, especially in conjunction with a large number of diagnoses. For the purpose of statistical computing we stored only the 237 services that occurred more than 10 times in our data. Moreover, SAVOD, SPSS and BMDP do not allow process analyses of the rendering of services.

Other than in the case of the services, there is no standard language regulation for the documentation of d i a g n o s e s by ambulatory physicians.

A. Standardization

Infinite possibilities: The range of possible diagnostic entries is virtually without bounds. In our study 7 722 different diagnostic texts were registered.

Nonidentity: There are no uniform guidelines for defining terms applied to complaints so that not even the postulated identity can always be ensured. At the same time there is no clear demarcation between diagnoses, problem descriptions and medical findings.

Unclear aggregation: The aggregation levels of the selected diagnoses vary widely.

Time-related influences: Secular tendencies interfer to an unknown extent. As the age structure of the physicians is not known, this problem appears to be a relatively serious one.

Interest interference: The most substantial distorting factor in the documentation process is the interference of interest in the diagnoses due to the following tendencies:

- Justification of services: Those diagnoses are selected that appear most relevant in terms of fees for the services rendered resulting in a generalization of diagnoses and a dramatization of ailments.
- Reference to sickness funds: In their communication with sickness funds physicians use different diagnostic terms than those they employ among themselves.
- Patient protection: Those diagnoses are documented for which services rendered can be financed. (For instance a general check-up for preventive reasons would be hidden behind some diagnosis.)

B. Differentiation

Apparent tautologies: Frequently several apparently redundant diagnostic designations are used.

Multiple diagnoses: A differentiation of ailments by means of multiple diagnoses - in our study up to 23 - is common, the relationship between the diagnoses remaining unclear.

Insufficient specifity: Only occasionally are statements made as to:

- Condition: i.e. the temporal context of the diagnosis in relation to the ailment as, for example, "condition after".
- Localization: i.e. the anatomical context as, for instance, information on the part of the body affected.
- Degree of certainty: i.e. a statement as to degree of clarification of the diagnosis such as "probably".

Course and intensity: Information on the severity of the disease, on duration, change, etc. is lacking almost as a rule.

C. Coding and data processing

In our case a text coding on the basis of the DVG (6) was selected, comprising over 22 000 diagnostic texts (7-digit on the basis of the ICD-E), with the aid of which 78 % of the diagnoses could be coded numerically. The remaining 22 % were stored as uncoded texts and roughly classified according to the ICD system. If available, additional data were coded on localization, diagnostic certainty, diagnostic condition and type of coding.

This approach permits the largest possible freedom of choice with regard to aggregation and combination. It probably leads, however, in comparison to a highly aggregated code, to a series of problems in data transfer, coding and mapping as a result of, among other reasons, frequent illegibility of the hand-written entries.

After 3 error-correcting loops our material retained an error rate of 9.9 % with reference to DVG (7-digit code with supplementary pointers) and 4.4.% to the 3-digit ICD.

D. Validity

The aforementioned error sources generate considerable interpretation problems. There are arguments (7) that the validity of the diagnostic data can be only roughly estimated, e.g.

- by comparing the diagnostic data of various physicians for the same patients,
- on the basis of the diagnostic means employed, which is only partly reflected in the fee-schedule. (There are no routine data available on the equipment used by a physician.)
- on the basis of drug prescriptions for which our data provide no information; this approach implies a circular reasoning due to the self-legitimizing character of the diagnostic entries.
- on the basis of knowledge regarding duration of illness and more frequent diagnoses. Our data are restricted only to one quarter.
- on the basis of rendering certain services in accordance with the fee schedule. We will deal with this matter in the following section.

Relation of services to diagnoses: It is basic to the evaluation of medical activity to imply reliability and validity of data, an objective and unambiguous relation of services to diagnoses and knowledge of effects of services on the course of an illness.

These conditions remain largely unfulfilled where routine data are concerned and cannot be fulfilled in view of the following facts:

- There are ex-juvantibus diagnoses and prima-vista diagnoses, since in ambulatory care there is often no necessity for the verification of diagnoses.
- The establishment of a diagnosis is often the chief service rendered by the physician.
- Services are justified by diagnoses and diagnoses by services.
- The quarterly diagnostic entries do not allow clearcut correlation to services in the case of multimorbidity.

FINAL CONCLUSIONS: The aforementioned sources of error indicate that practically all the findings with respect to diagnoses and services set out at the beginning are difficult to interpret, insofar as no epidemiological prevalence studies exist to indicate plausibility, and studies aimed at evaluating the relevance of error sources are not performed. At any rate one needs enough plausible arguments to relativize the

Table 1: Types of error according to variables

Types of error		Variables	Patient identific.	Age	Sex	Place of residence	Insurance scheme	Insurance status	Physicians' ident.	Medical discipline	District	Type of record	Date of service	Service	Diagnosis
Original records	Before documentation	Misidentification	x		x		x	x							
		Infinite possibilities													x
		Excessive scope												x	
		Nonidentity												x	x
		Insufficient differentiation												x	x
		Unclear aggregation												x	x
		Interest interference												x	x
		Justification of services													x
		Reference to sickness funds													x
		Patient protection													x
		Time-related influences													x
		Variability												x	x
	During documentation	Unclear documentation practice	x	x	x	x	x	x					x	x	x
		Lack of documentation interest		x	x	x									x[1]
		Lack of documentation	x	x	x	x		x						x	x
		Tautologies													x
		Insufficient specifity													x
		Condition													ⓧ
		Localization													ⓧ
		Degree of certainty													ⓧ
		No relation to disease episodes													ⓧ
		Intensity												x	x
		Course													x
	After documentation	Modification of entries												⊠	
		Informal entries												⊠	
		Problems in correlating data												⊠	⊠
		Insufficient reliability													
		Over time													ⓧ
		Across individuals													ⓧ
		Insufficient validation													
		Equipment													x
		Drug prescriptions													x
		Prima-vista diagnoses													x
		Vice versa justification of diagnoses and services												ⓧ	ⓧ
		Bias because of justification need													x
Transfer/Coding		Information losses through anonymization	ⓧ		ⓧ										
		Entries in free format												ⓧ	ⓧ
		Disadvantages of selected code													x
		Coding errors												⊠	⊠
		Limited storage												ⓧ	ⓧ
		Total of transfer errors												ⓧ	ⓧ
Analysis/Interpretation		Lack of control variables													

x Error should be considered, but can only be quantified in the framework of special examination

ⓧ Error can be indirectly quantified or checked

⊠ Error can be directly quantified or checked

---

1) medical interest lacking, economical interest present

above error sources. One should be extremely cautious in applying and interpreting complex multivariate methods, e.g. regression-models, log-linear models, etc. There are often subsets of variables that are uniformly affected by specific sources of error. Non-statisticians are apt to interpret these correlations as facts of empirical reality.
An evaluation based on our data will only permit an attribution of services to diagnoses in few cases, i.e. when diagnoses are marked individually and when the services listed in the fee-schedules correspond to external sociomedical standards.

5. THE RELATIVE SUITABILITY OF THE DATA

The types of error encountered are systematically compiled in table 1 according to the manner of handling these errors, namely:

- Error should be considered, but can only be quantified in the framework of special examination.
- Error can be indirectly quantified or checked.
- Error can be directly quantified or checked within the body of data itself, although occasional interpretative margins will have to be tolerated.

It is shown that the physician variables, i.e. the supply variables, seem most reliable, that the patient variables are only affected by the usual sources of error, which one cannot but tolerate in secondary analyses, and especially that service and diagnosis data entail problems that run counter to a naive interpretation.

REFERENCES

(1) Diagnosen in der ambulanten Versorgung. Edited by FW Schwartz, D Schwefel. Köln, Deutscher Ärzteverlag, 1980
(2) Hasford J, Redler E, Schuller A et al: Soziale Aspekte von Diagnosen und Leistungen in der Allgemeinpraxis. Beiträge zur Analyse der Wirtschaftlichkeit ambulanter Versorgung. Edited by D Schwefel, G Brenner, FW Schwartz. Köln, Deutscher Ärzteverlag, 1980, part 4, pp 9-44
(3) Verfahrensweisen zur Analyse der Wirtschaftlichkeit ambulanter Versorgung, Edited by J Boese, W van Eimeren, A Schuller et al. Beiträge zur Analyse der Wirtschaftlichkeit ambulanter Versorgung. Edited by D Schwefel, G Brenner, FW Schwartz. Köln, Deutscher Ärzteverlag, 1980, part 2, pp 11-179
(4) A strategy for evaluating health services. Edited by DM Kessner, CE Kalk. Washington, National Academy of Sciences, Institute of Medicine, 1973
(5) Senftleben HU: Die Qualität ärztlicher Verrichtungen im ambulanten Versorgungsbereich. Köln, Deutscher Ärzteverlag, 1980
(6) op cit (3), pp 37-46
(7) Probleme der Sekundäranalyse von Routinedaten der Gesetzlichen Krankenversicherung. Eine Expertentagung. Edited by W van Eimeren, E Redler (to be published)

HEALTH PROMOTION:

AN ALTERNATIVE ROLE FOR AUTOMATED HEALTH TESTING

E. M. Clark
Primary Medical Care
Southampton General Hospital
Tremona Road
Southampton, England

Summary

A hypothesis is proposed whereby an individuals susceptibilities to disease can be identified using Automated Multiphasic Health Testing techniques. These susceptibilities, matched to a general assessment of vulnerability would provide the basic information needed to predict the health or illness expectancy for an individual and form the basis to develop a personalized health promotion program.

Over the past few years at least in the United Kingdom, the controversy over Automated Multiphasic Screening has quietened. The round condemnation, based on the cost of case finding has had a telling effect on health care planners and administrators of the financially structured National Health Service[1]. Indeed, when the Health Service has difficulty meeting the overt demand then it would appear to be madness to go looking for covert disease. Nonetheless, private health organisations are increasing their facilities for health testing and evaluation. BUPA has recently opened two new centres and the National Coal Board operates routine health surveillance as do many other organisations.

A recent study[2] failed to demonstrate any benefit in morbidity or mortality arising from screening when compared to a similar non-screened population. For many years the Oakland MPS centre experienced a similar difficulty, although a recent article[3] suggests this may not be quite true now, reporting less disability from complications of hypertension, ischaemic heart disease and back trouble. Also each member spent about $2000 less on their health care.

Another study[4] indicated that mammography is valuable in women over 45 years of age, malignancy tending to be detected at an earlier stage compared to traditional methods.

However, these are lightweight arguments compared to those which raged a decade ago.

Hutchinson's model of illness[5], suggesting that patients with diseases which were treated at an early stage produced better results than those whose treatment starts later, has been challenged. There is little evidence to support it in the case of chronic diseases. For example, the natural history of 'in situ' carcinoma is uncertain, and it may be that the vast majority do not go on to become carcinomata.

In spite of this body of scientific and expert opinion people still want the reassurance of a 'check up'. They want to be told that everything is all right, whether or not such a positive statement can be justified. Have these people, who have been reassured a higher tolerance of symptoms or consulted their doctors less frequently? Perhaps the $2000 mentioned earlier is a reflection of this.

The concept of multiphasic screening developed from the traditional physical examination to which was added the benefits of high volume throughput and precision technology. It is more efficient, more accurate, more reproducible and more economical. It does the same things better but there are other considerations. Let us start from scratch by examining a few facts and see what alternative paths we may discover.

There are geographical pockets throughout the world where some diseases are more prevalent than others (Table I), and the same is true of industrial environments.

	Eng. & Wales	Japan
MALE		
Stomach	88	266
Lung/Bronchus	276	33
WOMEN		
Stomach	37	120
Breast	76	11

Mortality from Cancer (Ages 55 - 64) 1957-59
Rates per 100,000. (Ref.)

Table I

Fat people have a shorter life expectancy than slimmer people. Smokers are more likely to get lung cancer than non-smokers. Wearing a seat belt reduces injury and death in car accidents (Table II). American football players have higher uric acid levels

(Figure I) than the normal range. Medical students, mostly male, have higher uric acid levels than nursing students, mostly female (Figure II) and both have lower than average cholesterol levels (Figure III)[7].

	OCCUPANTS	
	Unbelted	Belted
Uninjured	27.5	42.2
Non life threatening	67.4	56.8
Life threatening	2.9	0.4
Died	2.2	0.6

Percentage of Injuries in Road Traffic Accidents. (Ref.)

Table II

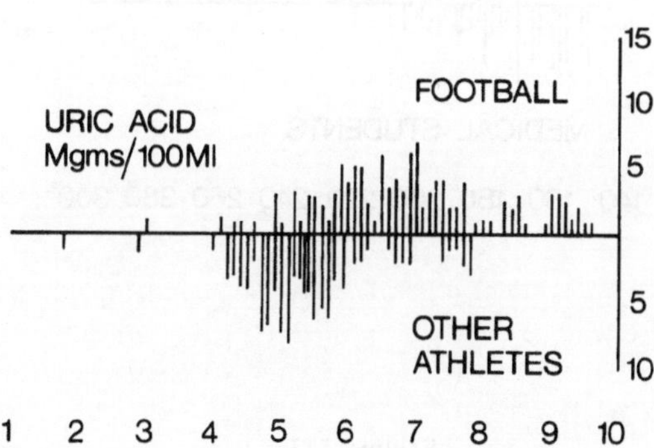

Figure I

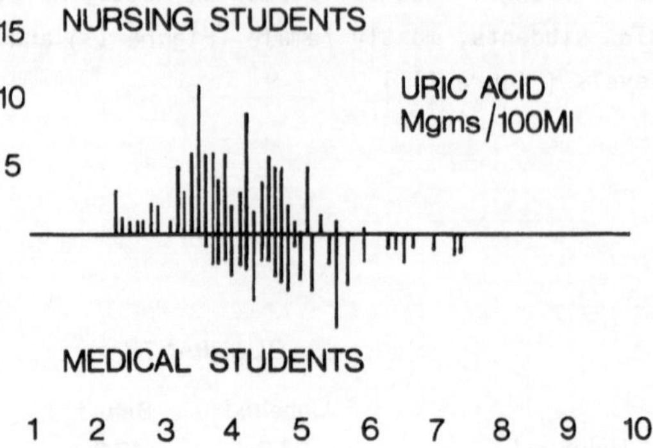

Figure II

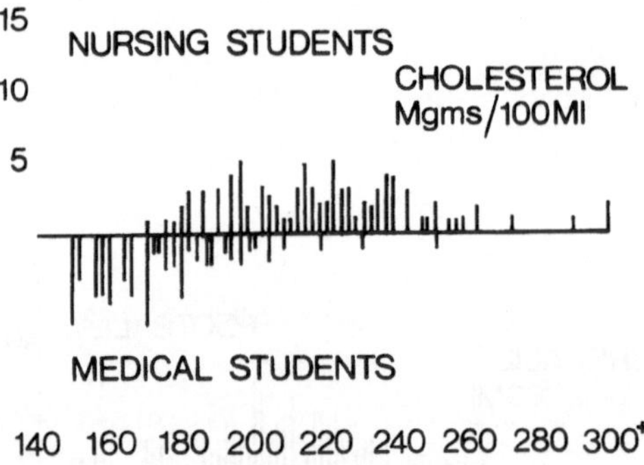

Figure III

Because of his bulk, his relatively hazardous occupation and, perhaps his high uric acid, the American football player is susceptible to a range of injuries and illnesses quite different to the lean, squash playing and "fairly fit", forty year old office worker. More specifically, a person with a kidney stone is more susceptible to urinary tract infections. A person with hypertension is more susceptible to ischaemic heart disease and cerebrovascular accidents. Each of us, by the nature of our genes, or past health experience, our environment and life style, has a pattern of susceptibilities, if not unique, then specific to ourselves.

Yet few of us manage to live up to, to fulfil our susceptibilities, and fail to meet our expectations of ill health. Most people who smoke do not die of lung cancer, most of us who drink do not suffer liver failure. While we remain susceptible, there is something which protects us. Some are more vulnerable than others.

A lot of evidence would suggest that our degree of vulnerability is governed by our reaction to stress. For example, children playing may give pleasure on one occasion and be irritating on another. Our reaction is determined less by the noise than by our frame of mind at the time. A series of experiments by Selye[8] demonstrated that stressed tissue, when subjected to a challenge later, showed clear evidence of ageing at a cellular level not present in the nonstressed tissue similarily challenged in the same animal.

Our ability to identify all the factors which are stressful remains incomplete. Nevertheless, Rahe and Holmes[9] have developed and scaled a questionnaire which gives an empirical measurement of stress. These Life Crisis Units present a useful, if imprecise, measurement of vulnerability.

This leads us to consider a model of health and illness proposed by Harold Wolfe[10] more than a decade ago, based on vulnerability and susceptibility.

Each individual has his own set of susceptibilities, but he is protected from stress by a defensive mechanism, his degree of vulnerability (Figure IV). As stress increases so is his vulnerability pushed back, exposing these susceptibilities which are most prominent at the time (Figure V). Thus, a businessman in difficulties who has suffered dyspepsia may well suffer the same symptom again as the first sign of his increased vulnerability.

It is not the stress itself but rather the reaction to it which is important. I think the model can be better represented by borrowing from Catastrophe Theory[11], using a simple cusp graph (Figure VI). Provided the individual has a positive reaction to stress his health will remain stable and satisfactory. However, should for some reason his reaction change negatively, then his health status will topple over the discontinuity edge and he will suffer illness.

This simplistic model implies a hierarchy of susceptibilities which is not intended. There are more factors than those represented here, and more dimensions than can be illustrated on a two dimensional surface. The model can be tested using longitudinal studies. First, by ascertaining the individual's susceptibilities, then at regular intervals, measuring his vulnerability, and so predict the appearance of symptoms and illness. This prediction I have called a Protodiagnosis[12].

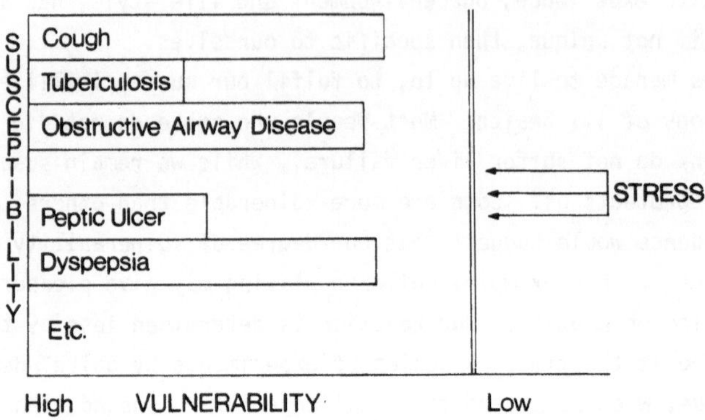

Figure IV

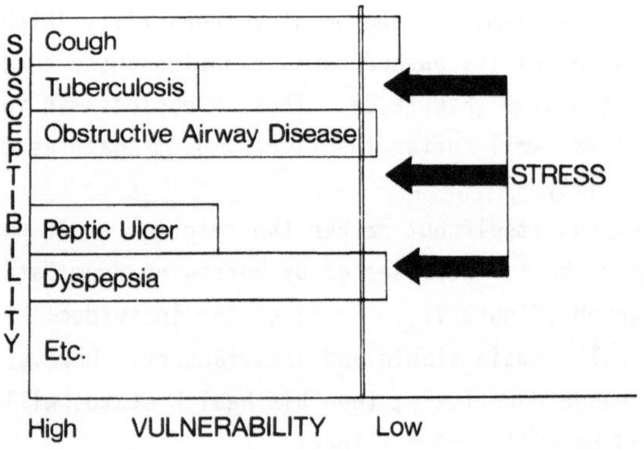

Figure V

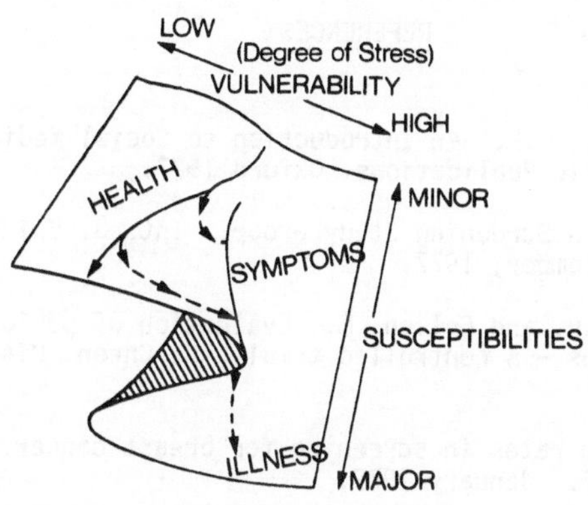

Figure VI

Clearly the accumulation of the necessary facts and measurements, and the calculation of the probabilities can best be done using automated testing methods and the computer.

The computer can select an exact matching cohort for comparison, so that deviations from this group norm would indicate the susceptibilities.

Sadusk and Robbins[13] have developed what they call a Health Hazard Appraisal. This indicates the risks of the individual inherent in his age and life style, and they demonstrate the statistical benefits associated with certain preventive actions. By extending this principle to each person's susceptibilities, a personalized health promotion program both in preventive terms and in the form of advice for the treatment of the minor symptoms could be provided. This protodiagnosis could give each person crude guidelines on how best to maintain his own health.

I would suggest that for automated health testing, this is a better thing to do, rather than doing the traditional examination better.

REFERENCES

1. McKeown, T. and Lowe, C.R. An Introduction to Social Medicine. Blackwell Scientific Publications, Oxford 1977.

2. The South East London Screening Study Group. Int. J. Epidemiology, 6 (4) 357-67. December, 1977.

3. Dales, L.G., Friedman, and Collen, M. Evaluation of periodic multiphasic health check ups - a controlled trial. J. Chron. Dis. 32 (5), 385 - 404, 1979.

4. Chamberlain. Error rates in screening for breast cancer. Clin. Oncol. 5 (2), 135 - 46. January 1979.

5. Hutchinson, G.B. Evaluation of Preventive Services. J. Chron. Dis. 11, 497 - 508, 1960.

6. WHO. Epidem. Vital Stat. Rep. 15, 308, 1962.

7. Coggins, W.J., Thomasson, G.O. and Clark, E.M. Multiphasic Screening of College Students. Jour. Amer. Coll. Health Assoc. Vol. 17, No. 5, 419 - 425. June 1969.

8. The Art of Predictive Medicine. Publ. Charles C. Thomas, Springfield, Illinois, 1967. (Hans Selye. Stresses in relation to disease pages 16 - 22, Chapt. I).

9. Rahe, R.H. and Holmes, T.H. Life Crisis and Disease Onset. I & II. Department of Psychiatry. Univ. of Washington, Seattle, Washington. 1964.

10. Stress and Disease. Harold G. Wolfe. Charles C. Thomas, Publ. Springfield Ill. 1968.

11. Structural Stability and Morphogenesis. Thom. R. Reading: Benjamin 1975.

12. Clark, E.M. A non automated Multiphasic Health Testing Program in a Student Health Service. Amer. Jour. Pub. Health. Vol. 63, No. 7. 610 - 618. July 1973.

13. Saddusk, J.F. and Robbins, L.C. Proposal for Health Hazard Appraisal in Comprehensive Health Care. J.A.M.A. March 25. 1968. Col. 203. No.13.

ANTENATAL CLINIC ANALYSIS AND EVALUATION OF PATIENT CARE FOR THE HEALTH CARE SYSTEM

D.D.F McColl
Health Computing Ireland Limited

R.F. Harrison
Department of Obstetrics and Gynaecology
Trinity College, Dublin

A.R. Unwin
Department of Statistics
Trinity College, Dublin

Summary

In an effort to improve antenatal care a pilot study of one year's attendance at the Rotunda Hospital, Dublin, Ireland has been undertaken. A measure of the value of examinations carried out during antenatal care has been developed. The usefulness of routine tests in mid-pregnancy was assessed.

1. Introduction

Although the perinatal mortality rate in Ireland has dropped in recent years, it remains higher than in most European countries (6). One of the reasons given for the lower rates in other countries is the high standard of antenatal care (11). It is believed that an improvement in the standard of antenatal care, particularly with early attendance, is followed by a drop in perinatal mortality and morbidity rates (15).

Antenatal clinics are available in Ireland for all mothers, where both community and hospital clinics and GP care are possible. Attendance is recommended every 4 weeks up to 28 weeks gestation, every 2 weeks up to 36 weeks gestation and every week after that.

At the first visit to a clinic the patient is given a thorough examination, her past medical and obstetric history is taken and certain investigations are carried out. This visit is the most important as most problems are then revealed (5). Each subsequent attendance can therefore be regarded as a "surveillance" visit.

There is general concern at the number of patients who attend late for their antenatal clinic (13) (10). In Ireland, it is estimated that over half the patients do not attend until after 20 weeks gestation (15). In spite of this low attendance, one of the logistical difficulties in running an antenatal clinic in Ireland is the large number of patients who have to be seen. At present, the resources of many clinics in terms of nursing, medical and administrative staff and as regards space are clearly stretched. If a policy were to be introduced which was successful in attracting patients earlier, these resources would probably be unable to provide an adequate service.

It has to be asked if all the investigations currently undertaken are absolutely necessary? (5). It could be that some of the more modern methods of diagnosis could actually replace older procedures. Also, although the first visit is essential, is it necessary to ask the patient to return every four weeks if she attends early enough and shows no adverse signs? It is acknowledged that these visits may be of some psychological value, which is however difficult to measure with any precision (5).

The primary objectives of the current pilot study are to evaluate the performance of the antenatal clinic and to recommend methodology for a fuller study. This study, while acknowledging the importance of social and psychological factors in antenatal care, concentrates on the investigations actually carried out in the antenatal clinic.

2. Population Studied

The antenatal clinic studied is in the Rotunda Hospital Dublin Ireland. Patients included in the study are all those who delivered at the Rotunda Hospital between 1st January 1979 and 31st December 1979. For these patients there is data available on their general identification, obstetric history, antenatal care, delivery and outcome of pregnancy.

These data have been collected for research studies in the prevention of perinatal mortality and morbidity, supported by the Friends of the Rotunda (3).

There is information on five antenatal clinic visits. These visits are the first visit, the last visit and the visits at approximately 20, 30 and 37 weeks gestation. Where there are no visits at these gestations, the nearest have been used. The information available is:-

(a) Gestation in weeks
(b) Proteinurea (Yes/normal)
(c) Abnormal BP (Yes/normal)

(d) Weight

(e) Number of cigarettes smoked

3. Methodology

A Assessing antenatal clinics.

The universal measure of the performance of the maternity services today is the perinatal mortality rate. This measure has been the most important measure in use over the last 30 years and in that time has been invaluable as a measure of progress in medicine (2). Chalmers, while describing the newborn baby's "... interaction and adaption during the perinatal period", refers to the perinatal mortality rate as "... that most extreme expression of maladaption - death" (4).

Alberman, who was an adviser to the British House of Commons Social Services Committee which recently published a report on perinatal and neonatal mortality (1), has said that she believes that all developed countries should now develop measures of morbidity - "even though this is so much more difficult" (1).

Neither the perinatal mortality rate nor a morbidity rate is a satisfactory measure of antenatal care. The perinatal mortality rate is well-defined, although there are international differences in its definition (6). It is not a measure of a condition over which the antenatal clinic staff have always some control. There are, included in perinatal mortality often deaths from congenital abnormalities (14). Morbidity is more difficult than mortality to define (1). Some cases, such as those resulting from spina bifida, are obvious at birth (14). Others suffering from less severe handicaps, may not be noticed at birth and may only develop symptoms later.

Two measures have been suggested specifically for antenatal care, 'Adequacy of antenatal care' (7) and 'Productivity of antenatal visits' (8). Neither of these meet the requirements of a good measure, which are that it should:

1. be sensitive to phenomena over which the staff have some control;
2. include conditions of pregnancy which affect the outcome of pregnancy or the management of the delivery and which can be detected and treated antenatally;
3. be well-defined.

In this paper a set of performance measures is suggested which assess the success of the clinic in detecting certain conditions of pregnancy. For each condition the measure is

$$\frac{100 \times (\text{number of patients with the condition detected antenatally})}{\text{Total number of patients with the condition}}$$

The usefulness of the measure lies in making comparisons from one year to the next and in comparing different clinics. Obviously not all conditions may be analysed in this way. Conditions which can be must meet the following requirements:

(a) The presence of the condition must affect the outcome of the pregnancy or the management of the delivery.
(b) The condition must be detectable antenatally.
(c) It must be known if the condition was not detected antenatally.
(d) The condition must be well-defined.
(e) The incidence of the condition must be sufficiently high so as to make its detection rate non-trivial.

B Evaluation of surveillance visits

For this pilot study all patients whose first visit was recorded as being before 16 weeks gestation and who made at least one other visit by the 28th week were considered. Only patients having solely hospital care were finally included in the study. The results of two tests regularly carried out at all antenatal visits were analysed to see how useful they were. This was done for all patients and for two 'low risk' groups identified by maternal and obstetric factors.

The first 'low risk' group was all the mothers who:

(a) were aged between 20 and 34 years;
(b) had a parity less than 4;
(c) were married.

These maternal risk factors were suggested by Chamberlain (1979).

The second 'low risk' group was a subset of the first, leaving out those whose previous obstetric history included:-

1. Early abortion
2. Late abortion
3. Previous deliveries with birth weight <2500 grams
4. Pre-term deliveries (<37 weeks)

5. Perinatal mortality
6. Perinatal morbidity
7. Neonatal death

4. Results

A Detection of conditions

As an example of the use of the measure in assessing the clinic's performance the condition singleton breech presentation was used.

Table 4.1 shows the detection of breech against the outcome of the pregnancy:

	Alive	Dead
Breech detected	59	3
Not detected	27	5

Table 4.1 - Outcome of breech pregnancies

Three out of 62 (5%) of the babies died when breech had been detected and 5 out of 32 (15%) died when breech had not been diagnosed. Although this difference is not statistically significant ($\chi^2 = 3.23$, $P < .10$), it does offer evidence that the outcome of pregnancy is affected by whether breech is detected antenatally or not.

The value of the suggested performance measure for breech is

$$\frac{100\ (62)}{94} = 66\%$$

B Tests at early visits

Table 4.2 shows (for all patients receiving antenatal care only at the hospital) the results of blood pressure and proteinurea tests at the first and subsequent visits. A patient was counted as 'normal' only if both tests were normal.

For the two 'low risk' groups tables 4.3 and 4.4 show corresponding results.

From tables 4.2 - 4.4 it can be seen that the percentages of patients who did not consistently show normal results at these visits were:

Other visits (≤28 weeks)	At first visit (<16 weeks)			
	ADVERSE	NORMAL	UNKNOWN	
ADVERSE	5	14	2	21
NORMAL	28	1553	37	1618
UNKNOWN	2	17	4	23
	35	1584	43	1662

Table 4.2 - All patients (hospital care)

Other visits (≤28 weeks)	At first visit (<16 weeks)			
	ADVERSE	NORMAL	UNKNOWN	
ADVERSE	1	6	2	9
NORMAL	19	1086	19	1124
UNKNOWN	1	11	3	15
	21	1103	24	1148

Table 4.3 - 'Low risk' from maternal factors (hospital care)

Other visits (≤28 weeks)	At first visit (<16 weeks)			
	ADVERSE	NORMAL	UNKNOWN	
ADVERSE	1	4	1	6
NORMAL	10	807	13	830
UNKNOWN	11	5	3	9
	12	816	17	845

Table 4.4 - 'Low risk' from maternal factors and obstetric history (hospital care)

All patients	6.6%
'Low risk' by maternal factors	5.4%
'Low risk' by maternal and obstetric history	4.5%

Percentages of patients who were not noted as having any adverse sign at the first visit and who subsequently showed an adverse sign can be summarised as:

All patients	1.0%
'Low risk' by maternal factors	0.7%
'Low risk' by maternal factors and obstetric history	0.6%

5. Conclusions and Recommendations

The measures of detection of conditions suggested in this paper have the properties required of good measures of antenatal care and complement existing measures of mortality and morbidity. Two tests commonly carried out through pregnancy, blood pressure and proteinurea, show a high degree of variability in their results in early pregnancy. This variability calls into question the efficacy of these tests during early pregnancy. The results of these two tests also suggest that it would be valuable to be able to identify at the first visit the approximately 90% patients who show no adverse signs up to 28 weeks. The 'low risk' definitions used in this paper go some way to meeting this aim but are far less successful than we had hoped. This tallies with the French experience (12).

This project was a pilot study for further work in evaluating antenatal care. It is intended to continue this research by evaluating the detection of breech and other conditions at the Rotunda clinic and elsewhere. It is also proposed to examine the early antenatal care visits in more detail.

Acknowledgement

We would like to thank Professor Alan Browne and the Friends' of the Rotunda for permission to use their data; Federated Dublin Voluntary Hospitals for financial support (D.D.F. McColl) and the Statistics and Operations Research Laboratory, Trinity College for assistance.

References

1. Alberman, E., Better perinatal health: prospects for better perinatal health, The Lancet, pp. 189-192, 26 January, 1980.

2. Baird, Sir D., The perinatal mortality rate as a measure of the efficiency of the maternity services, Health Bulletin, Scottish Home and Health Department, Vol. 35, pp. 234-242, 1977.

3. Browne, A.D.H., Computer assisted quality control in perinatal management, The International Cerebral Palsy Society Seminar on the Primary Prevention of Cerebral Palsy, Aosta, Italy, 1978.

4. Chalmers, I., Better perinatal health: the search for indices, The Lancet, pp. 1063-1065, 17 November, 1979.

5. Chamberlain, G., A re-examination of antenatal care, Journal of the Royal Society of Medicine, Vol. 71, pp. 662-668, September 1978.

6. Chamberlain, G., Better perinatal health: background to perinatal health, The Lancet, pp. 1061-1063, 17 November, 1979.

7. Gortmaker, S.L., The effects of perinatal care upon the health of the newborn, American Journal of Public Health, Vol. 69, pp. 653-660, July 1979.

8. Hall, M.H., Ching, P.K. and MacGillivray, I., Is routine antenatal care worth while? The Lancet, pp. 78-80, 12 July, 1980.

9. House of Commons: Social Services Committee, Perinatal and neonatal mortality, Vol. 1 Report, Her Majesty's Stationery Office, 19 June, 1980.

10. Kidd, G.M., The obstetric unit of the future, Irish Medical Times, pp. 21-26, 25 January, 1980.

11. Rooth, G., Better perinatal health: Sweden, The Lancet, pp. 1170-1172, 1 December, 1979.

12. Rumeau-Rouquette, C., Breart, G., du Mayaubrun, C., Crost, M. and Rabarison, Y., Evaluation de la pathologie perinatale et de la prevention en France: enquetes nationales INSERM 1972-1976, J. Gyn. Obst. Biol. Repr., Vol. 7, pp. 905-916, 1978.

13. Scott-Samuel, A., Delayed booking for antenatal care, Public Health, Vol. 93, pp. 246-251, 1979.

14. Scrimgeour, J.B. and Cockburn, F., Better perinatal health: congenital abnormalities, The Lancet, pp. 1349-1352, 22/29 December, 1979.

15. Stronge, J.M., A general review of the maternity services, Irish Medical Times, 25 January, 1980.

EVALUATION DES PROCESSUS DE SOINS AUX "PETITS POIDS DE NAISSANCE"

PRESENTATION DU SYSTEME

P. CINQUIN[+], L. DUSSERRE[+], J.B. GOUYON[++], A.M. CINQUIN[++], M. ALISON[++], J.L. NIVELON[++], D. TENENBAUM[++]

\+ Département d'Informatique médicale du C.H.R. de DIJON (Professeur ag. L. DUSSERRE) Hôpital du Bocage, 2 Bd Maréchal de Lattre de Tassigny, 21034 DIJON CEDEX Tél. (80) 65 81 23 poste 3335

++ Hôpital d'Enfants, C.H.R. de DIJON (Professeur M. ALISON et Professeur ag. J.L. NIVELON).

Summary

The creation of an evaluation process for the care of low birth weight infants in the Regional Hospital Center in DIJON made it necessary to deal with the medical records of the infants by means of informatics and to build up a follow-up medical record.

The essential cooperation between the physicians of public and private sectors is typical of this survey.

This paper presents the computerized medical record and the system supporting it.

INTRODUCTION

Les services des Prématurés et des Soins intensifs de l'Hôpital d'Enfants du Centre Hospitalier Régional de DIJON utilisent un dossier médical manuel qui donne toute satisfaction pendant le séjour hospitalier de l'enfant.

Mais la mise en place d'un système d'évaluation de la qualité des soins des enfants de "petits poids de naissance" a montré les insuffisances et les limites d'un tel dossier pour ce type d'étude : insuffisances quant à sa structure et limites quant à sa durée.

Il a donc fallu créer un nouveau dossier structuré, informatisé, complété par une partie "suivi" étalée sur une période d'au moins quatre ans. Un tel dossier permettra de juger de la croissance staturo-pondérale et de l'avenir psychomoteur, sensoriel et neurologique des enfants impliqués.

C'est ce système que nous présentons ici en considérant successivement :

- ses objectifs
- la population concernée
- sa place dans les autres systèmes d'information existants
- sa description
- le système informatique qui le traite.

La date de début d'exploitation de ce système est fixée au premier décembre 1980. La partie "suivi" du dossier sera mise en route au fur et à mesure. Les premiers résultats de l'exploitation statistique du dossier sont donc attendus d'ici un trimestre.

OBJECTIFS DU DOSSIER "PETITS POIDS DE NAISSANCE"

L'AUTOEVALUATION des services des Prématurés et de Soins Intensifs de l'Hôpital d'Enfants est le premier objectif de l'étude.

Il s'agit de définir des indicateurs de contrôle de la qualité des soins. L'édition, trimestrielle par exemple, de leurs valeurs permettra de suivre le bon fonctionnement des services et d'en ajuster la politique.

A côté de ces résultats obtenus à court terme, l'étude permettra à plus long terme d'évaluer l'efficacité des techniques utilisées en période néo-natale. On se demande par exemple quel pourcentage de surdités la méthode de dépistage néo-natal systématique de surdité de VEIT-BIZAGUET peut laisser échapper.

Il s'agit également d'aider à la gestion hospitalière en définissant, par exemple, les critères d'une répartition optimale des enfants entre les deux services concernés, selon la pathologie des enfants et les ressources disponibles en matériel et en personnel.

Le deuxième objectif du dossier concerne une RECHERCHE CLINIQUE destinée entre autres à définir et à évaluer des FACTEURS DE RISQUE.

Les études cliniques possibles avec le dossier préexistant étaient des études rétrospectives dont on connaît bien les inconvénients : recueil incertain des informations, choix limité des facteurs à étudier, populations hétérogènes, échantillons de taille réduite,...

Il est sûr que le dossier prévu permet des études prospectives multifactorielles plus précises : soit en confrontant les données péri-natales aux données du "suivi" pour définir des populations à haut risque, soit en utilisant seulement la partie périnatale. Ainsi J.D. KENNY (2) a établi dans une étude prospective ponctuelle que les hémorragies intraventriculaires des prématurés de 26 à 29 semaines sont plus fréquentes lorsque la P_{CO_2} est augmentée à la naissance.

La réalisation de ces deux objectifs implique le recueil d'informations sur toute la période péri-natale et au moins dans les quatre premières années de vie. Ceci suppose la coopération de plusieurs unités de soins des secteurs public et privé : maternité et services pédiatriques du C.H.R., cliniques obstétricales privées et également des pédiatres et médecins généralistes de la région.

Une telle opération nécessite un consensus médical et paramédical. Ce dernier a été acquis grâce non seulement à l'intérêt de l'étude mais aussi grâce au choix du circuit des informations, soigneusement organisé pour respecter la liberté de choix du médecin par les parents, le secret des informations, etc... Ce consensus sera entretenu par la diffusion périodique des résultats statistiques obtenus, diffusion respectant bien entendu le secret professionnel et d'une manière générale les règles déontologiques.

Cet objectif est réalisable par des moyens relativement modestes ; en effet l'informatisation du dossier néo-natal n'entraînera pas de surcroît de travail par rapport au dossier actuel. La saisie du dossier de "suivi" sera assurée par une secrétaire à mi-temps.

POPULATION CONCERNÉE

Le dossier présenté est rempli pour tous les nouveau-nés accueillis à l'Hôpital d'Enfants pesant moins de 2 500 g à la naissance, et/ou nés avant 37 semaines de gestation.

Ces nouveau-nés proviennent de la maternité du C.H.R. et des autres maternités (secteur public ou privé) de la région Bourgogne. La maternité du C.H.R. adresse tous les enfants de moins de 2 500 g, les autres établissements n'adressent qu'une partie de ces enfants.

Une étude préalable, menée grâce aux certificats de santé du 8ème jour, permet d'évaluer à 80% le pourcentage de "petits poids de naissance" de Côte d'Or accueillis à l'Hôpital d'Enfants. Ceci représente un flux d'environ 300 enfants par an.

Le recrutement des services de l'Hôpital d'Enfants est sûrement biaisé car les pathologies les plus graves sont bien souvent adressées au C.H.R.

SYSTÈMES D'INFORMATION EXISTANTS

Les systèmes d'information existants dans notre région sur la période néo-natale sont au nombre de quatre : le dossier hospitalier actuel, les statistiques hospitalières de morbidité, le certificat de santé du 8ème jour et les statistiques de mortalité de l'I.N.S.E.E..

Le dossier hospitalier actuel résume certaines données obstétricales et décrit complètement le séjour du nouveau-né à l'Hôpital d'Enfants. Mais les informations qu'il contient sont difficilement exploitables pour des études de recherche clinique ou d'évaluation qui imposent la manipulation de l'ensemble des dossiers. De plus il ne comporte pas de dossier de "suivi" structuré et systématique, ce qui limite considérablement le champ des études possibles.

Les statistiques hospitalières de morbidité fournissent peu d'informations utilisables pour l'étude en dehors du sexe et de la mortalité, elles sont d'ailleurs en complet remaniement.

Par contre les renseignements fournis par les certificats de santé ont l'avantage de concerner pratiquement toutes les naissances (97,6% de ces certificats sont remplis dans notre département). Ces certificats, qui donnent une description globale de la situation néo-natale du département, fournissent trop peu d'informations précises pour être utilisés seuls dans une étude d'évaluation telle que celle-ci. Toutefois ils peuvent servir de base à des enquêtes plus ponctuelles (e.g., étude par les services de la Protection Maternelle et Infantile (4) de juillet 77 à juin 78 du rôle du travail pendant la grossesse, des conditions de logement et d'autres facteurs dans la prématurité). Il existe en FRANCE un système national, GAMIN (1), de traitement de ces certificats, mais il n'est pas encore diffusé dans notre département.

Les statistiques de mortalité de l'I.N.S.E.E. apportent des éléments de description et de surveillance des mortalités néo-natale et infantile. Depuis 1975 on dispose, pour 74 causes de mortalité, de la répartition par sexe et par tranches de jours vécus, des enfants décédés de la période 0-1 an. Mais ces chiffres paraissent peu fiables : des études départementales menées par les services de Protection Maternelle et Infantile (4) en 1977 et 1978 semblent montrer qu'ils sont inférieurs à la réalité. De plus les causes de mortalité étudiées ne sont pas adaptées aux pathologies néo-natales. Tous ces éléments rendent difficile l'utilisation de ces statistiques.

Les insuffisances de ces systèmes existants nous ont donc amenés à développer un nouveau dossier "Petits poids de naissance", qui à notre connaissance, n'a pas d'équivalent en FRANCE.

DESCRIPTION DU DOSSIER "PETITS POIDS DE NAISSANCE"

La néo-natalogie, par définition, couvre une période limitée et les pathologies habituelles de cette période sont en nombre réduit. Il est donc possible de coder d'une manière précise les éléments du séjour hospitalier de l'enfant. Les données du dossier "suivi" sont par contre limitées à l'étude des développements neuro-psycho-sensoriel et staturo-pondéral de l'enfant.

Le dossier que nous présentons accorde donc une très large place aux pathologies du séjour hospitalier : il est volumineux (500 articles et environ 1 000 octets pour le support magnétique). Toutefois son utilisation quotidienne, à la place de l'ancien dossier tout aussi volumineux, ne majore pas le travail du service.

L'information à recueillir se divise en cinq parties :

- une première partie constituée d'un chapitre de renseignements généraux identifiant l'enfant et d'un chapitre d'antécédents familiaux.
- une deuxième partie relative aux événements antérieurs à l'arrivée de l'enfant dans le service (grossesse en cause, accouchement, transport de l'enfant jusqu'au service).
- une troisième partie consigne les données du premier examen et résume les renseignements généraux sur le séjour (courbe de poids, mode d'alimentation, tests de dépistages systématiques, ...).
- une quatrième partie concerne les différentes pathologies (pathologies métaboliques, infections, détresses respiratoires, apnées, pathologies digestives, hépatiques, hématologiques, neurologiques, cardiovasculaires, rénales, malformations et maladies héréditaires, pathologies cutanées, oculaires et endocriniennes).
- une cinquième et dernière partie constitue le dossier de "suivi' ; elle comporte des données cliniques simples qui résument au moins cinq examens (3ème mois, 9ème mois, 2ème, 3ème et 4ème année).

Les informations des deux premières parties, recueillies par les maternités, sont normalement transmises par le dossier de transfert. Celles qui manquent sont obtenues par examen du dossier obstétrical de la mère ou par téléphone. Elles sont suffisamment générales et importantes pour être toujours accessibles. On peut noter qu'elles sont compatibles avec les données collectées par le dossier commun "Grossesse" proposé par le Comité Consultatif d'Informatique médicale (3).

Tous les chapitres de la quatrième partie sont optionnels et ne sont remplis que si l'enfant présente effectivement la pathologie décrite.

Les quatre premières parties sont saisies au moment où l'enfant quitte le service. On dispose ainsi d'un recul suffisant (durée moyenne d'hospitalisation : 27 jours) pour corriger d'éventuelles erreurs de diagnostic ou pour voir se développer des pathologies qui échappent au certificat de santé du 8ème jour.

MISE EN OEUVRE DU DOSSIER INFORMATIQUE

Saisie des quatre premières parties du dossier

Elle est effectuée en temps réel sur un micro-calculateur HP 9845 B (159 K mots de 16 bits) par une secrétaire du service pédiatrique, à raison de deux vacations hebdomadaires.

L'intérêt du temps réel est évident pour une telle application : contrôle immédiat des informations saisies par le personnel du service qui connaît bien les dossiers, contrôles immédiats à plusieurs niveaux,...

Cette saisie qui, nous l'avons dit, s'effectue à la sortie de l'enfant, s'achève par l'édition du dossier sous une forme standard. Ainsi édité le dossier retourne à l'Hôpital d'Enfants où il est vérifié par l'interne ou l'assistant du service.

La lettre résumant les problèmes posés par l'enfant est éditée par le système et adressée au médecin traitant, au pédiatre et à l'obstétricien.

Saisie du dossier de "suivi"

L'originalité du "suivi" mis en place réside dans le coopération qu'il exige entre les secteurs publics et privés. Toutefois il est sûr que cette coopération complique la tâche du système chargé de vérifier que l'enfant est bien revu en consultation aux dates prévues.

Ce système de vérification fonctionne selon l'organigramme suivant :

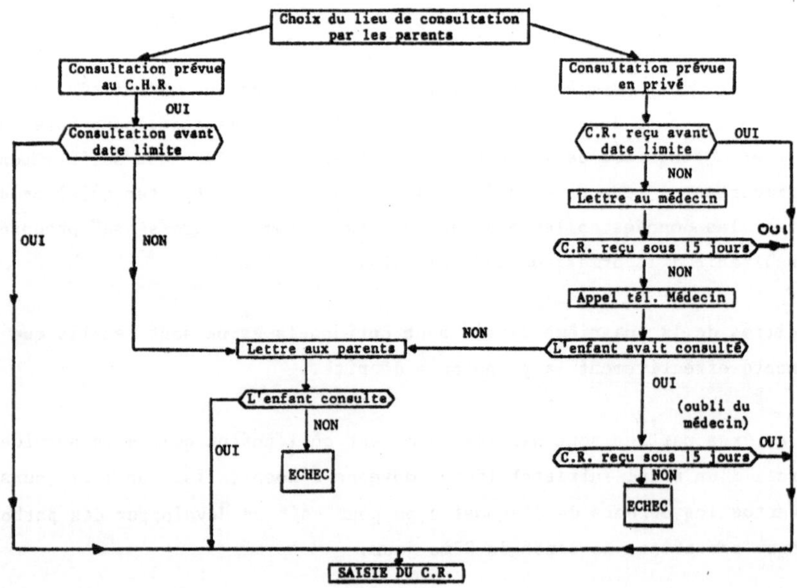

N.B. C.R. = compte rendu

Protection du secret du fichier

La protection du secret des informations a été ressentie d'emblée comme une nécessité impérative, car le dossier de "suivi" cerne de très près l'avenir neurologique des enfants.

Les dossiers enregistrés sont la propriété de l'Hôpital d'Enfants. L'ordinateur qui les traite appartient au Département d'Informatique Médicale, dirigé par un médecin. Le système informatique leur affecte un numéro d'anonymat qui assurera la protection lors de l'utilisation en routine du dossier de "suivi" : seuls le médecin traitant et le système pourront faire le lien entre un nom et un numéro et c'est sous ce numéro que les médecins traitants enverront les informations du dossier de "suivi". Par ailleurs la structure interne du fichier restera secrète.

Ces dispositifs de protection ont permis de vaincre les réticences des médecins, très sensibilisés à ce problème et très soucieux de préserver l'anonymat de leurs patients.

Exploitation du fichier

Une bibliothèque de programmes sera utilisable en temps réel par un personnel médical sans formation informatique particulière. La rapidité de réponse du système est assurée par la structure inversée des fichiers pour les articles les plus importants.

L'exploitation comporte deux volets :
- d'une part l'édition régulière d'indicateurs utilisables pour l'auto-évaluation des services, de renseignements d'ordre administratif (durée de séjour,...) éventuellement corrélés à des renseignements médicaux, d'indicateurs permettant de surveiller les évolutions des caractéristiques de la population étudiée.
- d'autre part les traitements utilisables à la demande pour des recherches cliniques précises, avec notamment les fonctions statistiques classiques (moyenne, variance, fréquence, corrélation, histogramme,...) et multidimensionnelles (analyse en composantes principales, analyse discriminante,...).

Conclusion

Ce dossier des "petits poids de naissance" constitue ainsi l'instrument de base d'un système d'information qui va permettre tout à la fois
- d'évaluer la qualité du processus de soins des enfants de "petits poids de naissance".
- d'effectuer les recherches cliniques destinées à améliorer cette qualité.

Structuré dans le but d'apporter un certain nombre de réponses aux problèmes de soins de la période périnatale il fera naître également, nous l'espérons, de nombreuses interrogations.

Références

1) Le système GAMIN ; projet GAMIN et débilité mentale
PRATIQUES, n°23 Juin 1978 p. 13-39

2) J.D. KENNY Pediatrics vol. 62 n°4 oct. 78, p. 465-465

3) Journées informatique et périnatalogie, organisées par C. SUREAU, SURESNES Mars 1980

4) Présentation par les services de Protection Maternelle et Infantile d'une enquête sur les prématurés de Côte d'Or entre juillet 77 et juin 78.
Journée régionale de Médecine périnatale. DIJON Oct. 78.

5) P. FERRARI
La prématurité - Aspects épidémiologiques - Problèmes psychologiques posés par l'enfant prématuré - Le devenir de l'enfant prématuré.
Revue de Neuropsychiatrie Infantile : n°9, sept. 1978 p. 407-449

6) OSBORNE C.E., THOMPSON H.C. - Criteria for evaluation of ambulatory child health care by chart audit : development and testing of a methodology.
PEDIATRICS, 56 : 4, 1975, p. 625-692.

CHILD : A COMPUTER SYSTEM FOR DATA ANALYSIS IN A SERVICE FOR PREVENTIVE SCHOOL CARE.

Luisa BERNARDINELLI (1), Carlo BERZUINI (2) and Giuseppe ROMAGNOLI (3)

(1) Istituto di Biometria e Statistica Medica,Universita'di Pavia, Via Taramelli 1, Pavia, Italy.
(2) Istituto di Matematica Applicata,Universita'di Pavia,Piazza Leonardo da Vinci,Pavia,Italy.
(3) Istituto di Igiene,Universita' di Pavia.

1.INTRODUCTION

About 4700 children are submitted each year to a visit comprehensive of an anamnestic questionnaire (family pathologies, physiologic anamnesis, pulmonary apparatus, gastrointestinal apparatus, infectious diseases, metabolism, cardiovascular apparatus, nutritional disorders), an objective examination, instrumental-clinical tests(blood pressure,schermography,ECG,visual acuity,audiograms), and laboratory tests in the Service for Preventive School Care of the District of Novara,Italy.

A data base of such information has been establishes,and is stored in computer-readable form. Since about 160 data items are generated at each visit, extraction of statistical information from the resulting considerable volume of data required the implementation of a computer-based system, named system CHILD. Either implementation and methodological problems were faced. The first aim of the system is to allow conducting a study of transversal type on the data base in order to (a) obtain descriptive group statistics over subsets of the collected population in order to derive standards (b) study the possibility of defining an optimal strategy to collect clinical information for assessing individual risk. The system CHILD is now operating in a fully conversational way under the Time Sharing System of a Honeywell 6040 computer through a typewriter-type terminal. It is entirely written in FORTRAN; it practically does not require user's knowledge of any control language at all.

2.METHOD

The system consists of programs for:

A - selection of classes of individuals of the data base through AND

OR combinations of recorded variables;

B - basic group statistics;

C - principal components analysis, adapted from (1);

D - unsupervised hierarchic cluster analysis via Ward's method,adapted from (2) ;

E - discriminant analysis by density estimation via a kernel method described in (3) ;

All the programs are functionally integrated: the output of each of them is structured in a way directly utilizable by another of them. Only one program at a time resides in central core during execution.

Program A requests the specification of a pathologic sector (ex.:cardiovascular), and then guides the user in defining, on the basis of a pre-specified set of synthetic variables relevant for the specified sector, classes of children distinct for diagnosis or degree of impairment. Such classes are called diagnostic classes. A label is assigned to each selected child corresponding to the diagnostic class he belongs to.

Program B allows a first insight into the data.

Program C is used to perform principal components analysis in the space of laboratory variables over separate diagnostic classes or combinations of them, and eventually transformation and reduction of coordinates for each examined child.

Program D produces a line-printer dendogram output representing the classification of the children in the space of laboratory variables;it allows cutting the dendogram at a desired level to obtain a partition of pairwise-disjoint clusters, and produces their scatter diagrams on requested projection planes, where each child is symbolized by the label of the class. The concordance between the clustering and the subdivision of the children in diagnostic classes is then studied, in order to evaluate the importance of laboratory tests as indicators of individual state. The analysis proceeds with an approach based on cluster analysis in conjunction with discriminant analysis : at first cluster analysis based on all laboratory variables is used to suitably partition each diagnostic class into disjoint subclasses. Then, using stepwise discriminant analysis to find a hierarchy of laboratory variables maximizing differences among diagnostic classes, inter-class misallocation rates via the leave-one-out technique,for different combinations of laboratory tests, are calculated through a subclass-by-subclass statistic rather than simply class-by-class. The following strategy for assessing individual state of a new child can then be devised: discriminant analysis yields a globally optimal combination of laboratory tests for each new child to be allocated in one of the diagnostic classes. Eventually, more tests are performed on the new child until the mean misallocation rate of the class found, say class I, falls under a desired threshold. At this point,laboratory variables already measured on the child are used via a nearest neighbour technique to allocate him to a subclass,say subclass J, within class I; use is made of previously computed misallocation statistics for each subclass,to determine the estimated probability that the child allocated in subclass J on the basis of already made tests,belongs to a class other than I. Such probability,instead of the mean error probability over class I, is used as termination criterium of the sequential test.Other tests can be suggested when corresponding variables give a high additional contribution to the distance between subclass J and most likely classes other than the I-th.

3.REFERENCES

(1) Lebart L, Morineau A and Tabard N. Techniques de la description statistique-Methodes et logiciels pour l'analyse des grands tableaux. Paris, Dunod, 1977.

(2) Jambu M, Lebeaux MO. Classification automatique pour l'analyse des donnees.2 Logiciels. Paris, Dunod, 1978.

(3) Habbema JDF, Hermans J. Selection of variables in discriminant analysis by F-statistic and error rate. Technometrics 19,487,(1977).

Prognostic Indicators of Survival in Intensive Therapy.

A Retrospective and Prospective study.

L. Dragsted, Qvist, J., Horwitz, O., Janstrup, F., Johansen, S.H.

Department of Anaesthesia and Intensive Care
Herlev Hospital, DK-2730 Herlev
Danish Institute of Clinical Epidemiology
Svanemøllevej 25, DK-2100 København Ø

The purpose of this work has been to study the mortality of patients, whose disease has been so severe that they have been in need of intensive care. We have studied the mortality both during hospital stay and during a follow-up period, in this paper I give the results for a 2 year follow-up period, but will at the meating give the results for another 2 year follow-up period.

The Intensive Care Unit (ICU) has received patients since the opening of Herlev Hospital May 1976 and our study includes all patients admitted to the Intensive Care Unit from June 1st 1976 to January 1st 1979 (this is the retrospective study). All patients from january 1st 1979 till december 31st 1980 comprises the prospective study.

The categories of patients received in ICU are:

1. Patients with developing or threatening respiratory insufficiency.
2. Patients in severe shock without regard to ethiology.
3. Other patients in need of special intensive treatment or observation.

Patients in the final stage of an incurable disease are not received in the ICU.

During the retrospective study, a period of 31 months 654 patients have been treated in ICU. Of these 223 died during their hospitalization. Vi have been special interested in certain groups of patients namely patients with sepsis an cronic lung diseas.

The National Heart, Lung and Blood Institute in a study on Extra corporal membrane Oxygenation showed that patients on a respirator for more than 24 hours requiring 50% or more oxygen had a mortality of 46%. In our study we found a mortality 72% using the same criteria . This made us interested in prognostic indicators of survival. It is known from other studies that mortality increases with failure of one or more organ systems and that the combination of respiratory failure and a acut renal failure gives a mortality of about 80%.

During the first study-period we had 119 patients with sepsis carrying a mortality of 68%, 32 of the patients survived the hospitaly stay, but one year after discharge only 20% are alive.

The highest mortality are found among those patients, who did require mechanical ventilation. The patients with cronic lung disease we found that 75% of the patients survived the hospitalization, but after one year only 59% are a live and we find again a higher mortality in the group of patients requiring mechanical ventilation. Together with The Danish Institute of Clinical Epidemiology we have study the mortality of all patients discharge. All danes have an identificationnumber consisting of 10 figures, the first 6 figures are birth date and the last 4 are a special identificationnumbers. All information concerning death date are collected in Datasystems and through the Danish Institute of Clinical Epidemiology we can ask this system, whether our patients are dead or a live and when they eventually have died. The three accompaning figures shows the mortality for surviving patients 2 years after discharge, the patients are divided in 3 agegroups: 1. less than 49 years, 2. between 50 and 69 years and 3. more than 70 years.

The expression cohort death mean the percentage of 100 new individuals that will be dead by the end of the follow-up period.

The death-area expresses the number of years lost through the follow-up period in percent of the maximum available number of years.

For the first group there is no expected mortality, but for our patients there is a mortality of 10% 2 years after discharge. In group 2 there are expected 4 to die out of 100, but of our patients 29 died during 2 years. In group 3 36 died out of 100 against the expected 15 out of 100 over 2 years.

These figures from the retrospective study have formed the background for a prospective study that started January 1st, 1979 also in cooperation with the Danish Institute of Clinical Epidemiology.

We have in this study try to find some easily recognisable prognostic indicators, that can help us in predicting the outcome for a patient in ICU. We have focused on 4 systems - the renal system, the hepatic system, the immunological system and the respiratory system. For each system we have made 4 function groups frem 0 to 3, from normal to no function.

Vi also note the diagnosis, especially if the patient have a malignant disease.

All surviving patients get every third month a questionnaire asking them if they are still under care, if they still are on leave because of illness, if they are in almost the same activity of if they are in the same activity as before their illness. Ontill now 95% of the patients have answered the questionnaires each time. In this fashion we try to measure the patients quality of life. By the end of 1980 the prospective study comprises a total of about 500 patients.

There have only been very few studies (1,3,5) on survival from Intensive Care but many studies (1,2,4,6) have tried to find indicators of survival. Cullen and co-workers from Massachusetts have very thoroughbly analysed groups of 226 consecutive critically ill patients. Cullen and co-workers also made a scoring system the so-called TISS score (Therapeutic Intervention Scoring System),(4). The system that have been used to determine appropriate utilization of intensive care facilities at the Massachusetts Generel Hospital, provide information on nurse staffing ratios for various patient care areas, quantitatively validate for clinical classification of critically ill patients into 4 categories thereby simplifying and organizing activities relating to patient care and analyse cost of intensive care relative to the extent of care offered. We find that the TISS score is a time consuming, too elaborate a system for daily use. In another work (2) Cullen and co-workers find that the Pao_2, cardiac index, acute renal failure are among diagnostic indicators that were significantly worse in patients who died within a year than in patients who survived with a succesfully recovery. They also found that acute renal failure was a primary predictor of death.

In one work (3) also by Cullen and co-workers there are a follow-up of patients and their quality of life after treatment in Intensive Care Unit. The same 226 patients which have been handled in other studies by Cullen, he found that 123 patients (54%) had died, 70 were still hospitalized and 31 were home. Only one of 103 survivers had fully recovered. By 12 months 164 patients (73%) had died, 10 were still hospitalized and 51 were home. 27 of 62 survivers had fully recovered. They also tried to make a cost benefit and analysis, but have excluded some costs.

If you try to make a cost benefit and analysis it is worth knowing that the expected life time of a patient who have been treated in Intensive Care are shorter than a normal person so that the cost by getting one patient through gives a higther cost per year for the shorting life spand.

$$\frac{\text{cost}}{\text{benefit}} = \frac{\text{cost per day x days in Intensive Care}}{\text{survival fraction x expected life time}}$$

From this it is easy to see that the determination factor is the expected life time as the survival rate is from 0 to 1. The results are giving in cost per year of expected life time. We vill be able to provide all the new results on survival rates and quality of life for patients after intensive care therapy at the meeting in March.

MORTALITY AFTER DISCHARGE FROM THE HOSPITAL.

AGE 15 – 49 YEARS (N = 111)

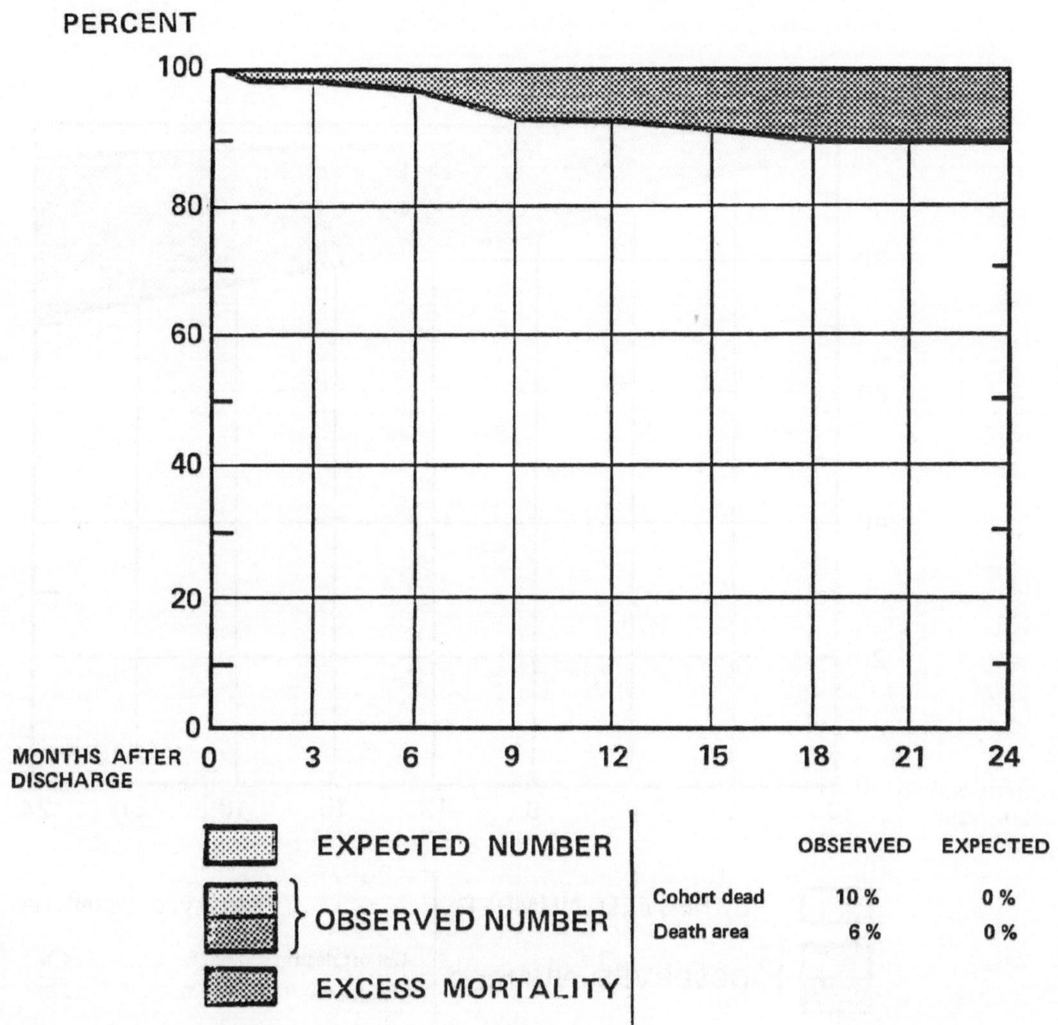

EXPECTED NUMBER

OBSERVED NUMBER

EXCESS MORTALITY

	OBSERVED	EXPECTED
Cohort dead	10 %	0 %
Death area	6 %	0 %

MORTALITY AFTER DISCHARGE FROM THE HOSPITAL

AGE 50–69 YEARS (N= 192)

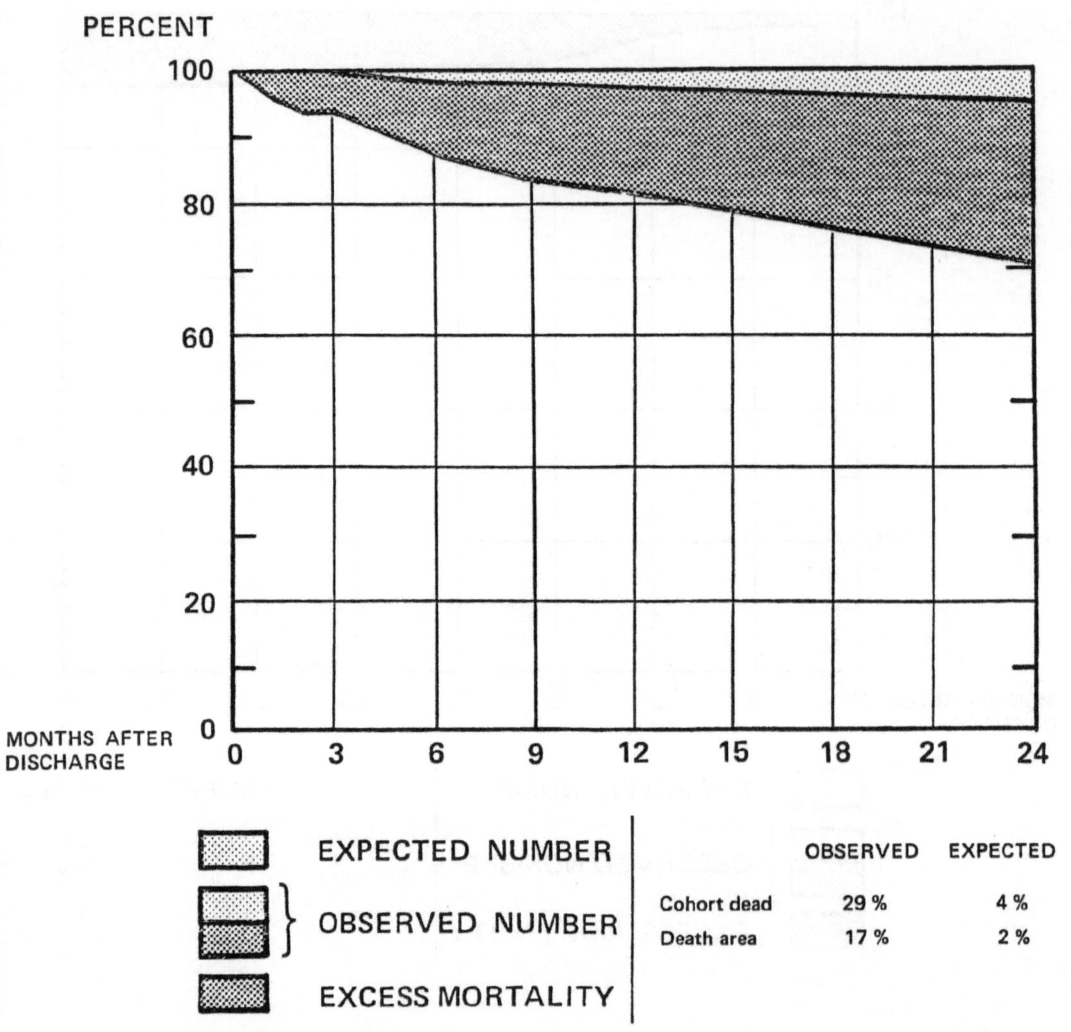

MORTALITY AFTER DISCHARGE FROM THE HOSPITAL

AGE 70 + YEARS (N= 100)

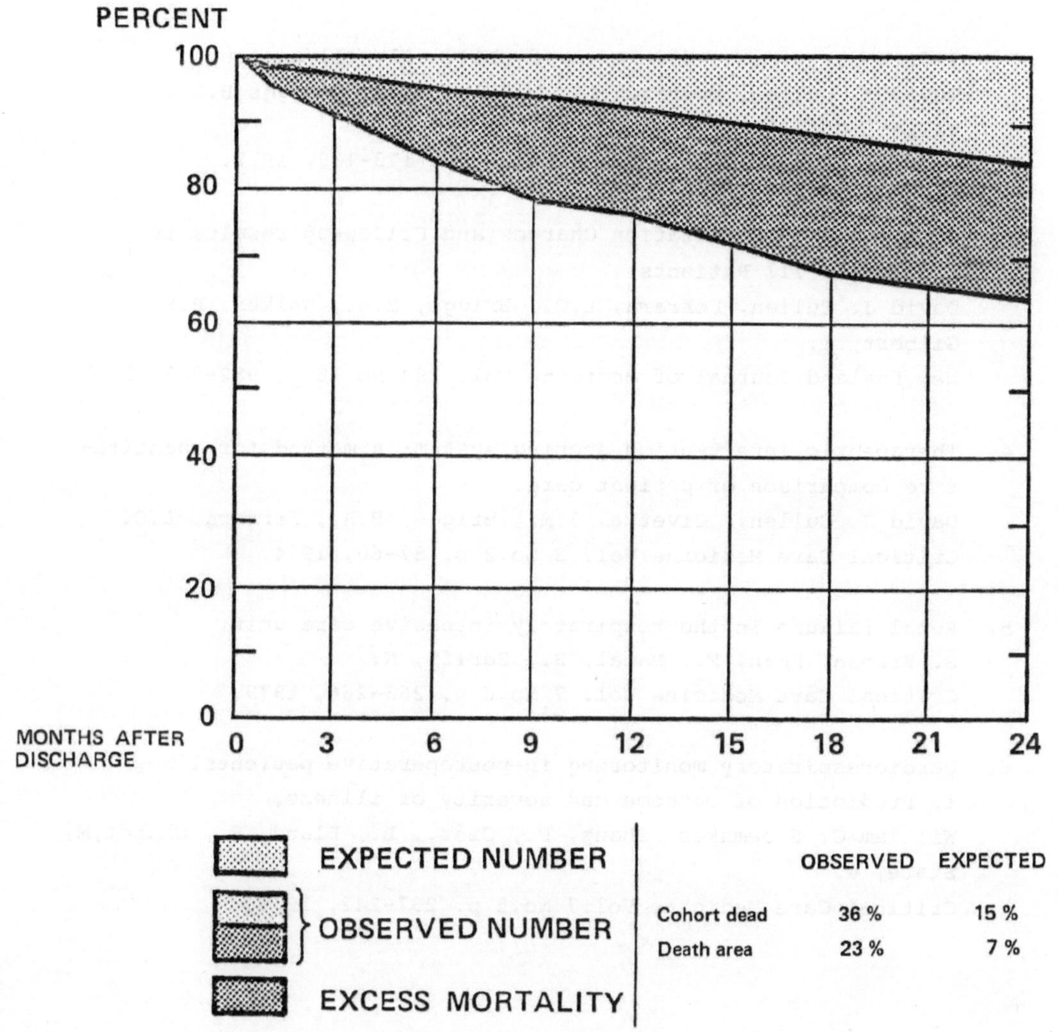

References

1. Mortality Prediction in Adult respiratory Insufficiency.
Robert H. Bartlett, Gazzaniga, A:B., Wilson A.F., Medley T., Wetmore N.
Chest 67: 6, June 1975. pp. 680-684.

2. Indicators of intensive care in critically ill patients.
David J. Cullen, Ferrara, L.C., Gilbert, J., Briggs B.A., Walker, P.F.
Critical Care Medicine Vol.5 No. 4, p. 173-179, 1977.

3. Survival, Hospitalization Charges and Follow-up results in Critically Ill Patients.
David J. Cullen, Ferrara, L.C., Briggs, B.A., Walker, P.F., Gilbert, I.
New England Journal of Medicine Vol. 294 No.18 p. 982-987, 1976

4. Therapeutic intervention scoring system: a method for quantitative comparison of patient care.
David J. Cullen, Civetta, J.M., Briggs, B.A., Ferrara, L.C.
Critical Care Medicine Vol. 2 No.2 p. 57-60, 1974.

5. Renal failure in the respiratory intensive care unit.
S. Kraman, Khan, F., Patal, S., Seriff, N.
Critical Care Medicine Vol. 7 No.6 p. 263-266, 1979.

6. Cardiorespiratory monitoring in postoperative patients.
1. Prediction of outcome and severity of illness.
William C. Shoemaker, Chang, P., Czer., L., Bland, R., Shabot,M, State, D.
Critical Care Medicine Vol.7 No.5 p. 237-242, 1979.

EVALUATION DE L'ETAT DE SANTE AVANT ET APRES HOSPITALISATION EN REANIMATION

JR LE GALL, J LATOURNERIE, D PLEVEN, P TRUNET, P CANDAU
Service de réanimation médicale,
Hôpital Henri Mondor, 94010 CRETEIL (F)

SUMMARY

To evaluate the results of a multidisciplinary intensive care unit (ICU) 228 patients (group I) have been prospectively studied and compared to a control group of 98 patients (group II) treated only in an intermediate unit. The health status (HS) was estimated A : good health, B : chronic and minor health problem with limited activity, C : chronic and major health problem with very decreased activity, D : institutionalized patient. Three months before ICU, then 1, 3 and 12 months after discharge, the HS was measured by physical examination or phone interview. Patients of group I had multiple organ failures and a level of therapy 4 times higher than in group II. Immediate survival rate was 67 per cent and 49 per cent after one year. Twenty per cent of surviving patients were still hospitalized three months after discharge. One year later 33 per cent of the 228 entering patients had a A or B health status level. All these results are significantly different from those of the control group.

En dépit de la multiplication des services de réanimation et le nombre croissant de patients traités, peu de résultats à court et long terme ont été publiés. Le but de notre étude était de suivre systématiquement pendant un an un échantillon de patients hospitalisés dans le service de réanimation de l'hôpital Henri Mondor à Créteil, et d'identifier les facteurs influençant les résultats obtenus.

METHODES

Le service de réanimation où se déroula l'étude est situé dans un hôpital universitaire et comporte 30 lits, et reçoit des malades médicaux et chirurgicaux. Il est divisé en 2 secteurs. Le secteur de réanimation proprement dite (14 lits) traite les patients les plus graves (médicaux : 70 pour cent, chirurgicaux : 30 pour cent) le rapport nombre d'infirmières/nombre de patient/24 heures est de 1.5/1. Le secteur de soins intermédiaires,ou de surveillance continue (16 lits) prend en charge les patients moins atteints (médicaux 90 pour cent, chirurgicaux 10 pour cent), le rapport infirmieres/malades est de 1/6.

La gravité des malades fut appréciée par le nombre de défaillances viscérales à l'arrivée. Sept grandes défaillances viscérales furent identifiées : neurologique, rénale, respiratoire, circulatoire, digestive, infectieuse et hématologique. Chacune d'elles fut définie par des critères précis (1).

L'intensité des traitements dans notre service fut jugée par le nombre de points TISS (Therapeutic Intervention Scoring System)(2). pendant les premières 24 heures. Ce cystème attribue de 1 à 4 points à quatre vingt gestes infirmiers pratiqués en réanimation.

L'état de santé fut apprécié 3 mois avant l'entrée en réanimation par l'interrogatoire de la famille ; 1 mois, 3 mois et 12 mois après la sortie du service par un suivi systématique, soit par l'exament clinique en consultation soit par l'interrogatoire téléphonique si l'état de santé semblait normal.

L'état de santé était classé en 4 groupes : A : bonne santé, B : problème de santé chronique et mineur diminuant l'activité habituelle, C : problème de santé chronique et majeur empêchant pratiquement toute activité, D : patient institutionnalisé, soit hospitalisé, soit en maison de repos soit à domicile mais nécessitant l'aide d'une tierce personne.

Un échantillon de trois cent vingt six malades a été étudié qui avaient été admis de façon consécutive de juillet 78 à juillet 79, une semaine sur deux.

Deux cent vingt huit malades avaient été hospitalisés primitivement dans le secteur aigu : ils constituent le groupe de malades de réanimation proprement dits ou groupeI. Quatre vingt dix huit malades ont été hospitalisés d'emblée dans le secteur intermédiaire. Ils forment le groupe II de contrôle.

RESULTATS

L'âge des patients ne différait pas dans le groupe I (moyenne 49.9, extrême : 15-82) ou le groupe II (moy. 51,3, extrême 19-90). De même la répartition entre hommes et femmes était similaire (femme 42 et 44%, hommes 58 et 56%).

La gravité des patients a été estimée par le nombre de défaillances viscérales pendant les premières 24 heures. Le tableau I montre que près des trois quarts des patients du secteur aigu (groupe I) avaient plusieurs défaillances, tandis qu'à l'inverse 80 pour cent des patients du secteur intermédiaire (groupe II) avaient une seule, ou moins d'une, défaillance.

L'intensité des traitements mesurée par le nombre de points TISS était significativement différente dans les deux groupes : dans le groupe I, 147 points par séjour en moyenne, 13.8 par jour, la durée moyenne de séjour était de 10.65 jours ; dans le groupe II 40 points par séjour en moyenne, 3.5 points par jour, durée moyenne de séjour : 11.42 jours.

L'évolution des 228 patients du groupe I est représentée sur le tableau II. Trois mois avant la maladie aiguë 73 pour cent des malades étaient dans la catégorie A et seulement 4 pour cent étaient institutionnalisés (catégorie D).

Le taux de survie immédiat est de 65.78 pour cent mais chute à moins de 50 pour cent à un an.

L'évolution de l'état de santé des survivants entre le 1er et le 12ème mois après la sortie montre que le pourcentage de survivants institutionnalisés (catégorie D) est élevé le 1er mois (41.45 pour cent), est encore de près de 20 pour cent le 3ème mois mais chute à moins de un pour cent à un an.

A l'inverse, la proportion de malades ayant une activité normale ou réduite double entre le 1er et le 12ème mois.

Sur le tableau III est représentée l'évolution des patients du groupe II (secteur intermédiaire). Alors que le profil de l'état de santé de cette population trois mois avant l'hospitalisation n'a aucune différence significative avec celui des patients du secteur aigue, l'évolution ultérieure est tout à fait différente. Le pourcentage de survie reste de l'ordre de 90 pour cent. Le pourcentage de patients des catégories A et B (activité normale et réduite) augmente plus vite. L'hospitalisation à la sortie du service de réanimation est plus brève et touche moins de patients que dans le groupe I.

DISCUSSION

L'état de santé des patients avant leur hospitalisation est rarement mentionné dans la littérature. THIBAULT et al (3) sur 2 693 patients hospitalisés dans un service de réanimation médicale à vocation cardiologique signalent un état de santé préalable médiocre chez le quart de leurs patients. Dans notre collectif l'état de santé 3 mois avant est satisfaisant (activité normale ou réduite) chez plus de 80 pour cent des patients et similaire dans les 2 groupes. Les malades hospitalisés en réanimation ne sont pas pour la plupart atteints de maladies chroniques.

Le taux de survie immédiate de 65.79 pour cent du groupe I est significativement différent de celui du groupe II (93.7 pour cent). Ce taux est proche de celui signalé par d'autres auteurs : NUNN : 67 pour cent (4), CULLEN : 52 pour cent (2), SPAGNOLO : 53 pour cent (5), PIERRI : 59 pour cent (6). D'autres auteurs ont des résultats moins bons : PESSI : 30 pour cent chez les patients de classe IV (7), ROSERS 37 pour cent chez les insuffisants respiratoires médicaux (8), CASALI 25 pour cent en cas d'insuffisance rénale aiguë (9).

Le taux de survie varie selon la gravité des patients. Les 228 patients de notre groupe I entrent dans les classes III et IV de CULLEN, ceux du groupe II dans les classes I et II.

La population du groupe I est caractérisée par une gravité plus grande, puisque la plupart des patients ont plusieurs défaillances, et une intensité de traitement en moyenne 4 fois plus élevée. Dans le travail de CULLEN, le nombre de points TISS par patient est de 23 en classe III et 43 en classe IV mais ces points sont mesurés le 1er jour et l'on sait qu'ils décroissent rapidement (2).

Pendant l'année qui suit la sortie du service de réanimation le taux de survie chute jusqu'à 49.12 pour cent chez nos patients. Dans la littérature le taux de survie à la sortie de l'unité et à la sortie de l'hôpital diffèrent notablement : NUNN et al (4) trouvent une mortalité supplémentaire de 17 pour cent dans l'hôpital chez les patients ventilés. Dans l'année suivante la chute du taux de survie est maximum chez les patients du groupe IV de CULLEN (de 73 à 27 pour cent).

L'état de santé des survivants est très différent dans nos deux groupes : dans le 1er des malades de réanimation le pourcentage des résultats satisfaisants (A et B) atteint 73 pour cent des survivants mais seulement 33 pour cent des 228 patients hospitalisés ; dans le 2èm groupe, 69 patients, soit 70 pour cent des 98 entrants sont dans le groupe A ou B. C'est dire que le retour à l'état antérieur est presque atteint dans ce groupe de patients intermédiaires, tandis qu'il en reste très éloigné chez les patients de réanimation. Les constatations de CULLEN sont analogues (2).

Beaucoup de patients sont traités en hôpital aigu ou en maison de convalescence après leur sortie de réanimation. 41 pour cent des survivants à un mois, 18 pour cent à trois mois n'ont pas regagné leur domicile. Dans le calcul des coûts du traitement de tels patients, celui de l'hospitalisation ultérieure doit entrer en compte.

CONCLUSION

Les malades traités dans un service de réanimation ont pour 80 pour cent une activité normale ou réduite trois mois auparavant. Atteints de défaillances multiples ils nécessitent un traitement 4 fois plus intense que des malades de secteur intermédiaire. Le taux de survie immédiat est de 67 pour cent mais seulement 49 pour cent un an plus tard. Vingt pour cent des survivants sont encore hospitalisés au 3ème mois après la sortie de réanimation. Un an plus tard 33 pour cent de l'ensemble des patients (n=228) a une activité normale ou réduite.

Tableau I : répartition des patients selon leur gravité, estimé par le nombre de défaillances viscérales pendant les 24 premières heures d'hospitalisation.

Nombre de défaillances viscérales	Groupe I secteur aigu (n=228) %		n	Groupe II secteur intermédiaire (n=98) %		n
O	4.2		10	34	80	35
1	22.2		51	46		47
2	23.6	73.1	54	12		12
3	20.1		46	6		6
4 et plus	29.4		67	2		2
	-------- 100 pour cent			----- 100 pour cent		

Tableau II : évolution des états de santé dans le groupe I (malades aigus n=228). Les pourcentages sont entre parenthèses.

	3 mois avant	Sortie service	1 mois après	3 mois après	1 an après
A	166 (78.6)		30 (22.9)	52 (41.6)	56 (50)
B	34 (14.9)		18 (13.7)	19 (15.2)	26 (23.2)
C	20 (8.8)		29 (22.1)	31 (24.8)	29 (25.9)
D	8 (3.5)		54 (41.2)	23 (18.4)	1 (0.8)
Total des survivants	228	150	131	125	112
Taux de survie		(65.79)	(57.45)	(54.82)	(49.12)

Tableau III : Evolution des états de santé dans le groupe II (malades intermédiaires n=98) Les pourcentages sont entre parenthèses.

	3 mois avant	Sortie du service	1 mois après	3 mois après	1 an après
A	71 (72.4)		38 (41.7)	48 (52.7)	47 (58.4)
B	14 (14.2)		10 (10.9)	17 (18.7)	22 (25.)
C	11 (11.2)		26 (28.5)	15 (16.5)	16 (18.2)
D	2 (2.04)		16 (17.5)	11 (12.1)	3 (3.4)
Total des patients	98	92	91	91	88
Taux de survie		(93.87)	(92.85)	(92.85)	(89.79)

REFERENCES

1 LE GALL JR, TRUNET P, LATOURNERIE J, and PLEVEN D
Is an intermediate unit close to an intensive one justified?
Crit. Care Med. 1979, 7:259

2 CULLEN DJ
Results and costs of intensive Care.
Anesthesiology 1977 ; 47:203-216

3. THIBAULT GE, MULLEY AG, BARNETT GO, GOLSTEIN RL, REDER VA, SHERMAN EL and SRINNER ER
Medical intensive Care : indications interventions and outcomes
New Engl J Med 1980 ; 302:938-942

4 NUNN JF, MILLEDGE JS and SINGARAYA J
Survival of patients ventilated in an intensive therapy unit
Brit Med J, 1979 ; 1:1525-7

5 SPAGNOLO SV, HERSHBERG PI and ZIMMERMAN HJ.
Medical intensive care unit : mortality experience in a large teaching hospital,
N Y State J of Med 1973 ; 754-7

6 PIERRI A.
Pazienti, impegno terapeutico, risultati e costi in un centro di rianimazione
Acta Anesth. Italica, 1980; 31:105-10

7 PESSI TT,
Experiences gained in intensive care surgical patients
Ann. Chir. Gynecol. Fenn 1973 ; S 185:3-72

8 ROGERS RM, WEILER C and RUPPENTHAL
Impact of the respiratory intensive care unit on survival of patients with acute respiratory failure.
Chest, 1972 ; 62:94-7

9 CASALI R, SIMMONS RL, NAJARIAN JS
Acute renal insufficiency complicating major cardiovascular surgery.
Ann Surg 1975 ; 181:370-5

A DATA PROCESSING STRUCTURE TO REGISTRATE DATA FROM GEOGRAPHICALLY DISPERSED CORONARY CARE UNITS.

Coen TUINSTRA (1), Jaap KOLFF (2), Arnoud vd LAARSE (2), Henk LIE (3), Gerard KAN (3), Frans van CAPELLE (3), Rolf MICHELS (4), Klaas BOM (4), Ruud VINKE (4)

(1)Dept of Medical Information Processing, Med Faculty, Leiden
(2)Dept of Cardiology, State University, Leiden
(3)Dept of Cardiology and Clinical Physiology, Univ. of Amsterdam
(4)Dept of Cardiology, Thoraxcentrum, Rotterdam

1.Ø SUMMARY.

The cardiology departments of six separate university hospitals of the Netherlands cooperate to collect data on diagnosis and treatment of all patients admitted to coronary care units, in order to be able to compare the effect of interventions in certain specified clinical entities . The paper describes some problems encountered during the early phases of data collection.

2.Ø INTRODUCTION

The Interuniversity Cardiological Institute embraces a collaboration between the departments of Cardiology of six university hospitals of the Netherlands. It stimulates and coordinates clinical as well as fundamental research in heart disease. Previous and currently ongoing projects concern evaluation of some automatic ECG-programs, evaluation of quantitative heart catheterisation and angiography, application of advanced echocardiography and electrophysiological research to gather insight into tachyarrhythmias. Participating members of the Institute are the Departments of Cardiology of the University of Amsterdam, Leiden, Nijmegen, Utrecht, of the Erasmus University of Rotterdam and of the Free University of Amsterdam.

Recently a new project has been started to evaluate the treatment , the prognostic significance of certain variables and the effect of interventions in patients with coronary heart disease(CHD). An important aspect of this project is the uniform way to register patient data, and the standardized manner to calculate infarction size. So as to get enough patient data which will allow for conclusions on a sound statistical basis within a reasonable observation period the patient data of the different

CCU's are pooled.

Clearly, the data to be collected in the different coronary care units (CCU) should contain the same type of information and should be based on the same definitions of clinical entities, accepted by each CCU. The number of semantic differences in the collected data should be kept to a minimum. Of even more importance is the necessity to identify these semantic differences before data collection is started. This seems to be a trivial point, but it turned out to be a source of major concern.

The present paper describes which data are registered and how the standardized way of data collection is initiated.

3.Ø ORGANISATIONAL DIFFERENCES IN CCU's

Although the purpose of and the medical functioning in the coronary care units (CCU) in the various hospitals are much the same, we yet have to recognize some quite substantial differences in patient management policy, which will influence the data on the patients to a considerable degree.

It is not obvious at all for instance, what is meant by the word "CCU". In some places it is a department in which patients are treated during the acute phase of myocardial infarction and the like only. This means that patient intake is based on a kind of prescreening, which excludes the admission of patients with (acute) non-cardial problems to a large extent. Discharge in these hospitals commonly is soon after the acute phase to a rehabilitation unit.

In other hospitals the CCU is a department where all patients are admitted with symptoms interpreted by anybody as signs of CHD, and all patients are kept there until they are well enough to go home.

Both the admission and the discharge policy have an influence on the collected data; not so much on the data of the individual patient, but certainly on the numbers for the CCU as a whole.

4.0 DATA TO BE RECORDED.

It had to be decided which data should be collected.So the purpose of the overall study namely to determine the effect of interventions in CHD should be kept in mind. But it is not clear as yet how this effect should be measured, nor is it possible to define exactly at this moment which parameters should be used to select matched cases required for the necessary test-sets.

However, there was one variable which was considered to be of crucial value, it concerns infarction size as measured by biochemical methods from the enzyme levels taken at various intervals after onset of infarction.

The total number of variables, including the biochemical measurements, amounts to about 300. The data recorded for each patient contain:

- admission information : time of arrival, onset of symptoms, where does the patient come from, etc.

- patient information : history, social circumstances, riskfactors, previous drug treatment, bloodpressure ,ECG, etc.

- management information : diagnostic procedures, type of monitoring, complications, etc.

- treatment information : administered drugs, cardiac assistance, surgical intervention, etc.

- discharge information : diagnosis, infarction size, cause of death, etc.

5.0 INFARCTION SIZE ESTIMATION

The importance of infarction size as estimated by biochemical methods was mentioned previously. A major effort by the participants was necessary to ensure that all centers would use the same methods to calculate infarcted area. Initially, the enzyme to be used in the present study, alfa hydroxybutyraat dehydrogenase (HBDH) (1)(2), was not currently in use in all centres, and when introduced , there proved to be rather large technical discrepancies between the laboratories of the participating centres. A quality control mechanism had to be instituted.(3)

6.Ø DATA REGISTRATION.

It was recognized that datacollection should be introduced in the CCU's in a careful way, because it meant deviation from used routine administration, causing extra work and attention, without immediate reward for the personnel involved.

6.1 ONLINE AND OFFLINE REGISTRATION

At present the data are registrated on preprinted forms, which are sent to Leiden where these are entered into a database.

From the outset, it has been our purpose to use the automated information systems as available to the participants for on-line input of the data. This should improve the data quality by checking the validity at entry and would enhance the completeness of the data. But some CCU's had had no experience with datacollection and other CCU's were accustomed to other sets of data to collect (4). Anyway, before much work could be spent on programs for online input, there should be some experience with the proposed set of input data. The use of forms provided a means for gradual introduction of the data collection system in the CCU's at relative low cost. These forms will also serve as part of the patient files (on paper) which are kept in the CCU's.

6.2 INTEGRATION IN HOSPITAL INFORMATION SYSTEMS

Online data collection will be executed at a later date by connecting input terminals to the local hospital information systems (ZIS) (5), which are either already available (Leiden, Utrecht and Rotterdam) or will be available by 1981 (University of Amsterdam, Free University). These hospitals apply the same informationsystem and cooperate in the developement and further introduction of ZIS. Nijmegen has its own information system which unfortunately is not compatible with the ZIS of the other centres.

The online input by way of the existing hospital information systems has the additional advantage that it will not be necessary to enter those data which are already available at the local database (patient-identification, laboratory results) . Also input check on the data can be made to be rigorously identical in all ZIS-using CCU's, because the programs are exactly the same.

6.3 DATA FLOW

In order to arrive at completeness of data which are to be analysed a database will be required containing cases from all participating centres during the study. The patient data are entered anonymously into this database for privacy protection. Connection of patient name and hospital number or CCU-number can only be carried out at the local CCU and not by the central database manager. But it is of course possible to search for patients with a certain data-profile and to select sets of patients who have a certain number of attributes in common.

The CCU's send their data to the database on the printed sheets or on magnetic tape. Mailing of paper will not be necessary once all CCU's have acces to online input facilities. It is not likely that in the early phase of the current project datatransmission through a datanetwork between ZIS-computers will be realized.

The ZIS systems are running on midicomputers (PDP11-70) and the available software is not readily suitable for statistical dataprocessing. Therefore at present all data are sent to Leiden where merging, processing, sorting and reporting on the collected data is performed on the university computer .

7.0 PRESENT STATUS

At this moment (november 1980) information on 1100 cases has been entered into the database with about 300 variables per case. The intake flow has increased to about 200 cases a month. The percentage of diagnosed myocardial infarction is about 60% of total intake. Infarction size can be determined in about 50 % of all patients with a discharge diagnosis of myocardial infarction.

8.0 REFERENCES

(1) Rosalki SB and Wilkinson JH :' Reduction of alphaketobutyrate by human serum.'
Nature (London), 1960; 188; 1110 -1111.

(2) Witteveen SAGJ, Hemker HC, Hollaar L, Hermens WTh: 'Quantitation of infarct size in man, by means of plasma enzyme levels.'
Brt. Heart J. ; 1975; 37; 795-803.

(3) Laarse A vd, Davids HA, Hollaar L, Valk EJM vd, Witteveen SAGJ, Hermens WTh : 'recognition and quantification of myocardial

injury by means of plasma enzyme and isoenzyme activities after surgery.'
Brt Heart J. 1979 ; 41 ; 660-667.
(4) Van Capelle FJL, Durrer D : 'A database management system for research applications'
Computers in Cardiology ; 1979 ; 233 -236
(5) Bakker AR, in:' MEDINFO 80', Lindberg/Kaihara Edts, Amsterdam. North Holland Publ., 1980; 505-509

Department of Anesthesia and Reanimation, Faculty of
Clinical Medicine Mannheim, University of Heidelberg
(Director: Prof. Dr. med. H. Lutz)

DATA RECORDING AND PRESENTATION IN THE DEPARTMENT OF ANESTHESIA AND REANIMATION, MANNHEIM

Hartung, H.-J., P.-M. Osswald, U. Böhner, H. Lutz

By introducing a computer convenient anesthesia record (6) could be realized, that the datas processing of a large numer of anesthesia records and connected with these records a lot of information were cleared up. And so the connections and the efficiency of anesthesias are more obvious.
First we used the edge punch card (7) which was soon replaced by the mark sense card (8). The informations and findings of these data carriers were read automatically and processed by computers. In 1976 these mark sense cards were revised and simplified because of the experiences. But it was too much work for both the documentation-secretary and the anesthesiologists. So in 1978 these data carriers were replaced. From this time the informations and datas were input off-line by a documentation-secretary over a terminal. In order to simplify and to shorten this work the anesthesia record and the software had to be changed.

The anesthesia record

The used anesthesia record includes all data and findings in a place sparing manner which had been documented on mark sense cards in earlier times. Data of the pre-, intra- and postoperative condition of the patient are registered. The back of the record is reserved to document the stay in the recovery room e.g. circulation data, treatment, fluid balance, condition, when coming in and leaving the room and the place of the patients' transfer.

Hardware

In the system proposed DIETZ computers are used. It is set up with a safety device as a double computer system. In the periphery a scope is present showing an alphanumerical and graph display of the data.
The intermediary data stores appear on two doublerecord store-mechanisms. The final stores are on tapes.

Software

For data registration, the Multi user system of DIETZ computers is used. The necessary time for data input of one anesthesia record requires three minutes and is done by one documentation-secretary. The processing and data presentation into the central unit is carried out in the formula language CBASIC. The choice of data presentation is simplified by a menue which shows the possibilities of the data presentation:

- Distribution of anesthesia services
- Distribution of parameters to the complete institute
- Distribution of parameters to single clinics
- Complications

The presentation of complications is done in various ways (Fig.) and it is possible to answer some questions of connections to preexisting diseases or to preexisting risks. Furthermore, we are able to present the data of records distinguished by complications.

COMPLICATIONS:

1 All complications

2 All complications of one anesthesiologist

3 Complications dependent on urgency

4 Complications and risks dependent on choice of anesthesia

Discussion

There is no doubt, that the data volume of a large number of anesthesia records (n: 20 000 per anno) can be processes only by computers (1, 2, 3, 4, 9, 10). Experiences - made by edge punch cards and mark sense cards in the last ten years - show that this data volume was only processed by an immense work and time. The cards used have to be proved and corrected. The time of control took as long as to fill out the cards.

Caused by the great stress of the anesthesiologists it was not efficient to give back each incorrect card, the analysis and processing could not be done in time (5). Further on the temptation was great to record and to process as many data as possible, without critical choice. In 1975 the annual statistics consisted of one hundred pages and it was very difficult to obtain a general view (5).

The final advantage of our new system is the clear arrangement of data and the simplicity of handling. A false marking or punching of cards is not possible, faults are minimized. The dialogue input of our program enables to control the plausibility of findings and data on the console. This is impossible using mark sense cards: the card has to be corrected by the related anesthesia record before read by the computer. The correction requires too much time. The required time for the new system is only one minute for checking off some rubrics, which is easier than the exact marking of a mark sense card (6). Therefore, the anesthesiologist is not turned away from surveillance of vital functions of this patient.

The data processing is made by the computer in our institute, which includes the advantage, that datas are available at each time. It is easy to change the program in a short time if there are different problems. By this system guarantees a maximum of flexibility.

The now used program enables us to solve some questions which are of special interest. We can demonstrate the relation of preexisting diseases, risks of anesthesia proceedings to intra- or postoperative complications.

Conclusions

The up to now extensive experiences with data carriers in the anesthesiology show that the now used system is most comfortable and very easy to handle and requires minimal time. Data presentation and processing is possible at any time. Furthermore we are able to demonstrate relations of preexisting risks and secondary diseases to complications.

References:

(1) Borchert K, Benad G, Thierbach F, Kampbehl H-J, Franke H, Bindernagel U. Erfahrungen mit einem EDV-gerechten Dokumentationssystems in der Anästhesie. Zbl Chir 1972 ; 97 : 1612

(2) Brückner JB, Bonhoeffer K, Mertens W. Planung und Organisation eines Anästhesiedokumentations-Systems mit maschineller Datenverarbeitung. Anaesthesist 1968 ; 17 : 135.

(3) Immich H. Problematik der Dokumentation in der Anästhesiologie. Z prakt Anästh 1970 ; 5 : 1

(4) Kleinheisterkamp U, Fassl H. Erfahrungen mit dem anästhesiologischen Dokumentationssystem der Universitätsklinik Mainz. Z prakt Anästh 1970 ; 5 : 35

(5) Kunze I. Rechnergestützte Patientenüberwachung in der Anästhesie und Intensivtherapie. Am Beispiel des Institutes für Anästhesiologie und Reanimation der Städt. Krankenanstalten Mannheim. Diplomarbeit der Universität Heidelberg, Fachhochschule Heilbronn, im Studiengang Med. Informatik 1979

(6) Lutz H, Peter K, Ahlborn E, Winnewisser W. Erster Erfahrungsbericht über den praktischen Einsatz des neuentwickelten Anästhesieprotokolls "Mannheim" zur maschinellen Datenverarbeitung. Anaesthesiol Inform 1970 ; 5 : 2

(7) Lutz H, Beimel R. Anästhesiedokumentation mit der Randlochkarte. Z prakt Anästh 1970 ; 1 : 28

(8) Lutz H. Direkte maschinelle Datenerfassung und Datenverarbeitung mit Markierungsbelegen und Markierungslesern. Z prakt Anästh 1970 ; 5 : 45

(9) Wawersik J. Datenverarbeitung in der Anästhesie am Beispiel eines dokumentationsgerechten Narkoseprotokolls. Z prakt Anästh 1970 ; 5 : 6

(10) Wawersik J, Köhler C, Bock B v. Datenauswahl und praktische Durchführung einer anästhesiologischen Basisdokumentation. Z prakt Anästh 1972 ; 7 : 14

HOSPITALISATIONS DUES A LA PATHOLOGIE IATROGENE DANS UN SERVICE DE REANIMATION MULTIDISCIPLINAIRE

P.TRUNET, JR. LE GALL HOPITAL HENRI MONDOR 94010 CRETEIL CEDEX

We prospectively studied all admissions to a multidisciplinary intensive care unit in order to determine how many were due to iatrogenic diseases and of these, what number were potentially avoidable. Iatrogenic disease was defined as a disease induced by either drug treatment, medical or surgical actions. We used precise criteria to determine the cause and effect relationship between the medical action, the patient's reaction and the severity. Of 325 patients admitted in the course of one year 41 patients (12.6 %) were hospitalized because of the iatrogenic disease. Many of these patients had concomitant serious illnesses. Nevertheless nearly half (19 patients or 46.3 %) of iatrogenic admissions were admitted with iatrogenic disease due to therapeutic or technical errors that were potentially avoidable. Iatrogenic disease was fatal in 8 cases, life threatening in 13, moderate in 20.

La pathologie iatrogène est considérée par certains auteurs comme un problème majeur du fait de sa morbidité et de son cout hospitalier. Une étude prospective a été réalisée dans un service de réanimation multidisciplinaire afin de déterminer la fréquence des hospitalisations dues à la pathologie iatrogène, et d'évaluer la gravité et la pathologie iatrogène évitable. MATERIEL & METHODES - Patients : Durant un an, un échantillon statistiquement représentatif de 325 patients hospitalisés dans le service a été analysé. - Définition : La pathologie iatrogène (P.I) a été définie comme la pathologie indépendante d'une éventuelle affection sous jacente et due au médecin. Elle comprend les affections dues à une prescription médicamenteuse, à un acte médical ou chirurgical, à visée prophylactique, diagnostique ou thérapeutique. Les intoxications volontaires ou accidentelles, les toxicomanies, l'aggravation des maladies par absence ou retard du traitement ont été exclues. - Pathologie iatrogène due aux médicaments : La relation de cause à effet entre le médicament et la pa thologie a été définie par 3 critères : 1. Intervalle de temps plausible entre l'administration du médicament et la réaction observée. 2. Réaction indésirable du médicament déjà connue dans la littérature médicale. 3. Accident non raisonnablement expliqué par l'affection sous jacente. La P.I due aux médicaments a été divisée en effets indésirables des médicaments et erreurs thérapeutiques. - Pathologie iatrogène due aux actes médicaux et chirurgicaux : La relation de cause à effet entre l'acte médical ou chirurgical et la pathologie a été définie par l'existence de 3 des 5 critères suivants : 1. Intervalle de temps plausible entre l'acte et la pathologie observée. 2. Pathologie due à l'acte déjà connue dans la littérature médicale. 3. Accident non raisonnablement expliqué par l'affection sous jacente. 4. Critères bactériologiques en cas de pathologie iatrogène infectieuse. 5. Critères anatomiques en cas de P.I mécanique. Les erreurs techniques dues aux actes médicaux ou chirurgicaux ont été établies selon des critères anatomiques. - Gravité de la P.I : La P.I a été jugée fatale si la mort est due directement ou indirectement à la P.I, toute autre cause étant exclue par la nécropsie. La P.I a été considérée comme sévère si des techniques thérapeutiques spécifiques à la réanimation ont été nécessaires, et si le patient a survécu. La P.I a été considérée comme modérée si seulement des techniques de surveillance ont été nécessaires.. RESULTATS : Parmi les 325 patients de l'étude, la P.I a été responsable de l'hospitalisation de 41 patients (12.6 %)(20 femmes,21 hommes,âge moyen 58 ans). La P.I était due aux médicaments dans 23 cas (7.1 %), aux actes médicaux dans 13 cas (4 %), et aux actes chirurgicaux dans 5 cas (1.5 %). La P.I était due à une erreur thérapeutique ou technique chez 19 patients (46.3 %). La P.I a été fatale dans 8 cas, sévère dans 13 cas, modérée dans 20 cas. La P.I était associée à une autre pathologie dans 15 cas (fatale 2, sévère 9, modérée 4) et à un cancer en évolution 5 fois. Parmi les 41 patients, 27 viennent d'un autre service hospitalier et 14 de leur domicile.

DISCUSSION : La fréquence de la P.I responsable de l'admission dans notre service est importante, quatre faits peuvent l'expliquer : 1. Le type prospectif de l'étude (1). 2. Notre méthode de surveillance (2). 3. L'origine de nos patients : 60 % de nos patients viennent d'un hopital, représentant en fait la P.I acquise au cours de l'hospitalisation. La sévérité de la P.I observée est due en grande partie à l'existence d'une affection concomittante sévère ou d'une affection maligne (20 patients). Ceci est retrouvé dans la littérature : les affections graves nécessitent des traitements non dénués de risques (3). Les erreurs thérapeutiques ou techniques représentent 46.3 % des admissions dues à la P.I. Par définition, ces erreurs doivent être diminuées ou éliminées par l'éducation des médecins (1, 4).

CONCLUSION : Les hospitalisations dues à la P.I. ont été étudiées de façon prospective dans un service de réanimation multidisciplinaire en utilisant des critères précis définissant la relation de cause à effet, les erreurs thérapeutiques ou techniques, et la gravité de la P.I. Les résultats montrent une fréquence importante d'hospitalisation dues à la P.I (12.6 %), et une haute fréquence d'erreurs thérapeutiques ou techniques (46.3 %). Ces erreurs thérapeutiques ou techniques représentent une P.I évitable. Cependant d'autres études multicentriques doivent être entreprises, calculer le rapport risque bénéfice de l'action médicale qui doit être prise en compte dans la décision thérapeutique.

REFERENCES : 1. Karch FE. Adverse drug reactions. A critical review. JAMA. 1975 ; 234: 1236-41

2. Cluff LE, Thornton GF, Seidl LG, Studies on the epidemiology of adverse drug reactions. JAMA. 1964 ; 188 : 976-83

3. Koch-Weser J. Fatal reactions to drug therapy. N.Engl J Med. 1974;291 : 302-3

4. Melmon KL. Preventable drug reactions. Cause and cures. N Engl J Med. 1971 ; 284 : 1361-8

SIMULATION AND QUEUEING MODELS TO ASSIST PLANNING OF ACCIDENT AND EMERGENCY SERVICES

D W Inman, J Henry, P Melville
North-East Thames Regional Health Authority
Management Services Division
The John Ellicott Centre
Cavell Street
London E.1
United Kingdom Telephone: 01 - 247 - 5454 x 611

ABSTRACT

A reduction in the number of accident and emergency units has long been a planning priority in the UK. And yet nationally, only broad planning guidelines exist to aid effective planning of accident and emergency care.

Two models have been developed to aid this planning process. The models allow analysis of an A & E department in some detail, and it is possible to experiment with changes in workload, staff/facility levels and operational policies.

The assumptions inherent in the models, and the model results are compared. A case study, using the models in one London health district, is outlined.

1 INTRODUCTION

In 1962, the Standing Medical Advisory Committee on Accident and Emergency Services in the UK recommended a substantial reduction in the number of accident and emergency units, advising that each unit serve a population of at least 150,000. More recently health services in the UK have been operating under tight financial constraints; this has resulted in hospital closures and rationalisation of health service provision. Closure of an acute hospital, or a change in role away from acute care, inevitably requires closure of any existing accident and emergency department, which typically provides about 10% of hospital admissions.

Adequate provision must obviously be found elsewhere. Questions must be answered as to where patients will transfer, and what changes are required, if any, in A & E provision at these sites. Whilst broad planning guidelines exist for A & E departments (1), (2), these relate to average dimensions within a department and to a broad range of catchment population. To answer questions about appropriate staff/resource levels and operational policies within a particular department, taking account of the needs of the local population, more detailed planning aids are required.

Two models have been developed to assist planning of A & E services, and these have been applied in one London health district. The models allow investigation of the effects of changes in workload, staff levels, facilities provided and operational policies within an A & E department.

This paper outlines these models, and a case study is presented in which these models were used to aid rationalisation of A & E provision.

2 THE PROBLEM

By early 1979, a decision had been taken to rationalise health service provision in one of the London health districts. An under provision of care for long stay patients had been recognised for some time against a background of acute provision above the national average. As part of the strategic plan it was decided to investigate the possibility of changing the role of one hospital in the district from acute to long stay care. This would result in closure of the existing A & E department, and concentration of A & E care at one hospital in the district. A study was set up to consider the resources and organisation required at this site, to meet the total A & E needs of the district. The study required two major elements of work; determination of the A & E workload that would attend at the one site in the district and the construction of models to translate this demand into staff and facility requirements.

3 ANALYSIS OF WORKLOAD

There are two main factors which determine workload; firstly the numbers of patients requiring care and secondly the resources required by these patients within an A & E department.

(a) Patients attending

Three elements of workload were considered:

(i) Catchment Areas

Closure of an A & E department implies transfer of work to nearby hospitals. A six week sample of attenders in the district, information from the local Community Health Council (3) and an analysis of the available transport network was used to estimate catchment areas and transfer of work. Sensitivity analysis, when running the model experiments, allowed the effect of assumptions inherent in this analysis to be investigated.

(ii) Trends and Future Requirements

The effect of general trends over the last five years, changes in primary care provision and possible future A & E closures were looked at. A further 10% increase in workload was allowed for.

(iii) Patterns of Attendance

These are shown in Figures 1 and 2 averaged over a four month period. For the purpose of modelling the arrival of patients, the day was split into four periods (0801-1300; 1301-1700; 1701-2100; 2101-0800).

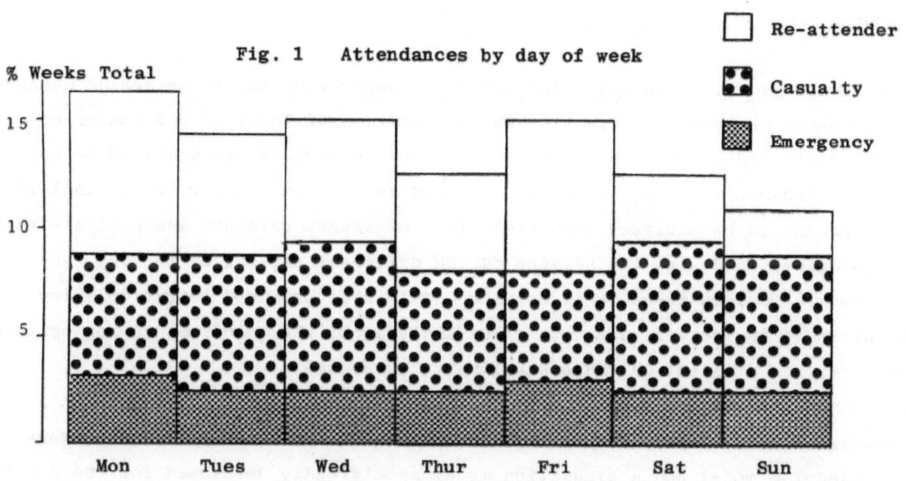

Fig. 1 Attendances by day of week

Fig. 2 Attendances by hour of day

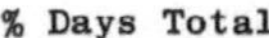

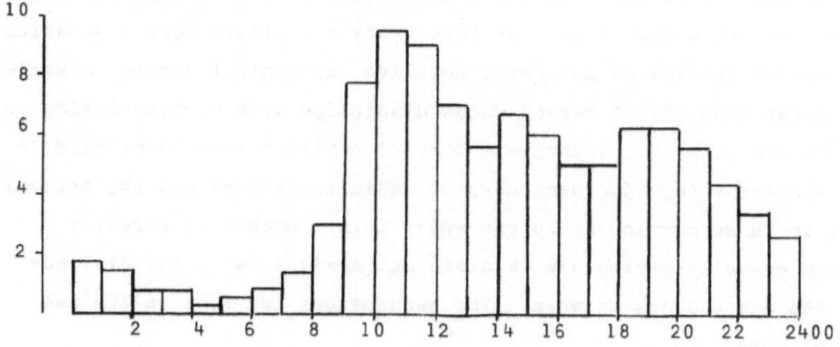

(b) <u>Resource Requirements</u>

A survey, recording the treatment of every patient over a one week period, was carried out to investigate the resources required by patients within the A & E departments. The facilities used, staff seen as well as treatment and waiting times were recorded. Fifty-eight patient flows through the departments, and twenty-one service entities which could cause the patient to wait were identified. Whilst the majority of patient flows involved fewer than four treatment episodes, a small proportion of patients required up to seven distinct episodes with up to four entities being used in any one episode. The complexity of some of the patient flows required care when modelling the department and resulted in two models being developed.

4 THE MODELS

One of the first stages in modelling the A & E department was to determine measures of performance whereby the effect of any combination of workload and resources could be evaluated. For this study, service to the patient, as measured by waiting times and throughput times, was used. The models allowed the service to individual patient groups to be analysed separately (eg. emergency patients and patients with minor injuries), and also the service during different periods of the day, and day of week. Besides these measures, the models also produced output to allow bottlenecks to be identified and to allow analysis of the requirements for waiting space; service utilisation and queue lengths were used.

Two models were developed, both using a computer for rapid analysis; a conventional queueing model and a simulation model specifically developed for the A & E departments in this London district.

(a) Queueing Model

Much has been written in the literature about models of queueing systems; (4), (5), (6) are some examples. For this study a multiple server queueing model with random arrival of patients, negative exponential service distribution and first come, first served queue discipline with no restriction on queue lengths was adopted. Twenty-one service entities were identified in the A & E department (eg. doctors, nurses, cubicles, X-ray) and the arrival of patients to these service areas was split into a number of streams; emergency and casualty patients with different arrival rates for distinct periods of the day and day of week. The assumptions inherent in the use of this model were:

- The service times were assumed to follow a negative exponential distribution; the evidence provided by the survey generally supported this assertion. An allowance was made for personal and administrative duties of staff.

- The arrival of patients to the service areas was assumed to follow a Poisson distribution. This fitted quite well with the observed pattern of arrivals at the department, but was questionable for services used later in the course of treatment (eg. X-ray).

- No restriction on queue lengths was assumed. Whilst this is not a valid assumption, theory predicts that provided utilisation of a service area does not rise above 80%, average queue lengths would not exceed five. However the use of this model for detailed analysis of bottlenecks is questionable.

- A specific assumption in this study was that combining two streams of patients (eg. pooling the work of emergency and casualty doctors) would result in a Poisson (combined) arrival process and a negative exponential service distribution; the former is theoretically valid but the latter is not.

A major limitation of the queueing approach was that a bottleneck at one service entity does not "spill-over" to other service areas. Furthermore, because the department was analysed for distinct periods of the day, taken in isolation, a build-up of patients waiting during one period of the day would not transfer to subsequent periods.

For these reasons, and because some of the assumptions inherent in the queueing model were in question, a simulation model was developed to more accurately reflect the operation of an A & E department.

(b) Simulation Model

A discrete, event step simulation model was developed. Twenty-one service areas formed the core of the simulation model. Each service area was described in terms of the number of patients that could be seen simulta- neously, for any hour during the week. This allowed staff rotas to be accurately respresented within the model. The time patients spent at any service area was described by the sum of a constant and a random variate from a negative exponential distribution, the distribution used being a function of the service area; this fitted the observed service distributions well for most service areas. As for the queueing model an allowance was made for personal and administrative duties.

The one week survey identified fifty-eight patient flows during the course of treatment. Each flow was treated as a separate arrival input stream to the department. As for the queueing model, a random arrival process was used for any one input stream, with different mean arrival rates by time of day and day of week; this corresponds well with the observed arrival patterns.

Two queue disciplines were investigated with this model. Currently patients are pre-assigned to a doctor on arrival by use of a ticket system. This was compared with a first come, first served discipline. In either case patient were given one of three priorities; emergency, casualty requiring urgent attention and minor injury. Patients in the course of treatment were given preference over patients of the same priority who had not yet received attention. The queue discipline operated only for patients of the same priority; emergency patients would always be seen before patients with mino injuries irrespective of time of arrival for example.

Because of the flexibility of the simulation model, a number of other aspect of the operation of an A & E department were incorporated. Patients could be directed to the same doctor throughout the course of treatment, and could occupy resources (nurses or cubicles) whilst waiting for treatment for example. It was also possible to model more accurately the pooling of resources than with the queueing model, and to investigate likely maximum queue lengths.

5 MODEL RESULTS

Detailed results of the model experiments are given in (7). In this section some of the results are outlined, and comparisons made between the two models.

(a) The effect of closure

The workload at the single remaining A & E department in the district was increased appropriately and bottlenecks identified. The models were used in an interactive process, increasing resources at the bottlenecks so as to restore service to the patients to current levels.

The results for key resources are shown in Table 1.

TABLE 1 Changes in Key Resource Levels

	Morning	Afternoon	Evening	Night
Medical Staffing	+80%	+50%	+50%	0%
Treatment Areas	+80%	+50%	0%	0%
X-Ray	+150%	+100%	0%	0%
Waiting Space	+30%	+30%	0%	0%

The two models gave similar results for the best estimate of work transfer. However the results were found to be sensitive to both the transfer of work and peaks in workload. Furthermore the model results diverged in these circumstances; the simulation model predicting the requirement for higher resource levels. This perhaps indicates how the queueing model ignores "spill-over" of work from one part of the day to another and inadequately models complex queueing systems with very high utilisation of the service areas.

The simulation model showed the necessity of changing staff rotas; an extension of cover in the evening and morning were shown to be necessary to keep queue sizes manageable.

(b) <u>The effects of the ticket system for casualty patients</u>

Using the simulation model, experiments were carried out to compare two alternative queue disciplines for patients with minor injuries; first come, first served versus the ticket system of allocating doctors to patients on arrival. The ticket system led to patients having to wait longer to see a doctor, to less even utilisation of the doctors' time and to greater requirements for waiting space (up by about 25%). It was therefore recommended that the ticket system be abolished.

(c) <u>The effect of pooling resources</u>

The purpose of pooling is to speed patient flow through the department by allowing any of the pooled doctors to examine and treat any patient, rather than some doctors being assigned only to emergency cases and others to patients with minor injuries. At present pooling only exists during evenings, nights and weekends, at the main A & E department in the district.

It was found that pooling improved the service to both types of patient. Initial waiting time was reduced by 20 - 30% and total waiting time by 30 - 45%. Pooling also reduced the queue lengths by up to 50%; both average and maximum queue lengths were reduced.

6 CONCLUSIONS

Using the results from the two models, recommendations were made on staff levels and facilities required to meet an increase in workload due to closure of one A & E department within this London health district. Experimentation on the models indicated that certain policies, currently in operation at the district's major A & E department, do not lead to the best service to the patient, and alternatives have been proposed. It is anticipated that it would be beneficial to implement these changes, irrespective of any increase in workload.

The models did not investigate the interaction of an A & E department with the rest of the hospital in any detail, and it is felt that this is a fruitful area for further work.

REFERENCES

1 Packwood T., The Organisation of Accident and Emergency Departments. Health and Social Services Journal. July 1974 1677-79.

2 Ministry of Health. Accident and Emergency Department. Hospital Building Note 22. London. HMSO. 1964.

3 The Use of Accident and Emergency Services in Harringay. (1). London. Harringay Community Health Council. 1979.

4 Cox D.R., Smith W.L. Queues. London. Chapman & Hall. 1971.

5 Benes V.E. General Stochastic Processes in the Theory of Queues. London. Addison-Wesley. 1963.

6 Riordan J. Stochastic Service Systems. Sussex. John Wiley and Sons. 1962.

7 N.E. Thames R.H.A. Study of Accident and Emergency Services in Harringay Health District. London. NETRHA. 1980.

EVALUATION D'UN PROGRAMME DE CHIRURGIE D'UN JOUR

A.P. Contandriopoulos, J.M. Lance,
M.L. McConnell-Bastian, R. Pineault*, M. Valois
Département d'administration de la santé
Université de Montréal, Montréal
H3C 3J7

One day surgery programs have developed rapidly in recent years, mainly as a result of government committments in several countries to contain hospital costs. This form of surgical care seems to be effective in reducing the length of in-hospital stay and consequently hospital costs. Our study objective is to evaluate by a randomized control trial (RCT), clinical results, patient satisfaction and costs associated with three surgical procedures, (tubal ligation, menisectomy, hernia repair) according to whether it is done in one-day surgery or hospitalization.

Face à une volonté des gouvernements de plusieurs pays de stabiliser le niveau des dépenses du secteur hospitalier, la chirurgie d'un jour connaît un développement rapide. Ce mode de soins apparaît comme un moyen de réduire les durées de séjour et donc les coûts hospitaliers. L'objectif de notre étude est d'évaluer au moyen d'un essai contrôlé aléatoire, les résultats cliniques, la satisfaction des patients et les coûts associés à trois interventions chirurgicales (ligature de trompes, ménisectomie, herniorraphie) selon que le mode de traitement est la chirurgie d'un jour ou l'hospitalisation.

1. INTRODUCTION

La chirurgie d'un jour ou "court-séjour" est le mode de soins selon lequel certains actes chirurgicaux effectués sous anesthésie générale et qui nécessitent habituellement l'hospitalisation peuvent être pratiqués efficacement sur une base ambulatoire. Cette définition exclut les actes mineurs pouvant être effectués en clinique externe ou au bureau du chirurgien.

La chirurgie d'un jour, se pratique depuis quelques décennies et son développement rapide au cours des dernières années est principalement relié au coût croissant de l'hospitalisation. Comme mode de distribution de soins pouvant constituer une alternative à l'hospitalisation, la chirurgie d'un jour est appelée à prendre de l'expansion tant du côté du volume des interventions que de leur complexité.

Certains avantages sont généralement associés à la chirurgie d'un jour. Au niveau des institutions, il est reconnu que des économies peuvent être réalisées si l'unité de chirurgie ambulatoire constitue une substitution à des lits d'hospitalisation déjà existants, ou si elle réduit les besoins en immobilisation. Selon le "Rapport du comité d'étude sur l'implantation des services ambulatoires spécialisés"(1), une unité de 12 lits de chirurgie d'un jour serait l'équivalent en productivité de 34

---

* Département de médecine sociale et préventive, Université de Montréal

lits d'hospitalisation. Le maintien du patient dans son milieu de même que la diminution du risque d'infection nosocomiale comptent parmi les avantages importants de la chirurgie ambulatoire.

Soulignons enfin que les autorités gouvernementales ont de plus en plus tendance à compter sur les soins d'un jour et même à privilégier ce mode de soins pour réduire ou tout au moins contenir les coûts toujours croissants de l'hospitalisation.

2. OBJECTIF ET DESCRIPTION DE LA RECHERCHE

L'objectif du projet d'évaluation de la chirurgie d'un jour est de réaliser une étude comparative de l'épisode de soins de certaines interventions chirurgicales selon deux modes: a) le traitement à l'unité de court séjour; b) le traitement par l'hospitalisation. La comparaison porte sur les trois aspects suivants: les résultats cliniques, la satisfaction et les coûts de l'épisode de soins. Les interventions retenues sont: la méniscectomie, l'herniorraphie et la ligature de trompes par laparoscopie.

Pour atteindre notre objectif, nous avons organisé un essai contrôlé aléatoire illustré au schéma 1. Chaque fois qu'un patient doit être opéré pour une des interventions retenues, le médecin évalue si le patient peut être traité en court séjour sans risques et conséquences pour sa santé. Ensuite, le chirurgien explique à ce sujet éligible à la chirurgie d'un jour que le mode de soins (court séjour, hospitalisation) lui sera communiqué lors de sa convocation pour les examens pré-opératoires. Si à ce moment le sujet exprime une préférence pour un mode plutôt que l'autre, il est non éligible à l'étude et fera partie des patients qui exercent leur choix. Enfin, tous les sujets éligibles à l'étude sont répartis au hasard entre le court séjour et l'hospitalisation. L'étude porte principalement sur ces sujets. Cependant, ceux qui exercent leur choix seront comparés au groupe des sujets répartis au hasard au niveau de la satisfaction. D'autre part, une analyse des dossiers des patients non éligibles dont l'état requiert l'hospitalisation, nous fournira des indications sur les facteurs empêchant une intervention en court séjour. Notre échantillon comporte 60 patients éligibles à l'étude pour chacune des interventions donnant un nombre total de 180 sujets répartis, aléatoirement entre le court séjour et l'hospitalisation.

SCHEMA 1: STRUCTURE DES GROUPES A L'ETUDE

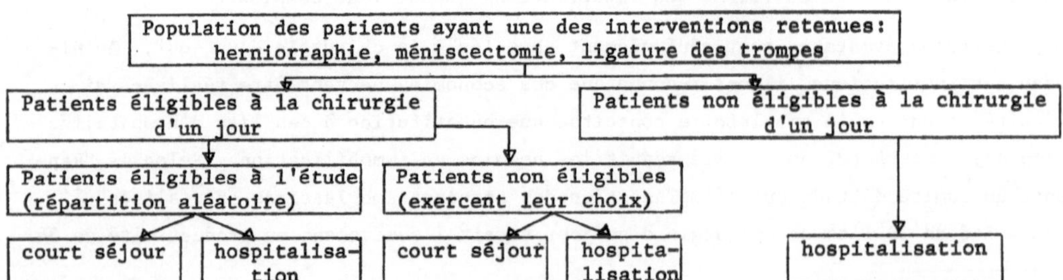

3. DESCRIPTION DES INSTRUMENTS DE MESURE

Les instruments de mesure que nous avons élaborées servent à la cueillette d'informations sur les coûts de l'épisode de soins, la satisfaction et les résultats cliniques. Les sources de données sont principalement: le patient, le dossier médical et le budget de l'hôpital. Les instruments évaluant les effets du mode de traitement et les dépenses personnelles sont administrés au patient à l'admission, 7 jours, 1 mois et 3 mois après l'opération tandis que les grilles des ressources utilisées en milieu hospitalier sont complétées à la fin de l'épisode.

3.1 Les coûts de l'épisode de soins

L'épisode de soins est défini comme étant la période de temps qui se déroule depuis la visite au chirurgien lors de laquelle la décision d'opérer est prise jusqu'à ce que le sujet reprenne ses activités normales après l'opération. Durant cette période, nous dénombrons tous les soins et services médicaux reçus par le sujet pour le traitement de son problème médical spécifique.

L'ensemble des coûts qui font l'objet de l'étude regroupe les coûts privés et les coûts sociaux, tel qu'illustré au schéma 2. Les coûts privés sont les dépenses encourues par le sujet pour l'aide à domicile, les déplacements, les pertes de salaire et autres dépenses. Les coûts sociaux, d'autre part, englobent les coûts faisant partie du budget de fonctionnement de l'hôpital et les coûts supportés par les régimes d'Assurance-Maladie et d'Assurance-Hospitalisation.

SCHEMA 2: COUTS DE L'EPISODE DE SOINS

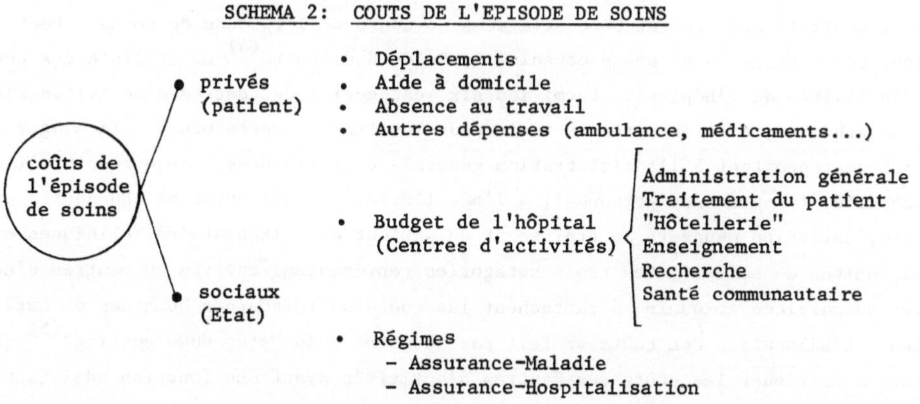

Les coûts sociaux sont établis en réalisant les étapes suivantes: identification des unités d'output; identification et valorisation monétaire des inputs faisant partie du budget de l'hôpital; identification et valorisation monétaire des inputs ne faisant pas partie du budget de l'hôpital; allocation des inputs par unité d'output.

Cette démarche rejoint l'approche du "disease costing"[2] qui nous amène à identifier des épisodes de soins qui utilisent une quantité de ressources dans le but d'aider à retrouver l'état de santé initial. Cette approche donne des résultats plus spécifiques que l'utilisation de coûts moyens des différents services hospitaliers reçus. Nous postulons alors que le produit "santé" s'apparente à la somme des ressources utilisées sur une période de temps pour retrouver la santé. Le schéma 3 adapté de Levy[3] illustre ce concept.

SCHEMA 3: COUTS DE RESTAURATION DE LA SANTE

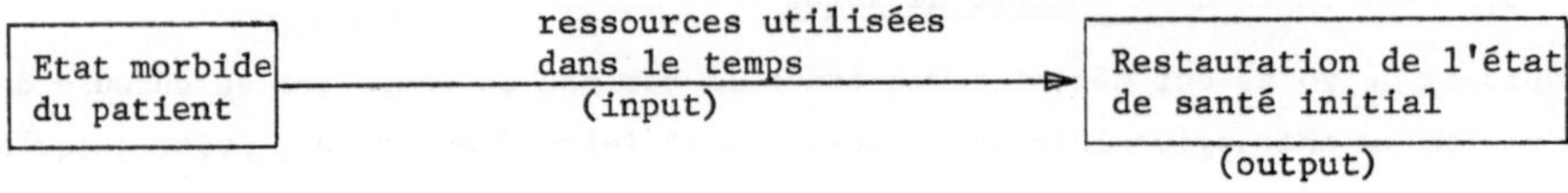

3.1.1 Identification des unités d'output

Dans notre étude les unités d'output sont facilement identifiées. Il s'agit des épisodes de soins de la méniscectomie, de l'herniorraphie, de la ligature des trompes. Ainsi le coût du produit "santé" est le coût de toutes les ressources utilisées durant l'épisode de soins dans le but de régler un problème de santé spécifique.

3.1.2 Identification et valorisation monétaire des inputs faisant partie du budget de l'hôpital

L'identification des inputs consiste à inventorier toutes les ressources (du budget de l'hôpital) qui peuvent être utilisées au cours de l'épisode de soins. Pour réaliser cette étape, nous avons consulté le Guide Budgétaire[4] et la liste des centres d'activités de l'hôpital. Parmi les six catégories de centres d'activités énumérées au schéma 2, nous en retenons trois pour les fins de cette étude. Il s'agit de ceux qui se rapportent à l'administration générale e.g. finances, ressources humaines, comptabilité, formation du personnel; à l'hôtellerie e.g. alimentation, buanderie et lingerie, entretien ménager; au traitement du patient e.g. laboratoire, cliniques externes, unités de soins. Ces trois catégories représentent environ 40 centres d'activités ou services auxquels se rattachent les coûts en ressources humaines et matérielles. L'allocation des coûts se fait par la méthode du "step down costing"[5] qui consiste à attribuer les coûts des centres d'activités ayant une fonction administrative ou hôtellière aux centres d'activités liés au traitement du patient. Le schéma 4 illustre le processus de valorisation monétaire à l'aide de deux exemples. Dans le premier cas, nous voulons établir le coût des soins infirmiers par patient. Pour ce faire, nous utilisons une grille adaptée de PRN 76[6] pour recueillir le temps consacré aux soins infirmiers par patient. Ensuite, nous appliquons un salaire horaire pour obtenir un coût/patient. Dans le deuxième cas, nous voulons déterminer les coûts de l'entretien ménager d'un service. C'est à l'aide du nombre de m^2 qu'occupe ce service et du coût/m^2 obtenu du budget de l'hôpital que nous pouvons obtenir un coût/service.

Cette démarche est répétée pour chacun des centres d'activités du budget de l'hôpital impliqué dans l'épisode de soins.

SCHEMA 4: VALORISATION MONETAIRE DES RESSOURCES

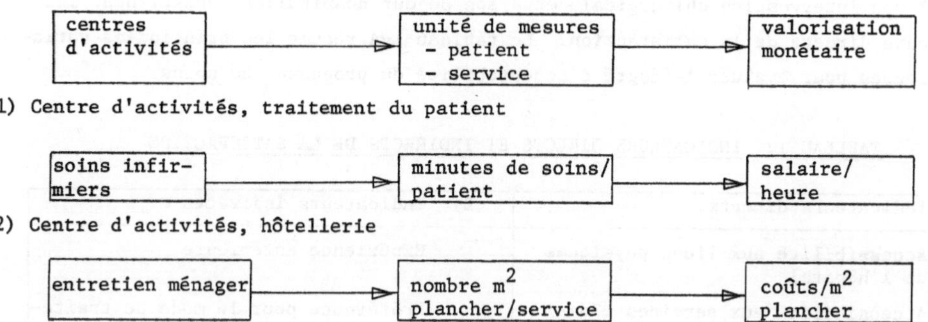

3.1.3 Identification et valorisation monétaire des inputs ne faisant pas partie du budget

Nous entendons par inputs ne faisant pas partie du budget toutes les ressources utilisées lors de l'épisode de soins qui sont financées par l'Etat mais qui ne font pas partie du budget de l'hôpital, e.g. visites chez le médecin, rémunération pour l'intervention chirurgicale. Les sources de renseignements pour la tarification de ces actes sont les manuels des différents régimes d'assurance santé du Québec[(7)(8)(9)].

3.1.4 Allocation des intrants par unité d'extrant

Cette étape consiste à faire la somme de toutes les ressources utilisées pour chaque épisode de soins donc pour chaque patient. Il s'agit d'une étape de réconciliation des ressources utilisées et de leur valeur monétaire, par épisode de soins.

3.2 Satisfaction

L'évaluation de la satisfaction des patients est une préoccupation importante, même s'il demeure difficile d'évaluer un tel sujet, compte tenu des problèmes de validité de mesure. Cependant, l'aspect comparatif de l'étude réduit les difficultés de validité interne car il s'agit de voir des différences entre les groupes pour certains critères établis plutôt que de construire une échelle de satisfaction.

En nous inspirant des études générales de la satisfaction[(10)(11)] et après une période d'observation pour tenir compte des particularités de l'hôpital, nous avons développé une série d'indicateurs visant à évaluer le niveau de satisfaction en relation avec le traitement reçu. Ces indicateurs ont constitué la première ébauche du questionnaire qui a été ensuite soumis à un jury pour l'évaluation du contenu. Les recommandations de ces juges nous ont permis d'élaborer la liste des indicateurs que nous avons définis comme: 1) indicateurs directs de la satisfaction; 2) indicateurs indirects de la satisfaction.

3.2.1 Indicateurs directs de la satisfaction

Les variables utilisées pour mesurer la perception du patient quant aux événements reliés à son intervention chirurgicale et à son séjour hospitalier, constituent les indicateurs directs de la satisfaction. Le tableau 1-A résume les principales variables retenues pour évaluer le degré d'acceptabilité du processus de soins.

TABLEAU 1: INDICATEURS DIRECTS ET INDIRECTS DE LA SATISFACTION

A) Indicateurs directs	B) Indicateurs indirects
Accessibilité aux lieux physiques de l'hôpital	Expérience antérieure
Accessibilité aux services médicaux	Préférence pour le mode de traitement
Organisation des services	Implication personnelle
Accueil et information reçue	Anxiété
Qualité des soins	Douleur

3.2.2 Indicateurs indirects de la satisfaction

Le degré de satisfaction du patient peut être influencé par d'autres facteurs que les services reçus pendant son séjour hospitalier. Pour cette raison, nous avons ajouté d'autres variables qui, même si elles ne mesurent pas directement le processus de soins, peuvent influencer le niveau général de la satisfaction face au traitement reçu. Tel que noté au Tableau 1-B, les expériences antérieures d'hospitalisation, la préférence quant au mode de traitement et l'implication personnelle, c'est-à-dire la perception des inconvénients reliés à l'intervention, ne sauraient être négligés dans l'analyse globale de la satisfaction.

Si la relation entre l'anxiété et le niveau de la satisfaction est peu documentée cette variable demeure importante dans le cas de bénéficiaires devant subir une intervention chirurgicale. Janis a démontré une corrélation élevée entre le niveau d'anxiété pré-opératoire et la période de rétablissement ainsi qu'un taux plus élevé de complications post-opératoires générales chez les patients anxieux[12]. Dans le cas présent, il sera intéressant au niveau de l'analyse de voir si le niveau d'anxiété varie en fonction du mode de soins (i.e. hospitalisation, court-séjour). L'instrument de mesure que nous avons utilisé est un questionnaire développé aux Etats-Unis par Spielberger et ses coll.[13]. Traduit et validé auprès d'une population francophone québécoise, ce questionnaire a l'avantage d'être facile à administrer et atteint des quotients de validité et de fidélité élevés (de l'ordre de .80).

Une étude de satisfaction menée auprès de patients de clinique externe a montré une relation entre le niveau de douleur perçue par le bénéficiaire et le niveau de satisfaction avec les services rendus[15]. Dans le cadre de notre projet, l'évaluation de cette variable chez les patients hospitalisés et de court séjour, nous permettra de voir si le niveau de douleur perçue varie en fonction du mode de traitement et dans quelle mesure celui-ci peut être associée au degré de satisfaction. L'instrument utilisé est le "McGill Pain Questionnaire"[16].

L'ensemble des indicateurs directs et indirects ont constitué une grande partie du questionnaire d'évaluation de la chirurgie d'un jour administré à domicile au 7ième jour post-opératoire.

3.3 Les indicateurs de résultats cliniques

Du point de vue méthodologique, les indicateurs de satisfaction peuvent être vus comme des variables de processus, c'est-à-dire tous les faits, actions ou événements reliés à l'intervention chirurgicale. Cette section porte au contraire comme son nom l'indique sur les variables de résultats de l'intervention. Pour ce faire, nous avons développé une série d'indicateurs provenant à la fois du bénéficiaire et des sources objectives retrouvées au dossier médical. Le Tableau 2 regroupe l'ensemble des indicateurs évaluant les résultats cliniques en fonction de leur source de provenance.

TABLEAU 2: INDICATEURS DE RESULTATS CLINIQUES

Bénéficiaire	Dossier médical
- Fidélité aux ordonnances médicales - Reprise des activités de la vie quotidienne - Perception de son état général - Présence de problèmes ou de complications - Nombre de consultations avec le chirurgien, un autre médecin à l'urgence - Reprise du travail	- Résultats chirurgical (réadmission, hospitalisation non prévue (court-séjour suelement), décès) - Complications (ex.: arythmie cardiaque, hypotension, choc) - Nombre de consultations avec le chirurgien, un autre médecin à l'urgence (identification du problème)

4. CONCLUSION

Les résultats de notre recherche permettront d'apprécier dans quelle mesure la chirurgie d'un jour est une alternative à l'hospitalisation au niveau des résultats cliniques, de la satisfaction des patients et des coûts, ce qui fournira des éléments au gouvernement pour planifier une meilleure utilisation des ressources hospitalières et aux administrateurs d'hôpitaux pour réviser la répartition de leurs lits. De plus, cette étude constitue une étape dans la détermination de critères d'éligibilité à priori par la connaissance qu'elle nous apporte des caractéristiques des patients, des interventions chirurgicales. Dans une étape ultérieure, on pourra préciser quel genre de patients bénéficieraient le plus de la chirurgie d'un jour et pour quels patients l'hospitalisation serait la plus indiquée. Les résultats de la présente recherche feront l'objet d'une communication ultérieure.

5. BIBLIOGRAPHIE

1)MINISTERE des Affaires Sociales. "Rapport du comité d'étude sur l'implantation des soins ambulatoires spécialisés", M.A.S., Québec, 1976.

2)BABSON, J.H., HEIDEMANN, E., and LAY, C.M. (1975). Disease costing applied to measuring the cost of treating patients undergoing surgical removal of the gall bladder (cholecystectomy), Working Paper No. 75-5, School of Health Administration University of Ottawa.

3)LEVY, E. et autres. Evaluer le coût de la maladie, Paris, Dunod, 296 p.

4)MINISTERE des Affaires Sociales. Guide budgétaire 1979-80 des Centres Hospitaliers, Editeur officiel du Québec, 1979.

5)EVANS, R.G. et autres. A Cost Analysis of Alternatives to Traditional Inpatient Care in a Children's Hospital, Surgical Day Care and Care by Parents, December 1978.

6)TILQUIN, C. et autres. "Determining nursing team size and composition", Dimensions in Health Service, December 1978, pp. 13-16.

7)ASSURANCE-MALADIE DU QUEBEC. Manuel des médecins spécialistes, régime d'assurance-hospitalisation, entente de novembre 1976 et amendements.

8)ASSURANCE-MALADIE DU QUEBEC. Manuel des médecins spécialistes, régime d'assurance-maladie, entente de novembre 1976 et amendements.

9)MANUEL DES MEDECINS OMNIPRATICIENS, régimes d'assurance-maladie et d'assurance-hospitalisation, entente de septembre 1976 et amendements.

10)HULKA, Barbara S. et autres. "Correlates of Satisfaction and Dissatisfaction with Medical Care: A Community Perspective", Medical Care, vol. 13, no. 8, August 1975, pp. 648-658.

11)WARE, John, E., et SNYDER, Mary K. "Dimensions of Patients Attitudes Regarding Doctors and Medical Care Services", Medical Care, vol. 13, no. 8, August 1975, pp. 669-682.

12)JANIS, Irving. Psychological Stress: Psychoanalytic and Behavioral Studies of Surgical Patients. New York: Academic Press, 1974, p. 439.

13)SPIELBERGER et autres. "Manual for the State-Trait Anxiety Inventory", 1970, Palo Alto, California.

14)BERGERON, Jacques, LANDRY, Michel. "La fidélité et la validité de l'adaptation française du questionnaire d'anxiété", 38ième Congrès International de la Psychologie Appliquée (1974).

15)STEWARD, Wankin (1978). "Direct and Indirect Measures of Patients Satisfaction". Journal of Community Health, vol. 13, Spring 1978, pp. 195-204.

16)MELZACK, Ronald. "The McGill Pain Questionnaire: Major Properties and Scoring Methods", Pain 1, 1975, pp. 277-299.

AIDE A L' ANALYSE D'ACTIVITE D' UN SERVICE DE CARDIOLOGIE A PARTIR DU TRAITEMENT PAR ORDINATEUR DES RESUMES D' HOSPITALISATION

Catherine TAINTURIER,+ Michel de HEAULME,+ Christian MERY,+ Yves GROSGOGEAT++.

\+ INSERM U 88 - 91, Boulevard de l'Hôpital 75634 PARIS Cedex 13 FRANCE

++ LA SALPETRIERE Service de Cardiologie H 47, Bld de l'Hôpital 75634 PARIS Cedex 13

Classical ways of Medical activity analysis meets some difficulties : choice of indicators, data categorisation, weak medical motivation etc... The paper presents an other approach from the daily discharge summaries, which becomes attractive an efficient provided data are collected through a controlled language allowing a text content analysis. Exemple is given with REMEDE supporting about 3500 discharge summaries in Cardiology.

L'analyse de l'activité d'un service de Médecine est un problème global qui peut s'aborder de plusieurs manières, dont les plus classiques sont l'audit et l'enquête. En ce dernier cas l'ordinateur sert essentiellement à effectuer les analyses statistiques sur les indicateurs retenus pour les enquêtes.

L'une des difficultés de cette approche est précisément d'avoir à choisir les données qui auront à être analysées, alors que bien souvent on ignore ce qui mériterait d'être recherché et évalué.

Une autre difficulté est que l'utilisation des questionnaires fermés nécessaires au recueil des données à usage statistique ne convient qu'à des études restreintes, sous peine de voir le nombre d'items nécessaires à une description étendue devenir trop important pour être utilisé dans la pratique médicale quotidienne.

Nous présentons aujourd'hui une approche complémentaire de l'analyse d'activité médicale à partir de l'exploitation par ordinateur des résumés du service de Cardiologie de la SALPETRIERE Paris (Pr. Y. GROSGOGEAT) (1).

1. PRINCIPE :

Il s'agit d'utiliser les résumés d'hospitalisation ou de consultation comme une mémoire collective reflétant la réalité de la pratique du service (2). En effet :

- ils contiennent normalement les faits principaux concernant les malades : signes cliniques majeurs, indications diagnostiques, examens lourds, types de traitement

- ils décrivent la combinaison des faits observés, qui échappe à un système de grille prédéterminée en particulier dans le cas des faits nouveaux

- ils contiennent l'évolution de la pratique au cours du temps : modifications des indications thérapeutiques, des investigations diagnostiques etc...

- Enfin, fait capital, leur exploitation correspond à un besoin médical et s'appuie sur une motivation quotidienne.

L'interrogation de ces résumés implique que l'ordinateur sache analyser leur contenu de façon pertinente, avec un minimum de faux positifs, et si possible sans faux négatifs. Pour ce faire les médecins utilisent directement un langage contrôlé, REMEDE (1, 3, 4, 5) développé par le Pr M. de HEAULME au CHU PITIE-SALPETRIERE.

Très brièvement ce langage permet d'utiliser les mots d'usage courant répertoriés dans un lexique, et de construire des "phrases" à l'aide d'une grammaire simple contenant une dizaine d'opérateurs. Le dossier d'un malade comprend un en-tête contenant les informations administratives indispensables précédant le texte du résumé proprement dit. Les dates figurent en marge gauche et caractérisent chaque évènement décrit.

Le suivi du malade se fait en ajoutant de nouvelles phrases datées.

Les résumés sont directement écrits par les Médecins et entrés par les secrétaires médicales à partir d'un terminal implanté dans le cardre du service.

Quatre remarques caractérisent l'utilisation de ce genre de langage :

1.1. Ce sont des langages faciles à manier pour les médecins qui s'expriment directement avec leurs mots habituels. L'apprentissage en est rapide, pour les médecins comme pour les secrétaires.

1.2. Un langage combinatoire permet une description ouverte des faits biocliniques, sans rester prisonnier d'une nomenclature figée. C'est la grande différence entre REMEDE qui atteint ce stade rendant acceptable une écriture directe par les médecins et des systèmes comme SNOMED dont l'utilisation directe paraît encore bien lourde au médecin (6).

1.3. L'exploitation en mode conversationnel est un aspect important du système :

- il facilite la tenue et la validation du fichier ;
- il rend le couple Médecin-Secrétaire responsable de la qualité des informations qu'il manipule ;

- l'interrogation disponible en permanence offre un système beaucoup plus efficace et attirant pour les Médecins.

  En effet :

  . elle répond au besoin ordinaire de sélection des dossiers

  . elle fournit à la demande des résumés dans un langage clair qui permet d'en apprécier le contexte

  . mais surtout elle permet l'interrogatoire pas à pas qui est le mode normal d'interrogation en Médecine, car une réponse unique du genre : "152 malades hospitalisés ont un rétrécissement aortique" est de peu d'intérêt en elle-même. A partir de ce premier résultat, il faut dépouiller le contenu des 152 cas pour en dégager les faits intéressants : examens demandés, intervention chirurgicale, complications etc... Bien souvent c'est au vu d'une réponse et de l'analyse des résumés correspondants que l'on pense à la question suivante. Le mode interactif est alors irremplaçable.

2. APPORT A L' ANALYSE DU SERVICE

La rédaction de résumés n'entraîne pas de soi une systématisation du recueil des données. Le médecin est seul juge de consigner ce qu'il estime intéressant. Il appartient à la communauté des utilisateurs de décider si certains faits doivent être recueillis systématiquement pour répondre à des besoins précis d'interrogation.

- tout d'abord on obtient un certain nombre d'indications classiques comme dans n'importe quel système : effectifs par âge, sexe, médecin, pathologies..., nombre et durée d'hospitalisation des malades par unité de soin etc...

- en ce qui concerne les pathologies rencontrées, un avantage original du système est de pouvoir les détailler à la demande sans être prisonnier d'une catégorisation contraignante, comme celle de l'OMS par exemple.

- REMEDE prépare également une certaine évaluation des procédures médicales en association aux pathologies les examens lourds et les traitements entrepris. Le fait capital est ici <u>l'analyse du contexte clinique qui seul fournit les éléments d'appréciation</u> des indications d'examens ou d'intervention.
  Ce contexte est obtenu :

  . soit par une question plus précise.

  . soit par la lecture au terminal des résumés qui met en évidence des relations ou des faits intéressants passés inaperçus.

- enfin le système peut attirer l'attention des médecins sur la fréquence et le type des complications d'examens ou de traitements.

L'exemple suivant illustre la potentialité d'exploitation des résumés REMEDE à des fins d'analyse d'activité médicale. Il s'agit de l'intérêt de la coronarographie chez les malades atteints de rétrécissement aortique sans valvulopathie associée. L'un des problèmes posés est de déterminer si les malades pourront bénéficier d'un pontage aorto-coronarien lors de la pose de la prothèse valvulaire. L'approche suivante a été obtenue en 2 heures de travail au terminal à partir des dossiers collationnés depuis 2 ans :

2.1. La conduite de tous les médecins du service est assez homogène : la coronarographie est le plus souvent pratiquée chez les malades pour lesquels on soupçonne une athéro-sclérose coronarienne : sexe masculin plus fréquemment, présence d'angor clinique (80 % des cas), association de facteurs de risque.

2.2. L'indication décroît après 70 ans et s'annule après 80 ans.

2.3. Les résultats de la coronarographie ont peu d'influence sur la décision opératoire : un seul malade sur 73 a été récusé pour des lésions coronariennes sévères.

2.4. La coronarographie a modifié le geste opératoire dans 3 cas (pontage associé sans décès post-opératoire) ce qui n'est pas négligeable. Dans 1 cas le malade ne présentait pas de douleurs angineuses.

2.5. Un seul examen sur 73 a été compliqué (anévrysme de l'artère fémorale) : l'examen est pratiquement sans danger dans ce contexte.

2.6. Un certain nombre de dossiers échappe à l'attitude générale parmi les 73 étudiés

. 10 malades présentant un angor clinique n'ont pas eu de coronarographie
. 16 autres malades ont eu une coronarographie alors qu'ils n'avaient pas d'angor.

L'étude de leurs résumés au terminal met aussitôt en évidence :

. que 5 malades du premier groupe ayant eu un angor avaient des raisons médicales de ne pas subir une coronarographie pré-opératoire. 3 parmi eux avaient un rétrécissement aortique très serré avec un retentissement clinique important et ont été opérés directement. Pour les 5 restants, le résumé de dossier n'est pas suffisamment explicite.

. que 13 malades du deuxième groupe ont subi une coronarographie sans raison exprimée dans le résumé.

3. DISCUSSION :

Le cadre de cet article ne permet pas de multiplier les exemples qui d'ailleurs se ressembleraient beaucoup. On peut retenir de la présentation faite les points suivants :

3.1. Les médecins ont à leur disposition un mode d'expression relativement simple, souple d'emploi, dont ils savent qu'ils tireront bénéfice sur le plan documentaire. On sait combien le recueil d'information sans motivation professionnelle peut lasser les médecins et biaiser considérablement les résultats.

3.2. En une séance de travail des faits médicaux déjà complexes sont mis en évidence et "dégrossis" jusqu'au moment où le manque d'information oblige à retourner au dossier complet, mais seulement sur un nombre de dossiers restreint et sachant ce que l'on cherche. On imagine le temps qu'aurait requis le dépouillement des 73 dossiers manuels, qu'il aurait fallu d'abord identifier et retrouver. A fortiori pour des études portant sur plusieurs centaines ou milliers de dossiers.

3.3. Les faits nécessaires à un audit interne sont accessibles en routine, mettant en lumière les conduites générales du service, en matière d'indication d'examens ou de traitements par exemple. De même l'absence de certaines données est mise en évidence et provoque la recherche de cette carence.

3.4. Toutefois cette contribution à l'analyse d'activité médicale a pour limite le manque de systématisation du recueil des données, à laquelle ne correspond d'ailleurs pas l'exploitation des résumés médicaux qui ont objectif et de décrire les faits tels qu'ils se présentent dans la complexité de la réalité observée.

Trois remarques peuvent être faites sur cette systématisation :

- certaines informations indispensables peuvent figurer sur une liste mnémotechnique : motifs d'hospitalisation, passages en réanimation etc... et rendre l'analyse d'activité beaucoup plus efficace.
- il en serait de même pour les informations principales caractérisant chaque pathologie, que chaque médecin s'engagerait à faire figurer dans ses résumés d'après des listes faciles à établir.
- il reste tout aussi important de comprendre que l'absence d'information dans les résumés traduit un élément dynamique du système, sachant que les faits principaux doivent y figurer et que leur absence n'est pas admissible.

  Par exemple l'examen des résumés montre que certains médecins notent : "ASPECT SINUEUX DES CORONAIRES" ou "EXTRACTION (ou INFECTION) DENTAIRE".

La discussion de la discordance de recueil à propos de ces informations facilement mise en évidence au terminal, détermine si tel fait mérite d'être indexé par tous ou s'il est inutile de poursuivre à moins d'une recherche personnelle.

Cet aspect dynamique nous paraît essentiel pour qu'un système d'information médical intègre de nouveaux schémas de connaissance et s'adapte en permanence au rythme rapide de l'évolution médicale. Il alimente avec des faits concrets la réflexions des utilisateurs et provoque la discussion de groupe qui reste indispensable à l'établissement d'un système d'information efficace.

4. CONCLUSIONS

En conclusion un système de comptes-rendus bio-médicaux s'appuyant sur un langage contrôlé du genre REMEDE satisfait deux buts complémentaires :

- répondre aux besoins documentaires quotidiens des secrétariats médicaux. L'évolution de la version actuelle vers un "style télégraphique médical" et l'intégration dans un schéma bureautique permettra de mieux répondre à cet objetif.

- fournir une "aide à la réflexion" à partir des faits réels observés, capable de dégrossir des éléments d'analyse et de fournir à l'évaluation les données qui mériteront de faire l'objet d'une enquête approfondie.

En effet les techniques d'aide à la décision présupposent le choix d'indicateurs pour caractériser une situation, d'hypothèse définissant des choix et des objectifs à atteindre. Dans le cas de l'analyse d'activité médicale on sait combien ces éléments font souvent défauts au premier stade de l'investigation et ne peuvent être projetés à partir de la seule intuition personnelle.

C'est précisément une des vocations d'un système d'information médicale (7) que d'être capable de prendre en compte les données telles qu'elles se présentent dans la pratique quotidienne et de permettre les mises en lumière et les rapprochements dont on devra faire la preuve à l'aide d'une méthodologie classique.

Encore faut-il que ces données puissent être analysées par l'ordinateur lui-même. D'où le recours à un langage médical contrôlé qui offre aux médecins un moyen commode de réaliser leur comptes-rendus quotidiens sous une forme qui en autorise l'analyse directe par ordinateur avec une pertinence acceptable que n'atteignent pas les systèmes documentaires usuels. La plupart de ceux-ci admettent un taux de pertinence global (bruit et silence confondus) de 60%-70%, insuffisant pour la pratique médicale quotidienne aussi bien que pour l'analyse d'activité.

REFERENCES

1 de Heaulme M, Tainturier C, Thomas D. Traitement par ordinateur des comptes-rendus médicaux : l'exemple du système REMEDE. Nouv Pr Med 1979 ; 40 : 3223-3226.

2 de Heaulme M, Tainturier c, Grosgogeat Y, Gremy F. Medical activity analysis : interest of medical languages like REMEDE. In : MEDINFO 80 ; Lindberg D, Kaihara S, Eds Amsterdam : North HOLLAND ; 1980 : 611-614.

3 Mery C, Menkes CJ, de Heaulme M, Delbarre F. Language artificiel permettant la mise sur ordinateur d'observations résumées. Rev du Rhumatisme 1975 ; 42 : 317-326.

4 de Heaulme M, Mery C. REMAID : an artificial medical reports on computers. In : MEDINFO 74 ; Anderson J and Forsythe JM Eds, Stockholm : GOTAB ; 1974 : 935-941.

5 REMEDE : An artificial language for clinical documentation. In : computational linguistic in Medecine . Schneider/Sagvall Eds. Amsterdam : North HOLLAND ; 1977 : 935-941.

6 SNOMED Systematized Nomenclature of Medecine ; COTE RA Eds,SKOKIE (Illinois): College of American Pathologist. 1979.

7 de Heaulme M. Conditions que doit remplir un système d'information hospitalier pour répondre aux projets d'analyse d'activité ; MIE Toulouse 1981 (sous presse).

EVALUATION D'UN SYSTEME INFORMATIQUE DE LABORATOIRE A PARTIR DE LA SIMULATION D'UNE JOURNEE DE TRAVAIL AU LABORATOIRE

B. HUET* – J. MARTIN**

* Informatique Médicale, UER de Bobigny, CHU Paris-Nord, 74, rue Marcel Cachin, 93012 BOBIGNY CEDEX.

** Informatique Médicale, Groupe INSERM 115, Faculté de Médecine (NANCY), B.P. 184, 54500 VANDOEUVRE-LES-NANCY.

Summary :

The estimate of an information processing system for a clinical laboratory, led us to realize a virtual system, this one has been elaborated during an experimental approach organized in two sequential phases : modelling and simulation from a configuration based upon a mini computer and data acquisition and preprocessing modules.

The resulting product is an analysis in processes and processors of one day's activity of the clinical laboratory with possibility of specializing each laboratory simulation.

The programs of simulation are written in SIMULA (process - oriented - language) and run on a large scale computer.

The parameters of this virtual system concern on one part Man-Machine relationship : global acceptability of the users face to the system, definition of Man Machine dialogues with sizing of VDUS ; on the other part technical specifications of the data acquisition + Preprocessing modules, estimate of the rate of the printer, estimate of REPROM and RAM, minimal estimation of disk storage.

The debate sets up around two subjects : are the parameters necessary and sufficient ? How will be the step going from the virtual system to the real system realized ?

The interest of this tool is large for the users.

1. INTRODUCTION

Evaluer un système informatique de laboratoire, c'est poser la question : tel système est-il adéquat pour telle application ?

Une évaluation suppose donc une analyse de l'application et une analyse du système. Les systèmes actuellement installés, donnant lieu à des degrés de satisfaction divers (1), il nous a semblé intéressant de reprendre dans son principe, l'informatisation du laboratoire, par une analyse en termes de fonctions se rapportant à l'information ; puis de la faire suivre, en interaction avec les utilisateurs, de la réalisation de maquettes informatiques, pour aboutir à un système virtuel servant de banc d'essai pour l'étude d'un système informatique de laboratoire. Ce banc d'essai s'appuie sur la modélisation du laboratoire de Biochimie de l'hôpital Avicenne (93000 BOBIGNY) (2). Il propose l'étude des paramètres du système.

En définitive, l'évaluation du système virtuel que nous avons élaboré va consister à soumettre aux utilisateurs les paramètres du système informatique pour les dimensionner, ce sont :

1) Les relations homme-machine : Acceptabilité du système par les utilisateurs, Définition des relations homme-machine, Evaluation des matériels de dialogue.

2) Les caractéristiques techniques : Configuration du laboratoire, définition des modules de saisie + prétraitement, évaluation du débit du périphérique de sortie, dimensionnement des mémoires mortes, dimensionnement des mémoires vives, dimensionnement du disque.

Sur une approche différente, LEROUDIER et PARENT ont utilisé la simulation dans l'évaluation des performances d'un système (3).

2. METHODE

Le produit a été défini au cours d'une approche expérimentale organisée en deux phases séquentielles : la modélisation et la simulation.

Par rapport aux quatre étapes classiques de développement d'un projet informatique (définition des objectifs, définition des spécifications externes, définition des spécifications internes, réalisation), la modélisation et la simulation se placent juste avant la réalisation (4).

La modélisation a débuté par le choix des concepts utilisés dans le modèle. La sélection de 3 concepts nous a permis de représenter la dynamique du laboratoire. Ce sont la notion d'objet (assimilable à une entité composite d'après BUNGE (5), les notions de processus et processeur et enfin une structure arborescente dans laquelle chaque niveau permet l'observation de l'activité du laboratoire à un certain grossissement.

Un processeur est défini comme une entité potentiellement porteuse d'activité vis-à-vis d'entités non porteuses d'activités (ex : un analyseur automatique, un microprocesseur sont des processeurs). Un processus est constitué dans le cas le plus simple du triplet suivant : processeur, objet de départ, objet d'arrivée (ex : analyse de l'urée, analyse de la glycémie...)

Au cours des nombreuses réunions entre concepteur et utilisateurs, les maquettes testées en simulation se sont révélées être de véritables "outils de dialogue" permettant, par ajustement, de dégager les paramètres d'un système informatique de laboratoire (6).

Le schéma défini en termes d'information est valable quelque soit le laboratoire, la modélisation d'un système informatique répondant à ce schéma aboutit à l'élaboration de modèles de base définis uniquement comme processus ou processeur, chaque modèle de base représente un objet du laboratoire (7).

Pour les utilisateurs, le système d'évaluation se présente comme une structure sur laquelle peuvent être choisis et créés, en nombre variable avec leurs paramètres, des modèles de base représentant des objets du laboratoire à différents niveaux de l'arbre du modèle avec quelques paramètres à définir. Il est donc possible de représenter le fonctionnement d'un laboratoire, en créant "à la carte" les processus et processeurs du laboratoire considéré à partir des modèles de base préexistants.

3. MATERIEL

Il a été fait appel à deux sortes d'outils : **1) Outils logiciels :** SIMULA 67 (8) (9) (10) est un langage "orienté processus", c'est-à-dire qu'il permet la simulation sur ordinateur d'un phénomène décomposé en processus et processeurs. **2) Outils matériels :** La simulation a été effectuée sur l'IRIS 80 du Centre de calcul de l'INRIA (Rocquencourt). La taille mémoire nécessaire à l'exécution des programmes varie entre 200 et 440 k octets, sur lesquels 140 sont occupés par le compilateur SIMULA.

4. DEROULEMENT D'UNE EVALUATION

Le système virtuel que nous avons élaboré pour le laboratoire de Biochimie de l'hôpital Avicenne a permis de mettre en évidence les paramètres suivants :

4-1. Vis-à-vis des relations Homme-Système

4-1.1. Acceptabilité vis-à-vis des utilisateurs

L'objectif est d'évaluer l'acceptabilité globale d'un système informatique vis-à-vis des utilisateurs.

Le moyen est constitué par l'outil de dialogue que constituent les maquettes informatiques paramétrées du système de laboratoire. Au cours d'entretiens avec le responsable du projet, les utilisateurs vont choisir les options et caractéristiques de leur futur système. In fine, ils auront donc a priori une acceptabilité globale satisfaisante du système réel, même si ce dernier nécessite en définitive un ajustement final vis-à-vis du système virtuel défini.

4-1.2. Définition des relations Homme-machine

Les relations Homme-Machine ont été modélisées dans plusieurs processus de dialogue, tels que : enregistrement des demandes d'examen, enregistrement des entrants depuis la veille...

La simulation déroule les dialogues sur un périphérique interactif virtuel selon deux organisations : automatique ou semi-automatique d'après la fréquence de demandes, au cours de ces dialogues, diverses options sont possibles telles que : circuit d'erreurs intégré ou non, enregistrement par profil ou par examen...

Les dialogues peuvent donc être élaborés à "la carte", selon les avis des utilisateurs et les spécificités du laboratoire, puis simulés car les programmes sont paramétrés (textes, pourcentage de réponse...) ; ils peuvent donc servir d'essai et d'évaluation des dialogues Homme-Machine dans les systèmes de laboratoire.

4-1.3. Evaluation du nombre de consoles de visualisation

Après définition des dialogues, trois paramètres doivent être étudiés pour une implémentation correcte : 1) Temps moyen approximatif d'exécution d'un dialogue défini sur une console de visualisation ; 2) Nombre (supérieur rencontré majoré de 15 % et non pas moyen) de dialogues à exécuter ; 3) Contraintes de temps pour un dialogue donné au niveau du laboratoire.

Ces données permettent de calculer le nombre de consoles de visualisation nécessaires au déroulement des dialogues dans les fourchettes horaires du laboratoire.

4-2. <u>Vis-à-vis des caractéristiques techniques</u>

4-2.1. Configuration informatique du laboratoire et modules de saisie et pré-traitement

Tous les matériels de base du laboratoire tels que : analyseurs automatiques, multiplexeurs, convertisseurs analogique/digital, microprocesseur ont été modélisés en processeur-objet avec des paramètres ainsi que les processus principaux se déroulant sur ces processeurs.

Nous simulons ainsi le fonctionnement (et même les pannes !) de la production, de la saisie et du prétraitement de l'information de n'importe quel laboratoire de Biochimie avec sa configuration propre.

La présentation dynamique de ce système virtuel, permet à l'utilisateur de choisir plus aisément la configuration en analyseurs et modules de saisie et prétraitement de l'information, en intégrant l'étude de configurations dégradées rencontrées dans divers cas de pannes.

4-2.2. Evaluation du débit du périphérique de sortie

La solution idéale consisterait en l'impression des résultats des malades au niveau des services demandeurs sur un périphérique local. Pour des raisons économiques, la solution actuellement choisie est l'impression de tous les dossiers au laboratoire ; pour un dimensionnement correct de l'imprimante, trois paramètres doivent être considérés : 1) Nombre moyen de lignes par feuille de malade ; 2) Nombre supérieur rencontré, majoré de 15 %, de feuilles de résultats à imprimer ; 3) Fourchette de temps de sortie des feuilles de résultats.

Ces données permettent de calculer le débit en lignes/minute de l'imprimante.

4-2.3. Dimensionnement des mémoires mortes des modules de saisie + prétraitement

Les fonctions à exécuter sur l'information fournie par un analyseur de marque donnée dans un laboratoire précis seront à sélectionner parmi onze fonctions inventoriées. Citons seulement : échantillonnage, lissage...

Chaque fonction est exécutée par un programme paramétré, implémenté sur un module de saisie et prétraitement.

A la suite des fonctions sélectionnées, la mémoire morte sera dimensionnée.

4-2.4. Dimensionnement des mémoires vives des modules de saisie + pré-traitement

Les analyseurs automatiques connectés sur les modules exigent une mémoire plus ou moins importante, selon leur degré d'évolution et d'intégration des fonctions de saisie et prétraitement.

4-2.5. Evaluation minimisée de la taille disque :

La modélisation du système informatique de laboratoire est allée jusqu'à proposer une organisation de fichiers dont les deux principaux sont le fichier état-civil et le fichier contenant les résultats biologiques des malades.

Le fichier Etat-Civil est constitué d'articles (1 article = 1 malade) de 50 octets.

Le fichier Biologique est organisé en une zone fixe et une zone de débordement.

La zone fixe doit être étudiée à partir des cahiers et des fichiers du laboratoire pour être optimisée pour chaque système de laboratoire. Deux paramètres de cette zone fixe sont à déterminer :

- le nombre de demandes d'examens à réserver systématiquement pour tout nouveau dossier (x).
- le nombre de paramètres biologiques à réserver systématiquement pour toute demande d'examen (y).

L'étude des fichiers d'un laboratoire doit être orientée pour en extraire :

- le nombre de demandes d'analyses par patient,
- la fréquence des demandes pour chaque paramètre biologique.

Divers calculs permettent alors à partir des paramètres représentant 85 % des analyses effectuées, d'obtenir plusieurs valeurs de x et y et de choisir la taille-mémoire la plus faible.

5. DISCUSSION

Cette discussion s'établit autour de deux pôles :

5-1. Les paramètres qui viennent d'être examinés sont-ils nécessaires et suffisants pour l'évaluation d'un système informatique de laboratoire ?

Les paramètres examinés se rapportent aux trois points suivants : 1) Etude des relations Homme-Machine pour garantir l'acceptabilité des utilisateurs vis-à-vis du système (11) (12). 2) Dimensionnement des entrées-sorties et de la capacité de stockage du système pour éviter les goulots d'étranglement dans les échanges et la limitation du stockage des informations. 3) Etude de la configuration avec les procédures de reprise et dégradées.

Ces paramètres englobent entre autres, les points déjà connus comme les plus facilement défaillants dans un système (13).

La configuration du système réel, tiré du système virtuel, avec les utilisateurs livrera peut-être un ajustement sur l'évaluation du système de laboratoire. Cet affinage de l'évaluation peut également provenir d'une amélioration de l'étude du schéma de l'information sur lequel s'appuie le système virtuel. Une nouvelle approche, proposée en 1970 par CODD (14), basée sur l'algèbre relationnelle a été reprise et améliorée par BERNSTEIN (15), TSICHRITZIS (16) et ROLLAND (17) qui a même proposé tout récemment un système de gestion des objets analysés (18) permettant ainsi une véritable maintenance au niveau de la phase conceptuelle de l'élaboration du système virtuel et par là même, un affinage possible du schéma informationnel.

5-2. Comment va s'effectuer le passage système virtuel ⟶ système réel ?

Le système virtuel dimensionné s'appuie sur un modèle établi en termes d'information à partir du "réel perçu" du laboratoire. Le passage du "réel perçu" au modèle s'effectue par une sélection de paramètres

Réel Inconnu ⟶ Perception du réel ⟶ Modèle

Le retour du modèle exprimenté (système virtuel) au réel perçu va s'accompagner implicitement de l'addition de nombreux paramètres.

Un même système virtuel peut donc faire aboutir à plusieurs systèmes réels possibles. Grâce aux paramètres qu'ils ont définis, les utilisateurs vont guider ce retour vers leur système réel.

6. CONCLUSION

La portée de l'évaluation d'un système est grande, car c'est la possibilité de fournir un système adapté aux utilisateurs et non l'inverse, et de réaliser ce système à un prix de revient plus faible.

En pratique, nous concluons que les paramètres actuellement dégagés par nous lors de l'analyse et la mise au point du système virtuel dans l'évolution d'un système informatique de laboratoire sont sans doute les plus significatifs dans l'évaluation d'un système informatique de laboratoire.

L'intérêt d'un tel outil de dialogue se manifeste à tous les niveaux des utilisateurs du système informatique : pour les cliniciens, il visualise le produit fini qui va être livré ; pour les biologistes, il est une garantie minimale des prestations fournies car les processus analysés et simulés seront implémentés sur le système réel, pour les personnels techniques, c'est la possibilité d'inclure dans le système réel certains desiderata d'organisation du travail.

L'informatique est un outil, forger un outil opérationnel nécessite la prise en compte de nombreux paramètres, certains sont exclusivement techniques, du domaine des informaticiens, d'autres nécessitent d'être évalués dans des conditions opérationnelles sur le lieu même de l'application. C'est dans ce dernier cas que réside l'intérêt de livrer aux utilisateurs un système virtuel avec quelques paramètres à définir.

L'évaluation des paramètres d'un système informatique au moyen d'un système virtuel est donc un procédé particulièrement fertile qui devrait être appliqué chaque fois qu'il s'agit d'implanter un système informatique dans un contexte opérationnel.

BIBLIOGRAPHIE

(1) PASTOR J., PAULI A.M. – "L'ordinateur en temps réel dans un laboratoire de biologie hospitalier" ; Techniques hospitalières, numéro spécial, le laboratoire et l'hôpital, Mai 1977, n° 380, 70-83.

(2) HUET B. – "Modélisation et Simulation de l'activité d'un laboratoire de biochimie clinique" ; Thèse de Biologie Humaine, 1980, Nancy.

(3) LEROUDIER J., PARENT M. – "Discrete event simulation modelling of computer systems for performance evaluation" ; Math. and Comp. in simulation (1979), 21, 50-79.

(4) SZYMANKIEWICZ J. – "Simulate before you act" ; Data processing (1976), May, 22-26.

(5) BUNGE M. – "Things" ; Int. J. of Gen. systems (1974), 1, n° 4, 229-236.

(6) DARMON I. – "Base de données, maquette et dialogue avec les utilisateurs" ; Inf. et gestion (1977), Mars, n° 85, 50-52.

(7) FRANTA W.R. – "The process view of simulation" ; Ed. North Holland, 1977.

(8) DAHL O.J., MYRHAUG B., NYGAARD K. – "The simula 67 common base language" ; Pub., 5-22, Norvegian Compting Ctr,Oslo, 1970.

(9) CII-HB – SIMULA – 1 – 1973 – "SIMULA sous SIRIS 7/SIRIS 8" ; Manuel d'utilisation, tome 2, Environnement et classes systèmes.

(11) SCHNEIDERMAN B. – "Human factors experiments designing interactive systems" ; comput. (1979), Dec. 9-19.

(12) STERLING T.D., LAUDON K. – "Humanizing Information Systems" ; Datamation (1976), 12, 53-59.

(13) MICHEL G. – "Eléments d'appréciation sur les systèmes informatiques orientés vers l'automatisation des laboratoires d'analyses biologiques" ; Rapport du S.T.I. (I.R.I.A.), Juillet 1975.

(14) CODD E.F. – "A relational model of data for large shared data bank" ; Com. A.C.M. (1970), 13, n° 6, 377-387.

(15) BEERU C., BERNSTEIN P.A., GOODMAN N. – "A sophisticate's introduction to data base normalization theory" ; Proc. IVth Int. Conf. on very large date bases, Berlin, 1978, 1978, pp. 113-124.

(16) BERNSTEIN P.A., SWENSON J.R., TSICHRITZIS D.C. – "A unified approach to functional dependencies and relations" ; Proc. ACM 1975 SIGMOD Conf. San Jose Calif, pp 237-245.

(17) ROLLAND C., FOUCAUT O. – "Concepts for design of an information system conceptual schema and its utilization in the REMORA project" ; Proc. IVth Int. Conf. on very large data bases, Berlin, 1978.

(18) ROLLAND C., LEIFERT S., RICHARD C. – "Tools for information system dynamic management" ; I.E.E.E. (1979), Aug, 251-261.

LA MULTIDISCIPLINARITE: UN INSTRUMENT DE POUVOIR DES PROFESSIONS

N. Allard-Breton; L.-H. Trottier; R. Pineault;
J.-M. Brodeur; F. Champagne
Département de médecine sociale et préventive
Université de Montréal
Montréal, P.Q.

This paper focuses on multidisciplinarity as one or the themes for organizing the work of various professionals in the context of a newly established general hospital. This theme has been put forward by the promoters of the centre and the study attempts to examine the relationships that have developed between the different professional groups involved in the operationalization of this theme. The general hypothesis is that the dominant profession is most determinant in shaping the content of multidisciplinarity work and in imposing its view on the other professional groups.

The research fits in the tradition of the case study which has been often employed in organization theory. Analysis of the data is predominantly of the qualitative type. The results presented tend to support the overall hypothesis.

La dominance médicale est de plus en plus contestée par les infirmières, les paramédicaux, les professionnels des sciences humaines et par des usagers insatisfaits des services médicaux. Cette contestation n'est-elle que le reflet de luttes corporatistes où des occupations professionnelles tentent d'accroître leurs privilèges et leurs pouvoirs? Ou est-elle le reflet d'une crise majeure devant les réponses médicales apportées aux problèmes de morbidité?

La volonté progressiste profonde qui a animé l'implantation d'un centre hospitalier à vocation communautaire au Québec et l'énergie qui y fut déployée pour instituer des pratiques novatrices afin d'assurer une organisation du travail qui palliait aux insatisfactions professionnelles, a suscité beaucoup d'espoir dans le milieu socio-sanitaire québécois. C'est en cherchant à actualiser des thèmes aussi nouveaux que la multidisciplinarité, la continuité des soins, la promotion de la santé et l'humanisation des soins, que les professionnels de cet hôpital ont tenté de réorganiser leur pratique en fonction de leur idéal professionnel. La réaction des usagers à la dominance médicale et aux pratiques professionnelles rencontrées dans cet hôpital ne fait pas l'objet de la présente étude.

Dans cet article, nous ne retenons que le thème de multidisciplinarité[1] pour illustrer comment les professions paramédicales[2] ont compris et interprété ce thème en fonction de leur projet particulier. Par l'évolution des pratiques hospitalières et des relations d'interdépendance professionnelle vécues dans cet hôpital, nous soulevons les obstacles qui ont compromis la réalisation de l'idéal multidisciplinaire des paramédicaux oeuvrant au sein de ce centre hospitalier.

Le centre hospitalier et son contexte d'implantation

Cette recherche se déroule dans un hôpital spécialisé, et non sur-spécialisé, né de la réforme québécoise des services de santé et des services sociaux (1971). Tant par ses objectifs que l'on peut qualifier d'avant-gardistes pour un centre hospitalier institué en milieu urbain (ouverture sur la communauté, affiliation universitaire exclusive à la médecine familiale et communautaire, privilèges de pratique importants accordés aux omnipraticiens) que par la thématique qui a stimulé son implantation et orienté la planification de ses services, ce nouvel hôpital indiquait sa volonté de se conformer aux dernières orientations du secteur sanitaire.

La réforme socio-sanitaire qui a marqué les années '70 au Québec visait à assurer une planification et une coordination intégrées des ressources sanitaires[3]. Les promoteurs de cette réforme se sont gagnés l'appui de larges couches sociales, dont les professions paramédicales, en suscitant les attentes et les espoirs les plus grands par une thématique empreinte des idéaux socio-démocrates modernes: "création d'une nouvelle médecine" (médecine globale), "cogestion des organisations de soins par les usagers et les travailleurs", "décentralisation et régionalisation des pouvoirs de décision", "une certaine égalisation du statut des professionnels de la santé.[4]

En 1973, par la réforme du Code des professions, le gouvernement québécois cherchait à trouver une solution aux problèmes provenant de l'expansion anarchique de la spécialisation du personnel technique et professionnel.[5] Cette réforme tentait, entre autres, de réduire les inégalités professionnelles en accroissant les privilèges des groupes professionnels les moins privilégiés. Par cette deuxième réforme, le gouvernement reconfirmait sa volonté de démocratiser les rapports professionnels.

Le centre hospitalier que nous étudions a été planifié dans ce contexte social où l'Etat "promettait de rationnaliser et de démocratiser en profondeur le secteur de la santé"[6] et où la population et les groupes professionnels étaient des plus mobilisés. En utilisant les thèmes les plus opérationnels de la réforme (promotion de la santé, continuité des soins, humanisation des soins et multidisciplinarité), les promoteurs de cet hôpital ont attisé les attentes des groupes professionnels qui aspiraient à l'égalité professionnelle et à une gestion hospitalière rationnelle et démocratique. Pour ces professionnels, tant médecins, infirmières que paramédicaux, ce nouvel hôpital devenait le lieu privilégié pour réorganiser leur pratique en fonction de leurs attentes respectives. Pour les omnipraticiens, cet hôpital leur offrait enfin une place importante dans un centre hospitalier universitaire. Cet hôpital offrait aux infirmières la possibilité d'organiser leur pratique pour assurer une prise en charge globale du patient sans avoir à conjuguer avec un personnel infirmier auxiliaire. Pour les paramédicaux, ce nouvel hôpital offrait la possibilité d'instaurer des pratiques novatrices pour augmenter leur participation aux décisions thérapeutiques et administratives. Toutefois, cet hôpital a ouvert (1978) dans un contexte de crise fiscale où les gouvernements (fédéral et provincial) cherchaient par tous les moyens à réduire les dépenses du secteur de la santé. Dès son ouverture, cet hôpital a fait face à des coupures budgétaires qui l'ont forcé à reformuler ses priorités.

Méthodologie

Dans cette étude de cas, nous avons utilisé une méthodologie qui nous permet de saisir la réalité organisationnelle de façon dynamique et "holistique". Il ne s'agit donc pas ici d'une analyse comparative où la population à l'étude doit être représentative de la population des centres hospitaliers, mais plutôt d'une analyse qu'on peut qualifier d'analyse interne (Lipset 1950), stratégique (Crozier, 1977), politique (Bacharah, 1980) ou encore ontologique (Freidson, 1975).[7]

Les données recueillies sont principalement de nature qualitative et descriptive. Elles ont été réunies sans catégorisation préalable, quoique de façon pré-déterminée et systématique. Nous avons utilisé quatre thèmes: multidisciplinarité, promotion de la santé, humanisation des soins et continuité des soins, afin de mener des entrevues dirigées auprès des cadres supérieurs et intermédiaires ainsi qu'auprès de représentants des médecins spécialistes et omnipraticiens, des infirmiers et des paramédicaux. L'observation participante et non participante, l'analyse de documents et un questionnaire portant sur les intérêts de carrière furent utilisés pour compléter les informations recueillies auprès des intervenants.

Une première analyse des données permet d'affirmer que chaque groupe professionnel n'a véritablement accordé d'importance qu'à certains thèmes. Ainsi, les omnipraticiens et les infirmières ont retenu les thèmes centrés sur le patient, i.e. la continuité et l'humanisation des soins. Les paramédicaux se sont concentrés sur les thèmes de multidisciplinarité et de prévention qui leur offraient des moyens pour restructurer et réorienter les services et les priorités de l'hôpital. C'est à travers la perception du groupe professionnel qui a accordé le plus d'importance à la multidisciplinarité que nous examinons l'idéal multidisciplinaire et les moyens mis de l'avant pour l'actualiser.

L'idéal multidisciplinaire: la collaboration globale

Les professions paramédicales, groupe qui accorde le plus d'importance à la multidisciplinarité, définissent ce thème comme un "modèle de collaboration globale".[8] Pour ces professionnels, la collaboration globale ne peut être effective sans travail d'équipe regroupant plusieurs spécialistes (paramédicaux, médecins, infirmières) ni sans un "respect mutuel" entre tous les membres de l'équipe face à la responsabilité thérapeutique et face à la reconnaissance de l'importance du champ d'expertise de chacun.

Les paramédicaux affirment que la morbidité est un phénomène complexe où les dimensions sociales, psychologiques et économiques sont, au moins, aussi importantes que les causes biologiques. Pour ces professionnels, une telle compréhension de la morbidité implique la nécessité de former des équipes multidisciplinaire où les diagnostics et les plans de traitement s'élaborent en fonction d'une problématique générale qui tient compte de l'unicité et de la complexité des individus. Cette conception s'oppose à l'activité médicale traditionnelle où diagnostics et plans de traitement ne sont élaborés que par les médecins et ne s'ébauchent généralement qu'en fonction d'un problème spécifique.

La complexité des phénomènes de morbidité justifie, pour les paramédicaux, la nécessité d'une approche globale où la collaboration interdisciplinaire se fait dans le respect absolu des connaissances scientifiques et techniques de chacun. Contrairement aux omnipraticiens et aux infirmières pour qui la collaboration interdisciplinaire signifie une complémentarité occasionnelle, i.e. modelée sur les relations qu'ils entretiennent avec les médecins spécialistes, les paramédicaux affirment que leur participation doit être usuelle et ce, non seulement dans certains cas, mais bien dans la très grande majorité des problématiques présentées par les bénéficiaires. Une telle participation implique une responsabilité thérapeutique partagée entre tous les membres de l'équipe, i.e. que les décisions se prennent collectivement et qu'il y a égalité professionnelle.

Par le modèle de collaboration globale, les professionnels paramédicaux questionnent la légitimité de l'hégémonie cognitive et technique de la profession médicale qui lui octroie une influence dominante dans l'orientation des priorités et des activités hospitalières. Pour que leur savoir scientifique et technique soit tout aussi considéré que celui de la profession médicale, les paramédicaux ont développé des moyens concrets qui cherchent à leur assurer une participation usuelle et continue aux décisions thérapeutiques et administratives.

Le projet des paramédicaux

Les modalités concrètes d'actualisation de la multidisciplinarité, instituées par les professions paramédicales,visaient à développer des mécanismes formels leur permettant d'influencer l'orientation et les pratiques hospitalières afin d'accroître leur autonomie professionnelle.

Pour atteindre une collaboration interdisciplinaire globale, les paramédicaux cherchaient à développer une gestion hospitalière décentralisée où les décisions seraient prises collégialement tant au sein des services, des directorats qu'au sein du Comité de Régie. On espérait ainsi assurer une plus grande participation de tous les intervenants à la définition des priorités hospitalières et, de cette façon, éviter qu'un groupe professionnel particulier s'accapare d'une trop grande partie du pouvoir. Pour ne donner qu'un exemple du type de réorganisation qu'ils ont tenté d'opérer notons que des démarches furent entreprises pour faire de l'orthophonie et de l'audiologie un service autonome au même titre que la physiothérapie ou que la psychologie. Etre reconnu comme service donne droit de participer aux réunions de la Direction des services hospitaliers (DSH) dont celles portant sur la répartition des budgets Une telle reconnaissance leur aurait donné un accès direct aux processus de décision et leur aurait assuré, simultanément, l'infrastructure nécessaire à l'organisation efficace de leur service.

Avant l'ouverture de l'hôpital, afin de stimuler la collaboration globale entre les professionnels, les paramédicaux, les infirmières et les omnipraticiens ont su faire reconnaître la nécessité de l'utilisation d'un dossier unique et par problème dans ce centre hospitalier. Ce dossier donne à tous les intervenants la possibilité de consigner leurs observations sur une même feuille d'évolution. Pour les paramédicaux, il s'agit là de la reconnaissance formelle que leurs observations ont autant d'importance que celles des médecins. Cependant, durant cette dernière phase de planification, les professions paramédicales n'ont pu obtenir le support des médecins et des infirmières pour jeter les bases nécessaires au fonctionnement des équipes multidisciplinaires. A l'exception de l'unité psychiatrique, les équipes multidisciplinaires n'ont pas fait l'objet de planifications préalables à l'ouverture de l'hôpital. Toutefois, pour atteindre le modèle de collaboration globale, d'autres modalités concrètes d'actualisation de la multidisciplinarité furent néanmoins construites mais en fonction, principalement de la logique interne de chaque service.

Par exemple, on créa un poste de coordonnateur administratif et technique aux laboratoires et à la radiologie afin d'assurer une cogestion médico-administrative des services diagnostics. Les techniciens qui assument cette fonction sont des cadres intermédiaires hiérarchiquement dépendants de la Direction des services hospitaliers (DSH)[9]. Cette situation est nouvelle dans la structure hospitalière, habituellement ce rôle est assumé par les chefs médicaux des laboratoires et de la radiologie qui relèvent de la Direction des services professionnels (DSP)[10].

Pour faciliter la collaboration entre les unités de soins et les services paramédicaux, plusieurs professions paramédicales ont ouvert des postes sur les unités de soins de médecine-chirurgie. Grâce à cette organisation ces professionnels s'assuraient un contact direct avec les bénéficiaires, par opposition à un rapport médiatisé par les demandes des infirmières ou par les références médicales, et jetaient ainsi des bases importantes pour stimuler la formation d'équipes multidisciplinaires.

Les modalités concrètes pour assurer l'actualisation de la multidisciplinarité permettaient, d'une part, d'assurer une présence continue des professionnels paramédicaux sur les unités de soins et, d'autre part, de leur assurer une plus grande participation aux processus de décision. Ces modalités relèvent d'une stratégie professionnelle qui vise à accroître l'autonomie de pratique des paramédicaux. Simultanément, ces modalités questionnent les relations traditionnelles qui gèrent l'interdépendance professionnelle en cherchant à développer une organisation du travail où les rapports professionnels sont plus égalitaires.

Dans la partie suivante, nous verrons comment se vit réellement la collaboration interdisciplinaire dans ce centre hospitalier. Nous examinerons par la suite les événements qui ont entravé la réalisation de l'idéal multidisciplinaire des paramédicaux.

Deux réalités d'interdépendance professionnelle

Selon la typologie développée par Brunet et Vinet,[11] la collaboration interdisciplinaire est vécue dans ce centre hospitalier, à travers deux modèles: le "modèle de subordination" et le "modèle de parallélisme disciplinaire". Le modèle le plus répandu est le modèle de subordination. Le travail n'y est pas organisé par équipe multidisciplinaire. Les interventions des paramédicaux auprès des bénéficiaires sont soumises aux demandes de consultation faites par le corps médical et la communication de l'information entre les professionnels se fait par les moyens habituels: notes au dossier, appels téléphoniques, rencontres informelles entre deux intervenants. Cette organisation hospitalière du travail professionnel est des plus classique et offre très peu de possibilité au développement et à l'utilisation de pratiques et de services novateurs.

Le second modèle d'interdépendance professionnelle rencontré dans l'hôpital se retrouve exclusivement sur deux unités spécialisés - psychiatrie, équipe d'évaluation et de réadaptation (EER) - et s'apparente au modèle de parallélisme disciplinaire. Ici, l'équipe multidisciplinaire existe et le chef d'équipe n'est pas nécessairement un médecin. Les décisions y sont généralement prises collectivement et la division des tâches reconnaît assez bien la spécificité de chacun. Les paramédicaux participent à l'évaluation des patients - évaluation qui doit être confirmée par le diagnostic médical - et à l'élaboration du plan de soins. Cependant, certains malaises subsistent quant à la responsabilité thérapeutique globale que détiennent les médecins. Pour les paramédicaux, il s'agit là d'une reconnaissance mitigée de la valeur et de l'importance de leur expertise.

En dépit d'une volonté progressiste réelle et malgré l'institution de pratiques novatrices, des relations d'interdépendance professionnelle des plus classiques se sont néanmoins développées dans ce centre hospitalier. Les paramédicaux n'ont pas réussi à imposer le modèle de collaboration globale qu'ils préconisaient. Confrontés aux réalités hospitalières, la multidisciplinarité n'a pu transgresser la dominance cognitive de la profession médicale ni les inégalités de statut et de pouvoir entre les professionnels.

Les événements qui ont compromis la réalisation de l'idéal multidisciplinaire

Durant la période de planification, les paramédicaux détenaient un certain leadership dans l'organisation des services qui seraient offerts. L'ouverture de l'hôpital, les restrictions budgétaires et les luttes professionnelles marquèrent un tournant décisif dans la prise de pouvoir par un groupe professionnel particulier au sein de cet hôpital.

L'ouverture de l'hôpital

L'ouverture de l'hôpital - l'arrivée massive des médecins spécialistes et omnipraticiens et la présence "soudaine" des bénéficiaires - fit surgir brutalement les difficultés d'articulation et d'interdépendance des services et des pratiques professionnelles. Un personnel jeune, mais pour la plupart expérimenté, devait relever le double défi de s'adapter à de nouveaux collègues de travail, à un nouveau milieu physique, à une technologie nouvelle et à des pratiques professionnelles novatrices, ainsi que d'assimiler de nouvelles procédures, de nouvelles techniques et une nouvelle forme de dossier. Il était aussi confronté à l'absence d'entente formelle entre les spécialistes et les omnipraticiens quant à leurs fonctions respectives, à l'inexpérience hospitalière de plusieurs omnipraticiens, à la duplication de tâches entre les paramédicaux et les infirmières. Cet imbroglio fut de plus accentué par des coupures budgétaires qui désorganisaient la planification interne de chaque service par des coupures de postes et des restrictions dans les programmes prévus.

Toutes ces difficultés combinées à la surcharge de travail nécessitée par les derniers préparatifs d'ouverture provoquèrent des tensions telles - particulièrement parmi le personnel qui avait minutieusement planifié les services en fonction des critères d'excellence actuels - que tous rejetaient la responsabilité des difficultés de fonctionnement dans le camp adverse et s'accusaient mutuellement de mauvaise foi et de manque de collaboration.

C'est donc dans une atmosphère de confusion et d'instabilité fonctionnelle que l'hôpital oúvrit ses portes. La logique "productiviste" introduite par la réforme du secteur de la santé et les inégalités de statut et de pouvoir entre les professionnels furent des éléments importants dans l'institution de règles organisationnelles et de relations d'interdépendance professionnelle des plus classiques.

La logique productiviste

La logique "productiviste" selon laquelle les ressources sont allouées en fonction de critères quantitatifs, i.e. en terme du nombre d'actes posés, plutôt qu'en fonction de justifications humanistes, s'est implantée dans le secteur hospitalier vers le milieu des années '70. La crise fiscale à laquelle l'Etat devait alors faire face, raffermit sa volonté de rationnaliser et de contrôler les dépenses hospitalières. Concrètement, cette volonté s'est manifestée par des coupures budgétaires importantes qui forcèrent les administrateurs et les professionnels à donner priorités aux services"efficaces" transformant ainsi la dynamique hospitalière de ce nouvel hôpital.

Dès l'ouverture de l'hôpital, confrontée aux coupures budgétaires, l'administration dutrapidement reviser ses priorités. Plusieurs services novateurs furent retranchés de l'activité hospitalière en raison de leur performance statistique qui ne répondait pas aux normes actuelles d'efficacité et de rentabilité. Toutefois, les services les plus touchés furent ceux qui questionnaient le plus profondément l'organisation traditionnelle du travail, les protocoles médicaux ainsi que certaines politiques administratives. Les psychologues attachés aux unités de médecine-chirurgie furent transférés à la clinique de planification familiale; les services offerts en externe par les ergothérapeutes, inhalothérapeutes, psychologues et orthophonistes furent soit drastiquement éliminés, soit réduits aux services traditionnellement offerts par les hôpitaux en ce domaine; les services d'audiologie et d'orthophonie n'acquirent jamais le statut de service autonome; le poste d'infirmière épidémiologiste fut éliminé; les postes d'infirmières chef d'équipes furent retranchés sur les unités de soins. Les coupures budgétaires affectèrent de plus les activités des services en réduisant au minimum les réunions intra-service et les réunions multidisciplinaires puisqu'elles diminuent la performance globale d'un service.

Par son droit exclusif sur les demandes de consultation et sur les prescriptions, le corps médical influence directement l'efficacité des pratiques et des services des autres professionnels. Aussi, est-il intéressant de constater que les services réduits ou éliminés correspondent à des services peu utilisés par les médecins et que les services retenus sont ceux qu'ils utilisent le plus: 1) parce qu'ils répondent à des besoins de diagnostic (radiologie, laboratoire) ou de traitement tel qu'exigé par les protocoles médicaux (pharmacie, physiothérapie); 2) parce qu'ils répondent à des problèmes auxquels les médecins, individuellement, ne se reconnaissent pas de compétence particulière (diététique, ergothérapie); ou encore 3) parce qu'ils assurent une plus grande rotation des lits (service social). Ainsi, l'efficacité statistique des services est directement dépendante de la demande médicale. La performance des services étant mesurée au nombre d'actes posés et au nombre de bénéficiaires rencontrés, chaque groupe professionnel cherche à faire reconnaître la supériorité de ses compétences auprès de la profession médicale. Dans ce contexte, le chevauchement de tâches entre les infirmières et certains paramédicaux devient une source majeure de conflits. Il s'en suit des luttes professionnelles, souvent très agressives, puisque l'accomplissement de ces actes justifie le nombre de postes alloué à chaque service et que les coupures budgétaires représentent, non seulement une diminution du pouvoir collectif de chaque groupe, mais aussi une menace individuelle.

Les luttes professionnelles

Les inégalités de statut et de pouvoir entre les professionnels jouèrent un rôle important dans l'établissement de rapports d'interdépendance des plus traditionnels au sein de ce centre hospitalier. A l'ouverture de l'hôpital, tout professionnel pouvait référer un bénéficiaire à un autre type de professionnel lorsqu'il le jugeait opportun. Les médecins s'opposèrent rapidement à cette règle "anarchique" et exigèrent que toute consultation soit prescrite par un médecin. Cette modalité, accompagnée du retranchement de certains paramédicaux sur les unités de soins retiraient à ces professionnels tous les moyens qu'ils avaient institués pour s'assurer une relation directe aux bénéficiaires et permettaient ainsi le retour à des relations professionnelles traditionnelles.

Les paramédicaux qui avaient d'abord cru que la présence des omnipraticiens favoriserait le recours fréquent à leur expertise, furent rapidement désillusionnés. Par suite d'ententes formelles et informelles entre les spécialistes et les omnipraticiens, ces derniers effectuent plusieurs tâches que les paramédicaux accomplissent généralement en milieu sur-spécialisé. Les luttes professionnelles n'en devinrent que plus agressives et, à l'instar des omnipraticiens, les infirmières et les paramédicaux, cherchant à s'assurer l'exclusivité de certains actes, effectuèrent des coalitions conjoncturelles avec les spécialistes.

Ces coalitions s'effectuent bien sûr en fonction des intérêts de chaque groupe et ce, même si elles provoquent, dans certains cas, des conflits entre les membres de la profession médicale oeuvrant dans des spécialités différentes. Grâce à ces alliances, les paramédicaux, supportés par des spécialistes, réussirent à évincer les infirmières concernant des actes délégués à ces deux groupes professionnels. Par contre, sur certaines unités de soins, d'autres spécialistes ont appuyé les infirmières et elles ont ainsi pu conservé la responsabilité d'autres actes délégués. Mais ces coalitions ne sont pas toujours possibles. Par exemple, en conflit avec les médecins spécialistes attachés aux services laboratoires, ne pouvant mobiliser d'autres membres de la profession médicale contre des confrères qui leur offrent un service diagnostic essentiel, affligés par le départ de certains cadres supérieurs qui les laissaient sans médiateurs influents au sein de l'administration, les paramédicaux ne purent conserver leur participation égalitaire à la gestion de ces services. Suite aux pressions soutenues des médecins spécialistes pour recouvrer leur autorité administrative traditionnelle, les fonctions du coordonnateur administratif et technique furent considérablement diminuées

Malgré un retour à des relations professionnelles fort classiques, certaines pratiques novatrices ont su résister aux coupures budgétaires et aux luttes professionnelles: le dossier unique et par problème (mais selon ses promoteurs - paramédicaux, infirmières, omnipraticiens - est fort mal utilisé); les fonctions intégrales du coordonnateur administratif et technique en radiologie (mais non aux laboratoires); la présence physique de certains paramédicaux sur les unités de soins (diététistes, ergothérapeutes). Bien que l'équipe multidisciplinaire psychiatrique subsiste sous sa forme originale et qu'une équipe ait été récemment formée en évaluation et réadaptation (EER) selon le modèle de parallélisme disciplinaire, les réalisations des paramédicaux ne sont cependant que mitigées. Les objectifs qu'ils poursuivaient ne sont pas atteints: pas de gestion décentralisée, pas de relation directe aux bénéficiaires, pas de responsabilité thérapeutique partagée égalitairement.

Bien que la réforme du secteur de la santé et la réforme du Code des professions, animées par des idéaux socio-démocrates, semblaient vouloir réduire les inégalités professionnelles, curieusement les moyens utilisés pour rationnaliser les priorités hospitalières et les inégalités professionnelles semblent, au contraire les exacerber.[12] Le nouveau type de gestion hospitalière introduit par la réforme sanitaire et les coupures budgétaires consolident, dans cet hôpital, le pouvoir médical et administratif et accentuent la subordination des professions paramédicales. Une telle symbiose d'intérêts entre les médecins et l'administration, combinée aux inégalités de statut et de pouvoir entre les professionnels ont permis d'instituer des rapports d'interdépendance professionnelle traditionnels dans ce centre hospitalier.

Conclusion

Malgré des efforts considérables déployés par les paramédicaux dans la planification de pratiques novatrices pour assurer une collaboration professionnelle globale, leur projet multidisciplinaire n'a pu se réaliser. Une situation confuse, au moment de l'ouverture de l'hôpital, de même que des coupures budgétaires entraînées par les politiques du ministère des Affaires sociales (MAS) ont conduit à l'institution de rapports professionnels traditionnels. Contrairement à ce qui fut vécu à l'ouverture de l'hôpital, le pouvoir et l'autonomie des paramédicaux furent diminués puisqu'en instituant des modèles traditionnels, leurs relations aux bénéficiaires sont redevenus indirects, i.e. qu'elles sont maintenant médiatisées par le corps médical et par les politiques administratives qui dictent les priorités hospitalières.

Dans les deux modèles d'interdépendance professionnelle en vigueur dans cet hôpital (subordination et parallélisme disciplinaire), les membres de la profession médicale déterminent, dans un premier temps, la clientèle des paramédicaux par le droit exclusif qu'ils détiennent sur l'hospitalisation. Dans le modèle de subordination, un second triage médical s'effectue sur la clientèle des paramédicaux par les demandes de consultation que les médecins leur prescrivent. Par ce <u>contrôle</u> sur la clientèle des paramédicaux, la profession médicale s'interpose dans la relation paramédicaux/bénéficiaires. Comme incitateurs des services paramédicaux, les membres de la profession médicale en deviennent les consommateurs.

Contrairement aux médecins pour qui la demande de services provient directement des bénéficiaires - groupe de consommateurs important, hétérogène et fragmenté - la demande pour les services paramédicaux dans un hôpital est stimulée par le corps médical, un groupe de consommateurs restreint et homogène. Ces situations différentes donnent des résultats diamétralement opposés dans l'autonomie de pratique et dans le pouvoir détenu par chacun de ces groupes professionnels. A cause du caractère hétérogène et fragmenté de la clientèle des médecins, les membres de la profession médicale, comme producteurs de service, ont la possibilité de définir les besoins des bénéficiaires et les moyens d'y répondre. Mais, comme groupe de consommateurs homogène et restreint, les membres de la profession médicale ont la possibilité de <u>définir</u> leurs besoins en services paramédicaux et d'<u>imposer</u> à ces professionnels la manière dont ils doivent y répondre.[13] D'un côté, ce sont les producteurs qui ont la possibilité de définir les besoins de la clientèle et les réponses à lui apporter en fonction de leur connaissance et de leur technologie. De l'autre côté, ce sont les consommateurs qui déterminent leurs besoins et la façon de les satisfaire. Ce pouvoir de la profession médicale sur le choix des bénéficiaires et sur l'utilisation des services paramédicaux est de plus accentué par la responsabilité thérapeutique globale que détiennent ses membres. Ce privilège donne à la profession médicale un moyen de plus pour imposer aux paramédicaux sa logique diagnostique et thérapeutique.

Dans ce contexte, il n'est pas exagéré de parler d'hégémonie de la profession médicale. Cette hégémonie médicale sur le choix des bénéficiaires, la demande de services, la définition des besoins et sur la détermination des pratiques paramédicales, réduit considérablement le contrôle de ces occupations sur la qualité de leur travail, leur autonomie de pratique et leur capacité à s'approprier une partie du pouvoir pour influencer les décisions hospitalières. Par ces moyens, la profession médicale contrôle le marché des services hospitaliers et impose sa logique scientifique et technologique à l'ensemble des pratiques professionnelles.[14]

Tout en oeuvrant à l'hôpital, les médecins demeurent des entrepreneurs indépendants. Au contraire, les membres des professions paramédicales sont des salariés soumis à l'autorité hiérarchique et ainsi, plus directement subordonnés aux politiques gouvernementales et aux instances administratives[15] qui dictent les priorités hospitalières.

Pour rationnaliser les ressources et les services hospitaliers, le gouvernement québécois a introduit un ensemble de normes bureaucratiques qui permettent de mesurer la rentabilité et l'efficacité hospitalière. Dans ce système, la performance globale d'un hôpital s'estime par des normes statistiques où l'efficacité de chaque service est déterminante. Ces normes bureaucratiques n'atteignent pas directement les activités médicales puisque la rémunération des médecins est gérée par un organisme gouvernemental central, la Régie de l'assurance-maladie du Québec (RAMQ). Ce sont les professionnels salariés, ainsi que leurs services qui sont le plus directement dépendants des fluctuations budgétaires du secteur hospitalier. La subordination des paramédicaux aux budgets hospitaliers fait en sorte que l'Etat, en déterminant les priorités hospitalières par ses politiques de santé, s'interpose, lui aussi, dans la relation paramédicaux/bénéficiaires.[16] Par le budget global accordé à chaque hôpital, l'Etat délègue certains de ses pouvoirs à l'administration hospitalière qui, pour répondre aux normes de performance imposées par le MAS, déterminent le nombre de praticiens par service ainsi que le nombre et le type de services qui seront offerts à la population. L'Etat et la profession médicale en médiatisant la relation paramédicaux/bénéficiaires, diminuent ainsi considérablement le pouvoir et l'autonomie de ces professionnels.

Les moyens utilisés par les paramédicaux pour atteindre le modèle multidisciplinaire qu'ils préconisaient - égalité professionnelle au dossier, accès direct aux bénéficiaires et aux lieux de décision - relèvent d'un idéal professionnel[17] dont la stratégie tend à les affranchir de la dominance médicale et bureaucratique[18] en accroissant leur autonomie de pratique et leur pouvoir[19] au sein de l'hôpital.

Bien que les professions paramédicales sont des occupations socialement privilégiées, leur double dépendance - aux pouvoirs médical et administratif - les place dans un rapport de subordination qui réduit considérablement leur capacité de déterminer leurs conditions de pratique. Ces occupations sont donc socialement privilégiées, dans le contexte général de la division du travail, tout en étant défavorisées dans le contexte de la division professionnelle du travail médical. Ceci nous mène à deux hypothèses analytiques qui apportent des éclairages différents sur la stratégie autonomiste de ces occupations.

Plusieurs auteurs, dont C. Wright Mills et Eliot Friedson[20], indiquent que dans nos sociétés post-industrielles, la structure d'autorité est dominée par les professionnels où leur pouvoir est justifié par leur connaissance. Dans cette même perspective analytique, Ivan Illich et John McKnight[21] montrent que, sous un masque altruiste, le professionnalisme ne tend qu'à accroître le pouvoir des professionnels en leur donnant la possibilité de définir les besoins de la population et les réponses à leur apporter. Le professionnalisme, par les droits et les privilèges qu'il octroie aux occupations, subordonne la population aux services professionnels en la désappropriant de ses moyens de survie. Une telle analyse suggère l'hypothèse que le projet autonomiste des professions paramédicales, dans ce centre hospitalier, n'est stimulé que par les intérêts mesquins de professionnels, au statut et au prestige déjà importants qui ne cherchent encore une fois qu'à augmenter leur pouvoir et leurs privilèges.

Toutefois, la dépendance des professions paramédicales à l'autorité hiérarchique hospitalière et à l'autorité médicale, vient questionner une telle hypothèse. Comme l'indique Eliot Freidson[22], les occupations professionnelles sont, de nos jours, aux prises avec deux types de contrôle social, le modèle bureaucratique et le modèle professionnel.[23] Par leurs privilèges corporatistes, les professions paramédicales jouissent légalement de l'autocontrôle professionnel, mais leur statut de salariés et leur dépendance à la profession médicale viennent réduire de façon importante cette prérogative professionnelle. La position subordonnée qu'occupent ces travailleurs dans la division professionnelle du travail médical, nous amène à émettre une seconde hypothèse. Comme le suggèrent Sarfatti Larson et Johnson[24], compte tenu de la double dépendance des professions paramédicales, la stratégie professionnelle qu'ils utilisent, pour accroître leur autonomie de pratique, comporte des éléments "révolutionnaires" ou, tout au moins, des éléments émancipatoires puisqu'elle questionne l'autorité hiérarchique et professionnelle. Par leur projet professionnel, les paramédicaux mettent en cause les droits d'hospitalisation, de diagnostic et de référence détenus par le corps médical ainsi que les protocoles thérapeutiques imposés par les médecins. Ce projet autonomiste met aussi en cause les bases de l'organisation du travail en cherchant à développer une gestion hospitalière décentralisée. Somme toute, un tel projet questionne et tend à changer les réponses actuellement fournies aux problèmes de morbidité ainsi que les règles régissant la division du travail. Comme l'indiquent les hypothèses que nous venons d'émettre, la stratégie professionnelle des paramédicaux

- accès direct aux bénéficiaires, gestion hospitalière décentralisée - qui vise à accroître l'autonomie et le pouvoir de ces professionnels salariés, correspond à un projet corporatiste mesquin mais simultanément à un projet socialement émancipatoire puisqu'il s'oppose à l'organisation du travail qui supporte la dominance médicale et administrative.

Références

1. La continuité des soins, l'humanisation des soins et la promotion de la santé feront l'objet de publications ultérieures.

2. Le groupe des professions paramédicales comprend: pharmaciens, techniciens de laboratoire et de radiologie, physiothérapeutes, inhalothérapeutes, ergothérapeutes, diététistes, psychologues, travailleurs sociaux, orthophonistes et audiologistes.

3. Gouvernement du Québec, Rapport de la Commission d'Enquête sur la Santé et le Bien-être social, Editeur officiel du Québec (1970), Vol. 4, Tome 2, pp. 25-69.

4. Renaud, M., "Réforme ou illusion? Une analyse des interventions de l'Etat québécois dans le domaine de la santé", Sociologie et Sociétés, Vol. 9, no 1 (avril, 1977), Les Presses de l'Université de Montréal, p. 128.

5. Rapport de la Commission d'Enquête sur la Santé et le Bien-être social, op. cit. p. 96

6. Renaud, M., op. cit. p. 128.

7. Lipset, S.M. et al., Union Democracy, The Free Press, New York, 1956.
Crozier, M., Friedberg, E., L'acteur et le système, Editions du Seuil, Paris 1977.
Bacharah, S.B., Lawler, E.J., Power and Politics in Organization, Jossey-Bass Pub. San Francisco, 1980.
Freidson, E., Doctoring Together: A Study of Professional Social Control, Elsevier Scientific Publishing, New York, 1975.

8. Brunet, M., Vinet, A., "Le pouvoir professionnel dans le domaine de la santé et des services sociaux".

9. La DSH regroupe tous les services offerts par les professionnels paramédicaux ainsi que le service d'Accueil, la Centrale de rendez-vous et une partie des cliniques externes. La DSH n'a pas la responsabilité de la qualité des actes posés par les professionnels, ses fonctions sont strictement d'ordre administratives.

10. La DSP est responsable de l'organisation du travail médical dans l'hôpital tandis que le Conseil des médecins et dentistes (CMD) est responsable de la qualité des actes médicaux posés au sein de l'institution.

11. Brunet, M., Vinet, A., op. cit.

12. Renaud, M., op. cit. pp. 150-151.

13. Johnson, T.J. Professions and Power, Studies in Sociology, MacMillan Press, London, 1977, p. 40

14. Ibid, pp. 41-47.

15. Sarfatti Larson, M., The Rise of Professionalism: A Sociological Analysis, University of California Press, 1977, pp. 19-52 et pp. 178-207.

16. Voir la notion de "mediative control" chez Johnson, Professions and Power, op. cit. pp. 77-86.

17. Vollmer, H.M., Mills, B.L., Professionalization, Englewood Cliffs, New Jersey, 1966.

18. Sarfatti Larson, M., op. cit.
Johnson, T.J., op. cit.

19. Freidson, E., Profession of Medicine: A Study of the Sociology of Applied Knowledge, Harper and Row, New York, 1970.

20. Mills, C. Wright, Les Cols blancs, François Maspéro, Paris, 1966.

21. Illich, I., Némésis médicale: l'expropriation de la santé, Editions du Seuil, Paris, 1975.
McNIGHT, J., Le professionnalisme dans les services: un secours abrutissant", Sociologie et Sociétés, Vol. 9, No 1 (avril 1977), pp. 7-19.

22. Freidson, E., Doctoring Together, op. cit.; Professional Dominance, op. cit.; Profession of Medicine, op. cit.

23. Dans le modèle professionnel, la pratique et les conditions de travail sont contrôlées par les travailleurs eux-mêmes. Dans le modèle bureaucratique, les conditions de pratique et de travail sont contrôlées par des superviseurs.

24. Sarfatti Larson, M., op. cit.
Johnson, T.J., op. cit.

Implementing Feedback and Tuning Facilities in a System for Patient Management Simulations.

Olle Rosin[1], Johan Elfström[2], Hans Holmgren[3]
Sture Hägglund[3] and Ove Wigertz[1].

Linköping University, Linköping, Sweden

ABSTRACT: Computerized patient management simulation systems are used to provide training of clinical decision making. Such systems face two kinds of users with different demands: teachers (problem authors) and students. The teachers, most often unexperienced as computer users, need easy-to-use author tools to handle the problems and the simulation results. The students want the system to be a practical aid for the acquisition of patient management knowledge. This paper describes the MEDICS system, especially its teacher support and student feedback facilities, which are designed to make patient management simulations as useful as possible.

1. INTRODUCTION.

In medical work it is essential to have knowledge about a number of facts but also to use a pattern for the management of the patients. Learning of and training in such management patterns are usually not included in the curriculum at the universities in Sweden, especially for the selection of invasive diagnostic methods and treatment ordinations. The patients' security is one obvious reason why this training can not be included in the basic medical training. This paper presents an attempt to use computerized patient management simulation [1, 2, 3, 4, 5] moments in the medical education. For this purpose we have developed a system for patient management training called MEDICS [6, 7, 8, 9].

The system, developed from the booklet technique for patient management problems (PMP:s) introduced by e.g. McGuire et al. [10], includes programs for simulation of patient management, tools for interactive construction, testing and editing of PMP:s and software for printing of formatted lists of the PMP database. MEDICS is also used for production of text booklets employed in surgery examination at our university and for automatic calculation of the students' examination results.

---

[1] Dept. of Medical Informatics, Linköping University, Linköping, Sweden
[2] Dept. of Surgery, Linköping University, Linköping, Sweden
[3] Software Systems Research Center, Linköping University, Linköping, Sweden
This work was supported by the Swedish Board for Technical Development under contracts 77-7535, 78-5269, 79-4958

Our approach is an experimental one, where we want to find out the possibilities and limits of computer support. This leads to an emphasis on modularity and extensibility. This paper will discuss the facilities implemented to provide feedback regarding PMP simulations both to teachers and students. The teacher needs a verification that the definition of the simulation problem corresponds to the intended pedagogical objectives, as well as he needs a documentation of the actual performance of the students' running the simulations. From the students point of view, it is also important that feedback mechanisms are built into the system, in order to make training with the system interesting and rewarding.

Section 2 of this paper will present a short introduction to the MEDICS system, with a more specific description of only those aspects of the system which are relevant to the topic of this paper. In sections 3 and 4 the implementation of feedback and tuning facilities for PMP:s are discussed from the viewpoint of teachers and students respectively. In these sections we will describe the facilities actually implemented during the development and test phase of the MEDICS project and then discuss design problems and experiences. The final section summarizes our experiences so far and presents some conclusions regarding the organization of the software system.

2. THE MEDICS SYSTEM.

The MEDICS programs are managing a database of simulation problems. Each problem contains a number of sections with information about a simulated patient. Such management sections are history taking sections, physical examination sections etc. Each section defines a context where a number of alternative actions are allowed, for instance one or more X-ray examinations may be ordered in an X-ray section. Each action is represented as an item with the attributes:

- TEXT: a text string describing the item.
- RESPONSE: a value or an answer that is returned in response to a selection of this item.
- SCORE: the score added to the score sums if the item is chosen.
- NEXT: a forced transfer of control to another activity section.
- TIME: the simulated time delay associated with the action.

The attribute value of an item can be stored in the database either as a constant text or as program instructions to make the simulation dynamic.

A management section is presented to the student as a screen picture containing a header and a menu. The header describes the activity in the section and instructions for entering decisions. The menu contains the texts of the items among which to choose. If there are too many items in a section it can be divided into subsections with separate screen pictures.

Some options defined in the context of a management section are not pure information gathering or simple treatment ordinations, but rather decisions to proceed to another section for continued work. These items are usually listed separately in a decision subsection to be considered when the activity within the section is completed.

The menu-printing routines are dynamic in two ways. a) Visiting a management section is allowed only once. Therefore the items branching to visited sections is removed from the decision list of the actual section. b) Different layouts may be used when appropriate. For instance when a simulation problem is rerun in a feedback mode, asterisks indicating previous selections and the scores of the items are printed out in the menus using the same menu-printing routine.

The representation of a management section is classified according to two independent aspects. We prefer to name these aspects the management type and the execution type of the section respectively. The management type declares what kind of activity is modelled in the section, and it is mainly used for generation of default data.

The data structures representing a management section are interpreted by a set of small programs, the execution monitors. The MEDICS system maintains exchanges between monitors to select different types of dialogues with the student. The execution type defines how control is executed at run-time, i.e. which execution monitor to use. Presently, execution type may be used to define whether management options should be selected from explicitly displayed menus or suggested in a free text format, whether a section is to be executed as a tree structure of subsections, e.g. depending on space limits of the screen when menus are used etc.

This view of a PMP as a data structure with attached descriptions of how it is to executed as a simulation, also simplifies interfacing of other facilities available in the MEDICS development environment, such as the PMP construction system, the booklet formatter, the scoring aid, the simulation editor, etc. [9].

3. SUPPORTING THE TEACHER.

We believe that it is essential that a good computerized system supporting PMP simulations should provide the PMP author with versatile and extensible tools for tuning simulation problems, both regarding overall structure and style as well as details of a specific PMP. For this purpose, the author needs information which can verify that the created simulations really satisfy his pedagogical requirements. Our experience is that a lot of ideas about what is useful feedback facilities are generated during actual use of the system. Thus we have better be prepared to introduce new facilities as system development proceeds rather than to assume that these demands can be completely specified in advance.

3.1 Tuning of PMP:s.

We want to use the computer as a tool to support construction and refinement of PMPs and not merely as a tool to implement a program realizing the finished specification of a simulation problem. The following set of facilities are the basic tools available in MEDICS supporting of PMP construction and tuning.

The main tool is the MEDICS PMP editing subsystem which allows the author to interactively create and modify PMP:s directly during test runs. Editing commands operate upon the data structure describing the PMP and the logical parts of screen layouts displayed to the students. Thus it works more in terms of changes of a specification than in editing of a program text. A central feature in MEDICS editing is the integration with test execution of the PMP, which means that the effects of a modification may be immediately inspected. Since properties of this subsystem are further described elsewhere [6, 9], we will not go into detail here but will only mention that it provides operations for entering and modifying items, as well as higher-level operations for e.g. automatic layout generation for multi-column menus.

An obvious but important tuning aid are formatted database listings, showing the contents and structure of a PMP in a perspicuous and manageable form. The way chosen to represent PMP:s as data structures benefits from allowing such reports to be produced with standard database report generator programs. A special case concerns decision aids for calibration of item scores, which is simplified by the possibility to request lists of items sorted on scores and presented section by section.

A related task concerning tuning of scores is assessing the appropriateness of various activity sequences, i.e. the order in which sections are visited. The scores assigned to decisions involving a transfer between two sections may be viewed as weights connected with the edges in the problem graph. Since a node may be visited only once, the optimal score (for decisions) is associated with the path having the highest total weight among the ones connecting a subset of the nodes (sections). In order to compare the scoring of different decision sequences, decision trees may be expanded with scores accumulated along each path from the root section to a leaf section representing an exit from the PMP simulation. By presenting paths sorted on accumulated score, verification that the scores really correspond to the recommended activity sequences is supported. The actual value of this facility is uncertain at present, and it seems that the pruning mechanisms needed to terminate low-scoring paths should be further improved in order to prevent excessive search in the problem graph.

3.2 Evaluating the performance of the students.

When a simulation is finished the simulation result is accumulated in a result file. The file also contains mean score, standard deviation of score and the number of simulation events of the actual problem.

The simulation result contains:

- the student's pseudonym
- a set of performance indexes calculated from the student's choices and the positive and negative score sums [10].
- a list of the visited sections
- a number of lists containing the items the student selected in each section
- time spent in each section
- the student's verbal suggestions
- the date of the simulation

This data, saved on the result files in a packed raw-data structure, is later converted to a more presentable structure in order to make it convenient for the teacher to read.

An interesting and typical feature of implementation of student performance monitoring facilities is the hypothesis logging activity. After using the system for some time, it was suggested that it would be interesting to collect responses from the students showing their working hypotheses regarding the present illness of the simulated patient. Thus it was proposed that such a response were to be requested immediately before each decision involving a transfer to another management section. Due to our organization of PMP programs, this facility was introduced by writing a small module performing the desired interrogation of the student and updating the execution monitors with one statement each. By adding a declaration, signalling hypothesis logging, all PMP:s, including those previously defined, could be executed with this hypothesis interrogation activity included.

4. STUDENT FEEDBACK.

It is usually desirable to provide a training student with an immediate feedback after a simulation run. It is for this purpose possible to produce just a simple judgement whether the result was acceptable or not. However, much is to be gained from utilizing the full power of the computer support in order to provide the student with a rich and varied feedback, conveying as much as possible of the intentions of the teacher. Besides the obvious possibility to store immediate feedback in the answers associated with items and a final explanation of the rationale behind the simulation, we have implemented back-tracking and review facilities.

Back-tracking means that when a simulation is run in a special mode, undoing of actions are allowed. Thus the student may try a specific treatment measure, inspect the effects and if realizing that the wrong track is being pursued, back-up an arbitrary number of steps and then resume the simulation from that point. While backtracking, every effect of undone actions are nullified and previous state values restored.

Another way to use the system in a training mode is to have scores and indexes immediately displayed after each action. Combining this feature with back-tracking presents an experimenting student, or a group of cooperating students, with a way to successively return to the optimal or near-optimal route through the simulation.

At the end of the simulation phase of a problem run, the student is offered the opportunity to return for a review of the problem. All sections of the problem are presented in a menu from which a choice of one or more is made, whereupon execution is transferred to the first of the selected sections. Execution now proceeds as in the simulation phase, with three important modifications: a) no book-keeping is done, b) transfers between sections proceeds sequentially through the list of choices made by the student at the beginning of the feedback phase and c) the menus include scores for each item and asterisks marking the choices made earlier.

When considering the pedagogical possibilities of reviewing a simulation for feed-back purposes, we decided to let the student literally return to the problem. We hypothesized that displaying scores for all items as well as indicating items chosen during the simulation phase would stimulate the student to confirm or reconsider earlier efforts. Scoring could be interpreted as rather eloquent teacher comments, at least of relative relevance of alternatives. Contrasting these comments with the alternatives actually selected should provide food for thought, which ought to go a long way towards meeting important pedagogical requirements.

"Return to the problem" sounds straightforward enough, but is it? It would be if simulation of a section were independent of context. But it is not, since, for some items of a particular section, evaluation of certain properties presupposes a history of selections of other items from the same section or of visits to other sections. We are thus led to see that, as well as repeat the presentation of relevant material from the problem database, we have to provide an environment. Our first intuition, which strongly guided the actual implementation, was to restore the environment as faithfully as possible to what it had been at a particular stage of the simulation phase.

One departure was made from the overall restoration strategy, and that consisted in displaying all decision alternatives defined for a particular section, rather than excluding those that are inaccessible through already having been visited.

5. CONCLUSIONS.

Our experience is that during use of a system like MEDICS, it is to be expected that a number of new needs will arise, calling for new facilities to be added to the system. The modular approach chosen for PMP representation in the MEDICS system seems to provide a good foundation for introduction of various services promoting powerful tuning of PMP specifications, as well as flexible feedback mechanisms both for authors and students.

In the present prototype system, it typically takes about ten hours of work to create and tune a new PMP, containing some ten sections and several hundred medical items. This work is done by a physician, usually without any programmer assistance.

The student feedback system has gradually evolved during the project period, with features added in response to actual demands. The addition of new feedback facilities have been achieved also for previously defined PMP:s without any need for modification of the data representing those simulations. The feedback subsystem is highly appreciated by the students, and it is entered by almost every student after the simulation proper.

REFERENCES:

1. Rimoldi, H.J.A.: The test of Diagnostic Skills. *J. Med. Educ., 36*, pp 73-79, (1961).
2. Friedman, R.B., Korst, D.R., Scultz, J.V., Beatty, E. and Entine, S.: Experience with the Simulated Patient-Physician Encounter. *J. Med. Educ., 53*, pp 825-830, (1978).
3. Harless, W.G., Drennon, G.G., Marxer, J.J., Root, J.A., Wilson, L.L. and Miller, G.E.: CASE - A Natural Language Computer Model. *Computers in Biology and Medicine, 3*, pp 227-246 (1973). Illinois (1972).
4. Nelson, C.D., Sajid, A.W. and Solomon, L.W.: Diagnose: A Medical Computer Game Utilizing Deductive Reasoning. *Med. Educ., 10*, pp 55-56, (1979).
5. Taylor, W.C., Grace, M., Taylor, T.R., Fincham, S.M. and Skakun, E.N.: The Use of Computerized Patient Management Problems in a Certifying Examination. *J. Med. Educ, 51*, pp 179-182, (1976).
6. Elfström, J., Gillquist, J., Holmgren, H., Hägglund, S., Rosin, O. and Wigertz,O.: A Customized Programming Environment for Patient Management Simulations. *Proceedings of the 3rd World Conf. on Medical Informatics*, pp 328-332, Tokyo (1980).
7. Elfström,J., Gillquist, J., Holmgren, H. and Hägglund, S.: Experience with a System for Training Medical Students in Patient Management. *Proc. of the 3rd int. conference of EARDHE*, Klagenfurt (1979).
8. Hägglund, S.: An Application of Lisp as an Implementation Language for the Domain Expert's Programming Environment. Report LiTH-MAT-R-79-39, Informatics Laboratory, Linköping University, Sweden (1979).
9. Hägglund, S., Elfström, J., Holmgren, H., Rosin, O., and Wigertz, O., Specifying Control and Data in the Design of Educational Software, Report Software Systems Research Center, Linköping University, Sweden, (to appear 1980).
10. McGuire, Ch., Solomon, L.M. and Bashook, P.G.: *Handbook of Written Simulations*. Center for Educational Development, University of Chicago,

COMMON STANDARDS FOR QUANTITATIVE ELECTROCARDIOGRAPHY : THE CSE PILOT STUDY

The CSE European Working Party

J.L. Willems (Project Leader), P. Arnaud, J.H. van Bemmel, P.J. Bourdillon, Ch. Brohet, S. Dalla Volta, R. Degani, B. Denis, M. Demeester, J. Dudeck, F.M. Harms, P.W. Macfarlane, A. Mariën, G. Mazzocca, J. Meyer, J. Michaelis, J. Pardaens, J. Peden, S.J. Pöppl, H.J. Ritsema van Eck, E.O. Robles de Medina, P. Rubel, M. Sajet, J.L. Talmon and Chr. Zywietz

1. SUMMARY

A four year concerted action project has been started in the European Communities (EC) with the aim of "Common Standards for Quantitative Electrocardiography" (CSE Project). Standards for computer derived ECG measurements are urgently required because more and more quantitative diagnostic ECG criteria are now being derived by ECG computer programs and in view of the existing differences, first of all with respect to time measurements of present computer programs.

A detailed protocol has been agreed upon by participating countries and a pilot study has been conducted, whereby several procedures and ideas have been tested out. Investigators from 18 different institutes of the EC participate actively, either in the visual analysis or computer processing of a common ECG library. Experts from North-America also collaborate in the project.

2. INTRODUCTION

In recent years there has been a rapid growth in ECG recording in general and the use of computer ECG processing in particular. There are at present, however, no standards for computer ECG analysis. There is a lack of agreed definitions of waves, of common measurements, of standardized criteria for classification and of common terminology for reporting. This has created a situation whereby large differences in measurements by different computer programs hamper the exchange of diagnostic criteria and make evaluation studies on the utility and performance of computer programs difficult (1-2).

To overcome these problems a four year concerted action has been started in the European Communities (EC) striving towards "Common Standards for Quantitative Electrocardiography" (CSE project) (3-5).

Through a concerted action project, Member States of the EC intend, as part of the rules and procedures applicable to their national programmes, to carry out research and agree to integrate these research activities at Community level (3). A list of the participating institutes can be found elsewhere (4). Active participants from the EC constitute the CSE European Working Party. In addition investigators from the USA, Canada, and soon from Japan, participate in the project, either as consultants or by processing data.

3. OBJECTIVES

The first and main objective of the CSE project is to study the problems of (i) standardisation of computerized ECG measurements, (ii) determining definitions of waves and (iii) reference points for the on- and off-sets of P, QRS and T waves. Ultimately when the same ECG would be given as input to programs A, B or C, the same results, for example of Q durations, should be printed, an objective which is at present not attained. At least, mean values and variances should fall within acceptable ranges.

After the objective of this project has been reached, the next step will be to strive at improving diagnostic criteria and algorithms. In order to reach these goals, a library of ECGs must be established. This library will assist research in attaining common standards in measurement, the goal of the running CSE project.

The CSE project does not aim at developing "one" European ECG interpretation package or at obtaining the official EC approval for some programs. Through the exchange of ideas and data during CSE, participating centers will definitely benefit and be able to improve existing programs.

4. CSE PROTOCOL AND STAGES OF THE CONCERTED ACTION

A Steering Committee, consisting of principal investigators from 6 key centers, has prepared a working document, which was discussed during three general workshops by delegates from 18 participating European institutes in November 1978, in May 1979 and in January 1980. Based on these discussions a scheme of action and an elaborate protocol emerged. During a pilot study, various procedures and ideas were tested on a limited scale, and the CSE protocol (4) was further refined.

After final approval (3) by the European Commission, the CSE project entered its first stage on June 1, 1980. During this stage (June 80 - Dec 81) an initial library of 250 ECGs will be processed by programs and five referees, whose task is to define initially individually and later agree collectively, the onsets and offsets of P, QRS and T waves. The results will be used as a data base for the discussion on Common Standards.

Based on the experience of the first stage, a larger set of more than 1000 ECGs will be analyzed during a second stage (Jan. 82 - June 83). The task of the referees will probably be to act as consultants for difficult cases, in which there are unacceptably large differences between the processing results from the participating centers. Subgroups of different problematic ECGs will be defined. Noise tolerance tests will be performed. The library will include records with 8, 10 or 12 simultaneously recorded leads.

Overall results will be critically reviewed in the third stage, during the fourth and final year of the CSE project, and a final report will be produced in 1984.

5. PILOT STUDY

A pilot study was started January 1, 1979. This stage was designed for testing ideas and procedures on a limited scale. The protocol and formats for transferring information to and from the coordinating center were established.

5.1. The CSE ECG library

During the pilot study a small set of 12 original and 12 "artificial" ECG were sent out to different centers and to the 5 referee cardiologists for testing. In a parallel way a larger library of 250 ECGs (Frank XYZ lead and 12-lead ECG recordings, recorded in lead groups with a minimum of 3 simultaneous leads) was assembled. This library was selected so as to consist of ECGs with different wave shapes and common rhythm disturbances. Five centers contributed to the library. The sampling rate was 500 Hz and a minimum quantisation level of 5 microvolts was required. Further technical details can be found elsewhere (4).

In view of the different techniques applied in various programs, it was decided, in addition to the original basic library, to construct an artificial ECG library. By picking one beat out of each of the lead groups of the original ECG recordings, strings of identical beats were composed with constant RR interval. The selected beats were chosen by eye in such a way as to be close to the dominant beat with a signal to noise ratio as high as possible. Beats were selected with as little as possible base line shift, noise or artefact.
The 250 original ECG recordings of the first phase and the corresponding artificial ECGs have been evenly divided into two data sets. The results obtained from the first

set will be released in detail for every individual ECG, whereas only the overall statistical results will be published for data set 2. In this way data set one can be used as a learning set, and data set two will serve as test set.

In order to study effects of beat-to-beat variability, out of 30 original recordings two additional beats were selected to form another 60 artificial records. The beats adjacent to the one first selected were taken. They have also been divided evenly into both data sets.

5.2. Analysis by the referees

Each of the five referees received a hard-copy on Mingograph paper of 5 beats per ECG, one for each lead group. The beats were enlarged five and ten times in scale and time, and a time reference channel was written on a fourth channel. Referees were asked to indicate point estimates as well as upper and lower confidence limits for the on- and off-sets of the P, QRS and T waves. In addition, the referees had to provide a wave morphology description e.g. P+QRSR'T+, i.e. positive P and T waves and a prime R after a QRS complex. Together with the beats written out at 500 mm/sec paper speed, recordings were delivered of low pass filtered ECGs (3 db point at 15 Hz and zero output at 35 Hz) at a paper speed of 250 mm/sec. A "standard" ECG recording of the whole tracing was given as well, with an indication of the selected beats. All markings of the referees had to be made on the beats recorded at paper speed 500 mm/sec, whereby sample indications in the 4th channel are at 1 mm apart. The time locations of these markings were manually read in the coordinating center and entered into a computer for statistical analysis.

In addition, programs were developed in the coordinating center for interactive analysis of the ECGs on a graphics display terminal. These programs were used by all referees individually in May 1980 for an interactive indication of fiducial points in only those pilot ECGs for which they differed too much in the first off-line analysis. All referees had to review all point estimates where at least two out of the 5 referees differed by more than Δ t msec from the median of the whole group . The Δt limits were respectively 10 msec for the on- and off-sets of P, 6 msec for QRS-onset, 8 msec for QRS-offset and 20 msec for T-end. In addition to the Δ t rule, they also had to review those cases whereby a 2 versus 3 opinion was given on the presence or absence of a Q or QS wave in a particular lead. By applying these rules it was found from the pilot data that the referees had to review between 10 and 15 % of the measurements in a second round.

Remaining differences in opinion were settled in a third round. For this purpose the referees were invited to the coordinating center to give their final opinion in a joint meeting for the 3 % of the cases for which the Δt rules were still not met after the second round. A final consensus was reached in the third round for the 12 cases. The median of the second round was accepted as final estimate in one third of the remaining problem cases.

In order to study the intraobserver variability, the referees are being offered the same enlarged beats of 25 ECGs on 3 occasions, randomly over a period of one year during the first stage of the project. This brings the total number of ECGs to be analysed manually during the first stage to 360 (250 + 60 + 50), whereas the programs have to process a total of 560 ECGs (250 original and 310 "artificial" recordings).

5.3. Data processing by the computer programs

Both the original and "artificial" ECGs of the pilot study have been processed sofar by 8 XYZ and by 7 standard 12-lead ECG computer programs developed in Europe and North America. These programs are the CIMHUB program (Brussels), the Lyon, HES (Hannover), Glasgow, Padova and the Giessen programs, the Modular System (Amsterdam), the Louvain program, the AVA, IBM (version 2), HP-78 and Telemed programs. In the first stage, ECGs will be analyzed in addition by the Halifax program, and probably also by the Siemens and Nagoya programs. Participation of the Marquette program is promised for the second stage as soon as a subset of ECGs is available with 8 or 10 simultaneous lead recordings. A description of these programs can be found in references 6 and 7. Parameters being measured are basic time measurements and amplitudes. Time locations with respect to the beginning of the record or of the reference beat are requested according to a certain format as well as a copy of the raw data for the modal or averaged beat if applicable.

Statistical analysis programs were developed in the coordinating center for ECG computer program to program comparison. Statistical descriptive data such as median and mean values and variances were computed, as well as minimum and maximum values and ranges for all measurements in each of the respective leads or lead groups. Differences were computed for each program compared to the median program values. Variance analysis, parametric and non-parametric tests were applied to the results.

5.4. Comparison of median referee to median program results

Median values derived from the referee data and the program results have been compared during the pilot study for the following measurements : P-duration, PR-interval, QT-interval and QRS-duration. Programs are under development by which a comparison can be made of the absolute time locations of the on- and off-sets of P, QRS and T as determined on the one hand by the referees and on the other hand by the programs. This comparison can only be made for the "artificial" ECGs composed by strings of identical beats selected out of the original leads.

6. DISCUSSION

In the CSE project, a pragmatic approach to standardisation, using a data base and the human reader as a referee for ECG wave recognition is being pursued. The European Working Party has the feeling that some logic and mathematical definitions for visual and computer coding of the so-called ECG "waves" may emerge from these efforts.

There are several reasons why a data base approach has been selected in the CSE project. Experiences of investigators working in pattern recognition have demonstrated that several mathematical algorithms may lead to the same solution in the average case. Some methods, however, may perform better under different conditions than other and vice-versa. The use of a data base for the development of algorithms is standard practice in various fields from automated character reading to computer- assisted chromosome and leucocyte typing. So far many ECG program developers have used this approach in the establishment of their algorithms. For this they used a local data bank and human wave recognition usually by a single reader from their team.

Furthermore discussions with cardiologists have revealed an unwillingness of the medical community to accept strict mathematical definitions, if they have not been tested against wave recognition results derived by human reading. These were the main reasons why the establishment of an internationally recognized, independent ECG library and an elaborate review by a group of referees was considered essential in the CSE project.

A library has therefore been selected consisting of ECGs with different wave shapes and common rhythm disturbances. Results obtained by different programs will be compared between each other and with the results of the human referees. These results will be discussed at several meetings and will serve as a basis for the implementation of guidelines towards standards for ECG measurement programs.

Successful completion of this study, will allow the establishment of an extended programme aiming at the evaluation and improvement of the diagnostic performance of ECG computer programs. Diagnostic criteria can only be exchanged when programs provide the same basic measurement results when identical ECG records are submitted for analysis.

One of the first results of the CSE project is the cooperative establisment of a data base with internationally accepted wave reference points. It is hoped that by joint efforts, the CSE project will result in standards that will be acceptable to both cardiologists and computer scientists engaged in developing computer ECG measurement and interpretation programs.

7. LIST OF CSE COMMITTEES

CSE Steering Committee : P. Arnaud (F), R. Degani (I), P.W. Macfarlane (UK), J.H. van Bemmel (NL), J.L. Willems (B) (CSE Steering Cee chairman), Chr. Zywietz (D).

CSE Board of Referees : P.J. Bourdillon (UK), G. Mazzocca (I), B. Denis (F), J. Meyer (D), E.O. Robles de Medina and F.M. Harms (NL), H.J. Ritsema van Eck, consultant (NL)

CSE Working Party : see list of authors

Consultants : J.J. Bailey and H.V. Pipberger (USA), P.M. Rautaharju (CAN)

CSE Concerted Action Committee (COMAC) : National Delegates for Belgium : M. Demeester, J. Pardaens; for Denmark : I. Christiansen, J. Damgaard Andersen, E. Sandoe; for France : Ph. Coumel, P. Rubel; for Germany : J. Meyer, Chr. Zywietz; for Italy : R. Degani, U. Manzoli, G. Mazzocca; for Ireland : I. Graham; for United Kingdom : P.W.Macfarlane, P.J. Bourdillon; for the Netherlands : E.O. Robles de Medina, J.H. van Bemmel (COMAC chairman).

CSE Project Leader : J.L. Willems

For the European Commission : K. Gerbaulet

8. REFERENCES

1. Willems, J.L. and Pardaens, J. : Differences in measurement results obtained by four different ECG computer programs, In : Computers in Cardiology, Rotterdam meeting, (eds.) G. Ostrow and K.L. Ripley, IEEE Long Beach, 1977, 115-121.

2. Willems, J.L. : A Plea for Common Standards in Computer Aided ECG Analysis, Comp. Biomed. Res. 1980, 13 : 120-131.

3. Council Decision of 18 March 1980 adopting a second research programme in the field of medical and public health research, consisting of four multiannual concerted projects (80/344/EEC). Official Journal of the European Communities 1980, N°L78 pp. 24-28.

4. Willems, J.L. (chairman), Arnaud, P., Degani, R., Macfarlane, P.W., van Bemmel, J.H. and Zywietz, Chr. : Protocol for the EEC Concerted Action Project : "Common Standards for Quantitative Electrocardiography" (Second Edition) Ref. N° CSE 80-06-00, Leuven, June 2nd, 1980.

5. The CSE European Working Party : "An approach to measurement standards in computer ECG analysis", in Optimization of Computer ECG Processing" (H.E. Wolf and P.W. Macfarlane, editors), North Holland Publ. Co, Amsterdam, 1980, pp. 135- 138.

6. van Bemmel, J.H. and Willems, J.L. (eds) "Trends in Computer-Processed Electrocardiograms", North Holland Publ. Co., Amsterdam, 1977, pp. 1-437.

7. Zywietz, Chr. and Schneider, B. (eds) : Computer Applications in ECG and VCG Analysis. Proceedings of the 2nd IFIP TC-4 Working Conference, held in Hannover, Germany, North-Holland Publ. Co, Amsterdam, 1973, pp. 1-583.

9. ACKNOWLEDGMENT

This research has been supported in part by the Commission of the European Communities, Second R & D Programme in the Sector of Medical and Public Health Research (Council Decision 80/344/EEC, Contract MR-7-B-(G)) and by local and national research funding to different institutes in 6 EEC Member States. Financial support to the coordinating center (Division of Medical Informatics, University of Leuven, 35 Capucijnenvoer, 3000 Leuven, Belgium) was given through FGWO grant # 3.0050.79.

UN SYSTEME INFORMATIQUE EN BACTERIOLOGIE CLINIQUE - UTILISATION ET EXTENSIONS POSSIBLES POUR L'AIDE A LA THERAPEUTIQUE ANTIINFECTIEUSE ET L'ECONOMIE DE L'ANTIBIOTHERAPIE

A. THABAUT, J.-L. DUROSOIR, P. SALIOU, A. GUILLOREAU
Hopital militaire Bégin. Saint-Mandé France

Summary

Resistance of bacterial agents to the most commonly used antibiotics is in close quantitative relationship with their use. Efficient control of that use requires permanent information on bacterial etiology of the principal infections, on sensitivity of the principal species to antibiotics. Such information can only been obtained by means of automatic treatment of laboratory results. A computer system has been in use in the Bacteriology Laboratory of a 800 bed hospital for a few years. That system uses optical cards for entry of data. Apart from the daily help thus given to the running of the Laboratory, it also gives monthly epidemiological records which allows the bacteriologist to inform and advise clinicians. Significant results have thus been obtained concerning the decrease in frequency of antibioresistant bacterial strains. An extention of any such system would lead to improving the economy of antibiotherapy.

1. Introduction

La chimiothérapie et l'antibiothérapie ont révolutionné le traitement des maladies infectieuses. L'utilisation des sulfamides, puis de la pénicilline ont connu dans ce domaine de très grands succès. Mais progressivement des échecs sont apparus et se sont multipliés, liés à l'émergence de souches bactériennes résistantes à ces agents antibactériens. Depuis, la recherche pharmaceutique a mis à la disposition du thérapeute de nouveaux antibiotiques. Devant chacun d'entre eux les succès initiaux ont fait place à des échecs de fréquence croissante. L'antibioticorésistance est devenue une règle dans les divers domaines de la pathologie. Très longtemps, le mécanisme de cette antibioticorésistance est demeuré chromosomique : sélection, sous l'influence de la pression sélective d'un antibiotique déterminé, de mutants résistant à cet antibiotique. Plus récemment, sont apparues des résistances de mécanisme plasmidique : toujours sous l'influence de la pression sélective d'un antibiotique, des bactéries porteuses de plasmides ont pu diffuser de malades à malades, ou par l'intermédiaire du milieu extérieur. Ces plasmides sont de petites particules d'A.D.N., porteuses de l'information génétique déterminant une résistance, en général de haut niveau, à un antibiotique déterminé. Ces plasmides diffusent eux-mêmes, de façon épidémique de bactéries à bactéries. Les dangers pour la Santé Publique de ce mécanisme de résistance sont évidents. On a ainsi vu apparaître en divers points du globe des épidémies de dysentérie bacillaire, de typhoïdes dues à des bactéries résistantes à plusieurs antibiotiques. De plus en plus fréquemment, les infections nosocomiales sont dues à des bactéries dites opportunistes et polyantibioticorésistantes par déterminisme plasmidique. Le caractère commun de l'apparition de ces caractères de résistance chromosomique ou plasmidique est d'être en relation quantitative étroite avec l'utilisation des antibiotiques. Or, des études récentes réalisées en particulier aux Etats-Unis ont montré que dans un pourcentage de cas variant de 19 à 64 % en fonction des milieux étudiés, les antibiotiques étaient prescrits de façon inadéquate ou abusive. Ces antibiotiques représentent une part très importante de l'ensemble des dépenses de santé (aux Etats-Unis, 19 % dans les hôpitaux universitaires les mieux surveillés, 34 % dans les hôpitaux communaux). Il s'avère donc indispensable que dans l'intérêt de la Santé Publique, les divers maillons de la "chaîne humaine" des antibiotiques, le chercheur qui découvre et met au point l'antibiotique, l'industriel qui le produit, le pharmacien qui le vend et le médecin qui le prescrit, exercent un contrôle efficace sur la mise à la disposition et l'utilisation des antibiotiques. Mais pour cela, l'information de ces différents maillons est nécessaire : information sur l'étiologie bactérienne actuelle des principales infections humaines, sur la sensibilité actuelle des principales espèces bactériennes aux antibiotiques commercialisés, sur l'évolution de cette sensibilité. Ces données acquises isolément dans divers laboratoires d'un territoire donné sont en général utilisées sur le plan individuel, ou même inutilisées, et dans la plupart des cas ne sont pas exploitées sur le plan épidémiologique. Leur complexité, leur multiplicité devraient au premier chef bénéficier d'un traitement informatique.

2. Méthodes

Le caractère qualitatif et descriptif des résultats obtenus en bactériologie a longtemps retardé la mise en place de systèmes informatiques par rapport aux autres disciplines biologiques comme la biochimie ou l'hématologie.

2.1. Objectifs. Les objectifs recherchés par de tels systèmes sont fonction des besoins du laboratoire de Bactériologie :

- Allègement des tâches de secrétariat, fort lourdes et très souvent réalisées par les techniciens eux-mêmes au détriment de leurs fonctions purement techniques.
- Rappel des résultats des examens antérieurs pratiqués pour le même malade afin d'en aider l'interprétation par le clinicien.
- Aide à la gestion : comptabilisation des actes pratiqués par les divers postes du laboratoire, codifiés en lettres clef (B).
- Enfin et surtout, dans le domaine qui nous intéresse ici, surveillance de la résistance bactérienne aux antibiotiques, afin d'en tirer des conclusions thé-

rapeutiques. Depuis quelques années, certaines réalisations en France (1), en Grande-Bretagne (2-3) aux Etats-Unis (4-5) ont atteint tout ou partie de ces objectifs. La plupart de ces réalisations utilisent soit pour l'entrée des données, soit pour la transmission des résultats aux cliniciens des systèmes "on line" qui exigent l'implantation de nombreux terminaux aussi bien dans les divers locaux du laboratoire que dans les services cliniques. Cette multiplication des terminaux, la complexité de la programmation nécessaire, expliquent le coût élevé de ces systèmes et aussi leur manque de souplesse. Voulant éviter ces écueils, nous avons mis au point et utilisons depuis quelques années dans le laboratoire de Bactériologie d'un hôpital de 800 lits, un système informatique qui devait modifier au minimum les habitudes des cliniciens et du laboratoire, qui devait conserver une grande souplesse d'utilisation et exiger le minimum d'investissements matériels (6).

2.2. Saisie des données. Pour satisfaire à ces objectifs, le recueil des données devait être effectué par le technicien lui-même, sans "intermédiaire humain" pour l'entrée dans la machine. Nous avons donc opté pour la carte optique. Nous avons créé un modèle de carte optique spécifique de chaque poste de travail correspondant en général à un ou plusieurs produits pathologiques (Exemples : coprologie, bactériologie des urines, bactériologie de prélèvements divers (hémocultures, pus, L.C.R., sérosités), bactériologie vaginale). Pour faciliter et guider le travail du technicien, le schéma de chaque carte optique suit d'assez près le plan de l'examen que celui-ci réalise : les premières colonnes sont réservées à l'identification. Les colonnes suivantes sont successivement réservées à l'enregistrement des renseignements cliniques, aux résultats de l'examen macroscopique et microscopique du prélèvement, suivent enfin les résultats qualitatifs et quantitatifs des cultures bactériennes. Le technicien enregistre ses constatations en cochant une ou plusieurs cases de chaque colonne. Certains résultats ou renseignements sont codés et leur saisie consiste à cocher dans les colonnes correspondantes, les chiffres correspondant au code choisi en fonction d'un thésaurus préétabli : renseignements cliniques, service d'hospitalisation, espèce bactérienne. Mais la plupart des résultats qualitatifs ou numériques sont enregistrés en cochant dans chaque colonne la case correspondant à chaque constatation et identifiés par un ou plusieurs caractères mnémoniques ou bien la quantification en clair.

- L'enregistrement des antibiogrammes. L'étude de la sensibilité aux antibiotiques des diverses souches bactériennes isolées et identifiées dans le laboratoire, est réalisé par l'un des postes de travail. Classiquement, l'activité de chacun des antibiotiques sur une souche bactérienne est quantifiée par la mesure de la Concentration minima inhibitrice (C.M.I.) de cet antibiotique pour cette souche, en mcg/ml de substance active. Dans notre laboratoire, nous déterminons cette C.M.I. par une méthode semi-automatisée de microdilution en milieu liquide (7). Cette méthode de microdilution est réalisée dans des plaques comportant 8 rangées de 12 cupules chacune. Chaque rangée contient des dilutions successives d'un des antibiotiques étudiés dans le milieu de culture approprié. On ensemence ensuite de façon automatique chacune des cupules par une quantité standardisée de bactéries de la souche bactérienne. Après 18 heures d'incubation, à 37°, la lecture de la 1ère cupule dépourvue de culture bactérienne dans chacune des rangées donne la C.M.I. de l'antibiotique de la rangée. La subculture d'une aliquote de chacune des cupules dépourvues de culture bactérienne, permettra après 18 heures d'incubation de déduire la concentration minima bactéricide de l'antibiotique (C.M.B.). Les cartes optiques destinées à l'enregistrement de ces résultats, représentent fidèlement le schéma de la plaque de microdilution. La première partie cependant de cette carte, est destinée à enregistrer les divers renseignements "d'état civil" de la souche bactérienne, à partir desquels seront réalisés les tris nécessaires aux différentes études épidémiologiques : un code identifie tout d'abord la séquence des 8 antibiotiques dont l'activité a été étudiée, cette séquence ayant évidemment été choisie en fonction de l'espèce bactérienne et de l'origine du prélèvement, viennent ensuite les renseignements permettant d'identifier le malade, le code indiquant le service d'hospitalisation, le prélèvement à partir duquel a été isolée la souche bactérienne, et enfin l'espèce bactérienne à laquelle elle appartient. L'enregistrement des résultats eux-mêmes consiste tout simplement à cocher sur la partie de la carte réservée à cet effet, la case correspondant à la première cupule où aucune culture bactérienne n'est visible. Après subculture, on enregistrera de même la C.M.B. en cochant l'une des cases réservées à cet effet.

2.3. Fonctionnement du système. Nous n'insisterons pas sur le fonctionnement quotidien du système et sur le traitement quotidien des données ainsi enregistrées : Lecture des cartes par un lecteur optique, impression des résultats destinés au clinicien après validation et signature par le biologiste, impression du "registre légal" du laboratoire. En ce qui concerne les résultats de l'étude de la sensibilité aux antibiotiques, la machine, en fonction de concentrations dites "critiques" qui lui ont été fournies pour chacun des antibiotiques, interprète les C.M.I. et les C.M.B. en termes de sensibilité, de résistance, ou de sensibilité dite intermédiaire, plus facilement assimilables par le clinicien. Nous n'insisterons de même pas sur les états périodiques fournis par la machine, et destinés à aider à la gestion du laboratoire : Bilan d'activité, répartition des actes réalisés au profit des différents services de l'hôpital.

2.4. Etats épidémiologiques. Mensuellement, l'ordinateur fournit la répartition des isolements bactériens pratiqués dans le laboratoire, en valeur absolue et en pourcentage en fonction des différentes espèces bactériennes, la répartition de ces isolements en fonction des différents produits pathologiques, enfin la répartition en fonction des différents services de l'hôpital, ou des malades "externes". A ce niveau, chaque souche bactérienne, avec la date de son isolement est accompagnée de son antibiotype, c'est à dire de la liste des antibiotiques auxquels cette souche est résistante. A partir de ces états mensuels, le bactériologiste rédige un bulletin "d'informations microbiologiques" par service de l'hôpital. Sur ce bulletin, adressé à chacun des médecins et à la surveillante du service, sont indiquées les répartitions des souches bactériennes isolées dans le service, en fonction du produit pathologique. et de leur sensibilité aux différents antibiotiques. Ces relevés sont accompagnés de commentaires attirant l'attention des médecins sur l'émergence d'une espèce bactérienne dans le service, ou sur l'émergence de la résistance à telle ou telle famille d'antibiotiques. Ces commentaires sont assortis de conseils sur l'emploi rationnel des antibiotiques. Il est évident que des programmes de tri, très simples, permettent d'obtenir à la demande la fréquence des diverses espèces bactériennes dans tel ou tel produit pathologique en fonction du temps, et donc de suivre l'évolution de l'étiologie bactérienne des infections ; ou bien dans un service déterminé, pour suivre l'évolution de l'écologie bactérienne du service et ainsi surveiller les infections nosocomiales ; ou encore les pourcentages cumulés des C.M.I. et des C.M.B. d'un antibiotique déterminé pour une espèce bactérienne déterminée, ce qui permettra de suivre l'évolution de l'activité de cet antibiotique sur cette espèce.

3. Résultats

Nous n'insisterons pas sur les résultats satisfaisants que nous avons obtenus quant au fonctionnement quotidien du laboratoire, la suppression du travail de secrétariat, et l'aide à la bonne gestion pour nous limiter à l'aide que nous a apporté ce système dans la surveillance épidémiologique et de la pharmacosensibilité des bactéries. Quelques exemples illustreront ces résultats.

. La comparaison de l'étiologie des infections urinaires observées chez les malades hospitalisés et chez les malades ambulatoires, a montré qu'"en ville", ces infections étaient déterminées essentiellement par Escherichia coli et Proteus mirabilis, et que les bactéries appartenant à ces espèces demeuraient sensibles aux principaux antibiotiques. Par contre, à l'hôpital, l'étiologie de ces infections était beaucoup plus polymorphe et représentée par des bactéries appartenant à des espèces souvent naturellement résistantes.

. L'étiologie des infections observées dans le service de chirurgie osseuse de l'hôpital s'est avérée surtout staphylococcique. Ceci a entrainé la mise en oeuvre d'une enquête épidémiologique, aidée des marqueurs sérotypiques et lysotypiques de cette espèce bactérienne. Cette enquête a permis de conclure que les malades le plus souvent transéatés d'autres formations hospitalières, arrivaient dans le service, porteurs de leur staphylocoque, et de dégager la responsabilité de porteurs éventuels appartenant au personnel.

. Les relevés effectués dans le service de réanimation de l'hôpital ont établi que les Pseudomonas aeruginosa et les Acinetobacter, bactéries opportunistes fréquemment à l'origine de surinfections dans ce service, appartenaient à des sérotypes différents, et qu'il n'existait pas d'épidémie hospitalière dues à ces espèces.

. La surveillance de la sensibilité aux antibiotiques des différentes espèces bactériennes nous a en particulier montré la fréquence des entérobactéries, des Escherichia coli, résistants aux ampicillines, antibiotiques à large spectre, d'usage fréquent. La restriction conseillée de l'utilisation de ces antibiotiques a permis d'obtenir une décroissance nette de cette résistance. Nous avons également observés à une certaine période, dans plusieurs services de l'hôpital, l'apparition de nombreuses souches de staphylocoques résistant aux antibiotiques de la famille des aminosides. Là aussi, la restriction conseillée de l'utilisation de ces antibiotiques a permis d'obtenir des résultats tangibles. Ce ne sont que quelques exemples de la surveillance permanente de la sensibilité bactérienne aux antibiotiques que ce système nous permet d'exercer, et des résultats que l'information ainsi portée à la connaissance des thérapeutes a permis d'obtenir. Dans l'ensemble, ces résultats sont concrétisés de façon éclatante par la diminution notable de la fréquence des isolements bactériens d'une part, et d'autre part par la diminution notable parmi ces isolements de la fréquence des espèces et des souches bactériennes antibioticorésistantes en fonction du temps.

4. Extension possible du système

Il est évident que la localisation de ce système à une formation hospitalière réduit d'autant son intérêt. Or il est facilement "portable" et en particulier transférable à de petits ordinateurs. Son extension aux autres formations hospitalières du Service de Santé des Armées est en cours. La carte optique de recueil des résultats de l'antibiogramme peut être facilement adaptée aux diverses techniques utilisées actuellement dans les différents laboratoires. Il sera évidemment nécessaire d'ajouter un code indiquant le laboratoire ou l'hôpital émetteur des données. L'extension de ce système ou de tout système semblable à l'échelon régional, puis national, et pourquoi pas international permettrait enfin une surveillance permanente de l'évolution de l'étiologie des infections bactériennes et surtout une surveillance permanente de la sensibilité des différentes espèces bactériennes aux antibiotiques. Les informations ainsi obtenues et diffusées périodiquement permettraient d'orienter les recherches des biochimistes vers tel ou tel antibiotique nécessaire dans telle ou telle zone géographique, d'orienter les thérapeutes vers l'utilisation préférentielle de tel ou tel antibiotique et l'abandon de telle autre famille. L'information permanente est le seul moyen efficace, non coercitif, d'obtenir la mise en oeuvre d'une antibiothérapie rationnelle et bénéfique aux malades et à la collectivité. Seules les méthodes informatiques peuvent permettre d'acquérir et de diffuser cette information.

BIBLIOGRAPHIE

(1) BRUN Y., FLEURETTE J., CHARLIEUX M., FALCOZ H., MOREAUX G. : Computerized management of a medical bacteriology Laboratory. Med. Informatics, 1979, 4,4.

(2) WILLIAMS K.N., DAVIDSON J.M.F., LYNN R., RICE E., PHILLIPS I.A. : Computer system for clinical microbiology. J. Clin. Pathol., 1978, 31, 1193-1201.

(3) MITCHISON D.A., DARREL J.H., MITCHISON R. : A computer - assisted bacteriology reporting and information system. J. Clin. Pathol., 1978, 31, 673-680.

(4) KUNTZ L.J. : Computerization in microbiology. Human Pathol., 1976, 7, 169 - 175.

(5) JORGENSEN H.J., HOLMES P., WILLIAMS W.L., HARRIS J.L. : Computerization of a hospital clinical microbiology laboratory. Am. J. Clin. Pathol., 1978, 69, 605-614.

(6) THABAUT A., DUROSOIR J.L., SALIOU P. : Un système informatique en bactériologie clinique. Proceed. 2 nd, Annual WAMI Meeting 1979, March, 520-523.

(7) THABAUT A., DUROSOIR J.L. : Semi-automatisation de la concentration minima inhibitrice et de la concentration minima bactéricide des antibiotiques isolés et associés. Méd. et Mal. Infectieuses. 1976, 6, 3, 90-100.

EVALUATION DE LA FIBROSCOPIE EN PNEUMOLOGIE
VALIDITE DES PRELEVEMENTS

P. LAMY, S. BRIANCON, K. KHALIFE, B. CANET, G. ETHEVENOT
Service de Pneumologie, Hôpital Villemin, 54037 NANCY CEDEX

SUMMARY

The authors try an assessment of technique and indications of flexible fiberoptic bronchoscopy in three studies. For oncology diagnosis true positivity rate is 0.75 and predictive value of negative result 0.88. Variations are indicated according to tumor's type and site and especially to indications, 20 percent of procedures seem to be useless. For diagnosis of tuberculosis a retrospective study shows worse results with bronchoscopy specimens than with expectorated sputum specimens. A prospective study has been begin for verfication. Preliminary results do not show any improvment of the bronchoscopy procedure in direct examination. For bronchoalveolar lavage, we assess lymphocytes populations expressed in percentage and immunoglobulines G and A expressed in mg/100 ml for discrimination of diffuse interstitial lung disease in hypersensitivity pneumonitis (HP) sarcoïdosis and other pulmonary pneumonitis and fibrosis (PF). The averages are significantly different, highest in HP, lowest in PF, but wide ranges do not allow to yield diagnostic limit values with high true positivity and negativity rate.

L'endoscopie à visée diagnostique a connu ces dernières années un grand développement en pneumologie. Le bronchoscope rigide, par son maniement difficile et lourd, limitait les indications de la technique ; l'apparition du fibroscope souple, avec sa facilité et son confort, a conduit à une multiplication des indications par le biais de nouvelles approches bronchiques et parenchymateuses, mais aussi d'une pratique plus large. Ainsi, la fibroscopie est devenue un examen simple, habituel, "de routine", qui s'inscrit dans le bilan pneumologique après la clinique et la radiologie, et parfois en dehors d'elles...

Nous avons tenté une évaluation à la fois de la technique et de nos indications dans deux études classiques, oncologique, microbiologique, puis dans le lavage broncho-alvéolaire d'apparition récente et pour lequel il serait intéressant de définir des critères diagnostiques. Cette étude fait appel à 573 malades qui ont été explorés sur une période de 6 mois.

I - LA FIBROSCOPIE A VISEE CARCINOLOGIQUE

400 malades sont concernés ; 24 d'entre eux ont été perdus de vue et non étiquetés de façon définitive, et en première approximation, nous les estimons se comporter comme les autres malades. La preuve d'un néoplasme a été apportée dans 100 cas par la fibroscopie (prélèvement histologique ou cytologique positif au 1er ou 2ème examen). Les cas non prouvés par la fibroscopie l'ont été par ponction transpariétale, chirurgie ou autopsie.

	NEOPLASME oui	non	Total
(+)	100	0	100
(-)	33	243	276
	133	243	376

Spécificité : 1
Sensibilité : 0.75
Valeur prédictive d'une fibroscopie négative : 0.88

Ces résultats indiquent la valeur de la fibroscopie et sont en accord avec la littérature (1, 2, 3). Deux chiffres sont intéressants pour nous ici :

a) que sont les 33 néoplasmes non diagnostiqués ?

b) pourquoi 64.5 % des malades ont-ils eu une fibroscopie à la recherche d'un cancer qui n'existait pas ?

a) Les 33 cancers se répartissent en 22 primitifs, 9 secondaires et 2 hémopathies. Les cancers secondaires sont moins bien diagnostiqués (47 %) que les cancers primitifs (81 %) ($p < 0.01$).

Le caractère topographique du cancer joue un rôle considérable ; 36 opacités radiologiques périphériques dont le diagnostic a pu être obtenu, se répartissent ainsi :

	NEOPLASME oui	non	Total
(+)	15	0	15
(-)	12	7	19
	27	9	36

Sensibilité : 0.75
Valeur prédictive d'une fibroscopie négative : 0.36

Ces images méritent donc que soit réalisée une fibroscopie dont les aspects peuvent être discordants, mais le faux-négatif est fréquent et ne doit pas faire reculer une indication chirurgicale indiscutable sur ce type d'images.

b) Le nombre considérable de fibroscopies "inutiles" nous a conduit à rediscuter nos indications, et nous avons revu tous les dossiers cliniques et radiologiques de nos patients, rétrospectivement, et à l'aveugle, par rapport aux résultats de la fibroscopie. Nous avons ainsi individualisé 3 catégories :

- catégorie 1 : indication d'évidence pour confirmation d'un diagnostic certain sur le tableau radioclinique,
- catégorie 2 : indication de nécessité pour établissement d'un diagnostic que ne permettait pas de prévoir le tableau radioclinique : hémoptysies quel que soit le tableau radiologique, image radiologique à type d'opacité ronde périphérique, médiastinale, abcès du poumon lobite rétractile, recherche d'un primitif après découverte d'un métastase de type épidermoïde, bilan d'extension d'un cancer oesophagien.
- catégorie 3 : indication de sécurité ou de luxe dont la nécessité n'apparaît pas clairement, et qui a été posée par déontologie, facilité ou scrupule.

Résultats

	Catégorie 1			Catégorie 2			Catégorie 3		
	Néoplasme		Total	Néoplasme		Total	Néoplasme		Total
	oui	non		oui	non		oui	non	
Fibroscopie (+)	42	0	42	58	0	58	1	0	1
Fibroscopie (-)	4	0	4	28	152	180	0	78	78
	46	0	46	86	152	238	1	78	79

Les 46 malades de la catégorie 1 ont tous un cancer : 45 fois primitif, 1 fois secondaire, toujours vu par l'endoscopiste qui ne peut cependant en faire la preuve histologique 4 fois. La sensibilité est de 0.91 et la valeur prédictive d'une fibroscopie négative est bien sûr de 0. La fibroscopie est ici un examen sûr qui ne fait que confirmer le diagnostic, mais cependant indispensable afin de voir la lésion, d'en préciser l'extension pouvant modifier l'attitude thérapeutique (élargissement ou contre-indication de la chirurgie) et d'en définir le type histologique (2).

La catégorie 2 est la plus intéressante ; c'est avec elle que se pose l'évaluation de la méthode dans les diagnostics difficiles. Les 24 perdus de vue sont tous de cette catégorie ; 13 sont des contrôles de néoplasme bronchique après traitement et ont été exclus. La sensibilité est de 0.67 et la valeur prédictive d'une fibros copie négative est de 0.84. Dans l'hypothèse du biais maximum où tous les perdus de vue seraient des néoplasmes, la sensibilité n'est plus que de 0.52. C'est dans cette catégorie que se retrouvent les néoplasmes à forme périphérique et les métastases broncho-pulmonaires.

Un seul cancer est diagnostiqué dans la catégorie 3. Pourquoi a-t-on fait la fibroscopie chez ce patient artéritique au stade IV, emphysémateux et qui présentait une altération de l'état général ? L'examen peut être qualifié de presque inutile.

En conclusion, au total donc, il est clair que la fibroscopie est un excellent examen utile et efficace à la condition que son indication soit correctement réfléchie après une démarche intellectuelle logique faisant intervenir les données cliniques et radiologiques. 20 % de nos examens pourraient être évités, diminuant le coût rendement de la méthode, l'aspect financier d'une telle extension n'étant pas négligeable et dépassant largement les 100 000 francs estimés chez ces 78 malades. Il n'en demeure pas moins que nous avons ainsi diagnostiqué un cancer plus précocémert que si avait été attendu le tableau radioclinique justifiant. Mais, est-il licite de poursuivre ainsi des examens abusifs ? Faut-il faire de la fibroscopie un examen de dépistage systématique ?

II - LA FIBROSCOPIE A VISEE MICROBIOLOGIQUE

Nous nous intéresserons ici à la recherche de bacilles tuberculeux, la recherche de germes banals ou opportunistes étant trop peu réalisée dans notre service pour en faire une évaluation.

Une fibroscopie a été réalisée 89 fois pour recherche de B.K. chez des sujets présentant une image radiologique suspecte. La technique de prélèvement consistait simplement en une broncho-aspiration du territoire incriminé, avec examen direct et mise en culture du prélèvement. Cette étude rétrospective nous permet de comparer les deux techniques de prélèvements que sont les crachats simples et la broncho-aspiration.

		BRONCHO-ASPIRATION					
		Examen direct			Culture		
		(+)	(-)	Total	(+)	(-)	Total
Crachats	(+)	7	2	9	16	7	23
	(-)	1	79	80	0	66	66
		8	81	89	16	73	89

Résultats concordants ($p < 10^{-9}$)
Coefficient de concordance 0.81
Pas d'amélioration décelable de la fibroscopie

Résultats concordants ($p < 10^{-9}$)
Coefficient de concordance 0.77
Supériorité des crachats sur la culture ($p < 0.05$)

Ces résultats d'une enquête d'observation où l'on ne connaît pas notamment le pourcentage exact de véritables tuberculoses, argumentant pour une inhibition éventuelle des cultures par la Xylocaïne utilisée à titre anesthésique (4), mais en contradiction avec d'autres études de la littérature (5, 6), nous ont conduits à entreprendre une enquête prospective pour répondre à deux questions : notre technique est-elle en cause ? faut-il préconiser l'arrêt de la fibroscopie pour la recherche de B.K. ? Dans des conditions standardisées sont effectués des prélèvements par broncho-aspiration et brossage du territoire intéressé, et ceci dans un ordre déterminé par le hasard chez des sujets dont le tableau radioclinique est suspect de tuberculose, mais dont les examens directs de crachats sont négatifs. Les 3 jours suivants, sont réalisés à nouveau des examens de crachats. Nous ne disposons à ce jour que de résultats préliminaires ; chez 15 sujets, la fibroscopie n'a jamais permis de trouver de bacilles tuberculeux à l'examen direct lorsque l'examen de crachats avait été défaillant. Mais bien sûr, il est trop tôt pour conclure de façon définitive.

III - LA FIBROSCOPIE POUR LAVAGE BRONCHO-ALVEOLAIRE (L.B.A.)

Avec cette technique, la fibroscopie ne se contente plus d'explorer la bronche, mais tente une approche du poumon profond. Dernier né des moyens d'investigations pneumologiques, facile dans sa réalisation technique, il demande que soient précisés des critères diagnostiques qui permettraient notamment de distinguer les pneumopathies diffuses en alvéolites allergiques extrinsèques (A.A.E.), sarcoïdose et autres pneumopathies et fibroses (P.I.D.). Nous ne reviendrons pas sur les conditions techniques qui ont fait l'objet de nombreux rapports et qui sont parfaitement codifiées (7). La particularité, l'originalité et la difficulté d'interprétation des résultats de cet examen résident dans le fait que les milieux biologiques broncho-alvéolaires recueillis sont dilués en proportion inconnue dans le liquide injecté puis partiellement recueilli.

Notre étude porte sur 115 L.B.A. de première intention : 20 témoins, 9 A.A.E., 51 sarcoïdoses, 20 P.I.D. et 15 diagnostics divers. L'exploitation statistique des résultats a été effectuée sur ordinateur HP 9825.

Les populations cellulaires recueillies sont composées de macrophages et de lymphocytes ; la présence de polynucléaires est pathologique et traduit soit un processus infectieux, soit une fibrose pulmonaire avancée. Nous nous intéressons ici aux variations de la lymphocytose exprimées en pourcentage de la totalité des cellules recueillies.

Témoins			A.A.E.			Sarcoïdose			P.I.D.		
n	m	s	n	m	s	n	m	s	n	m	s
20	5,12	3,9	9	60	26,1	51	32,7	19,8	20	10,9	10,2

Les témoins se comportent de façon particulière. Le tabagisme influence chez eux la lymphocytose. 4.2 % chez les fumeurs, 10.33 chez les nons fumeurs ($p < 0.01$) alors que nous ne retrouvons pas cette influence chez le sujet malade (analyse de variance avec ajustement sur le diagnostic ($F = 1.16$) non significatif).

La distribution de la lymphocytose paraît suivre une loi normale dans chacun des sous-groupes, cependant la variance dans la fibrose est inférieure à celle des deux autres groupes ($p < 0.002$). Alvéolite allergique et sarcoïdose n'ont pas une variance significativement différente ; la lymphocytose moyenne est différente dans les groupes ($p < 10^{-3}$).

Cependant, la variabilité est importante et il est difficile pour un sujet donné de fixer des valeurs diagnostiques seuils. Les meilleures valeurs discriminantes trouvées sont 15 et 50 % .

Lymphocytes	A.A.E.	Sarcoïdose	Autres	Total
L < 15 %	0	9	[13]	22
15 % < L < 50 %	3	[33]	7	43
L > 50 %	[6]	9	0	15
Total	9	51	20	80
Spécificité	0.87	0.66	0.85	0.73
Sensibilité	0.67	0.65	0.65	0.67

Ces résultats sont donc médiocrement satisfaisants ; ils apportent néanmoins un élément d'orientation appréciable confronté au contexte clinique et radiologique. Les recherches s'orientent actuellement vers l'appréciation d'éléments de surveillance dans la sarcoïdose traitée et non traitée afin de tenter de définir des critères <u>d'évolutivité</u> permettant l'arrêt ou la reprise d'une corticothérapie. Notons que nous ne mettons pas ici en évidence de lien entre le stade radiologique de la maladie et la lymphocytose (variance identique, $F = 0.13$), ni de différence entre la lymphocytose des sujets traités et non traités.

Stade 1			Stade 2			Stade 3		
n	m	s	n	m	s	n	m	s
18	34,5	18,3	24	31,4	22,3	9	32,7	17,3

Pour améliorer la sensibilité de la méthode, l'étude des composants biochimiques et notamment des protéines a été proposée. Les dosages sont réalisés par méthode immunonéphélométrique et les résultats exprimés en mg/100 ml. L'albumine est surtout utilisée pour servir de substance de référence à l'expression des résultats des immunoglobulines G et A (IgG, IgA).

	A.A.E. n = 9		Sarcoïdose n = 22		Autres n = 9	
	m	s	m	s	m	s
Protéine totale	57	28,9	33,35	20,7	16,1	6,8
Albumine	33,2	31,7	19,2	18,6	6,1	1,9
IgG	17,6	11,8	8,2	11,4	3,15	2,8
IgA	7,4	6,1	2,2	2,1	1,1	1

La distribution de ces valeurs ne suit pas une loi gaussienne ; la variance est sensiblement proportionnelle à la moyenne ; une transformation logarithmique permet de normaliser la distribution et d'égaliser les variances.

	A.A.E. n = 9		Sarcoïdose n = 31		Autres n = 12	
	m	s	m	s	m	s
Protéines	2,69	0,27	2,43	0,31	2,16	0,21
Albumine	2,36	0,43	2,12	0,39	1,72	0,27
IgG	2,14	0,33	1,67	0,47	1,36	0,35
IgA	1,74	0,35	1,16	0,41	0,89	0,38

Les différences sont hautement significatives ($p < 10^{-3}$) tant pour les protéines totales que l'albumine, les IgG, que les IgA et toujours dans le même sens valeurs supérieures dans les A.A.E., puis les sarcoïdoses, puis les autres pneumopathies donc évoluant dans le même sens que la lymphocytose. Il existe d'ailleurs une forte corrélation entre ces valeurs logarithmiques et la lymphocytose respectivement : r vaut 0.457, 0.473, 0.599, 0.506 ($p < 10^{-3}$) et enfin, il existe une forte corrélation entre ces différentes valeurs elles-mêmes (toujours $p < 10^{-3}$). Il apparaît donc au vu de ces résultats totalement illogique d'utiliser l'albumine comme substance de référence, et d'ailleurs toutes les liaisons disparaissent quand on utilise les rapports "classiques" IgG/Alb et IgA/Alb.

Ces évolutions dans le même sens et en fonction des diagnostics nous ont conduits à construire un indice qui permettrait d'améliorer la sensibilité diagnostique avec i = % de lymphocytes x IgG ; les meilleures valeurs seuils sont 0.25 et 50.

	A.A.E.	Sarcoïdose	Autres	Total
i < 0,25	0	6	8	14
0,25 < i < 50	1	20	4	25
i > 50	8	5	0	13
TOTAL	9	31	12	52
Spécificité	0.88	0.76	0.85	0.80
Sensibilité	0.89	0.65	0.67	0.69

L'amélioration n'est donc que médiocre et porte essentiellement sur les A.A.E. où la sensibilité devient satisfaisante. Par contre, tant la spécificité que la sensibilité restent médiocres dans les sarcoïdoses, principal point d'intérêt et d'exploration de cette technique. L'essai de construction d'indices plus complexes utilisant les logarithmes des immunoglobulines G et/ou A n'apporte pas d'amélioration sensible.

Cette étude nous a permis de retrouver l'ensemble des résultats de la lymphocytose de la littérature (7, 8, 9) ; nous confirmons l'absence de l'intérêt de l'albumine comme substance de référence (10). Par contre, HARF (10) ne trouve pas les mêmes répartitions des composants protéiques et signale des valeurs plus importantes dans la sarcoïdose que dans les A.A.E. Il préconise l'utilisation du potassium comme substance de référence ; nos résultats apportent une valeur discriminante satisfaisante avec l'utilisation du changement de variable. Au total, le lavage broncho-alvéolaire serait un examen intéressant dans les pneumopathies diffuses où il peut apporter une orientation diagnostique. Il garde cependant un intérêt essentiellement spéculatif et de recherche sans pouvoir entrer dans une pratique clinique courante. En effet, les imprécisions qui peuvent être liées à la technique, les importantes variations individuelles lui imposent des limites nettes. Les recherches doivent donc se poursuivre pour lui accorder une meilleure valeur diagnostique et surtout apporter des indices de surveillance dans la sarcoïdose.

BIBLIOGRAPHIE

1 - IKEDA (S.)
Flexible bronchofiberscope.
Ann. Oto-Rhinol.-Laryngol., 1970, 79, 916.

2 - JOB (Ch), PIERON (R.), OUSTRIERES (G.), BLANCHE (J.M.), JAGUEUX (M.)
Biopsie et fibroscopie dans le cancer bronchique.
J. Agrégés, 1975, 8, 105.

3 - PARAMELLE (B.), BRAMBILLA (C.), MACARY (C.), PARENT (D.), AUGUSSEAU (S.), RIGAUD (D.
Intérêt et validité des prélèvements en fibroscopie bronchique (à propo
de 1 200 examens).
Broncho-Pneumol., 1977, 27, 1-6.

4 - BARLETT (J.G.), ALEXANDER (D.), MAYEW (J) et coll.
Should fiberoptic bronchology Aspirates be cultured.
Am. Rev. Resp. Dis., 1976, 114, 73.

5 - DANEK (S.J.), BOWER (J.S.)
Diagnosis of pulmonary tuberculosis by flexible fiberoptic bronchoscopy
Am. Rev. Resp. Dis., 1979, 119, 677.

6 - De LABARTHE (B.), LE FRECHE (J.N.), KERNEC (J.), CORMIER (M.), KOMBILA (M.)
Exploitation microbiologique du brossage bronchique.
Nouv. Presse Méd., 1974, 3, 2413.

7 - VOISIN (C.), TONNEL (A.B.), LAFITTE (J.J.), RAMON (Ph.)
Les populations cellulaires des espaces aériens broncho-alvéolaires dans la sarcoïdose, les alvéolites allergiques extrinsèques et les cancers bronchiques.
Nouv. Presse Méd., 1977, 6, 2685.

8 - DANEL (C.), ARNOUX (A.), MARSAC (J.), BASSET (F.), CHRETIEN (J.)
Données cellulaires apportées par le lavage broncho-alvéolaire au cours de diverses pathologies interstitielles.
INSERM, 1979, 84, 489-498.

9 - REYNOLDS (H.Y.), MERRILL (W.W.)
Analysis of broncho-alveolar lavage in normal humans and patients with diffuse interstitial lung disease.
INSERM, 1979, 84, 227-250.

10 - HARF (R.), BIOT (N.), BIRON (A.), CHEVALIER (J.P.), FROBERT (Y.), PERRIN-FAYOLLE (M
Les composants protéiques du liquide de lavage broncho-alvéolaire.
Etude critique des modes d'expression des résultats.
INSERM, 1979, 84, 35-48.

EVALUATION DES PROCEDURES DIAGNOSTIQUES

DANS LES ACCIDENTS VASCULAIRES CEREBRAUX CONSTITUES

J.F. DARTIGUES*, J.J. PERE*, J.M. ORGOGOZO*, R. SALAMON**

* Unité de Pathologie Vasculaire Cérébrale, Hôpital Pellegrin-Tripode
Place Amélie Raba Léon - 33076 BORDEAUX CEDEX (France)

** Département Informatique, Université de BORDEAUX II
146 rue Léo Saignat - 33076 BORDEAUX CEDEX (France)

RESUME

Nous avons cherché à évaluer l'apport informationnel de diverses investigations pour le diagnostic d'accidents vasculaires cérébraux constitués.
A partir d'un audit nous avons établi que :
- l'examen clinique et biologique, le Doppler précoce et la tomodensitométrie étaient toujours nécessaires
- l'artériographie ne doit être prescrite qu'une fois sur deux
- la ponction lombaire et la scintigraphie n'ont plus leur place comme examens de première intention.

SUMMARY

Our study aimed to assess the contribution of different clinical and paraclinical investigations in the diagnosis of completed stroke in order to obtain an accurate and precise diagnosis.
Using an audit methodology we show that certain investigations are always necessary (clinical and biological investigations, Doppler, CT scanning), others are sometimes useful (angiography in 50% of cases) and that others are of no use (Lumbar Puncture, Scintigraphy).

EVALUATION DES PROCEDURES DIAGNOSTIQUES

DANS LES ACCIDENTS VASCULAIRES CEREBRAUX CONSTITUES

Les accidents vasculaires cérébraux (A.V.C.) constitués, c'est- à -dire impliquant un déficit neurologique persistant au delà de 24 heures (2) sont la troisième cause de mortalité en France et une des toutes premières causes de morbidité (1).

Ils représentent par ailleurs la moitié environ des admissions hospitalières neurologiques (3).

Jusqu'à ces dernières années ces malades étaient peu explorés du fait de nos limites thérapeutiques et de la faible efficacité des examens classiques.

L'implantation de techniques d'investigation de plus en plus sophistiquées scintigraphie, doppler, tomodensitomètrie) et l'amélioration de l'arsenal thérapeutique (chirurgie carotidienne et vertébrale, anastomose intra/extra cranienne, traitements antihypertenseurs, pace-maker cardiaques...) ont profondément modifié l'attitude des médecins.

On assiste à une tendance à l'accumulation d'informations par le biais de la prescription quasi-systématique d'examens qui outre qu'ils sont non sans risque ni coût, sont parfois inutiles et volontiers redondants.

C'est la raison pour laquelle nous avons essayé par une étude rétrospective d'apprécier la valeur informationnelle des différents moyens de diagnostic afin de dégager une stratégie d'investigations optimale.

I - MATERIEL et METHODE

A. PREALABLE

La notion de stratégie optimale doit faire référence à une décision débouchant sur une attitude thérapeutique qui sera la meilleure si son rapport coût-efficacité est le plus favorable.

Parfois, et tel est le cas des AVC, les progrès thérapeutiques vont de pair avec ceux qui concourent à améliorer la précision et l'exactitude du diagnostic.

C'est pourquoi notre objectif s'est limité à la recherche du diagnostic le plus précis et exact possible car dans le domaine pathologique qui nous occupe c'est incontestablement le meilleur guarant d'une conduite à tenir la plus adaptée.

B. POPULATION ETUDIEE

Nous avons étudié les dossiers de 119 malades hospitalisés dans le service de neurologie de l'Hôpital Pellegrin-Tripode entre juillet 1975 et décembre 1978 et ayant présenté un accident vasculaire cérébral constitué. Cet échantillon représente l'ensemble de tous les malades dont les caractéristiques, que nous allons décrire, permettaient d'étudier la valeur informationnelle des différents examens.

Notre échantillon comprend 82 hommes (69 %) et 37 femmes (31 %) dont les âges étaient les suivants :

Moins de 40 ans	: 6
De 40 à 50 ans	: 15
De 50 à 60 ans	: 61
De 60 à 70 ans	: 21
Plus de 70 ans	: 16

Les malades sont tous âgés de moins de 75 ans et ne présentent pas de contre-indication aux examens complémentaires (en particulier artériographiques), ils n'ont pas non plus un état clinique trop grave qui empêcherait un bilan complet.

Tous ces malades ont eu un bilan comprenant :

un interrogatoire - un examen clinique complet avec ECG, Fond d'oeil et radiographie pulmonaire, un bilan biologique sanguin et urinaire, un examen Doppler des artères du cou, une ponction lombaire, une scintigraphie cérébrale avec cinéangiographie, une artériographie et un examen tomodensitomètrique.

C. METHODOLOGIE

1) Dans le cadre des AVC la définition du diagnostic repose sur la détermination de différents facteurs que nous avons volontairement séparés ; ils sont :

- La nature (hémorragie ou ischiémie)
- Le volume
- La localisation
- Le territoire vasculaire précis
- Le mécanisme
- Les facteurs étiologiques

Nous présentons ici le résultat de notre étude que sur les cinq premiers facteurs ; l'étude du dernier est plus simple et repose particulièrement sur les résultats d'examens biologiques ; nous n'y reviendrons qu'au chapitre résultat.

2) Notre étude a été rétrospective et l'apport informationnel de chaque examen a été évalué par une méthode d'Audit par deux neurologues (J.M.O. et J.J.P.) qui appréciaient la valeur informationnelle de chaque examen pour chaque facteur diagnostique en terme de :

- Déterminant
- Adjuvant fort
- Adjuvant faible
- Intérêt nul

3) Nous avons décidé d'affecter à toute association d'examens un pouvoir informationnel égal au maximum de ceux de chacun des examens.
C'est-à-dire si 3 examens A, B, C apportent chacun pour un même facteur diagnostique l'information respective Adjuvant fort (pour A), Adjuvant fort (pour B), Adjuvant faible (pour C) nous avons retenu pour l'association (A,B,C) l'appréciation de Adjuvant fort.

Il nous était en effet impossible de considérer comme additives les informations de chaque examen.

4) Enfin un audit de contrôle en aveugle a été fait par un troisième neurologue (J.F. D.) pour apprécier la variabilité inter-observateur.

II - RESULTATS

1) Variabilité inter-observateur

L'audit de contrôle a montré une totale concordance de jugement pour la Nature, le Volume, la Localisation et le Territoire vasculaire.
Pour le facteur Mécanisme seuls 104 cas (sur 119) ont été jugés d'une manière analogue par les deux neurologues (soit 87 % de concordance).
Le facteur variabilité inter-observateur pour les différents facteurs diagnostiques est donc faible.

2) Le tableau I rapporte les résultats de l'Audit. N'y sont présentés que les valeurs informationnelles de chaque examen pris isolément pour chacun des facteurs diagnostiques.
Il faut noter la bonne performance :

- du Scanner pour nature, volume et localisation
- de la clinique pour la localisation
- du Doppler pour le territoire vasculaire
- de l'artériographie pour le territoire vasculaire et le mécanisme.

Notons également la médiocre performance d'ensemble de la scintigraphie et de la ponction lombaire.

3) Le tableau II rapporte les résultats pour les principales associations possibles d'examens.
Notons que la performance excellente de l'association clinique/Scanner pour la nature, le volume et la localisation n'est en rien amélioré si s'y ajoute un autre examen.
De même l'association clinique/artériographie est la meilleure possible pour apprécier le territoire vasculaire.
Enfin, aucune association n'a une bonne performance pour le mécanisme.

4) Une analyse analogue a été faite pour juger l'apport informationnel de la PL, du Doppler et de la Biologie qui montre :
- l'apport informationnel de la PL est quasi-nul
- le Doppler a un apport intéressant pour le territoire vasculaire mais cet apport devient faible devant l'association clinique/artériographie.
- la Biologie a une valeur informationnelle indiscutable pour le Facteur Etiologique.

5) CONCLUSION DES RESULTATS

A partir des résultats précédents nous pouvons proposer une stratégie optimale d'investigation devant un AVC constitué (en considérant que le diagnostic positif d'Accident vasculaire cérébral constitué se fait cliniquement (2,4)).

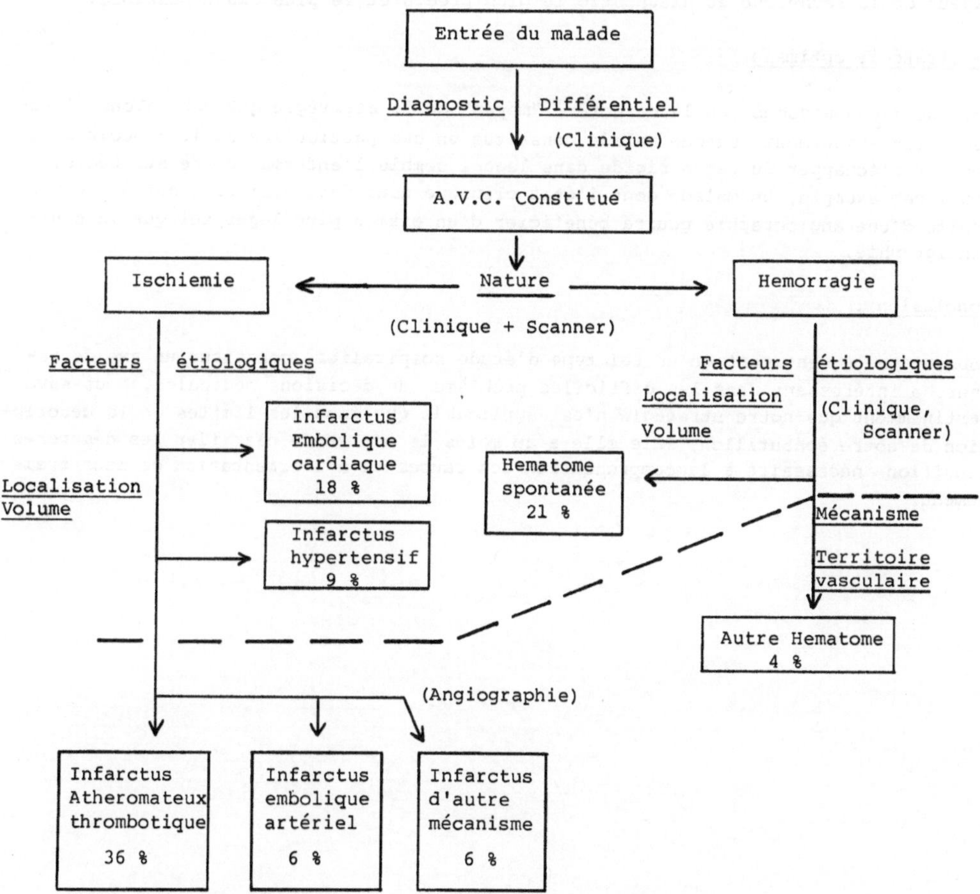

Il ressort de cette stratégie les points essentiels suivants :

. Nous ne faisons plus de Ponction Lombaire
. Nous ne prescrivons plus de Scintigraphie
. Un Doppler en fait systématiquement dans les premières 24 heures afin d'orienter ou d'éliminer une éventuelle investigation angiographique.

. Nous effectuons systématiquement un examen tomodensitométrique précoce
. L'artériographie n'est alors indiquée que pour un malade sur deux (52 % des cas).

III - DISCUSSION ET CONCLUSION

Représentativité de notre échantillon.

Le bilan clinique et paraclinique relativement lourd fait à nos malades implique que notre échantillon est représentatif de la population de malade présentant un A.V.C. constitué, âgé de moins de 75 ans, dont l'état clinique n'est pas trop grave, et hospitalisé dans un centre hospitalier disposant d'un service de neuroradiologie avec examen tomodensitométrique : il s'agit donc de malade pouvant bénéficier sans risque majeur de la recherche du diagnostic le plus précis et le plus exact possible.

La stratégie optimale

Nous ne méconnaissons pas le caractère "moyen" de la stratégie que nous avons élaborée. Bien évidemment, chaque malade constitue un cas particulier et le médecin doit pouvoir s'échapper du cadre rigide dans lequel semble l'enfermer notre stratégie. Ainsi par exemple, un malade dont l'état clinique nous fait hésiter quant à l'opportunité d'une angiographie pourra bénéficier d'un examen plus léger tel que la cinésintigraphie.

Conclusion :

Nous avons le sentiment qu'un tel type d'étude hospitalière constitue un axe de recherche intéressant dans les difficiles problèmes de décisions médicales. Nous savons pertinemment que notre stratégie n'est applicable que dans les limites de la description de notre échantillon, mais elle a au moins le mérite de clarifier les démarches condition nécessaire à la compréhension des causes et à l'orientation de leur traitement.

	A	H	S/S	B	D	P	T	G	A°
NATURE	O. 0.03 0.35 0.62	O.O3 0.20 0.45 0.32	O.O3 0.30 0.50 0.27			O.O5 0.08 0.72 0.15	O.78 0.10 0.10 0.02	O.1O 0.21 0.12 0.57	O.34 0.25 0.15 0.26
VOLUME			O.O5 0.60 0.30 0.05				O.77 0.10 0.07 0.06	O.13 0.39 0.10 0.38	O.O4 0.11 0.05 0.80
LOCALISATION			O.29 0.53 0.15 0.03				O.74 0.11 0. 0.15	O.27 0.25 0.10 0.38	O.O9 0.11 0.20 0.60
TERRITOIRE VASCULAIRE	O. 0. 0.10 0.90	O. 0.03 0.35 0.62	O.O3 0.21 0.64 0.12		O.21 0.12 0.30 0.37		O.O3 0.21 0.50 0.26	O.O3 0.11 0.37 0.49	O.48 0.20 0.21 0.09
MECANISME	O. 0.13 0.37 0.50	O.O3 0.14 0.40 0.43	O.O4 0.24 0.46 0.26	O. 0.14 0.58 0.28	O.O3 0.08 0.16 0.73				O.18 0.48 0.12 0.22

Tableau I audit - Données brutes. Dans chaque case sont représentés de haut en bas, le taux déterminant, adjuvant fort, adj. faible, nul. A Antécédent - H Histoire de la maladie - S/S Signes et Symptomes - B Biologie - D Doppler - P Ponction lombaire - T Tomodensitométrie - G Gammagraphie - A° Artériographie.

	C	CG	CT	CA°	CTG	CTA°	CGA°	CTGA°
NATURE	0.03 0.40 0.54 0.03	0.18 0.50 0.32 0.	0.83 0.14 0.03 0.	0.36 0.41 0.22 0.01	0.83 0.15 0.02 0.	0.87 0.11 0.02 0.	0.41 0.41 0.18 0.	0.87 0.11 0.02 0.
VOLUME	0.04 0.60 0.30 0.06	0.17 0.66 0.14 0.03	0.77 0.17 0.05 0.01	0.08 0.64 0.23 0.05	0.78 0.16 0.05 0.01	0.78 0.16 0.05 0.01	0.20 0.66 0.12 0.02	0.78 0.16 0.05 0.01
LOCALISATION	0.29 0.52 0.16 0.03	0.49 0.40 0.10 0.01	0.92 0.07 0.01 0.	0.36 0.59 0.14 0.01	0.94 0.05 0.01 0.	0.92 0.07 0.01 0.	0.57 0.37 0.05 0.01	0.94 0.05 0.01 0.
TERRITOIRE VASCULAIRE	0.20 0.27 0.49 0.04	0.20 0.28 0.48 0.04	0.22 0.36 0.40 0.02	0.52 0.29 0.17 0.02	0.22 0.40 0.36 0.02	0.52 0.33 0.13 0.02	0.51 0.29 0.17 0.02	0.52 0.33 0.13 0.02
MECANISME	0.08 0.45 0.42 0.05			0.20 0.55 0.20 0.05				

Tableau II : Associations d'examens

B I B L I O G R A P H I E

1. - A.M. BELLEVILLE SEJOURNE, M. BIENTZ, J. CHEVALLIER, C. DAGON, D. JOLLY
Morbidité et Mortalité dans les hôpitaux de Paris 1978 (à paraître)

2. - F. DONNADIEU - Exploration et classification des Accidents Vasculaires Cérébraux
Thèse n° 153 - Bordeaux 1978

3. - FISHER C.M., MOHR J.P., ADAMS R.D. - Maladies cérébro-vasculaires
In Principes de Medecines Internes pp. 1752-1785 Ed. Flammarion Paris 1972

4. - HARRISSON M.J.C. The investigation of Strokes in cerebral arterial desease,
Ross Russel R.W., Churchill-Livingstone - Edinburg 1976

LIMITES ET BIAIS DE L'EVALUATION RETROSPECTIVE D'UNE TECHNIQUE DE DIAGNOSTIC

A propos d'une étude de la scintigraphie cérébrale

A. Alpérovitch*, F. Cavaillolès**, C. Soussana**, B. Thébault**
B. Bok**

* INSERM - 94800 Villejuif - FRANCE
** HOPITAL BEAUJON - 92110 Clichy - FRANCE

Abstract

In order to assess retrospectively the diagnostic value of radionuclide brain scans, 399 cases which fulfilled the required diagnosis criteria were reviewed. These 399 cases constituted only 22 % of the scans performed during one year in the hospital. In this sample, the test overall accuracy was equal to 79.5. False positive errors (4 %) were less frequent than false-negative ones (16.5 %). By comparing scintigraphic diagnoses with preliminar clinical diagnoses, the main result appeared to be the following. When these two diagnoses were identical, the final diagnosis agreed with the preliminar clinical hypothesis in 97 % of the cases ; but when they were different, final diagnosis and preliminar clinical hypothesis agreed in only 15 % of the cases.

But limits and biases of such a retrospective study make suspectable this apparently positive conclusion. Indeed, they lead to i) overestimate the proportion of abnormal scans ; ii) under estimate the proportion of false-negative errors ; iii) over estimate, on the overall, the diagnosis value of this test. But it seems, unfortunately, that neither a prospective study nor a change in the efficacy criteria which are taken into account, can permit to eliminate important errors in assessment of diagnostic tests.

1. Introduction

La volonté d'évaluer les techniques de diagnostic ne s'applique pas seulement aux technologies nouvelles. Ce sont parfois des méthodes utilisées depuis un grand nombre d'années que les médecins veulent soumettre au regard critique d'une évaluation. Dans un tel cas, il est compréhensible que les cliniciens hésitent à entreprendre une étude prospective et essaient de tirer parti de données recueillies dans le passé. Quelles sont les difficultés de ces études rétrospectives ? Les conclusions de telles analyses ont-elles une grande portée ? Ce sont ces problèmes que nous voudrions discuter à propos d'une étude rétrospective de la valeur diagnostique de la scintigraphie cérébrale, étude préalable à l'installation d'un tomodensitomètre. Nous n'examinerons ici que deux des aspects de cette évaluation (3). La concordance du résultat de l'examen avec le diagnostic final permet d'apprécier la valeur diagnostique "absolue" de l'examen. La comparaison du diagnostic scintigraphique au diagnostic évoqué par le clinicien avant qu'il ait connaissance du compte-rendu du scintigraphiste permet de nuancer le jugement précédent en faisant intervenir la notion de valeur "relative" d'une technique de diagnostic.

2. Sélection des dossiers

1800 scintigraphies avaient été effectuées en 1976 dans le service de médecine nucléaire de l'hôpital Beaujon, pour des malades admis dans différents services de ce même hôpital ou consultants externes. Seuls les malades hospitalisés ou consultants en neurologie ou neuro-chirurgie, soit 702 cas, étaient retenus pour cette étude. Dans les autres dossiers, en effet, les renseignements concernant les symptômes neurologiques présentés par les malades et les hypothèses de diagnostic du clinicien étaient dans la majorité des cas imcomplets ou même absents.

Pour que le diagnostic final -référence majeure de toute évaluation- ait une certitude suffisante, il devait reposer soit sur une preuve histologique, soit sur un contrôle artériographique, soit sur une surveillance clinique de 6 mois. Ce n'est que pour 522 des 702 malades retenus à priori que l'un de ces critères de diagnostic était vérifié. Il faut souligner ici qu'en se limitant aux seuls diagnostics prouvés avec certitude (preuve histologique), l'échantillon n'aurait été constitué que de 135 sujets.

L'évaluation globale d'une technique de diagnostic tient pour l'essentiel en l'analyse de la répartition des sujets en 4 groupes, en fonction du résultat de l'examen (ici : normal ou pathologique) et de la réalité de l'anomalie (ici : présence ou absence de lésion cérébrale). Il faut donc pouvoir admettre sans contestation possible, que dans telle maladie, il existe -ou non- une anomalie susceptible d'être mise en évidence par la scintigraphie. Ainsi, pour le diagnostic "tumeur cérébrale", la réponse à une telle question serait oui ; pour le diagnostic "épilepsie essentielle", elle serait non. Pour une grande variété de maladies (sclérose en plaques, démence sénile artériopathique, etc ...), représentant au total 123 cas, les cliniciens ne pouvaient trancher entre ces deux alternatives, ce schéma trop sommaire se révélant inadapté et inapplicable.

Ainsi, au terme de sélections successives, l'analyse n'a-t-elle porté que sur 399 des 1800 scintigraphies effectuées en 1976.

3. Classification des scintigraphies

La scintigraphie cérébrale apporte deux types de renseignements. D'abord sur l'existence même d'une anomalie du cerveau. Ensuite, éventuellement, sur la nature de cette anomalie. Il doit donc y avoir deux niveaux dans l'évaluation de l'examen.

Le premier, celui de l'identification d'une anomalie, permet à priori le calcul des indices classiques mesurant la valeur diagnostique. Cependant, la conclusion du scintigraphiste n'a pas seulement deux modalités, anomalie présente ou absente ; elle parle aussi d'anomalie peu probable et d'anomalie probable. La sensibilité et la spécificité de l'examen vont dépendre du regroupement de ces 4 types de réponse en 2 classes. Nous soulignerons ici combien les qualités et la personnalité du lecteur peuvent influencer la formulation de la conclusion : une scintigraphie, c'est une image plus un lecteur et c'est ce couple indissociable que l'on évalue. Le choix fait dans cette étude, et qui a consisté à réunir absent et peu probable d'une part, présent et probable d'autre part, malgré son caractère "raisonnable" ne se justifie ni plus, ni moins, qu'un autre.

Pour caractériser les qualités de l'examen en matière de diagnostic étiologique (nature de l'anomalie), on peut calculer pour chaque catégorie de diagnostic le pourcentage de cas correctement identifiés, ce pourcentage étant exactement équivalent à la sensibilité. On peut aussi définir la valeur prédictive de chacune des hypothèses de diagnostic (5,6). L'analyse se complique ici du fait de l'existence de la réponse "indéterminée", correspondant à des anomalies dont la scintigraphie ne peut définir exactement la nature.

Nous préciserons que dans ce travail rétrospectif, il nous a semblé préférable d'utiliser le compte-rendu de la scintigraphie tel qu'il avait été rédigé au moment où l'examen avait été effectué, plutôt que demander à l'occasion de l'enquête une seconde lecture de l'image scintigraphique.

4. Comparaison avec les hypothèses cliniques

Aussi parfait que soit un examen, il n'a d'intérêt que s'il améliore les hypothèses de diagnostic que l'on peut évoquer en se référant à l'examen clinique et à quelques données biologiques simples. C'est de façon indirecte que l'on a tenté ici de cerner cette valeur relative de la scintigraphie, car une étude rétrospective se prête mal à cette évaluation. Nous avons, d'une part, comparé le diagnostic clinique (avant la scintigraphie) au diagnostic scintigraphique, selon les règles définies au tableau 1. Nous avons d'autre part, calculé la probabilité que l'hypothèse clinique soit exacte selon qu'elle est, ou non, confirmée par la scintigraphie. L'hypothèse clinique servant de référence était celle indiquée par le clinicien sur le formulaire de la demande d'examen. On ne peut cependant être sûr que ce diagnostic correspond à l'hypothèse réelle du clinicien. Il semble, en effet, que dans certains cas, c'est non pas le diagnostic le plus probable mais l'hypothèse qu'il veut éliminer que le clinicien inscrit dans sa demande. Par ailleurs, certaines hypothèses (comme hématome sous-dural) permettent de bénéficier d'une priorité et, bien naturellement, ce diagnostic est utilisé de temps en temps comme "laissez passer".

Diagnostic Scintigraphique \ Diagnostic Clinique	Exact	Faux	Indéterminé
Exact	SC = CL	SC > CL	SC > CL
Faux	SC < CL	SC = CL	SC < CL
Indéterminé	SC < CL	SC > CL	SC = CL

Tableau 1 : Confrontation des diagnostics cliniques et scintigraphiques : règles de comparaison

5. Résultats

Nous commenterons brièvement les résultats présentés dans les tableaux 2 à 5.

La sensibilité de l'examen est égale à .72, sa spécificité à .90. Les erreurs de type "faux négatif" représentent 16.5 % de l'ensemble des cas ; celles de type "faux positif" sont plus rares (4 %). Dans la catégorie "lésion cérébrale" sont réunies différentes anomalies (tableau 3) plus ou moins bien détectées par la scintigraphie. La sensibilité globale de l'examen est donc fonction de leurs proportions relatives.

Les valeurs prédictives positive et négative de la scintigraphie sont, sur cet échantillon, respectivement égales à .91 et .69.

	Diagnostique final: Lésion cérébrale	Diagnostique final: Pas de lésion
Scintigraphie pathologique	168 (42.1 %)	16 (4.0 %)
Scintigraphie normale	66 (16.5 %)	149 (37.3 %)

Tableau 2 : Comparaison du diagnostic scintigraphique au diagnostic final

Les tableaux 3 et 4 indiquent la valeur diagnostique de l'examen dans les maladies les plus fréquentes. On peut souligner le fort pourcentage de résultats "faux négatifs" observé pour les accidents vasculaires cérébraux. Cette observation appelle une remarque sur l'hétérogénéité de ce groupe allant de l'accident majeur récent à l'épisode transitoire datant de quelques jours. N'est-il pas alors excessif, pour certains de ces cas, de considérer une scintigraphie négative comme un résultat "faux négatif".

Diagnostic final	Résultat de la scintigraphie				
	Normal	Pathologique			
		Diagnostic V[3]	Diagnostic F[3]	Diagnostic X[3]	Total résultats pathologiques
Pas de lésion cérébrale					
(36)[1] Aucune pathologie cérébrale	36 (100)				
(129) Epilepsie ou Céphalées	113 (88)[2]		3	13	16
Lésion cérébrale					
(128) Accident vasc.cérébral	56	56 (44)	7	9	72 (56)
(28) Tumeur bénigne	2	13 (46)	8	5	26 (93)
(56) Tumeur maligne	7	35 (62)	2	12	49 (88)
(11) Hématome sous-dural	0	10 (91)	0	1	11 (100)
(11) Hématome intra-crânien	1	6 (55)	1	3	10 (91)

Tableau 3 : Valeur de la scintigraphie en fonction du diagnostic final

[1] Nombre de cas
[2] Pourcentage par rapport au nombre de cas
[3] V : Exact, F : Faux, X : Indéterminé

Hypothèse proposée par la scintigraphie	Nombre total de cas	Nombre de cas pour lesquels l'hypothèse est exacte	Valeur prédictive
Accident vasculaire cérébral	60	56	.93
Tumeur bénigne	16	13	.81
Tumeur maligne	49	35	.71
Hématome sous-dural	24	10	.42
Hématome intra-crânien	17	6	.35

Tableau 4 : Valeur prédictive de différents diagnostics scintigraphiques (sur 522 malades, cf paragraphe 2)

L'analyse du tableau 5 montre que le diagnostic scintigraphique est dans l'ensemble meilleur que le diagnostic clinique (χ^2(séries appariées) = 6.15). Il est cependant important de souligner que le diagnostic scintigraphique a pu s'aider, pour certains cas de doute, des informations cliniques figurant sur le formulaire de demande. Il faut d'autre part insister sur le fait que les erreurs ne sont pas de même nature, plus souvent de type "faux négatif" pour la scintigraphie, plus souvent de type "faux positif" pour le diagnostic clinique. Ce jugement comparatif doit donc être pondéré par la gravité relative des deux types d'erreur.

	Accident vasculaire cérébral	Tumeur maligne	Tumeur bénigne	Hématome sous-dural	Hématomes intra-crâniens	Epilepsie	Céphalée	TOTAL
SC = CL	60	31	12	7	7	55	14	186 (51 %)
SC > CL	24	11	9	3	3	44	11	105 (29 %)
SC < CL	44	14	7	1	1	3	2	72 (20 %)

Tableau 5 : Comparaison des diagnostics cliniques et scintigraphiques

Mais le résultat qui nous semble le mieux mettre en lumière l'intérêt de l'examen est le suivant : lorsque la scintigraphie confirme l'hypothèse clinique, cette hypothèse correspond au diagnostic final dans 97 % des cas, mais s'il y a désaccord entre clinique et scintigraphie, l'hypothèse clinique n'est juste que dans 15 % des cas.

On peut cependant se demander si cette dernière évaluation n'est pas trop optimiste. En effet, l'exactitude du diagnostic scintigraphique varie significativement selon le niveau de certitude du diagnostic final (tableau 6, χ^2 = 10.1, $p < 0.01$). Mais il est impossible à partir des données disponibles, ni de mesurer l'importance, ni même de prouver l'éventuelle existence du biais que l'on est conduit à suspecter en fonction de ce dernier résultat.

Diagnostic scintigraphique	Diagnostic final	
	Prouvé par histologie ou artériographie	Prouvé seulement par les arguments cliniques (examen et surveillance)
Vrai	83 (55 %)	137 (71 %)
Faux	49 (32 %)	38 (20 %)
Indéterminé	19 (13 %)	17 (9 %)

Tableau 6 : Valeur de la scintigraphie selon les critères de diagnostic

Discussion

Au terme de cette analyse, on serait assez enclin à conclure que le principal intérêt de ce travail est d'être une parfaite illustration de toutes les difficultés d'une évaluation rétrospective d'une technique de diagnostic (7).

Tout d'abord, cette étude surestime le pourcentage de scintigraphies pathologiques. Ceci est dû essentiellement au fait que pour tout sujet inclus dans l'échantillon, certains critères de diagnostic devaient être vérifiés : preuve histologique, ou artériographie, ou contrôle clinique au bout de 6 mois. Il est évident que chacun de ces critères a plus de chance d'être respecté lorsque l'examen scintigraphique est anormal. S'il est normal, le patient, en règle générale, ne sera pas opéré, n'aura pas d'artériographie, et dans un certain nombre de cas, ne sera pas revu au bout de 6 mois.

Cette étude sous-estime probablement la fréquence des erreurs de type "faux-négatif". En effet, une scintigraphie pathologique conduit le plus souvent à pratiquer d'autres explorations, artériographie en particulier, qui permettent de redresser une éventuelle erreur de type "faux-positif". Par contre, la démarche est différente si la scintigraphie est négative : il parait souvent alors raisonnable d'arrêter les investigations, la surveillance est peut être moins attentive et moins prolongée. Le proportion de perdus de vue dans ce groupe sera plus grande, certains processus à croissance assez lente (astrocytomes, par exemple), peuvent ne pas évoluer perceptiblement en 6 mois. On voit donc que tout ceci contribue à sous-estimer la fréquence relative des erreurs de type "faux négatif" par rapport à celles de type "faux positif" ; et par conséquent, à une surestimation globale de la valeur diagnostique de l'examen.

Le clinicien, pourtant, porte sur un tel travail un jugement moins sévère que celui du statisticien. Il retrouve dans cette analyse des intuitions non quantifiées, sa pratique lui permet quelques extrapolations de ces résultats fragmentaires à l'ensemble des patients (3), cette expérience l'aide à mieux cerner les limites et l'intérêt des travaux publiés sur le même sujet (1, 2, 4).

Il est important de souligner que les difficultés rencontrées dans cette analyse n'ont aucun caractère exceptionnel : ce sont celles d'à peu près toutes les études rétrospectives. Nous n'avons fait ici que les mettre en lumière, alors qu'il est habituel de les minimiser.

Mais les études prospectives sont-elles, quant à elles, exemptes de biais ? En fait, non. L'expérience personnelle que nous en avons nous a montré, comme à d'autres, que l'on y retrouve les mêmes problèmes que dans une évaluation rétrospective, mais à un moindre degré. Ces difficultés persistent quel que soit le niveau de l'évaluation de l'efficacité de l'examen (8) : diagnostic, choix des autres investigations et (ou) du traitement, influence à moyen et long terme sur l'état du patient. Nous poserons alors une question : en dehors de quelques situations privilégiées, peut-on vraiment évaluer une méthode de diagnostic ?

References

1 - P.O. ALDERSON, M. MIKHAEL, R.E. COLEMAN, M.GADO. Optimal utilization of computerized tomography and radionuclide brain imaging. Neurology, 1976, 26 : 803-807

2 - E.F. BERNSTEIN. The current place of non invasive diagnostic techniques in evaluating cerebrovascular disease. J. Roy. Soc. Med., 1978, 71 : 709-710

3 - F. CAVAILLOLES, A. ALPEROVITCH, C. SOUSSANA, B. THEBAULT, B. BOCK. Clinical usefulness of brain scintigrams. Int. J. Applied Radiat., (sous presse)

4 - G.H. BOULAY, J. MARSHALL. Comparison of EMI and radioisotope imaging in neurological disease. Lancet, 1975, ii : 1294-1297

5 - B.J. McNEIL, S.J. ADELSTEIN. Determining the value of diagnostic and screening tests. J. Nuclear Med., 1976, 17 : 439-448

6 - T. POYNARD, A. ALPEROVITCH. Evaluation des moyens de diagnostic - Etude critique des principaux indices mesurant la valeur diagnostique. Journal de Radiologie (sous presse)

7 - D. RANSOHOFF, A.R. FEINSTEIN. Problems of spectrum and biais in evaluating the efficacy of diagnostic tests. New Engl. J. Med., 1978, 299 : 926-930

8 - A study of the efficacy of diagnostic radiologic procedures. Report from the American College of Radiology, 1977.

EFFICACITE DIAGNOSTIQUE ET COUT DES EXAMENS RADIOLOGIQUES ET ENDOSCOPIQUES EN GASTROENTEROLOGIE

Miguel RODRIGUEZ, Geneviève MACQUART MOULIN, Jacqueline CORNEE, Jean-Pierre DURBEC, Patrice BERTHEZENE, Jean GUIOL : Equipe de Mathématiques Informatique U 31 de l'INSERM. André GREGOIRE : Cellule d'Analyse de Gestion de l'Assistance Publique. Henri SARLES, José SAHEL : Departement de Gastroentérologie de l'Hôpital Sainte-Marguerite

Marseille - FRANCE

SUMMARY

In Gastroenterology a great number of endoscopic and radiographic examinations performed on the hospitalised patients are expensive. It seemed of interest to study whether the diagnostic indications supplied by them duly compensate the expenses incurred.

This work intends to study for 8 radiographic and endoscopic examinations, the relations between the radiologic signs and the diagnostic indications (by means of a data screening method based on the Mutual Information theory) and the expenses incurred. The costs are calculated both from Public Health Management Organization statistics and accounting documents and from direct enquiries made within the Departments concerned.

The results show that the endoscopic examinations are, as a whole, very informational and, with the exception of the Wirsungography, less expensive than the radiographic examinations. On the contrary, the arteriography supplies little information for a high cost, and the plain film of the abdomen has the lowest mutual information for the lowest cost.

If only the economical aspect of the examination is being considered, the optimal sequence would be to give priority to practising the endoscopic examinations of the patients hospitalized in Gastroenterology, and, when necessary eventually the radiographic examinations.

1. INTRODUCTION

En Gastroentérologie les malades hospitalisés ont, de façon courante, un bilan radiologique et endoscopique qui tend à être de plus en plus complet. Un grand nombre de ces examens étant d'un coût élevé, il nous a paru utile d'étudier si les indications diagnostiques qu'ils fournissent sont à la hauteur des dépenses qu'ils entraînent. En effet, les budgets radiologiques et endoscopiques actuels sont très élevés et la question est de savoir s'il est possible de diminuer les coûts. Pour cela, il faut, soit pouvoir ordonner la séquence des examens proposés, soit même en supprimer certains. Ce travail se propose d'étudier, d'une part les relations entre les signes radiologiques et les indications diagnostiques, d'autre part les dépenses qu'ils entraînent. On cherche alors la séquence des examens les plus utiles pour le coût le moins élevé.

2. MATERIEL ET METHODES

Le travail a porté sur 1.500 malades hospitalisés dans le Service de Gastroentérologie de l'Hôpital Sainte-Marguerite à Marseille, et ayant tous subi leurs explorations endoscopiques et radiographiques dans le même Service d'Endoscopie Digestive et de Radiologie Centrale.

Les images radiologiques et endoscopiques sont interprétées par les spécialistes des deux services et décrites suivant un protocole normalisé systématique opérationnel depuis plus de trois ans (1). Chaque sujet est décrit par 142 variables relatives à la radiographie de l'abdomen sans préparation, le transit oesophagogastroduodénal, la radiographie des voies biliaires, la radiographie du recto-colon, l'artériographie, la wirsungographie, l'oesophago-gastroduodénoscopie et la colorectoscopie. Chaque variable a deux modalités suivant la présence ou l'absence d'un signe. Les affections étudiées portent sur : le cancer du pancréas, les pancréatites aiguës,les pancréatites chroniques, les ulcères gastroduodénaux, les tumeurs gastriques, les affections des voies biliaires, les cirrhoses du foie, les rectocolites hémorragiques, les tumeurs du rectocolon et un groupe de malades fonctionnels, soit au total 10 groupes diagnostiques. Le diagnostic a été posé en fin d'exploration clinique, biologique, radiologique et anatomo-pathologique.

- La relation entre signes et diagnostics a été étudiée par des méthodes de filtrage de données basées sur la théorie de l'Information Mutuelle (2).

- Le coût de chaque type d'examen radiologique et endoscopique a été estimé comparativement, d'une part à partir des données de la cellule d' Analyse de Gestion de l'Assistance Publique de Marseille et des documents comptables de l'Economat de l'Hôpital, d'autre part au moyen d'enquêtes directes au niveau des Services de Radiologie Centrale et d'Endoscopie Digestive.

3. ETUDE DES RELATIONS SIGNES - DIAGNOSTICS

Dans le présent travail, le recueil des données radiologiques et endoscopiques au moyen d'un questionnaire systématisé et leur stockage sur ordinateur aboutit à la collecte d'un très grand nombre de données sur un grand nombre de malades. Cependant, toutes les variables ne présentent pas le même intérêt pour l'etablissement d'un diagnostic donné. Certaines sont très informationnelles, d'autres sont sans intérêt. C'est la raison pour laquelle, afin d'étudier le degré d'association de ces variables avec les diagnostics, nous avons choisi d'utiliser les méthodes de filtrage des données. Ces dernières permettent de traiter très rapidement un grand nombre de variables et de sélectionner facilement les plus informationnelles pour un diagnostic donné (3). De plus, ces méthodes permettent les données manquantes qui sont inévitables, en particulier dans les examens radiologiques et endoscopiques où tous les examens ne peuvent pas être pratiqués systématiquement sur tous les malades.

3.1 METHODE DE FILTRAGE DES DONNEES

Les méthodes de filtrage des données son basées, d'une part sur les propriétés de l'information mutuelle (2,4) d'autre part sur le rapport des produits croisés des probabilités dans les tables de contingence .

L'information mutuelle permet d'étudier l'intensité de la liaison entre un ensemble de g groupes diagnostiques et une variable radiologique à q modalités (ici q=2).

- Si n_{ij} désigne le nombre de sujets du groupe diagnostique k présentant le signe i (i=1) ou ne le présentant pas (i=2), on montre que cette information mutuelle peut être estimées par la quantité:

$$I_N(X,Y) = \sum_{i=1}^{2} \sum_{j=1}^{g} \frac{n_{ij}}{N} \log \frac{N n_{ij}}{n_{i.}\, n_{.j}}$$

où N désigne la taille totale de l'échantillon considéré et où :

$$n_{i.} = \sum_{j=1}^{g} n_{ij} \qquad i = 1,2$$

$$n_{.j} = \sum_{i=1}^{2} n_{ij} \qquad j = 1,\ldots,g$$

- S'il n'y a pas association entre groupes diagnostiques et signes radiologiques on montre que la quantité : $\chi^2 = 2NI_N(X,Y)$ suit une loi du Chi2 à (q-1) (g-1) degrés de liberté (5). Cette propriété permet de tester la significativité des informations mutuelles estimées.

Une information mutuelle et un χ^2 élevés signifient une forte association très fiable. Par contre, une information mutuelle basse et un χ^2 bas correspondent à une faible association, peu fiable. Une information mutuelle élevée et un χ^2 bas décèlent une association apparemment forte, mais peu fiable étant donné qu'elle a été calculée sur un faible nombre de sujets. Une information mutuelle basse et un χ^2 élevé signifient une faible association, mais statistiquement fiable (par exemple parce que le nombre de sujets étudiés était grand).

Cependant, pour ce travail précis, il semble préférable de se fier plus à la valeur de l'information mutuelle qu'à sa significativité statistique.

En effet, dans l'étude des associations entre variables et diagnostics, l'information mutuelle rend compte à la fois de la fréquence de détection d'un signe et de l'association entre signe et diagnostic. On doit noter que la mesure d'une association entre variable et diagnostic n'influe pas directement sur son niveau de significativité.

3.2 RESULTATS :

Dans le présent travail l'information mutuelle entre chaque variable radiologique et les 10 groupes diagnostiques a été étudiée au moyen de la distribution de cette variable à partir du nombre de malades sur lesquels les examens ont été pratiqués. Toutes les variables étant binaires, l'information mutuelle portée par une variable ne peut être supérieure à Ln 2. Les 142 variables ont été classées par information mutuelle décroissante. La significativité de cette information a été testée. De cette façon on a pu apprécier la fiabilité qui peut être placée dans une information mutuelle estimée.

a) 55 variables ont une information mutuelle < 0.02, ce qui traduit une très faible association entre signes et les 10 groupes diagnostiques ou une sous représentation d'un diagnostic dans l'ensemble des patients soumis à un examen. De plus les χ^2 correspondant à ces informations mutuelles sont relativement faibles. Ces variables n'ont pas été retenues.

b) On a retenu toutes les variables dont l'information mutuelle est supérieure à 0.069, c'est-à-dire : information maximale apportée par une variable divisée par le nombre de groupes diagnostiques. 30 variables ont une information mutuelle supérieure à 0.069. Les 23 principales ont été rangées par information mutuelle décroissante (Tableau I). l'analyse de ce tableau montre que les variables ayant les informations mutuelles les plus élevées correspondent, dans l'ordre, aux examens suivants : rectoscopie, coloscopie, oesophagoscopie, radiographie des voies biliaires, wirsungographie, radiographies du colon, de l'estomac, de l'oesophage. On voit, en particulier, que les variables relatives aux examens endoscopiques du colon, du rectum, de l'oesophage et du duodenum ont une information mutuelle supérieure aux variables radiologiques correspondantes.

c) Parmi les variables ayant une information mutuelle comprise entre 0.02 et

TABLEAU I

Classement des principales variables par information mutuelle décroissante

Variables	Information Mutuelle	Nombre de groupes	χ^2	Nombre de degrés de liberté
Rectoscopie : tumeur rectale	0.250	7	57.78	6
Coloscopie : présence de polype	0.249	7	123.96	6
Oesophagoscopie : varices oesophagiennes	0.228	10	102.99	9
Coloscopie : polype non villeux	0.222	7	110.33	6
Lésions à la coloscopie	0.205	7	125.17	6
Coloscopie : rectocolite hémorragique	0.161	3	92.06	2
Anomalie à la radiographie des voies biliaires	0.159	10	159.42	9
Présence de polype à la rectoscopie	0.153	7	37.89	6
Duodenoscopie : présence d'ulcère	0.136	10	57.73	9
Anomalie à la wirsungographie	0.131	8	53.43	7
Radiographie des voies biliaires : calculs	0.129	10	138.07	9
Anomalie à la duodenoscopie	0.124	10	56.38	9
Rectoscopie : polype non villeux	0.124	7	31.91	6
Anomalie à l'oesophagoscopie	0.121	10	52.75	9
Duodenoscopie : ulcère du bulbe	0.117	10	51.91	9
Anomalie à la radiographie du colon	0.114	10	97.30	9
Anomalie à la radiographie de l'estomac	0.106	10	136.10	9
Anomalie du canal du Wirsung	0.104	8	44.22	7
Calcul vésiculaire à la radiographie	0.103	10	108.08	9
Gastroscopie : présence d'ulcère	0.094	10	60.52	9
Varices oesophagiennes à la radiographie	0.087	10	128.29	9
Coloscopie : présence de diverticules	0.080	7	64.71	6
Anomalie à la radiographie de l'oesophage	0.072	10	103.95	9
⋮				
Anomalie à l'artériographie	0.053	10	15.09	9
Calculs pancreatiques à la radiographie sans préparation	0.050	10	175.47	9

0.069 on trouve la radiographie de l'abdomen sans préparation et l'artériographie. Cette faible valeur de l'information mutuelle est liée au fait que le signe ne se retrouve fréquemment que dans des groupes diagnostiques de faible effectif. Cependant la présence de calcifications à la radiographie sans préparation (Information Mutuelle = 0.05 et χ^2 = 175.47) est caractéristique d' un groupe diagnostique déterminé,à l'inverse de l'artériographie (Information Mutuelle = 0.053, χ^2 = 15.09) (Tableau I).

Il faut cependant noter que le médecin peut disposer d'une information à priori qui l'oriente vers un type d'examen. En effet, il n'est pas toujours possible de pratiquer systématiquement tous les examens sur tous les sujets. Ceci explique que certains examens, comme la coloscopie, n'aient pas été pratiqués sur les malades atteints de cancer du pancréas.

Il semble donc possible de considérer qu'à information mutuelle égale, les signes les plus informationnels sont ceux concernant le plus grand nombre de malades. Toutefois, l'utilité d'un signe pour le médecin est bien caractérisée par la valeur de son information mutuelle, indépendemment du nombre de diagnostics finaux posés.

Le classement par information mutuelle decroissante des examens est donné par le tableau suivant (Tableau II).

TABLEAU II

Examens	Information Mutuelle
Coloscopie	0.225
Rectoscopie	0.175
Oesophago-gastroduodenoscopie	0.152
Radiographie des voies biliaires	0.130
Wirsungographie	0.094
Transit oesophago-gastroduodénal	0.083
Radiographie du colon	0.074
Artériographie	0.053
Radiographie de l'abdomen sans préparation	0.050

4. ETUDE DU COUT

On se propose d'estimer le coût moyen de chacun des huit examens radiographiques et endoscopiques étudiés.

Nous rappelons que la cotation de base en nombre de lettres clés de Z ou K d'un examen déterminé est fixée uniformément par la nomenclature générale des Actes Professionnels (Sécurité Sociale). Par contre, le prix de revient du Z et du K n'est pas fixe et doit être recalculé chaque année pour chaque établissement (6).

Le présent travail se propose d'estimer, à partir de deux sources d'information différentes, les prix de revient du K et du Z moyens pour un an de fonctionnement des Services de Radiologie Centrale et d'Endoscopie de l'Hôpital Sainte-Marguerite à Marseille et, à partir de cette estimation, d'approcher le coût moyen de chacun des huit examens étudiés.

Le calcul des dépenses a été évalué d'une part, à partir des documents statistiques et comptables de l'Assistance Publique de Marseille, d'autre part d'enquêtes directes menées dans les Services. On obtient ainsi deux estimation du Z et du K.

4.1 ESTIMATION DU PRIX DE REVIENT DES EXAMENS RADIOGRAPHIQUES

Calcul du Z moyen d'après les documents statistiques et comptables :

Les dépenses relatives au Service de Radiologie Centrale de l'Hôpital Sainte-Marguerite s'élèvent pour un an à : 8.227.271 Francs, ventilés de la façon suivante :

- Frais de fonctionnement	2.076.035 Frs.
- Frais de personnel	3.169.617 Frs.
- Prestations de service	302.480 Frs.
- Amortissement des bâtiments et du matériel et différentes charges (E.D.F., eau, impôts, taxes)	1.790.215 Frs.
Recettes à déduire	28.114 Frs.
- Répartition des services centraux	205.376 Frs.
- Charges générales des établissements	711.662 Frs.

Le nombre total de Z fournis par le Service de Radiologie Centrale en un an étant de : 1.573.340 on obtient un coût du Z moyen de :

$$\frac{8.227.271}{1.573.340} = 5.23 \text{ Francs}$$

Il faut noter combien cette évaluation du Z est globale et insuffisante pour approcher les dépenses spécifiques à chaque type d'examen.

La nomenclature de la Sécurité Sociale, en attribuant à chaque examen un nombre de Z plus ou moins important suivant son degré de sophistication, essai de compenser les différences entre les examens, mais ne peut prétendre à représenter leurs coûts réels.

Calcul du Z moyen par enquêtes directes auprès des Services concernés :

Les différences trouvées ont porté essentiellement sur : l'amortissement du matériel (770.883 Francs au lieu de 701.981 Francs à partir des données de l'Assistance Publique) et les frais de personnel (3.895.872 Francs au lieu de 3.169.617 Francs)

- Soit une dépense annuelle de 9.022.428 Francs pour 1.573.340 Z. On obtient un coût du Z moyen de :

$$\frac{9.022.428}{1.573.340} = 5.73 \text{ Francs}$$

Coût de chaque examen radiologique :

Il n'entre pas dans nos vues ici de discuter l'ecart entre le prix de l'examen fixé par la Sécurité Sociale et le prix réel. Cependant, la facturation d'un examen varie suivant chaque malade car elle comprend une valeur de base à laquelle peut s'ajouter une majoration. Pour avoir une cotation moyenne de chacun des examens plus proche de la réalité, il a été décompté, à partir des régistres du Service de Radiologie, l'ensemble des lettres clés unitaires correspondant à la catégorie en cause. La valeur moyenne en Z de chaque type d'examen a ensuite été obtenue en divisant le nombre de lettres clés comptabilisées sur un an par le nombre d'actes pratiqués. Les résultats donnent par ordre croissant : 32.70 Z pour l'abdomen sans préparation, 74.62 Z + 3 K pour les voies biliaires; 85.76 Z pour la radiographie du colon, 97.05 Z pour le transit oesophagogastroduodenal, 405 Z + 352 K pour l'artériographie.

4.2 ESTIMATION DU PRIX DE REVIENT DES EXAMENS ENDOSCOPIQUES

Calcul du K moyen d'après les documents statistiques et comptables :

Les dépenses relatives au Service d'Endoscopie s'élèvent pour un an à : 412.534 Francs pour 91.265 K fournis.

Coût du K moyen :

$$\frac{412.534}{91.265} = 4.52 \text{ Francs}$$

Calcul du K moyen par enquêtes directes dans le Service d'Endoscopie Digestive :

Les différences trouvées portent essentiellement sur l'amortissement du matériel (192.325 Fr. par enquêtes directes au lieu des 19.798 fournis par les états comptables) et les frais de personnel (372.209 Fr. au lieu de 264.010 Francs)

Le total des dépenses pour l'endoscopie digestive est de 693.614 Francs pour 91.265 K fournis, ce qui donne un prix de revient du K moyen de 7.60 Francs au lieu de 4.52 Francs.

Coût des examens d'endoscopie digestive :

Le nombre de K moyens par examen a été calculé comme pour la radiographie à partir des registres de facturation du Service. On trouve par ordre croissant : 10.96 K pour la rectoscopie, 45.28 K pour l'oesophagogastroduodenoscopie, 73.24 K pour la coloscopie, 100 K + 92.93 Z pour la wirsungographie.

Afin de pouvoir interclasser les valeurs unitaires de l'ensemble des examens, il a été procédé à une conversion des K en Z , en se servant du rapport :

$\frac{4.52}{5.23} = 0.86$ pour les estimations d'après les documents statistiques et comptables

$\frac{7.60}{5.73} = 1.33$ pour les estimations d'aprés les enquêtes

On obtient alors un interclassement de l'ensemble des examens (Tableau III).

TABLEAU III - Classement des examens par information mutuelle décroissante - Relation avec leur coût

Examens	Nombre de Z		Information Mutuelle
	Documents comptables	d'après enquêtes	
Coloscopie	62.99	97.41	0.225
Rectoscopie	9.43	14.58	0.175
Oesophago-gastroduodenoscopie	38.94	60.22	0.152
Radiographie des voies biliaires	77.20	78.61	0.130
Wirsungographie	178.93	225.93	0.094
Transit oesophago-gastroduodenal	97.05	97.05	0.083
Radiographie du colon	85.76	85.76	0.074
Artériographie	707.72	873.16	0.053
Radiographie de l'abdomen sans préparation	32.70	32.70	0.050

5. DISCUSSION

La valeur d'un examen pour la determination d'un diagnostic ne peut en toute rigueur se faire qu'au moyen d'une analyse préalablement planifiée. Ceci permettrait alors d'etudier avec plus de precision au moyen d'indices de spécificité et de sensitivité la valeur exacte d'un examen dans la pose d'un diagnostic. Dans le present travail, basé sur un fichier d'observations medicales systematiques informatisées, de telles analyses sont difficilement envisageables, tous les examens ne pouvant pas toujours etre pratiqués sur tous les sujets. La methode d'Information Mutuelle est bien adaptée pour surmonter ce type de difficultés.

Lorsque l'on compare la valeur des informations mutuelles de chacun des examens en relation avec leurs coûts (Tableau III), on voit que cinq types d'examens s'individualisent :

- Les examens endoscopiques : rectoscopie, oesophagogastroduodenoscopie, coloscopie, qui ont des informations mutuelles plus élevées que les examens radiographiques classiques correspondants, et cela pour un coût inférieur si la valeur du K est celle calculée à partir des documents comptables. Par contre, dans la réestimation du K après enquêtes (K = 7.60 au lieu de 4.52), le prix de la coloscopie est légèrement supérieur à celui de la radiographie du colon. Cependant, l'information mutuelle de la coloscopie est bien supérieure à celle de la radiographie du colon.

- Les voies biliaires ont une information moyenne pour un coût moyen.

- La wirsungographie a une valeur de l'information mutuelle assez élevée pour un coût élevé. Il s'agit donc d'un examen informationnel et coûteux.

- L'artériographie a une information basse pour le coût le plus élevé. Elle est donc peu informationnelle et très coûteuse.

- La radiographie de l'abdomen sans préparation a l'information mutuelle la plus basse pour le coût le plus bas. Il s'agit donc d'un examen à la fois peu informationnel et peu coûteux.

On pourrait résumer l'ensemble de ces résultats en disant que les examens endoscopiques sont très informationnels et, dans l'ensemble - mise à part la wirsungographie - moins coûteux que les examens radiographiques.

On pourrait alors se demander quelle serait, en tenant compte du coût, la meilleure séquence d'examens à pratiquer chez des malades hospitalisés en Gastroentérologie. Si on ne fait pas entrer en ligne de compte le confort du patient et si on ne considère que l'élément économique de l'examen, la séquence maximale correspondrait à pratiquer en priorité les examens endoscopiques et, éventuellement par la suite, les examens radiographiques. On aurait ainsi la meilleure chance d'aboutir plus rapidement à un diagnostic déterminé.

BIBLIOGRAPHIE

(1) CORNEE J, CHANON M, TROUVE C, RODRIGUEZ M. Computers management of medical records, external consultations and archives in a gastroenterology department. Meth Inform Med. 1977 ; 16 : 11-19

(2) CHAR-TUNG LEE. Information theory and data analysis. Math Biosci. 1971 ; 11 : 153-161

(3) DURBEC JP, CORNEE J, BERTHEZENE P. Data screening methods. Application to differential diagnosis in pancreatic pathology from radiological signs. Meth Inform Med. 1978 ; 17, No. 1 : 36-40

(4) STERLING TS, HABERMAN D, POLLACK S. Robot data screening an automatic search technique. Bio-med Comput. 1970 ; 1 : 61-74

(5) KULLBACK S. Information theory and statistics. John Wiley, New York, 1959

(6) CHAVALET S. Le prix de revient hospitalier. Editions Médicales et Universitaires Collection Economie et Santé No. 2. PARIS 1976

Aide au diagnostic des douleurs abdominales aiguës.
Nécessité d'une banque de données personnelle.

Y. Flamant, F. Lacaine, JM Hay, JN. Maillard.

Clinique Chirurgicale de l'hôpital Louis Mourier 92701 Colombes Cedex France*

En 1972 à Leeds, de Dombal (2) met au point une aide au diagnostic des douleurs abdominales dont la précision diagnostique dépasse de 10p cent celle des meilleurs cliniciens. En 1976 à Copenhague, Bjerregaard (1) se heurte aux difficultés d'utiliser, pour ses propres malades, le programme de Leeds. L'expérience ici rapportée est celle de l'échec du transfert de la banque de données de Leeds à une population Française, imposant la constitution d'une banque de données locale.

MATERIEL.

Entre le 1er mai 1977 et le 1er novembre 1978, 399 malades hospitalisés pour syndrome douloureux abdominal aigu ont été retenus, pour participer à l'étude multicentrique sous la direction de FT de Dombal. Les critères d'inclusion et les diagnostics discriminés sont donc superposables à l'étude de Leeds (2). En revanche le questionnaire a été détaillé pour empêcher toute ambiguité dans la réponse aux 36 signes d'interrogatoire et d'examen clinique et à deux examens complémentaires (leucocytose et abdomen sans préparation). Le diagnostic du clinicien est porté par un interne de 4è année dans les douze heures suivant l'admission. Le diagnostic final est porté à la sortie du malade sur l'histologie de la pièce d'exérèse ou sur les constatations opératoires ; en cas de traitement médical, une preuve formelle radiologique et/ou biologique a été exigée. Le diagnostic de l'ordinateur a été établi a posteriori sur les données de l'admission au moyen d'un programme Bayesien. Le vecteur de prévalence diagnostique et les probabilités conditionnelles (sensibilités) ont été recueillis prospectivement sur nos malades. Les prévalences se sont avérées superposables à celles d'une étude rétrospective faite sur les trois années précédant l'étude. La proportion d'informations manquantes dans les questionnaires prospectifs est de 0.7p cent.

RESULTATS.

1) L'analyse des 120 premiers malades par la banque de données de Leeds (JC. Horrocks et FT. de Dombal) a fourni une précision diagnos-

* Travail subventionné par la DRET et l'Université Paris VII

tique de 60p cent, très inférieure à la précision diagnostique des cliniciens (77p cent).

2) Le vecteur de prévalence diagnostique concernant 385 malades sur 399 est le suivant (en p cent) : Appendicite : 20.7 ; Cholecystite : 14.5 ; Occlusion : 9.1 ; Colique néphrétique : 7.5 ; Pancréatite : 3.9 ; Perforation d'ulcère : 3.4 ; Sigmoïdite : 1.3 ; Douleur non spécifiée : 39.6. 14 malades ont des diagnostics autres.

Sur les 385 malades classables, la précision diagnostique du clinicien est de 73.5p cent ; la précision diagnostique de l'ordinateur avec la banque de données de Colombes est de 79p cent. Sur neuf erreurs graves par défaut (le clinicien ne reconnait pas l'indication chirurgicale), l'ordinateur en aurait corrigé 29. En cas de concordance entre le diagnostic du clinicien et de l'ordinateur, le diagnostic est correct dans 85p cent des cas. En cas de discordance, le clinicien a raison 4 fois et l'ordinateur six fois sur dix. L'ordinateur ne peut classer les 14 malades dont le diagnostic diffère des huit affections exclusives considérées ; mais si l'on considère la décision opératoire résultant du diagnostic posé, l'ordinateur a tort une fois et le clinicien trois fois.

DISCUSSION.

Les performances des cliniciens n'ont été étudiées qu'à l'échelon du médecin des urgences, un interne de 4è année . Elles sont identiques aux performances des "house surgeons" (2). La banque de données de Leeds, capable de classer correctement 90p cent des malades Anglais, n'a pu classer que 60p cent des malades Français ; ce fait confirme -après Bjerregaard (1)- qu'il n'est pas possible de transférer geographiquement une banque de données sans perte de puissance. Le vecteur de probabilité a priori n'est pas superposable, la cholecystite, l'occlusion et la colique néphrétique étant deux à trois fois plus fréquentes dans notre population qu'à Leeds (4). Mais ce sont plus sûrement les variations dans les probabilités conditionnelles qui expliquent les 40p cent de mal classés : de Dombal a rapporté d'importantes différences sémiologiques inter-centres voire inter-races dans la pathologie abdominale d'urgence(3).

L'impossibilité de transfert d'une banque de données, si elle se confirme pour d'autres populations, est un handicap sérieux pour l'aide au diagnostic.

Avec 79p cent de diagnostics exacts, notre système dépasse un peu la performance des cliniciens ; avec l'aide au diagnostic, le risque de porter à tort le diagnostic d'occlusion passe de 20 à 3p cent ; le risque de porter à tort le diagnostic de douleur non spécifiée passe de 13.5 à 1.7p cent. Pour les malades de Colombes, le système travaille actuellement en temps réel, mais ce bénéfice n'a été obtenu qu'en recommençant localement la même étude prospective que celle de de Dombal. La banque de données de Leeds n'a pas supporté la traversée de la Manche ; il reste à étudier si une banque Française peut voyager sur dix, cent ou mille km à travers la métropole ou si chaque hôpital doit travailler deux ou trois ans avant de pouvoir bénéficier d'une aide au diagnostic.

REFERENCES

-1- Bjerregaard B., Brynitz S., Holst-Christensen J., Kalaja E., Lund-Kristensen J., Hilden J., de Dombal F.T., Horrocks J.C. : Computer-aided diagnosis of the acute abdomen : a system from Leeds used on Copenhagen patients. In de Dombal F.T. and Gremy F. Decision making and Medical care - Can information science help? North Holland Publishing Company (1976).

-2- de Dombal F.T., Leaper D.J., Staniland J.R., Mc Cann A.P., Horrocks J.C. : Computer-aided diagnosis of acute abdominal pain. Br. Med. J. 1972, 2, 9-13

-3- de Dombal F.T. : Communication to the World organisation of Gastroenterology Madrid June 1980.

-4- Wilson D.H., Wilson P.D., Walmsley R.G., Horrocks J.C., de Dombal F.T. : Diagnosis of acute abdominal pain in the accident and emergency department. Br. J. Surg. 1977, 64, 250-254.

PREVISION ET REGULATION DE LA DEMANDE DE SOINS INFIRMIERS A PARTIR D'UN SYSTEME D'INFORMATION AUTONOME*

M. Chokron et A. Haurie
Ecole des Hautes Etudes Commerciales de Montréal
5255 avenue Decelles, Montréal, P.Q., H3T 1V6
Tél: (514) 343-4370, 343-3801

SUMMARY

An autonomous data processing system has been designed for forecasting care demands in a hospital unit. An update of the patients in the unit and the state of their diseases is done every day. A forecast of the care demand by shift and nursing category is obtained for a maximum of seven days. This forecast is calculated from descriptions of the disease dynamics by semi-markovian processes. For each state of each disease, there is an associated distribution of work. The system can also help in planning the admission of elective patients.

At present the system is experimentaly used in an unit. It has been designed so as to maximize acceptance by nursing personnel. Its characteristics are: ease of utilization and autonomy of processing, so that control of the information remains in the hands of the nursing staff.

1. INTRODUCTION

Cet article a pour but de présenter un système de prévision et de régulation de la demande de soins infirmiers dans un département d'un hôpital. La prévision est établie à partir d'une modélisation de la dynamique des maladies à l'aide de processus stochastiques.

Le système réalisé est directement inspiré du modèle proposé par Collart et Haurie (1980) où une méthodologie de prévision et de régulation de la demande de soins était développée à partir d'une description par des processus stochastiques de la dynamique des maladies des patients traités.

Smallwood et al. (1969) ont, les premiers, proposé un schéma d'analyse du système constitué par un hôpital où la dynamique des maladies des patients traités était représentée par des processus semi-markoviens dont les états correspondaient à des régimes de soins caractéristiques. Un processus semi-markovien est caractérisé par une séquence d'états. Il existe des probabilités de passage d'un état à l'autre. Les durées de séjour dans un état ont des distributions qui dépendent de l'état de départ et de l'état d'arrivée. Ce type de processus permet donc une représentation assez fidèle de l'évolution des conditions d'un patient au cours de son traitement.

Kao (1972 et 1973) reprit ce formalisme pour analyser les systèmes d'hôpitaux à soins progressifs, c'est-à-dire où les patients sont déplacés d'une unité à une autre au cours de l'évolution de leur état de maladie. Kao obtint des formules de prévision du recensement des patients permettant d'anticiper l'occupation future des divers unités d'un tel hôpital compte tenu de l'occupation présente et des arrivées aléatoires de patients.

Collart et Haurie (1976, 1980) ont repris ces formules de prévision du recensement et les ont étendues au cas où une partie des admissions de patients pourvait être contrôlée et ont associé à chaque état de maladie une demande de soins aléatoire. Le formalisme de Smallwood et de Kao pouvait alors être utilisé pour construire un modèle de prévision et de régulation de la demande de soins au sein d'une unité de soins ou d'un

* Recherche subventionnée par le CRSNG-Canada, Subvention n^{o} A9368 par le fonds Alma-Mater de l'Université de Montréal et le fonds de soutien de l'Université de Montréal.

département. Nous référons le lecteur à ces articles pour plus de détails sur la formulation mathématique de ces modèles.

Les travaux décrits dans cet article ont consisté à réaliser un système opérationnel, basé sur cette méthodologie, qui pourrait être pris en charge et utilisé par le responsable du personnel infirmier d'un département ou d'une unité de soins pour l'aider dans sa gestion. En concevant ce système, nous nous sommes fixés trois objectifs:

(i) produire, sur demande, une prévision de charge de travail, par équipe (ou par quart) et par catégorie de personnel sur un horizon d'une semaine;

(ii) rendre minimal le fardeau supplémentaire créé par la procédure de recueil des données;

(iii) réaliser un système autonome complètement contrôlé par le personnel infirmier d'une unité de soins ou d'un département.

Un effort assez considérable de recherche et de développement a été consacré récemment au Québec dans le domaine des systèmes d'évaluation de la demande de soins infirmiers. En particulier le système PRN (Tilquin et al. (1978)) est implanté dans de nombreux hôpitaux du Québec. Ce dernier système permet de faire une évaluation de la demande de soins pour la journée en cours à partir du plan de soins établi chaque jour pour chaque malade. La demande de soins est établie après un traitement centralisé des journées. Ce système ne permet pas de faire des prévisions pour un horizon dépassant une journée.

Le système que nous avons développé paraît donc très complémentaire de ces grands systèmes d'évaluation en ce sens qu'il est résolument tourné vers la prévision, grâce à l'inclusion de la dynamique des maladies dans les données de base, et que, d'autre part, il est destiné à une utilisation très décentralisée comme un outil d'aide à la gestion à court terme des unités de soins.

2. OBJECTIFS POURSUIVIS ET CONTRAINTES SUR LE SYSTEME

Nous reprendrons dans cette section les trois objectifs principaux énoncés précédemment pour en dégager l'importance au niveau de la gestion des unités de soins et pour indiquer les contraintes qu'ils font intervenir sur le système informatique.

2.1 Prévision des charges de travail pour les sept prochains jours

La charge de travail pour le personnel infirmier, engendrée par la demande de soins d'un patient, évolue au cours du séjour du patient dans l'unité. Cette demande de soins évolue avec l'état du patient. Si l'on dispose d'une description correcte de la loi d'évolution de l'état de maladie de chaque patient, on peut envisager de prévoir la charge de travail engendrée par ce patient dans les jours futurs. Connaissant le recensement de la population de patients présents et les lois d'arrivée de nouveaux patients, une prévision sur la charge totale de travail peut être effectuée. Cette prévision pourra permettre une meilleure gestion prévisionnelle du personnel de l'unité lors de la construction des emplois du temps ou lors de demandes de personnel supplémentaire.

2.2 Fardeau minimal de recueil de données

Le système ne devrait pas occasionner une augmentation indue des travaux d'ordre administratif pour le personnel infirmier.

2.3 Système autonome entièrement contrôlé au niveau de l'unité ou du département

La technique de prévision adoptée requiert le recueil de peu de données quotidiennes mais nécessite des calculs complexes requérant l'utilisation d'un ordinateur. Les donnés pourraient être traitées par un ordinateur central et enregistrées à partir d'un terminal situé dans l'unité concernée. Cependant, une telle approche est susceptible d'engendrer de fortes résistances de la part du personnel concerné. En effet, le personnel infirmier est très soucieux de préserver une certaine autonomie d'action au niveau de l'unité de soins pour garantir une certaine qualité des soins. Un système où les données recueillies peuvent servir à produire de l'information utilisée à des fins de contrôle administratif est souvent perçu comme un danger par le personnel concerné qui tend alors à le délaisser ou même à le combattre. En donnant au personnel de l'unité de soins concernée la possession exclusive de l'instrument qui fournit l'information dont il a besoin pour améliorer sa propre gestion, on élimine cette source possible de résistance à des systèmes d'information plus formalisés.

2.4 Contraintes découlant des objectifs à atteindre

La méthode de prévision basée sur une description des dynamiques de maladie par des processus semi-markoviens requiert une grande capacité d'emmagasinage de données. Pour une unité où on retient vingt maladies différentes, chaque maladie étant décrite par un processus à cinq états avec une durée de séjour maximale, dans chaque état, de 20 jours, on doit être en mesure de conserver environ 60 000 nombres. L'obtention des prévisions à partir des méthodes de calcul exposées par Collart et Haurie (1976) demande environ 200 000 opérations. La recherche du nombre de patients électifs à admettre pour réaliser une régulation sous-optimale, selon la méthode décrite par les mêmes auteurs, nécessite 2 000 000 d'opérations arithmétiques.

Pour ne pas créer de surcharge de travail indue, le système doit être simple à utiliser et d'un apprentissage facile. Un mode de conversationnel s'impose donc. On veut pouvoir garantir l'obtention de prévisions de charge de travail avec moins de dix minutes de temps de calcul.

Enfin pour assurer l'autonomie du système, il faut que l'ordinateur et ses unités périphériques ne prennent pas plus de place qu'un bureau de secrétaire.

3. DESCRIPTION DU SYSTEME

3.1 Information produite par le système

L'information majeure produite par le système est illustrée sur le tableau 1. Ce tableau indique les prévisions de charge de travail réalisées le 10 juin 1980 pour les journées du 11 au 17 juin 1980. Un autre état présente une information plus complète avec les écarts-types des prévisions de charge de travail. Ce second état est obtenu après une dizaine de minutes de temps de calcul supplémentaire.

Pour obtenir ces prévisions, l'utilisateur du système devra avoir fourni un nombre prévu d'admissions de patients électifs pour chacun des sept prochains jours. Si l'utilisateur ne veut pas fournir ces prévisions d'admission, le système peut réaliser une prévision basée sur la recherche d'une régulation sous-optimale de la charge de travail.

3.2 Entrée de données nécessaires au fonctionnement du système

Après avoir mis en marche les différentes unités de l'ordinateur, c'est-à-dire l'unité centrale et l'écran cathodique, les unités de disques et l'imprimante, la séance de travail débute en indiquant la langue dans laquelle doit se dérouler la conversation. Ensuite, la date du jour est indiquée. Enfin, on présente à l'usager une liste des actions possibles (Figure 1).

Au cours d'une séance "normale", l'utilisateur va d'abord indiquer les congés, les admissions du jour et les changements d'état de maladie des patients présents dans l'unité. La figure 2 contient un exemple de mise à jour. Ensuite, il pourra obtenir soit les prévisions de charge de travail en indiquant les admissions envisagées pour les jours prochains, soit les prévisions de charge avec un programme d'admission calculé par le système.

Il est à noter qu'on peut obtenir en tout temps l'une ou l'autre, ou les deux types, de prévisions.

Une évaluation du temps total requis pour entrer les données quotidiennes nécessaires à la mise à jour du recensement de patients et pour obtenir le tableau 1 est d'environ 15 minutes.

3.3 Composition du système

La figure 3 donne une représentation générale du système. Pour obtenir les résultats escomptés, à partir de l'état observé des patients présents dans l'unité, il faut utiliser deux types de données:

(i) les données valides à long terme. Ce sont les données relatives à la capacité de l'unité de soins et à la dynamique des maladies. Ces données comprennent l'identification des maladies et des états qui leur sont associés ainsi que les probabilités de séjour dans un état et de transition d'un état à l'autre. Elles sont obtenues à partir d'une analyse statistique des activités de l'unité;

(ii) les données valides à court terme. Elles décrivent l'état des malades présents dans l'unité de soins. Ces données changent quotidiennement.

C'est pourquoi, le système comprend deux grandes parties:

a) un bloc de "long terme" qui a pour fonction d'établir et de mettre à jour les données à long terme. De plus, certains calculs nécessaires aux prévisions, et qui découlent de ces données, sont effectués une fois pour toute;

b) un bloc de "court terme" qui a pour fonction de mettre à jour les données à court terme et de calculer et d'imprimer les résultats de prévision.

De plus, un fichier historique permet de recueillir les données résultant des observations des transitions effectuées par les patients traités dans l'unité. Ces données pourront être complétées par les observations de charge totale de travail telle que fournies par le système PRN par exemple.

3.4 Configuration de l'équipement

Pour satisfaire aux contraintes indiquées en section 2.4, notre choix s'est porté sur un ordinateur Hewlett Packard HP35, photographié à la figure 4. Le coût de ce matériel est d'environ vingt mille dollars.

4. IMPLANTATION DU SYSTEME

Le système que nous venons de décrire est implanté de façon expérimentale dans le département de gynécologie de l'Hôpital Juif Général Sir Mortimer B. Denis.

Pour ce faire il a fallu choisir une année de base, en l'occurrence 1978, et établir les statistiques des maladies traitées dans le département. Cela nous a permis de sélectionner vingt maladies qui représentent quatre-vingt-dix pour cent des cas.

La loi de probabilité des dynamiques de ces vingt maladies a été construite à partir d'une estimation subjective des médecins et d'une confirmation ultérieure par analyse des dossiers des patients.

Un plan de soins-type a été élaboré pour chaque état de chaque maladie. Une distribution de la demande de soins a été établie à partir du plan de soins.

Les fichiers nécessaires ont été montés à partir de ces données. Depuis août 1980, le système est utilisé quotidiennement par l'infirmière chef. Les prévisions qu'elle obtient servent à vérifier ses impressions préalables quant aux surcharges de travail pour les jours à venir et à construire l'emploi du temps des infirmières.

5. EXTENSIONS

Les données de changement d'état accumulées chaque jour peuvent servir à corriger les lois de probabilités des dynamiques de maladie. En les exploitant on obtient un système qui s'adapte à l'évolution du traitement des maladies.

Si le système PRN ou tout autre système équivalent est utilisé concurremment pour évaluer la demande totale de soins observée au jour le jour, on pourra par analyse de régression estimer les demandes de soins par état de maladie. En effet si le recensement au jour t est donné par le vecteur:

$$x(t) \triangleq (x_i(t))_{i \in I} \qquad \text{où} \quad I \triangleq \text{ensemble des états.}$$

et $x_i(t)$ est le nombre de patients observés le jour t dans l'état i, et si y(t) est la charge totale de travail indiquée par une méthode du type PRN on aura le modèle linéaire:

$$y(t) = \sum_{i \in I} b_i x_i(t) + a + \varepsilon(t)$$

où le coefficient de régression b_i correspond à la charge de travail "expliquée" par un patient qui se trouve dans l'état i. Le terme ε(t) est l'erreur aléatoire du modèle de régression.

6. CONCLUSION

On peut déjà constater que le système est bien accueilli. L'infirmière chef l'utilise volontiers tous les jours. De plus, de sa propre initiative, elle en a disséminé l'usage aux autres infirmières du département.

Les résultats préliminaires de notre expérience semblent confirmer l'hypothèse que l'autonomie du système est un facteur de succès important dans l'utilisation de méthodes de gestion avancées dans le cadre d'une unité de soins hospitaliers.

7. REFERENCES

COLLART, D. et HAURIE, A., 1976, "On a Suboptimal Control of a Hospital Inpatient admission System", IEEE Transactions on Automatic Control, Vol. AC-21, pp. 233-238.

COLLART, D. et HAURIE, A., 1980, "On the Control of Care Supply and Demand in a Urology Department", European Journal of Operational Research, Vol. 4, n° 3, pp.160-172.

KAO, E.P.C., 1972, "A Semi-Markov Model to Predict Recovery Progress of Coronary Patients", Health Services Research, pp. 191-208.

KAO, E.P.C., 1973, "A Semi-Markovian Population Model with Application to Hospital Planning", IEEE Trans. Systems Man and Cybernetics, SMC-3, pp. 327-336.

SMALLWOOD, R.D., MURRAY, G.E., SILVA, D.D., SONDIK, E.F. and KLAINER, L.M., 1969, "A Medical Service Requirements Model for Health Systems Design", Proceedings IEEE, Vol. 57, pp. 1880-1887.

TILQUIN, C., 1978, "PRN 76, un système d'information pour la gestion des soins infirmiers", Rapport de recherche annuel 1978, EROS pavillon Ellendale, Univ. de Montréal.

REMERCIEMENT:

Nous remercions la Direction du "Montreal Jewish General Hospital" pour son aide dans la réalisation de ce projet ainsi que le docteur J. Schindler et Mmes A. Loyola et Wolfe.

DEMANDE DE SOINS INFIRMIERS 10 JUIN 1980
****

CATEGORIE DE PERSONNEL: INFIRMIERES/NURSES PATIENTS PRESENTS: 22

JOUR DE PREVISION	DEMANDE PREVUE (1) JOUR	(2) SOIR	(3) NUIT	Adm. Sug.	Ur.	Dep.	T
11 JUIN 1980	18 Hres	12 Hres 30 Mn	7 Hres 30 Mn	4	0	3	23
12 JUIN 1980	21 Hres	13 Hres 30 Mn	9 Hres	2	0	1	24
13 JUIN 1980	22 Hres 30 Mn	15 Hres	9 Hres 30 Mn	4	1	5	24
14 JUIN 1980	20 Hres	13 Hres 30 Mn	9 Hres	2	0	2	24
15 JUIN 1980	21 Hres	14 Hres 30 Mn	9 Hres	2	0	2	24
16 JUIN 1980	21 Hres	14 Hres 30 Mn	9 Hres	3	0	4	23
17 JUIN 1980	19 Hres 30 Mn	13 Hres 30 Mn	8 Hres 30 Mn	2	1	5	21

Adm. Sug.: Admissions Suggérées.
Ur.: Prévision du nombre d'Urgents.
Dep.: Prévision du nombre de départs (Présents, Urgents, Electifs).
T : Occupation totale des lits.

TABLEAU 1

LISTE DES OPERATIONS
****

1. CONSULTATION OU MODIFICATION DU DOSSIER D'UN PATIENT.
   Vous désirez faire une ou plusieurs des opérations suivantes:
   -Enregistrer le départ d'un patient
   -Enregistrer l'admission d'un patient
   -Enregistrer le changement d'état d'un patient
   -Consulter le dossier d'un patient
   -Corriger le dossier d'un patient

2. MODIFICATION DE L'OFFRE DE SOINS INFIRMIERS OU DE LITS.

3. PREVISION DE LA DEMANDE DE SOINS EN FONCTION D'ADMISSIONS SUGGEREES.

4. PREVISION DE LA DEMANDE DE SOINS EN FONCTION D'UN OPTIMUM CALCULE.

5. FIN DE VOTRE SESSION DE TRAVAIL.

QUEL EST LE NUMERO CORRESPONDANT A L'OPERATION QUE VOUS DESIREZ EFFECTUER ?

FIGURE 1

```
*** MISE A JOUR ***      DOSSIER DU PATIENT      LE  10 JUIN  1980
                         ******************
     1. LIT  :               5510A
     2. PATIENT  :           U-005485
     3. NOM:                 LAPORTE
     4. NOM DU MEDECIN:      PELLETIER
     5. MALADIE:             FIBROME UTERIN
     6. DATE D'ENTREE:       9  JUIN  1980    (MALADIE)
     7. ETAT DE LA MALADIE:  EXAMEN/INVESTIGATION
     8. DATE D'ENTREE:       10  JUIN  1980    (ETAT)

(1 = MODIFICATION A FAIRE, 2 = DEPART DU PATIENT, 3 = LE DOSSIER EST A JOUR) ?

 1 *
```

```
*** MISE A JOUR ***      DOSSIER DU PATIENT      LE  10 JUIN  1980
                         ******************
     1. LIT  :               5510A
     2. PATIENT  :           U-005485
     3. NOM:                 LAPORTE
     4. NOM DU MEDECIN :     PELLETIER
     5. MALADIE:             FIBROME UTERIN
     6. DATE D'ENTREE:       9  JUIN  1980    (MALADIE)
     7. ETAT DE LA MALADIE:  EXAMEN/INVESTIGATION
     8. DATE D'ENTREE:       10  JUIN  1980    (ETAT)

QUEL EST LE NUMERO DE LA LIGNE A MODIFIER (1 A 8) ?

 7 *
```

```
*** MISE A JOUR ***      DOSSIER DU PATIENT      LE  10 JUIN  1980
                         ******************
     1. LIT  :               5510A
     2. PATIENT  :           U-005485
     3. NOM:                 LAPORTE
     4. NOM DU MEDECIN :     PELLETIER
     5. MALADIE:             FIBROME UTERIN
     6. DATE D'ENTREE:       9  JUIN  1980    (MALADIE)
 --> 7. ETAT DE LA MALADIE:  EXAMEN/INVESTIGATION
 --> 8. DATE D'ENTREE:       10  JUIN  1980    (ETAT)
----------------------------------------------------------------------------
MALADIE DU PATIENT:  FIBROME UTERIN
LISTE DES ETATS DE LA MALADIE :                 1 .  EXAMEN/INVESTIGATION
******************************                  2 .  OPERATION
                                                3 .  POST-OPERATION
                                                4 .  COMPLICATIONS
                                                5 .  SOINS/CARE
                                                6 .  CONGE/DISCHARGE
NOTEZ LE NUMERO CORRESPONDANT AU NOUVEL ETAT DU PATIENT.

QUEL EST CE NUMERO ?

 3 *
```

```
*** MISE A JOUR ***      DOSSIER DU PATIENT      LE  10 JUIN  1980
                         ******************
     1. LIT  :               5510A
     2. PATIENT  :           U-005485
     3. NOM:                 LAPORTE
     4. NOM DU MEDECIN :     PELLETIER
     5. MALADIE:             FIBROME UTERIN
     6. DATE D'ENTREE:       9  JUIN  1980    (MALADIE)
     7. ETAT DE LA MALADIE:  POST-OPERATION
     8. DATE D'ENTREE:       10  JUIN  1980    (ETAT)

(1 = MODIFICATION A FAIRE, 2 = DEPART DU PATIENT, 3 = LE DOSSIER EST A JOUR) ?
 3 *
```

* Les chiffres soulignés sont les réponses de l'utilisateur.

FIGURE 2

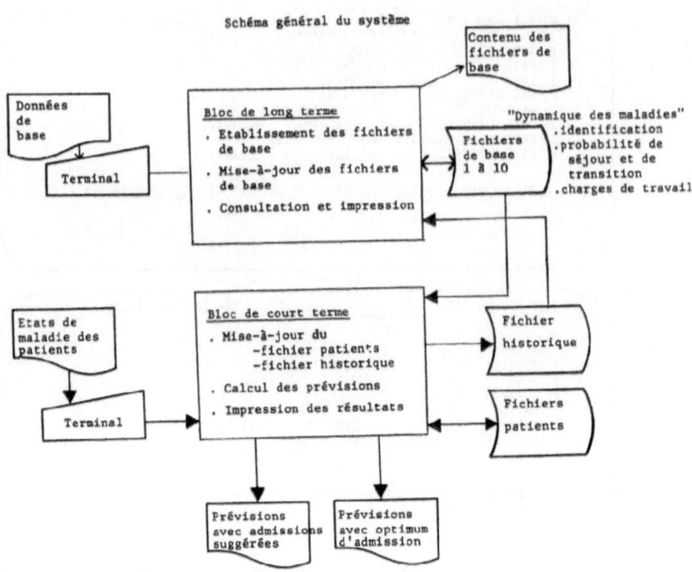

FIGURE 3

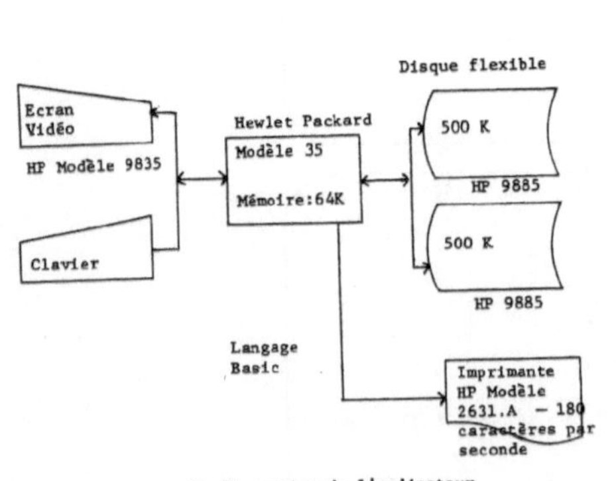

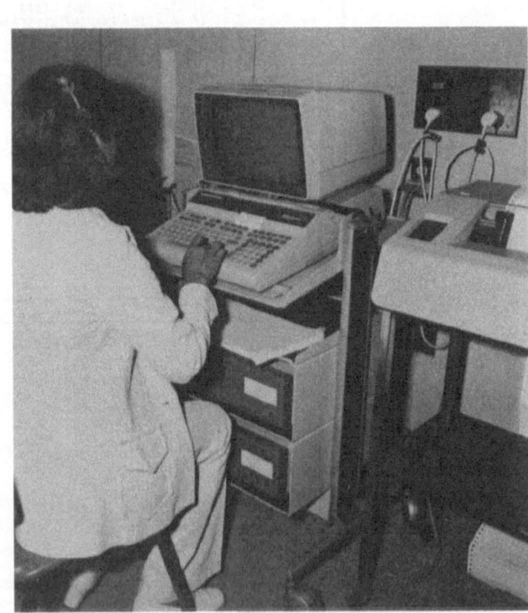

FIGURE 4

INDICATEURS DE L'ACTIVITÉ QUANTITATIVE DES MÉDECINS ANESTHÉSIOLOGISTES DANS LES BLOCS OPÉRATOIRES D'UN CENTRE HOSPITALIER REGIONAL

(Etude critique)

WEILLER-RACAMIER (J) [+], DUSSERRE (L) [++], CAILLARD (B) [+++], D'ATHIS (P) [++], LASSAUNIÈRE (J.M) [+], COULON (C) [+++], BOURDEIX-CHALMOND (I) [++].

[+] Département d'Anesthésie-Réanimation (Pr. Ag. M. WILKENING) - HOPITAL GENERAL - 3 rue du Faubourg Raines - 21033 DIJON CEDEX.

[++] Département d'Informatique Médicale du C.H.U. (Pr. Ag. L. DUSSERRE)

[+++] Département d'Anesthésie-Réanimation (Pr. B. CAILLARD) - HOPITAL DU BOCAGE - 2 Bld Mal de Lattre de Tassigny - 21034 DIJON CEDEX.

SUMMARY

QUANTITATIVE ACTIVITY DATA OF ANESTHESISTS IN OPERATING AREAS OF A REGIONAL HOSPITAL

In order to study the best distribution of anaesthesiologists in the different operating areas of a regional University Hospital we have analyzed different data gathered in our hospital : number of anaesthesia, number of hours spent in the operating area, number of "are K". (In France, the "K" is used for surgery and the "are K" for preoperative care, anaesthesia and postoperative care. Both -K and are K- are the result of a dialogue between the Health Insurance people and the doctors. This set number of are K allows anaesthesists to determine their fees.)

Of these these three criteria, the number of hours seems to be the most important but also the most difficult to estimate ; our study could not show any direct relationship between the two first criteria and the last one. Morever, we can go as far as to say that any notion of set standards would be difficult to achieve in this particular case.

INTRODUCTION

L'objet de ce travail est la recherche critique d'indicateurs d'activité des médecins anesthésiologistes de deux Départements d'Anesthésie-Réanimation dans un Centre Hospitalier Régional et Universitaire (C.H.U.), c'est-à-dire à l'intérieur d'hôpitaux de grande taille où il y a vocation de soins et d'enseignement.

Les tâches de ces médecins se sont progressivement et largement diversifiées : elles ont dépassé les actes directement liés à l'anesthésie d'un patient en vue d'une intervention, pour couvrir la surveillance d'unités de soins intensifs ou de réanimation et assurer le fonctionnement de la relève médicale et des urgences. Parmi cet ensemble de tâches, seule la mission en salle d'opération est facilement cernable car il est possible de la quantifier.

Apprécier correctement l'activité dans les blocs opératoires c'est, en fait, disposer de critères d'activité. Dans cette première approche l'objectif a été de définir une "quantité de travail", indépendamment des aspects qualitatifs sous-jacents. Les indicateurs d'activité habituellement utilisés en France sont le nombre d'interventions et le nombre de K, mais la durée d'activité apparaît également comme un indicateur souhaitable et c'est sur elle que nous avons centré nos efforts. Après l'exposé de la méthodologie et des résultats, la discussion se limitera à la recherche de normes permettant la répartition des effectifs d'un Département d'Anesthésiologie entre les différents blocs opératoires, en s'appuyant sur l'appréciation des trois indicateurs définis, et l'étude d'une éventuelle corrélation entre eux.

MÉTHODOLOGIE

Pour appréhender ces différents indicateurs, nous disposons :

- d'un cahier d'interventions qui collige depuis plus de cinq ans le nombre d'Aré K effectués dans les principaux blocs opératoires de l'un des deux hôpitaux concernés.
- d'un système informatique de recueil d'informations qui permet, depuis huit mois, de comptabiliser le nombre d'interventions, le nombre d'Aré K et d'évaluer le temps effectivement passé au bloc opératoire par le malade. Grâce à ce dernier système on est en mesure de connaître : le temps d'attente du patient (délai entre l'arrivée du malade au bloc opératoire et sa prise en charge par le médecin anesthésiste : délai I), le temps d'induction anesthésique (délai entre la prise en charge et le moment où le malade est devenu opérable : délai II), le temps d'installation du chirurgien (délai écoulé entre la fin de l'induction et le début de l'intervention : délai III), le temps d'intervention chirurgicale : délai IV, le temps de réveil (délai qui s'écoule entre la fin du pansement et la sortie du bloc opératoire : délai V).

Les problèmes pratiques posés par le recueil et la validation de ces informations ont fait l'objet de communications antérieures (1) (2).

RÉSULTATS

Ils concernent les trois indicateurs d'activité : durée, nombre d'interventions et nombre d'Aré K et l'étude de leurs liaisons.

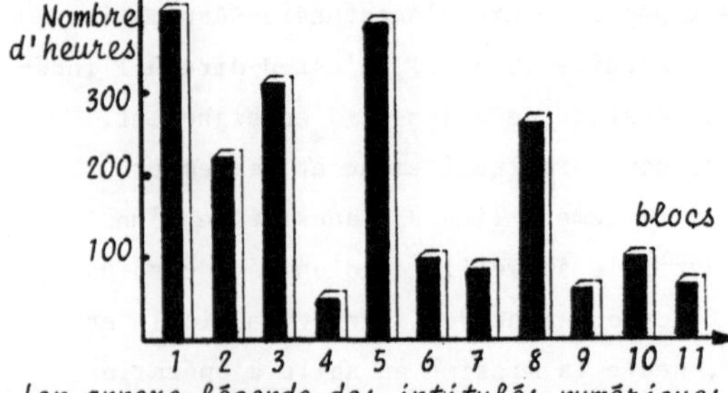

(en annexe légende des intitulés numériques des blocs opératoires). Fig.1

INDICATEURS DUREE : Rappelons qu'on entend par durée le temps de présence de l'anesthésiologiste au bloc opératoire. Sa présence n'est pas impliquée dans le délai I (attente du malade) et dans ce travail tous les temps sont donc mesurés à partir du délai II. L'activité en durée des anesthésiologistes dans chacun des blocs opératoires est donnée dans la figure 1 à titre d'exemple pour le mois de janvier 1980.

INDICATEUR NOMBRE D'INTERVENTIONS : On a dénombré les interventions pour l'ensemble de chaque hôpital au cours du mois de janvier 1980. En divisant par le nombre de salles (il n'a pas été pris en compte les salles d'activité très spécialisée et par ce fait d'utilisation infime) on a obtenu une moyenne de trente anesthésies par salle. L'examen des activités en nombre d'interventions effectuées par salle montre des écarts importants par rapport à cette moyenne de 30 (8 pour le minimum et 45 pour le maximum).

INDICATEUR NOMBRE D'ARE K : C'est l'indicateur habituel d'activité. A ce titre il mérite qu'on l'analyse successivement sur un mois (janvier 1980) et au cours d'une période de six mois (novembre 1979 à avril 1980). Au cours de Janvier 1980 l'activité en Arē K de chaque bloc opératoire est celle indiquée dans la figure 2.

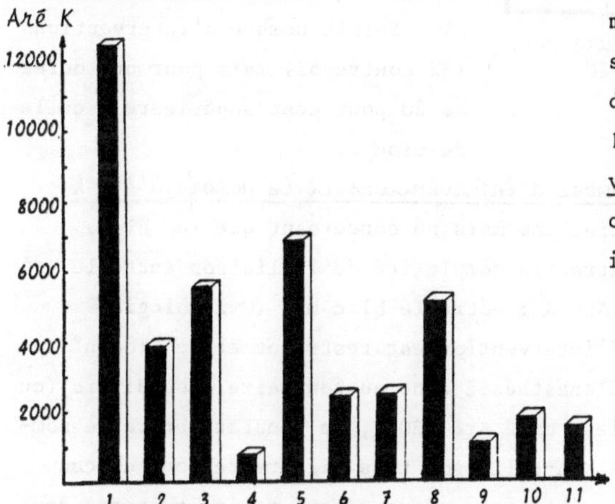

Fig.2 : Activité en Arē K des blocs opératoires en Janvier 1980. (En annexe la légende des intitulés numériques des blocs opératoires).

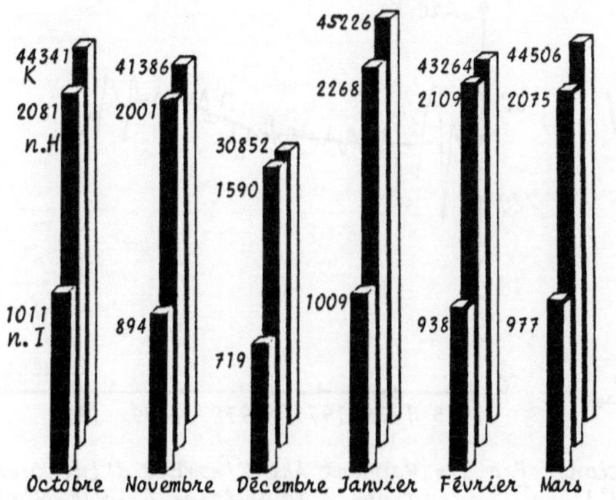

Fig.3 : Durée en heures (n.H), nombre d'interventions (n.I) et nombre d'Arē K (K) d'octobre 1979 à mars 1980 pour l'ensemble des blocs opératoires.

Pour la période de six mois il a paru intéressant de confronter sur un même graphique (figure 3), mois par mois et tous services confondus, l'activité en K, la durée et le nombre d'interventions.

ETUDE DES LIAISONS ENTRE LES INDICATEURS

1 - *Liaison entre le nombre d'interventions et la durée.*

SERVICES	NOMBRE D'INTERVENTIONS	DURÉE EN H	ARÉ K
BLOC 1	156	412	12219
BLOC 5	176	413	6867
BLOC 7	53	83	2497
BLOC 8 (sans neuro-radiologie)	32	104	2352

Tableau I : Valeurs des trois indicateurs dans quatre blocs en janvier 1980

La figure 3 comme le tableau I montrent, comme on pouvait s'y attendre, qu'aucune liaison simple n'apparaît entre le nombre d'interventions et la durée. Le tableau I est particulièrement explicite : si l'on compare les blocs 7 et 8, on constate que celui-ci réalise le plus faible nombre d'interventions (32 contre 53) mais pour une durée de 20 pour cent supérieure à celle du bloc 7.

2 - *Liaison entre le nombre d'interventions et le nombre d'Aré K*

Une étude portant sur cinq ans mais ne concernant que les blocs numéros 1 et 6 (annexe) permet d'illustrer la complexité de la liaison entre le nombre d'interventions et le nombre d'Aré K : entre le bloc n°6 (Gynécologie-Obstétrique) où l'éventail des types d'intervention est restreint et le bloc n°1 (Clinique Chirurgicale) où les types d'anesthésie sont au contraire très divers (du plus simple coté Aré K15 au plus complexe coté Aré K300), on constate entre le nombre d'interventions et le nombre d'Aré K une liaison très différente pour chacun d'eux. Cet effet apparaît sur les figures 4 et 5 qui représentent les rapports des nombres d'Aré K aux nombres d'interventions en fonction du mois et ceci dans les deux services pendant les cinq ans considérés.

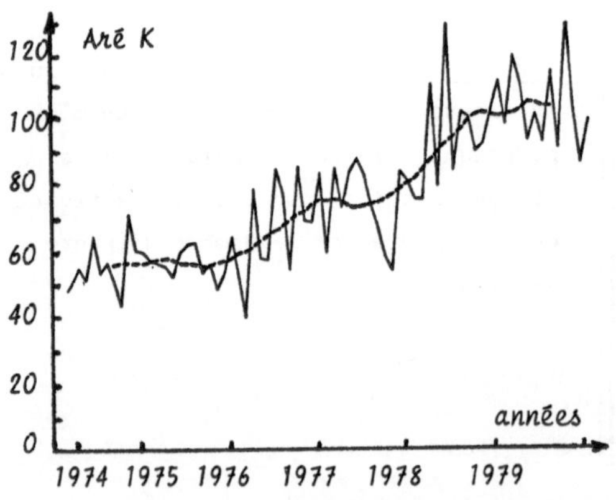

Fig.4 : Rapport Aré K/nombre d'interventions en Clinique Chirurgicale (BLOC N°1) pendant 5 ans.

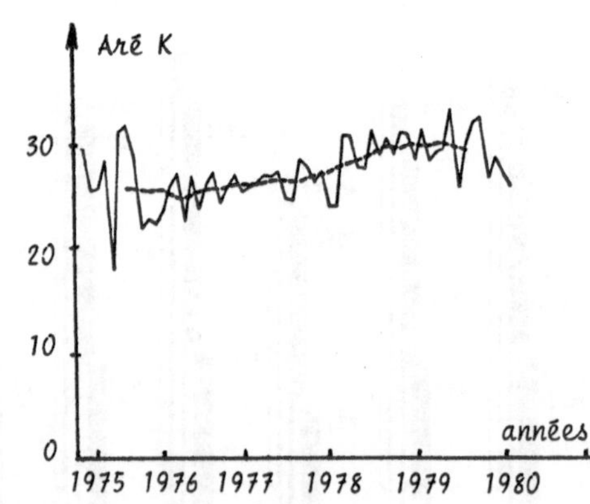

Fig.5 : Rapport Aré K/nombre d'interventions à la Maternité (BLOC N°6) pendant 5 ans.

Les lissages obtenus par la méthode des moyennes mobiles ont été superposés aux courbes brutes et représentés en traits discontinus.

Ces graphiques mettent en évidence des oscillations d'amplitude plus faible pour le bloc n°6 que pour le bloc n°1. Les lissages montrent une tendance apparemment négligeable pour ce même bloc, alors qu'elle est nettement croissante pour le bloc n°1.

3 - *Liaison entre le nombre d'Aré K et la durée*

Entre ces deux indicateurs, le calcul montre une liaison croissante significative mais non linéaire. L'analyse a montré que la liaison entre la durée et le nombre d'Aré K était la plus forte pour les interventions cotées plus de Aré K70 (figures 6 et 7).

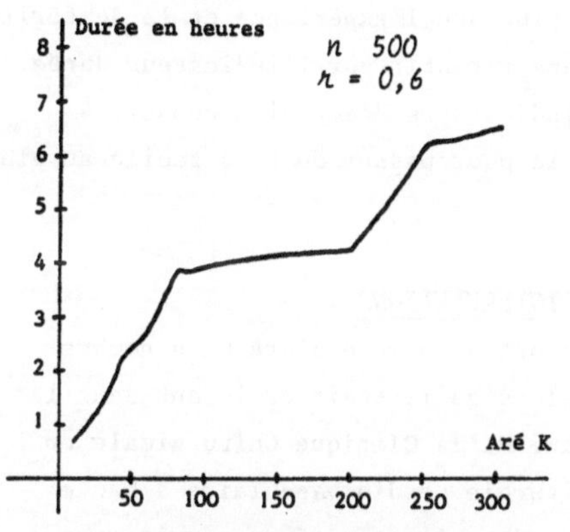

Fig.6 : *Représentation globale des durées en fonction des Aré K.*

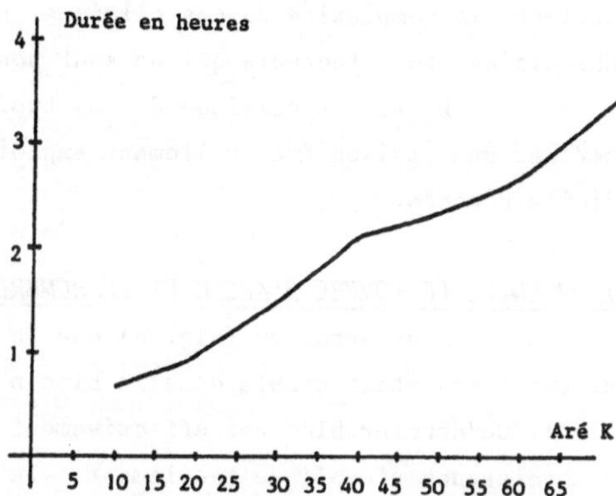

Fig.7 : *Représentation des durées en fonction des Aré K jusqu'à Aré K 70.*

Ni globalement ni à l'intérieur des différents intervalles d'Aré K considérés (moins de 25, de 25 à 40, de 40 à 70) on n'a pu mettre en évidence de liaison linéaire, elle est donc inutilisable en pratique.

COMMENTAIRES

La discussion des résultats est dominée par le souci d'aider à la répartition optimale des effectifs dans les blocs opératoires.

L'indicateur le plus sûr est la DUREE de présence de l'Anesthésiologiste au bloc opératoire. Cet indicateur a été peu utilisé jusqu'à maintenant car, si l'on veut des données objectives recueillies dans les meilleures conditions il faut disposer d'un système de recueil d'informations spécialement conçu à cet effet et situé le plus près possible de leur source. Si l'on ne se contente pas d'estimation (3), l'indicateur durée nécessite un appui logistique relativement lourd. Mais si ces conditions de précision sont respectées, il est légitime de l'utiliser comme indicateur de référence.

La signification de l'indicateur NOMBRE D'INTERVENTIONS est en revanche très limitée. Un bloc opératoire qui assure deux fois plus d'anesthésies qu'un autre ne travaille pas pour autant deux fois plus et il ne viendrait à l'idée de personne de mettre en équivalence une cure de hernie inguinale et une cure de malformation cardiaque sous circulation extra-corporelle ! La seule information que le nombre d'interventions peut fournir est une information ponctuelle, celle du temps passé à la consultation préopératoire, temps qui reste relativement constant quelle que soit l'intervention en cause. Ce type d'activité n'est pas évalué dans la présente étude.

L'indicateur NOMBRE D'ARE K est un indicateur officiel dont l'efficacité est souvent discutée. Dans sa conception même il fait intervenir la notion de forfait fondé uniquement sur le type d'intervention, sans prendre en compte l'état du patient, la complexité du cas clinique, pas plus que l'expérience et la dextérité du chirurgien, tous facteurs qui ne sont pas sans retentir sur l'indicateur durée.

L'analyse critique de ces trois indicateurs d'activité conduit à rechercher une liaison éventuellement exploitable pour passer du plus facile au plus difficile d'accès.

LIAISON ENTRE LE NOMBRE D'ARE K ET LE NOMBRE D'INTERVENTIONS :

Nous avons vu (Fig. 4) que le rapport du nombre d'Aré K au nombre d'interventions était stable dans le bloc n°6 alors qu'il était croissant dans le bloc n°1. Ce dernier bloc est effectivement celui de la Clinique Chirurgicale et cette croissance s'explique facilement : la chirurgie cardio-vasculaire à haute technicité prend une part de plus en plus grande dans l'activité du service.

Les oscillations constatées, amples pour le bloc n°1 s'expliquent, en dehors des variations saisonnières, par la grande dispersion du nombre d'Aré K. Il est évident que, dans un tel cas, la liaison entre le nombre d'Aré K et le nombre d'interventions est inutilisable pour la gestion. En revanche dans un bloc où l'activité est moins diversifiée (oscillations faibles observées sur la figure 5 pour le bloc n°6) on peut à la rigueur déduire le nombre d'Aré K à partir du nombre d'interventions, et inversement.

LIAISON ENTRE LE NOMBRE D'ARÉ K ET LA DUREE :

Entre le nombre d'Aré K et la durée, il existe une liaison multifactorielle dans laquelle interviennent probablement, étroitement liés, le facteur saisonnier, la structure de l'équipe chirurgicale, son degré de technicité, le taux de recrutement et les catégories de patients.

Le tableau I montre qu'on ne peut passer facilement de la notion "durée" à la notion d'Aré K : par exemple, pour une même durée en heure, l'activité en Aré K des blocs opératoires numéros 1 et 5 sont dans le rapport 0,56. De la même manière si les figures 6 et 7 mettent en évidence, à partir de Aré K70 une liaison entre la durée et le nombre d'Aré K, le calcul a montré que cette liaison est faible et inutilisable en pratique. Il n'est donc pas possible d'une manière générale de passer de l'activité en Aré K à une activité de durée.

CONCLUSION

Au terme de cette étude critique, le nombre d'interventions effectuées et la cotation en Aré K n'apparaissent pas comme des indicateurs valables de l'activité quantitative des Anesthésiologistes dans les blocs opératoires d'un C.H.U. ; et il n'est pas possible d'en déduire une juste répartition d'effectifs.

En revanche, l'indicateur durée est un paramètre quantitatif objectif dont l'efficacité est toutefois limitée par les caractéristiques suivantes :

- la durée de travail au bloc opératoire ne constitue qu'une fraction de l'activité anesthésiologique et cette fraction dépend de l'activité des services,
- elle présente une grande variabilité pour un même type d'intervention, cette variabilité étant due aux fonctions mêmes d'un C.H.U. : accueil des patients les plus complexes et éducation des futurs chirurgiens. Pour toutes ces raisons il serait illusoire de vouloir établir des normes de durées correspondant à des tâches bien définies : en tout état de cause elles ne seraient pas applicables hors du contexte local dans lequel elles ont été déterminées. En routine, où la mesure des durées fait défaut, seule une connaissance précise de la technicité et des hommes en présence, anesthésistes et chirurgiens, dans un cadre donné, permet de résoudre au mieux ce problème de la répartition des effectifs.

RÉFÉRENCES

1 - DUSSERRE L., CAILLARD B., D'ATHIS P., WILKENING M.
Evaluation de l'activité en bloc opératoire des médecins anesthésiologistes d'un groupement hospitalier universitaire. Etude critique de la motivation.
Systems Science in health care - 14,17 juillet 1980 - MONTREAL (Québec).

2 - CAILLARD B., DUSSERRE L.
Evaluation de l'activité des médecins anesthésiologistes dans les blocs opératoires du C.H.U. de Dijon.
Communication à la conférence "Informatique et évaluation de l'activité hospitalière" - Hôpital de la Pitié, PARIS, 5,6 Octobre 1979.

3 - HONTEBEYRIE P., de POUVOURVILLE G.
L'anesthésie-réanimation dans les Hôpitaux de l'Assistance Publique. Rapport d'étude de l'Ecole Polytechnique - Mai 1978.

ANNEXE 1

Légende des numérotations des intitulés des blocs opératoires :

N°1 - Chirurgie abdominale, thoracique et cardio-vasculaire,

N°2 - Chirurgie générale et d'urgence de jour,

N°3 - Chirurgie traumatologique et d'urgence de nuit,

N°4 - Chirurgie générale,

N°5 - Chirurgie infantile et orthopédique,

N°6 - Gynécologie-Obstétrique,

N°7 - Urologie,

N°8 - Neuro-chirurgie - Neuro-radiologie,

N°9 - Radiologie vasculaire, bronchoscopie, Cardiologie (cardioversions, cathétérisme cardiaque),

N°10- Stomatologie,

N°11- Otorhinolaryngologie.

Nous tenons à remercier Mesdames CLAIRGIRONNET et MAROLLEAU, Mesdemoiselles DAUDIN et LOYER pour leur contribution à ce travail.

AN OPTIMAL ALLOCATION OF NEWLY QUALIFIED NURSES TO WARDS

A. R. Shah * North East Thames Regional Health Authority

J. A. Hollowell Management Services Division,
St. Faith's Hospital, Brentwood, Essex.
United Kingdom.

* Now with Organisation and Manpower Planning Division,
Kuwait Oil Company (K.S.C.) AHMADI - 22, Kuwait
Arabian Gulf.

Abstract:

This paper describes a computer aided method of allocating newly qualified nurses to their preferred wards using the Hungarian Algorithm for the Assignment Problem. The principle advantage of the scheme described here is that it is extremely flexible, allowing various criteria to be taken into consideration for the allocation process. Moreover, it produces a complete solution which is optimal in terms of the numerical criteria specified.

1 INTRODUCTION

Trainee nurses in the U.K. have a dual role. They are students in training as well as employees of the hospitals which provide the necessary clinical experience. A substantial part of their training is spent in receiving clinical experience in different wards and/or specialties of the hospitals. As a result, trainee nurses develop individual preferences during the training period for wards and/or specialties to which they apply for jobs after completing training. This gives rise to what is essentially an allocation problem: that of matching preferences of the newly qualified nurses to the service requirements of the hospitals.

This allocation problem is common to most hospitals but its size and complexity obviously varies. Most teaching hospitals allocate between 30 and 100 newly qualified nurses three times a year. For such hospitals, allocation of nurses to wards 'by hand' is not only technically difficult but also very time consuming. In these circumstances, a computer-based system has obvious advantages over a manual system.

This paper describes a computer-aided procedure employing an 'assignment algorithm', which was developed for an optimal allocation of newly qualified nurses to wards in a teaching hospital in London.

2 CRITERIA FOR THE ALLOCATION PROBLEM

The nursing staff in a typical ward of a teaching hospital may be categorised into one of the following three broad groups: trained staff, trainee staff and auxiliary staff.

Of these, the trained staff usually constitute less than 30% in teaching hospitals. As a group they have a high turnover rate which could be reduced by allocating newly qualified nurses to their preferred wards.

Senior nursing administrators involved in solving this difficult problem usually employ one or more of the following criteria for the allocation process.

i) Preferences expressed by nurses:
This is perhaps the most important and commonly used criterion. An attempt is made to allocate all the nurses to one of their preferred wards.

ii) Ward-based assessments and/or preferences expressed by ward sisters:
For each clinical experience during the training period, the ward sister prepares an assessment of the training received by an individual trainee, which can be used, along with the sisters preferences, as a possible criterion for allocation.

iii) Interval between the date of promotion/appointment of a trainee and the date of vacancy in a ward:
The date of promotion/appointment of a newly qualified nurse depends on the annual or unpaid leave at the end of the training and also on any prolonged absence which may have occurred during the training period. The dates on which the vacancies arise within the wards also vary. As a result, there may be a period during which the ward will have additional trained staff or a deficiency of trained staff. Minimising the interval between the date of appointment and the date of the vacancy is sometimes used as a criterion for allocation.

iv) Period of Appointment:
In hospitals where applicants are asked to specify their intended period of appointment this can be used as a discriminatory criterion for allocation.

3 MATHEMATICAL FORMULATION OF THE PROBLEM

The problem may be stated as follows:
Determine an optional allocation of n nurses to m wards/posts according to some chosen criteria given the preferences of nurses for particular posts and the preferences of ward sisters for particular nurses.

The main steps in formulating this problem mathematically are as follows:

i) Ascribing scores to the choices made by nurses and ward sisters to compute preference matrices A and B.

ii) Computing on interval score matrix C.

iii) Computing an array W of weights for individual nurses.

iv) Computing an overall allocation matrix X by combining the matrices A, B and C and weights W and adding dummy rows or columns, where necessary to convert the matrix X into a square matrix.

Notation:

A is a nxm matrix in which

a_{ij} = the preference score of i th applicant for the j th job.

B is a nxm matrix in which

b_{ij} = the preference score of j th ward sister for the i th applicant.

C is a nxm matrix in which

c_{ij} = the interval score for i th applicant's appointment with j th job.

W is an nxl array in which

w_i = weight to be attached to the score of i th applicant.

Then, X is a nxm matrix in which

$$x_{ij} = w_i \quad (f_1 a_{ij} = f_2 b_{ij} + f_3 c_{ij}) \quad \text{for } i = 1,2....,n \quad j = 1,2....,m$$

Where f_1, f_2 and f_3 are the weights to be attached to the nurses' and ward sisters' preference scores and the interval scores

k is defined to be the larger of n and m

Defining $x_{ij} = o$ for all $i > n$ or $j > m$

gives a square kxk matrix X.

The elements x_{ij} form an overall allocation matrix of dimensions kxk where k takes the value m or n whichever is larger. Any element x_{ij} in this matrix is á measure of desirability of the i th applicant being placed in the j th job. The problem then is to make an assignment so as to maximise the sum of the assigned elements. This does not guarantee the assignment of a particular nurse to a particular ward even where such an assignment represents the largest number within the overall matrix X.

Stated mathematically, the problem then is as follows:

$$\text{maximise } z = \sum_{i=1}^{k} \sum_{j=1}^{k} x_{ij} \; y_{ij} \qquad (1)$$

where $y_{ij} = 1$ if i^{th} applicant assigned to j^{th} job. (2)

$= 0$ otherwise

such that the assignment variable y_{ij} satisfies

$$\sum_{i=1}^{k} y_{ij} = 1 \quad \text{for } j=1,\ldots,k \text{ and } \sum_{j=1}^{k} y_{ij} = 1 \text{ for } i=1,\ldots,k \quad (3)$$

Equations (2) and (3) ensure that only one applicant is assigned to any one job.

4 SOLUTION TO THE PROBLEM

The problem of optimum allocation of personnel resources has received a great deal of analytic attention for many years. The personnel assignment problem is a special case of the well known transportation problem (1). Several methods are available to solve this particular class of problem (2,3,4,5,6), the choice of method depending mainly on the size and nature of the problem.

Although an algorithm on the Ford-Fulkerson (4) network flow approach would have been appropriate for the size of the problem under consideration, the conceptually simpler approach of the Hungarian method (2,3) was used. An important feature of the Hungarian method is that of finding the maximal assignment that exists among the zero elements of the matrix. It was therefore decided to modify/improve this feature of the method in view of the size of the problem and the sets of identical elements expected in the assignment matrix. The modified version of the algorithm and its application to a similar sized problem for allocating medical graduates to pre-registration appointments has been described earlier (7).

5 IMPLEMENTATION AND RESULTS

Four criteria were described earlier which may be employed for the allocation of newly qualified nurses to their preferred wards. All these criteria were used as described below:

i) Preferences expressed by nurses
Applicants were asked to state five choices although many stated fewer than this. Some applicants also stated a preference for a group of wards based on specialty of site or sex.

Different policies were considered for assigning scores to their choices. A policy was adopted which increased the likelihood of higher ranking choices being allocated.

The scores ascribed to the choices were as follows:
1st choice - (28), 2nd choice - (21), 3rd choice - (15), 4th choice - (10), 5th choice - (6), (6th choice for a group of wards - (3)). No choice made but post acceptable (1), excluded choice (- 100).

ii) Ward-based assessments and/or preferences of ward sisters. Few ward sisters expressed their preferences for trainee nurses. In all cases only one or two choices were made. The scores assigned were 1st choice (28) and 2nd choice (21).

iii) Interval between the date of promotion/appointment and the date of vacancy.
Let d = (date of vacancy - date of appointment).
A positive value of d represents the number of days for which the ward will have additional trained staff while a negative value implies a shortage of trained staff.
The following scores were assigned for different positive values of d.
Similar scores were assigned for negative values of d.

d days	0 - 7	8 - 14	15 - 21	22 - 28	>28
score	50	30	15	5	0

Table 1: Scores ascribed for interval d days

iv) Period of Appointment
Applicants intending a longer period of appointment were favourably considered by using the multiplying factors in Table 2. This factor could be based on criterion other than the period of appointment.

Intended Period of Appointment (in months)	Multiplying factor, f_4
Less than 3	0.5
3	0.6
4 - 5	0.75
6 - 7	0.9
8 - 9	1.0
10 - 12	1.2
13 - 18	1.4
More than 18	1.5

Table 2: Multiplying factor f_4

Of the above four criteria, the preferences expressed by the nurses and the ward sisters were given the greatest weighting. The scores obtained from these two criteria were multiplied by 20. (i.e. $f_1 = f_2 = 20$). Similarly the scores obtained as a result of the application of the third criterion (of minimising interval dates of appointment and vacancy) were multiplied by 1. (i.e. $f_3 = 1$).

The scores thus obtained for the three criteria were added and then each applicant's scores survey multiplied by the factor derived from the length of appointment: this gave the 'final assignment matrix' for the allocation problem.

The modified version of the Hungarian Algorithm was applied to the final assignment matrix. A summary of results obtained is given in Fig. 1. in the appendix.

The effects of altering the weights f_1, f_2 and f_3 were examined. Fig. 2 gives the results obtained for $f_1 = f_2 = 1$, and $f_3 = 20$. Thus, the criterion of minimising interval between dates of appointment and vacancy was given greater priority. It can be seen that the solution obtained in this case differs significantly from the one previously obtained.

6 DISCUSSION

Results obtained from the computer aided procedure were considered satisfactory by the senior nursing administrators although some adjustments to the allocations were necessary. In future, the number of such adjustments could be reduced by encouraging all trainees to state preferences for five wards. In the problem described above some had stated only one or two preferences with the result that their allocations were frequently unsatisfactory if they did not obtain one of these choices.

The general procedure will be for the computer solution to be submitted to the Senior Nursing Administration responsible for making these appointments. A few adjustments may be required in order to take into consideration criteria other than those specified. However, the computer solution would provide a very satisfactory basis for a final solution. Since the problem of allocating newly qualified nurses to their preferred wards is a recurring one for most teaching hospitals, the method described here can save a considerable amount of the Senior Nursing Administrator's time.

The main disadvantage of the method is a technical one; the Hungarian method has limitations in terms of the size of the problem it can handle and the Ford-Fulkerson algorithm would be more appropriate if the size of the problem increased substantially

The main advantages of the computer based system over the manual system are as follows:

i) It is extremely flexible, allowing for the criteria for allocation to be easily varied.

ii) It allows a weighting of an individual applicant's preferences as well as of the various criteria used for allocation.

iii) It permits an easy withdrawal of any applicant at any stage. For example, candidates who have failed their examinations can be withdrawn.

iv) It provides a complete solution. In producing an optimal solution, it does not necessarily guarantee a few allocations with very high scores, particularly if the penalty incurred by others due to such high scoring allocation is prohibitive.

Moreover, by providing an optimum solution of the problem, the computer aided procedure described in this paper could help to reduce the turnover rate among the trained staff as well as increase the job satisfaction of the newly qualified nurses.

7 REFERENCES

1 Hitchcock F.L., The distribution of a product from several sources to numerous localities, J. Math. Phys., 2 (1941) pp 224-230.

2 Kuhn H.W., The Hungarian method for the Assignment problem, Naval Research Logistics Quarterly. Vol. 2 (1955), pp 83 - 87.

3 Kuhn H.W., Variants of the Hungarian method for Assignment problems, Naval Research Logistics Quarterly. Vol. 3 (1956). pp. 253 - 258.

4 Ford L.R. and Fulkerson D.R., Solving the transportation problem, Management Science, Vol. 3 (1956), pp 24 - 32.

5 Yaspan A., On finding a maximal assignment, Operations Research, Vol. 14 (1956) pp 646 - 651.

6 Munkres J., Algorithm for the Assignment and Transportation problems, Journal of the Society of Industrial Application Mathematics, Vol. 5., No. 1 (1957).

7 Shah A.R., An Optimal Assignment of Medical Graduates to pre-registration jobs, unpublished paper presented at Euro III Conference, Amsterdam, April 1979. European Journal of Operations Research. (in press).

APPENDIX

Figure 1 : Results $(f_1=f_2 = 20, f_3 = 1)$

POST	(DATE OF VACANCY)	NURSE	(DATE OF APPT.)	PREFERENCE	INTENDED PERIOD OF APPT.(MONTHS)
1. PRIVATE WARD	(12/11/79)	POOL	(2/12/79)	6	3
2. PRIVATE WARD	(20/11/79)	VERE	(3/12/79)	6	6
⋮		⋮	⋮		
15. DEVO	(9/12/79)	BUGG	(31/12/79)	2	12
16. DEVO	(1/12/79)	HUMP	(2/12/79)	1	0
17. TURN.	(10/ 1/80)	BELL	(10/12/79)	1	12
18. ROTH	(1/12/79)	HANL	(14/ 1/80)	2	12
19. ROTH	(20/12/79)	WASH	(10/12/79)	1	6
⋮		⋮	⋮		
70. MORR	(1/12/79)	COOP	(2/12/79)	3	0
71. ALEX	(1/ 2/80)	HUMP	(10/12/79)	1	6
72. A.&E		POST WITHDRAWN			

PREFERENCE 1 ALLOCATED TO 22 NURSES
PREFERENCE 2 ALLOCATED TO 14 NURSES
PREFERENCE 3 ALLOCATED TO 8 NURSES
PREFERENCE 4 ALLOCATED TO 5 NURSES
PREFERENCE 5 ALLOCATED TO 1 NURSES
PREFERENCE 6 ALLOCATED TO 13 NURSES
PREFERENCE 7 ALLOCATED TO 6 NURSES

TOTAL NO. OF DAYS OF OVERLAP = 1175
TOTAL NO. OF DAYS OF SHORTFALL = -296

Figure 2 ; Results shewing effect of altering weights $(f_1=f_2=1, f_3=20)$

PREFERENCE 1 ALLOCATED TO 10 NURSES
PREFERENCE 2 ALLOCATED TO 11 NURSES
PREFERENCE 3 ALLOCATED TO 11 NURSES
PREFERENCE 4 ALLOCATED TO 2 NURSES
PREFERENCE 5 ALLOCATED TO 2 NURSES
PREFERENCE 6 ALLOCATED TO 13 NURSES
PREFERENCE 7 ALLOCATED TO 20 NURSES

TOTAL NO. OF DAYS OF OVERLAP = 909
TOTAL NO. OF DAYS OF SHORTFALL = -104

ESTIMATION DE LA FIABILITE D'UN OPERATEUR EN ECHOGRAPHIE OBSTETRICALE

Isaël NISAND, Virginie MERCKX, Sylvie GUIKOVATY
Jean Pierre HOLTZ, Pierre DELLENBACH
Service de Gynécologie - Obstétrique
CMCO - SCHILTIGHEIM - Tél. : (88) 62 90 00
CHU - STRASBOURG, France

Summary

To evaluate antenatal ultrasounds reliability, fetal sex diagnosis has been selected as a performance indicator. This study has rewieved 4 000 pregnancies and for each pregnancy, 3.5 ultrasounds examinations have been computed.

Fetal sex diagnosis ability and correctness have been described as PENETRANCE and PRECISION. Both parameters are combined in one standardized coefficient which variations reflected individual and global improvements of the team aptitudes.

Coefficients interpretation does not require any ultrasounds specific knowledge ; this study is included in quality of care evaluation in obstetrics. Processing and diagnosis being simultaneous, the examination informative quality is linked to the operator competences.

Moreover, ultrasounds diagnosis is frequently an ultimate test before therapeutic decision in obstetrics. These coefficients should be helpful to prevent iatrogenic effects resulting from technologic abuses.

L'échographie obstétricale est un moyen inoffensif d'exploration du foetus. Son essor a modifié en quelques années la pratique obstétricale courante.

Prolongation de l'examen clinique, elle appartient à la catégorie des examens complémentaires dont l'interprétation est immédiate au cours de l'examen. La sélection de l'information utile se fait en temps réel et non sur documents.

La qualité de l'examen dépend donc non seulement de la qualité du matériel et des techniques, mais aussi et surtout de la qualité et de l'expérience de l'opérateur.

L'augmentation de la consommation échographique qui se fait parfois au détriment de la formation des échographistes donne son intérêt à cette étude. La fiabilité de l'échographiste sera d'autant plus importante que son intervention est souvent le dernier maillon dans le processus de la décision médicale.

Celui qui débute dans la pratique échographique doit affiner son acuité perceptive sous le contrôle simultané d'un opérateur plus anciennement formé. La transmission du savoir et l'auto-enseignement prennent des parts inégales d'un opérateur à l'autre. Aussi, l'évaluation de l'enseignement est difficile à réaliser si on ne dispose pas d'indicateur précis.

Ces constatations nous ont incité depuis plusieurs années à rechercher un moyen d'estimer la fiabilité d'un opérateur en échographie obstétricale.

Parmi les nombreux paramètres foetaux estimés et mesurés par l'échographiste, il nous fallait choisir une donnée simple, facile à contrôler et difficile à déterminer échographiquement. Après un premier essai où nous avions choisi comme paramètre de contrôle le diamètre bipariétal, notre choix s'est porté sur la détermination du sexe foetal et nous détaillerons dans la discussion les avantages de ce choix.

La méthode que nous proposons permet de quantifier non seulement les progrès d'un échographiste en formation mais aussi les fluctuations de qualité qui peuvent exister pour l'ensemble d'un département d'échographie. Les paramètres que nous proposons peuvent fonctionner au titre d'un contrôle permanent de la qualité des soins.

MATERIEL ET METHODES

Dans notre département d'échographie obstétricale travaillent 5 opérateurs d'ancienneté et d'expérience différentes. Les données ont été recueillies entre janvier 1978 et décembre 1979 avec une moyenne de 800 examens par mois. Cette population comprend les femmes enceintes dont la grossesse a été suivie par échographie de manière systématique ou sur indication. Pour chaque examen, les opérateurs ont été priés de noter le sexe foetal masculin ou féminin lorsqu'ils le voyaient. Le sexe véritable déterminé à la naissace a été enregistré sur le même document de saisie informatisée. Ce document est utilisé en routine pour le recueil de toutes les données biométriques et morphologiques établies dans le département d'échographie. Il est complété à la naissance avant d'être saisi et traité au Centre Régional d'Informatique Hospitalière des Hospices Civils de Strasbourg.

Le matériel échographique est constitué par 2 appareils en temps réel (ADR et COMBISON 100) de qualités inégales mais utilisés en alternance stricte par tous les membres de l'équipe.

Le nombre d'examens par grossesse a été de 3,57 pendant cette période. Ont été éliminés de cette étude tous les dossiers incomplets (accouchements dans un autre service, information mal transcrite, ambiguïté sexuelle à la naissance). Un programme d'analyse des dossiers a été constitué permettant d'étudier séparément les résultats globaux du département et les résultat de chacun des opérateurs identifiés lors de chaque examen.

RESULTATS

L'expression des résultats impose la définition au préalable des 2 termes de l'analyse qui sont : la PENETRANCE diagnostique et la PRECISION diagnostique.

La PENETRANCE correspond à l'expression en pourcentage des résultats (justes ou faux) rapportés au nombres examens effectués.

La PRECISION correspond à la proportion des diagnostics exacts par rapport au nombre de diagnostics effectués.

La PRECISION et la PENETRANCE varient en fonction de trois facteurs principaux : le sexe foetal, l'âge gestationnel et l'expérience de l'échographiste.

Elles varient encore avec la qualité de l'appareillage, la position du foetus, le caractère plus ou moins absorbant de la peau vis à vis des ultrasons.

Nous avons étudié l'évolution de la PENETRANCE et de la PRECISION en faisant varier séparément le sexe du foetus, l'âge gestationnel au moment du diagnostic et l'expérience de l'échographiste. Seront présentés ici quelques résultats portant sur les performances individuelles et sur l'ensemble du service.

1. Résultats d'ensemble du département d'échographie

	PENETRANCE	PRECISION
ANNEE 1979	1620 diagnostics/2022 grossesses	1554 diagnostics corrects / 1620 diagnostics portés
POUR LES 2 SEXES	80 %	96 %
SEXE MASCULIN	85 %	95 %
SEXE FEMININ	75 %	97 %

2. Résultats par échographiste

Nous avons considéré pour cette étude, non plus chaque dossier, mais chaque examen échographique effectué par un échographiste identifiable. Ceux-ci sont désignés par une lettre d'identification.

OPERATEURS	E	B	N	O
PENETRANCE GLOBALE	39	43	44	45
PENETRANCE MASCULINE	45	49	47	48
PENETRANCE FEMININE	33	36	41	42
PRECISION GLOBALE	96	95	84	94
PRECISION MASCULINE	97	93	76	89
PRECISION FEMININE	93	97	94	98
NOMBRE D'EXAMENS SUR DES FOETUS NES EN 1979	2 385	1 694	446	2 516

3. Coefficients diagnostiques

L'examen de ces données brutes nous a incité à utiliser des paramètres simples permettant de rendre compte de manière plus contractée de la fiabilité des opérateurs.

Le choix et l'établissement d'un coefficient pondéré qui sera discuté plus bas nous a permis d'exprimer nos résultats de manière plus simple. Ce coefficient varie de -1 à +1. Ainsi, l'on donne -1 à un opérateur qui se prononce au hasard, 0 à celui qui ne se prononce pas et +1 à celui qui se prononce toujours de manière exacte.

a. Evolution globale du service

MOIS DE 1979	POUR LES 2 SEXES	MASCULIN	FEMININ
JANVIER	0.52	0.71	0.29
FEVRIER	0.52	0.76	0.36
MARS	0.60	0.37	0.47
AVRIL	0.64	0.72	0.54
MAI	0.71	0.72	0.70
JUIN	0.68	0.67	0.69
JUILLET	0.62	0.55	0.71
AOUT	0.74	0.62	0.88
SEPTEMBRE	0.76	0.67	0.86
OCTOBRE	0.81	0.78	0.84
NOVEMBRE	0.71	0.55	0.88
DECEMBRE	0.79	0.77	0.81

b. Résultats détaillant les aptitudes respectives des échographistes

OPERATEURS	E	B	N	O
POUR LES 2 SEXES	0.32	0.34	0.16	0.33
MASCULIN	0.40	0.34	0.01	0.27
FEMININ	0.25	0.32	0.32	0.38
NOMBRE D'EXAMENS SUR DES FOETUS NES EN 1979	2 385	1 694	446	2 615

c. Coefficients détaillés de "O" en fonction du temps

	OPERATEUR "O"		
MOIS DE 1979	POUR LES 2 SEXES	MASCULIN	FEMININ
JANVIER	0.13	0.22	0.04
FEVRIER	0.14	0.22	0.06
MARS	0.13	0.24	0.02
AVRIL	0.30	0.33	0.26
MAI	0.33	0.39	0.28
JUIN	0.25	0.20	0.31
JUILLET	0.26	0.12	0.40
AOUT	0.44	0.33	0.55
SEPTEMBRE	0.41	0.26	0.58
OCTOBRE	0.50	0.34	0.65
NOVEMBRE	0.45	0.26	0.67
DECEMBRE	0.52	0.53	0.51

On observe des variations identiques pour chacun des opérateurs.

DISCUSSION

Le choix du diagnostic du sexe foetal comme indicateur de la qualité de l'interprétation échographique repose sur l'hypothèse suivante : les performances de l'échographiste s'améliorent lorsqu'il est capable d'augmenter la fréquence, l'exactitude et la précocité du diagnostic du sexe foetal.

La détermination du sexe comme indicateur de la compétence a été retenue pour 3 raisons. Il s'agit :

- d'une information difficile à recueillir qui nécessite de la part de l'opérateur un examen attentif et systématique du foetus, une connaissance suffisante des images trompeuses, une acuité perceptive qui ne peut être acquise d'emblée ;
- d'un caractère binaire qui divise en deux sous-groupes distincts la population ;
- d'un diagnostic vérifiable sans erreur, à terme, si l'on exclut du fichier les femmes n'ayant pas accouché dans le service.

On appréciera la sensibilité et la spécificité du test à partir de l'exemple suivant où l'on prend une PENETRANCE de 80 % et une PRECISION de 96 %, valeurs arrondies de nos résultats. Ainsi :

		LE SEXE DU FOETUS EST		
		EXACT	ERRONE	
L'OPERATEUR PEUT SE PRONONCER SUR LE SEXE DU FOETUS	OUI	77 soit 96% de la pénétrance	3	80(pénétrance)
	NON	1 chance sur 2 10	10	20
		87	13	100

Le calcul donne : SENSIBILITE 89 % (77/87) ; SPECIFICITE 77 % (10/13)

soit une bonne sensibilité et une spécificité satisfaisante. Un biais indéniable est introduit par la répartition paritaire du sexe dans la population du fait que, en se prononçant au hasard, l'on a une chance sur deux de se tromper. Ce phénomène renforce la sensiblité et minimise la spécificité. L'estimation de la validité du test soutient la notion déjà connue que l'échographie est un bon moyen de déterminer le sexe foetal ; mais elle ne suffit pas pour suivre la progression des compétences.

Afin de pénaliser la réponse fausse et la réponse au hasard par rapport à l'abstention, un score allant de -1 à + 1 a été établi en combinant la PRECISION et la PENETRANCE. Un coefficient de pondération a été calculé pour chaque type de réponse selon la formule suivante :

$$\text{score} = \frac{n\ (\text{réponses justes}) - 3\ \bar{n}\ (\text{réponses fausses})}{\text{total des examens pratiqués}}$$

On a pu suivre la progression dans le temps d'un échographiste grâce à l'évolution de son score pour l'ensemble des examens pratiqués. De même, on a pu établir les performances du service pour chaque grossesse en procédant à un calcul de score par dossier. Cette méthode permet de contrôler la fiabilité des diagnostics de sexe et de là, le recueil de l'ensemble des données échographiques, sous les deux perspectives suivantes :

- pour un opérateur donné, évaluation de la <u>phase d'apprentissage,</u>
- pour un service donné, évaluation des <u>éléments de variations</u> dans la vie du service (opérateurs nouveaux, changement dans les rythmes d'activité ...).

Cependant, deux questions demeurent :

- l'indicateur est-il toujours et également pertinent ?
- est-il possible de délimiter un seuil de compétence ?

La première question se justifie entre autre par le risque de voir l'échographiste débutant ne s'intéresser qu'à l'amélioration de son score, c'est-à-dire à la détermination du sexe.

En pratique, le diagnostic du sexe foetal n'est pas l'essentiel des préoccupations pronostiques de l'échographiste ; la détermination du sexe foetal ne peut se faire que si l'on a déjà acquis une bonne acuité sélective de l'ensemble des informations visuelles données par l'échographiste. Il n'en était pas de même lors d'un premier essai où le barême était établi à partir de la biométrie céphalique. Ce paramètre quantitatif utilisé comme contrôle avait entrainé une diminution très importante des écarts type observés.

La réponse à la deuxième question est plus délicate : l'observation des différentes courbes de progression, leur superposition, la comparaison des moyennes obtenues dans un service conduisent à apprécier un score minimal que doit atteindre un échographiste bien entrainé. Les résultats du service permettent de situer ce score minimal entre les bornes 0.2 et 0.3.

Dans la catégorie des épreuves diagnostiques non répétitives et non transmissibles, catégorie à laquelle appartient l'échographie, les critères de fiabilité des mesures ne sont pas faciles à élaborer. Durant la phase d'apprentissage, la réédition de l'échographie par un ou plusieurs opérateurs plus experts ou l'enregistrement d'un film dans le but d'une critique ou d'un enseignement ultérieur sont les seuls instruments d'évaluation possible.

A quel moment peut-on dire que l'opérateur est formé ? Comment ses capacités évoluent-elles ? Il n'existe pas de travaux dans ce domaine ; l'indicateur proposé permet une mesure "à distance" de la compétence ; mais outre ce caractère d'objectivité, le principal intérêt est d'être un révélateur ou un prédicteur d'autres aptitudes diagnostiques en échographie.

CONCLUSION

Il devient nécessaire de contrôler la qualité et la performance des départements d'échographie dont le nombre va croissant. Ce contrôle et cette évaluation sont difficiles du fait de la grande subjectivité due à l'interprétation des échographies.

Le test proposé a l'avantage d'être facile à réaliser et surtout d'être accessible à une personne étrangère à l'échographie. Mais sa limitation à un seul paramètre risque à long terme de diminuer sa pertinence.

Deux utilisations cependant se dégagent :

- la surveillance des fluctuations de qualité globale au sein d'un département d'échographie,
- le contrôle de l'évolution d'un seul opérateur ainsi que l'effet rétro-actif qui peut en résulter sur sa formation.

Ce test semble donc être un bon moyen d'améliorer la qualité de l'outil échographique.

REFERENCES BIBLIOGRAPHIQUES

(1) GUIKOVATY S. Le diagnostic échographique du sexe foetal. Thèse de Doctorat en Médecine. Strasbourg. 1980.

(2) HALER RS. The comparability of chest X.Ray interpretation and pulmonary function test results by differed observes. Journal of Ocupational Medicine. 1980 ; Vol.20; N°10 : 670-674.

(3) KASSIRER JP, PANKER SG. Should diagnosis testing be regulated ? N. England. J. Med. 1978 ; 299 ; N°17 : 947-949.

(4) LACAINE F, HUGUIER M, GREMY F. L'efficacité d'un examen à but diagnostique : de la donnée à la décision médicale. La Nouvelle Presse Médicale. 29 avril 1978 ; 7 ; N°17 : 1451-1453.

(5) MULLER P, NISAND I. Le diagnostic anténatal du sexe foetal. Entretiens de Bichat. Octobre 1979.

(6) ROSE G. Evaluation of the electrocardiogram ; Journées d'Etudes Internationales sur l'évaluation des activités et des services de santé ; Bruxelles, GERM ; 6-7 mars 1971 : p.53 - 58.

Simulation of Physician's Train of Thoughts:

A Heuristical Approach.

M. Haerringer, Universitaetsinstitut fuer Medizinische Physik und Biophysik, Harrachgasse, A-8010 Graz/Austria, M. Strobl, Institut fuer Angewandte Mathematik der Technischen Universitaet, Steyrergasse 17, A-8010 Graz/Austria, B. Leiber, G. Olbrich, Zentrum der Medizinischen Informatik - DOFONOS der Universitaet, Theodor-Stern-Kai 7, D-6000 Frankfurt/FRG

O. Summary:

Medicine possesses two faces. The one shows the use of higly developed material and techniques. The other thinks medicine to be an art, needing intuition, and a summing-up of associations to reach the correct diagnosis.

Because of the explosion of knowledge, it is impossibible to keep in one's mind all new findings in the medical sciences. Therefore, the necessity to broaden one's mind virtually should lead to the use of a computer. A model was sought to produce weighted results in accordance to the physician's train of thoughts and which would be a successful support to his daily routine work.

This paper deals with an approach to the simulation of the intellectual processes which produce a diagnosis out of the pattern of symptoms using algorithms implemented on a minicomputer.

Great value was placed on the use of a flexible model to allow both the implementation of its equivalent software on a minicomputer and the adaption to specific needs which cannot be covered by an oversimplified model.

The method is based on probability theory, allowing only the presence or absence of symptoms as input of the pattern. Out of this pattern originates the computation of the relative importance (or weight) of various symptoms producing automatically (i.e. after computation) an essential improvement of the pattern and a detailed prognosis of the probability of occurance of the syndrome.

Using a minicomputer, the development of special algorithms was necessary in order to efficiently use available storage space.

I. Introduction:

The process of medical diagnosis is a complex one. On the one hand, medicine is on the way towards an exact science, a virtually unreachable goal.

On the other hand, there is a great portion of largely intuitive medicine.

To be a good physician, you need luck (1). But luck without knowledge cannot prevent errors.

The explosion of medical knowledge justifies the introduction of models using the storage capacity and speed of a computer which makes available a lot of information without degrading the physician to a mere assistant to the computer desicions.

According to (2), there are 3 groups of diagnostic models:

1. Models of physician's train of thoughts.
2. Models of physical processes, and
3. Statistical models, based on Bayes' Theorem.

In this paper, there will be a presentation of an attempt based on the 1st model mentioned above.

II. Problem:

Because of the impossibility of keeping in one's mind more than a few of the most important clinical syndromes with their specific input patterns, there was a real need for a system which allows the input of symptom patterns and which as output produces out of them a list of syndromes ordered according to their specific medical importance. Through this, a useful support would be given to medical decision-making leading to a relevant diagnosis by paralleling the physician's train of thoughts. The train of thought is a complex interactive procedure (fig.1), which should be taken into consideration when developing a simple algorithmic equivalent.

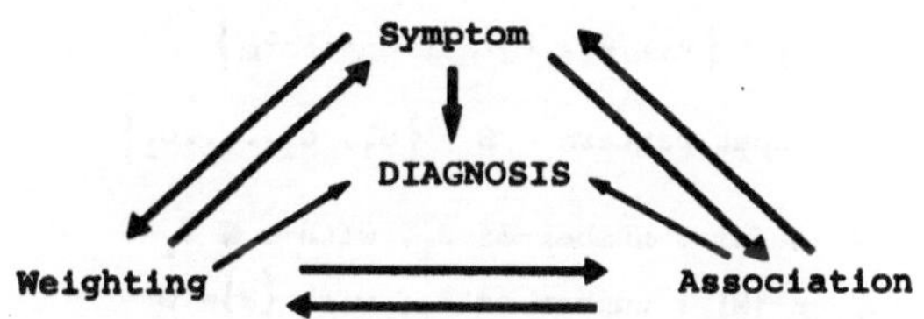

Fig. 1: Train of thoughts.

III. Model:

The above mentioned weighting is now extended from one to several symptoms. Out of this, there must be the demand on the model:

a. The more seldom a symptom or a pattern of symptoms is part of different syndromes, the more exact is the conclusion concerning the possible occurance of a specific syndrome.
b. If a symptom or a pattern of symptoms can be associated with high probability only with a single syndrome, than this does not necessarily imply the real presence of this syndrome.
c. The base for the valuation of a syndrome always is the intersection of the symptom pattern with the set of syndromes which describe the syndrome in question.
d. It must be made sure, that even unlikely results be recognized as as possible by the model.

The expected benefit of the model is to find (based on the input patterns of the symptoms) a most probable series of syndromes which are relevant for the case in question.

IV. Mathematical Statement:

To establish the relative weighting of the symptoms, the Laplace probabilities have been taken into account. This has been done although the computed weights are not real probabilities. Fig. 2 shows the definition of syndromes.

Symptoms : s, s_1, s_2, s_3 ......

Syndromes: S, S_1, S_2, S_3 ......

$S_i = \{s_1, s_2, s_3, \ldots\ldots\ldots s_m\}$

Input pattern $E = \{e_1, e_2, \ldots. e_l\}$

n (s) : number of S_i, with $s \in S_i$

n (M) : number of S_i, with $\{M\} \neq \emptyset$

g (S/M): weight of S with $M \subset S$

g (S/M) = 1/n (M)

Fig. 2: Definitions

The 1st formula of fig. 2 is the mathematical equivalent to the demand of III.a. Out of this, it is possible to define an indicating sign mathematically. Based on the Laplace probability, an indicating sign is only part of one single syndrome. Using other probabilities, the indicating sign has as its equivalent g(S/s)=1-Z with Z=0 or Z negligible. It can be deduced from the definition of an indicating sign, that the syndrome in question really occurs, if its weight is equal to one. That is, because the indicating sign does not include informations on whether or not there is a need for additional symptoms to get an exact determination of this syndrome. Based on the understanding of III.c, the probability is

$$g(S/E)=g(S/E \cap S)$$

The set $E \cap S$ is the set which contains the maximal number of symptoms, which are elements of both S and E.

$s_1 = \{a, b, c\}$

$s_2 = \{a, b, d, e\}$

$s_3 = \{c, e, f\}$

$s_4 = \{b, c, f\}$

$E = \{a, c\}$

	s_1	s_2	s_3	s_4	
<u>a</u>	<u>a</u>	<u>a</u>			n(a) = 2
b	b	b		b	n(b) = 3
<u>c</u>	<u>c</u>		<u>c</u>	<u>c</u>	n(c) = 3
d		d			n(d) = 1
e		e	e		n(e) = 2
f			f	f	n(f) = 2

Fig. 3: Symptom-Syndrome matrix

Using other words, the demand III.d asks to intersect all syndromes with the symptom patterns. This means that the syndromes and symptoms should be looked upon as matrix elements.

Fig. 3 shows an simplified example of a symptom-syndrome matrix. Let S1,...,S4 be syndromes with their symptoms a,...,f and E the input pattern, then this results in the right-hand matrix. Now, an intersection of the input pattern with every syndrome is carried out to get the weights:

$$g(S1/\{a,c\})=1$$
$$g(S2/\{a\})=.5$$
$$g(S3/\{c\})=.333$$
$$g(S4/\{c\})=.333$$

Based on this result, it is possible to construct a sequence which can become the starting-point to further investigations.

V. Implementation:

Implementing the model, care has been taken to make the use of minicomputers possible.

V.1 Dimensionning of the matrix:

Knowing the exact number of syndromes and symptoms, it is easy to find the maximum size of the essential storage capacity: Our data file consists of about 2.000 syndromes with approximately 20.000 symptoms. The required mass storage is about 40.000.000 matrix elements. But there is no simple rule to determine the number of the zero-elements within the matrix. This number can be calculated, if the powers of all sets of symptoms which are describing syndromes are summed-up and this number is subtracted of the number of elements of the matrix. This number, whichwhich can only be calculated, if the initial data are well-known. Practical measurements have shown that the number of zero-elements exceeds 97%. This means that it is obviously advantageous to optimize the matrix by using algorithms which eliminate the zero-elements.

V.2 Flow-chart:

Being content with a single processing of the input pattern, the oppertunities of using EDP-processing are made use of only in part. The starting point for writing the program was, that the physician does not collect all symptoms immediately, or thinks some of them to be unnecessary to establish the diagnosis. Therefore, a dialog between man and machine has been implemented, starting with the input of the first pattern, which is to be updated after every output of the computer by additional symptoms. Another feature of the dialog can be seen in the fact that it is possible to exclude syndromes which are looked upon to be possible by the machine, but impossible by the physician.

Terminating the dialog, it can be determined whether or not the symptom pattern in question corresponds with a syndrome or not, and if there is a result, this result is given.

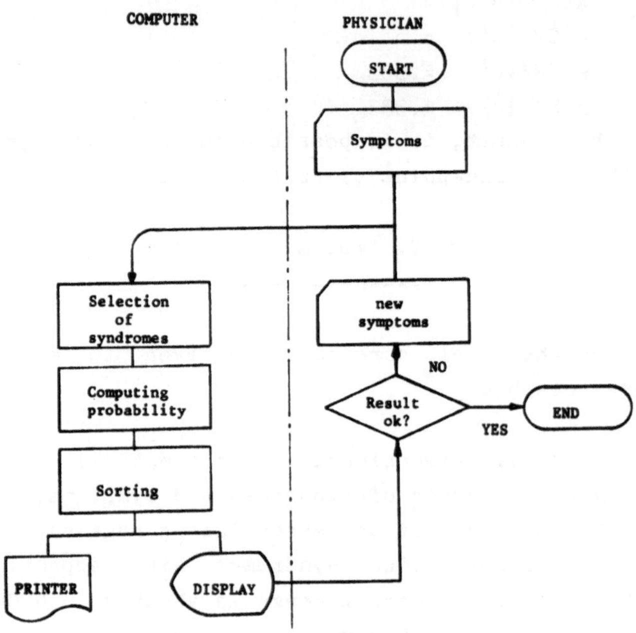

Fig. 4: Flow-chart

V.3 Output:

Based on the weights mentioned above, the computer constructs a sequence of possible syndromes at the end of each data input. The listing contains all syndromes, which describe the syndrome in question. Symptoms, which are part of the input pattern are indicated with a star.

The demand that even the most unprobable situation has to be taken into account, results in the fact that there are many syndomes listed in the output having only one or two symptoms identical with the symptom pattern of the syndrome in question. This leads to a very bulky output be which cannot made full use of. Therefore, there was the need for the introduction of an indicator which limits the output on the basis of probability. This indicator has to be fed in at the beginning of the program, and remains active until the end of the program. If necessary,it may be changed during the execution.

VI. Results:

The construction of a data matrix of about 2.000 syndromes has been successful. Using data reduction, there was a need for mass storage of about 10 Mbyte. The software written in COBOL has shown enough ease of use up to now. The calculation of the weights is working satisfactory. The software and the data has been tested and showed a good coincidence with the expected results.

VII. Discussion:

Concerning the minicomputer, the main problem is the external mass storage. This mass storage is needed to store the matrix and the names of both symptoms and syndromes. This requires about 10 Mbyte. A data base management system would be an advantage, but as far as we know, there is no system available for minicomputers. Therefore, the execution time is augmented. This will become the more important the more the input increases.

The validation of a symptom as part of a syndrome can be done in 3 different ways:

i. The symptoms are split into obligatory and facultative ones of which the obligatory are considered first.

ii. There are weights related to symptoms which show the frequency of their ocurrance with respect to a specific syndrome. Here, the weights are real probabilities, equal to one if the symptom is obligatory.

iii. The definition of the weight h of a symptom s can be determined using the Laplace-probability:

$$h(s/S) = 1/(n(s))$$

The comparison of these three possibilities shows the second one to both the best and the most exact. But there is a disadvantage, namely that the needed probabilities are not available. Therefore this model has to be looked upon as a theoretical one.

The disadvantage of the first suggestion is, that there is only a very limited possibility for graduation, although a stress is placed on the symptoms in constructing their sequence. The lack of more detailed graduatiuons is too large a problem to allow automatic weighting for practical and efficient use of this method.

Having favoured the 3rd possibility, we found a chance for graduation which is arbitrary up to a certain degree but fits excellently to the weights of the symptoms in simulating the physician's train of thoughts.

This graduation forms the basis for the introduction of a new indicator e, which limits the number of syndromes printed out. Of course this indicator allows a cutting-off of the most unimportant syndromes. This means that all symptoms s with h(s/S)<e are suppressed by the system. The value of e is variable and has to be fed in at the beginning of the program. Due to the nature of the model, considerable problems arise through the introduction of these artificial weights. These disadvantages can be eliminated however simply through a change-over to real probabilities, which can be done at any time. The result would be a more valuable sequence of weighted syndromes. As real probabilities are not available up to now, the use of Laplace-probabilities has to be looked upon as a useful equivalent. There is only a slight amount of man- and machine power necessary to transform these probabilities into real ones should there be enough information.

The greatest advantage must be seen in the fact that the user succeeds in finding a syndrome if it exists at all, based on an input pattern of symptoms found during an investigation of a patient. The syndrome is also suggested through a logical process very similar to the physician's train of thoughts without taking the final decision away from the medical specialist.

VIII. References:

(1) Olbrich, E.: Gefaehrdung der Dokumentation durch menschliche Unzulaenglichkeiten. Meth. Inform. Med. 4,135-136 (1965)

(2) Wardle, A. & Wardle L.: Computer Aided Diagnosis - A Review of Research. Meth. Inform. Med. 17,15-28 (1978)

ANALYSE DE L'ACTIVITE DE SELECTION DE L'INFORMATION DANS LA SURVEILLANCE OBSTETRICALE

Suzanne SEBILLOTTE
Groupe de Psychologie ergonomique
Institut National de Recherche en Informatique et en Automatique
Paris, France

ABSTRACT

In order to contribute to the design of computer systems which would aid obstetric surveillance, two studies were carried out to examine the operator's surveillance activities. These studies deal with the operator's knowledge acquisition process when he/she reads the patient's files. Consequently the technique used is the analysis of operators'recall of the information contained in these files. One experimental study shows that the differences in the operator's objectives direct the information selection and processing : for the doctor the objective is to diagnose and to select a pathological treatment ; for the midwife it is to monitor the evolution of a normal obstetric process. This is supported by results showing significant differences related to "profession" (doctor/midwife) and "experience gained" (experienced/trainee). An analysis of the patient's records processed by the operators shows on a same set of variables that the variables do not have the same relevance for the operators according to their hypothesis and the moment of the diagnosis. Besides, the processing of the main variables is different, that is, as a function of the hypothesis. This suggests for the design that the information should be displayed, that is classified, according to these factors : profession, experience, hypothesis, kind and moment of diagnosis.

INTRODUCTION

Dans une perspective de conception d'un système informatique d'assistance à la surveillance obstétricale ces études s'inscrivent dans le cadre des recherches sur les processus de représentation et de traitement de l'information (1). Actuellement, dans plusieurs centres hospitaliers(*), un même dossier périnatal structuré est utilisé pour assurer la surveillance obstétricale et pour des traitements informatiques a posteriori. Face à l'information très abondante du dossier, les opérateurs directement concernés par la surveillance de la grossesse et de l'accouchement procèdent à un filtrage et un codage, afin de constituer leur propre représentation. C'est une meilleure connaissance de ces processus de traitement qui pourra permettre de concevoir des moyens d'assistance informatiques. Nous présentons ici, deux études faisant partie d'un ensemble

---

(*) Ces études ont été menées dans le service du Professeur SUREAU. Maternité Baudelocque PARIS.

plus vaste.

- la première étude aborde expérimentalement la sélection et le traitement des informations par les opérateurs lorsqu'ils prennent connaissance du dossier,
- la seconde, analyse les synthèses (commentaires libres) contenues dans des dossiers réels en vue de rechercher les informations considérées comme les plus pertinentes par les opérateurs pour leurs hypothèses de diagnostic.

ETUDE EXPERIMENTALE : SELECTION ET TRAITEMENT DE L'INFORMATION

Des études récentes sur la mémoire (2) et en particulier sur la mémoire dite opérationnelle(3) (4) (5), ayant montré que le rappel des données mémorisées était un reflet assez fidèle des traitements et de la pertinence des informations traitées, l'expérience proposée aux sujets consistait en une épreuve de mémoire.

1. PROCEDURE EXPERIMENTALE

- la tâche demandée aux opérateurs était de prendre connaissance du dossier d'une femme, lors de son admission en salle de travail (pour accoucher). Quand les opérateurs estimaient connaître suffisamment le contenu du dossier, ils le rendaient à l'expérimentateur qui leur demandait alors de restituer sur une feuille blanche, ce dont ils se souvenaient concernant cette patiente. On a utilisé un dossier d'une femme suivie pendant toute sa grossesse dans le service et qui ne présentait pas de complications majeures. Dans les dossiers de ce type on peut distinguer :

  . des variables "simples" pour lesquelles une valeur est mentionnée (âge : 30 ans, hauteur utérine : 24cm) et des variables "complexes" représentant un ensemble plus vaste du dossier qui se décrit par une série de variables simples (variable complexe : col, variables simples adjointes : position, longueur, dilatation...),

  . des commentaires synthétiques libres faits par les opérateurs (3% des données fournies).

Ces variables ou commentaires se rapportent à trois moments de la grossesse : état initial, déroulement (objet de la surveillance) et état actuel de la femme.

- on a fait varier systématiquement les facteurs "profession" et "expérience acquise" : quatorze médecins et quatorze sages-femmes répartis en quatre groupes, ont participé à l'expérience,
- la passation était individuelle et les sujets ignoraient qu'il y aurait une épreuve de mémorisation à l'issue de la prise de connaissance du dossier,
- les mesures : on a relevé le nombre et la nature des informations écrites par les opérateurs en distinguant :

  . les informations élémentaires concernant un seul élément facilement identifiable, variable simple ou complexe du dossier (poids : 51kg, col dur) ,

  . les informations synthétiques se rapportant soit à plusieurs valeurs d'une même variable (poids stable, hauteur utérine toujours en rapport) soit à plusieurs variables simples ou complexes (grossesse normale).

2. RESULTATS

2.1. Analyse quantitative :

L'analyse des informations fournies par les opérateurs montre que :

. le nombre des variables du dossier qui sont rappelées est peu élevé : en moyenne 25% des variables dénombrées dans le dossier présenté. Il n'y a pas de différence entre les groupes expérimentaux, en ce qui concerne cette mémoire pure ,

. parmi ces variables rappelées, 50% sont relatives à l'état initial de la femme, 28% au déroulement de la grossesse et 22% à l'état présent de la patiente. Cette proportion diffère de celle du dossier étudié : les sujets rappellent proportionnellement plus de variables relatives à l'état initial, moins au déroulement de la grossesse et autant pour l'état actuel,

. le rappel des variables complexes est plus détaillé pour l'état initial que pour les autres parties du dossier ; pour cet état initial ce sont les débutants qui fournissent le plus de détails.

2.2. Transformation des données brutes :

Les opérateurs transforment les données brutes qui leur sont fournies : en effet, parmi les informations écrites par les sujets, 18% sont des synthèses contre 3% seulement dans le dossier présenté. Celles-ci concernent surtout la partie du dossier relative au déroulement de la grossesse (tableau I) et sont dans 60% des cas d'estimation de variables (col satisfaisant pendant toute la grossesse...) et pour le reste des diagnostics sur la grossesse ou l'état du foetus.

	Informations de synthèse	Informations élémentaires
Etat initial de la patiente	.14	.50
Evolution de la grossesse	.76	.28
Etat actuel de la patiente	.10	.22
TOTAL	1. (n=110)	1. (n=488)

Tableau I : fréquence des différents types d'informations fournies par les opérateurs (élémentaires ou de synthèses) selon les moments de la grossesse)

$\chi^2_2 = 89.65 \qquad S \leqslant .001$

- les facteurs "expérience acquise" et "profession" interviennent en interaction dans la fréquence de ces synthèses : les médecins expérimentés faisant proportionnellement plus de synthèses que les autres groupes qui ont un comportement identique (tableau II),
- dans les informations de synthèses la proportion entre estimation de variables et diagnostic est la même pour les quatre groupes d'opérateurs,
- en ce qui concerne les diagnostics posés par les opérateurs, les médecins expérimentés diffèrent encore des autres groupes, en faisant autant de diagnostics sur le foetus (tableau III).

	Médecins expérimentés	Autres groupes (non significativement différents) (*)
Informations élémentaires	.76	.84
Informations de synthèse	.24	.16
TOTAL	1. (n=147)	1. (n=451)

Tableau II : effet des facteurs "profession" et "expérience acquise" sur la fréquence des différents types d'informations fournies par les opérateurs.

$\chi^2_1 = 4.87 \quad S \leqslant .05$

	Médecins expérimentés	Autres groupes (non significativement différents) (*)
Diagnostic sur la grossesse	.53	.79
Diagnostic sur le fœtus	.47	.21
TOTAL	(n=15) 1.	(n=29) 1.

Tableau III : effet des facteurs "profession" et "expérience acquise" sur la fréquence des différents diagnostics posés par les opérateurs.

$\chi^2_1 = 3.30 \quad S \leqslant .10$

(*) médecins débutants, sages-femmes expérimentées et débutantes

2.3. Quelles sont les variables rappelées ? Les informations sélectionnées ?

On ne trouve que sept variables qui sont rappelées par la majorité des opérateurs (soit 75% des sujets). Il s'agit de variables élémentaires dont cinq sont relatives à l'état initial (parité, gestation, âge de la femme, résultats aux tests de la rubéole et de la toxoplasmose), les deux autres sont relatives à l'état présent (terme à l'admission et état des membranes). Les autres variables sont rappelées différemment selon les groupes expérimentaux :

- les médecins rappellent plus d'informations sur la surveillance obstétricale de la grossesse (hauteur utérine, col satisfaisant pendant toute la grossesse...) et sur des variables qui vont fixer un état permanent de la femme pour toute la durée de son accouchement (présentation, aspect du liquide amniotique...) ; les sages-femmes s'intéressent plus aux variables permettant de suivre le bon déroulement de la grossesse (poids, tension artérielle), ou de l'accouchement (dilatation du col, fréquence des contractions utérines),
- l'expérience acquise, en ce qui concerne l'état initial, intervient dans l'importance accordée aux informations se rapportant aux antécédents généraux, que les expérimentés rappellent plus souvent.

En RESUME, les représentations mentales qu'ont les opérateurs du cas obstétrical proposé coïncident avec les caractéristiques de l'image opérative décrite par OCHANINE (6) : image orientée vers les objectifs futurs ; elle est simplifiée, économique (ne contient que ce qui est indispensable pour l'action) et déformée (ce qui a une pertinence pour l'action est ce qui est le plus saillant dans l'image), déformation mise en évidence par l'auteur dans le diagnostic de maladie thyroïdienne et pour laquelle intervenaient les facteurs "profession" et "expérience"(7).

ETUDE DE DOSSIERS : UTILISATION DES VARIABLES AU COURS DE DIAGNOSTICS PRECIS

Dans l'étude précédente, le cas de la patiente qui était présenté aux opérateurs, était un cas pratiquement "normal" et l'ensemble des informations contenues dans le dossier était essentiellement relatif à la surveillance de la grossesse. L'objectif de cette deuxième étude est de mettre en évidence certains points clés dans l'élaboration d'un diagnostic précis et en particulier en utilisant les synthèses écrites par les opérateurs (commentaires libres). En effet, ces synthèses, qui jalonnent l'évolution clinique ont pour but soit d'attirer l'attention des opérateurs futurs sur certains états, soit de justifier une décision médicale. A partir de ces commentaires écrits en regard du recueil de données habituel (dossier structuré), il nous a semblé possible de déterminer les variables les plus pertinentes pour l'opérateur puisqu'il les prend plus particulièrement en compte et juge important de les mentionner.

1. PROCEDURE

Afin de faciliter l'étude et le traitement des données, on a choisi les diagnostics se rapportant à la croissance du foetus, pour plusieurs raisons :

- les variables choisies pour faire un diagnostic sont peu nombreuses,
- l'ensemble des diagnostics possibles est relativement restreint : quand des opérateurs constatent une anomalie relative à la croissance du foetus, les diagnostics qu'ils peuvent être amenés à faire seront principalement la normalité, une erreur de terme, une hypotrophie foetale ou l'association de ces deux derniers, hypotrophie et erreur de terme,
- enfin, ce type de diagnostic concerne un processus évolutif (la croissance physique du foetus). Les opérateurs doivent tenir compte de la variation des valeurs des variables leur permettant de suivre le déroulement du processus. Le facteur temporel intervient alors et le diagnostic ne pouvant être fait d'emblée, il semblait plus facile d'en suivre les différentes phases d'élaboration.

On a alors analysé les synthèses écrites par les opérateurs dans trente deux dossiers où un problème concernant la croissance foetale était soulevé.

2. RESULTATS

2.1. On a pu constater que l'élaboration des diagnostics se faisait en plusieurs étapes : simple constat d'une anomalie, formulation d'hypothèse et ensuite du diagnostic. Parmi les variables mentionnées sur le dossier par les opérateurs nous avons distingué :

- deux variables continues permettant de suivre l'évolution de la croissance du foetus : la hauteur utérine maternelle (HU) et les mesures effectuées sur l'image échographique du foetus(ETG),

- un ensemble contenant les autres variables : observations diverses, résultats d'examens complémentaires...

2.2. Fréquence d'utilisation des variables (figure 1)

. selon les étapes de l'élaboration du diagnostic (constat d'un élément anormal, hypothèse, diagnostic) : le premier constat d'un élément anormal concerne essentiellement la hauteur utérine dans 69% des cas. L'attention portée à cette variable relativement aux autres diminue ensuite régulièrement du moment de la formulation de l'hypothèse à celui du diagnostic,

. selon les hypothèses et les diagnostics formulés : nos analyses portent uniquement sur les hypothèses et diagnostics d'erreur de terme (e) et d'hypotrophie (h). On constate une différence entre ces deux cas aussi bien pour la formulation de l'hypothèse que du diagnostic.

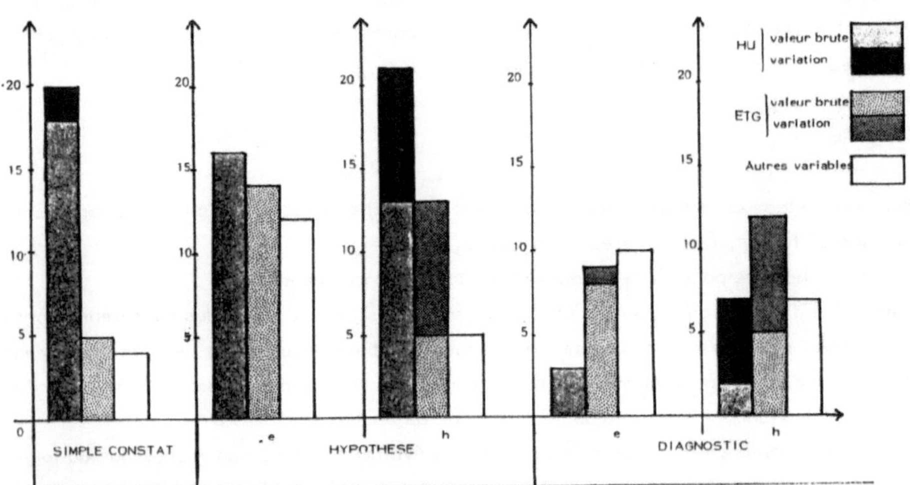

Figure 1 : effectifs des variables mentionnées par les opérateurs dans leur synthèse :

- types de variables : . selon les étapes de l'élaboration du diagnostic (simple constat, hypothèse, diagnostic) $\chi^2_4 = 18.34$ $S \leq .01$

. selon les hypothèses et les diagnostics formulés (erreur de terme (e), hypotrophie (h) $\chi^2_6 = 13.87$ $S \leq .05$

- mode d'utilisation des variables continues (valeurs brutes, variation) :

. selon les étapes de l'élaboration de diagnostic :

$\chi^2_2 = 8.74$ $S \leq .02$

. selon les hypothèses et les diagnostics formulés :

$\chi^2_3 = 33.18$ $S \leq .001$

2.3. Mode d'utilisation des variables continues (figure 1)

BARTHOLOMAY (8) critiquant certains modèles de diagnostic souligne l'importance des variables continues "dynamiques". Cette importance des variables continues ressort nettement ici, puisqu'elles représentent 76 % des variables mentionnées dans les synthèses faites par les opérateurs. Si ceux-ci détectent presque toujours une anomalie par la considération des valeurs brutes, selon l'hypothèse qu'ils émettront ensuite, ils s'intéresseront ou non aux variations. Pour le diagnostic d'hypotrophie ils privilégient l'estimation de la variation (HU et ETG) contrairement au cas des diagnostics d'erreur de terme basés principalement sur la considération des valeurs brutes.

En RESUME, il ressort de cette analyse que sur le même ensemble de variables utilisées pour différencier les diagnostics d'une même classe, celles-ci ont une pertinence différente pour les opérateurs, selon le moment de l'élaboration du diagnostic où ils interviennent : (simple constat d'anomalie, hypothèse, formulation du diagnostic) et selon les hypothèses qu'ils font. En ce qui concerne les variables continues, ce qui retient l'attention des opérateurs peut être soit la valeur absolue de la variable (valeurs brutes), soit la variation entre plusieurs valeurs de cette variable. Selon l'hypothèse ou le diagnostic considéré, le traitement des valeurs de ces variables est alors différent.

CONCLUSION

Nous terminerons en soulignant les limites de ces premières études et les perspectives ergonomiques qu'elles ouvrent. Il n'est pas encore possible de construire un modèle de sélection de l'information, car nous nous sommes limités à des cas relativement simples (dossier normal d'une part et diagnostics possibles peu nombreux d'autre part) afin de mieux cerner les problèmes. Il reste à poursuivre les recherches en étudiant plus finement le statut des informations retenues dans différentes situations et avec des dossiers plus complexes.

Du point de vue ergonomique, un système informatique d'assistance à la surveillance devrait tenir compte des facteurs mis en évidence. Cela supposerait entre autre une présentation des informations recueillies :

. qui permette une hiérarchisation et un regroupement facilitant les opérations de synthèse ,

. qui fasse apparaître les variations des variables continues,

. qui tienne compte de la représentation et donc des objectifs des différentes catégories d'opérateurs.

REFERENCES

(1) BISSERET A, BOUTIN P, MICHARD A. Eléments introductifs à l'ergonomie des systèmes

Hommes-Machines. Informatique et Sciences Humaines. 1980 (44) : 13-34.

(2) SCHONEN S de. La mémoire, connaissance active du passé. Mouton, Paris, 1974.

(3) BISSERET A. Mémoire opérationnelle et structure du travail. Bull. de Psycho. 1971 ; XXIV (5-6) : 281 - 294.

(4) SPERANDIO JC. Compléments à l'étude de la mémoire opérationnelle. Travail Humain, 1975 ; 38 (1) : 41 - 62.

(5) MICHARD A. Représentations opératoires et modèles du processus dans les tâches de diagnostic. Thèse 3ème cycle. Université Paris VIII. 1978.

(6) OCHANINE DA. The operative image of a controlled object in "man automatic machine" systems. XVIIIth International Congress of Psychology. Moscou 1966.

(7) OCHANINE DA. Le rôle des images opératives dans la régulation des activités de travail. Psychologie et Education, 1978 (2) : 63 - 72.

(8) BARTHOLOMAY AF. Some mathematical aspects of the medical diagnostic process. Bull. Math. Biophys. 1971 (33) : 413 - 424.

COMMUNITY NURSE RECORDS - PRIMARY HEALTH CARE NURSE.

Joyce Wiseman,
Senior Nursing Officer, Research and Planning,
Lancashire Area Health Authority, Blackpool District, U.K.

1. SUMMARY.

The paper has been formulated from a literary search into the primary health care (PHC) nurse's record, which was commissioned by the Department of Health and Social Security for England & Wales with the purpose of discovering the state of literary knowledge surrounding the health visitor and district nurses' records.

The literature search has centred itself on literature published in the United Kingdom, United States, Canada and Europe from 1970 to 1980.

Publications have been included in the search which relate to nursing records in both Community and Hospital; the General Practitioner Records and Health Care Information Systems.

2. THE AIMS AND PURPOSE OF THE LITERATURE SEARCH.

To define the meaning, purpose and need for a PHC nurse record; to discover common weaknesses and gaps in recording mechanisms with a focus on the PHC nurse recording; to learn of the correct criteria for record maintenance; to make recommendations to improve the status of the PHC nurses' record, together with recommendations for a future research programme for PHC nurse recording.

3. INTRODUCTION.

A total of approximately 170 literary references are included in the search, of which 21 refer specifically to PHC nurse records.

The literary search revealed a lack of publications related to nurse recording and community nurse recording in particular. Literature relating to health care records maintains an emphasis on hospital recording to the neglect of community health records which is also reinforced by comments from several authors and by Madeley and Metcalfe (1) in particular, who draw attention to the fact that health care planning should stem from the community environment.

4. DEFINITIONS OF THE TERMS "COMMUNITY NURSE" AND "RECORDS".

4.1 A "Community Nurse" in the United Kingdom is a primary health care nurse; a term which refers collectively to the "District Nurse" and "Health Visitor", and who are both members of the Primary Health Care Team together with a General Practitioner.

4.2 A "District Nurse" is a State Registered Nurse with a District Nurse Certificate which qualifies her to give skilled nursing care to all persons living in the community. She is a counterpart to the hospital nursing sister, and has responsibility for delegating nursing tasks to the nursing members of her district nursing team.

4.3 A "Health Visitor"(HV) has the basic State Registered general nursing qualification together with the additional qualification of "health visitor" obtained by 1 year's post registration course at a College of Further Education or University, and must have some knowledge of midwifery to undertake health visitor training. She is a family visitor and an expert in child health care, who is concerned with the promotion of health and the prevention of ill health through giving appropriate education, advice and support.

4.4 Records.

Sheldon (2) defines "records" as holding data on individual patients, whilst "information systems" hold data on population of patients". And Vuori (3) reminds us that it is often a misplaced belief that computers are synonymous with the term information systems.

The Concise Oxford Dictionary (4) describes a record as "a state of being recorded or presented in writing especially as authentic legal evidence; something established as fact by being recorded".

A King's Fund Project Paper, "A Handbook for Nurse to Nurse Reporting" (1979) describes the nursing record as a "primary legal document" which is "the only continuous account of patient care and may provide information which is not available elsewhere. It is a source of information on a patient's background and problems, includes care plans, and is a detailed guide to the planning, implementing and evaluating nursing care".

4.5 Health Care Records.

A text-book edited by Benjamin B. (5) contains subject matter which is pertinent to all health care records, and yet the book is entitled "Medical Records". The accuracy of the term "medical records" is drawn into question, which appears to place an emphasis on curative medicine rather than preventive health and, thus, total health care. "Health Care Records" would, therefore, appear to be a more balanced and correct title than the frequently used term, "Medical Records".

The book is possibly reflective of the lack of status and consideration which is given to the "Nursing Record", allocating 8 lines consisting of approximately 91 words to the subject of nursing records.

5. EDUCATING NURSES ON CORRECT RECORDING PROCEDURES.

From the literary search it would appear that criticism is directed in many instances at the quality of the nurses' record maintenance in both hospital and community. Criticism is directed at the lack of education which is provided to nurses during training and in post-graduate courses. McIntosh (6) is particularly critical of the apparant lack of recognition given to the importance of records during the District Nurse Training Programme, and she believes that this is because there are insufficient guidelines to nurse recording. Dingwall (7) discussed Health Visitor record keeping in some depth, acknowledges that the importance of record maintenance is taught to HVs during their Course but appears critical of some "individual styles" of recording.

6. THE LEGAL OWNERSHIP OF THE PATIENT'S RECORD.

The legal ownership of patient records is with the Secretary of State, and the hospital medical records officer acts as the custodian of the hospital records. A hospital when admitting a patient "enters an implied contract to render services... there is an implied contract that the record is confidential".

At the same time, compulsory disclosure of knowledge could be compelled by law on a subpoena or witness summons.

Literature discusses the legal status of the "hospital record" and "the patient" record thus highlighting the focus of interest into hospital records.

7. STEP-BY-STEP PROGRESS THROUGH THE "TIERS" OF THE PRIMARY HEALTH CARE NURSES' RECORD.

Record maintenance can be described as a process of "tiers", with the first record tier occurring prior to nurse and client/patient contact.

The following table helps to illustrate the step-by-step progress of community nurse recording. It will be seen that the individual client/patient's record has, ultimately a direct link to the Planning and Policy Divisions of the Department of Health and Social Security (DHSS).

A Table Indicating a Step-by-Step Progress Through

The Recording Process of the Primary Health Care Nurses.

(This is illustrated in the Paper Presentation as a Total of 7 Slides).

	STAGE OF RECORDING PROCESS	PURPOSE	PLACE/ACTION
Slide 1	1. Prior to client/patient contact.	Knowledge of patient	Office/doctor's surgery
Slide 2	2. Individual client/patient contact in home/clinic	To record care/advice given, plan of care & evaluation of care	Patient/client's home/clinic
Slide 3	3. Total client/patient daily contact record	To record the PHC nurse's daily activity	Office base
Slide 4	4. Weekly/monthly activity record	Statistics ⟶	Forwarded through to the Nursing Officer who sends them to the Area Health Authority Statistical Unit
Slide 5	5. Collation of the local PHC nurse statistics	• Local Examination • Breakdown • Analysis • Distribution	Results returned to: eg. Local Health Authority Regional Health Authority and DHSS
Slide 6	6. DHSS Statistics and Research Division	National collation of PHC nurse statistics	Distribution to → DHSS Planning & Policy Division & other sources, eg. Office of Population and Census.

Slide 7 - The Total Table.

The descriptive term of "tiers" to describe the Health Service Information System, is also given by Poulton K.R. (1979) in her conference paper, Medical Informatics, Berlin, in which she presents a diagram to illustrate a different need for information from records and/or total information system. She comments that "currently there is no standard system of recording, although all records deal with either clinical or nurse manpower information, which should be integrated into a total regional nursing information system".

During the step-by-step search, it became noticeable that district nurses and health visitors frequently duplicate their recordings, and the health visitor particularly, has a wide range of referral forms to consider for completion.

PHC Nurses were found frequently to be inconsistent when completing their statistical returns, and their diaries were completed in a haphazard manner, in limited space. Storage facilities were not seen, but varied depending upon the nurses' work base; lack of storage facilities could have a detrimental effect upon the completion of the record and on the maintenance of confidentiality.

8. SOME PRACTICAL ADVANTAGES TO BE GAINED FROM RECORDS.

Records which adhere to correct criteria and which are systematically maintained assist with the teaching to learners. The search has also revealed records which have been used as a research technique to evaluate various nursing procedures for clients/patients, and are a potential source in assisting the practising nurses and their managers with the care of the clients/patients.

Records can also be used to carry out an audit to assess the quality and quantity of nursing care delivery. This is more commonly carried out in the United States where private insurance companies insist on accountability to them by receiving evidence of health care delivery before payment of monies. There is a potential value for the increased use of nursing audit in the U.K., but for a nursing audit to be successful, the nursing records must be standardised and systematically maintained.

The report of the Government's White Papers on Public Expenditure : The Social Services (8) states in its' Summary of Recommendations, Para.55, No.4:- "The DHSS should give high priority to developing a comprehensive information system which would permit this Committee and the public to assess the effects of changes in expenditure levels, or patterns on the quality and effects of changes in expenditure levels, or patterns on the quality and scope of services provided".

9. FACTORS IN RECORDS WHICH ADVERSELY AFFECT STATISTICS AND AGE-SEX REGISTERS.

Vuori states that currently managers make a low demand for data off existing records for the following reasons which make records unreliable to managers:-

- Planners are unaware of the existence of data gathered by various statistical services.
- Available data are irrelevant.
- Lack of uniformity of definition in records.
- Lack of co-terminous data collection periods.
- Inflexibility in data retrieval.

Skidmore (9) states that errors and omissions on recording forms prevent reliable Hospital Activity Analysis data, whilst in the community, lack of definitions and the subsequent misinterpretation of forms give comparative figures little credibility. The total accuracy of the present for indices of health performance are questionned by the author, who urges for the rapid development of a standardised computerised community system.

10. METHODS OF MAINTAINING THE NURSING RECORD.

A nursing record is maintained by either :-

- The Kardex,
- A4 Sheets of Paper,
- Computer.

(Reference Source - The King's Fund Project Paper, "Nurse to Nurse Reporting).

10.1 Standardisation.

Continuity of recording is aided by standardisation, which applies to record card size, the design of the record card and the system of recording client/patient details.

The A4 size of recording sheet is advocated by both nursing and medical personnel together with Weed's (10) Problem Oriented Recording System which helps to provide a unified approach to record maintenance.

10.2 The Integrated Health Care Record.

It is shown that practical and ethical problems are being encountered by the primary health care team when endeavouring to implement the "integrated" health care record. Problems involve:- the recording space and access to the record by the various disciplines together with the issue of confidentiality and the need for the PHC nurse to maintain a separate record for the Local Area Health Authority.

Recording methods have to be evolved which enable the PHC nurse to record client/ patient details which satisfies the primary health care team of their adequacy and informative value, and spontaneously maintains the regard for confidentiality.

The solution could be a nucleus record, common to all members of the primary health care team, whilst other, more descriptive recording data, is retained by the individual nurse or doctor. This type of record organisation appears to be a feasible proposition with computer usage, because record data can be stored in the computer memory, and only be retrieved and shown on a screen through the knowledge and use of a code word.

11. THE COMPUTER AND CONFIDENTIALITY.

Conversely, it is with the introduction of a computer for client/patient record maintenance that the subject of "confidentiality" has become a topical issue for debate, and the rights of the individual for privacy.

11.1 Practical Aspects to Implementing Computer Security.

Barber B., et al (11) discuss policies and procedures which should be developed for computer confidentiality so that a balance is met between computer security and practical implementation, so making a computer a feasible proposition for use by health care personnel. They maintain that computer systems are usually more confidentially secure than their manual counterparts.

Holdich R.J. (12) suggests that if people are to receive the level of medical care to which they feel entitled, then they cannot have the level of confidentiality that they would like, and believes the whole thing can be resolved with a combination of competently framed laws and evolving social attitudes.

11.2 Computers and Data Protection.

Literature shows that the growth of computer data banks is a potential hazard to the individual through misuse, and if access is gained to the data it can be used for other purposes than originally intended, which contravene the person's rights to privacy, and so there is a need for measures to be taken which safeguard security of confidentiality. A Data Protection Committee appears to be synonymous with computer usage and the Exeter Community Health Services Computer Project have a Data Protection Committee, with a sub-group called the Computer Users Ethical Sub-Committee, which has made recommendations to safeguard computer confidentiality. The Council of Europe and British Computer Society have also laid down principles for confidentiality.

11.3 Computer Data Protection - An Emotive Issue ?

Serious and proper consideration and rulings have been, and are being given to confidentiality and the computer, but it can become an emotive issue and contra to organisational progress, as demonstrated in sections of "Privacy - The Information Gatherers" by Hewitt P. (13) on behalf of the National Council for Civil Liberties. Computer security rulings have to be made tempered with common sense, and if used correctly in conjunction with Barber's belief, computer systems are more secure than their manual counterparts.

12. COMPUTERS AND COST IMPLICATIONS.

A further disadvantage cited is the high cost to the 'on line' computer for patient recording purposes. Rivett (14) questions the high cost compared to its related value to assisting with patient care, and advocates that Health Authorities should make more use of Regional computer linkage which is cost-effective. Is the microprocessor going to remove the disadvantage of high cost and other practical disadvantages to computer use? Dingwall (15) asks "Are Nurses Ready for the Micro-chip?".

13. COMMUNITY COMPUTER PROJECTS.

13.1 The Two Major Uses of the Computer.

The computer has two major uses; one use is to the organisation, and the other to the caring of patients. Uses to the nursing organisation are given as, help with:- sickness and absence, learner allocation, learner training schedules, nursing plans. Uses with patient care are aiding with:- nursing records, nurse dependency and drug administration.

13.2 Assets to Computer Use.

It is gradually becoming a practice for computers to be used in the community setting both by general practitioners, themselves, and by administrators. Computers are claimed to aid efficiency by preventing misfiling and lost cards, and to help with increased accuracy to the data because of improved legibility.

13.3 The Exeter Community Health Services Project.

The community computer project which appears to have been most well documented is the Exeter Community Health Services Project, sponsored as part of the DHSS Experimental Computer Programme. Papers describing the scheme have been written by either general practitioners or computer specialists. Disappointingly, similarly to other community computer projects currently no systematic evaluation appears to have been carried out to establish the value and effect of a computer to the PHC nurses. In the Exeter project, the patient's record is maintained by on-line computer, the computer screen is in the doctor's surgery, and the patient record details immediately appear on the screen by the doctor's use of a code word. All the authors claim that the computer system provides:-

- better management of health delivery,
- better clinical research,
- better patient care.

The authors are so overwhelmingly enthusiastic about the scheme, only presenting the advantages, that the papers would appear to lose something of their learning value and credibility by not presenting some disadvantages to the practicalities of the computer system.

13.4 Nottingham University - Community Computer Developments.

Metcalfe et al and Sheldon of Nottingham University, School of Community Medicine, write about their computer developments for general practice, sponsored by the King's Fund Centre. Sheldon describes modules planned for general practice computer systems. The Health Visitor Package is capable of the:-

- collection of visit data,
- automatic projection of weekly and monthly summaries,
- integration of child health data onto overall record,
- production of priority and geographical visit lists.

And the District Nurse Package as capable of:-

- collection of visits data as per form 2257 and 2253,
- automatic projection of lists and weekly and monthly summaries,
- production of priority follow-up lists,
- production of summary/turn around document on referral.
- eventual automatic or semi-automatic production of visit lists,
- method of entering additional data onto the computer record.

14. IMPLEMENTATION OF THE COMPUTER - Implications to Staff.

14.1 Apprehensions to the Computer.

Comments are made in the literature that the workforces apprehension prior to computer use are unfounded, but emphasis is frequently made on the importance of educating staff and preparing them for the introduction of a computer.

A series of letters, editorial comments and articles which appeared in the Health Visitor Journal between December, 1976, and March, 1979, shows the concern of health visitors to the use of computers and their effect on the security of confidentiality.

14.2 Gaining Staff Commitment.

The letters help to show the importance of involving the practising field worker with the implementation of any new recording schemes, in order to make the scheme workable and to gain the commitment of field staff. One literary source says that home nurses feel "taken over by the computer" who appear to forget the computer is following their instructions for appointments and home visits.

14.3 Educating Nursing Staff for the Computer.

The Editorial, Journal of Community Nursing, May 1980, recommends that computer knowledge and awareness should become part of a nurse's mental equipment. This must be in conjunction with an agreed criteria by all health care personnel to principles and practice of recording policies and procedures.

15. TO SUMMARISE. (Illustrated in the Paper Presentation by 8 Slides).

A research programme is recommended with the objectives of:-

15.1 Promoting the continuous community/hospital record.

15.2 Reducing duplication of recording by community nurses.

15.3 Developing a "nucleus" record for the primary health care team.

15.4 Designing a record format which provides legal protection to the community nurse, provides a plan of care and will accommodate to computer use.

15.5 Performing an exercise of nursing audit through standardised record format.

15.6 Promoting an education programme on recording for community nurses.

15.7 Performing a monitoring exercise to evaluate the value of the community nurse record to the community nurse and nurse managers.

REFERENCES:-

(1) MADELEY RJ & METCALFE DHH. Doctors' Attitudes to Information Systems : A Survey of Derbyshire GPs. Jnl of the RCGP. 1978 : 28 : 654-658.

(2) SHELDON MG. Notes on Medical Records and Information Systems. Paper of Lecture Northern Consortium : 1979.

(3) VUORI H. The Use of Automated Health Information Systems in the Management and Planning of Health Services. Pub.Hlth.Jnl.London 1977 : 91 : 33-43.

(4) THE CONCISE OXFORD DICTIONARY. Oxford University Press. 1964. Fifth Edition.

(5) BENJAMIN B. Medical Records. 1977 : Heinemann : London : 24.

(6) McINTOSH JB. Record Keeping-A Boon or a Bind. Nursing Mirror Jnl.July 1978.

(7) DINGWALL R. The Social Organisation of Health Visitor Training.Croom Helm 1977.

(8) THE GOVERNMENT'S WHITE PAPERS ON PUBLIC EXPENDITURE : HMSO:UK:1980:Vol.I.

(9) SKIDMORE S. Time to be Ruthless. Hlth & SS Jnl. July 1977 : 1111.

(10) WEED L. Medical Records, Medical Education and Patient Care. Med.Publ.Inc., Chicago, 1969/70/71.

(11) BARBER B. et al. The London Hospital Computer Project (Confidentiality and Computer System) Taylor & Francil Ltd., 1976 : 327-337.

(12) HOLDICH RJ. The Importance of Patient Care Records. Nursing Times Jnl. July, 1978 : 1159-60.

(13) HEWITT P. Privacy Report. Nat.Council for Civil Liberties. 1977.

(14) RIVETT CC. Health Services and the Computer. Health Trends. 1977:7.

(15) DINGWALL R. "Are you ready for the Microchip?". Nursing Times Jnl. June 1979.

LA DOTATION DU PERSONNEL SOIGNANT EN FONCTION DES VOLUMES DE SOINS REQUIS DANS LES DIFFERENTS SERVICES: LE SYSTEME PRN 76

C. Tilquin, J. Carle, D. Saulnier, P. Lambert
Equipe de recherche opérationnelle en santé (EROS), Département d'administration de la santé, Université de Montréal,
C.P. 6128 Montréal, H3C 3J7, Canada

ABSTRACT

The PRN 76 System is a management information system for nursing. Its first component is a Care Plan Form by means of which the nursing staff can identify the patient's needs and plan nursing interventions in order to fullfil these needs. This initial form is completed by a Measurement Form of the Level of Care Required, designed to allow for determining the quantity (measured by the time required of the staff) of direct and indirect care required by each patient during the following twenty-four hours. Knowing the level of nursing care required by a patient, his class can then be determined using a classification diagram comprising six classes. These classes have been given a weighting specifying the quantity of care required by the "average" patient from each of the classes at each work shift. This weighting, in addition to the other norms relative to staff activities other than those associated with care, were used to construct evaluation tables for staff required. These tables help in determining the number of nursing staff members required in each care unit at each work shift, knowing the number of patient of each class present in this unit at this shift.

LE SYSTEME PRN 76

Le système PRN 76 est un système d'information pour la dotation du personnel soignant en fonction des volumes de soins requis dans les différents services de l'hôpital. Ses différentes composantes sont les suivantes:

1. Module d'identification et d'évaluation des besoins
   - 1.1 formule de plan de soins
   - 1.2 recueil de plan de soins de référence
   - 1.3 formule de contrôle de la planification des soins
2. Module de mesure des volumes de personnel soignant requis
   - 2.1 formule de mesure du niveau des soins requis par le patient
   - 2.2 schème de classification pondéré
   - 2.3 autres normes
3. Module d'aide à la décision et au contrôle de gestion

Dans ce texte, nous traiterons seulement du module de mesure des volumes de person-

EROS
Equipe de Recherche Opérationnelle en Santé
Département d'Administration de la Santé
Université de Montréal (Septembre 1978)

FORMULE DE MESURE
du niveau des soins infirmiers requis

PRN 76 - Projet de recherche en nursing 1976
Santé et Bien-Etre Social Canada, Projet no. 605-1233-45

Prodiguer des soins infirmiers / Prodiguer des soins sous ordonnance médicale

Besoins	Facteurs		
Hygiène & confort	Soins d'hygiène: bénéficiaire 0-4 ans	die	3
	Soins d'hygiène: bénéficiaire 0-4 ans	bid & plus	6
	Soins d'hygiène: bénéficiaire autonome	die	2
	Soins d'hygiène: bénéficiaire autonome	bid & plus	4
	Soins d'hygiène: bain partiel	die	4
	Soins d'hygiène: bain partiel	bid & plus	6
	Soins d'hygiène: bain comp. (pr.c.) (lit)	die	7
	Soins d'hygiène: bain comp. (pr.c.) (baig.)	die	9
	Soins d'hygiène: bain comp. (pr.c.) (lit/baig.)	bid & plus	16
	Soins d'hygiène: hydrothérapie: brûlé (prép.)		6
	Soins d'hygiène: hydrothérapie: brûlé (pr.c.)	die	11
	Soins d'hygiène: hydrothérapie: brûlé (pr.c.)	bid & plus	19
	Hygiène buccale	4-11 fois	1
	Hygiène buccale	12 fois & plus	3
	Rasage de la barbe		2
	Lavage de tête (lit/évier)		3
	Friction & installation (1-2 exécutants)	4 fois & plus	7
	Friction & installation (3 exécutants & plus)	4 fois & plus	16
	Lever et/ou marcher avec aide (1-2 exécutants)		4
	Lever et/ou marcher avec aide (3 exécutants & plus)		9
	Exercices passifs & actifs (pr.c.)		4
	Inst. et/ou surv.: traction(s)/prothèse(s)/bas/bandage(s)		2
	Application de contraintes physiques		4
	Application: sac(s) de glace ou eau chaude	(1-2 sacs)	2
	Application: sac(s) de glace ou eau chaude	(3 sacs & plus)	6
	Application de technique d'isolement		5
	Application de technique d'isolement (stérile)		10
Alimentation & hydratation	Alimentation et hydratation sans aide		2
	Alimentation et hydratation avec aide		5
	Alimentation et hydratation complète par personnel		11
	Hydratation per os	12 fois & plus	3
	Biberon et purée	6 fois & moins	12
	Biberon et purée	7 fois & plus	18
	Biberon et purée avec précautions spéciales		24
	Gavage en permanence	24h/24h	4
	Gavage en goutte-à-goutte ou à la seringue	6 fois & moins	6
	Gavage en goutte-à-goutte ou à la seringue	7 fois & plus	10
	Gavage (pr.c.)		12
	Perfusion courte durée (soluté)		2
	Perfusion en permanence (1 V.O.)	24h/24h	6
	Perfusion en permanence (2 V.O. & plus)	24h/24h	12
	Perfusion courte durée (sang & dérivés)	1 ou 2 unités	6
	Perfusion courte durée (sang & dérivés)	3 unités & plus	15
	Perfusion: hyperalimentation	24h/24h	12
	Perfusion: intra-péritonéale		40
	Dosage ing. et/ou exc.	14 fois & moins	1
	Dosage ing. et/ou exc.	15-24 fois	2
	Dosage ing. et/ou exc.	25 fois & plus	7
Elimination	Couches (bébé)		6
	Urinal et bassin de lit		3
	Bassin de lit (f)		5
	Incontinence et/ou condom		8
	Soins externes sonde vésicale et bassin de lit		2
	Installation: sonde ou cathéter	1-2 fois	3
	Installation: sonde ou cathéter	3 fois & plus	6
	Sonde(s) ou tube(s): ouvert(s)/fermé(s) et/ou tube rectal		1
	Drainage libre (ouvert)		1
	Drainage sous l'eau (circuit fermé)	1 tube	3
	Drainage sous l'eau (circuit fermé)	2 tubes & plus	6
	Drainage: succion continue	1-2 tubes	3
	Drainage: succion continue	3 tubes & plus	6
	Manipulation drains thoraciques		3
	Irrigation (toutes sortes)	2 fois & moins	2
	Irrigation (toutes sortes)	3-6 fois	4
	Irrigation (toutes sortes)	7-12 fois	6
	Irrigation (toutes sortes)	13-19 fois	8
	Irrigation (toutes sortes)	20 fois & plus	10
	Irrigation gastrique avec eau glacée (4000 cc)		24
	Irrigation colostomie		4
	Irrigation colostomie (pr.c.)		7
	Entretien stomie:	1 stomie	6
	Entretien stomie:	2 stomies & plus	15
	Extraction de lait		10

Besoins	Facteurs		
Respiration	Exercices respiratoires (prép. & inciter)		2
	Exercices respiratoires (pr.c.)	6 fois & moins	4
	Exercices respiratoires (pr.c.)	7 fois & plus	12
	Aérosol (prép. & inciter)		4
	Aérosol (pr.c.)		12
	Aspiration des sécrétions	6 fois & moins	3
	Aspiration des sécrétions	7-19 fois	6
	Aspiration des sécrétions	20 fois & plus	13
	Soins au trachéotomisé ou intubé		4
	Soins au trachéotomisé ou intubé avec respirateur		8
	Humidificateur et/ou éventail		1
	Administration O_2 (cathéter, masque, etc.)		3
	Administration O_2 (croupette ou tente complète)		6
Communication	Communication sociale		3
	Communication préventive		6
	Communication thérapeutique		12
	Enseignement au bénéficiaire et/ou à la famille		3
Surveillance & observation	Signes vitaux	4 fois & moins	1
	Signes vitaux	5-14 fois	4
	Signes vitaux	15-24 fois	8
	Signes vitaux	25 fois & plus	12
	Signes vitaux (T.A. d./a./c.)	6 fois & moins	3
	Signes vitaux (T.A. d./a./c.)	7 fois & plus	7
	Signes neurologiques	11 fois & moins	2
	Signes neurologiques	12 fois & plus	6
	Tension veineuse centrale	11 fois & moins	3
	Tension veineuse centrale	12 fois & plus	8
	Evaluation du coeur foetal et/ou cont. utérines		2
	Surveillance	10 fois & moins	1
	Surveillance	11-40 fois	4
	Surveillance	41 fois & plus	12
	Surveillance continue (pr.c.) partagée	2 bén. & plus	38
	Surveillance continue (pr.c.) exclusive	1 bén.	76
Thérapie	Méd. (P.O.-I.R.-Ovu.-Ong.-Gttes)	4 fois & moins	1
	Méd. (P.O.-I.R.-Ovu.-Ong.-Gttes)	5-14 fois	3
	Méd. (P.O.-I.R.-Ovu.-Ong.-Gttes)	15-24 fois	4
	Méd. (P.O.-I.R.-Ovu.-Ong.-Gttes)	25 fois & plus	5
	Méd. (S.C. ou I.M.)	3 doses & moins	1
	Méd. (S.C. ou I.M.)	4-7 doses	3
	Méd. (S.C. ou I.M.)	8 doses & plus	6
	Méd. (I.V.)	4 doses & moins	2
	Méd. (I.V.)	5-11 doses	5
	Méd. (I.V.)	12-19 doses	9
	Méd. (I.V.)	20 doses & plus	18
	Rasage	20% & moins	3
	Rasage	25-65%	6
	Rasage	70% & plus	12
	Asepsie	20% & moins	2
	Asepsie	25-65%	4
	Asepsie	70% & plus	8
	Application d'onguent	30% & plus	8
	Application d'onguent 30% & plus avec enveloppement		17
	Mèche et/ou pansement à enlever		1
	Points ou plâtre à enlever		3
	Plaie à l'air: nettoyage et/ou inst. lampe	8 fois & moins	2
	Plaie à l'air: nettoyage et/ou inst. lampe	9 fois & plus	6
	Pansement sec ou humide	1-2 fois	2
	Pansement sec ou humide	3 fois & plus	4
	Pansement avec écoulement	1-2 fois	3
	Pansement avec écoulement	3 fois & plus	8
	Pansement de régénération de la peau	1-2 fois	6
	Pansement de régénération de la peau	3 fois & plus	14
	Débridement de plaie(s)		6
	Appl. d'onguent et/ou pansement: brûlé	20% & moins	14
	Appl. d'onguent et/ou pansement: brûlé	25-45%	28
	Appl. d'onguent et/ou pansement: brûlé	50-70%	54
	Appl. d'onguent et/ou pansement: brûlé	75% & plus	72

Contribuer aux méthodes diagnostiques

Facteurs		
Collecte: selles et/ou expectorations		1
Collecte: urine		2
Prélèvement: sécrétions et/ou selles et/ou urine (an. simple)		1
Prélèvement: urine (culture)		2
Prélèvement: sang	3 fois & moins	2
Prélèvement: sang	4-8 fois	6
Prélèvement: sang	9 fois & plus	13
Pesée et/ou mensuration (1 exécutant)		1
Pesée et/ou mensuration (2 exécutants & plus)		2
Analyse simple à l'Unité	8 fois & moins	2
Analyse simple à l'Unité	9 fois & plus	6
Ass.: examen ou R.X. (pr.c.)		2
Ass.: M.D.: test à l'Unité (pr.c.)	1 fois	8
Ass.: M.D.: test à l'Unité (pr.c.)	2 fois & plus	16

Figure 1

nel soignant requis, les autres modules du système étant à un stade de développement moins avancé.

LA FORMULE DE MESURE AU NIVEAU DES SOINS REQUIS PAR LE PATIENT

La méthode de mesure retenue dans le système PRN est quelque peu en marge de l'approche traditionnelle selon laquelle la demande de soins infirmiers du patient est qualifiée par un vecteur constitué d'un certain nombre d'indicateurs (d'"état" de santé, de services requis ou "socio-démographiques" comme l'âge, le sexe) sélectionnés en fonction des "caractéristiques" de l'individu, à l'intérieur d'une liste limitée d'indicateurs, et quantifiée par le poids du vecteur établi statistiquement à priori sur la base de mesures de temps de soins infirmiers donnés (mesures obtenues par chronométrage ou par observations instantanées).

Ainsi dans le système PRN:

- la demande est qualifiée par un vecteur constitué de la liste exhaustive des éléments de service infirmier requis par l'individu

- elle est quantifiée par le poids du vecteur obtenu par addition des poids de chacun des éléments de services qui le constituent. Ces poids ou valeurs rendent compte du nombre de minutes du personnel soignant requises pour "exécuter" le service élémentaire correspondant pendant les prochaines vingt-quatre heures. Ces poids ont été déterminés à priori, non pas par mesures de temps, mais par des comités d'experts procédant selon une démarche systématique inspirée de la méthode de Delphi.

La formule de mesure PRN est donc une liste d'éléments de services infirmiers pondérés en points (un point = 5 minutes) selon le temps que prend leur exécution sur une période de vingt-quatre heures. Le premier instrument, mis au point en 1974 était uniquement adapté à la mesure en pédiatrie. En 1976, cet instrument a été "étendu" pour permettre aussi la mesure en médecine et chirurgie adulte, en gynécologie et obstétrique, en soins intensifs prématurés, enfants et adultes. Ce dernier instrument a été révisé annuellement depuis 1976 par des comités dont les membres ont changé chaque année (figure 1). Enfin, en 1980, l'instrument a subi une nouvelle extension. Cette dernière version est aussi utilisable en soins prolongés, en hébergement et en psychiatrie. Elle sera disponible au début de l'année 1981.

Le poids de chacun des éléments de service (dans la suite de ce texte, nous les appellerons FACTEURS) de la formule rend compte du temps requis pour exécuter sur une période de vingt-quatre heures, la ou les actions de soins infirmiers que lui confèrent sa spécificité, mais aussi les actions qui supportent ces actions spécifiques, à savoir:

- vérifier l'ordonnance médicale

- se laver les mains
- préparer le matériel
- identifier le patient
- expliquer l'action au patient
- observer systématiquement le comportement, les attitudes, les réactions physiques et psycho-sociales du patient pendant l'action de soins infirmiers
- communiquer verbalement et/ou non verbalement avec le patient pendant l'action de soins infirmiers
- isoler et installer le patient
- ranger la chambre et le matériel
- faire la relance

Il s'ensuit donc que le poids ou valeur d'un facteur rend compte du temps consacré à tous (tel que décrit ci-dessus) les actes recouverts par l'(les) action(s) de soins qu'il représente, que ces actes soient posés en présence (soins directs) ou non (soins indirects) du patient, et que ces actes soient physiques ou mentaux. Cette règle souffre une exception. Parmi les actes de support d'une action de soins, on retrouve souvent des déplacements. Or, les déplacements n'ont pas été considérés lorsqu'il s'est agi d'accorder une valeur aux facteurs. Cette exclusion a été motivée par le fait que le temps des déplacements varie avec la disposition physique des lieux; de ce fait, on ne pouvait en tenir compte dans la valeur des facteurs à moins que d'admettre que celle-ci varie aussi avec le contexte de dispensation des soins. On a cependant tenu compte des temps de déplacement ailleurs dans le module de mesure.

Lorsqu'un patient est admis, l'infirmière qui le prend en charge, après avoir rédigé son plan de soins, procède à la mesure de son niveau de soins en identifiant et additionnant (mentalement) la valeur des facteurs qui rendent compte de ses besoins pour les prochaines vingt-quatre heures. Chacun des ensembles de facteurs correspondant à un même besoin spécifique des patients constitue un ENTREFILET de la formule de mesure. Lorsqu'on procède à la mesure du niveau des soins requis par le patient, on n'a le droit de choisir qu'au plus un facteur par entrefilet, le facteur qui rend le mieux compte des besoins du patient.

Pendant toute la durée du séjour du patient, son niveau de soins est mesuré quotidiennement. Cette procédure est facilitée par l'inscription de la valeur des facteurs attribués au patient, en regard des actions de soins apparaissant dans son plan de soins. Le temps requis pour cette procédure est négligeable, si elle s'effectue en même temps que la mise à jour du plan de soins. La mesure quotidienne du niveau des soins requis par les patients prend place vers la fin du quart de jour;

vers la fin du quart de soir, on procède à une revision de ce niveau pour les patients dont le plan de soins a été modifié ainsi qu'à la mesure du niveau des soins requis par les patients nouvellement admis. Enfin, vers la fin du quart de nuit, on procède de la même manière qu'au quart de soir.

Pour garantir l'utilisation fiable de la formule de mesure, un guide de l'utilisateur a été préparé. Chaque facteur y est défini de façon très détaillée et les modalités de son utilisation y sont très précisément expliquées.

LE SCHEMA DE CLASSIFICATION PONDERE

Le niveau des soins infirmiers requis pourrait être utilisé tel quel dans le calcul de la dotation du personnel soignant (cela pose cependant un problème puisque ce niveau est établi pour les prochaines vingt-quatre heures alors qu'on a besoin de le connaître par quart de travail). Cependant nous avons pu nous rendre compte, en procédant par simulation, qu'il n'y avait pas perte d'information - du point de vue du calcul de la dotation - en substituant à la notion de niveau, le concept de classe. Le système PRN a six classes de patients: les patients dont le niveau est inférieur ou égal à 25 points appartiennent à la classe 1, ceux dont le niveau est compris entre 26 et 43 points appartiennent à la classe 2, entre 44 et 61 points à la classe 3, entre 62 et 106 points à la classe 4, entre 107 et 151 points à la classe 5. Au-delà de 151 points, les patients appartiennent à la classe 6. Le niveau n'est donc qu'un indicateur pour déterminer la classe du patient.

PONDÉRATION DES CLASSES (MINUTES)

Classe	Soins directs et indirects exceptés les CSB et les déplacements	CSB (communications au sujet du bénéficiaire)	Pondération de la classification (24 heures)	Pondération de la classification par quart de travail		
				Jour	Soir	Nuit
1	89	24	113	61	34	18
2	172	37	209	104	66	39
3	252	57	309	146	96	67
4	417	90	507	200	165	142
5	639	120	759	265	252	242
6	978	133	1111	379	371	361

Figure 2

Les classes ont reçu une pondération (figure 2) qui spécifie les temps de soins requis par le patient moyen de chaque classe. Les poids des classes ont été estimés à partir de deux échantillons, l'un de 2600, l'autre de 3000 plans de soins de patients recueillis un jour choisi au hasard dans leur séjour à l'hôpital. On a d'abord déterminé pour chaque patient, le niveau des soins qu'il requérait le jour où son plan de soins a été observé. De cette façon on a pu déterminer la classe de chacun à l'aide du schéma de classification précité.

Dans une deuxième étape, on a travaillé avec une formule de mesure similaire en tout point à celle présentée à la figure 1, à une exception près: on y a réparti pour chaque patient en particulier, la valeur (exprimée en minutes sur la base de la règle: 1 point = 5 minutes) de chaque facteur pour vingt-quatre heures entre les trois quarts de travail selon la façon dont toutes les activités afférentes à ce facteur se répartissaient entre ces trois quarts dans le cas de ce patient particulier. On était ainsi en mesure de calculer pour chaque patient, non plus le niveau de ses besoins pour 24 heures mais bien le niveau de ses besoins à chaque quart de travail. A partir de ces trois données et de la classe des patients déterminée dans la première étape, on a pu calculer les minutes de soins directs et indirects reliés aux actions représentées par les facteurs, requises en moyenne par le patient de chaque classe à chaque quart de travail. Pour obtenir les poids des classes, il restait encore à ajouter, respectivement, à ces moyennes, le temps moyen requis par patient de chaque classe à chaque quart de travail pour effectuer toutes les autres activités de soins qui peuvent être imputées à chaque patient individuellement et n'avaient pas été prises en compte (pour des raisons qu'il serait beaucoup trop long d'expliquer ici) par les facteurs de la FORMULE DE MESURE DU NIVEAU DES SOINS REQUIS. Ces activités que nous désignons par le vocable: "Communications au Sujet du Bénéficiaire - CSB" consistent en la rédaction du dossier, l'élaboration du plan de soins et les autres communications, au sujet du bénéficiaire, des membres du personnel infirmier entre eux, avec les médecins, avec les autres services et avec les proches du patient. Les temps de "CSB" ont été obtenus par consensus d'experts. L'explication détaillée de la procédure utilisée dépasse la portée de ce texte.

LES AUTRES NORMES

Connaissant les classes des patients dans une unité de soins un quart de travail donné et la pondération des classes, on est en mesure de calculer le nombre total de minutes requises pour prodiguer les soins (directs et indirects) à ces patients et pour les communications au sujet du patient (C.S.B.). Le personnel soignant consacre cependant une partie non négligeable de son temps à des activités autres que les soins et les C.S.B.. Des normes ont donc été aussi développées, toujours par consensus d'experts, pour mesurer le temps de ces activités. La pondération des classes est donc complétée par des normes relatives:

- aux activités administratives, à l'entretien et aux déplacements qui y sont reliés à l'intérieur de l'unité de soins (figure 3),

STANDARDS (EN MINUTES) POUR LES ACTIVITÉS ADMINISTRATIVES, L'ENTRETIEN ET LES DÉPLACEMENTS QUI Y SONT RELIÉS À L'INTÉRIEUR DE L'UNITÉ DE SOINS

Quart de travail		Minutes par unité de soins				
		Unités de soins intensifs		Autres unités de soins		
		10 bénéficiaires et moins	11 bénéficiaires et plus	20 bénéficiaires et moins	21 à 40 bénéficiaires	41 bénéficiaires et plus
Jour	semaine	240.5	341	264	334	411
	fin de sem.	121	171.5	142.5	196.5	261
Soir	semaine	63.5	115.5	75.5	104.5	145.5
	fin de sem.	58.5	106.5	70.5	98.5	137.5
Nuit	semaine	42	75.5	47	62	88.5
	fin de sem.	41	74.5	46	61	87.5

Figure 3

- aux déplacements à l'intérieur de l'unité de soins avec et/ou reliés aux patients,

- aux déplacements à l'extérieur de l'unité de soins avec et sans les patients,

- à la formation, aux réunions administratives et au temps non productif.

Une fonction mathématique simple, combinant toutes ces normes, permet de calculer le personnel soignant requis à chaque quart de travail dans chaque unité de soins. Pour aider les utilisateurs du système, des tables sont disponibles qui donnent directement le personnel requis connaissant le nombre de patients de chaque classe présents dans l'unité de soins.

EVALUATION DE LA VARIABILITE INTER-OBSERVATEURS DANS L'INTERPRETATION DE L'EXAMEN TOMODENSIMETRIQUE

P. BARBERGER-GATEAU*, J.F. DARTIGUES*, J.M. CAILLE**

* Département d'Informatique Appliquée - Université de Bordeaux II
146, rue Léo Saignat - 33076 BORDEAUX CEDEX (France)

**Service de Neuro- Radiologie, Hôpital Pellegrin-Tripode, place Amélie Raba Léon
33076 - BORDEAUX CEDEX (France)

L'apport d'une nouvelle technique diagnostique, comme l'examen tomodensitométrique (TDM) peut être évalué de deux façons : dans l'absolu, ou par rapport aux techniques existantes. Cette évaluation pose trois types de problèmes :

- tout d'abord, une technique est généralement évaluée en termes de précision ou d'exactitude diagnostique, par rapport à des critères anatomo-pathologiques (1) ou à d'autres méthodes de diagnostic (2) mais rarement d'un point de vue décisionnel. Or il importe également d'évaluer dans quelle mesure cette nouvelle technique va modifier la stratégie diagnostique ou la conduite à tenir (3).
- ensuite se pose un problème de méthodologie, d'une façon assez voisine de celle des essais thérapeutiques comparatifs, avec des contraintes de tirage au hasard et de double-aveugle difficilement réalisables en pratique.
- enfin et surtout, il est difficile de savoir exactement ce que l'on évalue : une technique pure, ou bien un ensemble d'éléments comprenant la technique plus ou moins associée à celui qui l'interprète, et à tout le contexte de la demande d'examen.

Ceci amène à se poser deux questions : dans la réalité, l'objectif n'est-il pas d'évaluer une technique replacée dans le contexte d'un service de façon pragmatique plutôt que sa valeur dans l'absolu ? et ensuite, comment apprécier la part de cet environnement ?

Dans le cadre de l'évaluation de l'examen TDM du cerveau, nous avons donc cherché à appréhender quelle était la variabilité de l'interprétation devant une même image, dans un même service de neuroradiologie, et le coût de l'erreur de diagnostic.

I - MATERIEL

100 dossiers ont été tirés au hasard parmi 6000 examens effectués avec un tomodensitomètre ND 8000 dans le service de neuroradiologie de l'Hôpital Pellegrin à Bordeaux (Pr J.M. CAILLE). La ventilation des diagnostics est représentative de l'ensemble des pathologies rencontrées dans ce service.

Le critère diagnostique a été défini par la conjonction d'arguments cliniques, paracliniques et éventuellement anatomo-pathologiques, mais ne porte que sur l'image : une image est classée comme "normale" si la pathologie correspondante ne donne pas de modifications au Scanner.

II - METHODE

Deux neuroradiologues d'un même service, A et B, ont analysé séparément les clichés de ces 100 patients, sans en connaître aucun renseignement clinique ni d'état-civil. Pour chaque dossier, chacun notait son diagnostic et précisait si des renseignements cliniques lui paraissaient indispensables pour l'étayer.

D'autre part, la ressemblance potentielle d'images entre elles a été évaluée empiriquement par un neuroradiologue, à partir de son expérience personnelle, dans une matrice qui apprécie par une note entre 0 et 10 la similitude entre les images correspondant au diagnostic I et celles du diagnostic J. Plus la note est élevée, plus la ressemblance est grande.

Le coût de l'erreur de conclure au diagnostic J alors que le vrai diagnostic est I a été estimé dans une matrice construite comme la précédente : plus l'erreur est grave, plus le coût est élevé.

III - RESULTATS

	lecteur A	lecteur B
nombre de diagnostics exacts	85	67
" " " faux	15	33
score pondéré par la ressemblance des images (maximum théorique: 680)*	606	470
coût total des erreurs*	91	206
nombre de demandes de renseignements cliniques	46	53

réponses identiques : 71 (65 exactes et 6 fausses)

IV - DISCUSSION

La concordance entre juges fait partie de l'évaluation globale d'une technique diagnostique. Ici, au sein d'un même service elle apparait médiocre.

Elle traduit en fait divers éléments :

. la différence d'expérience des deux médecins : un chef de service de neuroradiologie ayant derriere lui une expérience de plusieurs milliers d'images de Scanner, et celle d'un attaché nécessairement plus limitée. Ce facteur est très difficile à pondérer, et il se retrouve au niveau du score d'exactitude de chaque médecin, du coût de l'erreur, ainsi que de la quantité de renseignements demandés.

. l'absence volontaire d'information clinique : or, en pratique, celle-ci joue un rôle fondamental dans la réalisation de l'examen et son interprétation. Ici intervient un autre élément de fiabilité d'un examen : sa réalisation et sa lecture dans des conditions optimales, grâce aux renseignements fournis pas le neurologue par exemple.

Il est donc impossible en pratique, et d'un intérêt limité, de chercher à évaluer une technique indépendament de son environnement, de l'information apportée tant par les demandeurs de l'examen, que celle provenant de l'expérience individuelle du lecteur. Il reste l'exigence d'une certaine homogénéité au sein d'un même service, favorisée par la collaboration avec les neurologues et la participation des expériences de chacun, au diagnostic final.

* Ces scores n'ont été calculés que pour les 68 dossiers dont le diagnostic était univoque et figurait parmi les 12 plus fréquents.

BIBLIOGRAPHIE

1) - JACOBS L., KINKEL W.R., HEFFORER R.R. :

Autopsy correlations of computerized tomography : expérience with 6000 CT scans.
Neurology, 1976 ; 26 : 1111 - 18

2) - GREITZ T.

Computer tomography for diagnosis of intra-cranial tumours compared with other neuro-radiologic procedures.
Acta Radiol. (Suppl.) 1975 ; p 14

BAKER H.L.

The impact of computed tomography on neuro-radiologic practice.
Radiology. 1975 ; 116 : 637 - 40

CONDITIONS QUE DOIT REMPLIR UN SYSTEME D'INFORMATION HOSPITALIER POUR REPONDRE AUX PROJETS D'ANALYSE D'ACTIVITE

Michel de HEAULME
INSERM U 88, 91 bd de l'Hôpital, 75634 Paris Cedex 13

Medical activity analysis requires current information on the daily practice. Five groups of principal data are examined : equipment, patient identification, pathologies, medical acts, medical procedures, leading to define the minimal conditions required by an efficient development of a medical information system.

Il y a plusieurs approches pour tenter d'évaluer les institutions et les activités de soins, l'audit et l'enquête étant pratiquement les deux seules techniques à pouvoir être utilisées aujourd'hui en l'absence d'un système hospitalier d'information médicale.

Le but de cet article est de montrer qu'un tel système d'information est indispensable à une mise en oeuvre efficace des différentes approches analytiques et d'en esquisser les caractéristiques principales.

Deux faits s'imposent :

- On ne peut projeter d'évaluation sans <u>se donner les moyens d'acquérir l'information nécessaire</u>. Cette affirmation ne serait qu'une lapalissade si l'on avait constaté trop souvent que les nombreux débats sur l'évaluation des systèmes de soins escamotaient la partie pratique de l'acquisition des informations.

  La vanité de cette situation apparaît clairement quand on sait combien il est difficile d'acquérir une information médicale fiable, et a fortiori, toute une série d'informations répondant à un schéma d'évaluation, comme le montre un article sur les PSRO (1).
- En supposant acquise la possibilité de recueillir une information correcte, on constate qu'un processus d'analyse requiert rapidement une <u>information suffisamment détaillée</u> si l'on veut que les conclusions aboutissent à une rétroaction efficace sur la pratique médicale. Il ne suffit pas de dire que x % des cardiopathies valvulaires subissent des examens apparemment redondants comme le cathétérisme, l'échographie et le phonomécanogramme. Il faut pouvoir vérifier si la demande des trois examens était justifiée par les nécessités cliniques ou ne provenait que d'un réflexe routinier.

I. <u>LES INFORMATIONS AU MOINS NECESSAIRES</u>

Finalement, la mise en oeuvre d'un processus d'analyse d'activité en milieu médical requiert; dans sa forme la plus générale, la posssssion d'au moins cinq principaux groupes d'informations :

. des données structurelles sur les équipements mobiliers et immobiliers ainsi que sur les dotations en personnels des services, afin de rapporter les faits à des structures comparables. Ces données sont extérieures au système des informations médicales proprement dit et ne sont qu'évoquées ici dans cet article pour mémoire.
. une identification des sujets et des événements médicaux les concernant : hospitalisations, consultations, etc ...
. une identification des faits bio-cliniques et des pathologies.
. une identification de la nature des actes pratiqués.
. une identification des procédures utilisées par les médecins.

1.1. L'identification des sujets doit permettre de suivre leur trajectoire médicale. Elle implique donc un système permanent d'identification, qui, pour éviter les déterminations erronées ou multiples, doit nécessairement faire appel à une référence centrale. Ce fait est inéluctable pour maintenir la cohérence des données et du suivi des malades ou pour permettre l'analyse dans le temps des maladies et de leur thérapeutique.

Que ce besoin pose des problèmes au niveau de la protection des données individuelles est un autre fait irrécusable qui oblige à ne pas faire paraître l'identité des malades dans les études d'activité. Mais cette exigence a des solutions techniques, et elle n'enlève rien à la nécessité de pouvoir suivre le malade dans sa maladie et les conséquences des thérapeutiques appliquées si l'on veut effectuer une analyse d'activité qui ait un sens.

1.2. L'identification des faits cliniques et des pathologies pose les plus grands problèmes. Pourtant il faut bien admettre que la critique des procédures et des coûts n'a de sens que par rapport à la pathologie et à son évolution. On constate ici combien le seul décompte financier fourni par les informations de gestion hospitalière est impuissant par lui-même à fournir des arguments acceptables sur le plan de la santé. La conclusion doit en être fortement soulignée : la clé de l'interprétation des résultats de gestion dans le domaine de la santé est une information médicale sur les faits biocliniques et leur évolution. Or la description de ces faits n'est pas réductible à une ou plusieurs étiquettes nosographiques accolées aux coûts. Il s'agit bien plutôt de l'ensemble des faits qui fournissent le contexte clinique de chaque malade, son tableau clinique particulier. Certes il existe des cas typiques qui ne posent pas trop de problèmes. Mais dans le cas général, il faut pouvoir décrire l'ensemble des principaux faits biocliniques dans leur complexité et leur variabilité individuelle pour pouvoir ensuite choisir à bon escient les malades qu'il faudra regrouper dans la même étude pour obtenir des résultats pertinents.

Si l'on veut promouvoir l'évaluation, il faut donc disposer d'une identification des pathologies et des contextes cliniques qui rende aisés et efficaces l'inventaire et la sélection des groupes de sujets à partir des données recueillies sur le tout venant.

La grande difficulté est que la description des faits bioclinïques se fait mal au travers d'une représentation par les classifications hiérarchiques qui sont utilisées actuellement. Les défauts généraux en sont bien connus :

- c'est une représentation catégorisée a priori,qui fige la description médicale d'une façon qui ne correspond pas toujours aux besoins, et rend difficile l'évolution pourtant rapide des concepts médicaux.
- c'est un mode de représentation qui ne peut que conduire à une prolifération d'étiquettes si l'on veut préciser les descriptions. Dans le cas contraire, l'identification reste trop grossière pour être utile.
- la structure hiérarchique possède un défaut intrinsèque : le choix des ramifications dépend du point de vue auquel on se place. Non seulement ce choix a un caractère arbitraire que l'on devra imposer à tous les utilisateurs, mais il provoque des situations inextricables lorsqu'il s'agit de représenter des points de vue différents comme en clinique : classification selon les signes, selon les appareils, selon l'évolution, etc ... De plus, à partir d'un certain degré de finesse la même information pourrait aussi bien être rangée en des endroits différents, ce qui rend la classification encore plus arbitraire et oblige à des renvois incessants.

Toutes ces difficultés apparaissent clairement dans la Classification Internationale des Maladies (CIM). L'utilisation des codes numériques ne fait qu'aggraver la difficulté d'emploi pour les médecins. En conséquence, lorsqu'il s'agit uniquement d'une obligation administrative, bien souvent les codes sont fournis sans aucune motivation professionnelle et contiennent des erreurs de digits qu'il est très difficile de détecter ensuite.

Une amélioration considérable a été apportée par des systèmes organisant les notions médicales en classes indépendantes ayant chacune sa hiérarchie propre : symptomatologie, étiologie, topographie, etc ... la description médicale se fait en combinant les termes de chaque classe selon les faits observés.

Cette voie a été suivie dès 1965 par SNOP puis par SNOMED (2), qui cependant maintiennent des codes numériques pour les termes, et n'autorisent que des combinaisons élémentaires d'un terme de chaque classe. Une variante déjà plus souple est utilisée en routine à l'Hôpital Cantonal de Genève (3).

REMEDE (4, 5), développé au laboratoire à partir de 1972, permet d'utiliser directement les termes médicaux courants selon un jeu d'une dizaine de liens grammaticaux qui suffisent dans la plupart des cas et sont rapidement appris par les médecins et les secrétaires. Le prototype actuel fournit ainsi le premier exemple d'un véritable langage médical directement utilisable par le personnel soignant sans recours incessant à des lexiques volumineux, tout en restant analysable dans son contenu par l'ordinateur.

1.3. L'identification des actes doit se faire par nature. Il est bien connu que la notation du genre K, B, Z ... ne permet en aucune façon d'estimer si les dépenses ont été engagées de façon saine. Encore, moins de proposer aux médecins une modification (sélective) de leur pratique. Seul un détail de la nature de ces actes, rapportéé à un contexte clinique également détaillé, mettrait en valeur les pratiques abusives ou les stratégies diagnostiques les plus efficaces.

Finalement, la représentation des actes par nature rencontre la même difficulté descriptive que celle des tableaux cliniques. Elle doit recevoir une solution du même genre qi l'on veut éviter les surcoûts dus à la multiplicité des procédés d'indexation.

En particulier, la saisie des actes en salle, aujourd'hui inexistante en pratique, ne s'effectuera efficacement que si le personnel infirmier peut facilement transcrire en clair les indications du cahier des prescriptions, et non pas chercher puis transcrire (sans erreur) le code numérique d'une classification des actes médicaux ou chirurgicaux.

1.4. L'identification des procédures médicales, c'est à dire des conduites diagnostiques ou thérapeutiques usuelles, est un stade important de l'analyse d'activité. C'est à partir de l'identification de ces conduites et de leur discussion médicale que naîtront les possibilités d'évaluation au sens strict, c'est à dire de comparaison d'une pratique à une référence afin d'en juger l'intérêt.

Il importe donc au plus haut point qu'un système d'information médicale soit apte à refléter ces conduites avec un détail suffisant pour qu'on puisse les repérer efficacement et suivre leur évolution. Finalement, on retombe dans la même problématique rencontrée pour la saisie des faits cliniques et des actes pratiqués.

II. CONCLUSIONS

Les considérations précédentes conduisent à penser qu'une généralisation des méthodes d'évaluation, qu'elles concernent la gestion ou la pratique médicale, ne pourra pas dépasser le stade des analyses ponctuelles sans la mise en place d'un système hospitalier d'information médicale capable de fournir les informations utiles aux diverses étapes de la réflexion médico-administrative.

2.1. Un tel système ne peut avoir pour but la seule évaluation administrative, qui n'intéresse pas ou même fait peuraux médecins. Poursuivre en ce sens sans entraîner la motivation médicale ne peut conduire qu'à des désillusions répétées.

2.2. La motivation médicale provient essentiellement d'une possibilité de recueillir et de traiter en pratique quotidienne l'information médicale nécessaire aux différentes fins d'archivage, de consultation de dossiers et de recherches diverses. Il faut donc fournir aux médecins les moyens de traiter ces informations qui les intéressent et qui fourniront en même temps la source ordinaire des données d'évaluation.

2.3. L'information utile ne peut être collationnée à l'aide d'un seul système de représentation. Pour être efficace le système d'information doit donc comprendre :

2.3.1. La possibilité de décrire les informations principales sur le tout venant. Les divers comptes rendus biomédicaux contiennent bien ces informations et sont donc les documents qui doivent nourrir la première composante du système. Leur traitement par ordinateur permet :

. de discuter du fonctionnement et de la pratique du service (analyse d'activité médicale interne)

. de fournir aux audits le matériau de base de leur réflexion, n'ayant en général au départ aucune idée de ce qui pourrait être intéressant.

. de faire naître les hypothèses à partir desquelles seront construites les enquêtes ponctuelles. On sait combien il est difficile, par exemple, d'imaginer ce que pourraient être de bons indicateurs d'activité.

Ce n'est pas une projection a priori qui peut les déterminer, mais une réflexion sur la pratique quotidienne des services, reflétée au départ par les informations contenues dans les comptes rendus biomédicaux.

L'indexation de ces comptes rendus suppose une représentation combinatoire des faits biocliniques et des actes pratiqués aboutissant à un véritable langage médical compris par l'ordinateur.

2.3.2. La deuxième composante du système d'information est un système permettant de recueillir des informations spécifiques, soit à des fins de soins ou de recherches sur groupe de malades donnés, soit à l'usage d'enquêtes ponctuelles déterminées par exemple pour les besoins de l'évaluation.

En conclusion, la mise en pratique de l'évaluation de l'activité médicale ou de la gestion ne pourra passer dans la pratique courante que lorsqu'un système hospitalier d'information médicale aura pris naissance avec les composantes qui ont été soulignées. Le développement d'un tel système est aujourd'hui techniquement possible à un coût raisonnable et résoudrait en premier lieu bien des problèmes d'archivage et de communication qui paralysent aujourd'hui la vie des services. En second lieu, il fournirait un flux dynamique d'information reflétant la réalité de l'activité médicale quotidienne, permettant à la demande une réflexion pertinente sur les conditions de cette activité, et indiquant des enquêtes précises pour évaluer ce qui vaut la peine de l'être.

L'argument le plus souvent opposé au développement d'un tel système est son coût et "l'inflation informatique" qu'il risquerait de provoquer.

Plusieurs directions de réponse peuvent être apportées à cet argument :

- le coût du matériel qui était encore certainement prohibitif avec la technologie informatique de ces dernières années, atteindra un niveau tout-à-fait acceptable avant 1985. Ainsi, certains traitements linguistiques autrefois réservés aux centres de recherches peuvent entrer dans l'usage courant et répondre aux besoins exprimés.
- "l'inflation informatique" est limitée d'elle même par l'effort qu'il faut fournir pour produire une information correcte, et extraire ensuite des résultats intéressants.
- la mise en place d'un circuit d'informations médicales, répond à des besoins profonds quotidiennement exprimés par les équipes médicales, quant à leur secrétariat, le suivi des malades, la communication habituelle des informations, la recherche d'informations ou de dossiers, etc... Aucune évaluation n'a été faite du temps perdu (c'est-à-dire de la perte de productivité) caractérisant le système actuel, ou plus exactement l'absence de tout système. Des entretiens avec des chefs de clinique montrent qu'il peut atteindre 20 % de leur temps de travail, sans parler de celui des secrétaires.

  On peut évaluer le coût de l'implantation d'un système hospitalier d'information médicale, mais rien ne permet aujourd'hui de connaître le montant du gaspillage correspondant à la situation actuelle. Est-on sûr qu'il ne dépasse pas, et de loin, le montant qu'il faut investir pour obtenir une information utile ?
- Il faut se donner les moyens de ses objectifs. Si l'on veut mettre en place un système d'évaluation, il faut mettre en place des procédures de recueil de l'information. Autant faire d'une pierre deux coups et instaurer un système d'information médicale avec des procédures cohérentes pour l'ensemble des besoins.
- L'évolution des sociétés se fait vers une informatisation progressive des moyens de communication :
  - . pourquoi le secteur médical serait-il l'un des derniers à en bénéficier, alors qu'on a pu dire que la Médecine était une véritable "industrie de l'information" en elle-même ?
  - . à trop tarder les équipes médicales s'équiperont sans directives communes. La conséquence est claire : au moins sur le plan du langage, sinon des matériels, une situation de type Babel naîtra et rendra la communication et l'évaluation encore plus difficiles à réaliser.

REFERENCES

1 Demlo LK, Campbell PM, Spaght Brown S. Reliability of information abstracted from patients' medical records. Medical Care 1978 ; 16 : 995-1005.

2 In : SNOMED Systematized Nomenclature of Medicine ; Cote RA (ed.), Skokie, Illinois : College of American Pathologist.

3 Frütiger P, Rossier Ph, Scherrer JR. Automatic ICD/SNOMED codification of symptoms using a tree-branching logic. In Medinfo 77, Shires Wolff Eds, Amsterdam : North Holland, 1977.

4 de Heaulme M, Tainturier C, Thomas D. Traitement par ordinateur des comptes-rendus médicaux : l'exemple du système REMEDE. Nouv Pr Med 1979, 40 : 3223-3226.

5 Tainturier C, de Heaulme M, Mery C, Grosgogeat Y. Aide à l'analyse d'activité d'un service de Cardiologie à partir du traitement par ordinateur des résumés d'hospitalisation. In : MIE Toulouse 1980 (sous presse).

EVALUATION OF DOCUMENTATION AND RETRIEVAL QUALITY: FREE TEXT VERSUS CODING

Günther GELL and Wolf-Dieter SAGER
Universitätsklinik für Radiologie
A-8036 Graz, Auenbruggerplatz 9, Austria

SUMMARY

The reports of the Department of Radiology of the University of Graz are documented by the free text system AURA. A study was launched to assess the quality of retrieval when using this system. During a limited period parallel to free text processing the findings of all CT-examinations were also manually coded. Superior results for recall and precision of retrievals using a search for keywords in comparison with a search for codes were obtained.

1. INTRODUCTION

At the Department of Radiology of the University of Graz the free text documentation system AURA is in operation for nearly ten years (1,2). Radiologic reports are written on a terminal, and the text is processed and stored on the computer. For long-time storage the descriptive part of the reports is discarded. The clerical information and the textual information about the examination and the diagnosis (summary) are used for documentation and retrieval. The system serves as an index or catalogue to the films, allowing for rapid selection of relevant cases, therefore providing the basis for scientific work. Besides case finding AURA performs also feedback functions by regular correlation of the results of different kinds of examinations.

While general acceptance of and satisfaction with the system is very good no objective and sufficient data to assess the quality of documentation and retrieval were available. Reactions range from: "very good, all cases I could remember off hand have been retrieved" to "very poor, case XY, who had a carcinoma of the breast was not retrieved"; on investigation it turned out that no carcinoma was mentioned in the radiologic report, but indeed a carcinoma had been found in a subsequent operation - a fact that never came to the computer.

To gain more reliable data therefore a prospective study has been started with parallel coding and free text processing.

2. METHOD AND MATERIAL

2.1 Computed tomography

Computed tomography was selected as the field of the study for several reasons: This section has always shown great interest in documentation and is the most intensive user of the AURA facilities. The section has already experience with the use of codes because the CT-hardware allows for a ten-byte characterisation of each examination, which is stored with the picture files. This string is entered at examination time and contains in coded form information about the region of the examination (head, neck, thorax, abdomen etc.) the diagnosis (or question) of the referring physician, the technical settings of the machine (e. g. high resolution) etc. Over 5000 examinations per year are performed on two scanners.

2.2 Coding

Our CT-section has a very high workload and therefore only a short and easy to use code could be considered. The actual code has two facets, localisation and diagnosis. Localisation has two bytes, one of them is the region code from the examination (cf. above), the other is added together with two bytes for the diagnosis by the radiologist. Several codes can be used for one report. The codes are dictated by the radiologist at the end of the report and written together with the text of the whole report on the AURA computer terminal. The reports are then printed for distribution to the wards and stored on magnetic disc for documentation and retrieval.

Diagnostic code (examples)

T Tumor

TA Astrocytoma	TE Ependymoma	TK Craniopharyngioma
TC Carcinoma	TG Glioblastoma	TL Lymphoma
TD Dermoid cyst	TH Pituitary adenoma	TM Medulloblastoma
etc.	....	....

G Vascular lesions

GA Aneurysm	GH Inf. (haemorrhagic)	GS Sclerosis
GI Infarction (ischemic)	GM Malformations	GØ others

Localisations (examples)

C, S Head

C Skin	F Facial bones	A Pituitary gland
E Epiphyses	H Hemisphere	I Cerebellum
G Vessels	S Brainstem	K Bones
etc.	.....	.....

A Abdomen

B Pancreas	A Biliary tract	N Lymph nodes
C Skin	G Vessels	E Mesenterium
D Intestine	H Liver	L Spleen
etc.	....	.....

Examples of report - summaries with codes

Left frontal meningioma HTQ
Multiple metastasis in the liver, dilated bile ducts and gall bladder HTR, AXG

2.3 Implementation

The study started on first of August. Normal results or reports with only marginal findings were not coded although the code lists an item for "normal". For this preliminary study 1693 reports were collected until November 15. 1390 of them are from the head region. Only about one fourth of the reports (412) had been coded.

2.4 Selection of retrieval requests

To allow for an unbiased evaluation (as far as possible), all the retrieval requests concerning CT-examinations, that had been asked during the last four months were reconsidered and if possible reevaluated using both methods, search for keywords in the text and search for codes. From the 13 questions four had no corresponding code. Examples are a request for reports with Sturge-Weber-syndrome (the search had produced 13 reports out of 15.200), a request for pinealis-tumors (73 out of 15.700) or for instances of phacomatosis (7 out of 15.200). The necessity to keep the code as short as possible to limit the overhead for documentation of course prohibits the selective coding and retrieval of rare and very specific findings. Two questions were found to be independent of the diagnostic codes, looking for instances of high resolution head scans and for patients from a certain ward respectively. The seven remaining requests have been reevaluated and three more added, which were thought to be especially adapted to exploit the possibilities of the code.

2.5 Retrieval quality criteria

Intuitively one wants a documentation system to be complete and precise. For a given retrieval request all relevant documents (completeness) but no irrelevant documents (precision) should be produced. These claims are somewhat antagonistic and difficult to fulfill simultaneously. The criteria are formalized by the concept of recall and precision (3), recall being defined as the ratio of the number of all retrieved relevant documents to the number of all stored relevant documents, precision as the ratio of the number of all retrieved relevant documents to the number of all retrieved documents. Both recall and precision range from zero to one.

Recall one means that all relevant reports have been retrieved, precison one that all retrieved reports are relevant.

Recall and precision are not constants of a documentation system. They may be different for different retrieval requests or classes of retrieval requests.

3. RESULTS

3.1 Reevaluation of retrieval requests

In this section we will discuss the results of the reevaluation of questions that were already asked to AURA during the last few months, using both methods, text processing and codes for retrieval. We start with some examples.

3.1.1 Infarction

The original free text retrieval was based on a search for the words infarction or vascular lesion. Applied on the test file it produced 101 reports out of 1390 stored CT-reports, 2 of them were redundant (irrelevant). A search based on the corresponding code produced 73 reports, one of them redundant. Only 32 relevant reports had been found by both methods, free text missed 40 reports and code missed 67. On closer investigation it was found that the misses in the free text search were mostly due to the use of combined words (Multiinfarkt, Hirninfarkt), where the keyword "Infarkt" was part of the word. The free text question was therefore modified, to look also for instances where the term "Infarkt" was part of a combined word. This modified search found 184 reports, two of them again redundant. Only two reports found by the code search were missed because the diagnosis was termed "ischemic lesion". The results for recall and precision are shown below. They are calculated under the assumption, that all relevant reports have been found, if the results of both methods were combined.

	Recall	Precision
original free text retrieval	0.53	0.98
code retrieval	0.39	0.99
modified free text retrieval	0.98	0.99

Misses of code retrieval are due to the fact that a large part of the positive diagnoses was not coded at all, especially during times of high workload (e. g. holidays, when only one radiologist alone had to run the CT-section).

3.1.2 Lesions of the spine

19 reports out of 303 stored CT-examinations of the body were found by the free text search with 14 of them redundant and 5 positive findings. No reports were found by the code request - spinal lesions were never coded. The low precision 0.26 of free text search in this instance is caused by dictating habits. Spinal segments are frequently used to describe the localisation of lesions outside of the spine, e. g.: "paraaortic nodal mass at the level of lumbar segment L3". The original (real life) search was used to find 86 reports out of 2500. If we assume the same low level of precision as in the test file it means that about 60 reports were redundant and had to be thrown out by hand. Still a minor effort compared with a manual search through 2500 reports without documentation system. In this connection it should be mentioned that the computer prints the diagnosis (summary) of all reports found during a search. The radiologist therefore only has to scan the computer output and mark the really interesting before going to the archive for films etc.

3.1.3 Summary

During this study, seven "real-life" search requests have been reevaluated, following the pattern described above. Using free text, recall as defined in the previous sections was usually above 0.9 (that means over 90 percent of all stored relevant reports are retrieved), while precision had a much wider range from 0.25 to 1.00. Using code, recall was always poor (this will be discusses later), precision was higher, comparable with the precision of free text retrieval. In three instances out of seven questions, the formulation of the free text question had to be changed after comparison with code retrieval, in two instances the evaluation resulted in a modification of the codes used for the search. The modifications of the free text question were all of the same kind to look also for the keyword within a combined item. This option was introduced in the system after the first evaluations during this study.

3.2 Evaluation of special requests

Three additional questions were added, asking for items with a direct equivalent in the code: positive findings related to the kidney, positive findings related to the pancreas and pancreatitis. The results are not representative, because of the small numbers, but it is interesting to note, that just in these questions which were explicity designed for code retrieval the results were rather poor.

	text retrieval		code retrieval	
	reports found	correct	reports found	correct
kidney	4	2	0	0
pancreas	8	7	7	3
pancreatitis	2	2	1	1

The poor precision of code retrieval in the case of pancreas findings is an exception, due to a similarity between the codes for normal and for pancreas which led to misspellings.

3.3 Recall and precision

Taking together all the questions we may calculate overall values for recall and precision. The figures below represent the summary of ten retrieval requests with about 750 retrieved reports:

	recall	precision
free text retrieval	0.97	0.93
code retrieval	0.27	0.88

One question asked for cerebral atrophy. In this case it is very difficult to decide, whether a positive finding is normal, marginal or important. Therefore all retrieved reports, where atrophy was mentioned or coded were considered correct. This may be unfair to code retrieval, because marginal atrophies were probably mentioned but not coded. If we omit this question we get the following results:

	recall	precision
free text retrieval	0.96	0.90
code retrieval	0.37	0.86

4. DISCUSSION

Although interest in and use of free text processing for the documentation of medical data is increasing, very few quantitative studies about the quality of retrieval are available (4, 5). The present study tried to evaluate the retrieval quality of an existing free text system based on a search for keywords by parallel manual coding for a limited period. The underlying assumption was that coding would be complete and nearly error free. The preliminary results are summarised in the previous paragraphs show a different picture which is somewhat difficult to interpret. The most serious problem was the low percentage of coded reports, resulting in poor recall of code retrieval. This is certainly to a great part due to a policy error in the setup of the study - we should have asked to code every report - combined with the well known reluctance of physicians for manual coding and cannot be generalised. On the other hand, even if we extrapolate for complete coding, the recall of free text retrieval is high - more than 90 percent of the relevant reports are retrieved.
Concerning precision, free text retrieval values vary considerably, from about 0.25 (only a quarter of the retrieved reports) to 1.00 (all retrieved reports are relevant). We were surprised by the fact, that in our study overall precision of free text retrieval is slightly superior to that of code retrieval.

5. CONCLUSION

The preliminary results of a comparison of free text retrieval versus code retrieval seem to indicate that the overal quality of free text documentation is at least not inferior to the quality of documentation by manual coding. Parallel coding for limited time periods is valuable to gain deeper insight into the factors influencing retrieval quality and to improve the documentation system. Parallel coding as a routine procedure seems to be unnecessary because no significant improvement results.

6. ACKNOWLEDGEMENT

We wish to thank the following institutions for their support: Österreichischer Forschungsfonds, Österr. Krebsliga, Sektion Steiermark.

7. REFERENCES

(1) Gell G, Oser W, Schwarz G: Experience with the AURA Free-Text Documentation system. Radiology 1976; 119: 105 - 109

(2) Gell G: Free Text Analysis: An Attempt to solve the Documentation Problem. In: Lecture notes in Medical Informatics Vol. 1, Berlin - Heidelberg - New York, Springer, 1978: 83 - 89

(3) Vickery BC: Dokumentationssysteme. München - Berlin, Verlag Dokumentation, 1972.

(4) Köhler CO, Wagner G, Wolber U: Computer-assisted Writing of Medical Reports - A Bibliography. Meth. Inf. Med. 1979; 18: 98-102

(5) Kricheff II, Bender A, Chase NE, Korein J: Computer Processing of Clinical Data. In: Computers in Radiology, Basel - München - Paris - New York, Karger; 1970: 306 - 316

RECOMMENDATIONS FOR COMPARABLE MEDICAL RECORD SUMMARIES AMONG HOSPITALS IN THE EUROPEAN COMMUNITY

Francis H. ROGER, MD, MS. [1]
Centre d'informatique médicale de l'Université Catholique de Louvain, Clin. Univ. St-Luc, 10 Avenue Hippocrate, B-1200 Brussels, Belgium.

ABSTRACT

The biomedical information working group of the EEC recommended to restrict medical record documentation to a limited program to be coped with at an international level. A minimum basic data set (13 items) has been selected following the concept first formalised in the US and in the line of results from an enquiry by the WHO in Europe. The present state of availability and of comparability of the MBDS has been investigated. Such data abstracted from inpatients medical records should assume an increasing role in comparative studies of morbidity and health care patterns, clinical and epidemiological research, hospital cost containment, and planning and monitoring of services at all levels. Ten recommendations have been issued as a result of the EEC enquiry.

INTRODUCTION

At a time when most countries are concerned with cost containment in medical care, valuable sources of information are needed for the efficient management and development of health services.

As stated by a WHO report (1), "apart from notification of disease, the most readily available source of extensive data on morbidity is statistics on hospital in-patients. Most countries have hospitals, which almost invariably keep records of each in-patient. Statistical abstraction from such records is fairly readily possible". It is therefore a reasonable function of the EEC to encourage and assist the extension of this aspect of health information.

---

[1] The views expressed in this paper are those of a Consultant and do not necessarily reflect the views of the Commission.

THE EUROPEAN MINIMUM BASIC DATA SET

Since 1975, the BM_3 subgroup of the Biomedical working group (BMWG) of the CIDST (DG XIII) has been involved in developing a Minimum Basic Data Set (MBDS) for hospital information in the nine countries of the EEC.

The set has been selected following the MBDS concept first formalised in the USA (2), and in the light of results from an enquiry by the European Office of WHO on the availability of several items among hospitals in Europe (3).
Thirtheen items have been included in the European MBDS :

1. hospital identification
2. patient's number
3. sex
4. age
5. marital status
6. area of residence
7. month and year of admission
8. duration of stay
9. discharge status
10. main diagnosis
11. other diagnoses
12. surgical and obstetric procedures
13. other significant procedures

This set could be modified by subsequent agreement or expanded locally. Department identification and source of admission are two other important items to be considered.

For international purposes, it was accepted that the MBDS should not contain information which identifies directly a patient. It is desirable, however, that a local identifying number is provided in order to facilitate access to case records through the physicians responsible for the patient's care.

At the European level, the data required for comparative studies do not need to be as detailed as those used locally. A "bottom up" approach was recommended, implying that larger data bases such as extensive medical record summaries developed at the local level could provide a source from which an international, anonymous MBDS could be abstracted.

For example, computed age (item 4) may replace the date of birth, and month and year of admission (item 7) may replace the complete date of admission available in the hospital data base.
Given that these information systems are valuable for local use (clinical research, evaluation, hospital monitoring and management) as well as for regional and national use (population-related morbidity statistics, planning, epidemiologic research, resource allocation), common

definitions would add the advantage to enable international comparisons.

PRESENT STATE OF AVAILABILITY OF THE EUROPEAN MBDS

Following a meeting held in Edinburgh (4) and recommendations from a symposium organized by the Council of Europe (5), the BM_3 subgroup established a questionnaire in order to explore the adequacy, the availability and the degree of comparability of the 13 items selected. Results from the questionnaire were completed by interviews in each country. The purpose of the enquiry was not to cover all ongoing projects in Europe but to assess main differences between representative inpatients data systems for the MBDS in the nine countries. Hospital information systems which did not cover multiple specialities or did not collect any morbidity data were excluded. Table 1 shows the number of answers to the questionnaire by country.

TABLE 1 Number of answers by country

Country	Nber of answers	Country wide population base
Belgium	11	-
Denmark	1	>90 %
France	11	-
W. Germany	9	-
Ireland	3	>83 %
Italy	8	-
Luxembourg	1	-
The Netherlands	8	>90 %
United Kingdom	6	>90 %
TOTAL :	58	

1) Four countries aim at nationwide inpatients morbidity statistics :
- Denmark has a national coverage of non psychiatric data with only three hospitals not participating to the system (one University affiliated and two post-therapeutic institutions for rheumatic diseases).
- In Ireland, the Hospital inpatient enquiry (HIPE) covers 76 % of the Irish beds or more than 83 % of hospital discharges. Only district hospitals (small size) and some private hospitals (non teaching) do not participate to the HIPE. Psychiatric data as well as maternity data are collected separately.
- In the Netherlands, the Stichting Medische Registratie covers 80 % of 250 hospitals, or 90 % of all admissions. 70 % of private hospitals (70 % from 30 % of all hospitals) are excepted as well as a large tea-

ching hospital.

- In United Kingdom, several regions have to be considered. Psychiatric data and maternity data are collected separately.
  - In England and Wales the HIPE gives a 10 % sample from 100 % of non psychiatric inpatients in the National Health Service (NHS). 5 % of beds (private beds) are not covered by NHS.
  - In Scotland 100 % of non psychiatric data are covered, with the exception of 0,5 % of private beds.
  - In Nothern Ireland, 50 % of non psychiatric data are collected through the HIPE. Exceptions (50 %) are made of small hospitals, only non-University hospitals.

2) In five countries, nationwide hospital statistics are not yet available.

In Belgium, present university systems collect data following a uniform input and output required by the Ministry of Health. Discharge summary systems are in development and could be nationwide in the next future (25 % coverage now : all teaching hospitals, and arrays of regional hospitals in Flanders, Charleroi and Antwerpen).

In France, there is a national statistical return which is based on aggregated tables from hospitals. In this system, morbidity data are of low reliability. Beyond that, localized hospitals (some grouped and some isolated) have developed their own information system, that can serve to aggregate some data required by the Ministry. Private hospitals are missing (50 %).

In the Fed. Rep. of Germany, only the largest sickfunds organisations collect some medical data at the Federal level, but of low reliability (admission diagnoses, or diagnoses in relation with reimbursement criteria). Regional efforts to collect morbidity statistics are limited to public hospitals. Private hospitals remain out of scope. Localized hospitals, some grouped and some isolated have developed their own hospital information system including morbidity data.

In Italy, the Central Institute of Statistics collects in principle 1/4 of 1/4 of all Italian inpatients (one record out of 4 is processed for the 7 first days of each month). The last national tables date of 1974. Regions are encouraged to collect their data, without interregional coordination up to now. These efforts are limited to public hospitals and Nothern Italy. Private hospitals are out of scope (more than 40 %).

In Luxembourg, Hospital morbidity statistics are not covered by computerized systems yet. In some hospitals, physicians keep track of the cases through manual indices.

PRESENT STATE OF COMPARABILITY OF THE EUROPEAN MBDS

The elaboration of the questionnaire proved to be an original task in itself. The nature and extent of inconsistencies within the MBDS had to be preidentified and presented in the form of alternatives of definitions and classifications.
The degree of variations among the 13 items of the MBDS from general hospitals in the 9 EEC countries has been discussed elsewhere (6). Medical information systems appear to be strongly linked to health care systems concepts. Among each European country, a better uniformity is reached if nationwide systems have been developed or are in development. Population-based statistics are only available now in the four countries where national statistics are obtained. These countries are therefore in a better position to evaluate hospitals needs, to understand the dynamics of health care costs and to obtain epidemiologic studies.
In the five other countries, however, locally initiated systems are often more extensive, with less omissions of diagnoses, in order to reach the requests of local physicians and hospital administrators for clinical research, the evaluation of the quality of care, as well as for hospital management. A main incentive for the development of the MBDS in Europe is the variety of purposes that can be reached with it, all countries having diverse experiences that could benefit to others. It is given that these information systems are valuable for local uses as well as for regional and national uses, that common definitions in the EEC would add the advantage to enable international comparisons. Hospital inpatients MBDS should be considered as a first step toward a better coordination of medical information systems in Europe. A further step should consider factual data about health care delivered outside hospitals (general practice, outpatient visits, preventive medicine) as soon as they will be more widely available.

RECOMMENDATIONS

Following this EEC enquiry, the following guidelines have been proposed :

1. <u>The European MBDS concept</u>

Any hospital information system (inpatients) currently in operation or in development in the EEC should contain at least the minimum basic data set, e g the core of information with the most commonly available set of items and the most extensive range of usages.

2. <u>Uniformity of the definitions of the variables</u>
All data elements must be defined to promote uniformity but definitions must be sufficiently broad and flexible to accomodate multiple users. There is much to be gained from intra- and international comparability of items collected on hospital inpatients, including discharge diagnoses. Developing a common language of communication is a major objective of the CIDST.

3. <u>Coverage</u>
To serve its purposes, the MBDS should refer to some comprehensive data sources that are common to a broad category of hospitals. The splitting of psychiatric data from non psychiatric data has to be considered as it is common to several European countries and because of particular features applying to that speciality (particular set of hospitals, long stay patients, handicaped or diseased,...). This issue appears more important than the splitting of maternity data.

4. <u>Linkage</u>
The value of hospital inpatient medical record abstracts would be enhanced by the ability to link separate spells of stay for individual patients (spells in a department, hospital stays at different times in the same hospital or in different hospitals). Attention should be given to the incorporation of some mechanisms whereby such linkage could be achieved (unique number by hospital, soundex code, national number,...). Hospital information systems should allow the possibility to link administrative (identification, days of admission and discharge,...) and medical data (diagnoses, operations, other procedures,...) where these are separated for individual patients. Only the elements that are needed for linking different data sets to the same patient should be common to these data sets.

5. <u>Clinical feedback</u>
Those responsible for the development and management of health information systems should seek to ensure that the system is capable of responding to the requirements of individual physicians. The encouragement of a clinical interest in hospital information systems should, as a consequence, help to improve the quality of the clinical data.

6. <u>Population-based system</u>
Hospital information systems in which well defined and currently recorded population censuses are not available suffer a major handicap as they cannot produce rates. Countrywide morbidity statistics should be encouraged in the EEC countries where population-based hospital sta-

tistics are still missing. Attention should be given to limited geographic area with a known population when all hospitals in these areas could provide a MBDS.

7. Sampling

When a total system is not possible, eg the systematic collection of hospital discharge summaries for all inpatients, sampling techniques are recommended.

8. Clearing house

The EEC should establish a clearing house at which would be maintained a list of all the centers where hospital inpatients statistics are held. This list (preferably on computer file) would contain some standard account of each system (type of hospital, information scale, array of variables,...). This recommendation provides a mean of communication that should help to solve remaining problems (applicability of definitions, computer standards, output formats,...).

9. Exchange of data through pilot studies

The mechanisms of exchange of hospital data could hardly be solved without well-designed studies of international data collection and analysis. The EEC should support pilot studies to promote and coordinate uniform data collection and to examine, analyse and make meaningful interpretations of data comparisons. Initial projects might well be limited to hospitals of a similar standard where local agreement could be obtained. Attention should be given to indepth studies of a small set of hospitals versus larger comparisons of country-wide statistics.

10. Workshop

The EEC should sponsor a conference on "Hospital statistics for population-based health care and epidemiology", in coordination with the WHO European Office and European Scientific societies in order to submit the present recommendations to potential exchangers of hospital data, to set up priorities for further work in the use of hospital information systems for management and epidemiology, and to determine who could further agree to cooperate with whom about what in European countries.

REFERENCES

(1) World Health Organisation (1968). Morbidity statistics. Twelfth Report of the WHO Expert Committee on Health Services. Technical Report Series N° 389, Geneva.
(2) United States National Committee on Vital and Health Statistics (1972). Uniform hospital abstract : minimum basic data set. DHEW Publication N° (HSM)73-1451, Washington D.C.
(3) Regional Office for Europe of the World Health Organization (1976). Uses of hospital discharge summary forms in the European Region. ICP/SHS/ 029. Copenhagen.
(4) Kool GA Editor (1976) Hospital statistics and minimum basic data set. Report on a EEC seminar in Edinburgh. November 1975.
(5) Council of Europe (1975). Symposium on Information Systems in the Field of Health. Paris, 1-5 December 1975. Mimeogaphed.
(6) Roger FH. Role of comparable medical record summaries among hospitals in the European Community. Second International Conference on Systems Science in Healthcare, July 14-17, 1980, Montreal, Quebec (in press).

MINIMUM BASIC DATA SET FOR TUMOUR PATIENTS IN THE FEDERAL REPUBLIC OF GERMANY

Gustav WAGNER and Hans WIEBELT
Deutsches Krebsforschungszentrum
Heidelberg, Bundesrepublik Deutschland

SUMMARY

The authors introduce the program of a Minimum Basic Data Set for Tumour Patients developed in 1977/78 which has meanwhile been declared as the obligatory basic program for a coordinated tumour documentation for all tumour centers in the Federal Republic of Germany by the "Arbeitsgemeinschaft Deutscher Tumorzentren - ADT" (Association of German Tumour Centers). The program consists of three parts, a questionnaire for the first examination, a form for follow-up examinations and a final questionnaire. The German data acquisition program is comparable with other national and international projects of a basic documentation of malignant tumours.

INTRODUCTION

In view of its extreme complexity, genuine progress in solving the cancer problem can only be expected from national and international cooperation of scientists. This applies to basic research as well as to experimental and clinical cancer research and also to cancer control in the widest sense. This knowledge has, during the last few years, led to the development of tumour centers or oncological working groups in many countries. In the Federal Republic of Germany this development has been promoted by the Deutsche Krebshilfe e.V. at some German Universities (e.g., Cologne, Essen, Hamburg, Munich).

Within the framework of the tumour centers and oncology-oriented hospitals, the necessary collaboration must extend to all sectors of the cancer problem, i.e. cancer prevention and early detection, cancer diagnostics and therapy, cancer follow-up and rehabilitation. It is indispensable that, in spite of inevitable regional differences in the premises and structures, the therapeutic centers to be set up should strive for as much uniformity and concordance as possible in important functions and activities. The fate of a cancer patient - regardless as to where he may be resident - must in future not depend on the more or less random choice of the primary place of treatment. In this connection let us, for example, refer to the "Guidelines for Developing a Comprehensive Cancer Center" (1978) of the International Union against Cancer (1). Already in 1972 the National Cancer Advisory Board of the USA developed a catalog of criteria to be fulfilled by a tumour center if it strives for recognition as a so-called comprehensive cancer center (2).

Both guidelines place great emphasis on the problems of documentation and data processing. Experts all the world over today largely agree that a uniform clinical documentation with acquisition, storage, processing and evaluation of really comparable data with the aids proffered by modern data processing technology forms the basis of any progress to be made in diagnostics, therapy and follow-up of the cancer patient. Of course, it is necessary, first of all, to ensure the comparability of the data collected, i.e. to see to it that a uniform and generally applicable nomenclature and histopathological classification and also identical criteria for staging the tumours and judging the success of therapy are used.

Realizing the necessity of a standardized clinical documentation for any cooperation on the cancer sector, the representatives of 16 German tumour centers and oncological working groups gathered together in Heidelberg in November 1977 at the initiative of the German Cancer Research Center, agreed to set up, as a first step towards a future cooperation within the framework of the "Arbeitsgemeinschaft Deutscher Tumorzentren" (ADT), a binding basic program for the primary coverage and follow-up of tumour patients. In several meetings a committee under the chairmanship of G. Wagner (Heidelberg), consisting of 42 clinicians, statisticians and data processing experts from the institutions involved, worked out the so-called "Basic Documentation for Tumour Patients" (3). This program integrates local experience as well as the preparatory work of the German speaking TNM Committee and the practical experience gained in three comparable national and international projects (WHO (4), UICC (5), Comprehensive Cancer Centers, USA (6)).

The so-called Version 0 of the program was tested in a pilot study on roughly 1,200 patients in the course of the year 1978. Based on this experience, Version 1 was developed which has been in use in numerous hospitals since the beginning of 1979. At the meeting of the Working Group of German Tumour Centers (ADT) on September 3, 1979 it was decided to take over this version into routine and to call a further revision conference at the beginning of 1981 which should then work out a possibly improved Version 2. For the test phase of Version 1 the forms are printed in Heidelberg and sent to interested hospitals free of charge upon request. The same goes for the brochure "Basisdokumentation für Tumorkranke" (Basic Documentation for Tumour Patients) which contains exact coding instructions.

THE PROGRAM

As an obligatory multicentric program the "Basic Documentation for Tumour Patients" represents but a minimum basic data set; the initiators of the program restricted themselves quite consciously to the acquisition and processing of the most essential data.

The program for the Basic Documentation for Tumour Patient uses three types of questionnaires - 1. the questionnaire for the primary examination of the patient (white), 2. the follow-up questionnaire to be completed at each follow-up examination of the patient (yellow), and 3. the final questionnaire to be completed when the patient ceases to be monitored (red). The first five items serve patient identification; they are identical on all three questionnaires.

The three sets of questionnaires are blocked, prepunched and printed on NCR paper which permits copies being made without the use of carbon paper. The questionnaires are completed by the participating hospitals of follow-up institutions. The original is meant for the central data acquisition institution; the first copy is incorporated into the patient's medical record, the second copy serves to inform the medical practitioner involved in the patient's aftercare.

The questionnaire for the primary examination (Figure 1) of a new cancer patient contains 20 items. Subsequent to the identification features, there follow patient data, e.g., the date of the first diagnosis, the tumour localization, the histological diagnosis, the pretherapeutic and the definitive (postoperative) TNM code, the activity index (according to Karnofsky), the date of the onset of the specific therapy as well as some general information on the kind of therapy. Finally, the date of the first follow-up examination is recorded.

Basisdokumentation für Tumorkranke **Ersterhebung**

1. **Kartenkennzeichen** ☐☐ 2
2. **Klinik-Nr.** ☐☐☐☐ 6
3. **Patientenidentifikation** ☐☐☐☐☐☐☐ 13
4. **Geburtsdatum** Tag, Mon, Jahr ☐☐☐☐☐☐ 19
5. **Geschlecht** (1 = ♂, 2 = ♀) ☐ 20

6. **Staatsangehörigkeit** (Schlüssel siehe Rückseite) ☐☐ 22
7. **Anlaß der Erfassung** ☐ 23
   1 = Patient kommt von selbst, 2 = Krebsdiagnose bei Vorsorge, 3 = Krebsdiagnose durch Hausarzt, 4 = Röntgenreihenuntersuchung, 5 = Zufallsbefund bei anderweitiger Untersuchung, 9 = f.A.
8. **Datum der ersten Diagnosestellung** Tag, Mon, Jahr ☐☐☐☐☐☐ 29
9. **Ersttumor?** (0 = nein, 1 = ja) ☐ 30

10. **Tumorlokalisation** (nach Lokalisationsschlüssel DTNMA) ☐☐☐☐☐ 35
11. **Seitenlokalisation** ☐ 36
    0 = kein paariges Organ, bzw. nicht zutreffend, 1 = nur rechtes Organ, 2 = nur linkes Organ, 3 = beide Organe befallen, 9 = f.A.

12. **Tumordiagnose** (nach ICD-O-DA) ☐☐☐☐☐ 41

13. **Histopathologische Ausdehnung (P)** (nach TNM) ☐☐ 43
14. **Malignitätsgrad (G)** (nach TNM) ☐ 44
    1 = gering, 2 = mittel, 3 = hoch

15a. **Befund prätherapeutisch** ☐☐☐☐☐☐☐☐☐ 53
15b. **verwendeter Code** (Schlüssel siehe Rückseite) ☐ 54

16a. **Befund definitiv** ☐☐☐☐☐☐☐☐☐ 63
16b. **verwendeter Code** (Schlüssel siehe Rückseite) ☐ 64

17. **Allgemeiner Leistungszustand** (Schlüssel siehe Rückseite) ☐ 65

18. **Anderweitig vorbehandelt?** (0 = nein, 1 = ja) ☐ 66

19. **Beginn der spezifischen Behandlung** Mon, Jahr ☐☐☐☐ 70

20. **Art der Behandlung**

	(0) nein	(1) ja	(9) f.A.	
Operation	O	O	O	☐ 71
Strahlentherapie	O	O	O	☐ 72
Chemotherapie	O	O	O	☐ 73
Hormontherapie	O	O	O	☐ 74
Immuntherapie	O	O	O	☐ 75
sonstige:	O	O	O	☐ 76

21. **Termin der ersten Nachuntersuchung** Tag, Mon ☐☐☐☐ 80

....
Unterschrift des Arztes

Version 0

Figure 1: Basic Documentation for Tumour Patients - Initial Questionnaire

Basisdokumentation für Tumorkranke **Folgeerhebung**

1. Kartenkennzeichen ☐☐ 2
2. Klinik-Nr. ☐☐☐☐ 6
3. Patientenidentifikation ☐☐☐☐☐☐☐ 13
4. Geburtsdatum Tag, Mon, Jahr ☐☐☐☐☐☐ 19
5. Geschlecht (1 = ♂, 2 = ♀) ☐ 20

6. Datum der Nachuntersuchung — Tag, Mon, Jahr ☐☐☐☐☐☐ 26
7. Wievielte Nachuntersuchung? ☐☐☐ 29

8. Tumordiagnose (nach ICD-O-DA) ☐☐☐☐☐ 34

9. Allgemeiner Leistungszustand (Schlussel siehe Rückseite) ☐ 35

10. Remissionsgrad ☐ 36
1 = komplette Remission, 2 = partielle Remission, 3 = keine Änderung, 4 = Progression
11. Resttumor ☐ 37
0 = keiner, 1 = <2cm ϕ, 2 = >2cm ϕ
12. Rezidivtumor ☐ 38
0 = keiner, 1 = <2cm ϕ, 2 = >2cm ϕ

13. Rest-Lymphknoten ☐ 39
0 = keine, 1 = einer, 2 = mehrere
14. Rezidiv-Lymphknoten ☐ 40
0 = keine, 1 = einer, 2 = mehrere

15. Rest-Fernmetastasen ☐ 41
0 = keine, 1 = ein Organ, 2 = mehrere Organe
16. Rezidiv-Fernmetastasen ☐ 42
0 = keine, 1 = ein Organ, 2 = mehrere Organe

17. RNM-Befund ☐☐☐☐☐☐☐☐☐ 51

18. Tumorbehandlung seit letzter Nachuntersuchung (bzw. Erstuntersuchung)

	(0) nein	(1) ja	(9) f.A.	
Operation	O	O	O	☐ 52
Strahlentherapie	O	O	O	☐ 53
Chemotherapie	O	O	O	☐ 54
Hormontherapie	O	O	O	☐ 55
Immuntherapie	O	O	O	☐ 56
sonstige:	O	O	O	☐ 57

19. Nächster Nachsorgetermin — Tag, Mon, Jahr ☐☐☐☐☐☐ 63

....
Unterschrift des Arztes

Version 0

Figure 2: Basic Documentation for Tumour Patients - Follow-up Questionnaire

The follow-up questionnaire (Figure 2) serves to fix the findings at the follow-up examinations. The follow-up questionnaire contains 22 items to be covered at every follow-up examination of the patient. Any change in findings is to be recorded on these forms as accurately as possible. Since the date of the follow-up examination is recorded at the same time, it becomes possible to set up a documentation of the course of the disease for any patient and at any time.

Basisdokumentation für Tumorkranke **Abschlußerhebung**

1. Kartenkennzeichen ☐☐ 2
2. Klinik-Nr. ☐☐☐☐ 6
3. Patientenidentifikation ☐☐☐☐☐☐☐ 13
4. Geburtsdatum (Tag, Mon, Jahr) ☐☐☐☐☐☐ 19
5. Geschlecht (1 = ♂, 2 = ♀) ☐ 20

6. Datum des Abschlusses (Tag, Mon, Jahr) ☐☐☐☐☐☐ 26
7. Grund des Abschlusses ☐ 27
   1 = Patient ist verstorben, 2 = Patient ist nicht auffindbar,
   3 = Patient ist aus der Nachsorge ausgeschieden,
   4 = Patient ist anderweitig in Nachsorge, 9 = f.A.

x Bei Verstorbenen:
8. Sterbedatum (Tag, Mon, Jahr) ☐☐☐☐☐☐ 33
9. Todesursache ☐ 34
   1 = tumorabhängig, 2 = tumorunabhängig,
   3 = Tumorabhängigkeit ist nicht auszuschließen, 9 = f.A.
10. Autopsie ☐ 35
   (0 = nein, 1 = ja, 9 = f.A.)

....
Unterschrift des Arztes Version 0

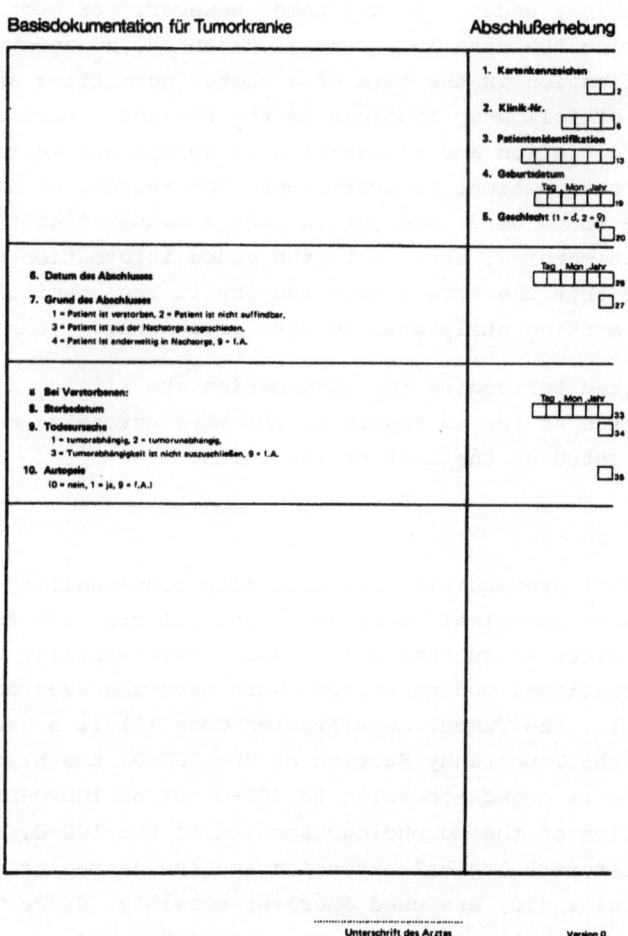

Figure 3: Basic Documentation for Tumour Patients - Final Questionnaire

The final questionnaire (Figure 3) is filled up when the patient is dismissed from monitoring. It contains 11 features and covers the reason for the patient leaving the supervision and - in the case of death - the date of death, the cause of death and the question whether or not an autopsy was carried through.

The vacant field in the left upper corner of every form is to take in each patient's personal data with the aid of an addressette.

For the purpose of clinical follow-up examinations, it is necessary to cover the patient under his full name. However, for storing and further processing the data in a central database, an anonymized patient identification in the form of a number permitting an exact record linkage of follow-up findings to the patient's medical record as well as the detection and elimination of double and multiple reports on the same patient is sufficient. For reasons of data protection, the forms were laid out in such a manner that the perforated right marginal strip with the coded information can easily be separated so that the form itself remains in the hospital and only the anonymized marking strip goes to data processing.

The codes required for coding the information are already printed on the questionnaires as far as possible, the more extensive codes being partly printed on the back of the forms.

DISCUSSION

The most essential prerequisite for attaining comparability of the data is the use of identical codes and identical criteria for evaluation. In order to guarantee as broad a comparability as possible, international coding systems were used wherever possible. Thus, for example, the Tumour Localization Code (7) is a German translation of the Topography Section of the ICD-O; the histological tumour diagnosis is coded according to ICD-O (8) or ICD-O-DA (9), the German translation of the Morphology Section of the ICD-O. For the grading, the histopathological extension and the degree of malignancy the TNM rules (10) are used wherever possible. Since TNM rules do not yet exist for all organ tumours, some other codes must be used for certain tumours, for instance the Evans Classification for the neuroblastomas, the Ann Arbor Classification for the lymphomas, etc. In each case it must be noted which code has been used.

The "Basic Documentation for Tumour Patients" is to be considered as a catalog of items which should be covered by all German cancer centers under any circumstances. Of course, it is left to the discretion of every center to cover additional information facultatively - according to the special sphere of interest. It should merely be safeguarded that in a more extensive program the items of the basic documentation are included and covered according to the coding rules agreed upon. A standardized basic program in the sense described would be an approach towards an exchange of comparable data on a regional, national and international level.

As a second step, a more detailed documentation, differentiated by type of tumour, is to be developed. Within the framework of this additionally envisaged tumour-specific special documentation, questionnaires have meanwhile been worked out for mamma tumours and colon-rectum carcinomas; forms for lung and stomach carcinomas and M. Hodgkin are underway.

REFERENCES

(1) UICC - CICA:
Guidelines for Developing a Comprehensive Cancer Centre.
Geneva: UICC 1978.

(2) Conference on Planning for Cancer Centers.
Cancer 1972; 29: 819-923.

(3) Wagner, G. (Hrsg.):
Basisdokumentation für Tumorkranke, 2. Ausgabe.
Heidelberg: Deutsches Krebsforschungszentrum 1980.

(4) WHO:
Handbook for Standardized Cancer Registries.
Geneva: World Health Organization 1976.

(5) UICC - CICA:
International Cancer Patient Data Exchange Project - Data Manual.
Geneva: UICC 1977; Edit. Geneva 1978.

(6) Centralized Cancer Patient Data System:
Data Acquisition Manual. Seattle, WA: Statistical Analysis and Quality Control Center 1977.

(7) Wagner, G. (Hrsg.):
Tumor-Lokalisations-Schlüssel
2. Auflage. Berlin-Heidelberg-New York: Springer Verlag 1979.

(8) WHO:
ICD-O International Classification of Diseases for Oncology
1st Edition. Geneva: World Health Organization 1976.

(9) Jacob, W., Scheida, Dorothea, Wingert, F. (Hrsg.):
Tumor-Histologie-Schlüssel (ICD-O-DA).
Berlin-Heidelberg-New York: Springer Verlag 1978.

(10) UICC:
TNM-Klassifikation der malignen Tumoren.
Dritte überarbeitete und erweiterte Auflage.
Berlin-Heidelberg-New York: Springer Verlag 1979.

ETUDE DE LA VARIABILITE INTRA ET INTER MEDECINS DANS L'UTILISATION D'UN DOSSIER STANDARDISE DE SURVEILLANCE DES MALADES HYPERTENDUS

Patrice DEGOULET (1), Gilles CHATELLIER (2), Claude DEVRIES (3), Pierre-François PLOUIN (2), Jean-Claude HIREL (3), Joël MENARD (2)

(1) Service d'Informatique Médicale, Hôpital Pitié, 91 boulevard de l'Hôpital, 75634 Paris Cedex 13, France
(2) Hôpital Saint Joseph, Paris
(3) Centre Interuniversitaire de l'Information 2 (CITI 2) et INSERM, Paris

Inter and intra-physician variability were analysed from the computerized ARTEMIS records for 1 260 patients referred to and followed up by the Saint Joseph Hypertension Clinic in Paris, between January 1st, 1978 and December 31st, 1979. For all the clinic's six permanent physicians, the mean response rate in these records to 29 important questions was 98.9 %. The mean rate per individual physician varied from 97.2 % to 99.7 %, and was negatively correlated with physician age. For questions concerning patient interviews (past history, symptoms at the first consultation,etc.), a positive correlation was observed between the proportion of positive answers and physician age. On the other hand, a negative correlation was found between physician age and the proportion of abnormalities recorded during clinical examination. The pulse rates and blood pressure noted were very different, depending on the physician, despite the random allocation of patients to doctors. Throughout 4 successive years of practice, intra-physician variability was only observed with respect to questions which did not require obligatory answers and did not directly concern therapeutic decisions. For all answers, intra-physician variability was far less important than inter-physician variability.

1. INTRODUCTION

La notion de variabilité dans les résultats et l'interprétation des examens de laboratoire est parfaitement admise dans la pratique médicale courante. Devant un résultat biologique le médecin s'interroge autant sur les conditions du prélèvement et la technique utilisée (variabilité liée à la mesure) que sur les caractéristiques du patient (variabilité liée au patient). Au contraire, la notion que le médecin lui-même agisse au cours de son interrogatoire et de son examen clinique comme un instrument de mesure est négligée. Les résultats de toute activité médicale sont cependant conditionnés par cette variabilité de la mesure : subjectivité de l'interrogatoire, qualité de l'examen clinique, expérience individuelle du médecin conditionnant le diagnostic et la thérapeutique (1), fatigabilité du médecin au cours de son exercice...

A côté de la variabilité des malades, quelle est l'importance relative de la variabilité intra et inter médecins ? Quels en sont les facteurs déterminants ? Cet article essaie de donner quelques éléments quantitatifs de réponse à partir de l'analyse statistique des informations recueillies dans le dossier standardisé ARTEMIS des malades hypertendus.

2. MATERIEL ET METHODES

2.1. Evaluation de la variabilité inter médecins

L'évaluation de la variabilité inter médecins est basée sur l'analyse des dossiers informatiques de 1 260 hommes hypertendus adressés en 1978 et 1979 à la consultation d'hypertension artérielle de l'Hôpital Saint Joseph (Paris) et examinés par six médecins. Elle ne concerne que les informations recueillies par ces médecins, lors de la première visite de chaque malade dans le service. Lors de cette visite, d'une durée de 45 minutes, le médecin remplit trois bordereaux informatiques, un bordereau "histoire clinique" contenant essentiellement les données d'interrogatoire (antécédents,recherche de contre indications médicamenteuses), un bordereau "consultation" permettant de décrire l'état clinique lors de cette visite, enfin un bordereau "traitement" contenant les principales décisions thérapeutiques (décision d'un bilan d'hospitalisation, renvoi au médecin traitant, décision de surveillance par le service..). Le mode d'utilisation de ce questionnaire a fait l'objet d'une description détaillée (2, 3).

41 variables ont été considérées(tableaux I à III).

- 20 variables qualitatives, à réponse obligatoire en tout ou rien, codées oui = 1, non = 2. L'absence de réponse positive ou négative est appelée non réponse.

- 12 variables, qualitatives en tout ou rien, mais ne nécessitant une réponse que lorsque le signe recherché est présent (codées oui = 1). L'absence de réponse (non réponse) ne peut dans ce cas être distinguée de la réponse négative.

- 9 variables quantitatives d'interrogatoire ou d'examen nécessitant une réponse obligatoire du médecin (poids, pression artérielle, ...).

Les calculs sont effectués sur chaque variable et pour chacun des six médecins du service : calcul du taux de non-réponses pour les questions à réponse obligatoire, calcul de la moyenne et de l'écart-type pour les variables quantitatives, calculs du taux moyen de réponses positives et valeurs extrêmes pour les variables qualitatives. La comparaison globale des taux de remplissage du médecin est effectuée par le X^2 de Friedman (4). L'existence d'une tendance entre les taux de réponses positives et l'âge des médecins (30 à 47 ans) est recherchée par le X^2 de tendance (5).

2.2. L'évaluation de la variabilité intra-médecins

Elle est effectuée par comparaison chez les 4 médecins présents dans le service depuis 1976 des résultats observés en 1976-1977 à ceux observés en 1978-1979. La méthode d'analyse de variance utilisée (5) permet d'analyser le facteur médecin (variabilité inter médecins), le facteur année (variabilité intra-médecins) et l'interaction médecin-année (variabilité différente des médecins dans le temps).

3. RESULTATS

3.1. Analyse de la variabilité inter-médecins.

3.1.1. Taux de remplissage des questions obligatoires

Le taux moyen de remplissage, calculé pour les 29 questions obligatoires des tableaux I et III, est de 98.9 % (E. T. = 1.3, Minimum 97.2 %, Maximum 99.7 %). La différence globale entre les 6 médecins est significative (X^2 Friedman : 33.6 à 5 DDL, $p < 0.001$). Les taux de remplissage bien que très élevés, sont corrélés négativement et significativement avec l'âge des médecins (n = 6, r = 0,90, $p < 0.01$). Les taux de remplissage aux questions obligatoires ne varient pas ou peu en fonction de la nature des questions (variables qualitatives ou quantitatives, données d'interrogatoire ou données d'examen clinique).

3.1.2. Variables qualitatives : taux de réponses positives

Les taux moyens de réponses positives pour les variables qualitatives en tout ou rien figurent sur les tableaux I et II. A l'exception des questions pour lesquelles la prévalence des réponses positives est faible (inférieure à 5 %), des différences significatives sont habituellement observées entre les médecins.

La fréquence de 5 des 12 signes d'interrogatoire (antécédents personnels, mode de vie, signes fonctionnels) ayant une prévalence supérieure à 10 % est corrélée positivement et significativement avec l'âge du médecin, . Au contraire, la fréquence de 3 des 4 données de l'examen clinique cardiovasculaire (anomalies à l'auscultation cardiaque, présence de souffles sur les trajets vasculaires, anomalies à la lecture de l'électrocardiogramme) est corrélée négativement avec l'âge du médecin.

3.1.3. Variables quantitatives

La moyenne des variables quantitatives obtenues par interrogatoire (âge, poids maximum au cours de la vie, âge lors de la découverte de l'hypertension artérielle, pression artérielle systolique la plus élevée connue) ou reposant sur une mesure précise (poids lors de la première consultation, indice SV1 + RV5 à l'électrocardiogramme) ne diffère pas significativement en fonction du médecin (Tableau III).

TABLEAU I : Variables à réponse obligatoire. Taux de réponses positives en 1978-1979 (-1260 dossiers, 6 médecins)

Age du médecin (années)	Réponses positives (%)	Variabilité Inter-Médecins Min 30	Max 47	X^2_{TOT} (1)	X^2_{TEND} (2)
ANTECEDENTS PERSONNELS					
Prise régulière de tabac	58.9	45.0	71.4	***	N. S.
Insuffisance cardiaque	1.6	0.0	2.3	N. S.	N. S.
coronarienne	4.0	1.8	5.3	N. S.	N. S.
Antécédents neurologiques	11.5	6.4	16.8	*	** (+)
psychiâtriques	10.2	6.8	19.5	*	* (+)
pulmonaires	18.8	15.2	26.3	*	N. S.
digestifs	24.5	20.4	28.4	N. S.	N. S.
Infections urinaires à répétition	2.7	0.0	5.6	*	N. S.
Antécédents uro-néphrologiques	27.5	21.9	35.1	**	*** (+)
Hyperuricémie ou goutte	19.7	12.9	23.7	N. S.	N. S.
(Taux de remplissage moyen (%))	(99.2)	(98.3)	(99.7)		
BILAN DE PREMIERE CONSULTATION					
. Données d'interrogatoire (± Examen Clinique)					
Activité physique régulière	30.6	17.7	38.4	**	*** (+)
Prise régulière de tabac	38.1	28.9	44.3	*	N. S.
Insuffisance cardiaque	0.7	0.0	1.5	N. S.	N. S.
coronarienne	4.8	3.8	6.5	N. S.	N. S.
Artérite des membres inférieurs	3.8	2.2	7.2	N. S.	N. S.
Problème psychiâtrique	6.4	1.4	12.7	***	*** (+)
(Taux de remplissage moyen (%))	(99.1)	(95.7)	(99.8)		
. Données d'examen					
Anomalie auscultation cardiaque	23.3	13.7	57.5	***	*** (-)
Souffle Vasculaire	18.6	8.8	27.7	***	** (-)
Abolition pouls périphériques	5.3	2.3	11.4	***	N. S.
Anomalie à l'ECG	41.2	37.6	55.2	***	*** (-)
(Taux de remplissage moyen (%))	(99.7)	(97.0)	(99.8)		

(1) X^2 total entre les 6 médecins. N. S. = non significatif. * = $p < 0.05$, ** = $p < 0.01$, *** = $p < 0.001$.

(2) X^2 de tendance. (+) = tendance positive en fonction de l'âge des médecins. (-) = tendance négative.

TABLEAU II : Variables à réponse non obligatoire. Taux de réponses positives en 1978-1979 (1 260 dossiers, 6 médecins)

	Réponses Positives (%)	Variabilité Inter-Médecins Min	Max	X^2_{TOT}	X^2_{TEND}
ANTECEDENTS PERSONNELS					
Asthme	6.0	4.4	6.5	N. S.	N. S.
Ulcère gastro-duodénal	5.2	3.5	6.1	N. S.	N. S.
Dépression	8.9	7.6	13.3	N. S.	N. S.
BILAN PREMIERE CONSULTATION					
. Signes fonctionnels					
Dyspnée d'effort	9.4	3.5	17.7	***	N. S.
Précordialgies	11.9	1.8	19.7	***	*** (+)
Angor d'effort	1.8	0.9	2.6	N. S.	N. S.
Céphalées	28.9	18.5	36.8	***	N. S.
Vertiges	12.4	2.7	24.8	***	N. S.
. Examen Clinique					
Souffle carotidien	8.2	2.6	13.7	**	N. S.
Souffle fémoral	5.1	1.7	8.8	**	** (-)
Abolition pouls pédieux	4.4	1.8	8.9	**	N. S.
Abolition pouls tibial postérieur	4.0	2.5	7.2	N. S.	N. S.

TABLEAU III : Variables quantitatives à réponses obligatoires : valeurs moyennes ± ET en 1978-1979 (1 260 dossiers. 6 médecins)

	Variabilité inter médecins m ± ET	Min	Max	F (1)
ANTECEDENTS. HISTOIRE CLINIQUE				
Age	46.0±14.8	44.2±14.9	47.1±14.9	N. S.
Poids Maximum (kg)	81.1±13.4	80.7±15.0	82.0±14.4	N. S.
Age de découverte HTA (années)	39.1±14.5	36.1±15.1	40.2±13.8	N. S.
P. A. S. Maximum Connue (mmHg)	200.4±29.4	199.7±27.2	201.8± 32.4	N. S.
(Taux de remplissage moyen (%))	(99.0)	(96.9)	(99.9)	
BILAN DE PREMIERE CONSULTATION				
Poids (Kg)	77.1±12.3	76.6±13.3	77.7±14.3	N. S.
P. A. S. (mmHg)	160 ±26.5	145.6±24.5	171.8±24.8	***
P. A. D. (mmHg)	93.4±16.1	84.2±12.7	102.5±14.9	***
Pouls (/mn)	74.0±11.6	69.4±12.6	75.6±10.7	***
E. C. G. (SV1 + RV5) (mm)	27.5± 9.5	27.2± 9.1	28.5± 9.7	N. S.
(Taux de remplissage moyen (%))	(99.0)	(97.1)	(99.8)	

(1) Analyse de variance. NS = Non Significatif. *** = p < 0.001.

Au contraire, la pression artérielle systolique ou diastolique et le pouls diffèrent très significativement en fonction du médecin examinateur. L'intervalle entre le chiffre moyen le plus bas et le chiffre moyen le plus élevé est de 16.2 mmHg pour lapression systolique, de 18.3 mmHg pour la pression diastolique et de 5.1 pulsations/minute pour le pouls.

3.2. Etude de la variabilité intra-médecin

3.2.1. Variables qualitatives

Les fréquences des réponses positives analysées chez les 4 médecins permanents du service, ne diffèrent pas significativement chez les malades examinés en 1978-1979 de celles mesurées en 1976-1977 pour les variables à réponses obligatoires et pour les variables à réponses non obligatoires concernant les antécédents personnels (asthme, ulcère gastro duodénal, dépression) ou l'examen clinique (souffles sur les trajets vasculaires, abolition des pouls). Au contraire, la fréquence de 4 des 5 signes fonctionnels cardiaques ou neurologiques notés à la première consultation (dyspnée d'effort, précordialgies, céphalées, vertiges) est plus basse en 1978-1979 qu'en 1976-1977. L'analyse de variance à deux facteurs (facteur médecin et facteur année) confirme l'existence d'un facteur médecin significatif ($p < 0.001$) pour la dyspnée d'effort , les céphalées et les vertiges et d'un facteur année significatif ($p < 0.05$) pour la dyspnée d'effort et les céphalées. En aucun cas l'interaction médecin-année n'est significative, ce qui montre la constance dans le temps des différences entre chaque médecin.

3.2.2. Variables quantitatives

L'analyse de variance à deux facteurs (médecin et année) effectuée sur les variables quantitatives du tableau III et pour les 4 médecins permanents du service, confirme l'existence d'un facteur médecin significatif pour la pression artérielle systolique ou diastolique de première consultation et le pouls ($p < 0.001$). Elle met en évidence un facteur année significatif pour la pression artérielle systolique et diastolique ($p < 0.001$) et l'indice SV1 + RV5 à l'ECG ($p < 0.05$), paramètres dont les moyennes sont plus faibles en 1978-1979 qu'en 1976-1977. L'interaction médecin-année est significative pour le pouls ($p < 0.05$), les pressions artérielles systoliques ($p < 0.01$) et diastolique ($p < 0.10$).

4. DISCUSSION

4.1. La qualité du remplissage d'un dossier informatique

Les données recueillies par le système ARTEMIS le sont grâce à l'utilisation par différents médecins d'un dossier médical standardisé qui a complètement remplacé le dossier médical traditionnel. L'évaluation de la fiabilité des informations enregistrées est une étape essentielle de l'évaluation d'un tel dossier informatique.

Des taux moyens de remplissage de 98 % pour les questions à réponses obligatoires avaient été observés dans les premières années d'utilisation (2). Ces résultats se maintiennent parfaitement au cours des années suivantes, et aucune lassitude n'apparaît chez les quatre premiers utilisateurs du dossier, tandis que deux nouveaux utilisateurs ont un coefficient de remplissage de 99.6 et de 98.9 %. Néanmoins, autour d'un taux moyen de remplissage de 98.9 %, les différences sont très significatives entre les médecins, et l'on retrouve pour la seconde fois une corrélation négative statistiquement significative entre l'âge du médecin, et le taux de remplissage du dossier (3). Néanmoins, les taux de remplissage sont largement suffisants pour répondre à l'objectif fixé initialement : prendre en compte avec la même certitude les réponses positives et les réponses négatives, en éliminant le risque d'oubli des questions que le médecin doit formuler.

4.2. Variabilité inter-malades et variabilité inter-médecins

Il est évident qu'à l'intérieur d'une même maladie, l'hypertension artérielle, existent des différences importantes entre les malades : âge, poids, passé pathologique, état de santé actuel. La répartition aléatoire des malades entre les différents médecins dans un service public dépourvu de consultation privée permet d'attribuer à chacun des 6 médecins des groupes d'hypertendus comparables. Sur les données d'interrogatoire, les valeurs numériques permettant une définition de la maladie sont identiques entre les malades vus par ces médecins : poids maximum au cours de la vie, âge de découverte de l'hypertension, pression artérielle systolique maximale connue. Le jour de la consultation, les variables indépendantes de toute influence du médecin (poids, indice SV1 + RV5 sur l'électrocardiogramme) ne diffèrent pas significativement. Par contre, des différences très importantes existent entre les malades vus par les 6 médecins, quant à leurs chiffres de pression artérielle systolique et diastolique, et à leur rythme cardiaque. La répartition au hasard des malades entre les médecins rend peu vraisemblable une orientation préférentielle des malades en fonction de leur gravité vers l'un ou l'autre des médecins. Que les différences puissent être dues à l'influence du médecin lui-même sur le pouls et les chiffres tensionnels est par contre un phénomène bien connu et qui s'intègre avec les difficultés multiples de définition de la maladie hypertensive (7).

Pour les variables qualitatives à réponses obligatoires, huit fois sur vingt, il existe des différences très significatives entre les médecins. Les phénomènes pathologiques retrouvés par l'interrogatoire sont d'autant plus nombreux que le médecin est plus âgé, les anomalies d'examen sont retenues d'autant plus souvent que le médecin est plus jeune. La variabilité entre les médecins est certainement dépendante d'une multitude de facteurs, dont le plus important est sans doute l'interaction médecin-malade, mais trois fois au cours de ce travail, l'âge du médecin semble influencer les résultats : le remplissage du dossier, la découverte d'antécédents pathologiques, la mise en évidence d'anomalies d'examen.

Pour les variables à réponses non obligatoires, les différences entre les 6 médecins sont importantes lorsque le symptôme est fréquent dans le groupe des malades (céphalées, vertiges, dyspnée d'effort et précordialgies) et sans influence majeure sur la conduite thérapeutique. La variabilité entre les médecins est bien moindre et non significative pour les 4 données d'interrogatoire ayant une influence directe sur le choix des thérapeutiques (asthme, ulcère gastro-duodénal, dépression et angor d'effort). La plus grande rareté de ces troubles par rapport aux désordres fonctionnels peut expliquer l'absence de différence significative entre les médecins. Néanmoins, les anomalies d'examen clinique (souffles vasculaires, abolition des pouls...) dont la prévalence est voisine sont-elles très influencées par le médecin. On peut donc suggérer que toute variable reconnue par le médecin comme étant susceptible d'avoir une influence certaine sur le choix thérapeutique est analysée de telle sorte que les différences entre les médecins sont atténuées. Ce n'est pas le cas lorsque les signes ou les symptômes étudiés sont plus reliés à une description conforme à l'enseignement reçu qu'aux modalités pratiques de l'intervention thérapeutique.

4.3. Variabilité des médecins dans le temps

L'analyse des taux de réponses positives observés de 1976 à 1979 est rendue possible par la qualité constante du remplissage des dossiers informatisés. Elle ne met pas en évidence de facteur année significatif, sauf pour quelques symptômes fréquents et d'importance pratique discutable pour la décision thérapeutique (céphalées, dyspnée). Les variations dans le temps des chiffres moyens de pression artérielle notés par les médecins sont associées à la variation simultanée d'un paramètre objectif : la moyenne de l'indice SV1 + RV5 sur l'échocardiogramme est plus faible chez les malades examinés en 1978-1979 que chez les malades examinés en 1976-1977. Le classement des médecins suivant les valeurs du pouls et de la pression artérielle est le même en 1978-1979 qu'en 1976-1977. Très probablement les différences observées, lorsqu'elles existent, sont plus le reflet d'une gravité moindre des malades vus en 1978-1979 par comparaison à 1976-1977 que de modification dans le temps des comportements des médecins. Dans tous les cas, la variabilité intra médecin apparaît plus faible que la variabilité inter médecins.

4.4. Les conséquences de la variabilité des médecins

Que les malades soient différents les uns des autres est une donnée indiscutable. Que les examens complémentaires aient une variabilité qu'il faille prendre en compte dans l'interprétation des résultats est un concept relativement récent, mais bien accepté. Que les médecins diffèrent les uns des autres au moment où ils sont placés devant les mêmes problèmes, est un concept que l'on suspecte raisonnablement, mais que ni les médecins ni leurs malades ne sont prêts à accepter facilement. Le dossier médical standardisé du système ARTEMIS a permis de mesurer cette variabilité entre les médecins. Les résultats obtenus l'ont été dans les conditions optimales de standardisation de l'exercice médical : répartition aléatoire des malades entre les médecins, entrainement uniforme des six médecins sur la maladie hypertensive deux ans et plus avant la réalisation de cette évaluation, utilisation d'un plan de consultation et d'un recueil de l'information standardisés. On peut donc penser que la variabilité mesurée ici a toutes les chances d'être minimisée par comparaison à ce qui serait observé chez des médecins de formations très diverses et exerçant dans de multiples centres. Les conséquences de cette variabilité entre les médecins sont multiples. Pour les malades, un fait rassurant apparaît : lorsque le problème a une importance majeure, les médecins diffèrent moins les uns des autres. Mais toutes les variables qui sont influencées par le médecin vont modifier les soins du malade. Par exemple, la découverte de souffles cardiaques ou carotidiens conduit au minimum à la pratique d'investigations complémentaires, dont la fréquence va donc être inéluctablement influencée par le médecin, indépendamment de règles médicales apprises de façon identique. C'est finalement sur la mesure tensionnelle elle-même, critère majeur du diagnostic et de la surveillance qu'apparaît une variabilité inter médecins susceptible d'influencer directement la conduite thérapeutique. Une méthode de mesure qui serait indépendante de la relation médecin-malade permettrait certainement dans de nombreux cas d'éviter la décision, ou au contraire de corriger l'abstention, d'un traitement médicamenteux à vie.

REFERENCES

(1) Shapiro AR. The evaluation of clinical predictions. A method and initial application. N Engl J Med. 1977 ; 296 : 1509-1514.

(2) Degoulet P, Ménard J, Berger C, Plouin PF, Devriès C, and Hirel JC. Hypertension management : the computer as a participant. Am J Med. 1980 ; 68 : 559-567.

(3) Degoulet P, Ménard J, Devriès C, Berger C, Hirel JC. Computerized evaluation of medical activities in hypertension care. in : Lindberg DAB and Kaihara S. Medinfo 80. Amsterdam : North-Holland, 1980 ; 607-610.

(4) Siegel R. Non parametric statistics for the behavioural sciences. New York, Tokyo : Mc Graw-Hill. 1956 ; 166.

(5) Armitage P. Statistical Methods in Medical Research. New York : John Wiley & Sons. 1971 ; 362-393.

(6) Lebart L, Morineau A, Fenelon JP. Traitement des données statistiques. Paris : Dunod. 1979 ; 215-236.

(7) Pickering G. Hypertension : definitions, natural history and consequences. Am J Med. 1972 ; 52 : 570-582.

COMPUTER-AIDED CLASSIFICATION OF CHRONIC DISEASES

R. Thurmayer, E. Eberle and H. Tyrell

Institut für Medizinische Informatik und Systemforschung der Gesellschaft für Strahlen- und Umweltforschung mbH., München, W. Germany

Summary

Methods for computer-aided classification of severity grades for the following three chronic diseases were developed: chronic bronchitis, chronic ischemic heart disease, chronic diseases of the joints and connective tissues.

A team of physicians assigned one out of four severity grades to each patient taking part in the study. Simultaneously, a computer program calculated severity grades when a certain combination of items in a questionnaire applied to a patient.

The so-called accuracy rate was determined by dividing the number of patients with the two resulting severity grades in agreement by the total number of patients. The accuracy rate amounted to 81.0% in chronic bronchitis, 91.9% in chronic ischemic heart disease, and 91.5% in the chronic diseases of the joints and connective tissues.

Introduction

In this paper we would like to present computerized methods for determining severity grades in chronic diseases. These methods have been developed in our institute in cooperation with the German social security agencies Verband Deutscher Rentenversicherungsträger (VDR) and Bundesversicherungsanstalt für Angestellte (BfA). The diseases under investigation were chronic bronchitis, chronic ischemic heart disease, and the chronic diseases of the joints and connective tissues ((1),(2),(3),(4)).

The purpose of a computerized severity grading is to facilitate the assessment of a disease, and allow comparisons between different cases.

Moreover, it is possible to derive admission criteria for rehabilitation therapy on this basis.

Methods

Questionnaires for each of the diseases were developed, enabling the pertinent clinical data of a patient to be filled in. In field tests a number of physicians had to file such a questionnaire whenever the proper diagnosis applied to a patient seeking rehabilitation therapy. The questionnaires were used by a team of experts in our institute to assign one out of four severity grades to the patient.

Simultaneously, symptoms and signs pertaining to one severity grade on the basis of clinical considerations, were put in the form of Boolean equations. A computer program was written to assign the appropriate severity grade to a patient in case such a Boolean equation applied. Figure 1 shows an example of the Boolean equations in the FORTRAN-like form used as an input in the computer program.

```
V080  Condition Related to Prev.Myoc.Infarction
V081  Condition Related to Prev.Myoc.Re-infarct.
V082  Cardiac Aneurysm
V108  ST Segment > 0.2 during Rest
V109  ST Segment > 0.2 during Exertion

Y(01) = IF (V080 EQ 2) THEN 3 ELSE 0
Y(02) = IF (V081 EQ 2 OR V080 EQ2 AND (V108 EQ 2
        OR V109 EQ 2)) THEN 4 ELSE 0
```

Figure 1: Boolean equations for severity grades in myocardial infarction

Results

As the computerized severity grading is based on physician-made Boolean

equations, we feel it is warranted to speak of rebuilding a physician's decision by means of a computerized method. Thus, any measure recording the accordance of the two methods of severity grading should mirror the quality of the computer-aided classification. We used the so-called accuracy rate as such a measure. This was determined by dividing the number of patients with the two resulting severity grades in agreement by the total number of patients taking part in the study.
In our early attempts we used a maximum of items in the questionnaires of importance for the grading to formulate the Boolean equations. They amounted to 39 in chronic bronchitis, 44 in the chronic ischemic heart disease, and 112 in the chronic diseases of the joints and connective tissues. The resulting accuracy rates were 97.5%, 98.6% and 99.2%.

We then tried to reduce the items involved in a stepwise manner until the accuracy rate declined to about 60% to 70%. For such an accuracy rate, a number of 10 to 20 items proved to be sufficient. Ultimately, a collection of 26 items, 21 items, and 32 items was selected to describe the severity grading in the three diseases under investigation. The corresponding accuracy rates were 81.0%, 91.9 and 91.5%.

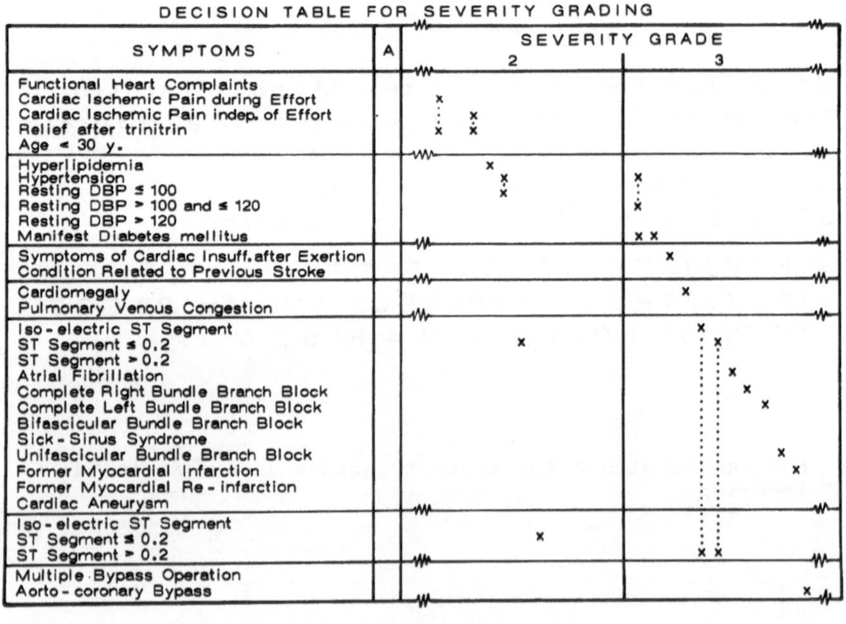

DECISION TABLE FOR SEVERITY GRADING

SYMPTOMS	A	SEVERITY GRADE 2	SEVERITY GRADE 3
Functional Heart Complaints			
Cardiac Ischemic Pain during Effort		x	
Cardiac Ischemic Pain indep. of Effort		x	
Relief after trinitrin		x x	
Age < 30 y.			
Hyperlipidemia		x	
Hypertension		x	x
Resting DBP ≤ 100		x	
Resting DBP > 100 and ≤ 120			x
Resting DBP > 120			
Manifest Diabetes mellitus			x x
Symptoms of Cardiac Insuff. after Exertion			x
Condition Related to Previous Stroke			
Cardiomegaly			x
Pulmonary Venous Congestion			
Iso-electric ST Segment			x
ST Segment ≤ 0.2		x	x
ST Segment > 0.2			
Atrial Fibrillation			x
Complete Right Bundle Branch Block			x
Complete Left Bundle Branch Block			x
Bifascicular Bundle Branch Block			
Sick-Sinus Syndrome			
Unifascicular Bundle Branch Block			x
Former Myocardial Infarction			x
Former Myocardial Re-infarction			
Cardiac Aneurysm			
Iso-electric ST Segment			
ST Segment ≤ 0.2		x	
ST Segment > 0.2			x x
Multiple Bypass Operation			
Aorto-coronary Bypass			x

Figure 2: Decision table for severity grading

To ease the grading procedure, decision tables were developed using the above mentioned final set of items. Our decision table, as shown in figure 2, deviates from the usual form. It consists of several columns. The A-column is for the user to enter the symptoms and signs he observes in a patient. Columns 1 to 3 contain specific combinations of symptoms marked by dotted lines which are intercepted by X's. To use the table one makes entries into column A, and goes on to the columns 1 to 3 until a combination of symptoms and signs in column 1,2, or 3 applies. The patient is then given the severity grade of the appropriate column.

Moreover, an easy-to-use severity-grading device was constructed in the form of a modified slide-rule (figure 3). It is made up of a cover and a tongue. The tongue can be moved underneath the cover making combinations of symptoms and signs appear in a column-shaped window on the cover. When a certain combination applies one can read the appropriate severity grade in another window on the cover.

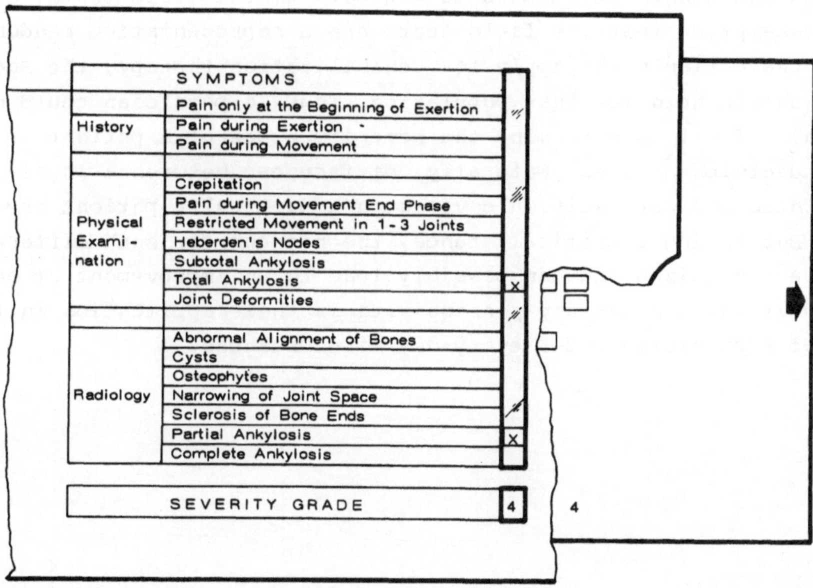

Figure 3: Slide-rule for severity grading

Discussion

The severity grading in the form of Boolean equations is based on clinical considerations. The validity of the equations was checked in field tests. The results showed that some needed completion or correction. Some of the items had rarely been filled in in the field tests, and were removed from the equations to avoid the problem of missing values.

In practice, a severity grading using some 100 items would certainly not be feasible. But the very high accordances between the computerized and the physician-made severity grading, suggest a reduction of the number of items involved in the determination of the severity grades. Feeling that one should not go below an accuracy rate of 80% we are inclined to regard 20 to 30 items as the best result obtainable with our data.

The Boolean equations are adapted to the data of the field tests, and with the assumption that the field tests are a representative random sample of the patients who apply for rehabilitation therapy, the Boolean equations should hold for that population. Thus, a physician could be aided in his effort to determine the severity grade of a patient by using our decision devices. Naturally, differences between a physician's opinion and our decision devices on a particular patient are possible. But taking a critical stance, the reasons for such differences will be recognized and can possibly lead to an improvement of our decision devices. A necessary prerequisite is their application in the practice of a physician under every-day circumstances.

References

(1) Thurmayr R, Schütz I, Kaliebe R, Schnieders H, Karl K, Fürnthaler E. Computer-aided classification of chronic bronchitis in comparison with other diagnostic tools. In: Lecture notes in Medical Informatics Europe 78 - First Congress of the European Federation for Medical Informatics, Proceedings, Cambridge, England, 4.-8.9.1978 (Ed.: J. Anderson), Berlin-Heidelberg-New York: Springer, 1978; 293-302.

(2) Thurmayr R et al. Computerunterstützte Bestimmung des Schweregrades bei der chronischen Bronchitis. In: Informationsverarbeitung in der Medizin - Wege und Irrwege. Bericht über die 22. Jahrestagung der GMDS, 3.-5.10.1977 (Ed.: C.Th. Ehlers) F.K. Schattauer, Stuttgart 1978.

(3) Thurmayr R, Schütz I, Kaliebe R, Schnieders H. Computer-aided classification of chronic bronchitis. Abstracts of the 1st. Annual WAMI Meeting (Annals of the World Association for Medical Informatics) Symposium on Medical Informatics, Toulouse, France, 14.-17.3.1978, 14, 1978.

(4) Schnieders H, Kaliebe R, Laux S, Schütz I, Thurmayr R, Fürnthaler E, Karl K. Praxisbezogene Vorschläge zur Diagnostik und Schweregradeinteilung der chronischen nichtspezifischen Atemwegserkrankungen (CNSRD). Praxis und Klinik der Pneumonologie 1979; 33: 917-933.

Acknowledgements

This work was done under the sponsorship and in cooperation with the Bundesversicherungsanstalt für Angestellte (BfA) in Berlin and the Verband Deutscher Rentenversicherungsträger (VDR) in Frankfurt. We gratefully acknowledge our indebtedness to Dr. med. Kaufmann, Prof. Dr. med. Mäurer, Dr. med. Neuhäuser, Dr. med. Schulz, Dr. med. Josenhans, Dr. med. König and Dr. med. Schütz for their continuous help and advice. Thanks also to Prof. Dr. med. H.-J. Lange for his support in the statistical methodology used in the study.

QUE DOIT CONTENIR LE DOSSIER D'UN MALADE CHRONIQUE ?

Jean-Marie MARTIN and Jean MARTIN
Groupe INSERM U115
Facultés de Médecine - Université de Nancy I
BP 184 54500 Vandoeuvre les Nancy - FRANCE

SUMMERY

Our aim is the automatic processing of the complete original medical record. This record is characterized by :

- the evolutivity of medical notions
- the problem of medical and administrative content of any record

We essentially study the problem of informational content discribing the patient's state of health.

Thus, we propose some methodological principles which help us to obtain a more complete content being more representative with the reality of each clinical case. We think that these processes are necessary in order to apply the epidemiological method.

I - INTRODUCTION

Il semble raisonnable que le dossier médical soit l'image la plus représentative possible de l'état de santé du malade au cours du temps.

"La pratique du dossier médical en milieu hospitalier est d'une extrême médiocrité" affirment GREMY et Coll.

Nous avons fait, comme beaucoup d'autres, la même constatation. La plupart des dossiers, lorsqu'ils sont repris, sont soit incomplets, soit mal remplis ou soit même peu lisibles. Juger un dossier "incomplet" suppose implicitement que l'on puisse constater une "différence" avec ce que devrait être un dossier complet. Ce dernier n'existe évidemment pas ; d'où le problème de ce que devrait contenir chaque dossier.

La confection, en fonction de ses contenus, d'un dossier quelconque se fait par approximations successives, au fur et à mesure de l'avancement de la connaissance médicale du malade, au long de la période de suivi.

Au total, pour remédier à la médiocrité des dossiers existants, il faut proposer des modes opératoires dont la mise en oeuvre apporte une aide efficace aux cliniciens.

II - LE CONTENU DU DOSSIER - DELIMITATION DU PROBLEME

Le problème du contenu du dossier médical peut être envisagé selon plusieurs points de vue. Nous ne faisons que signaler certains d'entre eux, pour insister sur trois méthodes de détermination de contenu. Ces trois méthodes sont envisageables et réalisées (au moins les deux 1ères), parce qu'elles s'inscrivent dans le cadre de l'informatisation du dossier.

2-1 Contenu documentaire

Il s'agit dans ce cas d'analyser le dossier selon les divers documents qu'il contient, indépendamment des informations consignées sur ces documents. Cet aspect du contenu débouche sur une évaluation des volumes (poids) de documents archivés et donc sur les moyens matériels à mettre en oeuvre pour les stocker et les manipuler plus facilement. Bien qu'intéressant, nous n'envisageons pas cet aspect ici.

2-2 Contenu informationnel

2-2-1 Définition

Le contenu informationnel peut être considéré comme la collection des informations consignées dans le dossier pour atteindre certains objectifs tels que :

- aide-mémoire pour les soins
- recherche médicale
- évaluation économique.

2-2-2 Contenu et variations selon le référentiel.

On pourrait envisager le problème du contenu sous l'angle des variations selon que l'on fait intervenir :

- plusieurs observateurs pour le même malade
- la manière différente de poser les questions selon les observateurs
- l'intervalle de temps séparant deux observations du même malade, par le même médecin
- etc

Dans la plupart des études qui ont été menées dans ce sens et que nous ne considérons pas ici, les auteurs tentent de montrer que la prise d'observation médicale est sensiblement objective et reproductible. Les variations selon le référentiel, bien que non nulles, peuvent être minimisées [4] [5]

III - METHODES DE DETERMINATION DE CONTENU

3-1 Contenu et questionnaire d'enquête

Le questionnaire d'enquête (q. d'e.) consiste à extraire un certain nombre de notions d'un champ d'activité. Cette opération conduit la plupart du temps à un nombre de notions limité à quelques centaines. Le choix qui est fait pour chaque notion (acceptation ou refus) solutionne radicalement le problème du contenu d'un dossier.

Les notions retenues dans le questionnaire le sont en général de manière très empirique : elles apparaissent "importantes" aux utilisateurs dans la perspective de travaux de recherche ou d'objectifs cliniques ou biologiques.

3-2 Contenu et dossier minimum

Définition : le dossier minimum peut être considéré comme un ensemble de notions à occurrence unique durant toute la vie du malade, qui contribuent à décrire son état de santé et sa situation administrative.

3-2-1 Dossier à transcription

Parmi d'autres, une manière d'acheminer le dossier médical en ordinateur consiste à utiliser un langage de transcription manuelle. Evidemment, cette opération aboutit dans le meilleur des cas à un dossier machine, au plus égal au dossier réel.

Pour remédier à l'absence de renseignements, nous éditons automatiquement et de façon personnalisée la liste des renseignements appartenant au dossier minimum théorique et n'appartenant pas au dossier réel correspondant. La figure 1 représente une feuille de demande de renseignements manquants. Les renseignements retrouvés sont inclus sans les dossiers informatisés en utilisant des procèdures de mise à jour existantes.

3-2-2 Collecte conversationnelle

Sa mise en place actuelle permettra d'arriver au même résultat mais dans des délais beaucoup plus courts, des contraintes pour la validation et la correction beaucoup moins lourdes que par des procédés en temps différé.

3-3 Contenu et évolutivité

Soient r visites (consultations ou hospitalisations)

$$V_1, V_2, \ldots\ldots, V_r$$

au cours desquelles le médecin a noté, pour le malade X, différentes notions

$$N_i, \ (i = 1, 2, \ldots, k)$$

représentées dans le dossier par leurs occurrences

$$N_i^l \quad (l = 1, 2, \ldots, r) \text{ au cours du temps}$$

NO. ARCHIVES le 27/07/78

PRIERE DE REMETTRE CES 2 FEUILLES

AU SECRETARIAT OU

AU DR POINTEL - MERCI

NOMBRE D'ENFANTS NES VIVANTS : 7

DATE DE NAISSANCE DE LA FILLE

DE LA FILLE

DE LA FILLE

DE LA FILLE

HEREDITE : NOMBRE TOTAL D'ONCLES PATERNELS ?

D'ONCLES MATERNELS ?

DE TANTES PATERNELLES ?

DE TANTES MATERNELLES ?

DE FRERES ?

DE SOEURS ?

DE FILS ?

DATE DU MARIAGE ?

FIGURE 1

A chaque visite l, le dossier présente un certain contenu, noté C_1.

Nous utilisons les r contenus C_1, C_2..... C_r déjà aquis, pour aider à l'élaboration du contenu C_{r+1} d'une nouvelle visite.

<u>Exemple</u> : (volontairement schématique) (cf Figures 2 et 3)

. Un malade X est venu consulter par deux fois : V_1, V_2

. Lors de la visite V_1, on a noté dans son dossier :

$$C_1 = \left| \begin{array}{l} \text{T.A. max = 17,5} \\ \text{Urée sanguine = 2,30} \\ \text{Léger bloc de branche partiel à gauche} \end{array} \right| \begin{array}{l} n_1^1 \\ n_2^1 \\ n_3^1 \end{array}$$

. Lors de la visite V_2, on a noté dans son dossier :

$$C_2 = \left| \begin{array}{l} \text{T.A. max. = 16} \\ \text{Bloc de branche partiel à gauche} \\ \text{Atteinte réno-vasculaire} \end{array} \right| \begin{array}{l} n_1^2 \\ n_3^2 \\ n_4^2 \end{array}$$

. Le malade X est hospitalisé, soit V_3

Au début de V_3 le contenu du dossier est :

$$C_1 \cup C_2 = \left\{ n_1^1,\ n_2^1,\ n_3^1,\ n_1^2,\ n_3^2,\ n_4^2 \right\} = C_{1,2}$$

Ce contenu $C_{1,2}$ édité en clair, ou mieux visualisé sur écran cathodique, suggère que durant l'hospitalisation V_3 le médecin observe et note dans le dossier au moins les deux notions N_1 et N_3. Selon son appréciation de la plus ou moins grande normalité de la notion N_2, notée n_2^1 lors de la visite V_1, il pourra ou non redemander une mesure de la notion N_2 et de même pour la notion N_4.

De plus, le médecin aura la totale liberté d'inclure toute autre notion N_5,N_6.. qui ne serait pas encore apparue lors des visites précédentes.

IV - <u>DISCUSSION</u>

. La méthode décrite au § 2-2 est mise en place pour plus de 3000 dossiers déjà introduits en ordinateur. Nous arrivons à un remplissage quasi-exhaustif de tous les dossiers informatisés par rapport au dossier minimum. Ce résultat n'a été possible que parce que le dossier minimum présente, par nature, un contenu fixe.

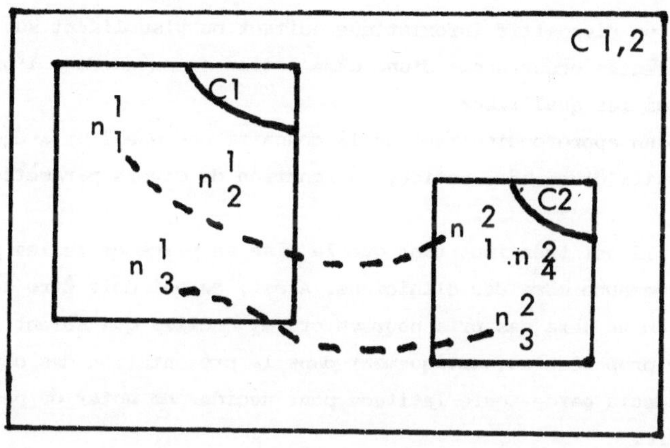

FIGURE 2

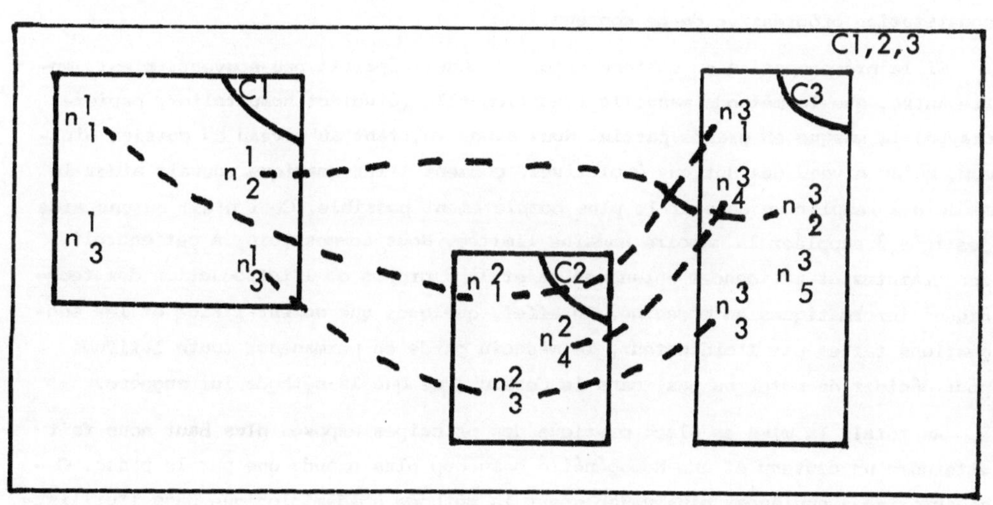

FIGURE 3

La méthode décrite au § 2-3, la plus intéressante, nécessite la réalisation de deux conditions préalables:

- un dispositif informatique éditant ou visualisant sur écran cathodique les différentes occurrences d'une même notion, rangées dans l'ordre croissant des dates qui les qualifient
- un approfondissement de la connaissance que l'on a des différents profils évolutifs d'une même notion, en fonction de divers paramètres

. Il est très important que la mise en place de telles procèdures se fassent à la demande même des cliniciens. Ainsi, ce qui doit être considéré comme une suggestion ne sera pas pris pour un ordre. Quelles que soient l'aide et les suggestions proposées automatiquement dans la présentation des données par ordinateur, le médecin garde toute latitude pour décider de noter ou pas ce que la méthode lui suggère.

. La plus grande homogénéité obtenue dans le contenu des dossiers peut encore être améliorée. Il faudra pour cela jouer sur les intervalles de temps, à l'issue desquels, telle catégorie de malades doit être revue systématiquement. Il s'agit du problème beaucoup plus vaste de la re-convocation semi-automatique des malades chroniques sur critères diagnostiques, biologiques, administratifs et autres.

V - CONCLUSION

Il est fondamental et indispensable que le médecin ait le souci du contenu d'un dossier quelconque et que l'informatique lui procure les moyens d'aide à la constitution progressive de ce contenu.

Si la préoccupation du contenu informationnel apparaît peu souvent, c'est, entre autre, que la méthode manuelle traditionnelle (étudiant hospitalier, papier-crayon) la masque en grande partie. Nous avons vu, tant au niveau du dossier minimum, qu'au niveau des notions évolutives, comment l'informatique pouvait aider le médecin à remplir un dossier le plus complètement possible. Ceci n'est qu'une aide destinée à suppléer la mémoire humaine limitée. Nous sommes loin, à cet endroit, des craintes et réticences entendues çà et là à propos de l'introduction des techniques informatiques en médecine. En effet, quelques que soient l'aide et les suggestions faites par l'ordinateur, le médecin garde en permanence toute latitude pour décider de noter ou pas, dans le dossier, ce que la méthode lui suggère.

Au total, la mise en place pratique des principes exposés plus haut nous fait atteindre un contenu et une homogénéité beaucoup plus grands que par le passé. Ceci autorise à envisager plus valablement la méthode épidémiologique dans l'utilisation des données recueillies. Où ailleurs qu'en milieu hospitalier, l'épidémiologie peut elle être pratiquée ?

BIBLIOGRAPHIE

1 - L. BARDIN
L'analyse de contenu
PUF Ed., Collection le Psychologue, Paris, (1977)

2 - Hospital Statistics and a Minimum Basic Data Set
Seminar under the auspices of the CEE
Ed. G.A. KOOL, Netherlands Institute for Preventive Care, Edinbourgh (1976)

3 - P. HENRY, S. MOSCOVICI
Problèmes de l'analyse de contenu
Langage, 11, Sept. 1968

4 - P.W. GILL, P.J. LEAPER, P.J. GUILLOU
Observer variation in clinical Diagnosis - A computer-Aided Assenssment of its Magnitude and Importance in 552 Patients with Abdominal Pain
Meth. Inf. Med., Vol 12, n° 2, pp.108-113, 1973

5 - de DOMBAL, F.T; LEAPER, D.J; STANILAND, J.R.
Pattern recognition : a comparison of the performance of clinicians and non-clinicians with a note on the performance of a computer - baser system
Meth. Inf. Med., Vol 11, n° 4, pp 32-37, 1972

A METHODOLOGY FOR DATA BASE SOFTWARE SELECTION IN HEALTH CARE SYSTEMS

F.J. LEVEN

Studiengang Medizinische Informatik
Universität Heidelberg/Fachhochschule Heilbronn
7100 Heilbronn, FRG

SUMMARY

The complex decision process of data base software selection in a health care system is structured by breaking it down into a number of steps comprising 1 analysis of the user requirements, 2 matching user requirements to data base functions and applying weights, 3 identification of candidate data base software systems and evaluating them against needs, and 4 calculating figures of merit and benchmarking best candidates. The different steps are discussed respecting the peculiarities of health care systems as to this problem area, and features of available database software systems.

1. INTRODUCTION

Designing a health care information system may lead to the decision to implement a data base system, because eg a need has been specified for shared access to data by several users under different application-specific views. Such a decision is higly irreversible with respect to eg the organizational, the sociological and medical impacts of a data base in a health care system, may they be highlights - as eg the availability of consistent patient data for chronic diseases in longitudinal records - or be drawbacks - as the problem of identification of personal records and retrieval of dossiers from a statistical data base (1).
The majority of medical databases in use today do not apply a DBMS (Data Base Management System), but it is likely that the usage of DBMS will increase, because standard data base software today is more and more able to cope with the various and variable requirements for

problem adequacy, user orientation, and cost-effectiveness.
The question, however, which general DBMS or specialized medical data base software is problem adequate is a highly complex task because of the difficulty to precise the user requirements and of the vast and heterogeneous range of candidate systems. They vary from structurally complex programmer oriented procedural systems to flat file end user oriented non-procedural systems. As to the state of the art of general DBMS today we speak of data base systems of generation 3 and 4 (figure 1). In generation 3 systems - following the CODASYL DBTG approach or IMS or MUMPS - the application programmer has to know in detail the data paths in order to navigate through the data base. In generation 4 systems - following the relational approach - however, access path control os totally the subject of the data base processor. In this way from generation to generation, there is an ever increasing conceptual distance between the low level memory access functions and the high level unser's functions, which has to be bridged by more and more complex data base management systems.
In order to achieve as much independence as possible of the application programs from the storage representation and description of

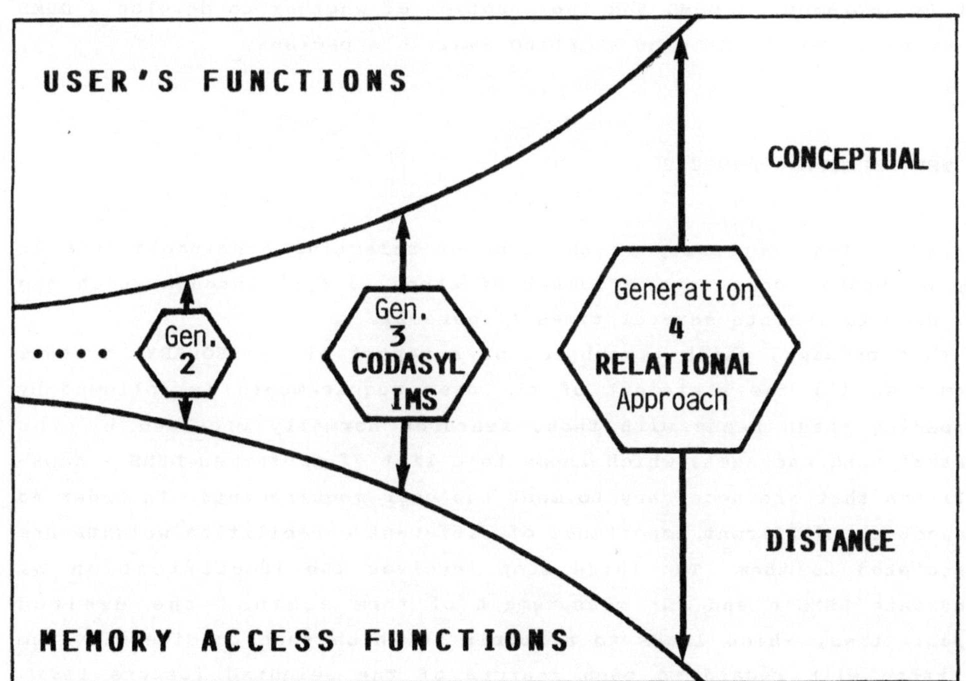

Figure 1. Generations of Data Base Management Systems

data structures the systems architecture of may data base systems today is multilevel and reflects the ANSI/SPARC 3-Schema approach, according to which

- the Internal Schema describes the physical data organization
- the Conceptual Schema describes the real world view of eg the hospital to be modelled in the data base
- the External Schemata describe the data as it is viewed by the various users of the data base, eg the doctors, the wards,...

One reason why the number of successful medical data base operations today is still quite small (2) probably lies in the fact that data bases are defined too much in computer-oriented terms rather than in medically-oriented terms. In this way the selection process described now must be primarily oriented on <u>what</u> the users need, though an abstraction from individual user requirements is necessary in the sense in which the conceptual schema describes an <u>overall</u> view of the data.

Not discussed in the following are the initial decision of whether or not to implement a DBMS and the question of whether to develop a DBMS in-house or to purchase an existing available package.

2. THE SELECTION PROCESS

To reduce the complexity of the task of selecting a suitable DBMS it may be broken down into a number of steps (3,4,5) through which one may need to iterate several times (figure 2).

In this process, which is subject of a report of the CODASYL Systems Committee (3) the statement of the user requirements is followed by comparing these needs with those features normally provided by the general DBMS packages, which leads to a list of preferred DBMS - capabilities that are necessary to meet the user requirements. In order to respect the different importance of different capabilities weights are associated to them. The third step involves the identification of candidate DBMS's and the measurement of them against the desired capabilities, which leads to a matrix in which each candidate system is rated with regard to each feature of the weighted feature list. With that matrix a figure of merit can be calculated for each

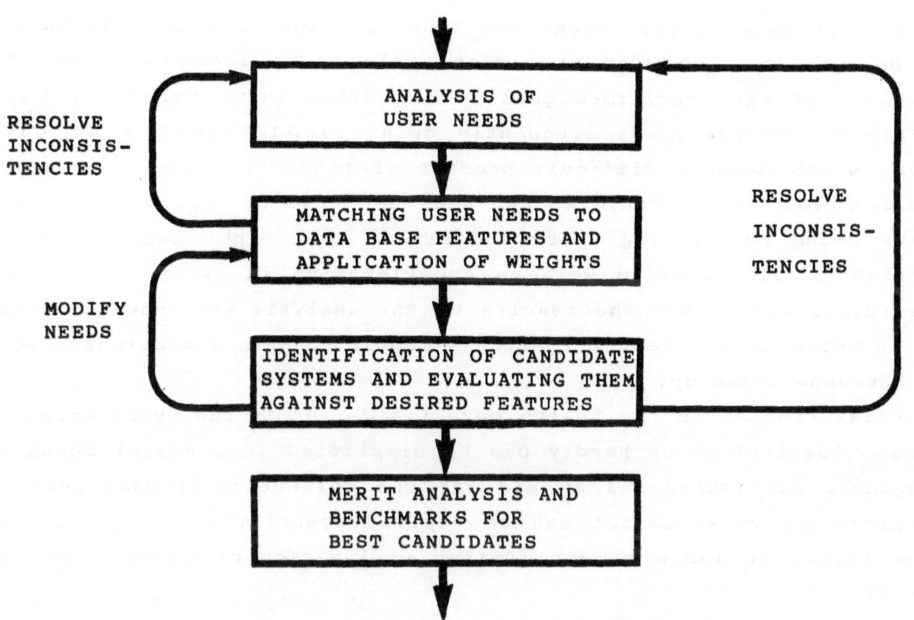

Figure 2. Process of data base software selection (modified after (3))

candidate, which probably leads to "best" systems, for which benchmark and further special testing can be done. The final phases not discussed in this paper then involve financial considerations, contract negotiation, and installation and acceptance testing.

An essential point in the selection process is the formation of the "selection team", which according to some salesmen's opinion should contain "all people of the enterprise who can say "No" to the purchase" (5).

Though this is certainly an oversimplification, it is essential that the selection group - a cross- section of all the user and application system implementor communities - has sufficiently great authority to eventually enforce changes in operating budgets, organization, and the way of doing business.

2.1 Collection and analysis of user needs

The first - and probably most difficult - step in the selection process deals with generating a consistent set of user requirements. This is a highly complex task, because users seldom know what they want and even more seldom what they need, furthermore because they often do not distinguish between real needs and functions that are "nice to have", and because the knowledge of hidden goals is as important as the knowledge of the proclaimed goals. Very often there exists a wide variety of diverse needs frequently being inconsistent with each other, which means a difficult process of tradeoff and refinement of requirements. As a technique that has been used to achieve some consensus among nonagreeing users and others the Delphi Method (3) is referred to according to which a questionnaire is answered by the articipants and, after the results of the analysis are known to them, is answered once more until after a couple of such iterations a sort of consensus comes up.

A special problem in the health care field lies in the overcomplexity of eg a hospital which hardly can be simplified in a useful model of manageable complexity. As an aid for the collection of user needs a questionnaire or checklist can be applied comprising at least the items listed in table I; for further explanation of these items see (3,4,5).

Once the set of user needs has been collected, it must be analyzed. The aim is to resolve inconsistencies due to misunderstanding and conflicts due to contradicting requirements.

2.2 Translation of user needs into desired capabilities and the application of weights

Input to this procedure (figure 3) are the list of user needs from step 1 and a list of all worthwhile features of available DBMS as described in database literature as eg (6).

The output is a matrix in which to each feature a weight is assigned with respect to each need indicating the urgency of the capability in order to meet the requirement.

Mandatory (M) eg is the availability of a DC-version (Data Communications) of the DBMS, if online interactive use is required. "Mandatory" means: without the feature the DBMS is not going to fit the tasks.

Rather important (eg I7o) may be the capability of report generating for administrative applications. "Important" means: there is a value of having this though it does not really have to be present. Undesirable (eg U5o) may be the feature of binding the data to the application programs at compile time whereas there is a strong need for

1. OVERALL CHARACTERISTICS

eg data management in
- a doctor's office
- a hospital
- a disease specific data base
- clinical research
- non patient data bases
- health maintenance organization

2. END USERS

* Types of end users:
  - data base administrator
  - application programmer
  - generalized function user
  - parametric user
* Number of users with respect to the diversity of needs and concurrent access
* Experience, qualification and turnover of users
* User interface
  - procedural vs nonprocedural
* Geographical dispersion of end users

3. DATA CHARACTERISTICS

* Data volume
* Volume change
* Growth in data volume
* Data volatility (rate of change of the values of data)
* Degree of data sharing
  - small (great) variety of users
  - horizontal data sharing (users are of the same organizational level)
  - vertical data sharing (users are of different organizational levels)
* Data structures
  * structure types
    - linear structure
    - hierarchical structure
    - network structure
  * structural complexity
  * structural volatility
  * conversion of current data

4. SYSTEM USE

* Mode of data access
  - insert, delete, update
  - retrieve
  - one record at a time
  - multiple records a time
* Directness of data access
  - batch use
  - online interactive use
* Response time
  - ultra fast:up to 1 second
  - fast:up to a few seconds
  - medium:up to a few minutes
  - slow:up to a few hours
  - deferred:up to a few days
* Reliability of data
* Availability of data
* Security, privacy of data
* Integrity of data
* System scheduling

5. APPLICATION PROGRAMS

* Number of programs
* Functions of programs
* Type of programs
  - batch oriented
  - transaction oriented
* Complexity of programs
* Size of programs
* Volatility of programs
* Growth rate of programs
* Implementation languages
* Modularity of programs
* Correctness of programs
* Documentation of programs
* Transportability of programs

6. SYSTEM REQUIREMENTS

* Systems personnel
  - systems programmer
  - application programmer
  - data base administrator
* Existing software to be interfaced with a DBMS
* Recoverability of system and data
* HW-capabilities

7. IMPLEMENTATION SCHEDULE

* Stages of realization
  - actual activities
  - long range plans

Table I. Checklist for collection of user needs

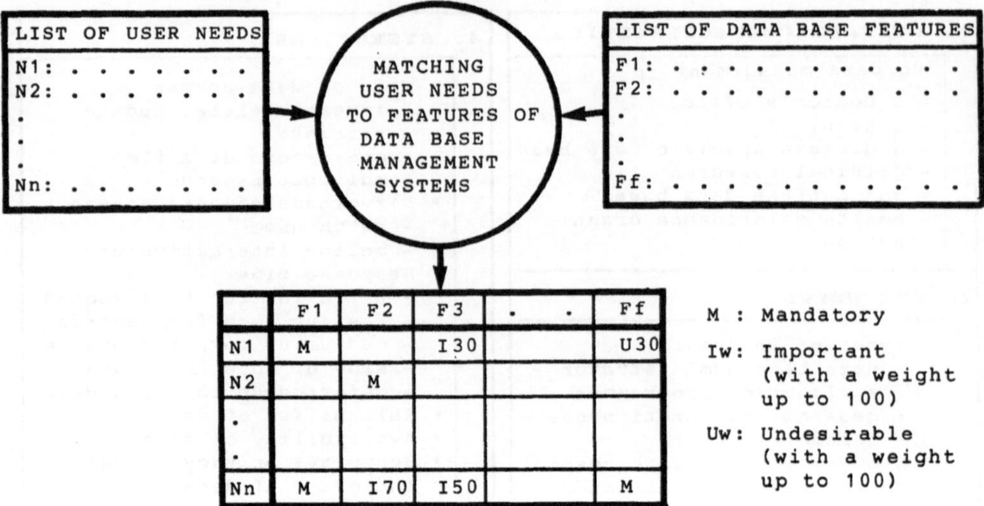

Figure 3. Translation of needs into desired capabilities

flexibility in changing data structures. "Undesirable" means: the value is negative; it may even eliminate the DBMS from consideration unless the feature can be turned off.

Spaces in the matrix mean "don't care" or: it is neither worth nor undesirable.

The above classification technique can be considered as a first step to identify required DBMS functions on the user needs.

As a second - more sophisticated - technique the method of "multilevel weighting" (3) can be applied: Whereas "mandatory" features are absolute which means that their absence disqualifies a system, "important" features are listed and grouped into some basic components. The result is a hierarchy of important capabilities, as shown in figure 4. According to this method a relative weight, which is a fraction of 100, is assigned to each node the total weight for all elements emanating from any one node is made 1oo percent. This breakdown of a need into its components helps the evaluator see the relative importance of each component. The relative importance eg of the feature "histograms" in figure 4 is 60% of 50% = 30% of the total evaluation weight for "report generator".

"The idea of this hierarchical structuring is to make the team consider weighting in an organized fashion. Rather than think of many

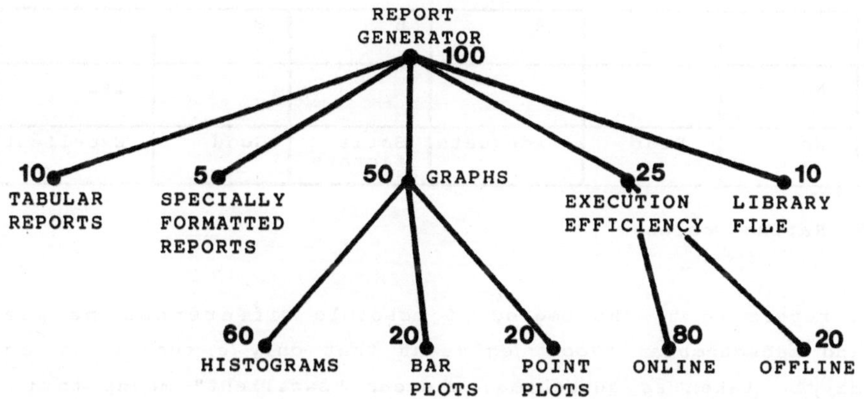

Figure 4. Multi-level weighting of important capabilities

parts in competition for points, each major part is evaluated against the other major parts, and so on down the tree." (3).

2.3 Construction of profiles of candidate DBMS

In this step the possible candidate DBMS's are identified from the large heterogeneous set of available systems eg by distributing a "Request for Proposal" to the vendors. The response of vendors then may be used as a basis for measuring the candidates against the desired capabilities. The result is a "feature profile", a list which rates each candidate DBMS with regard to each feature of the weighted feature list described above.
There may arise problems as eg to the case that no candidate provides the mandatory features, which possibly means modifying the requirements. Another problem is the rating task because not all features can be rated by the same rating scale.
If we take eg the following features

* F1 Complex network data structures
* F2 Subschema availability

we see that they must be evaluated in different ways, eg by applying scale S1 to F1 and S2 to F2 (figure 5).

scale	0	2	4	6	8	10
S1	No					Yes
S2	No	Poor	Adequate	Satis-factory	Good	Excellent

Figure 5. Rating Scales

Scale S2 refers eg to the degree of possible differences between schema and subschemata. "Poor" eg means that only a subset of one schema may be taken as subschema, whereas "excellent" means that a subschema may be derived from several schemata differing from them in various respects.

2.4. Merit analysis

According to the weight described in 2.2 and the rating profile described in 2.3 a merit or worth analysis (7) can be done by multiplying these and summing over all user needs.
There however must be warned of relying too heavily on small differences in the figure of merit derived by this technique; the primary goal is to uncover major differences between the candidates.
Once figure of merit values have been generated by the evaluation team, it may be possible to select one or several of the candidate systems and eventually run benchmark test.

3. CURRENT DATA BASE SOFTWARE AND FUTURE TRENDS

General DBMS today may be classified according to the underlying data model (8) into network systems (eg CODASYL DBTG systems), hierarchical systems (eg IMS or MUMPS) and relational systems, or, according to the following list of data base controversies:

DATA INDEPENDENCE	**versus**	**PROCESSING EFFICIENCY**
SELF CONTAINED SYSTEMS	**versus**	**HOST-LANGUAGE SYSTEMS**
NON-PROCEDURALITY IN DATA MANIPULATION	**versus**	**PROCEDURALITY IN DATA MANIPULATION**
MULTIPLE-RECORDS-AT-A-TIME LOGIC	**versus**	**ONE-RECORD-AT-A-TIME-LOGIC**
SET OPERATIONS	**versus**	**ACCESS PATH PROCEDURES**
CONTENT ADDRESSING	**versus**	**POINTER TECHNOLOGY**

It is obvious that eg relational systems fit into the left of these two categories, whereas most systems of DBMS generation 3 belong to the second class. Whereas with relational systems there are still performance problems, drawbacks of the other category of systems eg are (9): the overcomplexity of existing procedural data manipulation languages, the access path dependency and very often an insufficient orientation to the non programmer who does not understand trees or networks.

There are various general DBMS that are applicable to health care (2), among them systems that are run on midi- and minicomputers, and one system which was originally developed for and in a medical environment and now is being marketed for general minicomputer management: MUMPS.

Besides the aspects described above the selection of a DBMS also should consider future trends in data base technology (9): the shift of software functions to (data base machines), trends in conceptual schema design and data base semantics specification, and the approach to adequate non-procedural user interfaces and method base systems.

4. CONCLUSIONS

The selection of DBMS for application in a health care system must primarily be medically-oriented, rather than computer-oriented. The methodology described emphasizes this aspect by the approach of translating user needs into data base capabilities, a task however, that may be quite complex.

REFERENCES

(1) Schlörer J. Identification and retrieval of personal records from a statistical data bank. Meth. Inform. Med. 14, 1/1975, 7-13.

(2) Wiederhold G. Databases in healthcare; preprint of CS Report STAN CS 80-790, Standford, 1979.

(3) CODASYL Systems Committee. Selection and acquisition of data base management systems, New York, ACM, 1976.

(4) Sibley EH. Evaluation and selection of data base systems; in: Data base systems, Maidenhead, Infotech, 1975, 573 - 592.

(5) Carter AJT. Evaluation of data base management software; in: ibid., 265 - 310.

(6) Wiederhold G. Database design, New York, McGraw Hill, 1977.

(7) Helm H, Rienhoff O. Systematization of systems-selection-a worth analysis model for computerized medical reporting systems; in: Lindberg DAB, Kaihara S. (Eds). Medinfo 80; Amsterdam, North Holland 1980, 625 - 629.

(8) Sauter K. Databases in medical information systems, ibid., 444 - 452.

(9) Leven FJ. Trends in data base technology and their impact on medical data base applications, ibid. 475 - 479.

THE REPRESENTATION OF MEDICAL LANGUAGE-BASED DATA:

A REVIEW OF REFERENCE LANGUAGES & THEIR APPLICATIONS

B.J. Kostrewski
Centre for Information Science
The City University
Northampton Square
London EC1V OHB

and

J. Anderson
King's College Hospital Medical School
Denmark Hill
London SE5

Abstract

Reference languages have evolved to incorporate linguistic mechanisms for the representation of meaning. Standardization of terminology and the incorporation of semantic mechanisms and their definition for different applications are reviewed.

1. Introduction

The recent expansion of the concept of medicine is a corollary of increased understanding of physiological processes and the application of findings from other areas eg nuclear science and electronics to the practice of medicine. Clearly such very different subjects increase the conceptual complexity of medicine and its subsequent encoding for all levels of application (1).

The principal use of language based information in medicine are for:

i) The encoding of patient information in medical records which subsequently may be put to a variety of different uses, each making different demands on a reference language.

ii) The representation of medical concepts contained within published documents for Bibliographic database storage and retrieval.

Clearly both these applications place different demands on the structure of reference languages. Accurate clinical recording, is rooted in precise terminological representation. Reference languages are a relatively new development, incorporating the experiences of earlier bibliographic and disease related classifications, the descendants of Hippocratic Aphorisms. Thus one of the earliest fully recorded medical classifications is that of Fancois Boissier de Sauvages de la Croix, Nosologica Methodica (2). The growth of the recording of medical information was emphasized by the proliforation of classifications and terminologies; Kennedy & Kossman list some 130 different reference languages. In this context reference language refers to any systematic system for the representation and recording of language-based medical information.

All reference languages represent an attempt to standardize medical terminology. However, a special effort has been made by CIOMS, The Council for the International Organization of Medical Sciences (3) to derive a universally acceptable terminology for medicine. The International Medical Information Association, IMIA, has also been working towards this end. The Standard Nomenclature of Diseases and Operations (SNOD) (4) was compiled in 1933 and periodically updated. As with all reference languages the representation of the current evolution of concepts was a permanent issue. To overcome this the Current Medical Information and Terminology (CMIT) (5) became available in 1972. These computer produced listings allowed for frequent revision. The International Anatomical Nomenclature (6) was published in 1977 as was the facet structured TDM theasurus (7). The German language KDS thesaurus is structured along similar lines to the ICD schedules.(8)

2.0. The use of Reference Language in relation to Patient Data

2.1. Medical Records

The systematic recording of the course of disease together with the consideration of man as a total entity, are a legacy of Hippocratic medicine to present day practice. However, the adoption of the scientific method to the practice of medicine precipitated several changes, the major impact being the fragmentation of medicine into specialities, with a resultant loss of totality. The communication problem was further emphasized, firstly by increased population mobility and secondly by the introduction of group practice when a physician no longer ministered to a patient throughout a lifespan. Thus unambiguous communication assumed paramount importance. Furthermore the loss of continuity through the dispersion of documentation hindered good medicine in the sense that the totality of the human organism became lost. Some compensation for this has been attempted through the Record Linkage Studies which do attempt to bring together dispersed documents relating to an individual.(9)

Patient data within a record has several uses. The primary purpose is the recording of an individuals episode of illness and, through time, to build up a picture of the human organism. Secondly records are used for the collection of statistics, at regional national, and international levels, relating to mortality and morbidity (10). Recently the development of disease registers has become increasingly dependent upon the medical record (11). Moreover the derivation of statistics for planning at all levels are best based on the patient record. Clearly such varied applications place different demands on a reference language. The development of SNOMED, Systematized Nomenclature of Medicine (12) specifically for the encoding of patient data allows for more accurate representation.

2.2 Statistical Data

The original aim of the International Classification of Diseases (ICD) was to classify world wide, statistics, relating to all aspects of disease. The classification, originally conceived in the 1930's, was therefore strictly application orientated (13). Its origins maybe traced by the work of William Farr (1836) who devised a classification of the effect of disease on the population (14). Earlier (15) we have demonstrated the the relative generality of ICD, particularly suited to the statistical requirements of WHO. Although the recent, 9th revision, of ICD has increased the specificity of terminology the original framework has been retained. Integration and inter-convertibility between ICD & SNOMED allows for both detail of description of an episode of illness relating to a patient and also for the collection of statistics and linkage of data (16) Clearly the complimentary capacity of both systems of classification extends the application parameters of a system. Moreover the introduction of structured terminologies has contributed to the design of information systems based around their capabilities. Thus Jeanty (17) has utilized the capabilities of SNOMED to design a system for the exploitation of information contained in medical records.

2.3 Reference Databases

The medical record, in being the primary document of medical experience, is the primary reference tool for both education and decision support in diagnosis, therapy, management and prognosis. Thus the developments of Jeanty (17) and Rosati (18) at Duke University North Carolina extend the application of records into the reference domain traditionally occupied by the medical literature. In both cases the experience contained in medical records has been collated and synthesized into a specialist reference knowledge base the latter in hypertension and the former in gastroenterology thus utilizing the wealth of information and experience at a primary care level, much quicker than it otherwise could have been available through conventional publication. However, to utilize this intellectual wealth to its fullest capacity, the definition of boundaries of meaning is paramount. This also demands the standardization of terminology in order to further increase the potential and performance of the system.

2.4 Disease Registries

Another extension of the application of the medical record is the introduction of disease registries. This epidemiological research is centred upon the disease, and attempts to define a network of associated interrelationships. The strict definition of the goal, restricts the semantic demands placed on a reference language. However, geographical dispersion demands the definition of the parameters of meaning through the use of a structured controlled terminology needed for consistent documentation systems and subsequent statistical analysis. (Kayser 11). Thus it can be seen that the role of the medical record has been extended beyond the traditional function of recording of the course of disease. This repository is now being drawn upon for hypothesis formulation and as decision support. The clear definition of meaning, is central to the efficient functioning of such systems.

2.5 Consistency of Encoding

Consistent representation of concepts is the underpinning of a semantic system, and demands a consensus in physician encoding. The use of an available standardized terminology is one solution to the problem. However, the discipline imposed on a physician in the use of standardized terminologies is enormous, and may not be ultimately effective. To overcome this dilemma support systems employing medical documentation personnel to translate the physicians terminology into the structured terminology appropriate to the system have been implemented. Clearly this demands a comprehensive thesaurus with a comprehensive mapping of synonyms. When clinic or context linked this becomes a manageable proposition. The principles underlying this approach have been adopted in different ways by Thurmayr (19) and Griesser (20) who use this approach for the encoding of medical specialities. Gabrielli (21) has put forward 9 criteria for a medical lexicon in man/computer systems, emphasizing correspondence with natural language and economy of representation while Cox (22) has emphasized the need for a vocabulary which cuts across disciplinary boundaries. The terminology derived by Gabrielli (21) is partitioned into

7 categories, anatonic, physiology, measurement, clinical medicine, etiologic, clinical therapy, biomedical concepts. These cut across traditional boundaries, yet link the symptoms with body systems. The increased use of drug therapy coupled with increased legislation in drug development has resulted in a new demand being placed on patient recording and documentation. The strict monitoring of drugs at clinical trials stage and during post-marketing surveillance demands a strict definition of observations. Towards this end FDA have developed the "COSTART" The National Adverse Drug Reaction Directory. (23)

3.0 The representation of bibliographic information

3.1 Bibliographic Information

The major computer based databases were originally derived as a by-product of the production of several published secondary services, eg "freetext," Chemical Abstracts, (24), Biological Abstracts, (25) and "controlled" Index Medicus, (26) (27) these have assumed a function in their own right and although content representation has been extended for computer use, through the introduction of semantic mechanisms eg MeSH (27, 13, 14) this legacy still remains. European needs are being reflected on databases such as Cancernet (28) with particular emphasis on European Cancer work and Heclinet (29, 30) relating to hospital data. Excerpta Medica is currently available on Lockeed. The advent of Euronet (31) will make this information readily available throughout Europe.

The representation of bibliographic data for information storage and retrieval systems presents different demands on the structure of reference languages. While the literature may act as decision support its primary aim is both the extension and accumulation of knowledge and in a practical sense to lay the foundations for original research. The "controlled" terminology used for The encoding of cancer data is based on the original statistical derivations based on text, by Wolf-Terroine (32) and subsequently extended by Henzler (33). Pragmatic considerations demand that the description of document content should represent meaning in the most cost-effective manner and yet allow for heuristic interaction. Thus the dependence on statistical methods for the derivation of structured vocabularies introduces a quantitative, objective approach systems design, which traditionally had been based on subjective criteria of usage.

Bibliographic searching of "free-text", has been based on the physical representation of document content in surrogate form. Thus, titles, abstracts or keyword indexing without thesaural control, are the vehicle for the transfer of meaning. Clearly such systems are dependant upon user understanding of both the system and a thorough knowledge of the domain in which information is being sought. Thus at best only a definition of context is possible. The message contained in a document as represented by the surrogate is rarely completely captured by the search statement. The adequacy of surrogates for the transfer of the information content of documents has been investigated (34). The need for guidance at searching, ie. an expression of a network of associations generally at the level of synonymy or generic relations, has been introduced in "Biosis" through the Biosis Search Guide (35). An element of structure and relation is introduced through the introduction of a high level classification code incorporating some 650 biological categories. BIOSIS is now incorporating an increased element of medically related material (25). Both the 'controlled' and 'free-text' approaches can at best identify the context and not the actual information needed. For research purposes, this does not precipitate any great loss.

3.2 The Contribution of Bibliometrics

Initially the link between bibliometrics and content representation appears to be weak and yet it is fundamental to the representation of knowledge as it really is. Bibliometrics when transposed to the derivation of a reference language within a domain shows that the journals contributing the most pertinent terminology are also the core journals since they are most representative of current trends. Analysis of the Cancernet data has demonstrated world trends in cancer research, both experimental and clinical and allowed for qualitative associations between cancer and the principal therapies (36). A further practical implication is that strictly subject defined collections of documents may be encoded using unstructured terminologies eg as in IRBEL, Indexed References to Bioengineering Literature (37). Here the context is defined and document content is dependant upon representation by terms selected from alphabetical listings. Clearly document representation for bibliographic searching places different demands on reference languages than the representation of the content of patient records. Briefly a high degree of specificity is required for the representation of patient data while the representation of bibliographic data demands the definition of levels of context - backed by the awareness that we have an insufficient understanding of language and linguistic mechanisms to convey real meaning in mechanized retrieval.

3.3 "Knowledge Databases"

More recently the advent of "knowledge databases", has placed a new demand on the representation of knowledge within a particular domain. One such database is being developed by the National Library of Medicine, in the field of Hepatitis, drawing on the expertise of some 20 specialists eminent in this field (38). The aim is to retrieve information and not a bibliographic reference, demanding a representation for total relevance of output. By contrast bibliographic reference output may be ranked in order of relevance and relatively straightforward mechanisms for ranking have been introduced (39). Obviously there is a close link between "knowledge databases" based on expertise and reference databases based on information in medical records (18). Clearly, to be truly effective the reference terminology must play a central role in query formulation matched by an equal control of word usage within the "knowledge base". At each stage 'total' information is presented which reflects the interaction of the structure of the domain and the information structure. Each element of information will have to represent all information in the sense that what is retrieved is a structure composed of a well defined components (notion) and the interrelationships whose interaction contribute to the systhesis of an information unit.

4.0 The Function of Models

Models encapsulate scientific theories. Indeed the value of models is judged by their predictive capacity. To be truly effective reference languages should encapsulate within their structure the framework of the subject related model. Shneider (40) rightly draws our attention to the lack of an adequate formalism for both human biological and behavioural systems and for health-care systems. Such formalization determines the distribution of terminology and the allocation of documentation. Models partition concepts and their interrelationships. Classification is a process of modelling and abstraction and as such reflects knowledge at a present point in time. The notion that a classification reflects the structure of the domain is central to the derivation of a good application linked classification. Therefore, such classifications while being up-dated in the sense of inclusion of terminology still, in their board framework, reflect the structure of medicine which prevailed at the time of their conception.

4.1 Theoretical Considerations

It has been assumed that the incorporation of linguistic theories into the design of reference languages for information storage and retrieval systems would improve their performance. Reference languages without structure have limited use since their implicit framework can only be truly effective in narrow, well defined subject areas. In the integration of Saussure's (41) parameters of structure and generation of meaning, paradigmatic relations represent classes of entities as we know them within the accepted framework of knowledge while the syntagmatic relations represent levels of syntax. This classification with a strong hierachical structure eg ICD have a strong paradigmatic element while faceted classifications eg SNOP & SNOMED have a strong syntagmatic element (15).

4.2 Semantic Analysis

This results in the definition of classes of terms and their interrelationships. The two principal approaches are:

i) The explicit definition of relations together with a controlled terminology.
ii) The incorporation of rules for text analysis which recognize the linguistic elements used to express certain relationships.

Superficially these two approaches seem quite different however, their theoretical underpinnings are the same and both approaches demand the formalization of understanding by the definition of relations and the derivation of a dictionary.

The first example is based on intellectual analysis and definition of structure as in REMEDE, (42) through the introduction of symbolic operators between terms. Similarly the the definition of needs for diagnostic and therapeutic support systems, eg MYCIN (43) is an extension of the relational framework. This approach reflects the reliance on the subject related model and the linguistic components for its representation in the processing of knowledge. The realization that a special approach to the encoding of patient data was needed precipitated the development of SNOMED. (Systematized Nonmeclature of Medicine) which evolved from the original foundations laid by SNOP. Clearly this development appears to work well, allowing for a simulation of syntax based on a faceted system in the encoding of each item of information. This is based on the faceted principle partitioning the domain into interdependant categories which reflect its structure and relationships (44,45,46,47). The principal facets, Topography, Mororphology Etiology & Function, of SNOMED must be cited in that order. The two facets Diseases and Procedures complete the division. The tree structure of MeSH (27) show a partially faceted approach since they are not mutually exclusive.

Work on the automatic analysis of medical text has always been contextually defined. In Artificial Intelligence (AI) terms this defines the importance of 'frames' in the definition of meaning. Such analysis has been carried out on two levels: (i) the phrase or sentence level, as in the analysis of pathology (45,46,47,48) and radiology reports (49, 50,51) and (ii) the word level where word roots, prefixes and suffixes have a defined meaning in medicine and furthermore when restricted to a defined domain of medicine (52, 53,54) this approach has the nenefit of economy of storage.

Recently an analysis of patient records, as the primary document of the medical experience, has contributed to a further understanding of the medical reference framework. The four basic classificatory parameters are Diagnosis, Therapy, Management and Prognosis (55). Furthermore the information structure was revealed to be more complex for the patient record than for published papers. This was shown as the outcome of an analysis of language and linguistics and its theoretical contributions to meaning. Current linguistic theories are largely concerned with the mechanics of language and the axiom that syntax, at the sentence level, is an attribute of semantics. It is now realized that the construction of meaning is concerned with larger units of texts (56), and Information Retrieval systems may be developed towards that end; clearly this is already true in the case of "knowledge databases". In the case of the representation of documents the contribution of units of meaning, semantemes, and their role in structured representation has been postulated (55,57). The use of 'blocks' of meaning and their relative positions total meaning should, theoretically, be constructable. Moreover it defines 'blocks' of information classifying by both generality and specificity and simulates the goal directedness inherent in all medical activity. In terms of language representation the resultant partitioning is positional, both in relation to the document content and its linkage to the overall domain. The problem of language processing in medicine has been stressed by Blois (58) who recognized the diverse functions of identical and related words in medical text. The unit of information in terms of a meaningful unit, ie a unique concept has been emphasized in terms of concept representation (55). This has been incorporated both into thesaural design and testing (59). The foundation of these formalisms are embedded in the principle that co-occurent terms encapsulate related notions; this word clustering was done by Spark-Jones (60) with the aim of generating semantic structures for thesaurus compilation.

5.0 Conclusion

Earlier reviews (61,62) presented a comprehensive survey of medical classifications and and thesauri. The representation of meaning in computer systems for language based data has so far been dependant upon the application of classification and linguistic theories to the structure of reference languages. Representation tended to be linear; SNOMED introduced an element of multidimensionalty through the faceted approach.

Subsequent developments in the development of reference languages must take into account future developments both in terms of application and capabilities of current computer systems. For example the application of Viewdata (63) to medical information processing has introduced another dimension into the definition of a reference language for content representation. Clearly classes need to be strictly defined and the structure needs to allow for a step-by-step homing in on the required information with structural levels of representation. Such semantic structures must, of necessity be application related and reflect different levels and facets of the overall structure of medicine and yet be automous within themselves. "Knowledge databases", demands total representation of information and not just definition of context, for the retrieval of current concepts within a given domain. This contrasts with bibliographic retrieval where definition of context is dependant on the conceptual retrieval base.

Thus it is becoming apparent that the structure of reference languages must take into account not only linguistic mechanisms for the transfer of meaning but also allow flexibility for different applications. This evolution must allow both for changing and expanding terminology and for adaptation of structure to application.

REFERENCES

(1) ANDERSON, J. The Computer: Medical Vocabulary and Information Brit. Med. Bull. 1968 ; 24, 3 : 194-198.

(2) KENNEDY J, KOSSMAN LE. Nomenclature in Medicine. Bulletin of Medical Library Association. 1973 ; 61 : 238-252.

(3) WAGNER, G. The CIOMS project for international standardization of medical terminology. Proc. of the 17th Annual Conference of the Deutsche Gesellschaft für Medizinischen Dokimentation und Statistik. FK Schattauer Verlag, München. 1973 ; 129-133.

(4) American Medical Association Standard Nomenclature of Diseases and Operations. American Medical Association, Chicago. 1961.

(5) GORDON, BL. (ed). Current Medical Information and Terminology (CMIT) American Medical Association. 1972.

(6) International Anatomical Nomenclature Committee (ed). Nomina Anatomica, 4th Edn. Amsterdam. 1977.

(7) HÖPKER WW, KAYSER K, & RAMISCH W. Thesaurus der Medizin (TDM) an internationally compatible diagnostic system. Methods of Information in Medicine. 1977 ; 16, 1 : 28-31.

(8) IMMICH, H. Be merkungen zum Klinischen Diagnosenschlussel. Methods of Information in Medicine. 1966 ; 5 : 40-142.

(9) ACHESON, ED. Linkage of Medical Records. British Med. Bull. 1968 ; 27 : 206-209.

(10) ALDERSON, MR. Health Information Systems. Medinfo '77. 1977 ; 595-602.

(11) KAYSER K, & BURKHARDT H-U. Documentation in Pathology and its approach to epidemiologic research. WAMI Proceedings May 1980 ; 58-62.

(12) CÔTE, RA. Systematized Nomenclature of Medicine (SNOMED). College of American Pathologists, Skokie, Illinois. 1976-1979.

(13) International Classification of Diseases WHO, Geneva. 1978.

(14) ROBB-SMITH, AHT. International Classification of Diseases. Classification Society Bulletin. 1970 ; 2 : 3-22.

(15) MAJOR P, KOSTREWSKI BJ, & ANDERSON J. Analysis of the Semantic Structures of Reference Languages. Part II. Analysis of Semantic Power of MeSH, ICD and SNOMED. Medical Informatics. 1978 ; Vol. 3 (4) : 269-281.

(16) FRUTIGER P, ROSSIER P. et al ICD/SNOMED Nomenclature for encoding pathology reports of tumours. WAMI Proceedings ; 1980 ; 278-284.

(17) JEANTY, C. The Computerized Medical Record in Gastroenterology. Medinfo '77. 1977 ; 283-287.

(18) ROSATI, RA. A new Information System for Medical Practice. Arch.Int.Med. 1975 ; 135 : 1017-1024.

(19) THURMAYR RJ, SCHOEFFEL RJ, & THURMAYR R. Use of text Processing in Surgery Reports. WAMI Proceedings ; 1980 ; 291-297.

(20) GRIESSER G, & JAINZ M. Computerized Support of Activities and Identification of related Data. Kiel KIS in MIE '78. 1978 ; 767-773.

(21) GRABRIELLI, ER. Logic of a Computer based Medical Lexicon. Medinfo '77. 1977 ; 257-260.

(22) COX, EB. Towards a Medical Language. Medinfo '77. 1977 ; 25-256.

(23) COSTART. National Adverse Drug Reaction Directory. US Dept. of Health, Education, and welfare.

(24) DAYTON DL, IZENBERG AC, & SNYDER AM. Searching the Chemical Abstracts Service Information base for Biological Activities. Medinfo '77. 1977 ; 325-330.

(25) MARCHISOTTO, R. Biosciences Information Science (IOSIS): A comprehensive Biometical Information System. Medinfo '77. 1977 ; 341-348.

(26) LEITER, J. Online Systems of The National Library of Medicine. Medinfo '77. 1977 ; 345-349.

(27) Medical Subject Headings. National Library of Medicine, Bethesda, Maryland. 1980

(28) WOLFF-TERROINE, M. CANCERNET (Sabir - C): An European Network for Cancer Literature, Medinfo '77. 1977 ; 301-306.

(29) SCHNEEMAN, R. HECLINET - Specialized International Documentation for Hospital care. Proceedings MIB '79. 1979 ; 853-861.

(30) Thesaurus Krankenhauswesen. Compiled by Deutches Krankenhaus Institut, Dusseldorf Institut für Krankenhausbau der U.T.U. Berlin. 1978.

(31) Euronet DIANE Inaugurated 1980, Euronet News, Luxembourg 1980.

(32) WOLFF-TERROINE M, RIMBERT D, & ROUALT B. Improved Statistical Methods for Automatic Construction of a Medical Thesaurus. Methods Inform. Med. 1972 ; 11, 2 : 104-113.

(33) HENZLER, RG. Free or Controlled Vocabularies, International Classification. 1978 5, 1 : 21-26.

(34) BOTTLE RT, & SEELEY CR. Information Transfer Limitation of Titles of Chemical Documents. J. Chem. Doc. 1970 ; 10 : 254-259.

(35) BIOSIS Search Guide. Biosciences Information Service, Philadelphia. 1978.

(36) HENZLER RG, SANDOR L, & WAGNER G. Bibliometric Studies for the Evaluation of Scientific Literature in Cancer Research, in: Medinfo '77. 1977 ; 317-324.

(37) IRBEL. Information Retrieval in Bioengineering Literature. 1975.

(38) Information Transfer for Practioners. National Library of Medicine, Fact Sheet, December 1978.

(39) LANCASTER, FW. Evaluation of the Medlars demand search service, National Library of Medicine, Bethesda Maryland. 1968.

(40) SCHNEIDER, W. Impact of CL and AI Techniques on Modelling in Medicine, in Computtational Linguistics in Medicine edited by W. Schneider and Sagvall Hein. North Holland Publishing Company, Oxford. 1977.

(41) de SAUSSURE, F. Course in General Linguistics (Fontana, London). 1974.

(42) de HEAULME, M. Artificial Medical Languages, a Solution for Clinical needs in Documentation, example using REMEDE Systems, MIE '78. 1978 ; 63-72.

(43) SHORTLIFFE, EH. Computer Based Medical Consultations: MYCIN, Elsevier, New York. 1977.

(44) VICKERY, BC. Faceted Classification, Aslib, London. 1960.

(45) COLES EC, & SLAVIN G. Evaluation of Automatic Indexing of Pathology reports. Journal of Clinical Pathology. 1976 ; 29, 7 : 621-625.

(46) PRATT, AW. Use of Categorized Nomenclatures for representing Medical Statements in Computational Linguistics in Medicine ; 45-54. Editors W. Schneidner & Sagvall Hein. Proceedings of IFIP Working Conference on Computational Linguistics in Medicine. Uppsala, Sweden, 2-6 May 1977.

(47) PACAK, MG, PRATT AW, & WHITE WC. Automated Morpho - syntactic Analysis of Medical Language, Information Processing and Management. 1976 ; 12 ; 71-76.

(48) DUNHAM GS, PACAK MG, & PRATT AW. Automatic Indexing of Pathology Data. J.AM.Soc. Inf.Sci. 1978 ; 29 ; 81-90.

(49) GRISHMAN R, & HISCHMAN L. Question Answering from Natural Language Databases. Artificial Intelligence. 1978 ; 11 ; 25-43.

(50) HISCHMAN L, & GRISHMAN R. Fact Retrieval from Natural Language Medical Records. Medinfo '77. 1977 ; 247-252.

(51) SAGER N, GRISHMAN R, & INSOLIO C. Computer Programmes for Natural Language Files. Proceedings of ASIS Annual Meeting. 1977 ; Vol.14 ; 17.

(52) WINGERT, F. Morphosyntactic Analysis of Compound Word Forms, in Computational Linguistics in Medicine edited by Scheider, W & Sagvall-Heim, AL. North-Holland Publishing Company. 1977.

(53) WINGERT, F. Medical Language Data Processing, in Reichertz, PL & Goos, G. (eds.), Medizinische Informatick und Statistik: 3 Informatics and Medicine: An Advanced Course. Springer-Verlag, 1977 ; 579-646.

(54) WINGERT, F. A Model for the Segmentation of Medical Compound Words. Medinfo '77. 1977 ; 241-246.

(55) KOSTREWSKI BJ, & ANDERSON J. Structual Considerations for the Encoding of Medical Data: A Formalism for Medicine. Proceedings Medical Informatics Berlin '79. 1979 ; 841-852.

(56) VAN DIJK, TA. Complex Semantic Information Processing. In Walker, DE., Karlgren, H. & Kay, M. (eds) Natural Language and Information Science. FID Publication 551. Stockholm: Skriptor 127-163 ; 1977.

(57) KOSTREWSKI, BJ. Structural Considerations for the Derivation of Applications linked Reference Languages for Medical Information Systems in The Analysis of Meaning. Informatics 5 ed. M. MacCafferty & K. Grey. Aslib, London. 1979.

(58) BLOIS, M. The Structure of Descriptive Information in Medicine in Proceedings of 2nd Annual WAMI Meeting. 252-254 ; 1979.

(59) KAYSER K, RAMISCH W, von KENNE H, & HÖPKER W-W. Thesaurus and new volume Information, Medical Informatics. 1980 ; 5 ; 2 : 155-166.

(60) SPARK-JONES, K. Automatic Keyword Classification. (Butterworths, London). 1971.

(61) MAJOR P, KOSTREWSKI BJ, & ANDERSON J. Languages for Medical Information Systems. Medical Informatics, Vol.2 ; 1 : 35-46 ; 1977.

(62) PACAK MG, DUNHAM GS. Computers and Medical Language. Medical Informatics. 4 ; 1 : 13-28. 1979.

(63) FEDIDA, S. ROACH, ME. Viewdata and its Application to Medical Informatics. Proceedings Medical Informatics Berlin 1979, 718-778 ; 1979.

RELATIONAL DATABASE CARDIOCOD: A TOOL FOR CLINICAL RESEARCH IN CARDIOLOGY

by
Piotr J. JASIŃSKI, Bogumiła TALKOWSKA
Regional Computer Centre
Technical University of Poznań, Poland
and
Henryk KRUG
Institute of Cardiology
Medical Academy, Poznań, Poland

SUMMARY

The project of computer database for supporting research in clinical cardiology has been presented in this paper. The relational model of data is used to design a logical, problem–oriented structure of patient data. An adeqately designed relational query language for direct physician – database interactions has been presented through examples of query formulation, Computer database CARDIOCOD has been implemented and introduced in two clinical wards of Institute of Cardiology, Poznań in October 78.

INTRODUCTION

Large quantities of patient data readily available for analysis may assist physicians in clinical research. This view was recognized as the reason to initiate research and development of database for clinical cardiology. Primary objectives were that the project should have well grounded and reasonable computer science foundations and that according to present database design priorities the resulting system should be user-oriented (or so called user-friendly). Therefore we concentrated our efforts on:

– adequacy of data modelling to clinical reality;

– easy and convenient, direct usage of the system by the cardiologist.

RELATIONAL STRUCTURE OF CLINICAL DATA

The most important and commonly acknowledged advantages of relational model of data (q.v. relational databases) rely on that that logical structures of data can be seen and manipulated by the casual, non-technically trained user of the database in extremely simple, familiar forms.

According to the framework of relational model of data applied in the project, data entries are grouped in multicolumn tables; such database tables satisfy some set-theoretic properties and therefore are called (synonymously) relations [1, 2]. A set of conceptually simple algebraic operations stands as a formal basis for database processing. In our approach, focused on question-answering database interactions, we use 3 primary operations [3]. Two of them are monadic (i.e. applied to any single database relation) operations:

<u>projection</u> – allows to obtain all values of given columns (synonymously attributes) from a specified relation;

This work is a part of research which is sponsored by Polish Academy of Sciences (PAN).

selection – allows to retrieve data rows (entries) from relation, which rows satisfy given attributes value condition.

The third and most characteristic mechanism for relational databases is the dyadic operation:

join – allows to put together data rows from a pair of database relations.

In our proposal the last operation is limited to natural version only [4], i.e. performs equijoin on those columns which are common to both relations. Moreover, we introduced the concept of relationships between database relations. The join operation is now performable only on those pairs of relations for which relationship has been defined in external schema of the database. Limitation to the natural join together with the relationship concept makes possible the simplification of query structure (demonstrated in next section of this paper).

Problem-oriented logical structure of relational database for clinical cardiology is shown in Figure 1; named ellipses represent relations in the sense of the applied data model. Detailed description of relations in database for clinical cardiology is summarized in Table I.

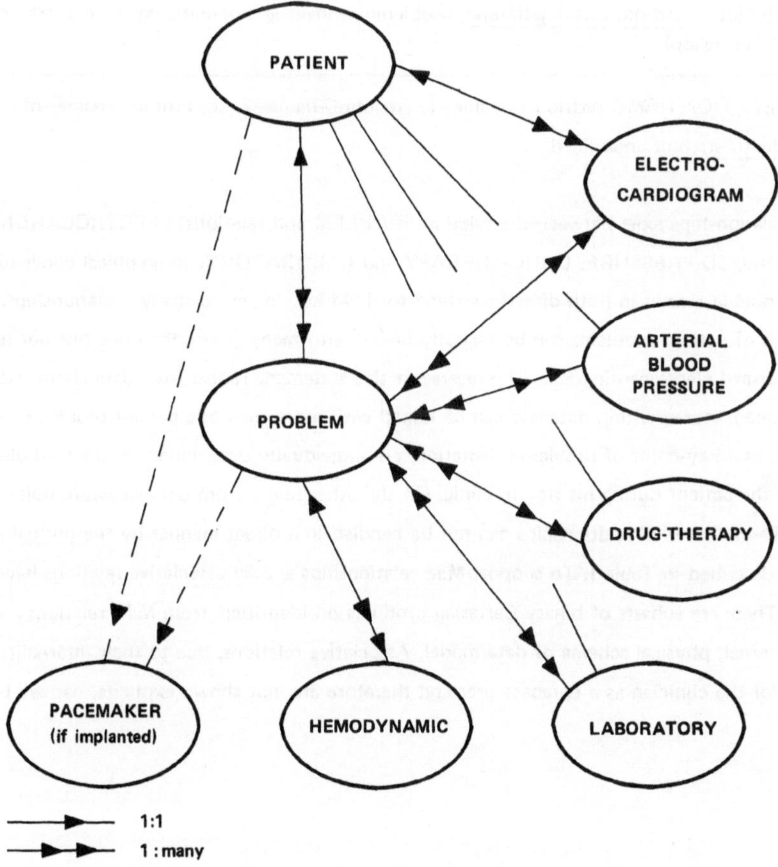

Figure 1. Logical structure of relational database for clinical cardiology

Table I. A database for clinical cardiology: relations description

PATIENT (pat-no, admission-data, previous-no, sex, age, marital-status, job-class, professional-activity, admission-overall-state, discharge-date)
PROBLEM (pat-no, problem-no, discovery-date, problem-code, clinical-status, plan, discharge-state)
ELECTROCARDIOGRAM (pat-no, ecg-no, registration-date, 26 elementary data items according to markedly modified Robles de Medina coding method [9])
ARTERIAL-BLOOD-PRESSURE (pat-no, test-no, measurement-date, method, systolic-pressure, diastolic-pressure)
DRUG-THERAPY (pat-no, therapy-no, start-date, drug-name, drug-administration-mode, days, daily-dosage, dosage-unit)
LABORATORY (pat-no, analysis-no, analysis-date, biomaterial-code, analysis-name, result, result-unit)
PACEMAKER (pat-no, problem-no, implantation-date, stimulation-type, electrode-type, pacemaker-type)
HEMODYNAMIC (pat-no, investigation-no, problem-no, investigation-date, co, sv, esv, edv, ci, ef, lvedp)

notation: RELATION-NAME (attribute—name—1, atrribute—name—2,....., atribute—name—n)

identifiers are underlined

Important relationships exist between the relation PROBLEM and relations: ELECTROCARDIOGRAM, ARTERIAL-BLOOD-PRESSURE, DRUG-THERAPY and LABORATORY. In graphical convention used in Figure 1, double arrows in both directions stand for M:M i.e. "many to many" relationships. For instance, each of patient problems can be logically linked with many (more than one but not necessarily all) performed electrocardiograms. The reverse of this statement is also true: data about each electrocardiogram stored within database can be linked with more than one patient problems. Such relationships, as a key-point of problem-orientation, are individually determined by the cardiologist who attends the patient during his stay in clinic. On the other hand, from data structure point of view it is evident that M:M relationships can not be handled in a direct manner by the normalized relations, as described in Table I. To support M:M relationships special associative relations have been introduced. These are subsets of binary Cartesian products on identifiers from M:M relations and are related to internal, physical schema of data model. Associative relations, due to their internality, are transparent for the clinician as a database user and therefore are not shown explicite, namely by ellipses in Figure 1.

QUERY LANGUAGE AS A USER INTERFACE TO CLINICAL DATABASE

The question-answering access to the database is provided by nonprocedural query language based on algebraic operations disccussed in previous section. In the designed language projection is recalled by "attribute names FROM" language construct, selection is recalled by "WHERE condition" construct and join operation is declared through an asterisk (*) symbol. Owing to the relationship concept the linguistic declaration of (natural) join operation now consists exclusively of the names of "joinable" relations. In other words the names of appropriate attributes (exactly identifiers), as shown in Table I, conditions for equality of their values and/or internal associative relations in case of joining M:M relations have been eliminated from the user declaration of join operation. Basic capabilities of the designed language are demonstrated through examples of query formulation. Numbers of symbols used in queries are not separately explained; they arise from applied coding schemas and adequately express the items which appeare in natural language questions (requests).

EXAMPLE 1

List the jobs performed by men patients, aged between 30 and 65, admitted to hospital in 1979 when seriously ill.

GIVE job-class FROM PATIENT WHERE sex = m AND age IN ⟨30;65⟩ AND
admission-date IN ⟨01/01/79; 31/12/79⟩ AND
admission-overall-state = 4.

EXAMPLE 2

In what state have the non-maried men with heart infarct been discharged and how old were they?

GIVE age, discharge-state FROM PATIENT WHERE sex = m AND marital-status NOT = 3 * PROBLEM
WHERE problem-code = 010.

EXAMPLE 3

In how many cases of patients with heart infarct the procainamide prevention was not applied?

COUNT PROBLEM WHERE problem-code = 010 * DRUG-THERAPY WHERE drug-name
NOT = procainamide.

EXAMPLE 4

What was the average age of patients who died suddenly in the course of heart infarct?

PERFORM AVERAGE ON age FROM PATIENT * PROBLEM WHERE
problem-code = 010 AND discharge-state = 7.

note: AVERAGE is a mnemonic name of special, non-relational operation. Examples of others, equaly important aggregation operations are MINIMUM, MAXIMUM, MINIMAX.

EXAMPLE 5

What is the frequency of all co-occurence complete AV block and heart infarct cases in function of heart infarct localization?

PERFORM HISTOGRAM ON ihd FROM PROBLEM WHERE problem-code = 010

* ELECTROCARDIOGRAM WHERE conduction = 5.

note: attribute ihd (ischeamic heart disease) has 13 distinct coded values — 11 of them represent heart infarct localizations. HISTOGRAM — like in previous example — is a mnemonic name of special operation. In this example the cardiologist obtains not only summary of data but a graphical output which allows convenient, visual interpretation of the received data.

EXAMPLE 6

What are the numbers of source clinical documents, age and sex for patients treated with propranolol in period longer than 9 days; also, for what problem(s) propranolol has been applied, in what dosage and in what state patients have been discharged?

The solution in this example is obtained in two queries because data which should produce output table are spread into three database relations. First query takes a from:

SAVE PATIENT * DRUG-THERAPY WHERE drug-name = propranolol AND

days > 9 AS PROPRANOLOL-PATIENTS.

and organizes a temporal (intermediate) relation PROPRANOLOL-PATIENTS which stores adequately selected and then joined rows from database relations PATIENT and DRUG-THERAPY. Then, the next query should have a from:

GIVE pat-no, age, sex, problem-code, daily-dosage, discharge-state

FROM PROBLEM * PROPRANOLOL-PATIENTS.

IMPLEMENTATION

Computer database system CARDIOCOD (CARDIOlogical COmputer Documentation) has been designed and implemented on ODRA 1300 (compatible to ICL 1900 series) computer [5]. CARDIOCOD database is maintained on disc storage. Each relation of data model is implemented as physically separate indexed file; one data record in a given file represents one row of data from corresponding relation. For statistics of first hundred patients stored in database see Table II.

Operational CARDIOCOD software consist of 3 structurally written COBOL programs (summary core size approximately 140 Kbytes). Two of these programs are for database updating and reporting (in batch processing mode). The third program is for interactive query processing and, according to Wiederhold design recomendations for statistical inference category of databases [6], offers some facilities to the clinical user (presentation of the data in scattergrams to examine possible correlation between attributes, histograms like in example 5). Storage of intermediate results in form of temporal relations (see directive SAVE in example 6) may avoid multiple reprocessing large portions of database.

Simple queries, containing projection and/or selection operations are executed through linear processing of entire files. Join operation however, turned out to be a major performance problem in relational databases implementation [7]. We chose collating as a implementation technique because:

Table II

CARDIOCOD[1)] DATA MODEL RELATION	Relations implemented as sequenced flat files record size (in bytes)	observed occurence per patient min	max	mean[2)]	storage area per patient
PATIENT	36	–	–	–	36
PROBLEM	20	1	8	2.95	59.00
ELECTROCARDIOGRAM	44	0	6	2.27	99.88
ARTERIAL-BLOOD-PRESS.	20	0	11	2.47	49.40
DRUG-THERAPY	44	0	31	5.85	257.40
LABORATORY	40	0	19	8.84	353.60
PACEMAKER optional	48	–	1	0.07	3.36
Σ Storage areas per patient					859.64[3)]

1) Statistics covers first hundred patients recorded in CARDIOCOD database since the begining of operation (October 78). Relation HEMODYNAMIC was added in the end of 79 and therefore is not included.

2) That figures seem to be relatively low but not all clinical facts are stored in database. For example, cardiologist selects only those electrocardiograms which represent clinically significant changes in patient state.

3) 860 bytes is the average requirement of storage space for patient clinical data. Approximately 160 bytes should be added for storage which is used to keep M:M relationships (by means of associative relations).

– all database files can be kept permanently after being sorted on the joining attributes (identifiers);

– in constant database volume growth collation, when compared with other techniques, offers moderate influence on processing time increase, and consequently on system response parameters.

The system has been in use in two clinical wards (approximately 60 beds including ICCU) of Institute of Cardiology, Poznań since October 1978. At present (October 1980) CARDIOCOD system contains data about 1700 patients.

DISCUSSION

The presented project involves long-term collection of data. Actual clinical population stored in database is still too small and too heterogenous for clinical research works. However, it seems obvious that CARDIOCOD system will act as a powerful tool in clinical studies on so large populations that are not available for analysis in a traditional manner. Such benefits of our system are expected in forthcoming future, because relational methods used in CARDIOCOD project have already proved to be both clinically applicable and useful.

Firstly, 2-years experience of storing patient data in the structure of CARDIOCOD database shows that clinical realms can be gathered within relational framework with adequacy level accepted by clinical community. Relational database in clinic, when compared with fixed-format computerized reports (for example [8]) offers much higher flexibility. In particular, in CARDIOCOD database the total volume of data per patient, and patient's occurence numbers of relational data rows (like electrocardiograms or drug-therapies) are highly variable and practically unlimited. A minor clinical drawback of CARDIOCOD system is the oversized, time consuming method used for coding electrocardiogram exercises [9]. Therefore, a more concise method, adopted from [10] is under development.

Secondly, our preliminary trials show that the necessary understanding of the relational database structure and, consequently, physician's practical usage of proposed language is possible after a couple of hours training. That is the basic condition to achieve one of our primary targets i.e. availability of a tool which enables direct interactions between clinical researcher and computer database system.

Relational approach to medical data, however less evident than in our project, has been reported by others (for example announcement health statistics application of PRTV system [11], normalized tabular data structures in TOD system [12]). In this paper, besides distinctly formulated cardiological application, we exposed results concerned with relational join operation and corresponding simplification of query structure. We aim at achieving the same results as the Medical System Hannover [13], but in a strictly relational environment of data. Currently MSH method is more advanced due to the definitive elimination of join construct from user queries. Also, the apparent advantage of MSH Descriptive Query Language is that we have not yet developed a mechanism for supporting equaly simple and straightforward form of queries for requests of the type as example discussed in Sauter et al. work [13].

In future, we shall work upon the problem of integrity constrains in clinical databases and their effective build-in into the next generation of CARDIOCOD system. Works concerning query interfaces to clinical databases and their more effective implementations will also be continued.

REFERENCES

[1] Codd E.F.: A Relational Model of Data for Large Shared Data Banks. Comm. ACM 1970; 13: 377–387.

[2] Codd E.F.: Recent investigations in relational data base systems. Information Processing 74, North-Holland, 1974, 1017–1021.

[3] Jasiński P.J.: Relational model of data intended for clinic's patients database design. Ph.D. Thesis (in Polish), Technical University of Poznań, Electrical Engineering Faculty, Poznań 1979.

[4] Aho A.V., Beeri C., Ullman J.D.: The Theory of Joins in Relational Databases. ACM Trans. on Database Systems 1979; 4: 297–314.

[5] Jasiński P.J., Krug H., Zerbe F., Kierzkowski Z., Jasiński K.: Kardiologiczna Komputerowa Dokumentacja (KARDIOKOD). Kard. Pol. 1979; 22: 695–704.

[6] Wiederhold G.: Database Design, Mcgraw-Hill, 1977.

[7] Todd S.: Implementation of join operator in relational data bases. IBM UK Scientific Centre, Peterlee, TN 15, Nov. 1974.

[8] Kennelly B.M., Vader C.G.: A Computerized Report Form for the Cardiac Intensive Care Unit. Intens. Care Med. 1980; 6: 9–17.

[9] Zerbe F., Dziamski R., Jasiński P.J., Krug H.: Metoda kodowania i komputerowego gromadzenia opisów badania elektrokardiograficznego. Kard. Pol. 1980; 23: 873–880.

[10] Brower R.W., Ten Katen H.J., Meester G.T.: Interim Data Processing in the Netherlands Study on Coronary Artery Bypass Graft Surgery. Computers and Biomedical Research 1980; 13: 87–101.

[11] Todd S.J.P.: Relational Database Research at the IBM United Kingdom Scientific Centre, Peterlee. A Survey 1970–1977. Report UKSC–0093, IBM Peterlee, Dec. 1977.

[12] Wiederhold G., Fries J.F., Weyl S.: Structured organization of clinical databases. National Computer Conference 1975, AFIPS; 44: 479–485.

[13] Sauter R., Weingarten W., Klonk J., Reichertz P.L.: A Multi-Level Approach for Data Description and Management of a Large Hierarchical Database Supporting a Hospital Patient Information System. In: Information Systems Methodology (ed. G.Bracchi and P.C.Lockemann), Lecture Notes in Comp. Sc. 65, Springer Verlag 1978: 367–379.

CHAINAGE CHRONOLOGIQUE DE DOSSIERS
APPLICATION A L'EVALUATION DU RISQUE DE LA DEFAILLANCE D'UN STIMULATEUR CARDIAQUE PAR ETUDE DE LA DERIVE DES PERIODES

CHAU N.[a], VALANTIN G.[a], KUBLER L.[b], MARTIN J.[a] et DODINOT B.[b]

Aide technique : Melle AUER M.C.[b] et Mmes KAUFMANN F.[b] et LEROY M.[b]

[a]Section de Statistique et d'Informatique Médicale, Groupe INSERM U115, Faculté de Médecine, B.P. 184, 54500 Vandoeuvre-les-Nancy.

[b]Service des Stimulateurs Cardiaques (Dr DODINOT), CHR de Brabois, Nancy.

SUMMARY

The follow-up studies of patients require the representation of the "chronological axis" of some data. In this paper, we describe a chronological chaining method of records which is a natural generalization of the structure of records having the "fixed format". This technique is easy to use. The program which we have conceived for a mini-computer Mitra 15/125 has already enabled us to answer many investigations. However, its structure allows the easy addition of new general or specific sub-programs. Besides, the running time of interrogation is shorter because it does not require any to and fro movements of the read head. We finally present its application to evaluate the risk of pace-maker failure by studying the temporal variation of the stimulation period.

1. INTRODUCTION.

Si les exemples d'application médicale de l'informatique se multiplient chaque jour, peu nombreuses, en revanche, restent les démonstrations d'un suivi chronologique véritable des malades. Une telle situation est due souvent au refus des équipes médicales de se lancer dans une étude informatisée prolongée. Mais à cet obstacle, il faut ajouter les difficultés croissantes auxquelles on va sans cesse se heurter depuis le recueil et le contrôle de données jusqu'à leur exploitation finale. Parmi les problèmes informatiques rencontrés, une place importante doit être accordée à celui de la reconstitution chronologique des évènements qui fera donc l'objet de cet exposé. Dans ce qui suit, nous exposerons d'abord, une méthode de chaînage chronologique de dossiers utilisable sur des mini-ordinateurs et facile à mettre en oeuvre. Nous présenterons ensuite son application à l'évaluation du risque de défaillance d'un stimulateur cardiaque (pace-maker) par étude de la dérive des périodes de stimulation.

2. CHAINAGE CHRONOLOGIQUE DE DOSSIERS.

L'étude de suivi des malades nécessite la représentation de "l'axe chronologique" d'un certain nombre d'informations. Le procédé est simple quand la structure des données est identique pour tous les sujets. Le problème que nous nous proposons d'étudier ici est beaucoup plus complexe. En effet, chaque individu I_k dispose de $n_{k1}, n_{k2}, \ldots, n_{kp}$ dossiers (ou articles) de p types fixés $T_1, T_2, \ldots, T_p$. Un dossier représente ici l'ensemble de données (quantitatives et qualitatives) concernant une opération déterminée pour un individu donné. Les nombres n_{ki} peuvent être très variables d'un sujet à l'autre.

En classant tous les articles par catégorie, nous obtenons p fichiers distincts $F_1, F_2, \ldots, F_p$; le fichier F_i correspond aux dossiers de type T_i. Chaque fichier F_i est un fichier dit à "structure fixe" c'est-à-dire tel que, pour chacun de ses articles, une donnée quelconque occupe toujours un même emplacement. Le chaînage chronologique de dossiers ainsi recueillis consiste à construire un "super-fichier" E tel que tous les dossiers appartenant à un même sujet y soient regroupés ensemble et classés dans l'ordre chronologique.

Structure du super-fichier E :

Chaque sujet est identifié par un numéro (1) et ce numéro doit être porté sur tous les dossiers. Nous appelons "super-dossier" ou "super-article" l'ensemble des informations dans E appartenant à un même sujet. Sa longueur peut être très variable d'un sujet à l'autre. E contient en son en-tête un catalogue dans lequel on trouve des renseignements descriptifs tels que le nombre p de fichiers F_i, le code et la longueur des F_i, l'emplacement du numéro de dossier et de la date dans chaque dossier, etc .... Chaque super-article contient un catalogue propre servant à mettre des informations précisant sa structure.

Création et mise à jour de E :

Dans E, chaque type de dossier T_i est représenté par un code caractère. Une mise à jour de E consiste à inclure dans E, un certain nombre de dossiers d'un type donné. La création d'un super-fichier peut être alors considérée comme une mise à jour d'un super-fichier initialement nul.

En fait, dans E, tous les super-articles sont ordonnés par ordre de numéro croissant. Si nous appelons E_0 l'ancien super-fichier, F l'ensemble de dossiers à ajouter à E_0, la construction du nouveau super-fichier E_f se décompose en deux phases suivantes :

- triage des dossiers de F suivant l'ordre de numéro croissant,
- et puis transcription de E_f par balayage séquentiel des trois fichiers E_0, F et E_f.

On note que ce procédé peut être très long car il faut copier à chaque fois tout l'ensemble E_f. Il existe d'autres procédés (2), (3), (4), (5) plus ou moins courts. Un procédé couramment utilisé consiste à copier F au bout de E_0 et ã établir ensuite la liaison entre E_0 et F par des pointeurs. Mais cette méthode exige que E soit sur un organe périphérique à accès direct alors que, pour notre méthode, E_0 et E_f peuvent être sur un organe à accès uniquement séquentiel. Cependant, il existe trois autres raisons qui expliquent le choix de notre méthode :

- le temps de réponse d'une interrogation est plus court car elle ne demande aucun mouvement de va-et-vient de la tête de lecture;
- on peut transformer tous les super-dossiers en des articles d'un même format fixe en complétant certains d'entre-eux par des dossiers vides; ceci nous permet alors d'utiliser des programmes généraux d'interrogation de fichiers à structure fixe dont nous disposons;
- et pour le problème qui nous préoccupe actuellement, il n'est pas indispensable d'inclure immédiatement dans le super-fichier les nouveaux dossiers; on peut donc regrouper ensemble ces derniers et reporter les mises à jour à des moments creux.

Difficultés rencontrées - Programmes et traitements employés :

Comme la forme de dossiers pour lesquels le recueil de données s'étend sur plusieurs années, celle des dossiers destinés à un chaînage chronologique doit souvent subir des transformations. L'expérience montre que, bien que le choix soit soumis à chaque fois à un examen attentif et malgré l'existence des "zones de réserves" pour des informations nouvelles, la durée de vie de chaque modèle est assez limitée. De ce fait , nous devons disposer d'un programme de transcodification très général.

Chaque dossier est soumis à deux contrôles successifs :

- un contrôle intra-dossier que l'on fait subir séparément à chacun des dossiers avant le chaînage;
- et un contrôle inter-dossier qui vérifie ensuite la concordance entre les informations des différents dossiers d'un même sujet.

Ces deux contrôles automatisés sont basés sur des critères sémantiques. Bien que le programme que nous ayons mis en oeuvre accepte des critères très généraux et complexes, il reste des erreurs non détectables automatiquement et il nous faut alors adjoindre un contrôle manuel supplémentaire.

Tous les traitements précités ainsi que les interrogations statistiques sont assurés essentiellement par le programme LOGIST (6) que nous avons conçu de façon à ce que l'adjonction de nouvelles procédures générales ou spécifiques telle que celle de constitution d'un axe chronologique des informations soit très aisée. Tous ces programmes sont paramétrés et écrits exclusivement en Fortran IV (ils sont par conséquent transportables). Leur mise en oeuvre a duré environ 4 ans. Ils sont actuellement utilisés en routine sur notre mini-ordinateur Mitra 15/125.

3. APPLICATION A L'EVALUATION DU RISQUE DE LA DEFAILLANCE D'UN STIMULATEUR CARDIAQUE PAR ETUDE DE LA DERIVE DES PERIODES.

Le problème qui est à l'origine de notre étude est celui des pace-makers. Le recueil de données est effectué au service des stimulateurs cardiaques (Dr DODINOT) du CHR de Nancy. Il a débuté, il y a environ 10 ans.

Au début, nous avions créé trois types de dossiers : le dossier "Primo-implantation" (P) qui correspond à la 1ère implantation d'un pace-maker chez un malade; le dossier "Hospitalier" (H) et celui de "Réintervention" (R) qui correspond à une réintervention chez un malade déjà porteur d'un appareil. Depuis environ 3 ans, nous avons supprimé le dossier H et ajouté 2 nouveaux : le dossier de "Consultation" (C) et celui de "Exit" (E) pour le cas où l'on est informé du décès du malade. Notons que, depuis leur création, la structure de chacun des dossiers P, R, C et E a subi plusieurs modifications.

La structure du super-dossier d'un malade peut être schématisée par la chaîne suivante :

PCC ... CRCC ... CRCC ... E

dans laquelle, chacun des dossiers R, C et E peut être absent. L'information étudiée (la période de stimulation) figure sur chaque dossier. Le délai séparant deux dossiers successifs est très variable.

Actuellement, ce système de dossiers concerne environ 2000 individus et, dans l'ensemble, a un volume approximatif d'un million de caractères. Certains individus disposent de plus de 15 dossiers. Pour le moment, nous travaillons en temps différé avec des bordereaux d'encodage. Mais nous attendons tous avec impatience la possibilité de passer à un système en temps réel sur console.

Ces fichiers ont permis déjà de répondre à de nombreuses évaluations sur la fiabilité de différents types de pace-makers, sur la qualité des électrodes, etc .... Le problème que nous allons envisager dans la suite est celui de l'évaluation du risque de la défaillance d'un pace-maker par étude de la variation de la période de stimulation $p(t)$ en fonction du temps t.

En principe, p(t) devrait être maintenue constante et égale à une valeur bien choisie pour chaque malade. Cependant, l'usure de l'appareil se traduit par un certain accroissement et il faut le remplacer dès que sa valeur dépasse un certain seuil. D'autre part, théoriquement la courbe de p(t) devrait faire partie des caractéristiques de l'appareil. Mais en pratique, celle-ci reste difficilement prévisible et varie beaucoup d'un type d'appareil à l'autre. L'accroissement de p(t) présente parfois des sauts et en fin d'évolution, un allongement rapide peut amener l'équipe médicale à intervenir sans plus attendre. p(t) apparaît donc comme le paramètre qui doit faire l'objet d'une surveillance très étroite.

Résultats :

Le but de notre étude est, connaissant la valeur de p(t) en m points quelconques $t_0, t_1, \ldots, t_{m-1}$, de déterminer l'instant t_f pour lequel la valeur de p(t) atteint un seuil préfixé et d'estimer le risque d'une défaillance avant cet instant t_f. La détermination de t_f apparaît donc comme un simple problème de lissage et d'extrapolation curviligne. Toutefois, le problème pratique est plus complexe car il faut tenir compte du fait que : la valeur de $p(t_0)$ dépend du malade et pour un malade donné, de la vraie valeur de t_0 ; l'évolution de p(t) varie avec la marque et le type de l'appareil (dont il existe une très grande variété), avec son état (neuf ou réchapé) et avec son mode de fonctionnement (mode sentinelle ou à émission permanente) ; et à chaque instant t_i, on peut modifier artificiellement la valeur de $p(t_i)$ (cas des pace-makers dits programmables).

Devant cette difficulté, nous avons choisi de recourir à une technique de mise en évidence typographique des variations temporelles de certaines variables (quantitatives et qualitatives). Elle consiste à présenter, dans une même figure, à droite, le graphique de p(t) en fonction du temps t et, à gauche, des renseignements complémentaires (voir figure 1). Ceci fournit en quelque sorte, une certaine représentation de l'histoire de chaque malade.

Présentons un exemple. Dans la figure 1, chaque ligne non vide concerne un dossier et le 1er caractère représente son code. A droite, nous trouvons le graphique de p(t), t étant exprimé ici en mois. A gauche, nous affichons pour chaque dossier la date réelle de l'opération et la valeur de p(t). Pour les dossiers P et R, nous ajoutons, en plus de ces 2 données, la marque et le type du pace-maker implanté. La 1ère ligne indique que le 19/8/1977, on a implanté chez le malade n° 3047, un pace-maker de marque 03 et de type 190A (un appareil programmable) en fixant $p(t_0)$ à 650 ms. Le 22/9/1977, on a programmé p(t) à 730 ms. Puis le 15/12/1977, on l'a ramenée à 646 ms. Le 17/1/1980, un épuisement brutal du stimulateur a amené l'équipe médicale à changer sans délai l'appareil. Nous ne donnons pas ici plus de détails; le lecteur désirant les obtenir peut se référencer à l'article de la référence (7). Notons que les données affichées sont paramètrées et que normalement, on a besoin de beaucoup plus d'informations.

Les documents ainsi obtenus peuvent être utilisés pour le contrôle manuel des données après chaînage, pour vérifier des hypothèses faites a priori et pour bâtir de nouvelles idées.

Citons deux autres problèmes. Le 1er est celui des contrôles de qualité des appareils. Le 2ème ressemble à celui de la détermination de t_f. Il peut être formulé comme suit : connaissant la valeur de p(t) en s points $t_0, t_1, \ldots, t_{s-1}$, déterminer l'instant t_s de la prochaine consultation (ou contrôle). Ce problème peut se prolonger naturellement en celui de l'établissement d'un calendrier de consultation par ordinateur.

Actuellement , nous sommes encore au stade de début de notre étude. Les résultats obtenus seront communiqués ultérieurement.

4. CONCLUSION.

La constitution d'un fichier rassemblant de nombreux modules est un outil simple et commode de surveillance évolutive de malades. Il faut porter une attention soutenue à la qualité des informations et à l'identification de chaque document.

La méthode de chaînage chronologique de dossiers que nous venons de présenter est une généralisation naturelle de la structure des dossiers à format fixe. Elle est facile à mettre en oeuvre. Le programme que nous avons conçu pour notre mini-ordinateur Mitra 15/125 permet de répondre à de nombreuses interrogations en mettant le fichier obtenu sous la forme d'un fichier à format fixe. La structure du logiciel permet une adjonction aisée de nouvelles procédures générales ou spécifiques tout en bénéficiant des possibilités existantes. En outre, le temps de réponse à une interrogation est plus court car celle-ci ne nécessite aucun mouvement de va-et-vient de la tête de lecture.

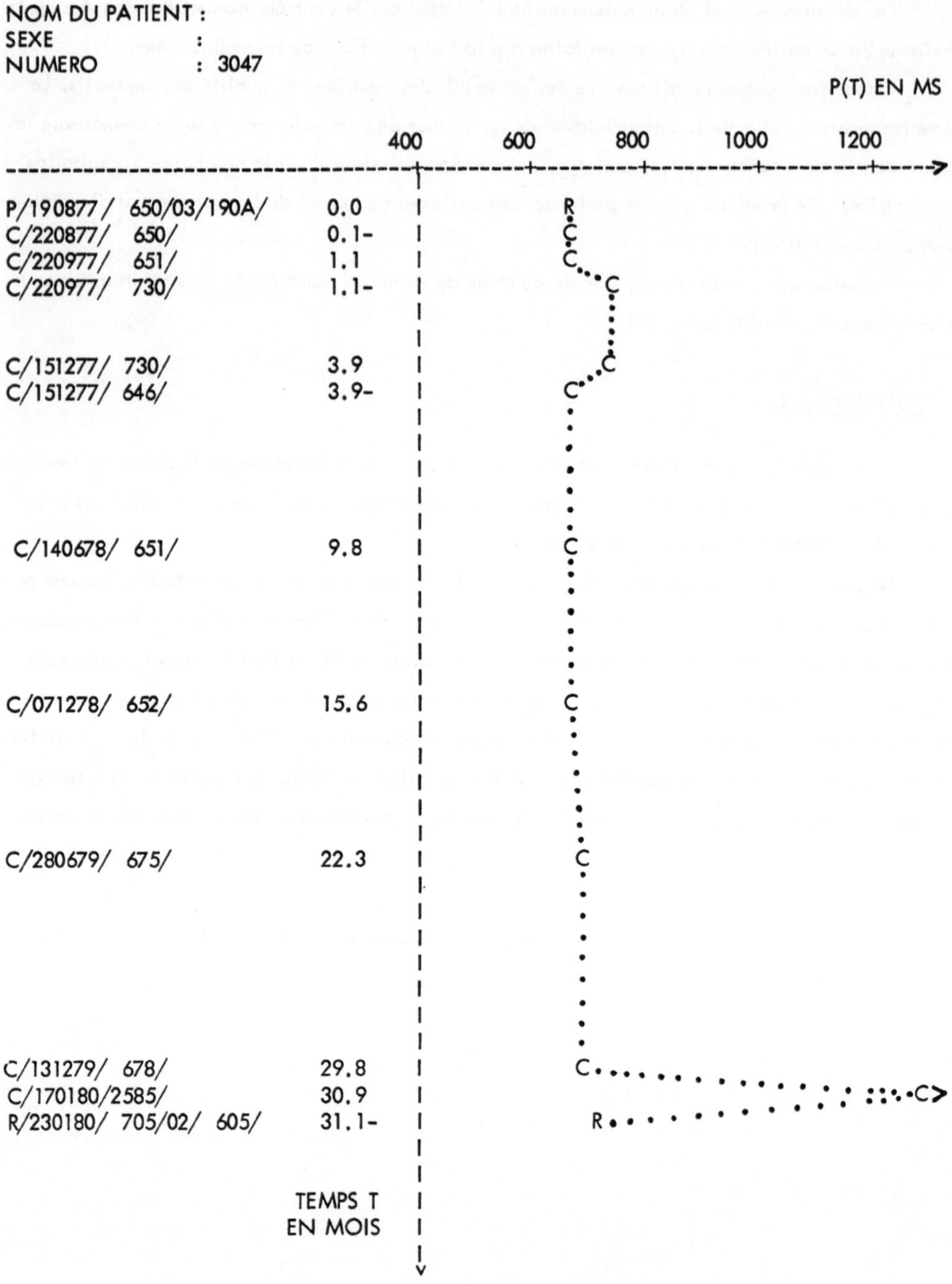

NOM DU PATIENT :
SEXE :
NUMERO : 3047

P(T) EN MS

400 600 800 1000 1200

P/190877/ 650/03/190A/	0.0	R
C/220877/ 650/	0.1-	C
C/220977/ 651/	1.1	C
C/220977/ 730/	1.1-	C
C/151277/ 730/	3.9	C
C/151277/ 646/	3.9-	C
C/140678/ 651/	9.8	C
C/071278/ 652/	15.6	C
C/280679/ 675/	22.3	C
C/131279/ 678/	29.8	C
C/170180/2585/	30.9	C>
R/230180/ 705/02/ 605/	31.1-	R

TEMPS T
EN MOIS

Figure 1 : Graphique de la période p(t) avec affichage de la valeur des informations complémentaires.

BIBLIOGRAPHIE

(1) Mur JM, Viard D, Mathieu JL , Martin J. Identification ability of the first five letters of christian name and surname. Méd Inform. 1979. vol 4. n°3, 199-202.

(2) Chantalou JP. Interactive Programming Language for Validation and Interrogation of Evolutive Data. In Anderson J (Edt). Medical Informatics Europe 78. 261-267.

(3) Goupy F. Le système Chronos, Réalisation d'un système de gestion de base de données médicales, orienté vers le traitement des données évolutives. Thèse de Doctorat d'Etat en Biologie humaine. Paris. 1978, Dact.

(4) Martin JM, Pointel JP, Martin J, Debry G. Long Range Medical Follow-up and Updating of Computerized Records. Meth Inf Med. Vol 19, n° 1,1980.

(5) Tardieu H, Nanci D, Pascot D. Conception d'un système d'information. Construction de la base de données. Les Editions d'Organisation, Paris, 1979.

(6) Chau N, Martin J, Cocco A, Legras B, Potdevin M. Concept and implementation of a program for treatments and statistical or logical interrogations of a file : Logist. Int J Bio-Médical Computing, vol 11, n° 2, 1980, 129-143.

(7) Dodinot B. Complications et pièges de la stimulation cardiaque. Stimucoeur Médical, vol 8, n° 1, 1980, 77-80.

HUIT ANNEES DE GESTION AUTOMATISEE DE DOSSIERS MEDICAUX HOSPITALIERS EN LANGAGE CLAIR

Alain GUILLOREAU AND Nathalie BOULARD

Centre de Traitement de l'Information
Médicale des Armées
69, Avenue de Paris - 94160 SAINT-MANDE (FRANCE)
1/374.12.40 - Poste 45.40

The Bégin military hospital automatism system's goes for 1973. He supports actually 125000 admissions and consultations corresponding with the observation of 85000 patients.

His periodic or variable exploitation allow

- **to have access to the médical record in natural langage**
- **to make record selection's corresponding with the documentary research modality**
- **to product epidemiology statistics job.**

The asked product analysis in connection with the theoric possibilities of the system shows that practitioners do not make the best use of the system, they enjoy; probably non conscious they are of the constraints and benefits inherent in use of a documentary automatism system.

Dans le cadre d'une expérimentation de gestion hospitalière médico-administrative automatisée lancée en 1972, *le Service de Santé des Armées* avait retenu la possibilité d'un suivi automatique du dossier médical pour les malades hospitalisés et si possible les consultants externes.

L'application commencée en septembre 1973, fonctionne depuis cette date sans interruption à *l'HIA Bégin à SAINT-MANDE* qui regroupe 680 lits répartis en 13 services cliniques. Des données médicales sur 125 000 hospitalisations et consultations sont ainsi disponibles sur supports magnétiques, correspondant au suivi de 85 000 patients.

Par rapport aux possibilités initiales restreintes, le système a évolué et permet actuellement la fourniture périodique ou aléatoire :

de données médicales individuelles
de données épidémiologiques dépersonnalisées
de données statistiques diverses (activité, clientèle etc)

Cependant l'analyse des produits demandés en regard des possibilités du système, montre que les médecins hospitaliers n'utilisent pas à plein l'outil dont ils disposent.

Seront abordés successivement :

- le choix et la collecte des informations médicales entrant dans le système et leur évolution dans le temps
- les principales caractéristiques des logiciels, des matériels et des procédures informatiques développées
- le coût de fonctionnement
- les résultats épidémiologiques obtenus
- les conclusions qui peuvent être dégagées sur la participation médicale aux procédures automatisées.

1. Choix des informations

Les spécifications intiales du collège de médecins et d'informaticiens qui avait jeté les bases du système étaient les suivantes :

- utilisation du langage naturel
- structuration du dossier magnétique superposable à celle de l'observation clinique classique.
- conservation possible tant des données qualitatives que quantitatives (résultats biologiques)
- protection et indépendance des informations relatives aux passages dans chaque service hospitalier (accès inter service interdit en utilisation épidémiologique)
- utilisation libre du système, en fonction des besoins et des possibilités de chacun, avec cependant conservation au minimum d'un diagnostic de sortie
- validation des informations qualitatives par le personnel médical le plus qualifié possible.

L'utilisation du langage naturel devait permettre d'éviter les contraintes d'une codification initiale, toujours cause d'une perte d'information, et donner la possibilité d'enregistrer des données à priori, sans présager de leur utilisation future. Cependant afin de permettre une exploitation automatique plus facile, une indexation par mots clés était adjointe systématiquement à chaque texte fourni. En 1975 fut rajouté la possibilité d'une codification complémentaire se reférenciant à la nomenclature OMS. Cette codification peut être soit donnée par le médecin, soit réalisée automatiquement par analyse des textes proposés. Elle fait référence actuellement à la CIM 75.

La structuration du dossier magnétique parallèle à celle de l'observation clinique donne la possibilité de ne traiter que certaines parties du dossier (suites opératoires, antécédents, résultats biologiques etc).

Cependant la masse des données biologiques relatives à chaque hospitalisation a conduit rapidement à restreindre cette possibilité, et à ne conserver d'une manière systématique que les résultats jugés significatifs par les cliniciens. Les archives biologiques restent donc stockées dans un sous-système spécifique du service technique commun, parallèle au dossier médical.

L'indépendance des informations relatives à chaque service est toujours respectée en exploitation courante. Elle permet d'éviter les conflits voire les contradictions entre les résultats fournis par les différentes unités et respecte les orientations sémantiques propres à chaque spécialité.

L'utilisation libre du système, limite la richesse des informations enregistrées, et conduit parfois à des «silences» et à des «bruits» difficilement supportés en exploitation.

Environ 10 % des hospitalisations n'ont pas de données médicales, et 40 % des diagnostics de sortie se révèlent plus que succints, par contre l'aspect contraignant est supprimé.

1.2. Collecte des informations

D'une manière générale toutes les données cliniques sont recueillies à la sortie du malade du Service hospitalier, à partir d'un document soit pré-établi automatiquement lors des formalités d'admission, soit réalisé manuellement. Une même hospitalisation peut donc conduire en cas de transfert inter-service à plusieurs enregistrements séparés.

Pour le laboratoire d'anatomo pathologie les informations sont saisies dès leur apparition, quelque soit la situation du malade (hospitalisation en cours, examen à titre externe, hospitalisé déjà sorti).

2. CARACTERISTIQUES TECHNIQUES

2.1. Généralités

Tous les documents concernant les données cliniques sont regroupés au «*Centre de Traitement de l'Information Médicale des Armées*» qui procéde : au contrôle manuel de la cohérence de l'indexation et à son homogénéité puis les saisit (encodage magnétique). Pour l'anatomo pathologie toutes ces opérations sont effectuées directement par le Service.

Les données sont ensuite traitées et mises en forme pour leur exploitation, après recyclage éventuel des anomalies détectées lors des contrôles automatiques (validation des mots clés par rapport au thésaurus). Ce thésaurus qui sert de référence pour l'utilisation du système comporte actuellement 4300 termes suivant les différentes spécialités médicales de l'hôpital (pas de service de psychiatrie). Après une utilisation ouverte au départ il est actuellement fermé. L'adjonction de termes nouveaux n'est réalisé qu'après avis d'une commission médicale.

2.2. Environnement

L'application de gestion du dossier médical est intégré dans le système de gestion administrative de l'hôpital, comme d'ailleurs tous les sous-systèmes de traitement des données techniques (laboratoires, pharmacie etc).

Cette intégration facilite le repérage des malades subissant des réhospitalisations successives ou venant en consultations externes en ne laissant aux médecins que la charge des informations techniques.

La reconnaissance des enregistrements propres à chaque individu se fait :

- soit par un numéro spécifique du malade
- soit par un numéro d'hospitalisation
- soit automatiquement à partir des données d'identification habituelles.

Le système d'identification administrative permet d'obtenir une grande sûreté dans la reconnaissance des enregistrements médicaux successifs d'un même individu (moins de 4 % d'anomalies) et libère les personnels médicaux de cette contrainte. Il permet de fournir en outre, automatiquement, des données administratives complétant le dossier médical (état matrimonial, nombre d'enfants, lieu de naissance etc).

2.3. Caractéristiques spécifiques

Les traitements particuliers aux dossiers médicaux relèvent de la conjonction de trois sous-systèmes :

- une gestion de banque de données
- un sous-système d'exploitation documentaire
- un sous-système d'exploitation statistique et épidémiologique.

2.31. Le système de gestion de banque de données :

C'est une application faisant référence à des fichiers classiques, intégrant toutes les informations :

- d'identification
- statistiques
- et médicales relatives à chaque séjour ou passage des malades dans l'ensemble hospitalier.

Il sert d'archive aux données médico administratives hospitalières.
Suivant le type d'exploitation demandé :

- travaux périodiques ou aléatoires
- travaux statistiques et épidémiologiques
- recherche documentaire
- périodes et/ou services à analyser,

les données sont extraites des archives pour être traitées par les autres sous-systèmes.

Le volume moyen d'un enregistrement relatif à un malade représente 850 caractères, le plus grand atteint 9000 caractères pour une hospitalisation. Toutes les informations sont datées.

2.32. Le sous-système statistique et épidémiologique :

Il fonctionne périodiquement pour la fourniture

- de relevés épidémiologiques relatifs aux hospitalisations de chaque service, pour chaque service, pour chaque mois considéré, avec un regroupement annuel, et pour l'hôpital dans son ensemble.

- de documents d'aide au secrétariat
  . récapitulation des malades hospitalisés au cours du mois avec code diagnostic OMS
  . récapitulation des examens anatomo pathologiques avec leur numéro de laboratoire et la liste des mots clés utilisés.

Il peut être utilisé aléatoirement pour tout travail statistique utilisant des données dont le repérage est simple, et qui n'entrent pas dans les textes traités en langage naturel, les mots clés, les codes OMS font partie du cadre de ces traitements.

2.33. Le sous-système documentaire

Il est utilisé chaque fois qu'il est nécessaire, pour affiner une recherche, de prendre en compte des données contenues dans les enregistrements en langage naturel (recherche avec troncature, recherche avec proximité) pour compléter l'insuffisance de l'indexation ou lorsqu'il est nécessaire d'utiliser des synonymes et/ou des hierarchies entre les mots clés.

2.34. Matériels et logiciels

Le système est opérationnel sur un ordinateur CII-HB IRIS 55. En fonctionnement normal il nécessite 64 K octects de mémoire, deux drivers de 50 mega octets et 1 à 3 dérouleurs de bande magnétique.

La phase de mise à jour hebdomadaire dure une heure environ. Les éditions périodiques mensuelles demandent deux heures de traitement.
La durée des travaux aléatoires : épidémiologie, recherche documentaire demandent de 20 minutes à 3 heures suivant leur complexité.
Une recherche documentaire standard dure 30 minutes.
Tous les traitements sont effectués par lots sans utilisation de terminaux.
L'ensemble des archives depuis 1973 est stocké sur six bandes magnétiques.

Les logiciels de traitement de base, épidémiologiques et statistiques ont été réalisés par le *«Centre de Traitement de l'Information Médicale des Armées»*. ils regroupent une soixantaine d'unités de traitement.

Le logiciel documentaire est la version V2 du progiciel MISTRAL de CII-HB

2.35 Coût de fonctionnement

La gestion du dossier médical revient à 1.65 F par jour soit 16 % du coût global des dépenses informatiques ramenées à la journée d'hospitalisation.
Le coût des travaux aléatoires ne peuvent être chiffrés que pour les interrogations documentaires, il est de l'ordre de 400 F par demande.

3. LES RESULTATS OBTENUS

«UN SYSTEME NE RESTE OPERATIONNEL QUE S'IL EST UTILISE». Or les treize services hospitaliers fournissent toujours depuis sept ans des informations, plus ou moins complètes ou significatives il est vrai, et interrogent périodiquement le système, d'une façon cyclique dans le temps (début et fin d'année).

Les relevés périodiques systèmatiques (pathologie de chaque service, répartition des entrants par catégories diverses) sont utilisés de façon variable par chaque Chef de Service.

Les demandes de travaux aléatoires concernent presque toujours la recherche de dossiers répondant à certains critères plus ou moins complexes afin de faciliter la préparation d'études qui feront référence aux informations des archives papier, de rassembler des données pour des cours ou des conférences. 40 demandes de ce type sont satisfaites chaque année.

Quelquefois la recherche du dossier complet d'un malade est sollicitée (une a révélé la présence de 43 séjours sur 3 ans pour un même individu.

Pour les demandes relevant directement des études épidémiologiques elles sont relativement rares, mais permettent de montrer que le système peut donner rapidement satisfaction (une journée pour la production des durées moyennes d'hospitalisation chez des sujets rapatriés d'Outre-Mer, atteints d'hépatites virales et par catégorie de personnel).

Enfin pour les travaux statistiques faisant appel aux méthodes mathématiques le système fournit des fichiers de travail qui sont repris dans un second temps.

4. LA PARTICIPATION MEDICALE

Après huit ans de fonctionnement on peut observer que les services se répartissent en trois groupes :

- ceux qui fournissent des informations peu significatives et relevant souvent d'une procédure réglementaire.
- ceux qui fournissent des données, par habitude mais les utilisent peu.
- ceux qui font appel régulièrement aux possibilités du système.

Parmi ceux-ci on peut relever le service d'anatomo pathologie et les services chirurgicaux, peut être du fait qu'un texte écrit (résultats d'ana - path ou compte rendu d'intervention) est chaque fois produit par les médecins ou chirurgiens et qu'il fournit souvent une information riche, fiable et structurée; ce qui corrobore les conclusions d'autres équipes qui ont abordé le problème.

Enfin les éditions récapitulatives des différents enregistrements propres à un malade, permettent d'obtenir un dossier médical raccourci mais relativement significatif de la pathologie d'un individu en montrant parfois des contradictions dans le temps entre les conclusions de la première hospitalisation et celles des suivantes. Cette possibilité est rarement exploitée du fait d'une certaine réticence des responsables à autoriser la consultation de la partie du dossier relevant de leur service, mais son exploitation s'intensifie et permet d'aborder les problèmes relatifs à la qualité des soins (les esprits s'y accoutument).

CONCLUSION

Le système présenté montre qu'il est possible de gérer de façon opérationnelle sur une longue période des éléments sélectionnés du dossier médical. Si l'exploitation de ceux-ci ne fournit pas toujours de résultats très évolués et d'intérêt général, elle permet cependant d'apporter une aide appréciable aux médecins qui font l'effort, et qui en ont la possibilité, de fournir des informations fiables.

Son maintien aprés huit ans démontre ainsi que le corps médical prend progressivement conscience que l'utilisation des techniques informatiques peut lui apporter quelque chose dans sa pratique quotidienne, mais que cette intégration d'un outil nouveau est longue et coûteuse à obtenir peut être du fait d'un manque d'information sur ses possibilités réelles.

BIBLIOGRAPHIE

- **«L'hôpital des Armées et l'Informatique» Guilloreau A. Médecine et Armées - 1969 / 3 / 211 / 221**

- **«Expérimentation d'un système autorisant la saisie en langage naturel et l'exploitation des données médicales» - Hertz, Delacroix, Fromantin, Guilloreau, Chabannes, Couturier. GEN. BIOL. MED. 1970 / 1 / 3 / 147 / 151**

- **«Gestion de l'Information Médicale» - Philip B., Guilloreau A., Informatique et gestion - 1972 / 1 / 34 / 93 / 96**

- **«Le dossier médical magnétique» - Sa constitution et ses utilisations - Bon, Denjean, Guilloreau, Chonez, Médecine et Armées - 1973 / 1 / 4 / 73 / 78.**

Software Systems Supporting Medical Registers

Dieter Schreiter, Claus-Dieter Donat, Rainer Koch and
Hans-Georg Vater

Computer Center, Medical School "Carl Gustav Carus" Dresden, GDR

Abstract

Parts of MADIS [1], the hospital information system of the clinics and institutes of our Medical School, are the subsysteme

- MADRIS - which is a register information system (long- and short-term storage of patient records and data)
- MADRAS - which is a search and evaluation system on the basis of descriptive and mathematical statistics.

Both these subsystems are developed in order to support medical care, medical research and the management and long-term planning of health care systems.

In the planning phase we had to decide whether and to which extent existing software components were useful for our objectives. This was possible, but we must solve both some interface problems between the software components and some problems of user-computer interaction (in terms of a problem-oriented language).

For some years we have used MADRIS and MADRAS in an effective manner. The preparation and generation of a new register in general needs less than four weeks in case of a problem analysis which has been finished before.

1. Introduction and aim

In 1976 we had to execute the order to establish a register of bone diseases. For this single case the required programs in PL/1 were written for data input, data check, data management and processing. The expenditure was ample. For more than two years the system is routinely applied and attains the planned aim in respect to standard requests [2]. Problems arise with individual evaluations of patient data on the basis of mathematical statistical methods.

In 1977/78 we were within a short time requested to establish registers for diseases like mucoviscidosis, tumors of the jaw-face region, broncho-pulmonary diseases and for further about ten diseases resp. disease groups.

Thereby, it had to be decided how this great number of registers could be established within a short time, and how effectively be managed in the computer centre. Besides the standard evaluations for patient care should preponderably be supported the individual evaluations based on relevant statistical methods for medical research, epidemiology and planning of health care facilities and nursing homes. This is in accordance with the actual trend for the efficacious utilization of computers for this purposes [3], [4], [5]. Further development of individual solutions had to be rejected. Instead of this, it was decided to develop

1. a register information system for multilateral utilization for standard evaluations
2. a statistical search- and evaluation system for individual statements of the problem and universal usefulness.

Available standard software should be used resp. adapted to a highest possible extent. Either system had repeatedly been applied in the meantime.

2. Register information system MADRIS

An analysis of the required performance extent in respect to registers showed the following crucial points:

- storage of a representative data selection derived from outpatient, inpatient or dispensaire care in respect to an individual patient suffering from special disease
- rationalization of organizational procedures in dispensaire consultation hours for patients with chronic disease, for specific outpatient care and for monitoring of high risk groups
- variable evaluation of the data stock, in particular for the characterization of the epidemiologic development of the disease or disease group, and for the design of strategies for the struggle against them as well as for the assessment of the efficacy of diagnostic, therapeutic and organizational procedures.

  Meeting these requirements MADRIS realizes the following functions:

- support of data aquisition on punch card respectively punch tape
- description of a data stock by means of a simple data description language
- definition of the check conditions in respect to syntactic and semantic correctness of data by means of a simple language
- concentration, assessment resp. computation of selected data before storage
- data storage according to data bank principles (inverse model)
- retrieval of data in batch and conversational mode applying a user convenient search language
- support of data output for
  - journals, records according to different organizing principles
  - duty of notification (for instance carcinoma)
  - call up and appointment scheduling system
  - providing reports on the course of the disease

Use was made of a general data bank system [6] for some general input functions, for storage and management, for retrieval and for parts of the output. Special functions of input and output are realized by additional own program-technical solutions. On demand further elements of the program for processing may be added (figure 1).

3. Search- and evaluation system MADRAS

MADRAS was developed for medical research purposes and the long-term planning of health care facilities for chronic diseases. It works in connection with data bases but also with arbitrary files. Besides the selection of adequate statistical procedures, therefore two tasks to be performed during the development:

1) to provide interfaces and the necessary data compatibility,
2) to make available auxiliary means in order to increase the user comfort of the overall system.

As an algorithmic basis for performance of the tasks of users, already available individual programs, statistical program packages [7] , utilities of operating systems and other program sources are used. The management of this program base with different structure and display facilities is performed by a program base system (PBS).

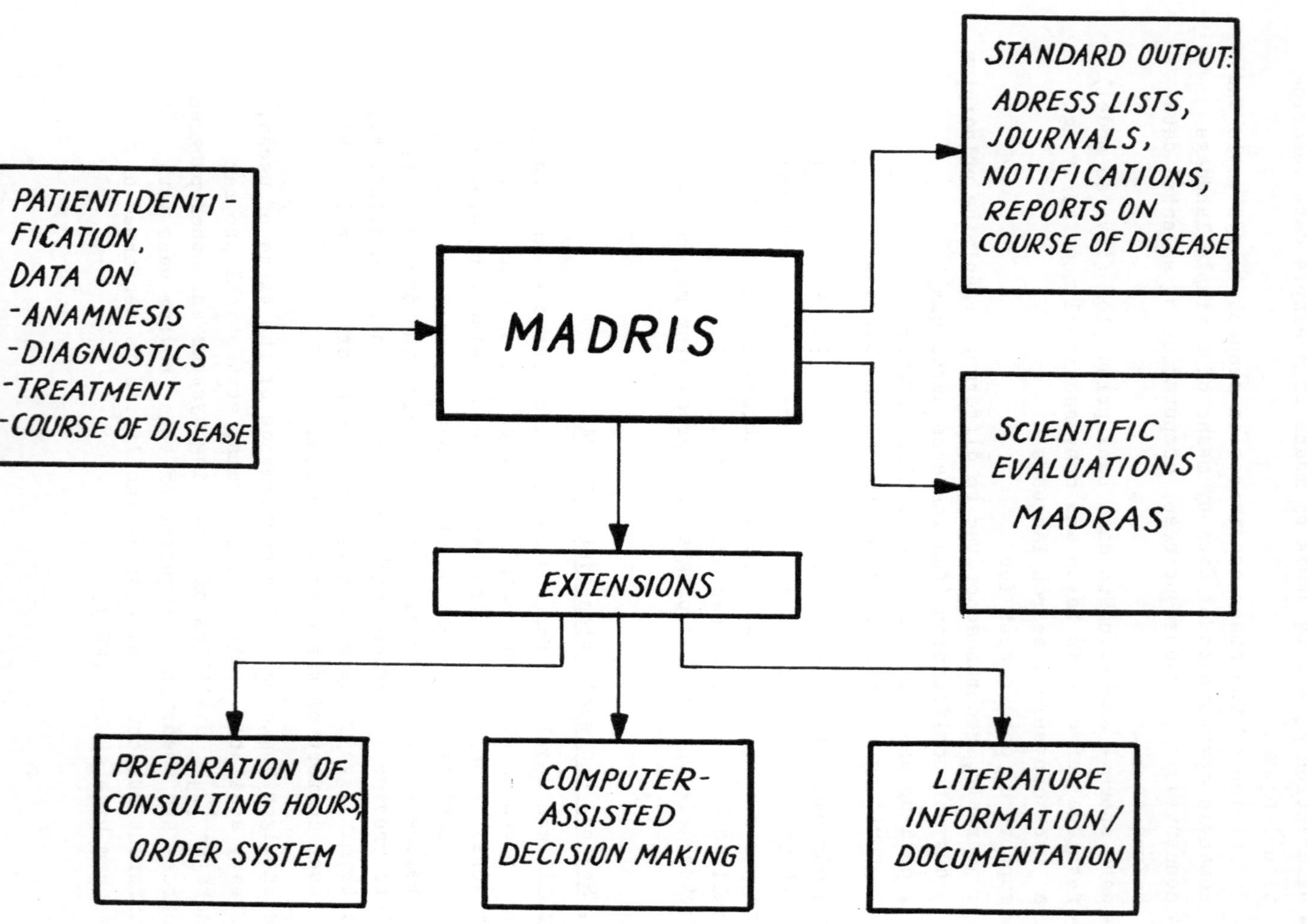

PATIENTIDENTI-
FICATION,
DATA ON
-ANAMNESIS
-DIAGNOSTICS
-TREATMENT
-COURSE OF DISEASE
MADRIS
STANDARD OUTPUT:
ADRESS LISTS,
JOURNALS,
NOTIFICATIONS,
REPORTS ON
COURSE OF DISEASE
SCIENTIFIC
EVALUATIONS
MADRAS
EXTENSIONS
PREPARATION OF
CONSULTING HOURS,
ORDER SYSTEM
COMPUTER-
ASSISTED
DECISION MAKING
LITERATURE
INFORMATION/
DOCUMENTATION

With it, the well-known principles of the management of files by data base systems are applied to the management of program structures. The establishing of a PBS is performed in the case of MADRAS by control systems in the kind of preprocessors or interpreters.

Especially for MADRAS the PL/1 macro interpreter as main component of the transformation of arbitrary text is used which from the input side represents a special language and on output side yields a job stream immediately to be performed.

The system conception leans upon the well-known 3 level architecture [8] . A separate language structure is assigned to each level.

1. External level: User oriented language terms for different user classes for wording the task.
2. Conceptual level: PL/1 macro texts for analysis of language terms of the external level and for synthesizing the structures of the internal level.
3. Internal level: Amount of all modes of expression of basis software (parameters, language terms, control statements, position parameters, keywords, and others).

Figure 2 shows the functional structure of the program base system

By the chosen kind of implementation MADRAS is an open system. With it, the extension or the replacement of parts of the basis software as well as the addition of new language elements is possible.
Two user groups are aimed at by MADRAS:

1. Occasional users (physicians, medical students and other members of hospital staff) who want to perform the inquiry and evaluation tasks themselves.
2. Skilled user (statisticians, members of the computer centre) who render inquiry and evaluation request service with extensive and - in mathematical respect - pretentious kind of evaluation on the basis of interdisciplinary cooperation of information processing and medicine.

MADRAS is designed as a system with dialogue possibility which is, of course, also suitable for batch processing. It assists both displays and type-writer-like terminals inclusive teletype-writers.

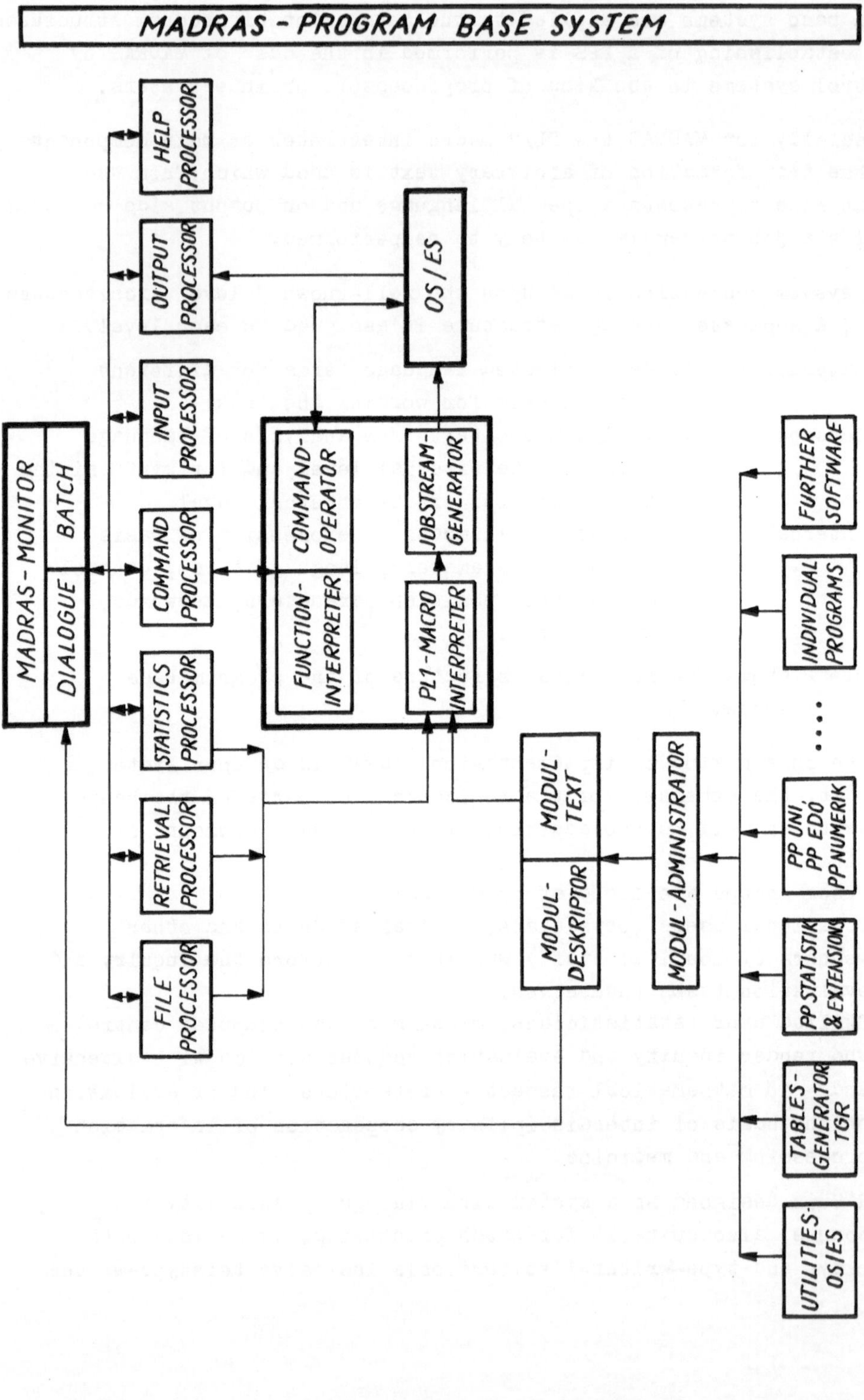

MADRAS - PROGRAM BASE SYSTEM

MADRAS - MONITOR
DIALOGUE
BATCH

HELP PROCESSOR
OUTPUT PROCESSOR
INPUT PROCESSOR
COMMAND PROCESSOR
STATISTICS PROCESSOR
RETRIEVAL PROCESSOR
FILE PROCESSOR

OS/ES

COMMAND-OPERATOR
FUNCTION-INTERPRETER
JOBSTREAM-GENERATOR
PL1-MACRO INTERPRETER

MODUL-TEXT
MODUL-DESKRIPTOR
MODUL-ADMINISTRATOR

FURTHER SOFTWARE
INDIVIDUAL PROGRAMS
....
PP UNI, PP EDÖ, PP NUMERIK
PP STATISTIK & EXTENSIONS
TABLES-GENERATOR TGR
UTILITIES-OS/ES

FIG. 2

According to the different user groups, two different modes of dialogue are employed:

1. program-controlled dialogue for the occasional user with the aim to instruct and assist the user in the display of the evaluation,
2. user-controlled dialogue for the experienced user with the aim of a rapid and convenient display of the evaluation request and its handing over to processing.

Whilst for the second user group the overall scope of mathematical-statistical procedures and extensive functions for data handling are provided, for the first user group are only such methods available which are applicable without instruction for the display of the evaluation and interpretation by a statistician. Of particular importance is the manner of communication of the experienced user with the program base. For this purpose a special language is provided. This language renders possible the display of the evaluation aim meeting users wishes. By the BPS a transformation of these language elements into the special coding rules of the basis software is performed. For this, the knowledge of the various display rules of the basis software by the user is no longer necessary.
The MADRAS language contains the main categories

- language terms for the manyfold file and record manipulations
- language terms for the investigation of autonomous data stocks
- language terms for the formulation of evaluations by means of mathematical statistical methods.

An additional available command language and further auxiliary functions serve the system control, respectively the provision of user's assistance in dialogue mode.

4. Conclusions and outlook

After having established a register by means of this software, now working on further registers, and experiences having gathered with more than one hundred evaluation requests, the following first conclusions can be drawn:
The systems have proven their practicability on principle. Either system renders possible a quick meeting of users wishes. The orientation - underlieing our development work - for the deliberate

utilization of delivered software, was obviously favorable in the projecting phase. A preliminary analysis of the hitherto existing applications naturally revealed the necessity of the improvement of some software parameters of the systems, a further increase of the customer's convenience and the extent of technological details. At the same time our investigation is aimed at the transferability of the system to other computer bases.

Reference

[1] Schreiter, D.: Rechentechnik in Medizin und Gesundheitswesen; Neue Technik im Büro 24 (1980) 4, S. 97 - 101

[2] Knoch, H.-G., Dominok, G.-W., Pape, K. and Schirpke, J.: Erfassung, Diagnostik und Therapie von Knochentumoren; Beiträge zur Orthopädie und Traumatologie 24 (1977) 10, S. 533 - 542

[3] Blum, B.J. and R.E. Lenhard Jr.: Experience in Implementing a Clinical Information System; MEDINFO '80, S. 38 - 42

[4] Ellsässer, K.-H. et al.: Instruction Concept in the System KRAZTUR; MEDINFO '80, S. 867 - 870

[5] Naito, M. et al.: ISCHEM: Information System for Coronary Heart Evaluation and Management; MEDINFO '80, S. 881 - 885

[6] System manual to PS AIDOS OS/ES, VEB Kombinat Robotron

[7] Programmer's Guide to PP STATISTIK, VEB Kombinat Robotron

[8] Schubert, D.: Stand und Tendenzen der rechnergestützten Programmsynthese auf der Grundlage problemorientierter Systemunterlagen; messen-steuern-regeln 21 (1978) 10, S. 585 - 588

A GRAPHIC MICROCOMPUTER SYSTEM FOR CLINICAL RENAL DATA

M. GORDON, H.E. de WARDENER, J.C. VENN, J. WEBB and H. ADAMS

Department of Medicine, Charing Cross Hospital Medical School, London W6 8RF, England

1. INTRODUCTION

The system improves utilisation of two major resources in dialysis and transplantation - clinical data and staff. Data is expensive to acquire, but in conventional records systems becomes obscured by necessary accumulations of new data, and cannot be seen in context. Staff must spend much time searching notes, or remain inadequately informed. In either case quality of care falls, especially with growing numbers of patients and changes of staff. The computer improves access to data and permits better care for more patients.

2. METHODS

2.1 Hardware summary: DEC LSI-11 microprocessor with twin 10-Mbyte cartridge discs, video generators, serial interfaces and electrostatic printer/plotter. Four remote user stations, each with VDU and video monitor, in dialysis ward office, transplant unit office, outpatient clinic, and ward clerk's office.

2.2 Software summary: Compact multi-user, multi-task executive. Simple, fast database. Reentrant run-time libraries and structured user sub-systems for retrieval, update, reporting and utilities, with password protection. Run-time configuration facilities. Automatic link to laboratory computers. Block-structured applications language with generalised reporting facilities.

2.3 Operation: The equipment runs 24 hours per day, unsupervised. Medical, nursing and paramedical staff control subsystems with the VDU numeric keypad, guided by a small dynamic 'map'. Tabular data appears on VDU and graphic data on video monitor. Access needs minimal typing. The data stored, organisation of access and display formats are configured for a particular Renal Unit. Typical organisations are:

2.4 Retrieval: Tabular - patient identification and status, diagnosis, GP details predialysis synopses, events history. Screen tests, tissue type and transplant data, transfusions, EDTA return data. Biochemistry, haematology and blood pressure/weight variables. Graphic - (with range indications, moveable cursor and read-out, variable time-scales, computed averages and optional plot modes): blood pressure/weight, haematology, calcium metabolism, protein metabolism, liver function. Experimentally, compressed digitised photographs have been stored.

2.5 Update: Manual VDU-update system for all variables above. Automatic link to acquire biochemistry and haematology data.

2.6 Reporting: Spooled tabular reports for: all data-sets above, new abnormal data, sorted creatinine list for waiting patients, transplant waiting lists, patient directories, reminders. Statistics of numeric data, data-base validation, and EDTA return. User-written reports via generalised reporting facility. Hard copy of all graphic displays.

2.7 Utilities: General utilities including: set system data, copy disc, index build, index sort, edit formats, archive data and generalised data edit.

3. RESULTS

The system has operated with successive improvements on a PDP-11 computer for more than four years (1,2) and for seven months on the LSI-11 microcomputer. It presently holds data for 247 patients on home and hospital dialysis and with transplants. The system has gained acceptance among medical and nursing staff, who use it regularly for daily ward rounds, group meetings and clinics, and for ad hoc data retrieval at any time. Manual data input is done by the ward clerk. Quantative measures of effectiveness are not available. However from observation, unskilled users take only a few minutes' instruction to learn the system; it is very much easier to obtain and interpret data from the computer than from written records; medical staff confirm they feel better informed and more relaxed on ward rounds after consulting the system; if the system is taken out of action there are usually complaints and protests within minutes from clinical or paramedical staff; and clinical staff are irritated by incompleteness in data. Figures 1 to 6 show typical data presentations.

4. DISCUSSION AND CONCLUSIONS

The system is available as a commercially supported package from about £25,000. Annual running costs are about 15% of this. These costs may be close to the point at which computer data-handling becomes cost-effective for a significant proportion of Renal Units in Europe. Costs may reduce with advances in hardware. The results indicate the computer is superior to conventional records systems. Data years old can be found readily and all data is seen in context. The graphic facilities allow dense clusters of data to be understood. The computer can also prepare statistics and print EDTA returns. An apparent drawback is the need for more discipline in updating the system with complete and accurate information. In reality, this only means better communication is demanded within the Renal Unit. The system is vulnerable to engineering and power failures, but these have not been a significant problem. We are not aware of any comparable microbased implementation.

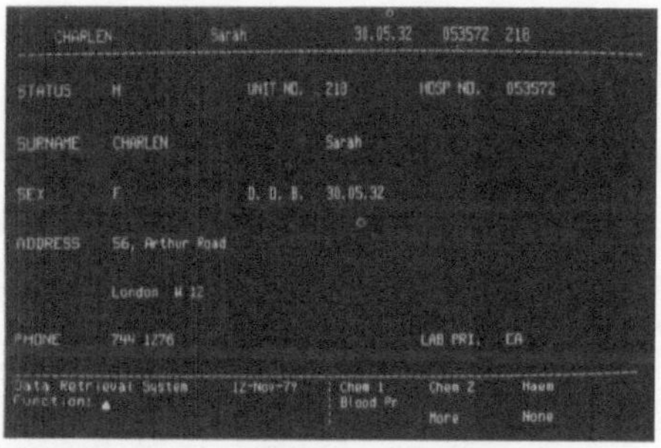

Figure 1 VDU identity display

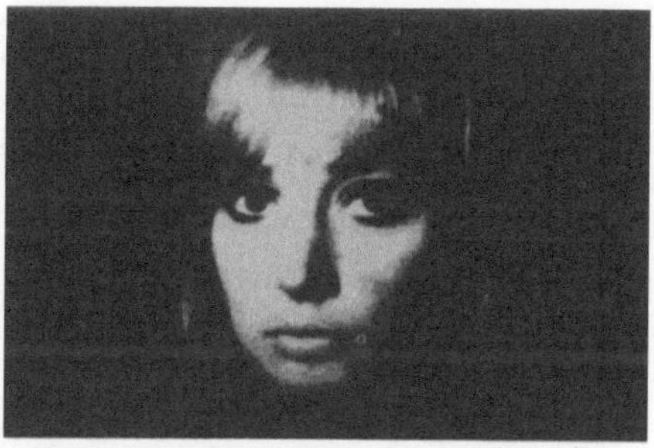

Figure 2 Digital photograph

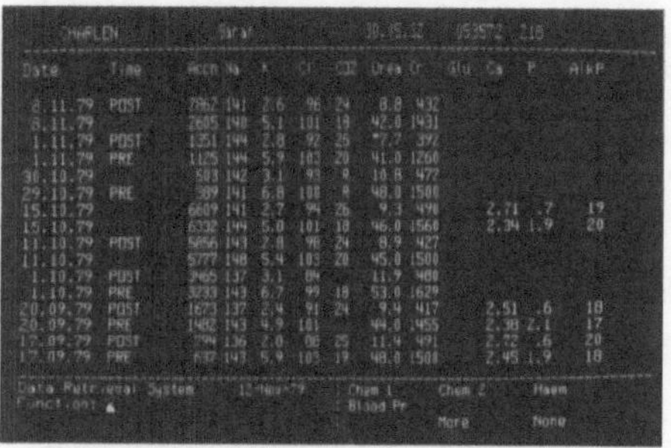

Date	Time	Accn	Na	K	Cl	CO2	Urea	Cr	Glu	Ca	P	AlkP
8.11.79	POST	2862	141	2.6	96	24	8.8	432				
8.11.79		2605	140	5.1	101	19	42.0	1431				
1.11.79	POST	1351	144	2.8	92	25	*7.7	392				
1.11.79	PRE	1125	144	5.9	103	20	41.0	1260				
30.10.79		503	142	3.1	93	8	10.8	472				
29.10.79	PRE	389	141	6.8	108	8	48.0	1500				
15.10.79		6609	141	2.7	94	26	9.3	490		2.71	.7	19
15.10.79		6332	144	5.0	101	18	46.0	1560		2.34	1.9	20
11.10.79	POST	5856	143	2.8	98	24	8.9	427				
11.10.79		5777	148	5.4	103	20	45.0	1500				
1.10.79	POST	3465	137	3.1	84		11.9	400				
1.10.79	PRE	3233	143	6.7	99	18	53.0	1629				
20.09.79	POST	1673	137	2.4	91	24	9.4	417		2.51	.6	18
20.09.79	PRE	1482	143	4.9	101		44.0	1455		2.38	2.1	17
17.09.79	POST	794	136	2.0	88	25	11.4	491		2.72	.6	20
17.09.79	PRE	632	143	5.9	105	19	48.0	1500		2.45	1.9	18

Figure 3 VDU biochemistry display

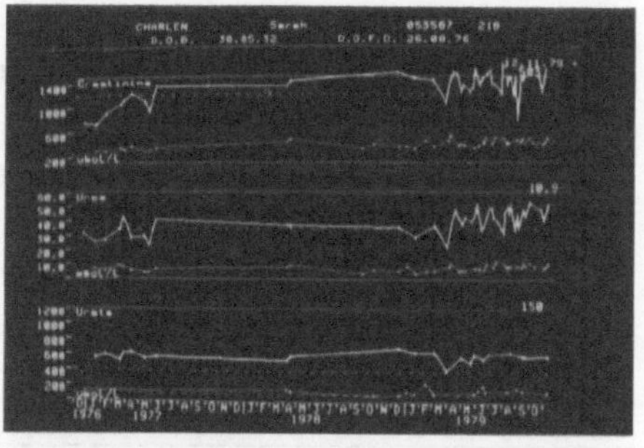

Figure 4 Creatinine graphs

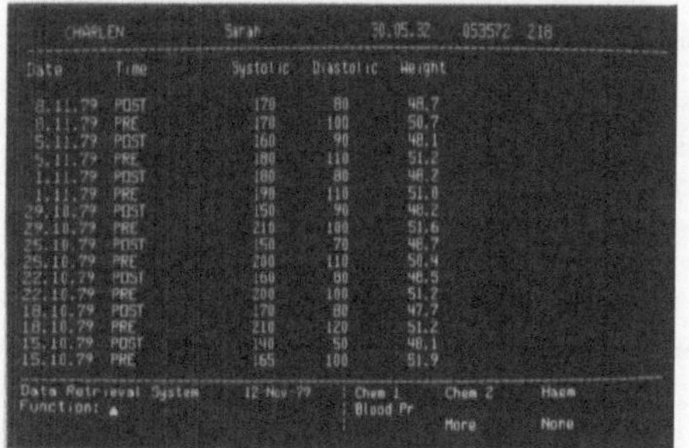

Date	Time	Systolic	Diastolic	Weight
8.11.79	POST	170	80	48.7
8.11.79	PRE	170	100	50.7
5.11.79	POST	160	90	48.1
5.11.79	PRE	180	110	51.2
1.11.79	POST	180	80	48.2
1.11.79	PRE	190	110	51.0
29.10.79	POST	150	90	48.2
29.10.79	PRE	210	100	51.6
25.10.79	POST	150	70	48.7
25.10.79	PRE	200	110	50.4
22.10.79	POST	160	80	48.5
22.10.79	PRE	200	100	51.2
18.10.79	POST	170	80	47.7
18.10.79	PRE	210	120	51.2
15.10.79	POST	140	50	48.1
15.10.79	PRE	165	100	51.9

Figure 5 VDU blood pressure display

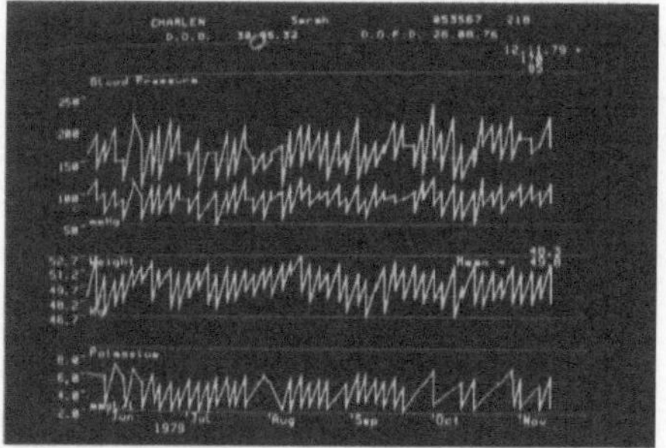

Figure 6 Blood pressure graphs

5. BIBLIOGRAPHY

(1) Gordon, M. An interactive graphical minicomputer system for the management and exploration of clinical renal data. Proceedings Medinfo 1977, World Conference on Medical Informatics, Toronto (1980).

(2) Gordon, M. An interactive graphical minicomputer system for the management and exploration of clinical renal data. Computer Journal 21, No.1, 91-93 (1978).

MISE SUR ORDINATEUR DE DOSSIERS HEMATOLOGIQUES ET REALISATION PAR ORDINATEUR DE COURBES DE SURVIE OU DE REMISSION SELON LA METHODE ACTUARIELLE

J. BINON - Cl. BELLENOT

Unité de Recherches sur les Maladies du Sang
Prof. G. SOKAL
Université Catholique de Louvain
Clos Chapelle-aux-Champs, 30 - U.C.L. 30.52
1200 Bruxelles - Belgique

SUMMARY:

Different steps are described, steps going from the regular collection of fundamentally scientific data on inpatients or outpatients in hematology, to the plotting of survival of remission curves following the actuarial method and on the comparison of curves by the logrank test and this by means of a desk computer and a plotting table.

Ce travail a été réalisé avec la participation de Mme K. DELEUSE, secrétaire scientifique, que nous remercions vivement de sa collaboration.

1. INTRODUCTION

Il importe souvent, en médecine, de connaître et de représenter la fréquence d'un évenement survenant dans une population bien définie.

Dans un service d'Hématologie, le problème de ce type le plus fréquemment rencontré est l'étude du taux de survie ou de rémission permettant l'évaluation de l'efficacité d'un traitement ou la découverte de facteurs de pronostics.

2. METHODES ET MATERIEL

2.1. Recueil des données

Au départ, il y a les dossiers des patients, sources de données. Les dossiers dont il est question sont ceux des patients hospitalisés ou consultants en hématologie dans l'ensemble hospitalier des Cliniques de Louvain-en-Woluwe, Mont-Godinne Jolimont et Auvelais.

Les données sont recueillies par un médecin, à une fréquence de trois fois par semaine, selon un code général, mais, suivant le type d'affection, certaines données sont recueillies d'autres ne le sont pas.

Ce code comprend :

1. des renseignements d'identification : nom, prénom, date de naissance, sexe, date de diagnostic ...
2. des renseignements concernant le diagnostic ainsi que des caractéristiques cliniques et biologiques : stadification des lymphosarcomes ou des leucémies lymphoïdes chroniques, localisations principales des lymphosarcomes ou des formes leucémiques tumorales, marqueurs de membrane, groupe HLA, paramètres biologiques initiaux, anomalies du caryotype, type de l'immunoglobuline monoclonale et présence ou non de protéinurie de Bence-Jones dans le myélome, nom du toxique en cause dans les affections hématologiques d'origine médicamenteuse, ...
3. des renseignements concernant la thérapeutique : type de schéma de chimiothérapie, type de traitement radiothérapique et dose appliquée, type et date d'intervention chirurgicale, ...
4. des renseignements concernant l'évolution : date d'évaluation du traitement et type de réponse à ce traitement (exemple 1 : rémission complète, rémission partielle ou échec pour l'évaluation du traitement des leucémies aiguës ou de la maladie de Hodgkin ...), date et type de rechute (médullaire, ganglionnaire, méningée, testiculaire ...), date d'acutisation ou de transformation d'une forme en une autre pour les désordres myéloprolifératifs, modifications apportées au traitement ou adoption d'un nouveau traitement, morbidité infectieuse ou autre présentée par le patient, date de décès et cause de décès, date de perdu de vue, ...

2.2. Entrée des données

Après le recueil, arrive l'étape d'entrée des données. Le service utilise un ordinateur de bureau de marque IBM 5110 comprenant :

- une unité centrale
- un clavier
- un écran
- un lecteur de cassettes
- une armoire à disquettes
- une imprimante.

Le système est relié en série à une table traçante de marque Tektronix 4662.

L'introduction des données se fait par un jeu de questions-réponses : méthode interactive de très grande facilité pour la secrétaire scientifique chargée de ce travail. De plus, le fichier est d'accès direct ; ceci permet une modification ou un complément rapide de la fiche d'un patient.

Le programme, écrit en APL, permet :

- la gestion du fichier (ajout de patients, mise à jour ...)
- le traitement des données

2.3. Traitement des données

En ce qui concerne cette dernière étape, le programme offre la possibilité :

1. de calculer certaines statistiques sur un groupe de patients correspondant à un critère précisé. (exemple : impression du nombre de cas retenus ainsi que la liste des âges au diagnostic; ensuite calcul de la moyenne et de la médiane de ces âges).
2. d'extraire du fichier des malades correspondant à des critères précisés, de les imprimer, de réaliser les calculs nécessaires -selon un intervalle choisi par l'utilisateur - aux courbes de survie ou de rémission et de dessiner ces courbes ainsi que les intervalles de confiance.

   Pour résoudre le problème lié aux inégalités qui se produisent dans la durée d'observation des patients, nous utilisons, pour le tracé de ces courbes de survie ou de rémission, la méthode actuarielle, qui permet de faire rentrer dans l'étude tous les patients quel que soit leur temps de participation à l'étude (1).
3. de superposer sur un même graphe plusieurs courbes de survie ou de rémission.
4. de réaliser le test de comparaison de courbes de survie ou de rémission.

   Le test utilisé est le test de logrank souple dans son principe et son calcul(1).

3. RESULTATS ET DISCUSSION : ILLUSTRATION PAR UN EXEMPLE

Lorsqu'on désire savoir si le sexe a une influence sur le pronostic de la survie dans la leucémie myéloïde chronique, il suffit :

1. de sélectionner, par ordinateur, les malades atteints de leucémie myéloïde

chronique, de sexe masculin d'une part, de sexe féminin d'autre part.

2. de rechercher, dans la mesure du possible, ce que fut le devenir des perdus de vue.
3. une fois ces dernières données introduites, il suffit de mettre en route le programme existant. La figure ci-dessus (photo effectuée à partir du graphe) montre les résultats obtenus, résultats en concordance avec ceux obtenus notamment par une équipe américaine (2).

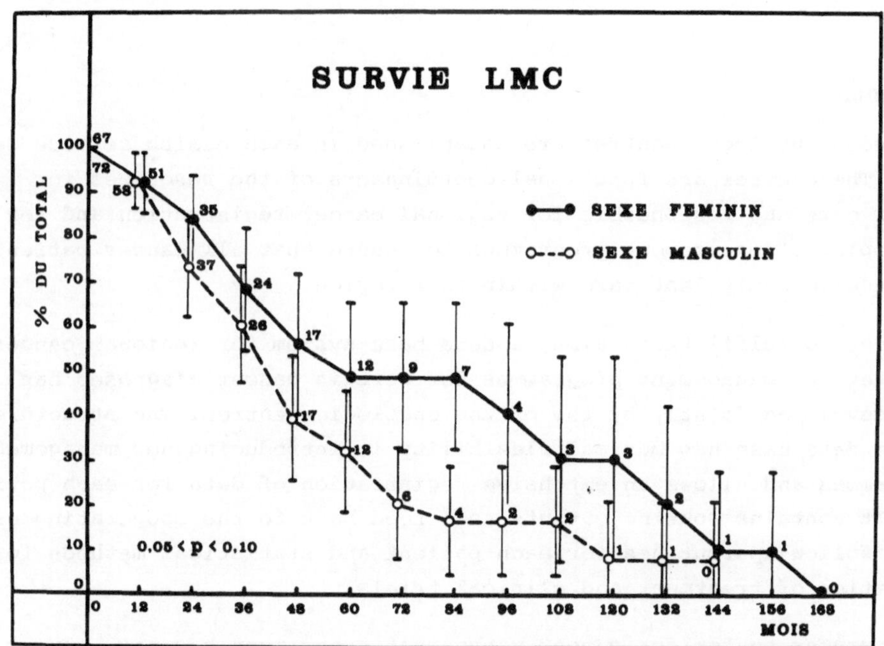

Il en résulte qu'à partir d'un matériel peu sophistiqué et peu coûteux, servant à 75% à d'autres tâches et de l'emploi de personnel régulier mais quantitativement peu important au point de vue temps (médecin, programmeur, secrétaire scientifique), il y a possibilité de traitement rapide de données pour des études rétrospectives autant que pour des essais prospectifs dès que ceux-ci sont terminés.

REFERENCES

1. PETO R., PIKE M.C., ARMITAGE P., BRESLOW N.E., COX D.R., HOWARD S.V., MANTEL N., Mc PHERSON K., PETO J., SMITH G., "Organisation et analyse des essais thérapeutiques comparatifs comportant une longue surveillande des malades", Rev. Epidém. Santé Publ., 27, 167-255, 1979 (Traduit par HILL C. et al)

2. SCHILLING R.F., CROWLEY J.J. "Prognostic signs in chronic myelocytic leukemia" Amer.J.Hematol., 7 : 1-10, 1979.

MANAGEMENT PROGRAMMES FOR CANCER DISEASES

Britta Mattsson, B.A.[1] and Hans E Peterson, M.D.[2]

[1] The Regional Cancer Registry in Stockholm, Karolinska Hospital, S-104 01 Stockholm 60,

[2] Health Care Information Systems, Hälso- och sjukvårdsnämnden, P.O.B. 9099, S-102 72 Stockholm, Sweden

1. SUMMARY

In Sweden oncologic centres are established in each health service region. The centres are functional coordinators of the resources for cancer care and responsible for regional cancer registration and for developing of management programmes to ensure that all cancer patients can receive equivalent care within that region.

In order to fulfil these aims, a data base system for regional cancer register and management programmes for certain cancer diagnoses has been developed, jointly by two of the oncologic centres. The structure of the data base has maximal flexibility in introducing new management programmes and allows an extensive registration of data for each patient. It contains routine outputs as a feed back to the cooperating clinics, follow-up routines for each patient and statistical methods for evaluation of treatment and clinical trials.

The computer system for cancer management programmes has now, almost without alterations, been adopted to programmes for chronic disorders, such as for pacemaker and arterial hypertension patients.

2. BACKGROUND

Sweden is administratively divided into 7 health service regions in which the resources for cancer treatment are organized by the county councils. Instead of building specialized cancer hospitals in each region the treatment of cancer patients is carried out in different departments within ordinary hospitals but coordinated by a so called oncologic centre in each region.

These centres are functional coordinators of the resources for cancer care in the various departments of the hospitals. The regional oncologic centres have administrative and organizational functions. These are defined as follows:

- To establish a regional cancer register.
- To develop and operate programmes of management, including follow-up routines with appropriate distribution of the work between the various units in the chain from district health centres to regional hospitals.
- Responsibility for advice and information on neoplastic disorders within the region and to provide training in clinical oncology for various categories of staff in the health service.
- To attend to the psychologic, psychiatric and sociomedical aspects of cancer care.
- To promote collaboration between basic oncologic and clinical research.

3. THE ORGANIZATION IN THE STOCKHOLM-GOTLAND REGION

The County of Stockholm and the island of Gotland together constitute a health service region. The population of this region is approximately 1.6 million, which is one fifth of Sweden's total population. Each year more than 6.000 primary tumours are diagnosed within the region. The region has 20 acute care hospitals, 13 of them large or fairly large.

The Stockholm-Gotland Oncologic Centre was instituted in 1976. The structure of the health services with a number of large hospitals responsible for different catchment areas, and somewhat varying character of corresponding departments within these hospitals, tend to obscure the demarcation of the regional clinic in certain specialities. On the other hand, the geographical closeness of these large hospitals is conductive to collaboration.

4. INFORMATION FUNCTIONS OF THE STOCKHOLM-GOTLAND ONCOLOGIC CENTRE

4.1. Management programmes

The activities of the Oncologic Centre are currently directed mainly to producing management programmes for patients with neoplastic disorders. It has been estimated that the total number of management programmes required for standardized cancer care in the Stockholm-Gotland region is about 40. Six programmes are now currently in use, while another two are under development. These programmes cover about 40 percent of the cancer patients treated in the region.

A programme of management is defined as a systematic schedule of agreed principles concerning referral network, diagnostic methods, treatment and follow-up of a patient with a particular disease. The aim of cancer management programmes is to ensure, that all cancer patients within a region can receive equivalent care, irrespective of where in the region they live and which doctor they have initially consulted. This care should further be optimal with respect to current knowledge and available resources.

A management programme can bring about increased medical reliability and, by simplifying communications between clinics, etc, minimize duplication of work. In addition, data extracted from the programme provides a basis for evaluation of treatments and for epidemiologic studies of particular diseases.

The contents of management programmes will vary according to the disease. Some fundamental data, however, should always be included in the written programme.

Outline of basic data in a management programme

General description of the disease: epidemiologic information, nature and course of the disease, results of previous studies (eg evaluation of methods of examination and treatment, clinical trials), developmental trends.

Referral network: referral from primary care units, etc, management conferences, treatment centres.

Diagnoses: methods for preliminary diagnosis, measures for checks of diagnosis.

Treatment: surgery, radiotherapy, chemotherapy, immunotherapy, other therapeutic measures.

Follow-up: intervals, responsible clinics, schedule for follow-up examinations.

Evaluation: "production control", methods for information and evaluation.

Within the context of a management programme it may become necessary to compare the values of alternative methods of investigation or treatment. Such comparisons will as a rule take the form of controlled clinical trials with random allocation of patients to treatment and control groups. The trial must first, in the usual way, be shown to satisfy ethical criteria.

4.2. Regional tumour data base

Since 1958 all malignant primary tumours diagnosed in Sweden are notified to the Board of Health and Welfare's Cancer Register. Regional Cancer Registers are progressively built up in each health service region (1). The regionalized tumour registers will supply processed data to the Central Register, which will have a coordinating function.

All doctors in clinics, hospitals, pathologic and cytologic laboratories and departments of forensic medicine must notify newly diagnosed cancer cases. All registration of patients is based on an identity number. The identity number, consisting of the date of birth and a unique four digit (serial) number, is given to every citizen at birth. All person registers in Sweden, containing information about individuals are based on this unique number which means that information easily can be transferred between different registers, eg cancer registers and death records (2).

The Regional Tumour Register in the Stockholm-Gotland region now contains data for about 135.000 cancer cases for the period 1958 - 1979. It provides a comprehensive survey of all the cancer cases in the region and is useful as base-line information in studies of specific management programmes.

5. COMPUTER SYSTEM FOR MANAGEMENT PROGRAMMES AND FOR THE REGIONAL TUMOUR REGISTER

Programmes of management for certain neoplastic conditions have been operative for some years. Large quantities of data have previously been collected and have been processed, mainly by manual methods such as punch cards. As the number of patients and consequently the volume of information have increased, a computerized administration and evaluation of the programmes' result have become increasingly desirable. At the Oncologic Centre a computer system that registers, stores and evaluates information from management programmes is now in operation.

This system also comprises the base for the Regional Tumour Register (3, 4).

5.1. Technical data

The computer system is implemented on a Cyber 172 and operating under NOS (Network Operating System). The programmes are written in FORTRAN Extended. All transactions can be run multiterminal interactive to the system.

5.2. Input data

Registration of data are made from forms specially designed for the respective management programmes. These forms will replace the cancer notifications and thus reduce duplication of work at the clinical level. The Stockholm-Gotland region has approximately 90 departments from which information is supplied to the Tumour Register. The annual number of tumour diagnoses is currently estimated to be about 6.300. Most of these patients will be treated according to one of the agreed management programmes with frequent follow-up. Tumours not included in any management programme will be recorded only in the Regional Tumour Register with baseline data.

5.3. Structure of the register

With the aim of attaining maximal flexibility in introducing new management programmes into the system, the Regional Tumour Register is organized as a data base. This offers direct access to all subroutines in the Register. The registration of data for each patient within the programmes is much more extensive than in the basic cancer registry. Figure 1 illustrates the structure of the data base in which each entry has ten segments. Only segment 1 is obligatory for all primary tumours. Segment 1 to 9 are common to all programmes while segment 10 is programme-specific. This construction implies that if new segments are required for further information this can be added without alteration of the existing structure.

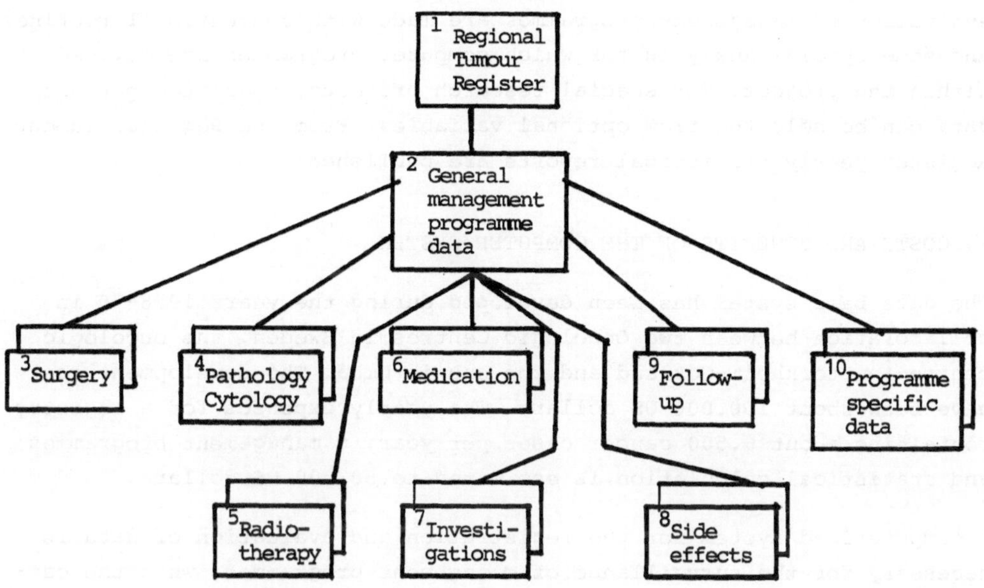

Figure 1. Structure of the data base.

5.4. Registration

The registration is made in direct access to the data base. Before the registration in the cancer register the identity number is checked against a population register, from which the name and address of the patient is retrieved. In the cancer register there is a check against the total data base in order to avoid duplicates. A patient is very often reported from several clinicians and pathologists depending on where the treatment is given.

All registered variables, eg date of diagnosis, treatment and death, coded diagnosis, hospital number and so on are validated within the system.

5.5. Output data

The computer system includes surveillance of follow-up visits to the clinics. Lists of future appointments and reminders following missed appointments can be supplied to clinics requesting them.

Evaluation of the collected data takes the form of periodic standardized output to be submitted to all collaborating clinics. Statistical evaluation of management programmes are made with conventional routines and some special analysis for which computer programmes are devised within the project. For special research projects, specified patient data can be selected from optional variables. From the Regional Tumour Register yearly statistical reports are published.

6. COSTS AND BENEFITS OF THE COMPUTER SYSTEM

The data base system has been developed during the years 1978-79 in collaboration between two Oncologic Centres in Sweden, the oncologic centre in Stockholm-Gotland and the one in Umeå. The development costs have been about 150.000 US dollars. The yearly expenses for a registry containing about 6.500 cancer cases per year, 6 management programmes and statistical calculation is estimated to 50.000 US dollars.

A computerized system for the registration and evaluation of data is necessary for the surveillance of management programmes, when the cancer care is organized on a multicentre basis. The base-line data and the follow-up information, supplied by the clinician or by linkage to other population registers, form the base for evaluation of current diagnostic and therapeutic procedures. The data, so far collected, has been widely utilized for various research projects on epidemiology, prognosis and treatment of neoplastic diseases. Administrative procedures, such as follow-up routines, have been much facilitated.

Based on the cancer management programmes development of programmes for other chronic disorders have been realized, such as for the pacemaker and arterial hypertension patients.

7. REFERENCES

(1) WHO Handbook for standardized cancer registries. Offset publ. No. 25. World Health Organization, Geneva 1976.

(2) Bolander AM. Linkage of census and death records to obtain mortality registers for epidemiological studies in Sweden. Proc. XI Int. Cancer Congress, Florence 1974. Excerpta Medica, Amsterdam 1975 ; vol. 3 : p. 36-39.

(3) Möller TR. Computer application in oncology. Department of Oncology, University Hospital, Lund 1977.

(4) Laszlo J, Cox E, Angle C. The hospital tumour registry. Cancer 1976 ; 38 : 395-402.

LA BASE DE DONNEES ANATOMO-PATHOLOGIQUES DE BOURGOGNE

P. DUSSERRE[+], H. BASTIEN[++], R. MICHIELS[+++], F. CABANNE[++]

+ Laboratoire de Pathologie Humaine et Expérimentale, 18, rue Sainte-Anne - DIJON

++ Centre de Lutte contre le Cancer, 1, rue Professeur Marion - DIJON

+++ Laboratoire d'Anatomie Pathologique, C.H.U. - DIJON

SUMMARY

Pathologists have to recognize the various lesions responsible for diseases whether they practise in public or in private hospitals. Thus, they daily give precise diagnoses and features of the development and probable courses of the diseases. All these investigations and controls of diagnoses concern a lot of chapters of pathology and make up a great deal of objective and available data for medical research and especially epidemiological research.

In the area of DIJON pathological laboratories have been equiped with mini-computers and the same information system. So pathologists have been able to create the first regional pathological data base by gathering the histological and cytological lesions of all their laboratories. Thus they are enabled to contribute to epidemiological studies and, for example, to work out regional registries of diseases.

Since 1976, lesions of breast, dysplastic and cancerous cytological and histological lesions of uterine cervix, malignant lymphomas have been especially studied.

A notable extension in the other French regions is to be expected : already a region larger in area than Burgundy is dealing with this pathological data base.

INTRODUCTION

Qu'ils exercent en milieu hospitalier ou en secteur privé, les anatomo-pathologistes ont à reconnaître les diverses lésions à l'origine de la maladie. Ils apportent ainsi quotidiennement le diagnostic précis d'une affection et ses caractéristiques évolutives et pronostiques.

Il en est actuellement ainsi de toutes les affections chirurgicales ou médicales, cancéreuses ou non, faisant l'objet de biopsies, d'analyses des pièces opératoires, de nécropsies, de prélèvements cytologiques. Toutes ces investigations et contrôles diagnostiques couvrent de multiples chapitres de la pathologie et constituent pour la recherche médicale, et pour la recherche épidémiologique, une masse d'informations objectives directement utilisables.

La création d'une base de données anatomo-pathologiques régionale à DIJON est une expérience qui résulte de la mise en place progressive d'un certain nombre de systèmes informatiques homogènes, complètement intégrés dans le fonctionnement des laboratoires en cause. A notre connaissance, aucune expérience équivalente n'a été tentée jusqu'à présent.

MATERIEL ET METHODES

1) SYSTEME INFORMATIQUE

Le système informatique choisi a été conçu en tenant compte des contraintes spécifiques du fonctionnement de tout Laboratoire d'Anatomie Pathologique. Il utilise actuellement des calculateurs SEMS SOLAR 16/40 auxquels sont adjoints une console de visualisation, une imprimante 200 l/minute et une unité disque de 2x5 Moctets.

Le système assure le contrôle sévère de l'identité du patient et du protocole d'examen ainsi que la rapidité et la sécurité de l'édition des résultats. Il fournit en sous-produit, une gestion intégrée automatique du Laboratoire.

Un tel système permet aujourd'hui à plusieurs Laboratoires d'Anatomie Pathologique, tout d'abord dijonnais puis régionaux, de fonctionner en temps réel, avec grande fiabilité, selon des critères de langage identiques, tout en préservant l'individualité la structure administrative et la personnalité de chacun d'eux. Il leur donne surtout, par simple entente, la possibilité de mettre en commun leurs différents fichiers pour disposer d'une base de données régionales.

2) CARACTERISTIQUES DES INFORMATIONS

A l'occasion de tout examen, les Laboratoires enregistrent pour chaque patient : des informations administratives (identité complète du patient, âge, sexe, numéro et date d'enregistrement de l'examen, code des Services ou Médecins prescripteurs), des renseignements cliniques et biologiques relatifs à ce malade. Ces dernières informations sont précises, homogènes et comparables car le code "organe lésion" est défini par un thésaurus qui résulte du consensus des utilisateurs.

Il s'agit d'un code facile à mémoriser car le numéro de la lésion est le même pour tous les organes comportant cette variété histologique. A cette codification propre au Laboratoire, sont rattachés les codes de classification internationale (CIM-O). La validité des informations est assurée par le fait même qu'elles sont utilisées en routine par les différents intervenants.

3) UTILISATION STATISTIQUE DES INFORMATIONS

Chaque Laboratoire est en mesure d'assurer automatiquement l'édition des résultats, le travail habituel de Secrétariat et de Comptabilité, la sélection des dossiers, sur des caractéristiques choisies, à la demande des Médecins traitants, ceci en temps réel.

Les Médecins peuvent ainsi estimer leur activité selon une périodicité donnée (nombre d'affections traitées, fréquences relatives par rapport à l'ensemble des maladies, répartition des sexes, des âges, etc...).

4) GROUPEMENT DES INFORMATIONS

A partir de ces informations recueillies de façon homogène et stockées sur bandes magnétiques, il a été possible de créer une base de données anatomopathologiques régionale. Ces informations sont centralisées au Centre Régional Informatique de Statistiques anatomopathologiques de DIJON. Des fichiers des maladies cancéreuses ou non, sont ainsi créés. Ils regroupent les patients provenant de tous les Laboratoires d'Anatomie Pathologique participant à cette collecte. Les examens redondants pour un même malade dans une pathologie donnée sont supprimés. On est alors en mesure de constituer des registres de malades porteurs d'affections cancéreuses ou non, utilisables pour des études épidémiologiques.

RESULTATS

Cette base de données anatomopathologiques permet de disposer, grâce à un langage normalisé, d'informations médicales d'une très grande fiabilité, recueillies à la fois dans le secteur public et dans le secteur privé d'une aire géographique déterminée. Il est donc possible, pour la première fois en FRANCE, d'aider efficacement à la mise en oeuvre d'études de morbidité et de registres épidémiologiques, au moins à l'échelon de la région Bourgogne.

Personne en France, actuellement, ne connaît avec précision l'incidence des tumeurs bénignes ou malignes, Les sources d'information dont on dispose sont représentées par les certificats de décès rédigés par les Médecins (on connait leur imprécision et leur manque de fiabilité), les statistiques de morbidité hospitalière qui ne sont pas toujours de meilleure qualité, et par l'"enquête permanente cancer" des Centres de Lutte contre le Cancer, mais qui ne concerne que les malades consultant dans ces établissements.

C'est pourquoi, la base de données anatomopathologiques est à l'origine, en Bourgogne, de travaux épidémiologiques comme le registre bourguignon des tumeurs digestives (5) ou d'étude d'évaluation du processus de soins du cancer intra-épithélial du col utérin (4). Elle apporte une aide à la réalisation du registre des cancers du Doubs, dont les malades des zones limitrophes peuvent être répertoriés dans notre région.

Un tel regroupement d'informations facilite la prise en compte d'un nombre élevé de sujets, en mortalité ou en morbidité, qu'il s'agisse de séries hospitalières ou de population géographiquement déterminée. L'intérêt de la base de données anatomopathologiques est accru par le fait que cette spécialité médicale explore l'ensemble des maladies (pathologie cancéreuse et pathologie non tumorale).

Depuis 1976, nous avons étudié les lésions du sein identifiées par l'examen histologique, les lésions utérines identifiées par les frottis cervico-vaginaux de dépistage (3), et depuis 1979 le processus de soins du carcinome intra-épithélial du col utérin (4).

1) LES LESIONS DU SEIN

Parmi les 1.577 cas répertoriés en 1976, les cancers du sein se remarquent par leur particulière fréquence : 399 cas soit 25,3 %. Les lésions bénignes se partagent entre les mastopathies (866 cas soit 55 %) et les fibro-adénomes (312 cas soit 19,7 %).

Ces affections étudiées par tranche d'âge montrent que le fibro-adénome est la lésion de la femme jeune entre 20 et 30 ans, que la mastopathie apparait plus tard avec un pic de fréquence maxima entre 40 et 50 ans et que le cancer du sein est surtout observé entre 50 et 80 ans (Figure I).

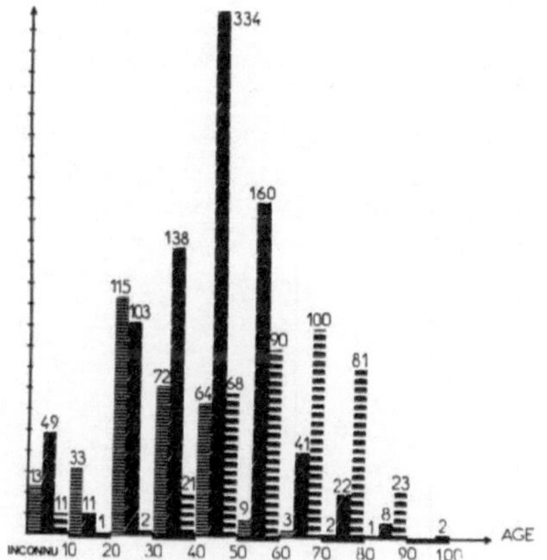

BOURGOGNE 1976

LES LESIONS DU SEIN . 1577 cas

Fibro-adénomes . 312 (19,7 %)

Mastopathies . 866 (55 %)

Carcinomes . 399 (25,3 %)

Figure I : Recensement des lésions du sein Répartition des malades par types de lésions et par tranches d'âge de 10 ans.

2) LES FROTTIS CERVICO-VAGINAUX

30.231 frottis cervico-vaginaux ont été dénombrés en 1976 parmi lesquels figurent 171 lésions dysplasiques et 157 cancers du col utérin.

Plusieurs constatations s'imposent montrant l'insuffisance du dépistage du cancer du col utérin dans notre région.

a/ Le nombre de lésions dysplasiques (5,6 °/°°) et des lésions cancéreuses (5,2 °/°°) du col utérin est encore trop élevé (Figure II)

b/ Sur une population de 1.574.540 sujets (recensements de 1975) figurent 799.295 femmes. Parmi elles, sont recensées 627.315 femmes âgées de plus de 15 ans. Si chacune bénéficiait d'un frottis cervico-vaginal de dépistage au moins tous les cinq ans, nous devrions réunir 125.000 examens environ par an, au lieu du chiffre actuel, insuffisant, de 30.000.

c/ Enfin, si le dépistage débute à 20 ans (Figure II) et s'il semble correctement effectué entre 20 et 50 ans, il se relache après la ménopause. Ceci est d'autant plus regrettable que c'est après 50 ans que les lésions graves du col utérin se signalent avec une fréquence maximale.

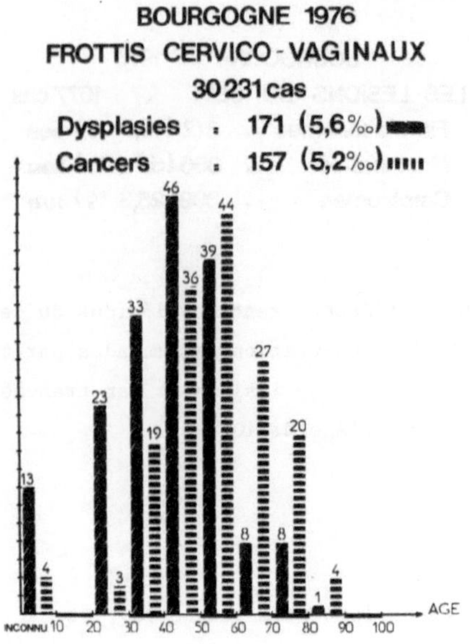

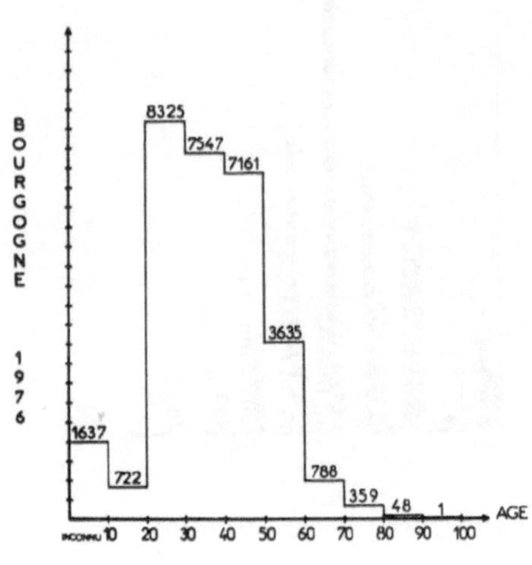

Figure II: Recensement des lésions dysplasiques et cancéreuse du col utérin dépistées par frottis cervico-vaginal (Région Bourgogne 1976).

Figure III : Recensement des frottis cervico-vaginaux de dépistage (Région Bourgogne 1976).

3) EVALUATION DU PROCESSUS DE SOINS DU CARCINOME INTRA-EPITHELIAL DU COL UTERIN

Une étude d'évaluation (4) relative au processus de soins du cancer intra-épithélial du col utérin, utilise comme source primordiale d'information la base de données anatomopathologiques de Bourgogne.

Cette étude poursuit les objectifs suivants : déterminer les critères épidémiologiques de la maladie en Côte d'Or (Figure IV) analyser les différentes étapes du processus de soins, évaluer l'incidence économique de la maladie selon les différents secteurs d'hospitalisation (Hôpitaux publics, centre anti-cancéreux, médecine privée) et mettre au point un outil méthodologique spécifique à ce type d'évaluation et utilisable pour d'autres maladies.

On conçoit qu'un tel travail n'est possible que dans la mesure où tous les malades présentant ce type d'affection, sont répertoriés dans tous les secteurs de la Médecine.

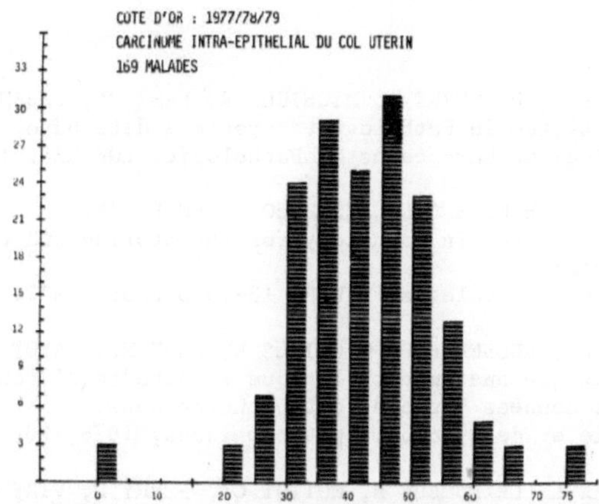

COTE D'OR : 1977/78/79
CARCINOME INTRA-EPITHELIAL DU COL UTERIN
169 MALADES

Figure IV : Cancer intra-épithélial du col utérin.
Répartition des malades par tranches d'âge.

DISCUSSION

L'anatomie pathologique fournit le plus souvent un diagnostic précis et surtout un diagnostic anatomo-clinique qui peut être répertorié dans une codification précise facilement utilisable par les Laboratoires qui s'y intéressent.

De plus, elle contrôle la presque totalité de la pathologie organique. En dehors des maladies infectieuses et des affections psychiatriques, la plupart des maladies font aujourd'hui appel à un examen anatomo-pathologique (histologie, cytologie, microscopie électronique, autopsie). L'archivage informatique d'un matériel aussi varié qu'abondant, sans cesse croissant, permet de constituer une base de données utilisable par tous les Médecins, en particulier les épidémiologistes.

Le regroupement informatique des dossiers histologiques et cytologiques des Laboratoires de la région Bourgogne aboutit à la constitution d'une base de données importante qui collecte environ 200.000 dossiers par an.

Cette base de données est commune à tous les centres hospitaliers, les centres de lutte contre le cancer et les Laboratoires des secteurs privés qui fournissent à eux seuls, plus de la moitié des diagnostics.

On peut prévoir que son extension géographique progressera au fil du temps : elle dépasse largement les frontières des quatre départements bourguignons.

REFERENCES

(1) BASTIEN H, DUSSERRE P, DUSSERRE L, MICHIELS R, LAMY ML, CABANNE F.
Use of a computer system in Pathology to create a data base.
6e Congrès de la Société Européenne de Pathologie, LONDRES, 17 septembre 1977.

(2) BASTIEN H, MOTTOT Cl, HORIOT JCL, JUSTRABO E, KNOPF JF.
The use of a mini computer in Pathology for the storing and the creating of a cytological data base.
7e Congrès Européen de Cytologie, LIEGE, 13-15 octobre 1977.

(3) BASTIEN H, MOTTOT Cl, DUSSERRE P, MICHIELS R, LAMY ML, CAYOT F.
La méthode informatique anatomopathologique : méthodes d'archivages et de création d'une base de données histo et cytopathologiques.
Archives d'Anatomie et de Cytologie pathologiques, 1978, 26, 2, 83-87.

(4) BASTIEN H, DUSSERRE L, LE RUMEUR N, MOTTOT Cl, FERRY D, VIRY B, CUISENIER J.
Exemple d'évaluation d'un processus de soins dans un département français (Côte d'Or). Le cancer intra-épithélial du col utérin.
Conférence internationale de la Science des Systèmes dans le domaine de la Santé. MONTREAL, 14-17 juillet 1980.

(5) FAIVRE J, KLEPPING Cl, MARTIN F, CABANNE F, MICHIELS R, DUSSERRE P.
Incidence des cancers digestifs dans une population bien définie. Bilan de deux années d'enregistrement dans le département de la Côte d'Or.

(6) MICHIELS R, DUSSERRE P et L, BASTIEN H.
La méthode informatique appliquée à l'Anatomie Pathologique. Ses conséquences d'ordre médical et économique à partir d'une expérience régionale.
Académie des Sciences morales et politiques, PARIS, Séance du 19 décembre 1977.

REMERCIEMENTS

Nous remercions de leur participation M. BORDES, B. VIRY et J. PENY du Laboratoire de Pathologie de DIJON, E. JUSTRABO, Cl. MOTTOT et J.F. KNOPF du Centre Hospitalier Universitaire de DIJON, M. LAMY, du Centre Hospitalier de NEVERS.

UNE EXPERIENCE DE DOSSIER MEDICAL INFORMATISE EN CARCINOLOGIE CERVICO-FACIALE; SON APPORT AU SUIVI DES MALADES ET A LA RECHERCHE CLINIQUE.

Vincent MORICE[+], Henri SZPIRGLAS[++], Claude CHASTANG[+],

(+) Département de Biomathématiques de la Pitié-Salpétrière
Groupe U 194 de l'INSERM "Méthodologie Informatique et Statistique en Médecine".
91, Bd de l'Hôpital - 75634 PARIS Cedex 13

(++) Clinique de Stomatologie de Chirurgie Maxillo-faciale
47, Bd de l'Hôpital - 75634 PARIS Cedex 13

The difficulties encountered before 1979 in the statistical studies (therapeutic evaluation, prognosis research, clinical epidemiology) concerning head and neck cancer led us to reconsider the medical record structure in this pathology. So, since january 1979, the oncology department uses exclusively a standardized medical record, identical for all the patients with an oral tumor whatever the treatment, and able to describe all the possible evolutions. The medical record is, on the other hand, computerized, which allows first, to help the patients follow up (medical summaries sent to the different physicians, new convocations of patients...) and second, to realize clinical studies. These two objectives - decision making help for a particular patient, clinical research for a particular pathology - are probably an original characteristic of this project. The resulting consequences are already numerous : medical record restructuration, physician education, decision making help, and tool for the clinical research...

Les données médicales, cliniques, biologiques, radiologiques, etc... recueillies dans un service hospitalier constituent le dossier médical : elles sont dans un premier temps confrontées pour établir le diagnostic et définir le traitement pour un malade donné, puis suivre son évolution.

Dans un second temps la confrontation des dossiers concernant le plus grand nombre possible de malades comparables permet la recherche épidémiologique, clinique et thérapeutique.

Ce papier analyse les difficultés rencontrées dans la constitution et l'utilisation du dossier médical classique en carcinologie cervico-faciale. Il présente ensuite les solutions apportées depuis le 1er Janvier 1979 pour y remédier.

1. LA SITUATION ANTERIEURE

1.1. Le dossier médical

Le rôle du dossier médical est avant tout de mémoriser des informations concernant un malade, d'en permettre la transmission entre médecins ou services pour faciliter le suivi du malade au cours du temps.

Le dossier hospitalier contient des documents de natures variées :

- Un cahier clinique comportant l'identification du malade; ses antécédents; l'histoire de la maladie; le bilan clinique initial; la décision thérapeutique éventuellement infléchie par les résultats; son évolution sous traitement; et les appréciations pronostiques successives.
- Un dossier d'examens complémentaires constitué des feuilles de résultats envoyées par différents services ou laboratoires.
- Différents documents tels que radios, photos, bilans isotopiques, etc...

En carcinologie le nombre de ces documents est particulièrement important :

- La nature à la fois aigüe et chronique de la maladie conduit à augmenter le dossier à chaque poussée évolutive. Mais, même en dehors de ces poussées, le bilan de surveillance et des séquelles est particulièrement lourd et complexe.
- D'autre part l'affection est multidisciplinaire : chirurgien, anesthésiste, chimiothérapeute, radiothérapeute, etc... doivent participer et accéder au dossier avec toutes les difficultés inhérentes aux transmissions d'un département à l'autre dès lors que les médecins ne sont pas regroupés autour du lit d'hospitalisation..

L'ensemble du dossier est contenu dans une pochette; elle peut contenir un nombre élevé de documents souvent non ordonnés, ce qui rend laborieuse la recherche d'un document ponctuel. En outre le risque de perte est important en raison des nombreuses manipulations.

1.2. La recherche clinique, épidémiologique et thérapeutique

En dehors de rares protocoles thérapeutiques, la confrontation de dossiers médicaux a permis de réaliser des études cliniques le plus souvent rétrospectives. Cependant l'information n'a pas été recueillie dans l'optique de telles études. En particulier sur un dossier non standardisé les médecins ne consignent pas les éléments sans intérêt immédiat pour le malade ce qui se traduit par un taux élevé de valeurs manquantes pour des paramètres finalement nécessaires à l'étude. Le rejet de ces dossiers incomplets conduit donc à des biais de mesure et d'échantillonnage importants.

De plus, la recherche des dossiers utilisables pour une étude est toujours une tâche longue et aléatoire. Cette recherche est pourtant souhaitable pour faire profiter un malade de l'expérience acquise avec les malades précédemment traités dans le service et si possible de pouvoir confronter cette expérience avec celle des autres centres de traitement.

La difficulté de réaliser ces études cliniques a conduit à critiquer l'organisation de l'information médicale, et en premier lieu le dossier médical. De plus, les limites de l'interprétation des résultats liées au caractère rétrospectif de ces études, ont amené à étendre les protocoles thérapeutiques qui , d'une part, standardisent l'attitude thérapeutique et, d'autre part, permettent l'interprétation causale.

2. LE DOSSIER MEDICAL STANDARDISE

2.1. Objectifs

La carcinologie cervico-faciale constitue un terrain de recherche clinique, épidémiologique et thérapeutique permanente. L'objectif premier a donc été de faciliter cette recherche. Il a donc fallu standardiser le dossier médical pour que les dossiers des malades soient plus homogènes et que le taux d'informations manquantes soit diminué.

Un second objectif a été de constituer un dossier médical assez général pour accueillir tous les types de situations carcinologiques se présentant dans le service et en suivre l'évolution. Il a donc fallu utiliser un grand nombre de variables. Ce dossier reste cependant un questionnaire fermé de taille limitée. Sa définition, qui est celle de l'information minimale nécessaire à l'action médicale, est évidemment imparfaite et implique des choix a priori. Cependant le questionnaire laisse la liberté d'exprimer sous forme de commentaire libre tout renseignement non explicitement prévu; l'étude ultérieure de ces commentaires pourra donner lieu à une modification de structure.

Si la standardisation a permis d'augmenter la qualité et l'ordonnancement des données une informatisation du dossier a été nécessaire d'une part pour en assurer la gestion, d'autre part pour pouvoir exploiter leur contenu et manipuler simultanément un nombre élevé de paramètres (analyses statistiques multidimensionnelles).

2.2. Le questionnaire

Le questionnaire actuellement utilisé est le fruit d'un long travail, d'un ensemble de compromis, mais aussi de modifications, le plus souvent mineures [1]. Il permet de décrire le bilan clinique et la décision thérapeutique quel que soit le moment de l'évolution. Chaque reprise évolutive est décrite par un document semblable qu'il suffit d'ajouter au précédent.

Ce questionnaire est divisé en chapitres :

- le premier (45 items) concerne l'identification du malade et ne sera rempli qu'une fois, lors de la première consultation. On y trouve la situation familiale et professionnelle, les facteurs de risque (professionnel, tabac, alcool, chocs psychologiques, antécédents familiaux tumoraux), les antécédents personnels non tumoraux, les antécédents tumoraux avec la nature de leur traitement et le résultat obtenu.
- la seconde partie (511 items) se subdivise en plusieurs chapitres et décrit un bilan

complet de la maladie cancéreuse : elle constitue donc la partie évolutive du dossier.

Le premier item permet de préciser le type d'évolution : bilan initial, récidive sur place, deuxième localisation, évolution ganglionnaire, récidive ganglionnaire, évolution métastatique, deuxième cancer.

Sont détaillés ensuite :

. les éléments du diagnostic
. la description de la tumeur (T)
. son extension : ganglionnaire (N) et viscérale (M)
. l'anatomie pathologique
. les examens complémentaires : tests immunitaires, hémogramme , radiologie, scintigraphie...
. le bilan préthérapeutique
. les séquences de traitement : avant intervention locale, traitement chirurgical de la lésion, avant intervention sur les ganglions, traitement chirurgical des ganglions, traitement post-opératoire.
Il est possible de décrire aussi un traitement exclusif de toute intervention chirurgicale et le traitement spécifique des métastases. Les éventuels protocoles suivis sont indiqués.
. l'évaluation des résultats
. la séquence de chimiothérapie ou d'immunothérapie.

Ce chapitre de chimiothérapie (336 items) permet de coder le déroulement et le résultat de plusieurs protocoles successifs au cours d'une même évolution.

L'importance de ce chapitre résulte de l'orientation oncologique du service : recherche de thérapeutiques adjuvantes efficaces, grâce à des essais randomisés.

- le dernier chapitre (8 items) permet de mettre à jour le dossier à chaque consultation en y portant la date de cette consultation, l'état du malade et la date du prochain rendez-vous. Le dossier peut être clos par la date du décès et sa cause (lié ou non au cancer).

Bien que le nombre d'items de ce questionnaire soit élevé, en raison de sa généralité, son remplissage n'est pas trop long puisque certains items sont mutuellement exclusifs et certains chapitres, comme la partie de chimiothérapie, sont sans objet pour certains malades.

2.3. Le système informatique

Le fichier des malades est supporté par un système informatique de gestion de questionnaires évolutifs général qui a été conçu et mis au point au sein de l'unité INSERM U 88 de méthodologie informatique et statistique en Médecine [2, 3]. Ce système permet de définir le questionnaire comme une suite d'items regroupés en chapitres. Un item est défini par un nom d'au plus 6 caractères (DATE, CENTRE, SEXE...) et par le type de valeurs qu'il peut prendre : oui ou non pour un item logique; une liste de valeurs particulières exclusives pour un item dit "à valeurs particulières" (ainsi l'histologie présentera l'une des modalités : carcinome épidermoïde, cyclindrome, adénocarcinome, muco-épidermoïde, etc...); un nombre pour un item numérique comme le nombre de globules rouges ou le PH; du texte pour une variable commentaire comme le nom. Des codes particuliers, ou valeurs spéciales, peuvent être utilisés pour traduire le manque d'information : B pour valeur manquante, S pour item sans objet, A pour item en attente d'une valeur.

L'archivage des dossiers peut s'effectuer soit en mode conversationnel, c'est à dire directement à partir d'un écran de visualisation, soit en mode différé lorsque les données ont été préalablement saisies sur cartes perforées où bandes magnétiques. Dans les 2 cas le système contrôle la cohérence des données et signale les anomalies, ce qui permet la validation des dossiers médicaux. Le fichier de données peut ensuite être interrogé à l'aide d'un langage spécifique qui permet la réalisation de tris à un nombre quelconque de niveaux, le calcul de paramètres caractéristiques (moyennes, variances,...), l'édition de listes répondant aux critères désirés, l'édition de dossiers en texte libre (résumés), l'extraction de sous-fichiers utilisables par la bibliothèque de programmes statistiques (analyses multidimensionnelles, courbes de survie...).

2.4. Le recueil des données

La réussite de ce projet de dossier médical informatisé est conditionnée par la qualité du recueil des données.

Le questionnaire se présente sous la forme d'un cahier sur lequel le médecin doit coder l'information concernant son malade. Il lui a donc fallu accepter de modifier sa pratique pour la normaliser et rentrer dans une structure plus logique, plus précise, mais plus rigide, qu'il s'agisse du codage proprement dit qui, par sa forme, peut impliquer des choix précis (différenciation cellulaire : 1 = différencié, 2 = peu différencié, 3 = indifférencié), ou de la signification même des termes utilisés qui a dû souvent être sinon modifiée, au moins clarifiée.

Le remplissage pose donc le double problème de la formation du médecin et de l'acceptabilité par celui-ci, d'autant plus que, comme la prise d'une observation, le remplissage reste un travail fastidieux. Le risque est alors grand de voir des items ou chapitres non ou mal remplis dans un dossier. C'est pourquoi ils doivent être validés : dans un premier temps, la secrétaire est chargée de rechercher les items manquants; puis le coordonnateur prend personnellement en charge les difficultés les plus importantes, vérifie certains dossiers, discute avec les autres médecins chargés du recueil, pour s'efforcer de maintenir le niveau de qualité des dossiers.

L'archivage et la correction des dossiers sont réalisés par une secrétaire une fois par semaine, en conversationnel. Le système informatique utilisé, AIDE, effectue une dernière validation des dossiers en indiquant les incohérences qu'il y trouve.

L'ensemble de ces opérations de saisie font de cette phase la partie la plus critique du système :

- l'acceptabilité est variable selon l'intérêt qu'y trouvent les médecins.

- la formation doit être continue.
- le départ de la secrétaire médicale peut conduire à un blocage rapide du système, même si l'archivage informatique est réalisé normalement.

3. BILAN DE DEUX ANNEES D' EXPERIENCES

3.1. La recherche clinique, épidémiologique et thérapeutique

Le fichier informatique, difficile à constituer, est au contraire d'utilisation aisée : il suffit de définir précisément une question pour que l'étude puisse être réalisée sans aucun recueil complémentaire d'information grâce aux différents programmes d'interrogation de la banque de données (PLD) et d'analyses statistiques.

Des protocoles randomisés de chimiothérapie et d'immunothérapie sont en cours (GIFA, vindésine, bestatine...) mais le recul de deux ans n'a permis que de premières évaluations qui n'ont pas encore montré de différence significative .

En revanche des dossiers rétrospectifs ont été introduits dans le fichier informatique afin d'effectuer plusieurs études pronostiques [4, 5]. Citons :

- Etude des facteurs pronostiques de la rémission et de la survie de 239 cas de tumeurs du maxillaire supérieur [6].
- Etude de 64 dossiers de cancers in-situ et 58 dossiers de cancers micro--invasifs [7]. Une étude plus poussée est en cours sur des données anatomopathologiques spécifiques complémentaires.
- Etude de 40 cancers muco-épidémoïdes.[8]
- Etude des adénopathies cervicales.

3.2. L'aide au suivi du malade

Les études statistiques faites à partir du fichier informatique ne constituent pas encore un apport important au malade : les dossiers prospectifs sont trop récents pour fournir des résultats utilisables et les études rétrospectives, nécessairement biaisées, permettent d'avancer des hypothèses à confirmer par des études prospectives. Mais la standardisation et l'informatisation du dossier médical constituent une aide immédiate au suivi du malade :

- L'obligation de remplir le questionnaire conduit le médecin à effectuer sur le malade un examen plus complet qu'il ne l'aurait sans doute fait naturellement. D'autre part, le contrôle autant humain qu'informatique effectué a priori sur le dossier constitue une forme d'évaluation de son travail, qui le pousse à l'améliorer. L'équipe médicale voit donc sa qualité augmenter, en même temps que s'améliore la qualité des données.
- Après chaque mise à jour hebdomadaire du fichier différentes éditions sont systématiquement réalisées : listes de malades et résumés des observations en clair.

Les listes sont de plusieurs types et peuvent être modifiées à la demande. Il s'agit principalement d'une liste par ordre alphabétique de tous les patients (environ 300 nouveaux malades par an) actuellement suivis dans le service. Sur cette liste apparaissent tous les items les plus importants (localisation, TNM, histologie, traitement, résultat du traitement). Au dernier bilan sont notés de plus la date de la dernière consultation, l'état lors de cette consultation et la date du prochain rendez-vous. Une autre liste importante concerne les seuls patients en cours de chimiothérapie. Cette liste décrit l'histoire simplifiée du traitement : indication, protocoles, nombre de cycles prévus, date et cause d'arrêt. D'autres listes, comme la liste des patients décédés peuvent être éditées à la demande. Ces différentes listes, par la facilité de leur consultation et le nombre de renseignements qu'elles contiennent, permettent une rapidité de réponse impossible à atteindre avec les dossiers médicaux non informatisés.

Les résumés des observations sont édités en clair. Ils sont utilisables, soit pour les besoins du service, soit comme document destiné au médecin traitant ou tout autre médecin appelé à s'occuper du malade.

Cette génération automatique de résumés libère donc les médecins d'un travail quelquefois long, et les rend plus disponibles pour les soins aux malades.

4. CONCLUSION

4.1. Les aspects positifs

L'expérience de dossier médical informatisé qui vient d'être décrite semble originale sur plusieurs points :

- l'analyse des problèmes posés par la situation antérieure a conduit à une critique de l'activité médicale et à prendre conscience de la nécessité d'une standardisation à plusieurs niveaux : dossier médical, séquences thérapeutiques, étapes de recherche. Ainsi les études cliniques impliquent :
  - des hypothèses précises, si possible une démarche expérimentale, des procédures standardisées (bilan initial, traitement, surveillance, évaluation des réusltats).
- la standardisation du dossier médical est bien acceptée par l'équipe médicale et son remplissage semble simple puisqu'il a pu être réalisé par des médecins extérieurs à la clinique de stomatologie.
- le recueil est réalisé de façon systématique depuis deux ans pour tous les nouveaux malades.
- la standardisation du dossier conduit à effectuer des examens cliniques plus complets et la validation de l'information recueillie à améliorer le niveau clinique.
- l'archivage systématique de tous les dossiers sur un système informatique assez général pour permettre des interrogations faciles, permet de réaliser des études ponctuelles sans imposer à l'activité médicale une surcharge de travail.
- bien que ce système n'assure pas la gestion de l'information médicale dans un

sens aussi général que MIS, les éditions systématiques sont d'une grande aide pour le suivi des malades.

- l'unicité de l'équipe médicale donne aux informations contenues dans le fichier une homogénéité qu'on ne peut obtenir dans des systèmes multicentriques ou multidisciplinaires comme la Mayo Clinic [9].

4.2. Les difficultés

En dépit des avantages précédents, ce projet reste par certains côtés très fragile.

- Son existence est liée fortement à la détermination du responsable médical.
- Le dossier standardisé est parfois perçu comme une tâche supplémentaire, en particulier lorsque la secrétaire médicale cherche à en éliminer les valeurs manquantes.
- Le recueil et la validation des informations est l'occasion pour les médecins de constater leur "fragilité" [10].
- Le projet implique nécessairement des dépenses qui sont partiellement prises en charge par l'institution hospitalière. Si le recueil de l'information fait partie de l'activité médicale, la secrétaire est financée sur des fonds privés. Les dépenses informatiques sont prises en charge par l'Assistance Publique, mais l'activité de recherche clinique n'est en général pas financée sauf pour les hospitalo-universitaires.

A côté de cette fragilité organisationnelle des difficultés informatiques gènent la marche du projet. Actuellement le projet utilise un ordinateur non accessible au service (centre de calcul universitaire). Cela a conduit à choisir un accès hebdomadaire au fichier pour la mise à jour et les éditions systématiques.

Mais ce délai paraît trop long à l'équipe médicale qui souhaite pouvoir accéder au fichier à tout moment pour effectuer directement les opérations de mise à jour, d'édition de résumés médicaux ou d'interrogations élémentaires. Il convient donc d'envisager un système informatique local. Seules les analyses statistiques complexes devraient alors être réalisées sur un ordinateur plus puissant. Une telle solution est désormais envisageable : des configurations suffisantes et les logiciels de base sont actuellement disponibles pour 100.000 F.

BIBLIOGRAPHIE

1 Baron M. Le dossier médical informatisé en carcinologie cervico-faciale. Thèse pour le doctorat en Médecine. 1979.

2 De Heaulme M, Chantalou JP. AIDE : a system for time dependent data collection and analysis. 2nd World Conférence Medical Informatics, MEDINFO 77, Toronto Ed DB Shires and H Wolf, NORTH HOLLAND Pub C°.

3 Chantalou JP. Interactive Programming Language for validation and interrogation of Evolutive Data. MIE 78 Proceedings, Cambridge England 1978 ; 261-267.

4 Armitage P, Gehan EA. Statistical Methods for the identification and use of Prognostic Factors. Int J Cancer. 1974; 13 : 16-36.

5 Peto R, Pike MC, Armitage P, Breslow NE, Cox DR, Howard SW, Mantel N, McPherson K, Peto J, Smith PG. Design and analysis of randomized clinical trials requiring prolonged observation of each patient. I - Introduction and design. Br J Cancer. 1976 ; 34 : 585-612. II - Analysis and examples. Br J Cancer. 1977; 35 : 1-39. Organisation et analyse des essais thérapeutiques comparatifs comportant une longue surveillance des malades. Rev Epidem et Sant Publ. 1979 ; 27 : 167-225.

6 Vaillant JM, Morice V, Bertrand JCh, Marneur M, Chantalou JP, Dilichen J, Chastang Cl, Szpirglas H. Cancer du maxillaire supérieur : étude rétrospective de 239 cas. Soc de Stomat. Nancy Mars 1979.

7 Szpirglas M, Morice V, Bertrand JCh, Chastang Cl, Marneur M, Tsamis JB,Mamelle G, Roth-Ghanassia V, Chantalou JP. Epidémiologie des cancers sur papillomatos orale floride, IVe Congrès Français de Stomatologie et de Chirurgie maxillo-faciale. Paris 4-8 Septembre 1979.

8 Bertrand JCh, Szpirglas, Brocheriou Cl, Bagot JL, Chastang Cl, Morice V. Tumeurs muco-épidermoïdes des glandes salivaires. Etude de 40 cas. Rev de Stomat et de Chir maxillo faciale 1980.

9 Kurland LT, Elveback L, Nobrega FT. Mayo Clinic records linkage system in the Rochester Olmsted Epidemiology Program Project. Uses of epidemiology planning health services, Ed A Michael Davies. Savremence Administracija, Belgrade. 1973 ;- 164-176.

10 Grémy F. Avenir et signification de la médecine informatique. IMIA Paris, Juin 1979.

A CANCER REGISTRY INFORMATION SYSTEM

K.-H. Ellsässer[***], C.O. Köhler[**], H.P. Meinzer[**], W. Zatonski[*]

[*] Maria Sklodovska Memorial Institute, Warsaw

[**] German Cancer Research Center, Heidelberg

[***] Oncological Center, Heidelberg-Mannheim

SUMMARY

A universal and economical information system is described which is adapted to the special needs of a cancer registry.

The system is used to collect, store, retrieve, evaluate and present data under epidemiological aspects. It was jointly developed by the German Cancer Research Center (Heidelberg), the Oncological Center Heidelberg-Mannheim and the Maria-Sklodovska-Memorial Institute of Oncology (Warsaw).

The system is implemented on a small PDP11/34 computer. The software was developed using MUMPS and the dialog and generator system KRAZTUR. The design of the system was chosen to be compatible with general cancer registry forms and to correspond to the recommendations of the WHO. For easy implementation, we made full use of the data storage facilities of MUMPS.

INTRODUCTION

In every tumor center regional cancer registries are to be kept, apart from optimal patient care. With the larger number of patients two aims - optimal patient care and the gaining of new knowledge from structured and standardized documentation - can hardly be attained without the use of modern information processing equipment.

All cancer registries work with large amounts of data which must be accessible to programs for epidemiological evaluation. In order to use small, economic computers it is, therefore, necessary to aggregate the data in a first step. The logic of the aggregation process is rendered flexible enough to select those data which are to be processed in a second step. After the first step of data reduction the results can be presented.

Having reduced the data, it is possible to apply statistical methods. These methods can be categorized on two levels. First, simple statistical methods to carry through basic epidemiological analysis and, second, more sophisticated algorithms used in special epidemiological studies. The results of all steps can be presented in the form of tables, histograms and graphs.

The whole system is running under MUMPS and has direct dialog access possibilities. The system KRAZTUR contains features for documentation and statistics. It will be implemented in several tumor centers in the Federal Republic of Germany and the Polish Cancer Center in Warsaw.

DOCUMENTATION

The data to be collected in the tumour documentation can be classified in 4 logical blocks:

- general personal data
- general medical data
- general oncological data
- special oncological data.

General patient data are preponderantly administrative data which principally have to be collected only once. General medical data include, for instance, height and weight. General oncological data are data which will have to be collected with any kind of dangerous disease, such as onset of the disease, definitive finding, histological confirmation, etc. Special oncological data differ with each type of tumour.

For the collection of data a special form has been developed. Providing the basic data is a minor problem, since the signs and symptoms as well as their manifestations for the items are binding. In general there are three different kinds of data input:

- initial data collection
- subsequent data collection
- final data collection.

In Warsaw all data is collected on one dataform. Updating of data is also done with the help of this standard form.

EPIDEMIOLOGICAL EVALUATIONS

In order to render accessible the great number of data acquired and stored for epidemiological evaluation, the data will have to be reduced as a first step. This means that, for one thing, the data is anonymized and the corresponding statistic programs must and can only access selected data. For the purpose of data reduction, the user only states the names of those items that are to be evaluated. In this procedure it is possible to transform this data by corresponding routines (e.g., standardization, calculation of age from birth date and actual date, etc.).

After this data reduction the data is available for the corresponding statistical routines. These routines can be divided as follows:

- simple epidemiological statistics

  These, for instance, include setting up frequency tables. In these tables different items are being compared (e.g., sex, age, histological diagnosis, localization, occupation, therapy, date of first diagnosis, date of death, etc.). If only one item is evaluated, the results can be presented in the form of a histogram.

- sophisticated statistics

  These include statistical routines which are applied, e.g., for statistics on survival rates, statistics on case-control studies, on multivariate analysis, etc. (1).

For drawing up and changing printed texts KRAZTUR also offers great advantages, since the flexibility of the system makes it possible to consider user's requests very simply and quickly.

DATA PRESENTATION

In order to present the values obtained by epidemiological evaluations to the user in such a way that he will understand the results without being familiar with EDP, it will be necessary to offer corresponding routines for data presentation. The system KRAZTUR offers routines which, for instance, print out histograms or frequency tables via terminal or printer. Via a connected plotter results may be printed out in a graphic form that these 'pictures' can be used for scientific work (2).

ORGANIZATION

A cancer registry can only work successfully if the data of all patients is completely covered. In order to attain this ideal state as completely as possible, the system checks as to whether the results of routine follow-up examinations are reported and covered for all patients. If there is no report for any one patient over a given period of time (in years), the system then automatically sets up a letter to the registry office. This is to clarify whether this particular case can be considered closed (death of patient) or whether an attempt must be made to obtain the required data by other means.

THE SYSTEM KRAZTUR

The above described modules in the information system have been realized with the system KRAZTUR (general documentation system supported by microcomputers with additional text and retrieval functions). With KRAZTUR it is possible to collect, store, process, evaluate and print out any data in any structure. The original system was developed in the language MUMPS 800 on a Philips computer P856 of the firm CHF-Mueller. The later version is operated under DSM-11 on a PDP-11 computer by DEC (3).

The entire KRAZTUR system is based on the instruction concept which is designed in such a fashion that certain recurring processing steps are standardized and combined. These individual steps are defined as instructions. The system includes few instructions which, in corresponding order, present the realization of a certain application (e.g., acquisition dialog) (4).

This instruction concept puts the user in a position to solve his problems with the system KRAZTUR without extensive knowledge of EDP. The requirements placed on a communication system of this type by the user can be roughly listed as follows:

- collect and store data
- search for, select and process data
- display data

To fulfil these tasks, the system KRAZTUR offers tools which enable the user to 'generate' the realization of his requirements in dialog with the system, taking his needs into account. The first step includes the definition of the items to be collected. For this purpose, the system KRAZTUR contains the dialog 'database description'. To begin with, it is stated under which name the data are to be stored.

The items to be stored are combined in data groups. Each item requires different specifications as follows:

- name of the item
- mode
- name of variables
- field number
- coding
- inversion
- correction number
- assistant text

If the above named information has been given for all items to be covered, an operable dialog version can be generated with the KRAZTUR function 'dialog generator'. The user need only indicate which items are to be used to identify the item carrier and which items are to be covered.

Before a user can call up the newly generated dialog, the permission for this user to apply this dialog must first be entered with the function 'user generator'. Following this step, the user may call up 'his' dialog.

Once the user has collected and stored his data with the aid of his dialog function, the 'retrieval' function of the KRAZTUR system will be used. To begin with, the user has to state which group of data he wishes to process. The user can restrict an earlier search by further conditions. Conditions for several items may be given in the search (any Boolean expression is possible). The result of such a retrieval run can be displayed.

The user can define in the dialog in which way he wants his data to be printed out or to be seen on the screen. He can choose the form of a list, a table, a running text or a histogram.

For the purpose of generating such a printing function by means of the KRAZTUR function 'printing generator', the user need merely indicate the names of the items to be printed. After the printing function for the corresponding user has been admitted, he can call up this function and obtain his output, according to his wishes, either via terminal or printer.

Before calling a statistical routine, the KRAZTUR function 'Data reduction' must be carried out. This system stores the selected data chosen by the user in dialog in a separate database. By this process it is guaranteed that the subsequent statistical routines work with anonymized data only.

The list of usable statistical functions (e.g., histograms, frequency tables, correlations, etc.) can be extended at any time according to the requirements of the respective user.

Since personal data are processed in the compound system of the Tumour Center with the system KRAZTUR, various modules for data protection and data safety are included.

FUTURE OUTLOOK

We have tried to solve the well known problem of the acceptance of any new system by timely information, training, motivation and maximum comfort of the system. Experiences were gathered during the pilot phase in Heidelberg. Here, in particular, the flexibility of the system with regard to its adaptability to users' wishes has proven very valuable.

REFERENCES

1) Rothman, K.J., Boice, J.D. Jr.:
Epidemiologic Analysis with a Programmable Calculator.
NIH Publications No. 79-1649, 1979.

2) Ellsässer, K.H., Hepperle, G., Hoenicke, E., Offenhäuser, K.H.:
Datenpräsentation und Verlaufsdarstellung im Arztbrief und am Bildschirm.
In: Möhr, J.R., Köhler, C.O. (Eds): Datenpräsentation.
Springer, Berlin - Heidelberg - New York, pp. 177-185, 1979.

3) Ellsässer, K.H., Hönicke, E., Offenhäuser, K.H.:
KRAZTUR. Techn.Rep. Nr. 3.
Integrierte Onkologische Einrichtung, Heidelberg-Mannheim, 1979.

4) Ellsässer, K.H., Hönicke, E., Köhler, C.O., Offenhäuser, K.H.,
Vogt-Moykopf, I.:
The Instruction Concept in the System KRAZTUR. In: Lindberg, D.A.B.,
Kaihara, S. (Eds): Medinfo 80, North Holland Publ. Co., Amsterdam,
pp. 867-870, 1980.

AUTOMATION OF DATA BASE

USED BY THE MISSOURI KIDNEY PROGRAM

Arthur E. Rikli, M.D., M.P.H.
Melissa A. Thomas, M.A.
C. Richard Evans, M.S.

Missouri Kidney Program
Columbia, MO 65201/USA

1. SUMMARY

When the Missouri Kidney Program decided to transform its manual data management system into an automated one, a review of the nature and scope of these systems was required. Initial review resulted in alteration of the original system and in revised expectations of the automated system. The program decided to retain the collection of epidemiological and service utilization data in the initial automated system and to defer inclusion of fiscal and facility data. Analysis of the need and use of the data reconfirmed the value of computerization for timely decision making. Preparation for automation of the system is described.

2. The Missouri Kidney Program (MoKP) was established by state legislation in 1968 to help end stage renal disease (ESRD) patients meet their medical needs. MoKP is a state-operated organization with a staff of 8 persons and an advisory council of 15. Since 1968 over $12 million was spent to help pay for dialysis, kidney transplantation and special patient needs such as drugs and transportation to and from treatment. Thirty ESRD facilities, which have treated over 2,000 patients, participate in the program.

3. The management of the program began by collecting standard patient information required on billing forms. The information was collected from representatives of dialysis facilities who had contracts for state funding. By 1976, dialysis had become a much bigger business than it had been in 1968, and the decision was made to expand the data collection system to include more items of information.(1) By 1980, another decision was made to automate the system since the number of patients monitored and the number of data elements collected on each patient had grown beyond the capacity of the program's small staff to handle them manually. This decision to automate a manual system led to a review of previous decisions on what data to collect and how to collect them. The structure and rationale of the data management

system had to be clearly conceptualized before the software essential for the automated data base could be developed.

4.1. To begin this retrospective review of the system, the need for the data was analyzed with reference to work done in Michigan and Minnesota. Through the years the system had grown to serve several masters, not just the Missouri Kidney Program. Health Systems Agencies, which are federally-funded regional planning and evaluation programs for all areas of health care, used the data to determine need for and appropriateness of ESRD services. When Missouri's dialysis units wanted to expand or diversify their operations, they came to MoKP for information on patient distribution and existing service capacity. When the federal government established a separate regional planning and review body for ESRD services, this new organization needed a model of data collection to minimize start-up efforts. These demands for information, in addition to MoKP needs, can be classified in four major categories:

1. epidemiological information (incidence and prevalence by demographic and geographic characteristics and ESRD diagnosis;
2. utilization of ESRD services (dialysis and transplantation);
3. facility capacity and configuration; and
4. treatment charges and reimbursement.

As the program approached computerization, each of these categories were closely investigated to ascertain whether or not the data were still relevant and still needed by users of the system.

4.2. Basic epidemiological data, ie, patient age, race, sex and diagnosis were used to describe the treated ESRD population and trends in that population.[(2)] It was discovered, through collection of this data, that more men than women find their way into the ESRD care system and that proportionately more nonwhites than whites required ESRD therapy. The difference in sex distribution may be linked to disease diagnosis, particularly the prevalence of glomerulonephritis in the male population. The reasons for this sex difference are still open to question. MoKP's data system gives researchers information to investigate this subject.

4.3. The difference in racial distribution may be more easily understood. Since blacks are more prone to hypertension, and hypertension is related to kidney disease, the higher prevalence of blacks in the

ESRD population is not surprising. The impact of public education efforts on the importance of early detection and treatment of hypertension may reduce the number of hypertension cases that culminate in renal failure.

4.4. Through the data base, a trend toward increased age of patients beginning dialysis was followed. Before government funding became available in 1973, hospital committees were forced to choose which patients would receive time on the few dialysis machines available. Generally, patients under the age of 55 who had no other complicating illnesses and who were judged to be capable to rehabilitation were selected for this expensive treatment. With the advent of public support, these restrictions were lifted, and older patients and patients with more serious illnesses were accepted for therapy.

5.1. The data system showed that the average age of treated patients climb to above 50 years. It is still climbing; in FY 1978/79, 36% of Missouri's new ESRD patients were over the age of 60. The impact of patient age on treatment costs will be significant in the future and a trend that should be monitored.

5.2. The occurence and distribution of patients by age/race/sex diagnosis was still significant in describing current and anticipated cases of reported ESRD and in directing efforts to reduce the number of cases that require treatment. Accurate collection of this data and their inclusion in the automated data base for forecasting need for facilities and services became an essential requirement.(3)

6.1. The tracking of patient use of services had always been one of the most successful features of the manual data management system. Each month, every dialysis unit was required to identify each of its patients, not only by basic epidemiological information discussed previously, but by specific designations showing the patient's status within the treatment system. The dialysis unit has a selection of well-defined classifications to choose from. Each of these categories either denotes entry into the system, exit from the system, or a maintenance status. Figure 1 conceptualizes movement of patients into and out of the two major treatment populations.

6.2. The circles represent (prevalence) the numbers of persons in each of these populations at beginning of time interval. The arrows

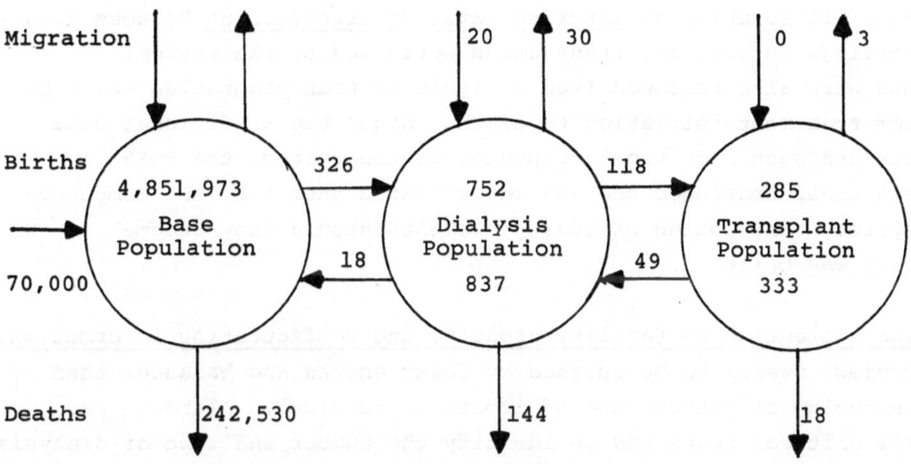

FIGURE I

Schematic Representation[3] of Patient Movement in ESRD System for a Specified Period of Time in a Given Geographic Location (Missouri 7/1/79 to 6/30/80).

represent (incidence) the numbers of persons who move from or to each circle during a specific period of time. The arrows describe the births, deaths, migration, and flow of patients from the base population to and from therapy. All transplant patients are assumed to pass through the dialysis population.

6.3. For example, migration in or out of Missouri or movement between two cities in Missouri, is classified by the unit from which the patient has moved as a "deletion." The unit that receives him will assign him as an "addition." In this simple manner, patients are added and deleted to the proper dialysis census. Since placement of expensive dialysis services depends largely on patient distribution, following patient movement between treatment settings is critical. Before the MoKP began to track patient physical movement, no one in the state had verified the number of treated ESRD cases or where they required treatment.

6.4. This illustration of tracking patients transferring between treatment settings is only one transaction performed by the system. Patients were also followed from dialysis to transplantation and back and from treatment initiation to death. Since the traditional data elements are such a critical component of the system, the MoKP endorsed their continued use and incorporated them into the computerized system. The option of adding elements should they become necessary was built in.

7.1. The collection of facility capacity and configuration information, upon review, seemed to be guarded by fewer checks and balances than the monitoring of patient use of treatment services. Although each dialysis unit was requested to identify the number and type of dialysis treatments it rendered, by type and setting, a methodology has not been incorporated for verifying this information. If a patient was recorded as receiving 13 home hemodialysis treatments during one month, the MoKP never verified that the patient had ever been recorded as trained for home care. Although each month aggregate totals of treatment distribution were calculated and probably reasonably accurate for the state, consistency on a patient-by-patient basis was missing from the system. As a result of this revelation, the staff decided to investigate the possibility that the interactive computer system would relate input on a patient's monthly services with previously entered data on that same patient to detect obvious inconsistencies. This capability might economically be prohibitive but the review has revealed a need for closer examination of patient treatment data. An audit of the facilities' records to detect less obvious inconsistencies in treatment or charges may be required.

7.2. As part of the long-range hope for the automated system the program would also like to include facility-specific data in addition to Missouri patient-specific data. Such information could include data on non-Missouri patients treated in Missouri facilities and the number of dialysis stations, by type, so that service capacity could be tied to the treatment information to calculate utilization rates. Knowledge of such rates is critical, not only in monitoring efficient use of expensive equipment, but in determining need for expanded or diversified services. Planning, financing and gaining approval for new services is a complicated process in such a governmentally-regulated industry and timely anticipation of service saturation points or service needs can conveniently activate this process. These and similar issues led not only to a review of the present data collection and analysis system for computerization, but to a review of future expectations.

8. The fourth component of the system, collection of treatment cost and reimbursement, received the greatest criticism during the retrospective study. The billing form required dialysis units to list the facility's charge against each patient for that month and the anticipated reimbursement of those charges from all payment sources. Anticipated reimbursement was requested since identification of actual payment is a delayed and untimely process. Frequent adjustments in this data in succeeding months made each monthly billing form inaccurate, with respect to fiscal data, shortly after it was filed. The cost and difficulty of entering such variable data in our initial automated system was considered and excluded. The review, however, did signal a need for in-depth analysis of reimbursement policies and the value of the fiscal information collected. It also reaffirmed previous impressions that adequate cost data are desirable, but difficult to obtain. As a result of the review, some resources were allocated to a University-sponsored cost flow identification study spearheaded by a health economist.(4)

9. After reviewing the benefits and drawbacks of the system, attention was turned to the mechanics of its operation. The accuracy of the epidemiological service and fiscal data depended largely on those facility personnel who completed the billing form. Their incentive for conveying correct data was that reimbursement from the program hinged, by stipulations in our contract, on successful completion of that form. This check on data accuracy, although reassuring, is not fool-proof. Some of the data elements, for example, numbers of treatments rendered to a patient during a month, defy verification by the staff. The computerized system, obviously, could not alleviate this problem. The solution depended upon improved working relations with the facility personnel who completed the form. Personal contact between the staff and these data entry people had to be reinforced through written and physical interaction. In the revised contract guidelines for FY 1980/81, a detailed explanation of the value of the data collected and its practical application was inserted. Decisions were reached by health planners, regulators and financiers on the fate of the ESRD system in Missouri based on the information provided by

each facility and that accurate data were essential if these decisions were to be in patients' and health providers' best interests.

10. The Missouri Kidney Program uses the facilities of the University of Missouri Computer Network which operates an Amdahl 470/V7 under MVS (Multiple Virtual Storage operating system) Release 3.8. The direct access computerized data base is stored on an IBM 3350 disc (with tape backup) which is accessed in interactive mode via Digital Equipment Corporation Decscope and Decwriter using TSO (Time Sharing Option) over dialup lines. The software is written in the PL/1 programming language and SAS (Statistical Analysis System) is used for statistical analysis. Estimated cost for conversion of the system from manual to automation on a mini computer is 3 years at $50,000/year.

11. In conclusion, the Missouri Kidney Program's plan to automate its ESRD patient information system cost $25,000 and led the program to a comprehensive review of that system, its uses and its mechanics. This review led to alterations and improvements in that system and to a more realistic concept of how it would weather the transfer from manual to automated storage and retrieval. In this process of "recreating" the principles and assumptions behind the system, the conclusion was that a computer could make the kidney program more efficient and one of the greatest benefits of automation would be, identifying specifically, where there are needs to improve the source data.

12. Acknowledgements with appreciation for the assistance provided with this paper, are extended to: Margie Ross, Dorothea Courtney, James Watson, David Austin and Michael Leonard.

13. BIBLIOGRAPHY

(1) Thomas MA. The Missouri Kidney Program patient information system. Dial & Trans. 1979 ; 8:12 ; 1203-7.
(2) Rikli AE, Thomas MA. Missouri Kidney Program annual report. 1978-79.
(3) Rikli AE, Leonard MS, Takasugi S. Renal model showing patients' needs and resource requirements. (Proceedings of MEDIS '78. Kansai Ins Info Sys. Osaka Japan. 1978) 1979; 18-21.
(4) Hicks L. Expenditures on ESRD in Missouri - 1979. Univ of Mo Mo Kid Prog (in progress).

A SELECTION AND FOLLOW-UP SYSTEM FOR ORGAN TRANSPLANTATION

Q.P. Lansbergen
CDIV, University Hospital, Leiden
EUROTRANSPLANT, Leiden

SUMMARY

In Western Europe there are more than 20.000 people with endstage renal diseases. Fifteen years ago, transplantation of unrelated cadaveric kidney became an alternative for heamodialysis.

The prognosis for renal graft survival can be improved by selecting a suitable recipient on the basis of immunological criteria. That fact was the motivation for the founding of Eurotransplant (ET) in 1967. It is a cooperative effort of over 200 dialysis centres in Austria, Belgium, Germany, Luxemburg and the Netherlands.

All renal patients considered for transplantation are registered in the database of the University Hospital in Leiden - presently approximately 13.000. Whenever a donor kidney becomes available, the pool of about 2700 patients waiting for transplantation is searched for the 40 best matched candidates.

Follow-up information on the 6700 transplantation, performed since 1967 under the auspices of ET are recorded on magnetic tape. Twice a year, the graft failures are reported by the centres, using the questionnaires printed by the computer. Death dates are supplied yearly on tape by the European Dialysis and Transplantation Association (EDTA).

Graft and patient survival are analysed mainly by actuarial survival statistics. The results of those analyses are used to optimize the matching algorithm for selecting donor-recipient pairs.

Since 1979 this system is also used for selecting patients for cornea transplantation and the analysis of the results.

1. INTRODUCTION

More than 20.000 people in Western Europe suffer from endstage renal disease. The classis treatment is haemodialysis, two or three times a week. An alternative is renal transplantation with a kidney from an unrelated cadaveric donor. The reaction of the immunological defence mechanisms of the patient against the donorkidney can end in the rejection of the graft. The prognosis of renal graft survival can be improved by transplanting a well matched kidney on the basis of immunological criteria. Because there are so mutch different HLA tissue types possible, the probability of finding a well matched kidney by random selection is very small. To increase this chance, the patients waiting for transplantation have to be pooled.

These facts were the motivation of the founding of EUROTRANSPLANT in 1967. Under its auspices a waiting list was set up of patients from Austria, Belgium, Germany, Luxemburg and the Netherlands, who were considered for a kidney transplantation. Whenever a donor-kidney becomes available, that list is searched for the best matched candidates.

Information on all transplantations, mediated in this way, are recorded by ET and added to a computer file. To keep this file up-to-date, questionnaires are filled in by the phycisian in charge. In the event of graft failure the patients return to local dialysis centres, therefore information about death is supplied by the EDTA, with which all dialyses centres cooperate.

The outcome of the analyses of the results of kidney transplantation is used to optimize the matching algorithm for selecting donor-recipient pairs. Figure 1. shows the result of an analys of the effect of well-matched kidneys according to HLA-tissue type on graft survival. It is a confirmation of the original idea on which ET was founded.

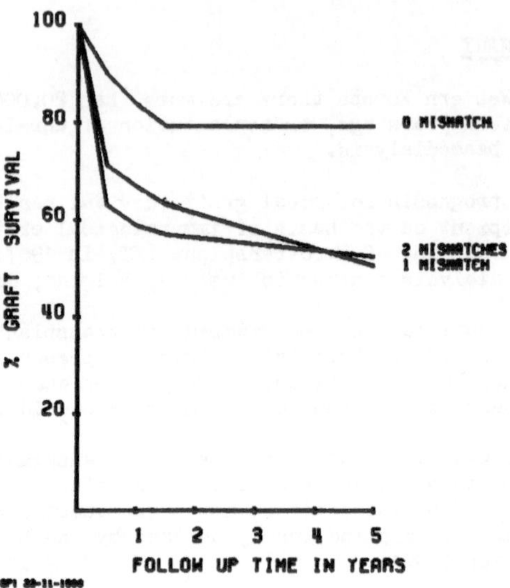

Figure 1.

2. THE EUROTRANSPLANT INFORMATION SYSTEM (ETIS)

Since the start of ET, we have used computers to fascilitate the tasks of registering patients, of matching and of analysing the transplant results. At first various small computers were used. In 1975, the decision was made to develop a new integrated information system. (ETIS)

Requirement for the system are:

- All information on renal patients, kidney donors and kidney transplantation must be recorded on disc and be available for on-line inspection.
- Selection of suitable recipients must be:
  a) rapid (within seconds)
  b) flexable with regard to the matching criteria
  c) done by the regional centres, using telex
  d) 24 hours availability
- Results of the transplantations, in terms of graft or patient survival, have to be analysed with appropriate statistics.

The system consists of four parts:

2.1 Patient and donor registration
2.2 Recipient selection
2.3 Transplantation registration and follow-up
2.4 Transplant analyses

The first three parts are operating under the Hospital Information System (HIS), an inhouse developed operating and database system(1,2), on the PDP 11/70 of the Leiden University Hospital.
Transplantation follow-up analyses are performed on the IBM 370 of the University.

ETIS global architecture is shown in figure 3, the end of the artical.

2.1 Patient and donor registration system

All renal patients in the ET region, considered for transplantation as well as all donor kidneys reported are registered centrally, in real time, in the HIS database. At present, personal and medical data, HLA tissue type and HLA antibody reactivity of more than 13.000 patients and more than 6700 donors are stored on disc.
For patients waiting for transplantation, an extract of the information recorded in the database is duplicated on a directly accessable file, called the WAITING LIST. All changes in the list are automatically reported to the phycisian on a mutation document printed by the computer.

2.2 Selection of recipients

An extract of the information, relevant for matching is kept up-to-date contantly in the waiting list file by the registrat ion system. Whenever a donor kidney becomes available the list is searched for the best matched candidates on the basis of immunological and clinical criteria.
Within seconds, the fourty best matched candidates are selected. To provide the local centres associated with ET, access to the computer, an interface between the computer and the public telex network has been developed.

In addition, every month, a list of all patients on the waiting list is provided with the information arranged in such a way that matching can be done without the computer.
Figure 4, at the end of the artical, shows the printout of a match reguest.

2.3 Transplantation registration and follow-up

Information about the transplantation is reported to ET, which adds it to the database. The follow-up information is kept up-to-date contantly. Questionnaires printed by the computer, are filled in regularly by the centres, in order to inform ET about the graft function. Because the patients return to local dialysis centres, ET depends on the EDTA registry for information on patient's death.
This information is inputted centrally in the database, either by hand or by magnetic tape.

2.4 Analysis system

The transplant analyses are performed on a different computer, an IBM 370/158 of the Leiden University, for the following reasons:

1. The system was already operating on this computer.
2. Many other statistical packages are available: SPSS, BMD, etc.
3. Rewriting the existing system for HIS gives problems with regard to core memory limitations.

At the start of a new serie of analyses all transplantationinformation, recorded in the database, is put on magnetic tape.
This tape forms the data file for the analyses on the University computer.
The analysis are done mainly with actuarial survival statistics, described by R. Pieto et all (3,4). Currently, a new analitic model, Proportional Hazards, is under investigation, in order to study the interrelation of the multiple factors on renal graft survival more clearly.

The outcome of the analyses, after confirmation by other groups or controlled experiments, are used to optimize the matching criteria.

3. DISCUSSION

The objectives of ET are to improve kidney graft prognosis. This is done by selecting well matched donor-recipient pairs. Figure 2 shows the overall improvement realised over the years. Per year of transplantation, the graft survival is plotted.

To efficiently handle the data ET requirs database oriented system. It provides an easy way for storing the many different information items. In addition, by keying in the data via an instructiv dialog, highstandard of quality is reached. Unfortunately, a database storage system is inefficient for matching.
For that reason, a summary of the information of only those patients actually waiting for transplantation is kept up-to-date constantly in a directly accessable file, the WAITING LIST. This scheme gives a simple, flexable, separate selection system with a maximum efficiency for searching. A disadvantage is that the information

has to be duplicated and kept up-to-date contantly.

ETIS has been implemented by parts and it replaced gradually the parts operating on the University computer.

from 1970 - the analysis system
1977 - patient registration
selection of recipients
1979 - donor registration
1980 - transplant registration
1981 - follow-up system

Since 1979, the system is also used for cornea transplantation.

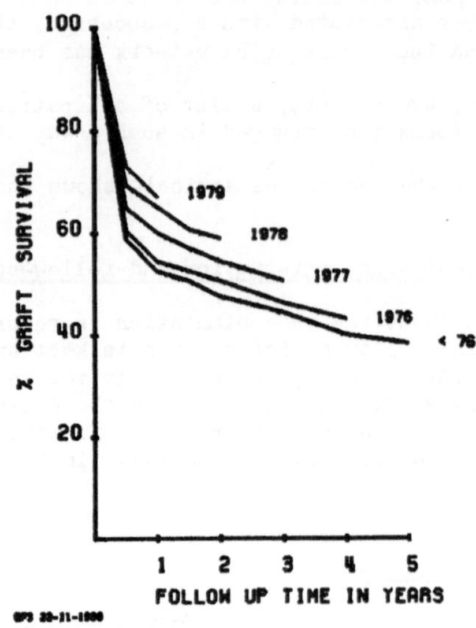

Figure 2.

4. CONCLUSION

Since 1976 ET has been using a new information system, ETIS, in order to improve kidney graft prognoses by selecting well matched donor-recipient pairs. By using the database concept, the data is stored in an efficient way. Via an instructiv dialog the data is put in, ensuring a high quality. For efficiency reasons, information necessary for matching is duplicated and is kept up to date constantly in a separate file. Within seconds the fourty best matched candidates for transplantation may be selected. Via telex, dialysis centres have access to the WAITING LIST for matching only.

Analyses are done on the large University computer that is best suited for the task. Many statistical packages are available, and core size is no problem. The transfer of data between the two computers is via magnetic tape, which presents problem.

Referenties

1. Bakker, A.R., Scope and limitations of a minibased centralized Hospital Information System. Proc. MEDINFO 80 (1980), p 505.
2. Bakker, A.R., Implementational approach and evaluation of the use of Leiden University Hospital Information System, Proc. MEDINFO 77 (1977), p 943.
3. Pieto, R. et all, Design and analyses of randomized clinical trials, requiring prolonged observation of each patients.
Introduction and design. Britisch Journal of Cancer (1976) 34, p 585.
4. Pieto, R. et all, Design and analyses of randomized clinical trials, requiring prolonged observation of each patients. Analyses and examples.
Britisch Journal of Cancer (1977) 35, p 1.

Figure 3 Global system architecture

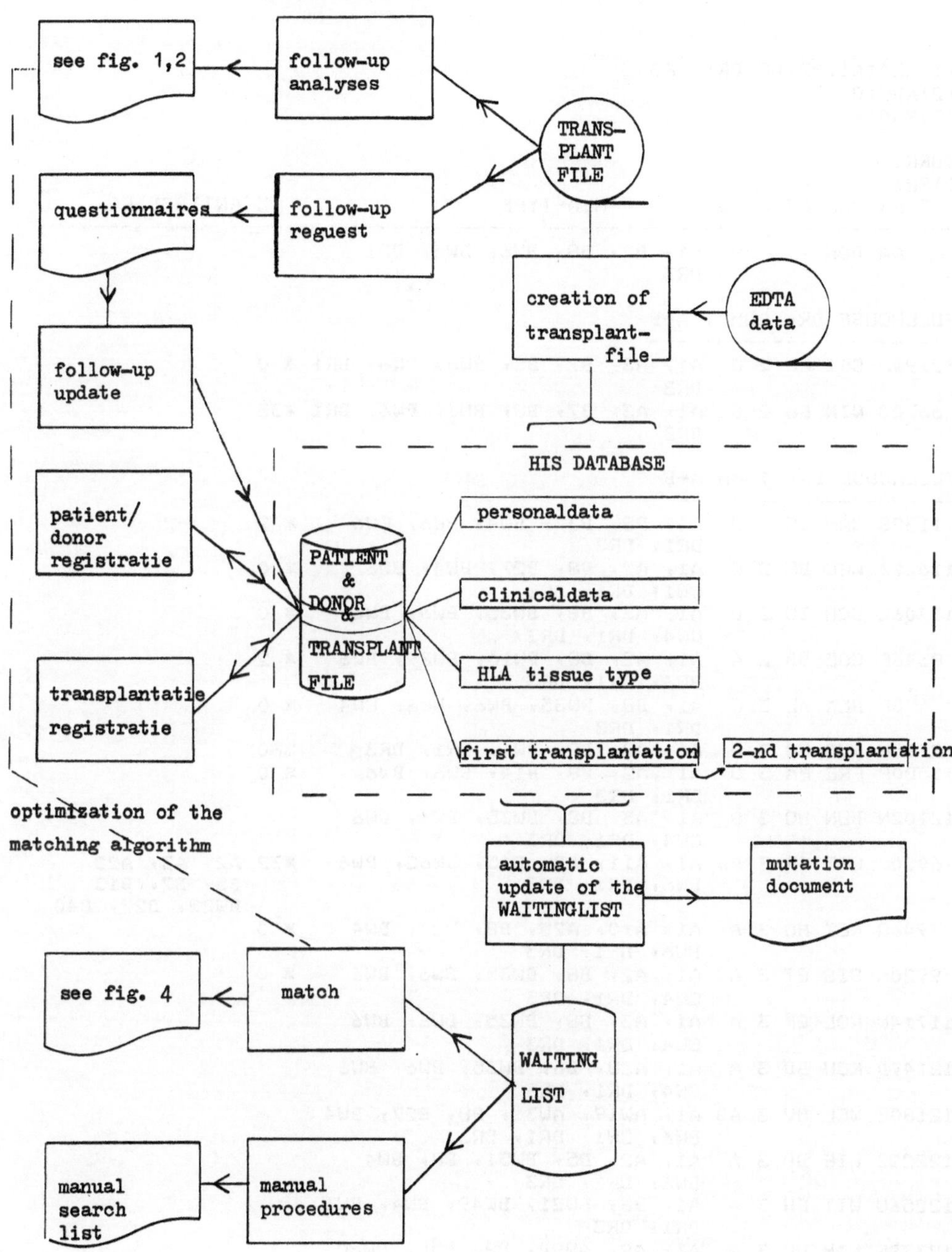

Figure 4 List of the 40 best matched candidates for transplantation

```
(1)HLA:A1,B7,B8,DR1,DR3
(2)ABO:O
(3)RHD:+

CORR:
DISP:
  ETNR NAM CC U AB        HLA-TYPE                        % ANTIBODIES
------------------------------------------------------------------------

    OA DON        O  A1, B7, B8, BW6, BW6, DR1
                     DR3

FULLHOUSE DR, COMP. A+B
-----------------------

12194N SEI ML 2 O  A1, A3, B7, B8, BW6, BW6, DR1 * O
                   DR3
 6670D WIN ES 2 B  A1, A3, B7, B8, BW6, BW6, DR1 *35
                   DR3

FULLHOUSE DR, 1 MM A+B
----------------------

11132S JAN DE 2 O  A1, B8, B37, BW4, BW6, CW6    * 2
                   DR1, DR3
11629Z WEL BE 2 O  A1, A2, B8, B27, BW4, BW6     * O
                   CW1, DR1, DR3
11706L SCH ZU 2 O  A1, A3, B8, BW35, BW6, BW6    * O
                   CW4, DR1, DR3
 8546F GOE DD 2 A  A1, A2, B8, BW16, BW39, BW6   * 2
                   BW6, DR1, DR3
  450F BLA AL 3 O  A1, B8, BW35, BW6, BW6, CW4   * O
                   DR1, DR3
 2795H RUD HO 3 O  A1, A2, B8, BW6, DR1, DR3     *60
11580P FRE MA 3 O  A1, A2, B8, B14, BW6, BW6     * O
                   DR1, DR3
12202N BUN HO 3 O  A1, A3, B8, BW35, BW6, BW6
                   CW4, DR1, DR3
 6020E OTT GR 3 AB A1, A11, B8, B15, BW62, BW6   *32 A2, A3, A28
                   BW6, DR1, DR3                     B5, B7, B13
                                                     BW22, B27, B40
 7946Q REI HO 3 A  A1, A10, A25, B8, B27, BW4    * O
                   BW6, DR1, DR3
 9920M SIS GT 3 A  A1, A2, B8, BW35, BW6, BW6    * O
                   CW4, DR1, DR3
11714W ROL GK 3 A  A1, A3, B8, BW35, BW6, BW6
                   CW4, DR1, DR3
12149D KOU BD 3 A  A1, A28, B8, BW35, BW6, BW6
                   CW4, DR1, DR3
12180E WEL GV 3 AB A1, AW19, AW31, B8, B27, BW4
                   BW6, CW1, DR1, DR3
12222Z LIE DD 3 A  A1, A2, B5, BW51, B8, BW4
                   BW6, DR1, DR3
12256U WIT EH 3 A  A1, B8, BW21, BW49, BW4, BW6
                   DR1, DR3
12338N KAM UL 3 A  A1, A9, AW24, B8, B40, BW60
                   BW6, BW6, CW3, DR1, DR3
```

L' EVALUATION DE LA QUALITE DES SOINS : L' EXPERIENCE DE L' HEMODIALYSE

François GOUPY(+), Patrice DEGOULET(+), Jean-Claude HIREL(++), Marcel LEGRAIN(+++).

(+) INSERM U 88 - Groupe de Recherche en Santé Publique
et Epidémiologie sociale et économique

(++) Centre Interuniversitaire de Traitement de l'Informatique 2 (CITI 2)

(+++) Service de Néphrologie - Groupe Hospitalier Pitié-Salpétrière

After reviewing concepts and methods for assessing the quality of medical care, we discuss the Programme Dialyse Informatique de la Société de Néphrologie. From the point of view of evaluations of medical pratice, we highlight the advantages of this system which was implemented 8 years ago, long before quality assessment was recommended by the French government as a part of an overall cost containment policy. We conclude that although quality assessment might have an economic impact in the long run, it is of critical importance to the medical profession.

1. INTRODUCTION

L'évaluation de la qualité des soins est-elle un mal nécessaire que les médecins doivent accepter pour répondre aux exigences des gestionnaires du système de santé ou bien est-elle une exigence nouvelle de la médecine en raison du développement scientifique des techniques ? Nous prendrons, en néphrologie, l'exemple d'un système utilisé en France depuis huit ans : cette expérience, qui illustre certains des aspects méthodologiques de l'évaluation de la qualité des soins, montre comment des médecins ont mis en place, de leur propre initiative, un système d'évaluation de leur pratique.

2. L'EVALUATION DE LA QUALITE DES SOINS : RAPPEL DES CONCEPTS ET DES METHODES

2.1. Objectif général. L'évaluation de la qualité des soins a pour objectif de vérifier que le système de soins apporte à la population tous les bénéfices possibles. Cette évaluation est faite en répondant à deux questions : les patients susceptibles de bénéficier des soins sont-ils pris en charge par le système de soins ? Les résultats obtenus pour les patients pris en charge sont-ils effectivement ceux qu'on peut espérer, compte tenu de l'état actuel des connaissances et des techniques? Ces deux questions sont liées à la distinction qui est faite entre les évaluations de programme et les évaluations d'institution.

2.2. Les objets de l'évaluation

Pour répondre à ces questions, l'analyse doit porter sur trois niveaux selon Donabedian : structures, processus, résultats [1]. Les évaluations de structures mesurent la densité et la technicité des installations (postes de dialyse par million d'habitants, importance de la dialyse à domicile), la densité et la qualification des personnels. Les évaluations de processus analysent les pratiques (fréquence et durée des séances de dialyse, fréquence relative d'utilisation des différentes techniques d'épuration extrarénale). Enfin les évaluations de résultats mesurent à l'aide d'indicateurs de santé l'efficacité des processus (taux de survie, taux de complications : incidence des accidents cardio-vasculaires, des hépatites, des polynévrites).

2.3. Les méthodes : 3 types d'approche sont possibles.

- L'exploitation des statistiques sanitaires permet de détecter les anomalies de résultats globaux. C'est l'approche d'évaluation de la qualité des soins qui est la plus ancienne. Par exemple, la mortalité périnatale, la morbidité du tétanos permettent de mesurer l'impact de programmes sanitaires ; les registres du cancer permettent d'apprécier les conséquences des actions de dépistage et de prise en charge de la maladie.

- Les études ponctuelles (audits nord américains) permettent d'identifier les insuffisances d'une institution ou d'une unité de soins [2]. Ces enquêtes analysent des résultats diagnostics (faux positifs, faux négatifs), des résultats thérapeutiques (récupération fonctionnelle, mortalité) pour des catégories homogènes de patients, ou bien vérifient que les examens et traitements prescrits correspondent aux normes de qualité admises par la profession. Les jugements peuvent être portés par les médecins responsables des soins des patients (audit interne) ou bien par des médecins experts du problème analysé (audit externe).

- Le contrôle de qualité est une garantie de la qualité des soins. C'est une procédure qui fonctionne en routine et qui concerne chaque patient individuellement : son caractère routinier le distingue des audits qui sont des études ponctuelles dont les conclusions conduisent le plus souvent à de simples recommandations. Différentes techniques peuvent être utilisées : la plus simple est par exemple le protocole de suivi d'un patient qui est la garantie pour chaque patient que le minimum indispensable d'informations sur ses antécédents, son état clinique et biologique aura été obtenu. Ces protocoles de suivi diffèrent des protocoles de recherche par les objectifs implicites qu'ils supposent : un protocole de recherche vise à documenter un patient, un protocole de routine vise à obtenir les variables les plus discriminantes, au moindre inconfort pour le patient et au moindre coût pour la collectivité, pour parvenir à la précision diagnostique justifiée par l'action thérapeutique. Dans certains cas, la qualité des soins peut être garantie par ordinateur. Une machine peut-être utilisée pour fournir des informations facilitant ou améliorant la fiabilité de la décision médicale : aide au diagnostic, signalement des incompatibilités médicamenteuses, aide au suivi d'un patient.

3. LE CAS DE LA DIALYSE : LE PROGRAMME DIALYSE INFORMATIQUE

3.1. Objectifs

A partir de l'expérience initiale du CMC Foch (Suresnes), la Société de Néphrologie prit l'initiative de développer le programme "Dialyse Informatique" auxquels participent aujourd'hui 40 centres de dialyse. En 1972, ce programme avait trois objectifs :

- améliorer le suivi médical des patients grâce à un dossier standardisé et des données statistiques mensuelles permettant à chaque centre de situer ses résultats par rapport à ceux d'autres centres de dialyse.
- développer un programme de recherche épidémiologique
- fournir aux autorités médicales responsables des données statistiques qui puissent aider à développer au mieux les moyens thérapeutiques requis par l'insuffisance rénale terminale.

3.2. Méthodes

Nous décrirons très rapidement la structure d'information recueillie et l'utilisation qui en est faite : une représentation et une discussion détaillées du programme Dialyse Informatique [3, 4, 5] ont déjà été faites.

Information recueillie : la constitution et la mise à jour d'un dossier est effectuée à partir de quatre questionnaires :

- l'identification rassemble les antécédents du patient, les conditions initiales du traitement par l'hémodialyse et les facteurs de risque ;
- le bordereau de séance, rempli lors de chaque séance, comprend l'ensemble des résultats cliniques et biologiques avant et après dialyse, les caractères techniques de celle-ci et un relevé des éventuels complications, troubles cliniques et incidents techniques survenus pendant la séance ;
- un bilan clinique est effectué tous les trimestres ;
- un bordereau de fin de dialyse est rempli à l'occasion d'un transfert dans un autre centre, d'une transplantation ou d'un décès.

Précisons que ces questionnaires informatiques sont intégrés dans le dossier médical : chaque bordereau comprend une partie informatique et une partie libre réservée à l'observation ; seul le double de la partie informatique est transmis à un secrétariat central qui en gère l'exploitation.

Information restituée : l'information recueillie est retournée aux centres de dialyse sous trois formes :

- des éditions par patient présentent chaque mois sous forme récapitulative, l'évolution pendant les six derniers mois des principales données cliniques et biologiques ;
- des statistiques comparatives intercentres permettent à chaque centre de se situer ;

- des statistiques nationales sont publiées annuellement dans un numéro spécial du Journal d'Urologie et de Néphrologie [6, 7, 8, 9, 10, 11]. L'information sur les problèmes ponctuels est apportée aux centres sous la forme de lettres d'information.

3.3. Le programme Dialyse Informatique est un outil d'évaluation de la qualité des soins

En prenant les trois types d'approche, qui ont été distingués dans le paragraphe 2.3., nous montrerons par des exemples comment le dossier informatique standardisé a apporté aux néphrologues un outil d'évaluation de la qualité des soins.

Sa fonction de registre a permis :

- une analyse annuelle du recrutement des patients dialysés : on constate qu'un nombre croissant de patients âgés et présentant une maladie générale (diabète, cancer...) est pris en charge;
- un suivi de la mortalité et morbidité et une analyse des facteurs de risque [12];
- une appréciation de l'importance des problèmes de la dialyse : la fréquence des hypertensions a justifié le développement d'un programme de recherche qui a eu pour conséquence la modification de la composition des bains de dialyse; la fréquence des polynévrites a suscité une enquête détaillée qui a précisé leur mode de survenue et leur évolution [13].

Sa fonction d'audit médical peut être illustrée par une analyse comparative des résultats biologiques avant et après dialyse qui fit apparaître 7 centres dont les valeurs de bicarbonates plasmatiques étaient très inférieures aux valeurs moyennes. Un audit fut alors organisé : une lettre d'information reproduisant de façon anonyme les résultats en question fut adressée à chacun des centres; en même temps, on leur demanda de bien vouloir mesurer les bicarbonates systématiquement pendant trois mois pour tous les malades et d'indiquer précisément la méthode de dosage utilisée par le laboratoire. La conclusion de cet audit prospectif fut que pour 4 centres, cette déviation n'était qu'apparente en raison de méthodes de dosage non uniformes; par contre 3 centres purent grâce à la lettre d'information être avertis de ce problème particulier et améliorer ainsi la qualité technique de la dialyse de leurs patients. Cette fonction est très appréciée des centres de dialyse qui téléphonent parfois au secrétariat central afin d'obtenir des statistiques complémentaires leur permettant d'expliquer certaines déviations observées.

Sa fonction assurance de qualité est le fait du dossier informatique standardisé qui est la garantie pour chacun des patients que le minimum indispensable d'information a été pris en considération par l'infirmière et le médecin (qui ont rempli le bordereau de séance) à chaque séance de dialyse ou par le médecin (qui complète le questionaire) à chaque bilan clinique trimestriel. Le dossier informatique standardisé a même été utilisé par les malades eux-mêmes ou leur famille dans le cas particulier de la dialyse à domicile [14]. Bien entendu la qualité d'un dossier médical n'est pas nécessairement le reflet de la qualité des soins [15].

4. DISCUSSION

4.1. L'insuffisance rénale terminale est un domaine favorable à l'évaluation de la qualité des soins

Les institutions : en raison du caractère récent de l'hémodialyse et de l'incidence faible de la maladie, les centres de dialyse sont en nombre réduit et surtout les néphrologues se connaissent bien. Enfin la Société de Néphrologie est active et représentative de la discipline et un registre européen de la dialyse et de la transplantation (EDTA) avait déjà été mis en place, et bénéficie d'une reconnaissance internationale [16].

La technique est extrêmement codifiée et son efficacité n'est pas à démontrer : ceci facilite la coopération entre les centres de dialyse qui ne redoutent pas une évaluation parce qu'ils se savent fort de moyens thérapeutiques d'une très grande valeur.

Les résultats sont faciles à mesurer. En effet les indicateurs de santé sont d'une définition précise (mortalité, complications de l'hémodialyse) et de plus le suivi des patients est simplifié du fait de leur dépendance thérapeutique.

4.2. Le volontariat est la garantie de la fiabilité des données

Les 40 centres participant au Programme Dialyse-Informatique n'assurent pas une représentativité puisqu'ils ne constituent pas un échantillon tiré au sort. Cependant, la continuité du recueil et la fiabilité des données apportés par le volontariat, assurent la validité du contrôle de qualité.

4.3. Les enseignements du Programme DI

Vers quels enseignements de portée générale, l'expérience décrite dans le cas très particulier de l'hémodialyse rénale peut-elle conduire ?.

- Les évaluations sont une exigence médicale avant d'être une exigence économique. Parce que les médecins sont intéressés par la comparaison des résultats médicaux de leur activité, les évaluations n'ont une chance de modifier des comportements que si elles sont menées par les médecins (à leur initiative et sous leur responsabilité) et si ces évaluations portent avant tout sur des résultats qu'ils comprennent en termes de morbidité et mortalité.
- L'évaluation de la qualité des soins est plus facile pour une technique d'utilité indiscutable. Parce que la technique médicale dans son ensemble est hétérogène et souvent culturelle [17], il est souhaitable, dans un premier temps tout au moins, d'évaluer les résultats de techniques bien codifiées dont l'utilité est reconnue unanimement. Cependant, on ne saurait s'arrêter aux évaluations faciles à entreprendre, ce qui pose le problème du choix des thèmes des évaluations [18]. Ce choix peut reposer sur des critères de risques évitables [19], parce qu'une action appropriée peut avoir des effets à court terme. Mais les critères de coût (importance du coût unitaire de l'acte ou importance de la fréquence relative

d'exécution de cet acte sont évidemment des critères importants à considérer, en sachant que 70 à 80 % des coûts correspondent à des dépenses de personnels : les solutions envisageables ici peuvent donc difficilement apporter des résultats à court terme ou moyen terme.

- Une tenue rigoureuse des dossiers médicaux et une organisation précise du suivi des patients sont des conditions préalables à toute évaluation. Pour les études rétrospectives, la tenue systématisée des dossiers est une condition quasi nécessaire; pour les études prospectives qui supposent un protocole utilisé par tous (et donc une tenue nécessairement rigoureuse des dossiers), la principale difficulté est d'obtenir un consensus sur les définitions des variables.

5. CONCLUSION

En Amérique du Nord, le principe d'une évaluation de la qualité des soins fut débattu dans la profession médicale à la fin des années soixante, et depuis 1972 une loi fédérale (PSRO), destinée à contrôler les dépenses de santé des Etats-Unis inclut dans ses dispositions l'évaluation de la qualité des soins [20]. Ce n'est donc pas un hasard si cette évaluation est proposée aujourd'hui à l'ensemble des médecins français par les responsables de la santé publique au moment même de la prise de conscience du coût de notre système de santé. Cela signifie-t-il que l'évaluation de la qualité des soins est un outil dont ont besoin les gestionnaires de notre système de santé ? Il est vrai que cette nouvelle démarche, qui ne peut-être faite que par les médecins eux-mêmes, devrait apporter aux responsables politiques des informations pouvant éclairer les conséquences de leurs choix (mais ces choix ont toujours été faits et continueront de l'être), par contre elle donne aux médecins un outil leur permettant de vérifier la qualité du service rendu (et de montrer éventuellement, mesuré en termes de santé, l'effet de restrictions budgétaires).

Nous avons présenté et discuté le Programme Dialyse Informatique, parce qu'en 1970, sous l'impulsion de la Société de Néphrologie, et bien avant que les concepts et les méthodes en aient été introduits et discutés en France, des médecins mettaient en place un système d'évaluation de la qualité des soins : nous avons ainsi voulu montrer qu'au-delà de la logique actuelle qui en fait une exigence économique (mise en rapport des résultats et des coûts de l'activité médicale), l'évaluation de la qualité des soins est avant tout une exigence des médecins qui sont, après les patients, les premiers intéressés à s'assurer qu'ils obtiennent les meilleurs résultats possibles.

Enfin, parce que l'évaluation de la qualité des soins est d'abord une exigence médicale, parce que les évaluations centrées sur une technique diagnostique ou thérapeutique ou sur une pathologie donnée sont les plus faciles et les plus gratifiantes, et enfin parce que les études les plus riches d'enseignements sont celles auxquelles collaborent plusieurs services de même spécialité, les Sociétés Scientifiques ont un rôle essentiel à jouer dans la conception, la réalisation et la diffusion d'études d'évaluation de la qualité des soins.

REFERENCES

1 Donabedian A. The quality of medical care : methods for assessing and monitoring the quality of care for research and for quality assurance programs. Science 1978 ; 200 : 856-864.

2 Brook RH, Appel FA. Quality of care assessment : choosing a method for peer review. N Engl J Med. 1973 ; 288 : 1323-1329.

3 Goupy F, Hirel JC, Legrain M. DIAPHANE : National data bank for kidney dialysis. In : Anderson J, Forsythe JM. : MEDINFO 74, North HOLLAND, Amsterdam 1974 ; 341-345.

4 Goupy F, Hirel JC, Degoulet P, Legrain M. DIAPHANE : Une banque de données sur la dialyse itérative. Bilan de deux ans d'une étude coopérative réalisée à l'échelon national. Journées d'Informatique Médicale, Toulouse 1975. IRIA, Le Chesnay, Tome I ; 1975 ; 291-298.

5 Goupy F. Le système CHRONOS : réalisation d'un système de gestion de base de données médicales orienté vers le traitement des données évolutives. Thèse de Doctorat d'Etat en Biologie Humaine Paris VI ; 1978.

6 Société de Néphrologie : Commission informatique. Programme Dialyse Informatique-Résultats statistiques d'une étude coopérative comprenant 20 centres de dialyse itérative. J Urol Nephrol. 1974 ; 80 : 989-1047.

7 Degoulet P, Goupy F, Proulx J, Bloch P, Berger C, Aimé F. Société de Néphrologie-Commission informatique. Programme Dialyse Informatique II, Etude statistique évolutive. J Urol Néphrol. 1975 ; 81 : 873-920.

8 Degoulet P, Proulx, Aimé F, Berger C, Bloch P, Goupy F, Legrain M. Société de Néphrologie-Programme Dialyse Informatique III. Données épidémiologiques. Stratégies de dialyse et résultats biologiques. J Urol Nephrol 1976 ; 82 : 1001-1042.

9 Degoulet P, Reach I, Aimé F, Berger C, Goupy F, Jacobs C, Rojas P, Legrain M. Programme Dialyse Informatique IV : Rapport Cumulatif, Epidémiologie des complications. J Urol Nephrol. 1977 ; 83 : 925-983.

10 Degoulet P, Lauwers E, Aimé F, André JL, Bouissou F, Broyer M, Delons S, Gagnadoux MF, Kermanac'h C, Landthaler G, Loirat C. Programme Dialyse-Informatique V. L'hémodialyse chez l'enfant. J Urol Nephrol. 1978 ; 84 : 895-934.

11 Degoulet P, Reach I, Rozenbaum W, Aimé F, Devries C, Berger C, Rojas P, Jacobs C, Legrain M. Programme Dialyse Informatique-VI. Survie et facteurs de risque. J Urol Nephrol 1979 ; 85 : 915-962.

12 Degoulet P, Reach I, Aimé F, Rioux P, Jacobs C, Legrain M. Risk factors in chronic haemodialysis. Proc EDTA, London : Pittman. 1980 ; 17 :(in press).

13 Rojas P, Degoulet P, Jacobs C, Legrain M. Enquête sur la polynévrite urémique. J Urol Nephrolo. 1977 ; 83 : 985-997.

14 Masselot JP, Adhemar JP, Laederich J, Degoulet p, Kleinknecht D. Utilisation du système informatique DIAPHANE pour la surveillance des patients traités par hémodialyse à domicile. J Urol Nephrol. 1979 ; 85 : 963-969.

15 Fessel WJ, Van Brunt EE. Assessing quality of care from the medical record. N Engl J Med. 1972 ; 286 : 134-138.

16 Relman AS, Rennie D. Treatment of end-stage renal disease. N Engl J Med. 1980 ; 303 : 996-998.

17 de Kervasdoué J. Les politiques de santé sont-elles adaptées à la pratique de la médecine. Soc du Travail. 1979 ; 3 : 250-273.

18 Fineberg HV, Hiatt HH. Evaluation of Medical Practices : the case for technolgy assessment. N Engl J Med. 1979 ; 301 : 1086-1091.

19 Rutstein DD et al. Measuring the quality of medical care : a clinical method. N Engl J Med. 1976 ; 294 : 582-588.

20 Lacronique JF. L'évaluation de la qualité des soins aux Etats-Unis. Cahiers Medicaux 1978 ; 3 : 1972-1977.

STATISTICAL SOFTWARE FOR EPIDEMIOLOGICAL STUDIES

Malte SUND, Allmut HÖRMANN, and Walter LEHMACHER
Society for Radiation and Environmental Research (GSF)

Institute for Medical Informatics and
Health Services Research (MEDIS)

München, Federal Republic of Germany

SUMMARY

The paper starts with emphasizing that most epidemiological quantitative methods are specialized applications of more general statistical concepts. For this reason the discussion of epidemiological software needs is first presented within the framework of the area of Statistical Computing. Basic statistical software functions are identified to form a basis for software evaluation. Sources of information about existing software are presented. Actual software suggestions follow, concentrating on general purpose packages, a numerical library, and some special application programs. These suggestions are discussed in more depth on the basis of data description and data analysis techniques specific to epidemiological research, pointing in particular to problem areas. The paper proceeds by discussing software requirements for the somewhat neglected topic of data handling and data manipulation.

EPIDEMIOLOGICAL QUANTITATIVE METHODS WITHIN THE GENERAL FRAMEWORK OF APPLIED STATISTICS

In order to be able to end up with software suggestions it is helpful to consider the relationship between quantitative methods in epidemiologic research and those used in other areas of applied statistics. Epidemiology is certainly an independent science as we may infer for instance, from the World Health Organization's definition, which calls for the study of 'factors determining frequency and distribution of disease in human populations'. The topics of its research are, however, very heterogeneous, and overlap with many other areas to the point where they become indistinguishable from other fields of research. Accordingly, epidemiological research uses methods from many other disciplines.

For example, the knowledge about the nature of measurement processes, especially the measurement of qualities which cannot be observed directly, are taken from the field of psychology and its discipline psychometrics. This is especially true for the concept of measurement error, the concepts of validity and reliability of measurements, and the principles for the development of measuring instruments, like questionnaires, and their scaling. Many methods for the presentation and the analysis of frequencies as in crosstabulations, the use of indices such as the cost of living index, and the methods of sample surveys have been taken from sociology and its discipline sociometrics. From the field of economics and its econometric methods for the analysis of time series and the identification of trends are used. From biology and biometrics, more exactly from agricultural research, methods for the design and analysis of controlled experiments have been introduced, which in medical statistics form the complex of clinical trials. The list could be extended. In epidemiology these methods are often referred to by a different name which describes a particular application as in the example of the 'clinical trial'. We methodologists, however, when acting as consulting statisticians, often are forced to look for the statistical and mathematical principal behind this name as to be able to utilize more general knowledge about these matters. This is even more true when we examine software aspects of these procedures.

For example, epidemiologists connect the concept of prevalence with the proportion of people from a population who suffer from a certain illness. The consulting statistician should then immediately think of general results about the properties of proportions (see for instance Fleiss 1973). When looking for suitable software he should then bear in mind properties of his computer and of the programming language used for deviding two numbers. This is an extremely simple example, but hints at all elements comprising the area of Statistical Computing we are working in (see Kennedy, Gentle 1980). Only from this point of view we are able to suggest for epidemiologists high quality software.

EPIDEMIOLOGICAL SOFTWARE REQUIREMENTS WITHIN THE FRAMEWORK OF STATISTICAL COMPUTING

All over the world there exist innumerable programs, program libraries, program systems for statistical calculations in all application areas, for all computer types, and written in all programming languages, which cost little or nothing and are easily available. A letter is often enough to receive a card deck! This flood of programs is highly redundant, however. Programs are being rewritten over and over again just because the output of an older program is considered to be poor; for a new method such as an asymptotic variance of an odds ratio a new program is immediately presented; if features of different programs should be made available to the user via an unified control language a new program package is developed.

Sadly enough it is often the case that other functions than those for which the program is written receive more attention and care. The output may now be beautifully compiled but the calculated numbers are of dubious quality; the variance might be accurately calculated, but the accompanying crosstabulation is illegible; the package may be easy to use, but permits no user extensions: all of which motivates someone else to write a new program whose code is constructed with so much 'artistry' that it is totally incomprehensible to the person who has to convert it to a different computer installation.

These few examples should make clear that when selecting an existing software product, many different areas must be evaluated, none of which taken by itself is of much value to the user. Some of theses areas are for example the communication between program and user, i.e. the reading and interpretation of control language by the program and the reaction of the program in form of messages and program steps (program control). An important area especially in statistics is the reading and storing of data and its preparation for calculations e.g. by selection of cases and variables, by transformation of variables and treatment of missing values (data manipulation). Actual calculations are especially critical (numerics). We already mentioned the output, i.e. the printing and plotting of results (presentation of results). Beside these tasks, which the program itself should perform other, items must be considered such as programming, program correction, portability and last not least documentation without which the other capabilities mentioned above exist only abstractly, so to speak. These areas generally require so diverse capabilities that one person alone cannot be proficient in all of them, at least not when one considers the required and readily achieved standards of today. Statistical software will, therefore, be the better, the more expert knowledge is exploited in all of the areas. In our opinion this is realized best when the software product is rigorously structured according to the above mentioned areas program control, data manipulation, numerics, and presentation of results. The numerical expert should program only the numeric algorithms and should not have to develop data concepts or even be concerned with the design of output (Victor, Sund 1977; Victor, Hörmann, Sund 1978). It is for these reasons that the great majority of existing programs is to be considered bad programs.

Luckily, however, some program collections, program packages, and program systems have evolved out of the vast pool of offered programs which although still far from being perfect, are in fact valuable tools. This process was enhanced by a number of factors. The most important factor certainly is that the awareness for the problems of statistical computing has increased enormously within the last ten years. This is true for all parties concerned like program suppliers as well as users and professional organisations.

For many years now the American Statistical Association (ASA) has a section on statistical computing which organizes annual meetings. There is a conference called 'Computer Science and Statistics: Symposium on the Interface' organized on behalf of the International Statistical Institute. In Europe the COMPSTAT symposia are attracting big audiences. Especially at COMPSTAT, which by the way will be held next year here in Toulouse, European users can gather invaluable information about statistical software, and program suppliers can inform themselves about user wishes and critique. ASA has formed a committee on evaluation of program packages some years ago, which prepared a very valuable suggestion for the evaluation of statistical software (Francis, Heiberger, Velleman 1974). In the meantime many such evaluations have been made and have generally been presented at these conferences. Therefore the proceedings of these three conferences are of special interest to those who seek information about statistical software (the latest proceedings of the 'Section', of the 'Interface', and of COMPSTAT are included in the references, see American Statistical Association 1980, Gentleman 1980, Barritt, Wishart 1980). The book 'A Comparative Review of Statistical Software' is a veritable gold mine. It was published on the occasion of the founding of the International Association for Statistical Computing (Francis 1979). In the Federal Republic of Germany the 'Gesellschaft für Medizinische Dokumentation, Informatik und Statistik' (GMDS) has concerned itself with these problems. In a subsection of GMDS a detailed list of requirements for modern statistical software was developed which has been discussed with various package producers (Hultsch, Jannasch, Krier, Sund, Victor 1978). For a thorough discussion of sort of a state of the art package you might want to look at Muller (1980).

In addition to this situation of being constantly evaluated some program producers experience a necessity for commercial success. Most of these producers always have been non-commercial, including universities whose public funding agencies are beginning to force upon them at least partial cost coverage in the last years such as the British Government upon NAG or the American National Institutes of Health upon BMDP.

Until now the user can profit quite a bit from this competitive situation, especially from general purpose program packages which have been developed in many years and by the investment of large manpower to cover a wide range of statistical methods. Terms such as 'Social Sciences' or 'Biomedical' in their titles remain purely historical references. Six systems have evolved as the leading general purpose packages: BMDP, GENSTAT, OSIRIS, PSTAT, SAS, and SPSS at least when one uses COMPSTAT meetings and other indicators as measures. According to a recent study (Failing 1981) medical statistics institutes in the Federal Republic of Germany use virtually only two systems, namely BMDP and SPSS. OSIRIS and PSTAT are not so well known here and offer no significant advantages over BMDP or SPSS.

Even a short description of the remaining four packages is impossible in the limited space of this paper (the FORTRAN-packages are of the order of 100 000 statements each). We would rather like to refer the reader to the comparative overview of Francis (1980). A short characterization, however, might be attempted as follows. SPSS (Statistical Package for the Social Sciences) is the oldest of the four and has become popular mainly because of its easily learned control language and its data handling capabilities (Nie, Hull, Jenkins, Steinbrenner, Bent 1975). BMDP (Biomedical Computer Programs, P-Series) has an even more comfortable control language and provides the by far widest range of statistical methods (Dixon, Brown 1979). SAS (Statistical Analysis System) is the most modern system. It is also very well suited to be used as a monitor for controlling extraneous modules (other packages and user programs) but it is only available on IBM hardware (SAS Institute 1979). GENSTAT is similarly modern while not so machine oriented as SAS. It might be called a statistical compiler but it is not easy to use, not even by the sophisticated statistician, because of its hard to understand documentation (Rothamsted Experimental Station 1977).

As a basis for a statistical program library for the epidemiologic researcher we would suggest the BMDP system for its superior range and quality of analysis methods. For IBM customers we additionally recommend SAS (BMDP can be called by SAS without having to leave SAS). Non-IBM customers might try GENSTAT in addition to BMDP and possibly use SIR as some sort of a SAS substitute (see below). Contact addresses and prices are given in a table at the end of this paper.

Generally additional software is needed, for example to fill gaps not supported by the packages, as replacement for poorly designed program sections, and for special applications. The most important instrument for supplementary user programming is a good numerical subprogram library. In this area the only choice, very strictly speaking, is the NAG library (Numerical Algorithms Group). It is at the present time the only numerical library, whose algorithms are collected from and programmed by experts in each field of numerics, which has been exhaustively tested and evaluated by other experts, and which by still others has been converted to different computers using the most demanding data sets. Its documentation is the best we have seen so far and employs a very efficient method of guiding the user to find 'his' algorithm (NAG Central Office 1980). NAG is, however, again a general purpose library which fact results in some numerical procedures to be missing. For filling in, it is suggested to refer to IMSL (International Mathematical and Statistical Libraries 1977)' or to use the published algorithms of the ACM (Association for Computing Machinery 1980).

A great variety of special purpose packages also exist (compare Francis 1979). These include for instance packages which cover special statistical areas as CLUSTAN (Wishart 1970) which is offering a quite exhaustive list of clustering techniques.

SOFTWARE REQUIREMENTS RESULTING FROM SPECIFIC EPIDEMIOLOGICAL ANALYTIC METHODS

So far we have stressed the aspect that many quantitative methods of epidemiology are specialized applications of general statistical procedures and, therefore, are in most cases preferrably dealt with using standard software packages. We would now like to go into requirements necessitated by specialized epidemiological methods.

The basic objective of epidemiologic research is a detailed description of the percentum occurrance of illnesses or the averages of certain medical or socioeconomic parameters (e.g. blood pressure or income) stratified according to certain population subgroups. That is to say that tables are required which for qualitative data list frequencies and percentages and for quantitative data present averages and variances, both of which are subdivided into groups. Since the occurrance of an illness often is dependent upon a complex multifactorial exposition, epidemiologic research needs efficient tabulation or survey programs which permit the ad lib stratification of data with respect to a multitude of factors like age, sex, housing, and diet. This is as desirable for the explorative steps at the beginning of an investigation of the data as it is for the production of camera ready tables for the final report.

The statistical aspect of this problem is trivial as is the implementation of its calculations. Basically all program packages provide solutions to this problem, but all of them leave certain things to be desired in terms of simplicity of command language (i.e. simple use and readability which can be achieved by syntax and symbols resembling a natural language, consistent semantics, concise specifications, or convenient programming features) or tabulating power (i.e. flexibility of arrangement, placing of subgroups on a page, labeling ability, and visual impact). According to a paper of Francis, Sherman and Heiberger (1976) the second point which is so important for information transfer, is adequately supported by only three of the examined packages (GENSTAT, RGSP, TPL). When taking into account the differences in command languages the only recommendable special package is TPL (Tabulating Programming Language) which is, however, supported on IBM machines only (Mendelssohn 1975). For further details we refer the reader to the original paper cited above. We should repeat, however, that no general suggestions can be given for the user, but that it rather depends upon the special requirements which standard program is adequate or which special program needs to be considered. It would certainly be necessary that producers of standard program packages such as BMDP, SPSS, and SAS include in their products these important requirements for a good survey program. Since all numeric information is contained in the existing program it would only be necessary that the output be improved in terms of readability and flexibility; i.e. an output editor (see Hultsch et al 1978) should be added which combines the productivity of the special software with the simple command language of a standard program package.

Aside from purely descriptive methods for observed data epidemiology uses analytical techniques from inferential statistics, mainly methods of analyzing categorical data (see Fleiss 1973). The capital objective of epidemiological research is the determination of the (correlative) relationship of an illness with one or more exposition factors. The description and analysis of these associations is done using 2x2 contingency tables with the help of suitable measures like for example cross product ratio and the Phi-coefficient. The source of most illnesses however is multifactorial. To analyze the complex exposition structure which may contain unknown confounding effects there are generally two methods for the control of extraneous factors: stratified analysis and multivariate statistical modelling.

Stratification (see Fleiss 1973) is done by forming subgroups, calculating the interesting ratios from each group and combining these by using Cochran, Mantel-Haenszel or similiar techniques to form a conclusion about the relationship between illness and exposition which is valid for all strata. Standard software can be used to calculate the single subgroup results, but the combination of these to a summary test statistic must be done by special programs. The most important multivariate techniques of statistical modelling are, on the other hand, available in standard packages. The analysis of the log-linear model is solved by BMDP in an outstanding fashion (since the ECTA program of the originators of this method was adopted very early). BMDP similarly contains programs for logit analysis (binary logistic regression) according to Cox. Aside from this, many analytical techniques can be realized indirectly by reducing them to their mathematical and statistical essentials and reprogramming them using programs designed for other methods. As an example we would like to mention the configuration frequency analysis (CFA) according to Krauth and Lienert (1973) which can be considered as special residual analysis of the log-linear model and therefore be calculated to a large degree using BMDP (see Lehmacher 1980, 1981). There are, however, a series of methods, which necessitate the use of additional special packages, as for example the Grizzle-Starmer-Koch procedures which allow a general linear analysis of the original or transformed contingency table. These examples may suffice to demonstrate the general situation of these multivariate procedures. None of the standard packages has integrated the multitude of currently available methods, the newest standard being represented by BMDP. It is necessary for the user either to stick to methods directly or indirectly integrated in the packages or to get special software from the developers of new statistical software or methods, where generally, however, the portability, numerical quality, and documentation do not correspond to professional standards.

SOFTWARE REQUIREMENTS RESULTING FROM DATA HANDLING NEEDS

So far we have discussed software requirements for epidemiological studies from the analysis point of view but we have not yet touched the very important data handling phase. Preparation of data for analysis is very often quite a demanding task and can even become the crucial point. Once again we can identify different phases like data collection, data input and structuring, data checking and correction, data retrieval and manipulation, each of which, for a given problem, can be of different complexity, can require different activities and, therefore, place different workload on software.

The analysis steps have developed into packaged tours through a program, i. e. into activating many computational steps by means of just one very simple command (STATISTICS ALL in SPSS is perhaps the most famous example). The trade-off is, of course, a certain loss of flexibility. Data handling has been tried to deal with in quite the same manner in order to keep this part of the control language as simple as that of the analysis part. But it seems that this is nearly impossible to do. Data handling requires much more control by the user than the analysis. That is why in packages the data handling part of the control language is the one that is more difficult to become sophisticated in, but it is usually still too simple to allow for more complex data situations. For many data problems, therefore, the user has to resort to additional tools like supplementary programming in a higher level language, for transposing data matrices, for instance; to excessive use of the file editor, e. g. for converting characters to numbers; to operation system commands for concatenating, sorting, merging files etc.; or he even has to learn a second package's data manipulation language, if he has to use this package for additional analyses. By using any combination of these tools one is, of course, very flexible for meeting the demands of most data problems and proceeding in this manner is exactly what is being done in routine work.

But this way of dealing with the problem can have serious drawbacks. It can require greater skills and experience in reliably exploiting the possibilities of these tools, than are available. To rely on these tools can mean that it takes too long until the data are ready to go into the analysis stage. Also, the whole problem can become rather messy if too many data files are derived for analysis from the same master file, thereby loosing track of the exact contents of the files. Therefore, many people advocate the use of a data base system. These systems have been constructed for the sole purpose of offering a unified treatment of handling data, at the same time creating the problem of how to interface them with the packages. The big data base systems, most of which have been developed for commercial applications, do not, however, seem to be what one really needs. Because they are meant for all conceivable data situations they are too big and too complicated in the great majority of applications in epidemiological research.

Perhaps for this reason a few data management systems have envolved which try to combine features of packages, like simplicity of language, with capabilities of data base systems like more complex data models. At the time being the most recommendable one of these systems, SIR (Robinson 1980), is especially designed for the researcher's needs in health science to manage very easily and comfortably both simple and complex data sets of any size. For example, by its comfortable handling of dates and times as separate data types, by its complex retrieval facilities aiding in the problem of selecting matched pairs, by incorporating data security aspects even on item or record level, SIR meets the data manipulation needs of epidemiological research. Due to its easy-to-learn, SPSS-like and therefore well-known powerful control language SIR can be used by the researcher himself without expert help. Favouring an interface concept towards statistical packages - BMDP and SPSS files can be both read and written - and being available on a variety of machine types, SIR presents itself to be a central system for data management open to all of those statistical analysis systems which can process BMDP and/or SPSS files. So an integration of statistical methods distributed over different packages as well as the exchange of data sets written in SIR defined structures could be achieved. This type of data exchange was realized by the concept of uniform basic data sets (Murnaghan 1978). A system comparable to SIR with similar features proves to be SAS which accomplishes this integration principle, too, but, as mentioned before, is restricted to IBM machines.

TABLE OF ADDRESSES AND LICENSE FEES

(Prices given apply to degree granting institutions/non-profit and governmental/commercial organisations. Figures in parentheses are for the following years)

BMDP	BMDP Statistical Software Health Sciences Conputing Facility USA-Los Angeles, Ca. 90024	$ 500/1000/1500
GENSTAT	NAG Central Office 7 Banbury Road Oxford OX2 6NN United Kingdom	£ 300/500/500
NAG	NAG Central Office 7 Banbury Road Oxford OX2 6NN United Kingdom	£ 700/858/858
OSIRIS IV	OSIRIS Special Order RM 4250 Institute for Social Research P.O. Box 1248 USA-Ann Arbor, Mich. 48106	$ 1400/1600/2400
P-STAT	P-STAT Inc. P.O. Box 285 USA-Princeton, N.J. 08540	$ 1000/5000/5000
SAS	SAS Institute Inc. P.O. Box 10066 USA-Raleigh, N.C. 27605	$ 700/4500/4500
SIR	SIR Inc. P.O. Box 1404 USA-Evanston, Ill. 60204	$ 2000/3500/5000 ($ 1600/2800/4000)
SPSS	SPSS Inc. Suite 3300 444 North Michigan Ave. USA-Chicago, Ill. 60611	$ 1500/5000/7000 ($ 1000/3000/3500)

REFERENCES

American Statistical Association (Ed). 1979 Proceedings of the 139th Annual Meeting of the American Statistical Association, Statistical Computing Section. Washington:

American Statistical Association, 1980.
Association for Computing Machinery (Ed). Collected Algorithms from ACM. New York: Association for Computing Machinery, 1980.
Barritt MM, Wishart D (Eds). COMPSTAT 1980. Proceedings in Computational Statistics. 4th Symposium held at Edinburgh 1980. Wien: Physica, 1980.
Dixon WS, Brown MB (Eds). BMDP-79. Biomedical Computer Programs P-Series. Berkeley: University of California Press, 1979.
Failing K. Lücken im Methodenspektrum von Statistikpaketen. Statistical Software Newsletter 1981; 7: in press.
Fleiss JL. Statistical Methods for Rates and Proportions. New York: Wiley, 1973.
Francis I (Ed). A Comparative Review of Statistical Software: The International Association for Statistical Computing Exhibition of Statistical Program Packages. Proceedings of the 41st Session of the International Statistical Institute, 1979.
Francis I. A Taxonomy of Statistical Software. In: Barritt MM, Wishart D (Eds). COMPSTAT 1980. Proceedings in Computational Statistics. 4th Symposium Held at Edinburgh 1980. Wien: Physica, 1980.
Francis I, Heiberger RM, Velleman PF. Report and Proposal of the Committee on Evaluation of Program Packages to the Section on Statistical Computing. Washington: American Statistical Association, 1974.
Francis I, Sherman SP, Heiberger RM. A Look at Languages and Programs for Tabulating Data from Surveys. In: Hoaglin DC, Welsch RE (Eds). Proceedings of the Ninth Interface Symposium on Computer Science and Statistics. Boston: Prindle, Weber & Schmidt, 1976.
Gentleman JF (Ed). Proceedings of the Computer Science and Statistics: 12th Annual Symposium on the Interface. Waterloo: Department of Statistics, University of Waterloo, 1980.
Hultsch E, Jannasch H, Krier N, Sund M, Victor, N. Requirements for Program Systems Used for Statistical Data Analysis. Statistical Software Newsletter 1978; 4: 5-30.
International Mathematical and Statistical Libraries. IMSL, Computer Subroutine Libraries in Mathematics and Statistics. Edition 6. Houston: IMSL, 1977.
Kennedy WJ jr, Gentle JE. Statistical Computing. New York: Dekker, 1980.
Krauth J, Lienert GA. Die Konfigurationsfrequenzanalyse und ihre Anwendung in Psychologie und Medizin. Freiburg: Alber, 1973.
Lehmacher W. Die Konfigurationsfrequenzanalyse als explorative Methode. In: Victor N, Lehmacher W, van Eimeren W (Eds). Explorative Datenanalyse. Frühjahrstagung der GMDS, München, 1980. Heidelberg: Springer, 1980.
Lehmacher W. A More Powerful Simultaneous Test Procedure in Configural Frequency Analysis. To appear in: Biometrical Journal 1981; 23.
Mendelssohn RC. The Development of Table Producing Language. Washington: Bureau of Labor Statistics, 1975.
Muller ME. Aspects of Statistical Computing: What Packages for the 1980's Ought to Do. The American Statistician 1980; 34: 159-168.
Murnaghan JH. Uniform Basic Data Sets for Health Statistical Systems. International Journal of Epidemiology 1978; 7: 263-269.
NAG Central Office (Ed). NAG Library Manual - Mark 8. Oxford: Numerical Algorithms Group, 1980.
Nie NH, Hull CH, Jenkins JG, Steinbrenner K, Bent DH. SPSS. Statistical Package for the Social Sciences (2nd ed). New York: McGraw-Hill, 1975.
Robinson BN, Anderson GD, Cohen E, Gazdzik WF. Sir Users Manual. Evanston: SIR Inc., 1980.
Rothamsted Experimental Station (Ed). GENSTAT. A General Statistical Program. Rothamsted Experimental Station: The Statistics Department, 1977.
SAS Institute (Ed). SAS Users Guide. Raleigh: SAS Institute, 1979.
Victor N, Sund M. The Importance of Standardized Interfaces for Portable Statistical Software. In: Cowell W (Ed). Portability of Numerical Software. Proceedings of a Workshop at Oak Brooks. Berlin: Springer, 1977.
Victor N, Hörmann A, Sund M. Portabilität statistischer Software. In: Reichertz PL, Schwarz B (Ed). Informationssysteme in der medizinischen Versorgung. Ökologie der Systeme. Bericht über die 21. Jahrestagung der GMDS. Stuttgart: Schattauer, 1978.
Wishart D. CLUSTAN. User Manual (3rd ed). Edinburgh: Program Library Unit, Edinburgh University, 1978.

THE MANAGEMENT OF MULTINATIONAL CANCER CLINICAL TRIALS AT THE EORTC DATA CENTER

M. BUYSE, M. VAN GLABBEKE, M. STAQUET
EORTC DATA CENTER, INSTITUT JULES BORDET, BRUXELLES;
FACULTE DE MEDECINE ET LABORATOIRE DE STATISTIQUE MEDICALE,
UNIVERSITE LIBRE DE BRUXELLES

SUMMARY

After a brief introduction to the EORTC and its Data Center, this paper presents the methodology used to run cooperative clinical trials on cancer treatments. The computer system is broadly presented in terms of hardware, file organisation and software. Examples of results include comparisons of toxicities to treatment, survival experience by treatment group, search for prognostic factors. Finally, some possible future developments are discussed.

1. INTRODUCTION

1.1 THE EORTC

The European Organisation for Research on Treatment of Cancer (EORTC) was founded in 1962 to conduct, develop, coordinate and stimulate European research on the experimental and clinical bases of cancer treatments and related problems (1-2).

The clinical research is mainly carried out by cooperative groups of clinicians interested in a particular site of disease and/or treatment modalities. Over 300 European institutions participate in these groups which meet at least twice a year to discuss trials, protocols, treatments and results of their research.

The essential activity of a cooperative group is to conduct controlled clinical trials. Most of these trials are multicenter (i.e. patients are treated in different institutions) and also multinational. As of November 1980, approximately 80 clinical trials are currently active among the EORTC cooperative groups. Since 1971, over 8000 patients from all over Europe have been entered in EORTC trials as indicated in Table I.

TABLE I: PARTICIPATION IN EORTC TRIALS AS OF NOVEMBER 1980.

FRANCE:	2531	THE NETHERLANDS:	1436
BELGIUM:	1322	UNITED KINGDOM:	817
ITALY:	523	DENMARK:	412
SWITZERLAND:	396	GERMANY:	352
SPAIN:	195	NORWAY:	89
ALL OTHERS:	182		
TOTAL OF PATIENTS = 8255			

1.2 THE DATA CENTER

Due to the fast development of EORTC trials, it was soon felt that the data processing and statistical treatment could hardly be supported by the groups themselves; therefore the decision was taken in 1974 to create a central organ, which would provide statistical and data management services to all EORTC cooperative groups (4).

This "Data Center" is located at the Institut Jules Bordet (Bruxelles); its present staff is highly multidisciplinary as it consists of 2 physicians, 2 statisticians, 2 mathematicians, 2 engineers, 2 nurses, 2 biologists, 2 sociologists, 1 chemist and 4 medical secretaries.

The aim of the Data Center is to collect, centralise and analyse data from the various trials, and to standardize protocol writing, methods of data evaluation, and publication of results at a European level.

1.3 CLINICAL TRIALS IN CANCER RESEARCH

The purpose of this paper is not to discuss the rationale of clinical trials (5-9) nor to show their key role in the research of cancer treatment (10-16). It may however be useful to briefly describe the various types of clinical trials and their characteristics. The development of new drugs and cancer therapies is generally conducted in three steps:

(i) the biochemical bases of these therapies are studied, and hypotheses are confirmed by <u>in vitro</u> experiments;

(ii) the therapies are tested on <u>animals</u> to predict activity levels and toxicities, a step called "screening";

(iii) the clinical experimentation is then carried out on <u>humans</u>.

It goes without saying that this last step must be carried out with extreme caution in order to ensure both the respect of fundamental ethics for the patients treated as well as the scientific quality of the results observed. These requirements are best fulfilled in clinical trials.

The first experimentation on humans of a new therapeutic regimen is carried out with so-called <u>phase I</u> trials, the main purpose of which is to determine the maximum tolerable dose.

The activity of the new regimen is then tested through so-called <u>phase II</u> trials, in which one is essentially interested in determining the rate of response to the regimen as well as the types of tumour on which the regimen is active.

The very last step is then to compare the new regimen (supposing it is indeed active) to the best available therapy for a specific cancer. This is done through <u>phase III</u> trials, in which the emphasis is generally put on overall survival of the patients and duration of response to treatment.

2. METHODS

2.1 COMPUTER FORMS

With some modifications, the following basic forms are used by all groups:

(i) the registration form, which is filled out when a new patient enters a clinical trial and is thus assigned at random to one of the treatment groups defined by the protocol. From the computer viewpoint, the registration form is the root of an individual patient's record.

(ii) the on-study form, which contains the basic patient information, in particular the characteristics which are thought or known to be of prognostic value, such as previous history, staging of the disease, performance status, etc...

(iii) flow sheets and treatment forms, which are filled out regularly (for example, every two months) by the attending physicians to enable a close follow-up of patients in terms of tolerance to the treatment and evolution of the disease.

(iv) the summary form, which is normally filled out either at the end of the treatment period or upon progression of the disease or death of the patient.

All these forms are completed within each institution and are sent regularly to the Data Center, where they are checked for correctness by the data managers, and then keypunched on cards. The punched cards are read and verified by the computer and stored in the appropriate permanent file.

2.2 HARDWARE

The Data Center has access to the Computer facilities of the Université Libre de Bruxelles, consisting mainly of a C.D.C. CYBER 170/750 computer, twelve disk drivers (200 million character disks), six magnetic tape drivers, and a CALCOMP plotter. Access to these central facilities is possible through card readers/line printers in batch mode or through video screens and portable teletypes in interactive mode. In addition, the Data Center has recently acquired two ISC 8052 microcomputers with graphic colour screens, which can be used both on-line with the main computers (for large computations and data retrieval) or off-line (for visualisation of results : survival curves, etc...)

2.3 FILE ORGANISATION

The permanent files containing all information pertaining to the different protocols are simply sequential files in which patient records are ordered by institution and by registration date. The various items stored for each patient are described in a special library file called the "variable description file" which is nothing else than a dictionary of items specifying the name of the item, its physical location in the record, the limits allowed, etc. This system was originally developed by Dr. M.Zelen of the State University of New York at Buffalo and implemented in Brussels in 1976 where it has been adapted to EORTC requirements.

2.4 SOFTWARE

A full description of our software would be out of place in this paper. The computerized tasks take care of the creation, updating and periodic checking of a data file as well as the printing of administrative and statistical reports. It is worth mentioning that the system has been geared to interactive usage by non-computer experts, so that access to, for example, the statistical programmes does not require much computer expertise, nor any knowledge of programming. This has been made possible by extensively using the very flexible and powerful job control language (JCL) of CDC computers.

3. RESULTS

Some typical results, obtained with the help of the statistical software at our disposal (17-26) are now presented.

3.1. TOXICITIES

In phase II trials, where essentially new drugs (or analogs of existing drugs) are being tested, the toxicities reported give first hand information on the aggressivity of the new treatment, which may eventually lead to dosage adjustments. In these trials, hematologic disturbances are usually the most crucial toxicities and are therefore followed closely through laboratory data.

Of course non-hematological toxicities or side-effects (digestive, renal, pulmonary problems, etc.) are sometimes equally important in the overall picture of treatment effects. Even when they do not endanger the patient's life, these toxicities must be reported quite regularly as their impact on the patient's comfort (e.g. in the cases of nausea, diarrhea, etc.) or on the patient's psychological well-being (e.g. in the cases of alopecia, anorexia, etc.) may be considerable.

3.2 TREATMENT COMPARISONS

Besides toxicity comparisons, the most common end-points of a phase III trial are to quantify the benefit of one or several treatments in terms of response rates (in the case of advanced diseases), prolongation of disease-free interval (in the case of adjuvant therapies), or prolongation of survival (in all cases). The key tool for the statistical analysis of survival-type data is the comparison of "survival curves", which estimate the proportion of patients surviving as a function of time (17-18). Figure 1 drawn by a CALCOMP plotter, enables a quick visual comparison of two treatments of gastric cancer after surgical resection of the primary tumour. These curves are complemented by the corresponding statistical tests, which in this particular case, showed a clear benefit of treatment 2 over treatment 1 on overall survival of the patients.

The burning question here is "how many trials have actually shown big differences between two treatments"? Although quoting percentages would be somewhat premature for the EORTC (many trials still being in progress), it is fair to admit that the percentage of trials showing significant treatment differences is low - but this is largely due to the ethical constraints on treatment comparisons which are inherent to the design of Phase III trials!

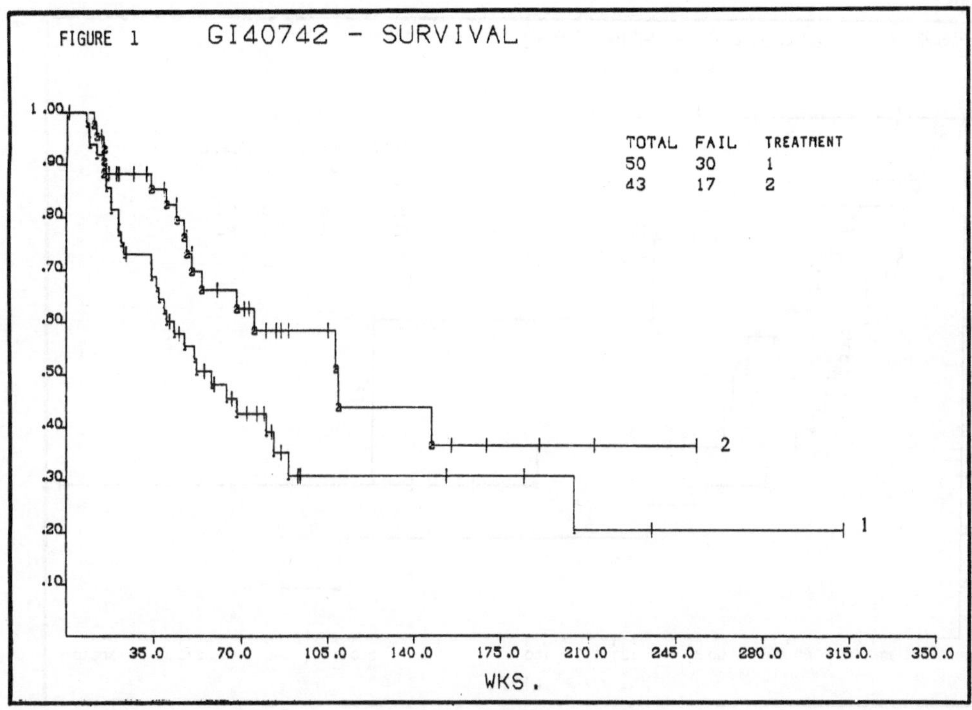

Naturally, treatment comparisons are not always as clear-cut as in this ideal example, so that other considerations must then be accounted for: the toxicities to treatment (see above), but also the possible influence of "prognostic factors" i.e. of variables which have a strong influence on the evolution of the disease. A recent example will clarify this point: in a study of stage III and IV non-Hodgkin's lymphomas, two induction chemotherapies were compared. One of the important prognostic factors was known to be the pathological classification of the tumour. While the overall comparison between the two treatments did not show any significant difference on survival, patients with a "high risk" pathological category clearly benefitted from the administration of the more aggressive chemotherapy, whereas the other chemotherapy appeared significantly better for the group of patients with a "low risk" pathology!

3.3 PROGNOSTIC FACTORS

It is thus essential to identify prognostic factors for a particular disease. This may be done by analysing contingency tables (if one is interested in responses to treatment) or by using the survival curve technique (if one is interested in durations); for example figure 2 shows that the survival experience of patients with gastric cancer heavily depended on the degree of penetration of the tumour in the gastric wall. One should thus adjust the treatment comparison made above to take account of the influence of this prognostic factor on the survivals in both treatment groups.

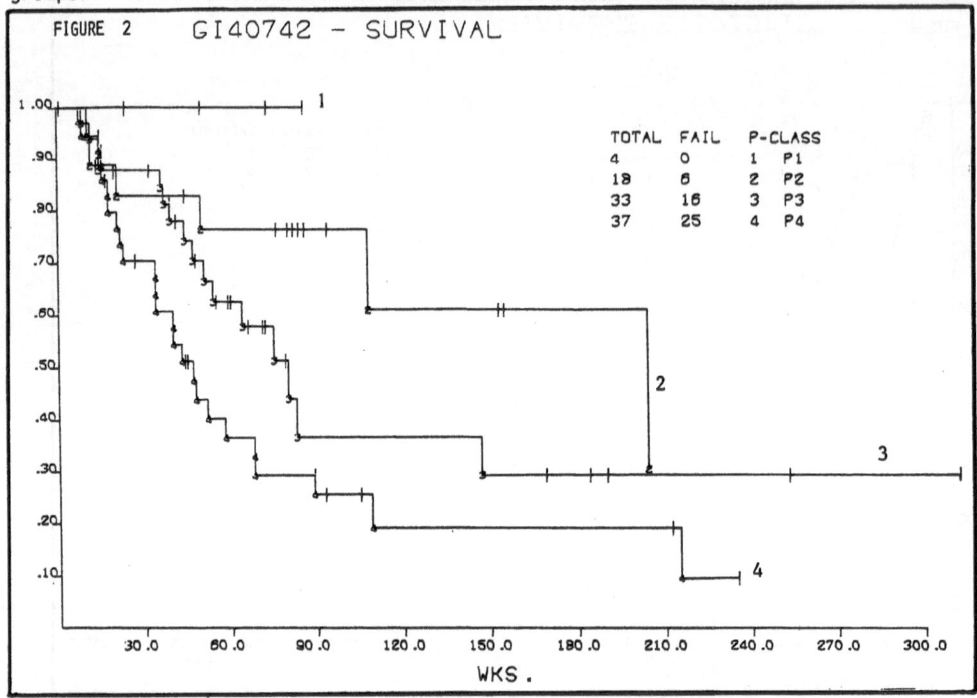

After identification of individual prognostic factors, multivariate models become necessary to select the most important ones: various regression models may be used to this effect (19-21)

4. DISCUSSION

There is little question about the usefulness of randomised trials in any kind of clinical research, in particular in the field of cancer treatment. Clinical trials have not only enabled the discovery of more effective treatment modalities in terms of remission rates or survival time, they have also shown quite clearly that in some cases standard treatments could be replaced by less toxic or less aggressive therapies, without any loss in efficacy. The EORTC Data Center's contribution to this slow but necessary progress in cancer treatment is apparent in over 50 annual publications made by EORTC groups in specialised journals or books.

That clinical trials gain from involving several institutions is a debated question, but apart from the obvious shortening of trial duration if several institutions participate, large multicenter trials always seem preferable to us to single center trials. There is in our experience considerable variation among institutions in almost all clinical trials. This variation inevitably throws a shadow on single center trials but also calls for careful attention in analysing the results of multicenter trials, no matter how large they are. Recently, in a study on the treatment of malignant gliomas,we showed that the survival time of patients was different in small institutions from that of patients in the larger institutions, which raised important questions about the selection of patients and the quality of their follow-up in the various institutions. It is quite unlikely that these problems would have been so easily revealed without the help of computers. More generally, it is fair to say that without some sort of computerized system, neither the data management nor the statistical analysis of large-scale clinical trials would even be possible.

The centralisation of data is not always well accepted by the individual investigators: to prevent problems of this nature, strict rules regarding the privacy of data and clear publication policies have been set up within the EORTC.

What future developments can one expect in the field of computerized clinical trials? First, the booming market of low-cost <u>microcomputers</u> will undoubtedly facilitate remote entry of data; institutions could put their own patient data on suitable storage devices (magnetic tapes, cassettes or diskettes) which would then be sent to the central Data Center. The second step would of course be a direct connection (e.g., via telephone line) between the Data Center and the remote institutions, both for the data entry and for file exploration by any physician. This development cannot be envisaged as yet, mainly because it would represent a very substantial investment, but recent developments of computer <u>networks</u> such as EURONET/DIANE give us confidence that it may become a reality in a not too distant future. Thirdly, there is an ever growing interest on the part of the medical body in the capabilities of computers. We therefore think that the access to and use of the computer must be made as simple as possible; this is why we strive to develop <u>user-orientated procedures</u> which can easily be understood and used by any non-expert. Lastly, the development of <u>sophisticated statistical softwares</u> - particularly for multivariate analyses (22-26) will make it possible to investigate in more depth the masses of information collected throughout clinical trials. This will hopefully enable the investigators to also address themselves to the more complex problems, such as the multiple biological effects of the treatments, the resulting toxicities, and eventually the effect of the various therapies on the quality of life of treated patients.

ACKNOWLEDGMENTS

This work is supported by Grant Number 5R10 CA11488-11 awarded by the National Cancer Institute, DHEW.

We would like to thank the following institutions and individuals for their software:

State University of New York at Buffalo (Dr. Zelen, now at Sidney Farber Cancer Center, Boston), M.D. Anderson Hospital and Tumour Institute (Drs.George and Gehan), University of Massachussetts (Dr. Hosmer), National Institutes of Health (Dr. Byar), Oxford University (Dr. Peto), Istituto di Biometria e Statistica Medica (Dr.Marubini), Westminster Medical School (Dr. Jones), Université de Liège (Drs. Albert and von Frenckell) and Université Libre de Bruxelles (Drs.Cantrenne and Coussaert).

REFERENCES

ON THE EORTC

1. TAGNON, H.J.: The EORTC - A European community project for the control of cancer. Biomedicine, 24: 18-19, 1976
2. SMITH, T.: The case for a European approach to cancer research. The Times, April 5, 1977
3. STAQUET, M.J.: Current Research of EORTC Cooperative Groups, Project Groups, Study Groups, Task Forces and Working Parties. Communication - January, 1980
4. STAQUET, M.J., SYLVESTER, R., MACHIN, D., et al: The EORTC Data Center. Europ.J.Cancer 13: 1455-1459, 1977

ON CLINICAL TRIALS

5. HILL, A.B.: The Clinical Trial. N.Engl.J.Med. 247: 113-119, 1952
6. SCHWARTZ, D.: L'essai thérapeutique chez l'homme. Flammarion, 1970
7. BYAR, D.P., SIMON, R.M., FRIEDEWALD, W.T., et al: Randomized Clinical Trials: Perspectives on some recent ideas. N.Engl.J.Med., 295: 74-80, 1976
8. PETO, R., PIKE, M.C., ARMITAGE, P., et al: Design and analysis of randomised clinical trials requiring prolonged observation of each patient: -
   I. Introduction and design. Br. J. Cancer 34: 582-612, 1976
   II. Analysis and examples. Br. J. Cancer 35: 1-39, 1977
9. STAQUET, M.J.: The Practice of Cooperative Clinical Trials. Europ.J.Cancer, 12, 241-243, 1976

ON CANCER CLINICAL TRIALS

10. CHALMERS, T.C., BLOCK, J.B., and LEE, S.: Controlled studies in clinical cancer research. N.Engl.J.Med., 287, 75-78, 1972
11. ARMITAGE, P., BLOCK, J.B., and SARACCI, R.: Report of the scientific meeting on some developments in the methodology of controlled clinical trials in cancer. Int. J. Cancer 14, 576-579, 1974
12. BRESLOW, N.: Perspective on the statistician's role in cooperative clinical research. Cancer 41, 326-332, 1978
13. MacLENNAN, R., CALUM, M., STEINETZ, R., et al: Cancer Registration and its techniques. IARC Scientific Publications No. 21, 1978
14. WHO Handbook for Reporting Results of Cancer Treatment. WHO Offset Publication No. 48, Geneva, 1979
15. TAGNON, H.J. and STAQUET, M.J.: Controversies in cancer: Design of Trials and Treatment. Masson Publishing, 1979
16. STAQUET, M.J.: Randomized Trials in Cancer, A Critical Review by Sites, Raven Press, New York, 1978

ON STATISTICAL SOFTWARE

17. PIKE, M.C., HOWARD, S.V., SMITH, P.G., et al: Survival Analysis Computer Program (Surv-C). DHSS Cancer Epidemiology & Clinical Trials Unit, Oxford, U.K., 1976
18. SMITH, T.L.: Explanation of coding for Survival or Remission Curves, University of Texas, M.D. Anderson Hospital and Tumour Institute, Houston, Texas, 1974
19. LEE, E.T.: A computer Program for linear logistic regression analysis. Computer Programs in biomedicine 4, 80-92, 1974
20. WANG, C.Y., HOSMER, D.V., LEMESLOW, D.: A users guide to MSLR: Multiple stepwise logistic regression. University of Massachussets, Amherst, Mass., 1977
21. LEE, E.T.: Program Documentation for Cox's regression model. University of Texas, M.D. Anderson Hospital and Tumour Institute, Houston, Texas, 1974
22. ALBERT, A.: Programme de dicrimination logistique pour 2 groupes. Université de Liège, Belgique, mai 1978
23. BAKER, R.J., NELDER, J.A.: The GLIM system release 3, generalised linear interactive modelling. Numerical Algorithm Group, Oxford, UK, 1978
24. DIXON, W.J., BROWN, M.B., et al: Biomedical Computer Programs P - Series, University of California Press, 1979
25. NIE, N.H., HULL, C.H., JENKINS, J.G., et al: Statistical Package for the Social Sciences, Second Edition, Mc Graw Hill Book Company, 1975
26. LEBART, L., MORINEAU, A., TABARD, N.: Techniques de la description statistique Méthodes et logiciels pour l'analyse des grands tableaux. Dunod, 1977

DEUX METHODES D'INDIVIDUALISATION DES POSOLOGIES, EXEMPLE DU LITHIUM

Anne GUILLAUME, Jean-Louis STEIMER, Alain MALLET,
Jean-François BOISVIEUX.
Inserm U.194, Département de Biomathématiques, 91 bd. de l'Hôpital
75634 PARIS Cedex 13.

SUMMARY

The determination of interindividual dosage regimen is not easy for drugs presenting toxicity risks and a large interpatient variability, such as lithium does. In that case two methods, using respectively the renal clearance and the 24-hour serum level as prognostic factor of the dosage requirement are proposed. Our purpose is to show how pharmacokinetics, statistics and numerical methods can be applied to compare these two prognostic factors.

INTRODUCTION

Le lithium, utilisé pour le traitement ambulatoire des malades amiaco-dépressifs, réunit deux propriétés qui rendent son emploi délicat. Tout d'abord, afin d'éviter les risques de toxicité, il est nécessaire que la concentration plasmatique en ion lithium ne dépasse pas 2.0 mmole/l, et pour garantir l'efficacité du traitement, qu'elle ne descende pas en dessous de 0.8 mmole/l(1). La marge thérapeutique est donc étroite et ces contraites sont d'autant plus importantes qu'il s'agit d'un traitement au long cours. Par ailleurs, des observations faites après administration d'une même dose à un échantillon d'individus montrent que la concentration plasmatique évolue de manière très différente d'un sujet à un autre. Cette grande variabilité interindividuelle, jointe à une marge thérapeutique étroite, fait qu'il est difficile d'utiliser une posologie standardisée pour traiter les malades. La procédure habituelle d'adaptation du traitement consiste à l'initialiser par des doses faibles, puis à augmenter celles-ci jusqu'à ce que la concentration plasmatique minimale(C_{min}) atteigne une valeur jugée acceptable (environ 1.0 mmole/l) ; C_{min} est facilement mesurable, par un prélèvement de sang effectué juste avant la première prise de lithium de la journée. Cette méthode assure un traitement efficace, mais les risques de toxicité ne sont pas complètement exclus puisque la connaissance expérimentale de la concentration plasmatique maximale (C_{max}) nécessite un grand nombre de mesures. Un autre inconvénient de cette méthode est la durée de la période d'adaptation, qui peut être longue puisqu'il faut attendre après chaque changement de posologie qu'un équilibre s'installe.

Aussi recherche-t-on des grandeurs facilement et rapidement mesurables qui permettent de fixer d'emblée la dose correcte pour chaque patient. Dans le cas du lithium, deux critères sont utilisés . C_{24}, concentration mesurée vingt-quatre heures après administration d'une dose fixe de carbonate de lithium, et u, la clairance rénale du lithium qui se détermine à partir de prélèvements sanguins et d'un recueil urinaire effectués dans les vingt-quatre heures suivant l'administration d'une dose fixe. Des simulations sur ordinateur utilisant des méthodes de modélisation et des données statistiques (2), nous ont permis d'évaluer l'intérêt prédictif de ces grandeurs ainsi que leurs rapports avec C_{min} et C_{max}. Ces résultats sont présentés dans la dernière partie. Les deux premières parties présentent respectivement le modèle utilisé pour le lithium et quelques résultats préliminaires de simulation.

1 - MODELISATION DE LA PHARMACOCINETIQUE DU LITHIUM.

Le modèle utilisé est le modèle ouvert à deux compartiment avec absorption du premier ordre (3) (figure 1).

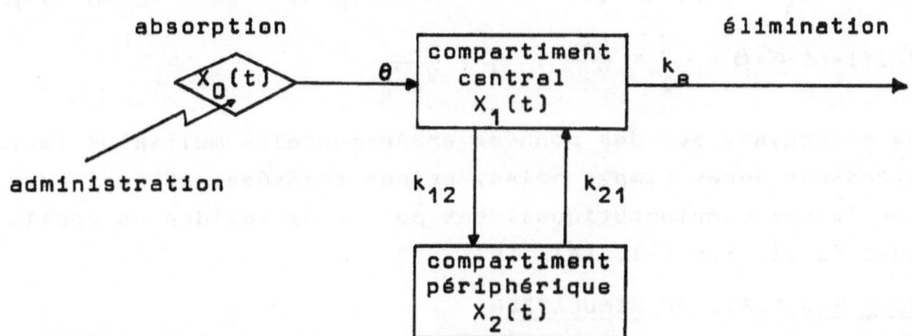

Figure 1 - $X_0(t)$, $X_1(t)$, $X_2(t)$, quantité de médicament à l'instant t respectivement, non libérée, dans le compartiment central, dans le compartiment périphérique. θ , k_e, k_{12}, k_{21}, constantes de vitesse respectivement d'absorption, d'élimination, de transfert entre les deux compartiments.

Le compartiment central figure le plasma et les organes qui s'équilibrent rapidement avec celui-ci. Le compartiment périphérique regroupe tout le reste de l'organisme. k_{12} et k_{21} schématisent les processus de transfert entre les compartiments, et k_e celui d'élimination. L'administration de lithium se faisant par voie orale, la cinétique d'entrée dans le plasma à partir du tractus digestif est traduite par une phase d'absorption de constante de vitesse. La formule très mathématique du modèle est alors le système d'équations différentielles suivant qui

traduit l'évolution des quantités de médicament dans les différents compartiments.

$$\frac{dX_0}{dt} = -\theta X_0$$

$$\frac{dX_1}{dt} = +\theta X_0 - (k_{12}+k_e)X_1 + k_{21}X_2$$

$$\frac{dX_2}{dt} = +k_{12}X_1 - k_{21}X_2$$

Pour la suite, des notations différentes seront utilisées, fondées sur le changement de paramètres suivant (2) :

$k_{12} = \frac{k}{V_1}$, $k_{21} = \frac{k}{V_2}$, $k_e = \frac{u}{V_1}$, où V_1 est le volume du compartiment central, V_2 celui du compartiment périphérique et u la clairance rénale.

Le modèle pharmacocinétique est défini par la donnée des cinq paramètres θ, k, u, V_1, V_2. La concentration à l'instant t dans le compartiment central après administration unique d'une dose D_o, C(t) est donnée par :

$$C(t) = \frac{X_1(t)}{V_1} = \frac{\theta D_o}{V_1} \left[\frac{(\frac{k}{V_2} - \alpha)}{(\alpha-\beta)\ (\alpha-\theta)} e^{-\alpha t} + \frac{(\frac{k}{V_2} - \beta)}{(\beta-\alpha)\ (\beta-\theta)} e^{-\beta t} + \frac{(\frac{k}{V_2} - \theta)}{(\theta-\alpha)\ (\theta-\beta)} e^{-\theta t} \right]$$

α et β vérifiant $\alpha+\beta = \frac{k}{V_2} + \frac{k+u}{V_1}$; $\alpha\beta = \frac{uk}{V_1 V_2}$

Des études s'appuyant sur des données expérimentales multiples (mesures de concentrations après simple prise, prises répétées, et ceci pour différentes formes pharmaceutiques) ont permis de valider ce modèle de la cinétique du lithium (2), (4), (5).

2 - QUELQUES RESULTATS DE SIMULATION.

Nous avons vu dans le paragraphe précédent que la concentration plasmatique dépend des cinq paramètres θ, k, u, V_1, V_2. La figure 2 donne plusieurs courbes de concentration obtenues par simulation du modèle. Elles correspondent à l'administration d'une même dose pour différentes valeurs possibles des paramètres.

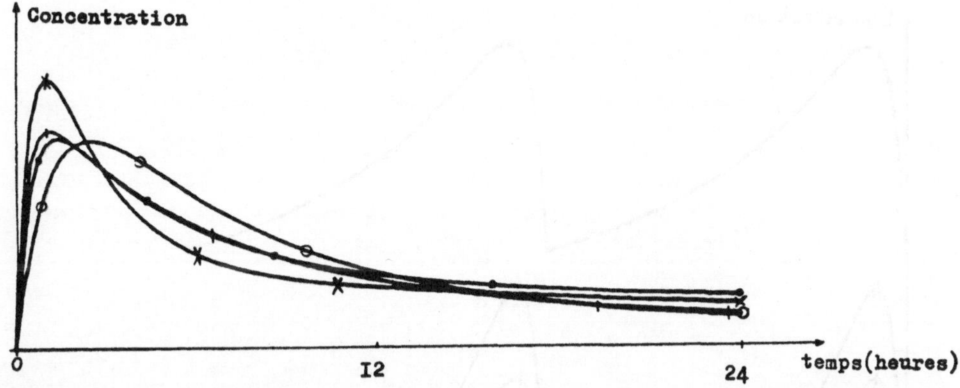

Figure 2 - Evolution de la concentration plasmatique au cours du temps après administration orale unique, pour différentes valeurs de paramètres pharmacocinétiques.

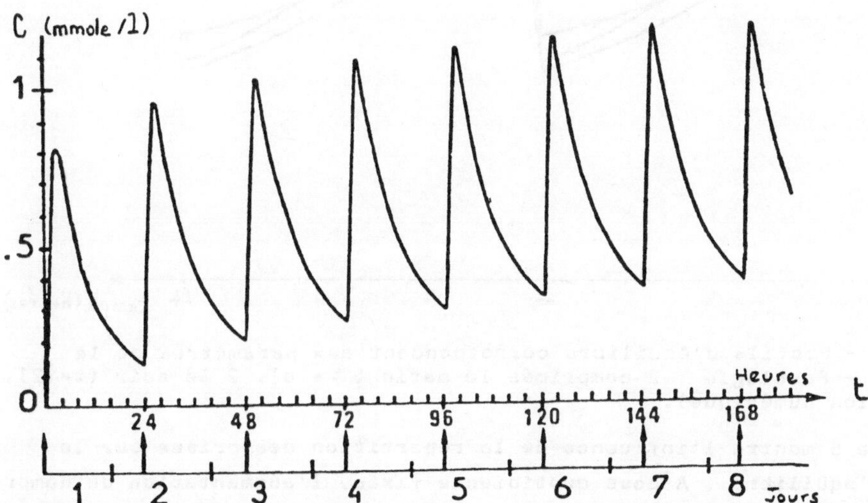

Figure 3 - Evolution temporelle de la concentration au début du traitement (simulation numérique)

La figure 3 montre que, lorsqu'un traitement chronique est instauré, le profil des concentrations évolue jusqu'à atteindre un état d'équilibre. Ce régime permanent est observé lorsque la quantité totale de médicament éliminée sur une journée, qui augmente en même temps que la concentration, compense exactement l'apport quotidien de médicament, le profil des concentrations est alors périodique. La figure 4 présente les profils d'équilibre correspondant aux paramètres de la figure 2. On notera que les deux courbes qui présentent les sommets les plus proches sur la figure 2 donnent des profils d'équilibre très différents.

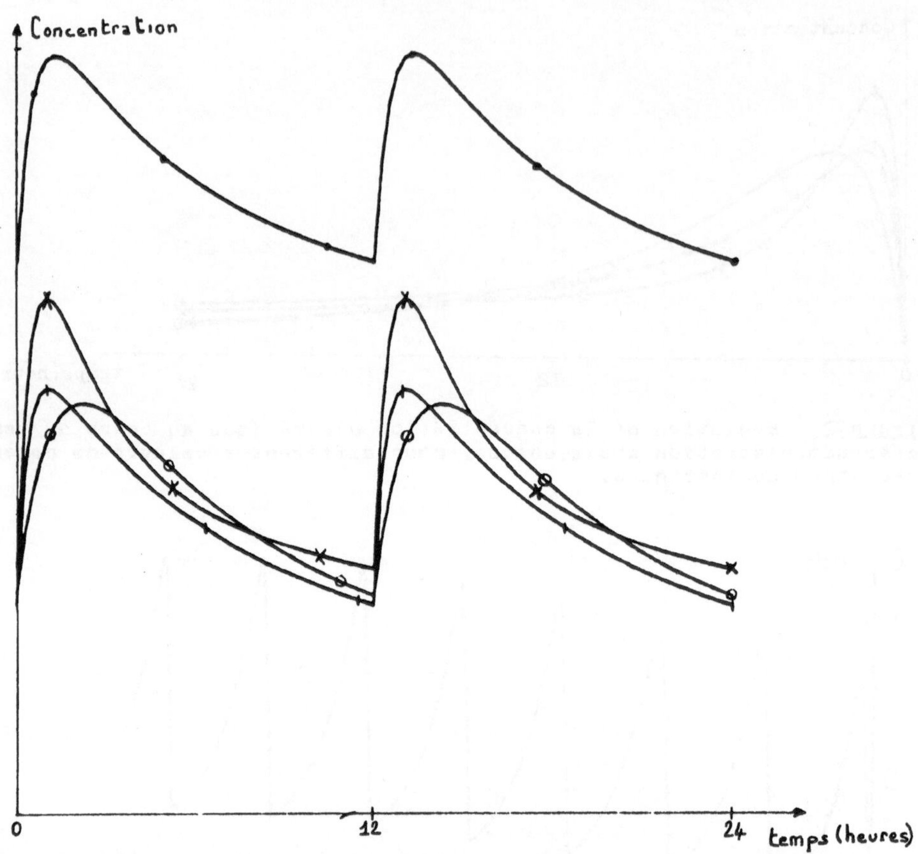

<u>Figure 4</u> - Profils d'équilibre correspondant aux paramètres de la figure 2 - Posologie : 2 comprimés le matin (t = o), 2 le soir (t=12). (simulation numérique).

La figure 5 montre l'influence de la répartition des prises sur le profil d'équilibre . A dose quotidienne fixée, l'augmentation du nombre de prises a pour effet de diminuer l'écart entre les concentrations maximale et minimale et donc de réduire le risque d'exursion en dehors de la marque thérapeutique.

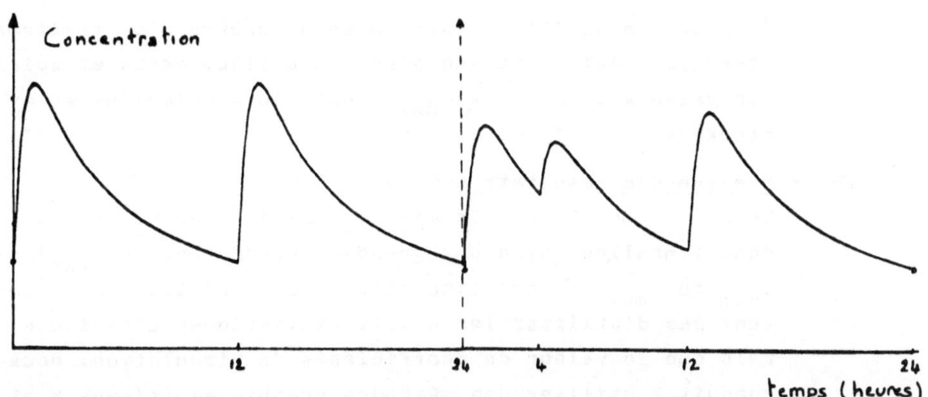

Figure 5 - Profils d'équilibre correspondant à l'administration d'une même dose Do, en deux prises (courbe de gauche) et en trois prises (courbe de droite).

3 - APPLICATION A LA COMPARAISON DE CARACTERES PREDICTIFS.

3.1 - Méthode utilisée.

La procédure de simulation utilisée comporte plusieurs étapes:

3.1.1. - Tirage au sort de 200 individus fictifs.

Un individu "fictif" est défini par le vecteur $\xi = (\;, V_1, V_2, k, u)$. La densité de probabilité de ce vecteur a été estimée sur la base d'un échantillon d'apprentissage (2) : il s'agit d'une loi multinormale dont la moyenne est le vecteur

$$\bar{\xi} = (1.85,\ 22,\ 37,\ 2.5,\ 1.26)$$

et la matrice de covariance est la suivante :

$$\begin{pmatrix} 1.59 & & & & \\ 0.82 & 32.7 & & & \\ -1.36 & 23.8 & 75.9 & & \\ 0.31 & 2.71 & -0.3 & 1.05 & \\ -0.07 & 0.91 & 0.88 & -0.11 & 0.12 \end{pmatrix}$$

Les méthodes de tirage aléatoire sur calculateur permettent de simuler un échantillon de 200 individus fictifs dont la distribution est identique à celle de la population.

3.1.2. - Simulation de la cinétique du lithium chez les 200 individus.

Pour chaque individu, sont obtenus par simulation :

a) le profil des concentrations sur 24 heures, après administration d'une dose fixe. C_{24} et d'autres grandeurs telles que la concentration maximale, sa date, etc, sont alors déterminées et stockées.

b) le profil d'équilibre après mise en oeuvre d'un traitement standard (administration d'une dose fixe, matin et soir). Les valeurs de C_{min} et C_{max}, sont alors calculées et stockées.

3.1.3. - Analyse des résultats obtenus.

Le but recherché est la mise en évidence de relations fonctionnelles entre une grandeur prédictive (u, C_{24}) et C_{min} ou C_{max}. La non linéarité de ces relations ne permettant pas d'utiliser les outils statistiques classiques tels que la valeur de coefficients de circulation, nous à conduit à utiliser des méthodes graphiques (figure 6 et suivante)

3.2 - Etude du caractère prédictif des différents paramètres.

La clairance rénale u conduit à des résultats concluants (figure 6)

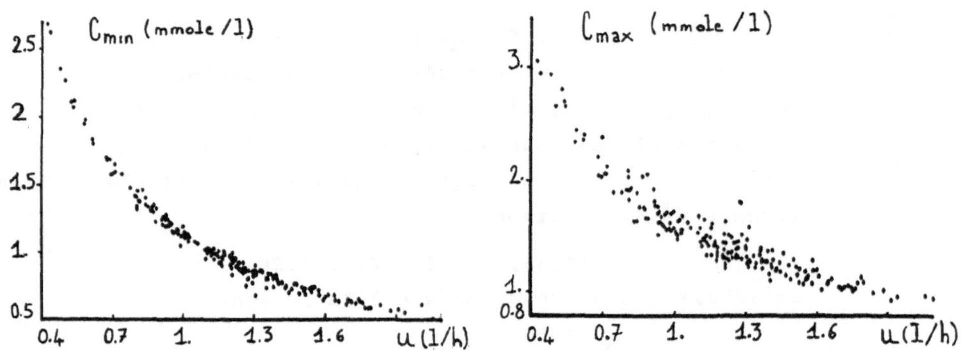

Figure 6 - Les concentrations minimales (C_{min}) et maximale (C_{max}) à l'état d'équilibre en fonction de la clairance rénale u.

La faible dispersion des points met nettement en évidence le caractère prédictif de u et permet d'établir une relation fonctionnelle de type hyperbolique entre u et respectivement C_{min} et C_{max}. Les même tracés pour (C_{min}, V_1), (C_{max}, V_1), (C_{min}, V_2), (C_{max}, V_2) montrent qu'aucune relation fonctionnelle n'est décelable entre C_{min}, C_{max} et les paramètres de volume. Ce résultat traduit le peu d'intérêt pratique des indicateurs morphologiques cliniques (poids, surface corporelle, ...), fait déjà souligné pour d'autres médicaments (7).

La dispersion plus importante des points dans la figure 7 montre que C_{24} est a priori moins prédictif que u. Cependant il faut souligner que dans ces simulations u et C_{24} sont des valeurs exactes. l'application de ces résultats en pratique courante nécessite donc l'évaluation des erreurs de mesure sur u et C_{24}. Le bruit de mesure, une fois quantifié, peut alors être introduit dans la simulation et permet d'obtenir une comparaison des caractères predictifs de u et C_{24} en pratique courante.

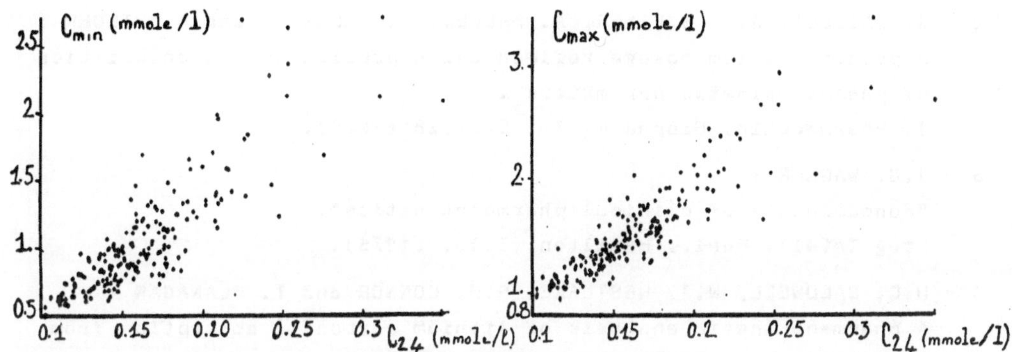

Figure 7 - Les concentrations minimales (C_{min}) et maximale (C_{max}) à l'état d'équilibre en fonction de la concentration C_{24} mesurée 24 heures après une prise unique de médicament.

Conclusion

L'analyse pharmacocinétique, la simulation numérique et l'analyse statistique constituent des outils d'aide à la décision précieux pour la définition de posologies individualisées dans le cadre de traitements au long cours. La mise en oeuvre combinée de ces techniques repose sur l'expérience clinique et une étude prospective préalable. La première conditionne la connaissance des seuils d'efficacité et de toxicité du médicament (3), (5), (6). La seconde aboutit à l'élaboration du modèle pharmacocinétique, à la mise au point de la simulation numérique et à la quantification de la variabilité interindividuelle. Le tirage aléatoire de patients conformément à la distribution statistique estimée des paramètres pharmacocinétiques de la population permet, sans expérimentation supplémentaire, d'évaluer de façon quantitative, les capacités prédictives de grandeurs mesurables en routine et partant, les performances potentielles des diverses stratégies d'individualisation des posologies.

REFERENCES

1 - P.E.E. BERGNER, K. BERNIKER, T.B. COOPER, J.R. GRADIJAN and G.M. SIMPSON :
Lithium kinetics in man : effet of variation in dosage pattern.
Br. J. Pharmacol. 49 : 328-339 (1973).

2 - J. GAILLOT, J.L. STEIMER, A. MALLET, J. THEBAULT and A. BIEDER :
A priori lithium dosage regimen using population characteristics of pharmacokinetic parameters .
J. Pharmacokin. Biopharm. 7 : 579-628 (1979).

3 - J.G. WAGNER :
"Fundamentals of clinical pharmacokinetics".
Drug Intell. Publ., Hamilton, Ill., (1975).

4 - H.C. CALDWELL, W.J. WESTLAKE, S.M. CONNOR and T. FLANAGAN :
A pharmacokinetic analysis of lithium carbonate absorption from several formulations in man.
J. Clin. Pharmacol., 11 : 349-356 (1971)

5 - A. AMDISEN :
Monitoring of lithium treatment through determination of lithium concentration.
Dan. Med. Bull. 22 : 277-291 (1975).

6 - T.B. COOPER, P.E.E. BERGNER and G.M. SIMPSON :
The 24-hour serum lithium level as a prognosticator of dosage requirements..
Am. J. Psychiat. 130 : 601-603 (1973).

7 - L.B. SHEINER, S. BEAL, B. ROSENBERG, V.V. MARATHE :
Fosecasting individual pharmacokinétics.
Clin. Pharm. Ther. vol. 26, n° 3, pp 294-305 (1979).

APPLICATION DU MODELE DE COX A L'ETABLISSEMENT D'UNE CLASSIFICATION PRONOSTIQUE DE LA DETERIORATION INTELLECTUELLE DANS LA MALADIE DE PARKINSON

Jean-Louis GOLMARD[1], Alain GUILLARD[2], Claude CHASTANG[1]

1 INSERM U 194 - Méthodologie Informatique et statistique en Médecine
91, bd de l'Hôpital, 75634 Paris cedex 13

2 Clinique de Neurologie, Hôpital de la Salpétrière
47, bd de l'Hôpital, 75651 Paris Cedex 13

L DOPA which reduces akinetic symtoms has also prolonged the survival time of Parkinson patients but as a consequence mental deterioration can be observed in some patients. Thus the aim of our study is to determine what parameters could allow a prognosis of Parkinson intellectual performances patients. For this purpose, 244 patients have been followed for periods ranging from 4 to 11 years after the beginning of the DOPA therapy. The statistical methodology involved both actuarial method and Cox's model for censored data. So far our main results can be summerized as follow : three classes of patients were determined :

i. a hight-risk group exhibiting transitory psychotic symtoms during the first year of DOPA therapy ;

ii. a low-risk group with only a tremor at the begining of the therapy or an age less than 60 years, and

iii. the remaining patients constitute the intermediary-risk group.

INTRODUCTION

L'apparition de la L DOPA en 1969 a considérablement modifié le devenir des Parkinsoniens : ce médicament a permis d'augmenter l'espérance de vie de ces malades, et surtout d'améliorer la qualité de cette survie. Mais, avec le recul du temps, il est acquis que l'amélioration substantielle apportée aux Parkinsoniens par la L DOPA ne se prolonge pas indéfiniment. Dans le plus grand nombre des cas traités on voit apparaître après quelques années des troubles divers, essentiellement des troubles moteurs, qui sont souvent différents de ceux observés au cours de l'évolution naturelle de la maladie, et, dans une proportion moins importante, des troubles psychiques, les uns aigus et transitoires, les autres insidieux et progressifs, conduisant à un tableau de démence plus ou moins prononcée.

Dans ce travail, nous nous sommes intéressés à ces troubles psychiatriques et nous avons essayé de préciser quels sujets traités par la L DOPA présentaient un haut risque de telles complications particulièrement graves. L'intérêt pratique de l'isolement d'un groupe de Parkinsoniens à haut risque psychiatrique est certain puisque sont apparus au cours de ces dernières années d'autres médicaments capables d'influencer heureusement, mais moins bien que la L DOPA, les troubles moteurs qui caractérisent cette maladie neurologique.

DONNEES

1. L'échantillon

Notre échantillon est constitué par tous nos patients atteints de la maladie de Parkinson dont le traitement par la L DOPA ou par l'association L DOPA inhibiteur de décarboxylase a été entrepris entre mai 1969 et mai 1976. 244 patients répondent à cette définition. L'état actuel de ces malades suivis par l'un d'entre nous a été apprécié au cours du deuxième trimestre 1980. Le recul d'observation pour les sujets encore vivants est donc de 4 ans au minimum, 11 ans au maximum.

2. Les variables

a. Les facteurs pronostiques potentiels

La majeure partie des facteurs de risque éventuels est constituée par des variables dont la valeur est connue dès l'instauration du traitement à la L DOPA : ces variables sont décrites au tableau I. Il nous a paru nécessaire d'y inclure deux variables dont la valeur n'est établie qu'après un an de traitement : le résultat global de la thérapeutique, apprécié cliniquement, et l'existence de troubles psychiques transitoires pendant la 1ère année de traitement (dépression, troubles psychotiques transitoires).

b. L'évolution de la maladie

Tous les faits évolutifs particuliers ont été consignés, mais les chapitres les plus importants sont :

- les troubles moteurs de modalités diverses,
- la détérioration intellectuelle,
- l'éventuel décès.

PREMIERE SELECTION DES VARIABLES PRONOSTIQUES

1. La méthode

La première étape de l'analyse est une étude des liaisons de chacune des variables retenues au départ (tableau I) avec la variable d'intérêt : temps d'apparition d'une détérioration intellectuelle (D.I.).

Comme tous les individus n'ont pas présenté effectivement une D.I. à la date à laquelle est réalisée l'étude, le principe de la méthode repose sur la méthode actuerielle (1) :

- chaque variable est divisée en 2 à 5 classes, soit de façon naturelle (sexe par exemple), soit arbitrairement par regroupement (âge) ;
- pour chaque groupe ainsi obtenu, une courbe dite "courbe actuarielle" est calculée. Sont considérés comme sujets "censurés" les individus :

- . décédés sans avoir présenté de D.I.
- . perdus de vue en cours d'étude,
- . sous surveillance au moment de l'étude, et n'ayant pas encore présenté de D.I.

- pour chacune des variables, le test de comparaison des courbes correspondant aux différents groupes est le test du LOG RANK (1).

2. Résultats

Au terme de cette analyse préliminaire, 9 variables ont été retenues, soit pour des raisons statistiques (tests significatifs), soit pour des considérations médicales. Ces 9 variables sont indiquées au tableau I.

SELECTION DES VARIABLES UTILISEES DANS LA CLASSIFICATION ET CLASSIFICATION

1. Principe

A ce stade de l'analyse, chacune des 9 variables retenues pourrait servir à établir une classification pronostique. Celle-ci pourrait être "améliorée" par la prise en compte simultanée de plusieurs variables, et le meilleur ajustement correspond à la prise en compte simultanée de l'ensemble des variables. Néanmois, une classification basée sur les 9 variables retenues n'est pas souhaitable, pour au moins 3 raisons :

- deux raisons pratiques : la procédure de classification d'un nouvel individu serait relativement complexe, et n'aurait pas une signification très claire pour le médecin,
- une raison théorique : si la classification est "trop ajustée" à l'échantillon, elle risque d'être peu généralisable à des échantillons provenant d'autres populations.

Le problème est donc de trouver un sous ensemble de variables qui réponde aux conditions suivantes :

- le nombre de variables doit être petit (de l'ordre de 2 à 4),
- l'ajustement obtenu avec ces variables doit être "presque aussi bon" que celui obtenu avec l'ensemble des variables,
- la procédure de classification proposée ne doit pas paraître absurde par rapport aux connaissances médicales.

Finalement, la procédure suivante a été adoptée :

a. utilisation d'un modèle mathématique permettant de prendre en compte simultanément l'ensemble des variables, de façon à obtenir un bon ajustement aux données.
b. classement des individus par risque croissant, et détermination arbitraire de 3 groupes, 1 groupe à faible risque, un groupe moyen, et 1 groupe à haut risque.
c. recherche des variables caractéristiques de chaque groupe.
d. établissement de la classification à l'aide des variables retenues.

2. Méthodes

a. le modèle mathématique utilisé est le modèle dit "à risques proportionnels", proposé par COX, en 1972 (2, 3).

Ce modèle repose sur les hypothèses suivantes :

- soient T le temps d'apparition d'un événement, Z un vecteur $(Z_1, \dots, Z_p)^T$ de p variables. La densité de probabilité de T s'écrit :

$$f(t ; t) = \lambda(t; z) \exp - \int_0^t \lambda(u ; Z)\, du$$

avec $\lambda(t ; z) = \lambda(t; 0) \exp\left(\sum_{j=1}^{p} \beta_j Z_j\right)$

où . $\lambda(t ; Z)$ est le risque instantanné de l'individu Z au temps t,

. $\lambda(t ; 0)$ correspond au risque instantanné au temps t d'un individu dont les variables Z_j, j = 1, ... , p, valent toute s zéro.

Le principal avantage de ce modèle, outre sa relative simplicité, est que $\lambda(t ; 0)$ n'est pas spécifié, ce qui permet d'obtenir un meilleur ajustement qu'avec un modèle complètement paramétrisé.

b. La recherche des variables caractéristiques de chaque groupe a été effectuée en examinant les distributions de chacune des variables selon les groupes sans utilisation de tests statistiques.

3. Résultats

Les 3 variables retenues pour établir la classification sont les suivantes :

1. forme clinique (forme tremblante pure ou non)
2. âge au début du traitement par L DOPA (âge inférieur à 60 ans, ou supérieur ou égal à 60 ans)
3. existence de troubles psychiques transitoires pendant la première année de traitement.

Finalement, la procédure de classification proposée est la suivante :

- le groupe à haut risque (groupe 3) est constitué par tous les individus ayant présenté des troubles psychiques transitoires pendant la première année de traitement. Les autres sujets se répartissent dans les groupes 1 et 2.
- le groupe à faible risque est constitué des sujets qui ont une forme tremblante pure ou qui sont âgés de moins de 60 ans au début du traitement.

Les courbes actuarielles des 3 groupes ainsi formés sont tracées figure 1.

VALIDATION DES RESULTATS (AJUSTEMENT)

Le terme de validation recouvre plusieurs problèmes. Pour "valider" la classification proposée, il est nécessaire de :

1. vérifier que les hypothèses du modèle de COX ne sont pas absurdes par rapport aux données,
2. étudier les ajustements obtenus à chaque étape de la procédure adoptée,
3. vérifier que la classification ainsi obtenue à partir d'un échantillon est généralisable à des individus provenant d'autres populations.

Nous ne pouvons pas, faute des données correspondantes , valider la classification au sens du 3. Nous reviendrons plus loin sur ce point.

Il n'existe actuellement aucun test rigoureux permettant de valider le modèle de COX au sens de 1. Les procédures les plus utilisées sont empiriques et graphiques : les individus sont regroupés en classes, et on vérifie en traçant les courbes de survie de chaque classe qu'elles ont à peu près la forme prévue par le modèle. Un exemple de telles courbes est présenté à la figure 1.

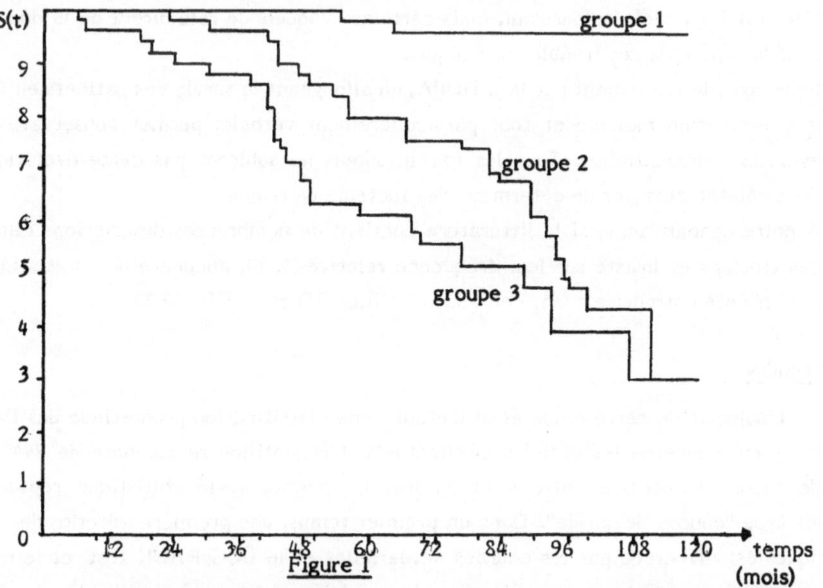

Figure 1

Les ajustements sont testés par le test du rapport de vraisemblance (8). TSIATIS (4) a démontré que les tests asymptotiques usuels restaient valides dans le cas de données censurées. Dans des conditions particulières, mais vérifiées en pratique, les résultats de ces tests sont présentés au tableau II. Ils confirment la validité de la classification proposée : les 3 variables retenues pour la classification ne diminuent pas significativement la vraisemblance de l'échantillon par rapport au modèle "complet" à 9 variables.

DISCUSSION

1. La division de l'échantillon en 3 groupes, effectuée après avoir rangé les individus en ordre de risque croissant,d'après les résultats obtenus par le modèle de COX, est

arbitraire. Ce fait poserait un problème si les distributions des variables dans chaque groupe étaient très différentes suivant les endroits où s'effectuent les séparations entre les groupes. Heureusement, l'analyse des ces distributions montrent que les résultats ne sont pas modifiés sensiblements par des décalages des endroits de séparations entre les groupes.

2. L'utilité pratique d'une telle classification est de bien classer des individus autres que ceux qui ont servi à l'établir. En l'absence des données nécessaires, nous n'avons pu valider la classification de ce point de vue. Les seuls arguments qui plaident en faveur de sa "robustesse" sont qu'elle repose sur peu de variables, ce qui diminue la probabilité d'avoir un échantillon biaisé par rapport à ces variables, et que la définition de celles-ci est simple : ce sont 3 variables binaires, faciles à coder pour le clinicien.

3. La détérioration intellectuelle des PARKINSONIENS a lontemps été un objet de controverse. Avant la période de la L DOPA, des grands auteurs niaient son existence. Ceci est impossible aujourd'hui, mais certains évoquent le rôle direct de la dopathérapie dans la génèse de ces troubles psychiques.

   Pour nous, le traitement par la L DOPA, en allongeant la survie des patients,en facilitant leur expression motrice et tout particulièrement verbale, permet l'observation de ces évolutions démentielles. Tous les Parkinsoniens ne subiront pas cette évolution, il est donc capital d'essayer de déterminer les facteurs de risque.

   A notre connaissance, si la littérature contient de nombreuses descriptions cliniques de ces troubles et insiste sur leur fréquence relative (5, 6), aucune étude statistique de ce type n'a été entreprise avant celle deA. GUILLARD et C. CHASTANG (7).

CONCLUSION

L'objectif de cette étude était d'établir une classification pronostique des Parkinsoniens en ce qui concerne les déficits intellectuels. L'échantillon se compose de 244 individus suivis de façon prospective entre 4 et 11 ans. La méthodologie statistique repose sur les méthodes type "courbe de survie". Dans un premier temps, une première selection des variables pronostiques est effectuée par les courbes actuarielles et le LOG RANK test, et le modèle de COX est utilisé pour achever la sélection des variables servant à établir la classification. Finalement, la classification suivante est proposée :

- groupe 3 (mauvais pronostic) : tous les sujets ayant présenté des troubles psychiques transitoires pendant la 1ère année du traitement. Le reste des individus se répartit dans les groupes 1 et2.
- groupe 1 : sujets de moins de 60 ans, à l'instauration du traitement, ou présentant une forme clinique tremblante pure.

REFERENCES

[1] Peto R, Pike MC, Armitage p, Breslow NE, Cox Dr, Howard SV, Mantel N, Mc Pherson R, Peto J, Smith PG. Traduit et présenté par : Hill C, Doyon F, Fohanno C, Campet

S. : Organisation et analyse des essais comparatifs comportant une longue surveillance des malades. Rev Epidem Santé Pub ; 1979 : 27, 167-255.

[2] Cox DR, . Regression models and life tables JR Stat Soc ; 1972 B : 34, 187-220.

[3] Kalbfleisch JD and Prentice RL. The statistical analysis of failure time data;1980,Wiley,NY.

[4] Tsiatis A. : A large sample study of the estimate for the estimate for the integrated hazard function in Cox's regression model for survival data. Tech report n° 562, department of statistics, University of Wisconsin. Madison (1978).

[5] Mardsen CD, Parkes SD. Success and problems of long-term levodopa therapy in Parkinson's disease. Lancet, 1977, 1 : 345-349.

[6] Sweet RD et al. Mental symptoms in Parkinson's disease during chronic treatment with levodopa. Neurology, 1976, 26, 4 : 305-310.

[7] Guillard A, Chastang C. Maladie de Parkinson. Les facteurs de pronostic à long terme. Rev Neurol (Paris) 1978, 134, 5 : 341-354.

[8] Kendall M and Stuart A. The advanced theory of statistics. Charles Griffin et Co Ltd, London, 4ème édition, 1978, vol 2, 240-245.

<u>Tableau I : liste des variables éventuellement pronostiques</u>

A. Variables dont la valeur est établie lors du bilan initial (jour de l'instauration du traitement à la L DOPA = temps zéro)

- ⁎ sexe
- ⁎ âge
- ⁎ délai entre la date du diagnostic et l'instauration du traitement
- ⁎ forme clinique (tremblante, autres formes)
- syndrome dépressif
- antécédents familiaux de maladie de Parkinson
- antécédents de thalamectomie (traitement antérieur)
- importance du tremblement
- ⁎ importance des troubles moteurs
- ⁎ autonomie
- ⁎ signe de Babinski (non, unilatéral, bilatéral)
- reflexe mentonnier
- troubles oculo-moteurs
- reflexe médian

B. Variables dont la valeur est déterminée après 1 an de traitment

- ⁎ résultat global du traitement (amélioration, inchangé, aggravation)
- ⁎ existence de troubles psychiques transitoires pendant la remière année de traitement (non, dépression, confusion)

Les variables marquées d'un ⁎ ont été retenues pour l'analyse multivariable.

Tableau II : Ajustements

	- 2 LOG L max
1. modèle à 0 variables	580,252
2. modèle à 9 variables	517,478
3. modèle à 3 variables	518,050

modèle 2 contre modèle 1 : $X_9^2 = 62{,}774$ p 0,001

modèle 3 contre modèle 2 : $X_6^2 = 0{,}572$ p 0,50

Le test utilisé est celui du rapport de vraisemblance (voir, par ex. (8))

AN EXAMPLE OF MODEL-BUILDING IN ANALYZING RELATIONS BETWEEN PRIMARY AND SECONDARY RISK FACTORS OF CORONARY HEART DISEASE

G.Welzl, Th.B.Ludwig, G.Rediske
Institute for Medical Informatics and Health Services Research (MEDIS) of the Society for Radiation and Environmental Research (GSF) Munich, Federal Republic of Germany

1. SUMMARY

An example is given for a modelling procedure which arises in statistical analysis of complex processes. Coronary heart disease (CHD) is associated with a hierarchy of risk factors, which requires consideration of a large number of different variables. Relations between selected and condensed variables and risk factors are analyzed by means of log-linear models. The models we use take into account interactions and are guided by established theories of CHD causation. This modelling procedure was applied to data collected in a study of CHD. The results of the first analyses are presented.

2. INTRODUCTION

The development of electronic data processing (EDP), e.g., by increasing the storage capacity and the development of more comfortable data base systems has obviously created new possibilities for the statistical analysis of epidemiological studies. The general availability of statistical program packages has encouraged the use of multivariate analysis methods even more. The use of such multivariate statistical methods led to a number of re-analyses of well-known epidemiological studies, e.g., the Framingham Study (1) or the Western Collaborative Group Study (2). These studies show that for the analysis of the pathogenesis of complex disease processes, confounding or interaction effects must be taken into consideration. This is particularly true for chronic disease processes such as CHD with its temporal changes and the mutual influencing of its risk factors. But despite the present analysis program systems and EDP possibilities the methodological and statistical problems which arise are considerable. It is intended to present such problems by an example of model-building in analyzing relations between primary and secondary risk factors of CHD.

3. PROBLEM

For the types of CHD - myocardial infarction, and angina pectoris - a multifactorial genesis is assumed, hypercholesterolaemia, hypertension, hyperglycaemia, overweight, smoking and lack of physical activity usually being considered among the most important somatic risk factors. Between these primary risk factors there are numerous correlations and interactions with regard to predicting the incidence of CHD (2). Besides these classical risk factors a number of psychosocial factors are investigated; approaches such as the investigations of behavior type A (3) or the life-event research (4) are well known. Even if such concepts are sometimes disputed, the significance of psychosocial stress for the genesis of CHD is widely accepted.

The effect of psychosocial variables on the final event of CHD through the known pathophysiological risk factors is described by Schäfer and Blohmke (5) in form of a pathogenesis model. This hierarchical model contains levels with variables of various degrees of abstraction. At the highest level there are variables of global nature like personality and heredity or social environment. These factors, together with 'secondary risk factors of the first order', such as social status, occupation or mobility lead to reactions of individuals like anxiety, worries, dissatisfaction, the 'secondary risk factors of second order'. These reactions determine the state of stress which, besides behavior characteristics, e.g., nutritional habits, physical activity and smoking, set up neural and hormonal processes which in turn affect blood pressure, blood lipids, blood sugar and blood clotting.

Preconditions for the empirical testing of such models are suitable measurements of the psychosocial factors as well as the somatic risk factors. In addition, the problem requires statistical methods which take into account both the previous contextual information and its complexity, i.e., large number of variables and non-linear relationships.

4. KIND AND ORIGIN OF DATA

The study was carried out from 1977 to 1979 in the medical center for heart and circulatory diseases Höhenried (6). Subjects were 1135 males and 630 females aged from 20 to 60 years who underwent residential preventive CHD care. By means of a standardized examination and assessment package suitable for EDP, data were obtained in the fields of, e.g., cardiological and angiological findings, resting ECG and exercise ECG, laboratory examinations of blood and urine, medical and social history and GIESSEN test (7). The variables were classified into primary risk factors for CHD, behavior, psychosocial stress indicators and social situation. Relations between these fields are to be investigated.

5. STATISTICAL METHODS

Statistical methods used to answer the present problem originate essentially in the field of analysis of multidimensional contingency tables. The data in a multidimensional contingency table is often described by log-linear models (8). Using log-linear models, the logarithms of cell probabilities are expressed as a sum of main effects and effects of higher order (interactions). Neglecting effects of higher order, a simple model arises. Taking into account many effects of higher order lead to very complex models. For the analysis of multidimensional contingency tables, therefore, many different log-linear models may be considered. For this reason a systematic method to select a suitable model is needed. By limitation to 'hierarchical' models several strategies are known. One method is based on building a hierarchy of submodels followed by an overall simultaneous test procedure (9). A different procedure consists of testing the individual effects of the log-linear models (10). A stepwise procedure for model-building was also conceived to ascertain diagnostic algorithms (11).

Procedures for model-building have to consider two essential requirements which can hardly be fulfilled simultaneously. The selected model should be as simple as possible, i.e. include as few effects as possible of lowest order and reproduce associations essential for the description of the data, even if this requires the consideration of the effects of higher order.

In our experience, simple models (as those underlying linear logistic regression) cannot satisfactorily describe the complex situation of the present problem. On the other hand, when investigating very complex models the danger of overfit arises. For instance, we could hardly reproduce effects of the 4th order. In addition, since the analysis programs usually use asymptotic test procedures (12), problems may turn up by estimating parameters when cells in contingency tables have small expected values.

The procedure used may be demonstrated in the following examples. The association between hypercholesterolaemia and work overload is to be studied. With regard to physiological aspects, characteristics from the behavioral field, e.g. overweight, must be taken into account. Figure 1 shows the prevalence of hypercholesterolaemia (cholesterol > 25o mg %) with respect to work overload in the total sample and in subgroups stratified by weight. An association between hypercholesterolae-

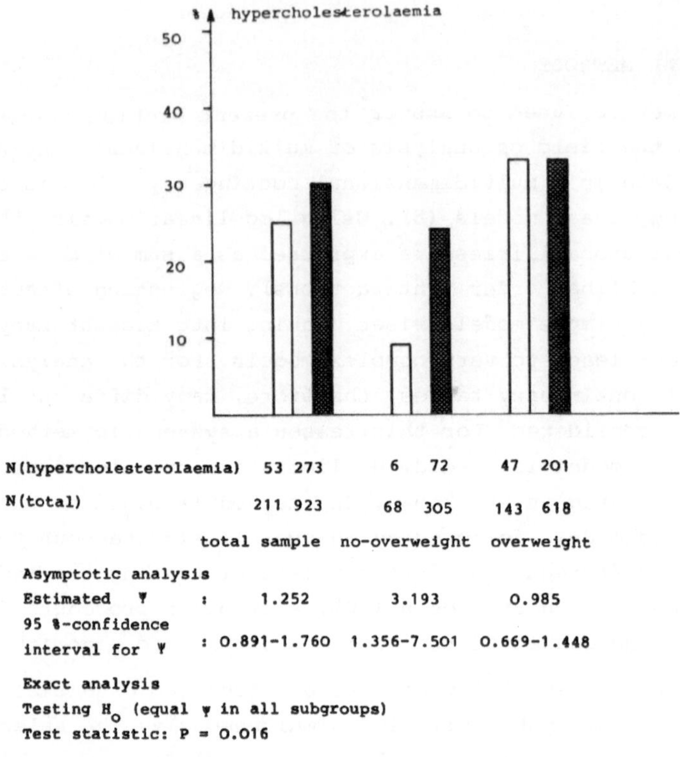

Figure 1: Relative frequency of hypercholesterolaemia in relation to 'work overload' (■ yes, □ no) in the total sample (N=1134) and in the subgroups 'no overweight' (N=373) and 'overweight' (N=761)

mia and work overload is only present in one subgroup. Therefore, an effect of 3rd order must be considered in model-building. For evaluating the parameter odds ratio for differences in strata both asymptotic and exact test procedures are available (13).

Figure 2 shows a different situation. There is an association between hypertension and hereditary taint in the total sample but no association in subgroups. This effect appears since the answer to the question :" Has your physician ever informed you of your having a high blood pressure?" - is associated with hereditary taint and with hypertension. The measure of association when combining tables in subgroups is called partial correlation.

To answer the present problem, the association between a primary risk

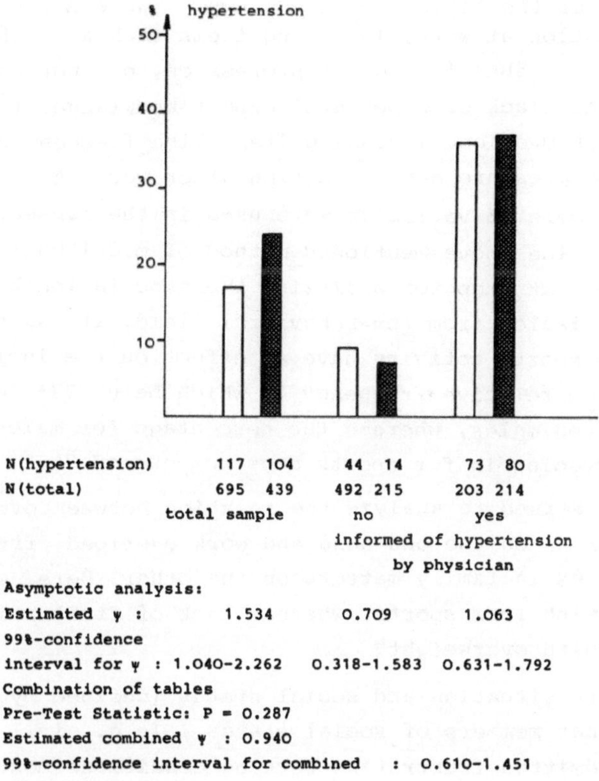

Figure 2: Relative frequency of hypertension in relation to hereditary taint (■ yes, □ no) in the total sample (N=1134) and in the subgroup 'informed of hypertension by physician' no (N=707) and yes (N=417).

factor and a contributory risk factor was analyzed by taking into consideration one further factor at a time. As a measure of association either the partial correlation or the different odds ratio in subgroups were systematically described. For the model-building, therefore, both confounding effects and non-linear associations are considered.

6. RESULTS

As an example some results from the investigation of the association between hypertension and behavior, psychological stress indicators and social situation are outlined with respect to the data of males. To assess the contributory factors about 200 items were collected. Before applying the model-building procedure, cluster and factor analyses were carried out. For instance, according to the results of both methods, items of the field 'strain at work' were arranged in two groups: frustration at work, including items such as lack of recognition, not 'getting ahead' in one's profession, pay not commensurate with performance, lack of superiors' expert knowledge, too many 'bootlickers', and work overload including items like frequent overtime, too much work, time pressure and exhaustion after work. As a result of the reduction procedure 25 variables were used in the subsequent statistical analyses. The above mentioned method of model-building was applied in the next step for analyzing the association between hypertension and variables from the behavioral field. It was shown that overweight and sports activity have an effect on the incidence of hypertension the relative frequency of which being 27% for not sporting, overweighted males, whereas the percentage for males having normal weight and going in for sports does not exceed 7%.

A further step served to analyze the relation between overweight and sports activity on the one hand and work overload, frustration at work, and worries in family matters on the other. Here, work overload is associated with less sports, whereas lack of frustration at work is associated with overweight.

Considering work situation and social status (defined by Janowitz (14)) it was found that members of social status I (e.g. civil servants of senior rank) admitted frustrating working conditions most frequently, however very seldom complained of work overload (Figure 3).

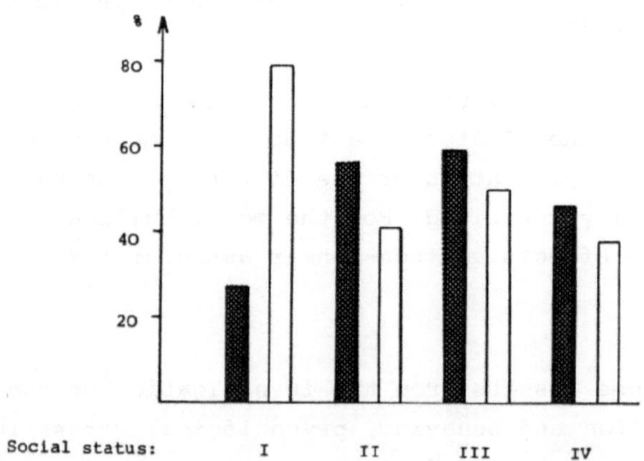

Figure 3: Relative frequency of 'work overload' (■) and 'frustration at work' (□) stratified by social status in the Höhenried cohort.

A greater proportion of work overload appeared in social status II and III (e.g. foremen and skilled workers). Evaluating the associations between hypertension, overweight, lack of sports activity, frustration at work , work overload and social status simultaneously, the essential associations are shown in Figure 4.

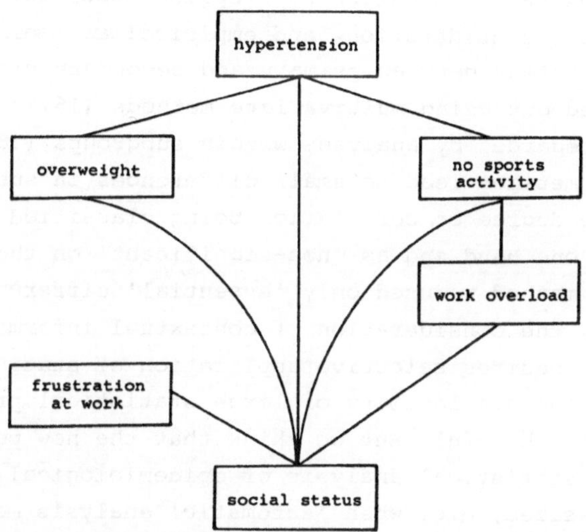

Figure 4: Associations between hypertension and secondary risk factors.

Thus, it may be realized that the association between frustration at work and overweight, as was previously shown, is perhaps explained by the associations 'frustration→social status' and 'social status→overweight'.

7. DISCUSSION

The examples shown originated from the investigation of associations between primary and secondary risk factors of CHD. Particularly with relation to hypertension a large number of psychological and social factors is often demanded to be considered, in order to explain the differing incidences in different populations and social groups (15). Especially when psychosocial factors are evaluated it should be noted that

(a) great interdependence of factors must be allowed for
(b) associations between primary risk factors and contributory factors may appear differently in subgroups, e.g., according to social status
(c) the variety of factors may be classified by contextual considera-

tions. For this reason an evaluation strategy suitable for the problem should (a) provide multivariate methods, taking into account partial correlations (b) enable the construction of a model corresponding to the complex data structure by inclusion of interactions of higher order (non-linearities) (c) take into consideration the pre-known contextual information by stepwise modelling while alternating contextual considerations and empirical analyses. More recent analyses of associations between primary and secondary risk factors of CHD were carried out using multivariate methods (16,17,18). Non-linearities are regarded by analyses within subgroups (18). Separate analyses may sometimes lead to small differences in subgroups in relation to the degree of correlation being classified as 'significant' on the one hand and as 'non-significant' on the other hand, whereas in the method we used only 'essential' differences were noted. Finally, the consideration of contextual information by stepwise modelling requires selective application of statistical methods. Here, the availability of large statistical program packages is certainly helpful. But we think that the new possibilities in EDP for the statistical analysis of epidemiological studies are often overemphasized, e.g. when 'automatic' analysis methods are the principle aim.

8. References

(1) Hully SB, Rosenman RH, Bawol RD, Brand RJ. Epidemiology as a Guide to Clinical Decisions. The Association between Triglyceride and Coronary Heart Disease. N Engl J Med. 1980; 302:1383-1387.

(2) Woodbury MA, Manton KG, Stallard E. Longitudinal Analysis of the Dynamics of Coronary Heart Disease in the Framingham Study. Biometrics. 1979; 35: 575-585.

(3) Dembroski TM, Weiss SM, Shields JL, Haynes SG, Feinleib M. Coronary -Prone Behavior. Springer, New York, 1978.

(4) Rahe RH. Life stress and illness. Thomas, Springfield/Ill., 1974.

(5) Schäfer H, Blohmke M. Herzkrank durch psychosozialen Streß. Hüthig, Heidelberg, 1977.

(6) Glawar I, Halhuber MJ, Hofmann H, Korschofsky A, Moosmüller M, Pesahl G, Höbel W, Perz S, Pöppl SJ, Rediske G, Roos G, Welzl G, Zock H. Entwicklung von Algorithmen zur Frühdiagnostik und Prädiktion koronarer Herzerkrankungen für die Anwendung bei Vorsorgeuntersuchungen. Konzept des Vorhabens. GSF-Bericht. 1978; MD 238.

(7) Beckmann D, Richter HE. Giessen Test. Huber, Bern, 1975.

(8) Bishop JMM, Fienberg SE, Holland PW. Discrete Multivariate Analysis. Theory and Practice. The MIT Press, Cambridge, 1977.

(9) Whittaker J, Aitkin M. A Flexible Strategy for Fitting Complex Log-Linear Models. Biometrics. 1978; 34: 487-495.

(10) Benedetti JK, Brown MB. Strategies for the Selection of Log-Linear Models. Biometrics 1978; 34: 680-686.

(11) Welzl G, Faus-Kessler T, Lajosi F, Ludwig TB, Raffler H, Scherb H, Schirm H. Anwendung von log-linearen Modellen zur Analyse der Diagnosevergabe in der Münchner Pädiatrischen Längsschnittstudie. In: Modelle in der Medizin - Theorie und Praxis. Bericht über die 23. Jahrestagung der GMDS, Köln, 1978.

(12) Dixon WJ, Brown MB. Biomedical Computer Programs P-series. University of California Press, Los Angeles, 1979.

(13) Welzl G, Siegerstetter J. Programm KA 2x2. In: Institut für Medizinische Datenverarbeitung der GSF: Programmsysteme und Einzelprogramme. Vol 2 MD 255, 1977.

(14) Janowitz M. Soziale Schichtung und Morbidität in Westdeutschland. Kölner Z f Soziologie u Sozialpsychol. 1958; 10:1 - 38.

(15) Pflanz M. Psychische und soziale Faktoren bei der Entstehung des Hochdrucks. Internist. 1974; 15: 124-128.

(16) Haynes SG, Levine S, Scotch N, Feinleib M, Kannel WB. The relationship of psychosocial factors to coronary heart disease in the Framingham Study. I. Methods and risk factors. Am J Epidemiol. 1978; 107: 362-383.

(17) Haynes SG, Feinleib M, Levine S, Scotch N, Kannel WB. The relationship of psychosocial factors to coronary heart disease in the Framingham Study. II. Prevalence of coronary heart disease. Am J Epidemiol. 1978; 107: 384-402.

(18) Haynes SG, Feinleib M, Kannel WB. The relationship of psychosocial factors to coronary heart disease in the Framingham Study. III. Eight-year incidence of coronary heart disease. Am J Epidemiol. 1980; 111: 37-58.

REMARQUES SUR LA DECISION PRONOSTIQUE

Jean Bernard
Institut de Recherches sur les Leucémies
et les Maladies du Sang (UER d'Hématologie
Hôpital Saint-Louis, 75010 Paris

La gnose, c'est la connaissance ; le pronostic, c'est la connaissance du futur ; plus modestement en médecine, c'est le jugement que porte un médecin après le diagnostic, sur la durée, le déroulement, l'issue probable d'une maladie, l'éventuelle action du traitement.

Ainsi le pronostic est-il l'acte central de la décision médicale, intimement lié aux deux autres actes dont il dépend. Du diagnostic presque entièrement (l'extrême bénignité, l'extrême gravité de certains états permettent pourtant parfois un pronostic sans diagnostic) du traitement, moins complètement pendant les millénaires d'inefficacité des thérapeutiques, fortement actuellement, les questions de pronostic s'alliant sans cesse aux questions de traitement.

Il suffit en effet d'énoncer les questions posées pour mesurer l'importance du pronostic, la diversité de ces questions.

L'importance du pronostic qui concerne l'homme au plus profond : ce malade va-t'il guérir ou mourir ? Va-t'il, s'il guérit, rester infirme ou se retrouver ingambe ? Sera-t'il ou non exposé aux récidives ? Quelle est son espérance de vie ?

La diversité des questions posées :

Question relativement simple lorsqu'il s'agit du pronostic des états aigus, du pronostic des urgences médicales, ce fut longtemps le seul pronostic possible. C'est celui qui nous reste le plus accessible parce qu'il s'agit d'un pronostic à court terme.

Facile aussi pour le pronostic d'une complication, tel celui de la septicémie à colibacille qui complique une aplasie, tel celui de l'encéphalite qui complique une fièvre éruptive.

Déjà plus difficile, lorsqu'il s'agit de pronostic d'un stade, d'un moment de l'évolution.

Il a longtemps été très malaisé de fixer le pronostic d'une maladie de Hodgkin. Il est devenu moins ardu de prévoir l'avenir d'un Hodgkin IA ou IIB.

Vraiment difficile lorsqu'il s'agit du pronostic d'un malade qui reste souvent très imprécis.

Ainsi un infarctus du myocarde, une leucémie aiguë peuvent tuer ou guérir complètement. Même pour une affection constamment fatale, comme la leucémie myéloïde chronique, la mort peut survenir trois mois ou quinze ans après le début clinique.

II

En dépit de cette diversité, il existe une constance, une unité de problèmes posés par la décision pronostique, une unité de ses méthodes. Ces méthodes, longtemps insuffisantes, ont beaucoup progressé en ces dernières années. Un double courant a uni le progrès thérapeutique et la décision pronostique. Le progrès thérapeutique suppose une indication thérapeutique, un choix dans une appréciation pronostique beaucoup plus rigoureuse que par le passé. Ce pronostic affiné facilite à son tour les progrès du traitement.

Cette orientation nous éloigne des données sentimentales (sentiment du médecin, sentiment de la famille) sur lesquelles se sont si longtemps fondées les décisions de pronostic. Récemment encore Siegler analyse l'attitude de ces médecins qui, en présence d'un cas grave, portent toujours un pronostic fatal (hang crepe) ; il en compare les avantages, les inconvénients, le rapproche du pari de Pascal.

III

La décision pronostique se fait nécessairement en deux temps, le temps de l'analyse, le recueil des données, le temps de la synthèse. Les progrès de la médecine ont grandement amélioré le premier temps, mais laissent incertain et souvent difficile le second temps.

A chaque étape, nous devrons tenir compte des méthodes et des faits. Les méthodes : 1) Méthode traditionnelle. Jusqu'à ces toutes dernières années, le pronostic procédait d'une intuition globale fondée sur une expérience personnelle. 2) Méthode moderne. La décision pronostique devient de plus en plus un modèle mathématique avec ses règles d'établissement, ses avantages, ses inconvénients. Les faits, avec les progrès constants de notre connaissance clinique, radiologique, biologique, remettent en question ou obligent à affiner les méthodes.

Je vous propose de suivre un médecin dans l'exercice de sa décision pronostique et je vous demande de m'autoriser à emprunter la plupart de mes exemples à ma discipline, l'hématologie.

IV

Analyse. Recueil des données.

Les données recueillies sont nécessairement de trois ordres, les premières liées à la maladie, les deuxièmes liées au malade, les troisièmes liées au traitement, c'est-à-dire au médecin.

La maladie d'abord. Longtemps, et depuis Hippocrate, cette partie du pronostic s'est fondée sur des impressions, des appréciations de la mine, du teint, du comportement, utiles certes, mais approximatives. A cette approximation s'est substituée actuellement l'analyse parfois encore imparfaite, mais aussi précise que possible, des phénomènes observés. Cette analyse porte sur la quantité, la qualité, la topographie, la chronologie de ces phénomènes.

Voici un malade admis à l'hôpital avec le diagnostic de leucémie aiguë. Le nombre des cellules leucémiques est un facteur important du pronostic. Nous ne savons pas encore déterminer exactement ce nombre mais nous pensons l'approcher en mesurant : 1) le nombre de cellules leucémiques présentes dans le sang, 2) les dimensions des organes, foie, rate, ganglions qui forment les cellules leucémiques.

A la prolifération des cellules leucémiques est associée l'insuffisance des cellules normales,. Il n'y a pas de corrélation nécessaire entre les deux désordres. L'importance de l'insuffisance des cellules normales, la diminution des globules rouges, des plaquettes, des polynucléaires sont mesurées et prises fortement en compte dans l'établissement du pronostic. Doublement 1) Pour le pronostic immédiat, ce qui est relativement simple : relation entre le thrombopénie et le danger hémorragique ; 2) pour le pronostic à moyen ou long terme, ce qui est beaucoup plus complexe : signification de la thrombopénie variant avec les formes de leucémie. L'étude de J.L. Binet a récemment montré que, pour les leucémies lymphoïdes chroniques, le classement, et pour une large part le pronostic, dépendaient de la thrombopénie.

Le pronostic d'une leucémie aiguë dépend pour une large part de la nature, de la qualité des cellules leucémiques. Une leucémie lymphoblastique est moins grave qu'une leucémie myéloblastique. Parmi les leucémies lymphoblastiques, certaines sous-variétés, à lymphoblastes B ou lymphoblastes T, ont une gravité particulière. L'appréciation de la qualité des cellules progresse ; elle a longtemps été purement descriptive, fondée sur des formes et sur des couleurs. Elle se fonde aujourd'hui sur les propriétés, les fonctions exprimées avec le langage de la biochimie. Elle ne sera vraiment exacte que lorsque nous saurons exactement définir la cellule leucémique, les diverses cellules leucémiques.

Dans toutes les maladies, la topographie des lésions est importante. Au cours d'une maladie hémorragique, l'hémorragie des centres nerveux et l'hémorragie de la peau n'ont pas la même signification. La thrombose d'une artère du muscle cardiaque et le thrombose d'une artère nourrissant un muscle de la jambe sont très différentes.

Mais l'analyse topographique va au-delà de l'importance inégale quoad vitam des différents territoires de notre temps. Certaines topographies ont en elles-mêmes des significations fâcheuses, l'atteinte de la moelle osseuse au cours d'un lymphome, des ganglions abdominaux, au cours d'une maladie de Hodgkin.

Il y a apparemment contradiction entre l'utilisation de données chronologiques et la décision pronostique, le pronostic ayant justement pour objet de prévoir la chronologie future. Les données fournies par l'anamnèse sont cependant utiles.

Ainsi l'appréciation aussi précise que possible de la croissance d'un cancer, de son "temps de doublement" apporte au pronostic des données utiles. Bien plus, dans certains cas, cette comparaison chronologique est seule efficace. Ainsi pour les aplasies médullaires assemblées par Y. Najean et son groupe, l'étude initiale ne permettrait pas de pronostic assuré. La comparaison des deux premiers bilans à intervalles définis apporte de fructueuses informations sur le pronostic, les indications thérapeutiques.

Le malade. Il est banal de rappeler le rôle du sexe, de l'âge, des maladies antérieures, du milieu socio-économique, des facteurs familiaux (ainsi l'hémophilie est également grave chez tous les membres d'une même famille).

Il est permis d'espérer de sérieux progrès de l'analyse de certains facteurs génétiques. L'étude des groupes sanguins et plus particulièrement du système de groupes HLA ne révèle pas seulement la prédisposition aux maladies. Certains de ces facteurs de groupe gouvernent très probablement l'évolution aiguë, subaiguë ou chronique de certaines maladies, la sensibilité ou la résistance à telles thérapeutiques. De nouvelles et très importantes données fort utiles au pronostic vont selon toute vraisemblance être acquises pendant les prochaines années.

Le médecin. "C'est notre inquiétude, c'est notre impatience qui gâche tout et presque tous les hommes meurent de leurs remèdes et non pas de leurs maladies" écrit Molière dans le "Malade imaginaire". Cette affirmation est probablement injuste. Longtemps les médecins n'on eu aucun pouvoir, pas même celui d'aggraver, en tout cas pas celui d'améliorer. Cette situation s'est profondément modifiée. Le pronostic d'une maladie, en cette fin du XXème siècle, dépend pour une large part de la thérapeutique. Ceci sur plusieurs plans.

D'abord sur un plan général, celui de l'état de la thérapeutique. Le pronostic de la tuberculose, de la maladie hémolytique du nouveau-né, du cancer du col de l'utérus, de la maladie de Hodgkin, a été, on la sait, transformé en ces trente dernières années. D'autres progrès sont espérés.

Une remarque préalable doit ici être faite. Le présent exposé concerne la décision pronostique ; la décision prise par le médecin au chevet d'un malade dans un cas défini (ou qu'il faut définir). Ce pronostic personnel est, tout à la fois, différent du pronostic général de la maladie considérée et pour une large part dépendant de ce pronostic général.

Dans chaque cas particulier, l'analyse des symptômes ébauchés ci-dessus doit être interprétée en fonction de la thérapeutique.

Ainsi il n'était pas très important en 1946 de savoir que les leucémies aiguës myéloblastiques tuaient en 1,5 mois, les leucémies aiguës lymphoblastiques tuaient en 2,5 mois. Il est très important en 1980 de savoir que les thérapeutiques sont différentes pour les lymphoblastiques et les myéloblastiques, que (pour se limiter à l'enfant) la guérison peut être espérée dans 50 % des leucémies aiguës lymphoblastiques, 10 à 15 % des myéloblastiques. Ainsi aussi le classement histologique des lymphomes en formes nodulaires et formes diffuses conduit à proposer des thérapeutiques toutes différentes à envisager un pronostic tout différent.

Ainsi encore, les divers classements topographiques de la maladie de Hodgkin gouvernent nos indications thérapeutiques.

Les médecins ont toujours souhaité adapter le traitement à la gravité de la maladie. La définition de classes pronostiques homogènes permet une thérapeutique rigoureusement adaptée, et aussi une organisation satisfaisante des essais thérapeutiques.

Dans un cas particulier, la promptitude du secours médical est un élément important du pronostic. Inégalement important. Fondamental par exemple pour l'appendicite aiguë d'un enfant. Important, mais pas seul important en matière de cancer. Il est grave de méconnaître un cancer à son début, de retarder le moment du traitement. Il serait plus grave encore de le traiter avec une rapidité approximative. Le pronostic dépend avant tout de la qualité, de la rigueur des indications thérapeutiques portées par un médecin, par un groupe de médecins, compétents, informés.

Cette donnée doit être analysée. les responsables des groupes coopératifs de traitement des leucémies aiguës assemblant des équipes traitant peu de malades et des équipes traitant de nombreux malades, ont souvent noté de notables différences de pronostic. 1) A certaines périodes le pronostic est meilleur pour les malades soignés par les petites équipes. 2) Dans l'ensemble, le pronostic est meilleur lorsque de nombreux malades sont traités.

Ces différences s'expliquent par le risque infectieux diminué fortuitement à certaines périodes mais dans l'ensemble mieux combattu dans les grands centres disposant des traitements symptômatiques utiles (transfusion de globules blancs, etc...)

Au pronostic statique du passé, se substitue pour un malade traité un pronostic <u>évolutif</u>, fréquemment ajusté en fonction des résultats de la thérapeutique. De nouvelles données apparaissent. Ainsi dans le traitement d'une leucémie aiguë, pour un médicament donné, nous connaissons les dates limites à partir desquelles une rémission ne peut plus être espérée. Pour une combinaison thérapeutique définie, nous connaissons certains critères, certaines réponses qui permettent, dans une certaine mesure, de prévoir l'évolution ultérieure.

Telle est cette étape initiale de recueil des données. L'informatique a beaucoup amélioré notre gestion de données, mettant à la disposition d'un seul individu à l'instant T les données recueillies à travers de nombreuses années par de nombreuses personnes. Par sa rigueur elle améliore la qualité de l'acte médical et de nos dossiers médicaux.

Le choix des données recueillies est très important et fait appel au départ dans les études rétrospectives à l'expérience clinique des médecins. Le danger demeure de méconnaître l'importance d'un paramètre clinique ou biologique. D'où la nécessité de constamment amender l'archivage des données avec l'arrivée d'informations neuves, de faits cliniques biologiques nouveaux.

V

Synthèse. Critique. Traitement des données.

Le deuxième temps est celui de la synthèse, de la critique, du traitement de ces données. Le pronostic va se fonder sur cette synthèse, cette critique, ce traitement.

Ce traitement comprend lui-même deux étapes : 1) Critique des paramètres pronostiques, 2) Appréciation globale du pronostic.

Critique des paramètres pronostiques.

Dans un premier temps, la valeur pronostique de chaque donnée ou paramètre ou variable pronostique sera étudiée isolément, ce qui permet une première sélection du sous-ensemble à étudier. Avec d'emblée des insuffisances, des difficultés.

Ainsi il est bon (pour continuer avec les leucémies aiguës) de tenir compte du nombre total des rechutes leucémiques. Il serait meilleur de disposer de méthodes assurées d'évolution. Il serait meilleur encore de mesurer non seulement le nombre mais la cinétique cellulaire, plus exactement les cinétiques cellulaires comparées des cellules leucémiques et des cellules normales. Les progrès dépendront plus ici des progrès de la connaissance que des méthodologies. Ainsi encore, la durée de la première rémission hématologique a longtemps été le critère de choix. On tend à lui substituer la durée de la rémission globale ou survie sans rechute qui reflète mieux les chances de guérison.

Appréciation globale du pronostic

Un malade est une somme de variables pronostiques. Pour tenter d'apprécier cette somme, ce groupement, deux méthodes peuvent être employées : méthode empirique, méthode d'analyse multifactorielle. Voici, à titre d'exemple, notre expérience personnelle, l'analyse multifactorielle ayant été faite grâce à l'aide de l'équipe du Professeur Grémy.

a) Méthode empirique. L'analyse rétrospective de 650 dossiers de leucémies aiguës nous avait permis de retenir un certain nombre de paramètres défavorables : âge supérieur à 15 ans, globules blancs supérieurs à 35 000, volume ganglionnaire supérieur à 3 cm, et/ou débord hépato-splénique supérieur à 6 cm, variété cytologique à grands lymphoblastes.

De façon empirique, nous avons défini une classe pronostic 1 : aucun signe défavorable, une classe pronostic 2 : un signe défavorable, une classe pronostic 3 : plusieurs signes défavorables. Les classes empiriques ont - de nombreuses études l'ont montré - une valeur pronostique supérieure à chacun des paramètres isolés. Cependant cette méthode empirique ne tient pas compte de la valeur différente de chacun des paramètres et de leur interdépendance. Ainsi le nombre et même la cinétique des cellules leucémiques n'ont pas de valeur absolue. Ils doivent être appréciés en fonction de deux autres paramètres : 1) la sensibilité de ces cellules leucémiques aux thérapeutiques choisies, 2) le pouvoir qu'a l'organisme de maîtriser la prolifération maligne plus ou moins tôt,plus ou moins complètement. Ces deux paramètres sont évolutifs, varient l'un et l'autre avec le temps. La sensibilité aux médicaments diminue en principe avec le temps. Les défenses de l'organisme sidérées par définition à la période initiale peuvent se reconstituer ensuite. Nous connaissons certains aspects de la relation cellules leucémiques-médicaments ; nous pouvons la mesurer ou au moins l'apprécier in vitro. Nous ne connaissons pratiquement rien de la relation hôte-leucémie.

Même si l'on suppose réglées les questions précédentes, même si nous savons mesurer correctement les divers facteurs gouvernant le pronostic, qu'ils dépendent de la maladie, du malade, de la thérapeutique, demeure notre ignorance de leur hiérarchie, de leur poids respectif.

b) Analyse multifactorielle

- La méthode de régression multiple permet d'apprécier l'apport de chacune des variables prises isolément à la prédiction du critère choisi, par exemple temps de survie sans rechute.
- Par la suite, les modèles prédictifs ont utilisé un critère plus caractéristique de la courbe de survie ou de rémission, la probabilité de décès ou de rechute sur un individu vivant à l'instant T. Si cette probabilité est constante au cours du temps, la durée de survie ou de rémission présente une distribution exponentielle.

La méthode de Cox ou modèle de Cox ne fait pas l'hypothèse d'une distribution particulière de la durée de survie, elle permet donc une prédiction vraisemblablement plus précise dans le domaine des affections malignes où les réactions de l'hôte sont probablement variables dans le temps, c'est ce que semble démontrer notre expérience dans les leucémies lymphoblastiques.

VI

Voici quelques années, le Professeur Grémy m'avait fait l'honneur de me demander une introduction analogue sur la décision diagnostique. Il peut être utile de comparer les deux grandes décisions qui inspirent toute la médecine. La décision diagnostique est le plus souvent rationnelle. La décision pronostique le plus souvent probabiliste.

La décision diagnostique est de plus en plus fondée sur la physiopathologie. Une anémie est due à la déperdition, à la destruction, à l'insuffisance de formation des globules rouges. D'où une série d'arbres dichotomiques ou trichotomiques. On sait combien a été féconde dans ce domaine l'alliance de l'hématologie et de l'informatique. La décision pronostique est définie par deux traits : 1) Elle est donc probabiliste. Depuis Hippocrate après tout, le médecin agit en se fondant sur des prédictions probabilistes antérieurement établies. Mais le nombre, la diversité des données recueillies rendaient sa tâche difficile, sinon impossible. Les méthodes de l'informatique récemment expliquées rendent ici des services inestimables. Pour le diagnostic, elles ont appris aux médecins la rigueur, mais elles n'ont rien apporté. Pour le pronostic, elles sont irremplaçables. L'élaboration étroitement liée du pronostic et des indications des applications thérapeutiques serait impossible sans l'informatique. 2) Au moins dans un nombre important de cas, car - et c'est le deuxième trait - la décision pronostique dépend étroitement et de plus en plus des progrès de la thérapeutique. Arrivent la streptomycine ou la vitamine B12, le pronostic de la méningite tuberculeuse ou de la maladie de Biermer ne se pose plus. Tout dépend du diagnostic et du traitement qu'il indique.

Plus exactement, l'histoire de la médecine depuis 40 ans nous a appris l'existence de deux sortes de progrès thérapeutiques, le progrès immédiat, le progrès lent, pierre à pierre. Le progrès lent est celui des traitements de la maladie de Hodgkin, des leucémies aiguës. Il n'est pas tant dû à l'arrivée de nouvelles médications qu'au meilleur usage des médications connues. C'est-à-dire, tout compte fait, à un classement correct des diverses formes de la maladie considérée, à une appréciation correcte des facteurs de gravité, à des indications thérapeutiques fondées sur cette appréciation. Le progrès ici dépend pour une large part de la décision pronostique.

RESUME

Le pronostic est l'acte central de la décision médicale entièrement lié aux deux autres actes dont il dépend. Du diagnostic presque entièrement, du traitement, moins nettement pendant des millénaires d'inefficacité des thérapeutiques, très fortement actuellement.

La décision pronostique se fait nécessairement en deux temps, le temps de l'analyse, le recueil des données, le temps de la synthèse,
1) Analyse. Recueil des données. Les données recueillies sont nécessairement de trois ordres :

a. liées à la maladie (la leucémie aiguë est prise pour exemple : nombre, nature des malades, topographie, chronologie) ;

b. liées au malade (sexe, âge, facteurs génétiques) et liées au médecin (sur le plan général, dans chaque cas particulier. Notion de pronostic évolutif).

2) Synthèse critique. Traitement des données. a) Critique des paramètres pronostiques. b) Appréciation globale du pronostic. - Méthode empirique ; - Analyse multifactorielle.

<u>Conclusion</u>. Comparaison de la décision diagnostique et de la décision pronostique.

SUMMARY

The formulation of a prognosis, a pivotal part of medical decision-making, is intimately linked to two other medical precepts on which it is ultimately dependent. The first of these is the diagnosis, on which prognosis is almost entirely structural ; the second is treatment, which has historically played a lesser role in prognostication (a consequence of the ineffectiveness of most remedies), but which offers an important contribution to prognosis today.

Prognostic decisions are formulated in two phases : a period of analysis, during which data is collected, and a period of data synthesis.

1) Analysis, data collection.

The information to be collected may be divided into three categories :

a. disease-related (taking acute leukemia as an example. The incidence, patient condition, topography, chronology).

b. patient-related (sex, age, genetic factors).

c. physician-related (in general and in particular cases). The notion of an evolution in prognosis.

2) Synthesis, formulation of a response to the information gathered.

a. a critique of prognostic parameters.

b. the overall appreciation of the prognosis. - empirical trial, multifactorial analysis.

Conclusion. Comparison of the diagnostic and the prognostic decisions.

REFERENCES

(1) Berry DA. Statistical inference and the design of clinical trials. Biomedicine 1980 ; 32 : 4-7

(2) Chastang C, Avavier A, Grémy F. Connaissance pronostique. intérêt et méthodes (Symposium : Jugement et Décision en Cancérologie clinique). Bordeaux 10-11 mars 1980 (sous presse)

(3) Cox DR. Regression models and life tables. J. Roy. Stat. Soc. B 1972 ; 34 : 220.

(4) Cox DR, The teaching of the strategy of statistics. Bull. Int. Stat. Inst. 1977, XLVII (1) : 552-558.

(5) Dannenberg AL, Shapiro AR, Fries JF. Enhancement of clinical predictive ability by computer consultation. Methods Inf. Med. 1979 ; 18 : 10-14.

(6) Freedman LS, White SS. On the use of Pocock and Simon's method for balancing treatment number and prognostic factors in the controlled clinical trials. Biometrics, 1976 ; 32 : 691-694.

(7) Gehan EA. Adjustment for prognostic factors in the analysis of clinical studies. In : Methods and impact of controlled therapeutoc trials in cancer. Paris, UICC Technical Report Series, 1978 ; 36 : 35)79.

(8) Gehan EA, Smith TL, Budzar AU, Keaying MJ, Freireich EJ. Knowledge acquisition from historical data. Application to cancer. Clinical trials. (Symposium : Jugement et Décision en Cancérologie clinique). Bordeaux 10-11 mars 1980 (sous presse).

(9) Kjöller E, Mortensen LS, Larsen ME. Evaluation of prognosis. Danish Med. Bull. 1978 ; 25 : 238-242.

(10) Mathé G, Belpomme D, Misset JL. Etude pluriparamétrique du pronostic des maladies et nouvelles formes cliniques. Nouv. Pr. Méd. 1979, 9 : 2265-2266.

(11) Nakache JP, Lorente P, Chastang C. Evaluation of prognosis and determination of therapy using multivariant method. Biomedicine, 1978 ; 28 : 19-24.

(12) Pocock SJ et al. Sequential treatment assignment with balancing for prognostic factors in the controlled clinical trial. Biometrics 1975 ; 31 : 103.

(13) Shapiro AR. The evaluation of clinical prediction. New Engl. J. Med. 1977 ; 296 : 1509-1514.

(14) Siegler M. Pascal's wager and the hanging of crepe. New Engl. J. Med. 1975 ; 289 : 853-857.

(15) Smith AH. The assessment of patient prognosis using an interactive computer program. Int. J. Biomed. comput. 1978 ; 9 :37.

DECISION THERAPEUTIQUE ETABLIE A PARTIR DE LA CONNAISSANCE PRONOSTIQUE - PROBLEMES METHODOLOGIQUES

Claude CHASTANG, Bernard ASSELAIN, Ariane AUQUIER, François GREMY

Groupe INSERM U88 : Méthodologie Informatique et Statistique en Médecine
CHU Pitié-Salpétrière - 91, Boulevard de l'Hôpital - 75634 PARIS Cedex 13

The phvsician has always had a great interest in prognostic knowledge : enability to predict the evolution, to better know the physiopathogical mechanism and to adapt treatment according to the prognostic status. This important medical need leads to perform numerous prognostic studies, sometimes coupled with clinical trials. Our experience in this field leads us to suggest the research of new prognostic factors easy to measure in the daily activity, and, to go further in the development of statistical methods well-adapted to the explanation of more complex response variables. In fact, first, the present prognostic explanation is weak for most diseases, and second the medical reality is often over simplified. Whatever the progress may be, though, the important prognostic variability (due to sampling, environment...) requires the validation of results of prognostic studies.

The use of prognostic knowledge for taking therapeutic decisions leads us to define a prognostic classification of patients into a small number of classes. In pratice, 3 classes often seem to be sufficient. This classification will serve as a background for setting up an experimental design the aim of which is to prove the interest of the therapeutic adaptation and also to show the efficiency of new therapeutic agents. This strategy leads us to include large numbers of patients.

De 1945 à 1970, d'importants progrès thérapeutiques ont été réalisés, expliquant l'actuelle prédominance de la pathologie chronique. Malgré le relatif piétinement de la recherche thérapeutique, une meilleure utilisation des ressources thérapeutiques permet cependant d'obtenir de substantiels progrès. L'une des voies est de chercher à personnaliser le traitement. En effet, un contexte pathologique définit un ensemble hétérogène de malades dans ses caractères comme dans son évolution. Ainsi, cette démarche vise à associer à la variabilité biologique une variabilité thérapeutique qualitative (thérapeutiques différentes) ou/et quantitative (posologie, fréquence).

Cette démarche apparaît quasi-spontanée si l'on dispose d'outils thérapeutiques efficaces, donc sans doute iatrogènes (e.g., on sait que les immuno-suppresseurs efficaces dans certaines affections rhumatologiques induisent des leucémies aigües). Par ailleurs, les progrès dans la connaissance physio-pathologique et les études pharmacologiques justifient cette approche en apportant des éléments rigoureux d'indications thérapeutiques. En outre, il est désormais nécessaire de prendre en compte l'aspect économique de la décision médicale : il est souhaitable de réserver les thérapeutiques coûteuses aux seuls malades pour lesquels elles sont nécessaires. Enfin, on notera que cette démarche est un fondement de l'éthique médicale qui exige que tout malade bénéficie du meilleur traitement.

La personnalisation du traitement est un problème trop vaste et trop difficile. Aussi, nous nous limiterons à l'examen des difficultés méthodologiques d'un sous-problème : comment adapter de façon rigoureuse le traitement à la gravité prévisible de l'affection ? En effet, si cette démarche est intuitive pour le médecin, force est de constater que sa mise en oeuvre spontanée ne repose pas sur des bases méthodologiques solides. L'objectif principal de cet article est de décrire les difficultés de cette approche et de proposer quelques concepts assurant une progression rigoureuse.

Tout d'abord, cette approche implique qu'à la connaissance diagnostique s'ajoute une connaissance pronostique, base de la décision thérapeutique (cette conception n'implique pas nécessairement une aggressivité thérapeutique croissante avec la gravité : par exemple, l'evolution systématiquement péjorative à brève échéance du cancer du poumon métastasé conduit à ne pas pratiquer une intervention chirurgicale, réalisée en l'absence de métastases diagnostiquées).

Une fois cette connaissance pronostique acquise, il convient de l'utiliser à des fins de décision thérapeutique et de démontrer l'intérêt de l'adaptation thérapeutique au pronostic.

I. ACQUISITION DE LA CONNAISSANCE PRONOSTIQUE

La connaissance pronostique provient de sources nombreuses et complémentaires : le jugement clinique, indispensable pour suggérer l'étude d'un paramètre, la littérature qui livre l'expérience d'autres équipes, les études rétrospectives qui ont l'avantage de permettre une approche pronostique à un coût faible et dans des délais brefs, mais surtout les enquêtes prospectives, réalisées ou non à l'occasion d'essais thérapeutiques, qui limitent, entre autres avantages, les biais d'échantillonnage et de mesure.

1.1. Problèmes liés à la réalisation d'une enquête pronostique

Une étude pronostique vise d'une part à identifier les éléments prédictifs de l'évolution, et d'autre part, à prévoir l'évolution d'un nouveau malade, issu de la même population et placé dans le même environnement, en particulier thérapeutique. Ces deux conditions ne sont pas de pures clauses de style et constituent des contraintes importantes qui renforcent la difficulté de cette approche thérapeutique.

1.1.1. Choix des paramètres dont on recherche la valeur pronostique

Les conditions d'utilisation en pratique médicale courante de cette information conduisent à en exiger les caractères suivants : définition simple, reproductibilité, recueil non traumatisant, facile et peu onéreux, obtention quasi-immédiate de la valeur, forte liaison avec l'évolution.

La faible explication pronostique de l'évolution, souvent constatée, doit encourager la recherche de nouveaux paramètres. Par ailleurs, l'évaluation des examens complémentaires devrait comporter une dimension pronostique.

1.1.2. Description de l'évolution : Choix du (des) critère(s) de jugement

Des affections qui conduisaient à brève échéance à une issue fatale ont vu en quelques décennies leur évolution transformée par les progrès thérapeutiques. D'où l'intérêt de prendre en compte le délai de survie grâce aux méthodes actuarielles [1]. En outre, l'étude des maladies chroniques fait intervenir de nouveaux critères de jugement, d'apparition plus précoce et/ou traduisant mieux le mécanisme physio-pathologique.

C'est ainsi que l'analyse de protocoles thérapeutiques dans la maladie de Hodgkin (maladie mortelle il y a 30 ans et pour laquelle on évoque la guérison dans certaines formes) privilégie la durée de rémission, état qui s'achève par une rechute, reprise évolutive de la maladie qui n'implique pas systématiquement le décès à brève échéance. Ainsi, la durée de rémission est un critère précoce et précis de l'efficacité thérapeutique. Au contraire, le décès peut être lié à une reprise évolutive de la maladie et/ou à l'action iatrogène du traitement (5 % de leucémies aigües induites à 5 ans) [2] ou à une cause intercurrente. Dans le but d'adapter le traitement à la gravité, il convient, d'une part, d'identifier les formes évolutives qui justifient une thérapeutique aggressive, et d'autre part, les formes moins évolutives pour lesquelles le risque iatrogène conduit à une réduction de l'aggressivité thérapeutique.

Ainsi, dans la maladie de Hodgkin, le critère de jugement optimal serait une variable tronquée à 3 issues : rechute décès iatrogène, survie sans rechute. Prentice [3] a proposé un développement du modèle de Cox [4] afin d'appréhender l'explication de tels critères à risques compétitifs.

1.1.3. Caractéristiques des études pronostiques en pathologie chronique d'après notre expérience.

Au grand nombre de paramètres qui détiennent isolément une valeur pronostique s'oppose le plus souvent le nombre réduit de facteurs pronostiques (au sens de l'analyse multidimensionnelle), témoin de la forte liaison des paramètres pronostiques. Aussi, on aboutit fréquemment à une explication pronostique faible, ce qui ne permet pas de prédire l'évolution de façon précise. Plusieurs éléments peuvent être avancés pour expliquer ce résultat qui contrarierait le développement de l'adaptation thérapeutique à la gravité s'il devait se maintenir : tout d'abord, il s'agit d'affections chroniques et l'on sait que la prévision est toujours plus facile à brève échéance qu'à longue échéance. De plus, le mécanisme physio-pathologique de nombreuses maladies est mal connu, et trop souvent, on l'appréhende par ses seules conséquences "superficielles" (fièvre, amaigrissement, VS, anémie...), d'où la nécessité d'un effort de réflexion qui permettrait de définir de nouvelles variables. En outre, les éléments pronostiques sont recueillis à un moment variable de l'évolution de la maladie qu'ils décrivent sans traduire la rapidité évolutive. En effet, la prise en compte de données évolutives améliore la prédiction [5], mais cette information est rarement disponible lors de la décision thérapeutique qu'elle peut seulement infléchir par la suite.

1.2. Difficultés méthodologiques dans l'utilisation de la connaissance pronostique.

La confrontation des résultats d'études pronostiques concernant la même affection montre une importante variabilité, qui est parfois même retrouvée au sein d'une même enquête, comme c'est le cas du Coronary Drug Project [6], vaste projet d'étude de la correction des troubles lipidiques chez des sujets ayant présenté un infarctus du myocarde.

Ces auteurs séparent les sujets ayant reçu le placebo en 2 échantillons selon leur origine géographique et sélectionnent pour chaque échantillon un sous-ensemble de 10 variables explicatives de la survie parmi 40 variables. Seules 2 variables sont communes (rang 5 et 1, 9 et 6). En fait, ces 2 sous-ensembles, apparemment différents, décrivent une information voisine puisque chaque sous-ensemble de paramètres permet de prédire correctement l'évolution de l'autre échantillon.

L'utilisation décisionnelle de la connaissance pronostique implique que l'on vérifie la généralité des conclusions, étape exceptionnellement envisagée jusqu'à présent.

1.2.1. Eléments de variabilité des résultats d'études pronostiques.

L'échantillonnage et l'environnement, avec en premier lieu l'incidence thérapeutique, constituent les 2 facteurs essentiels de cette variabilité.

L'expérience du groupe coopératif français d'étude de la leucémie lymphoïde chronique confirme l'importance de l'échantillonnage, dont le rôle est négligé à tort dans ces études pronostiques : en effet, le recrutement de certains services comporte quasi-exclusivement des formes à haute évolutivité biologique (médiane de survie : 24 mois) tandis que d'autres services drainent essentiellement des malades sans signes biologiques ou tumoraux (médiane de survie supérieure à 7 ans). Dès lors, il ne serait pas surprenant d'obtenir des résultats pronostiques différents si les effectifs permettaient des études séparées. En outre, on peut observer une modification de l'échantillonnage au cours du temps.

L'environnement regroupe un vaste ensemble de facteurs contribuant à la variabilité pronostique : mesure des paramètres, traitement, soins annexes, surveillance...

L'incidence thérapeutique est multiple : les traitements randomisés en constituent la partie évaluable, mais peuvent aussi intervenir une attitude thérapeutique systématique (antibiothérapie, transfusions dans le traitement d'induction des leucémies aigües myéloblastiques) ou des particularités thérapeutiques propres à un centre. L'impossibilité fréquente de disposer d'un groupe de malades non traités peut compliquer la mise en évidence d'interactions traitement- variables, condition nécessaire à l'adaptation thérapeutique. En effet, en l'absence de cette interaction (l'incidence thérapeutique est alors identique quelque soit le profil), la décision thérapeutique ne peut être qu'unique.

C'est ainsi que Byar et Corle [7] ont proposé une stratégie thérapeutique dans le cancer de la prostate en utilisant les résultats d'un essai thérapeutique randomisé comparant placebo et oestrogène : à partir d'un sous-ensemble de 7 paramètres, ils déterminent le traitement optimal, abstention ou hormonothérapie. Ces auteurs mettent en évidence un groupe de 113 malades (25 % de l'échantillon initial) pour lequel le bénéfice moyen calculé de cette adaptation thérapeutique est de 24 mois.

1.2.2. Généralité des résultats d'études pronostiques

L'utilisation de la connaissance pronostique à des fins de décision thérapeutique rend indispensable d'en montrer le caractère général. Cette nécessité a été soulignée par de nombreux auteurs [6], [7], mais les procédures suggérées requièrent des effectifs très importants. Ces procédures seront dites internes ou externes, selon qu'elles utilisent ou non l'échantillon étudié.

Les procédures externes permettent de valider les résultats d'une étude en utilisant d'autres données : données personnelles antérieures ou ultérieures, données d'autres auteurs. Les difficultés en sont : les biais d'échantillonnage non décelables, le recueil hétéorogène, le rôle de l'environnement. Ces difficultés sont moindres si l'on dispose de données recueillies successivement au sein de la même institution ou du même groupe coopératif, et surtout s'il s'agit de protocoles chaînés (protocoles successifs présentant un bras commun).

Les procédures internes intéressent le même ensemble de données. Rares sont les études, telles celles du Coronary Drug Project, qui permettent de scinder l'échantillon global en deux : l'échantillon de base qui fait l'objet de l'étude et l'échantillon-test qui en confirme les résultats.

Les procédures fréquemment utilisées qui appliquent les règles décisionnelles aux malades qui ont permis de les élaborer n'apportent pas la preuve rigoureuse de la validité des résultats.

D'où l'intérêt possible dans les études pronostiques de la méthode du "Jackknife" [8] [9], technique statistique qui permet d'estimer les paramètres et de calculer leurs variances en répétant l'analyse, un sujet ou un groupe de sujets étant éliminé. De même, l'utilisation des techniques bayésiennes dans les études pronostiques devrait aboutir à une meilleure estimation des paramètres et de leurs variances.

Dans cette perspective d'adaptation thérapeutique, il apparaît donc indispensable d'adapter, voire de développer des outils méthodologiques afin de s'assurer de la consistance des conclusions pronostiques.

II. UTILISATION DE LA CONNAISSANCE PRONOSTIQUE A DES FINS DE DECISION THERAPEUTIQUE.

2.1. Utilisation de l'information pronostique .

Une étude pronostique permet de déterminer les variables pronostiques et dans un second temps, peut aboutir à l'identification d'un sous-ensemble décrivant au mieux la totalité de l'information pronostique.

Cette connaissance n'est qu'un outil nécessaire, mais non suffisant de l'adaptation thérapeutique à la gravité. En effet, il faut prouver l'intérêt de cette démarche. D'autre part, il faut être capable de mettre en évidence d'autres progrès thérapeutiques. D'où la nécessité de protocoles expérimentaux afin d'atteindre ces deux objectifs. La mise en oeuvre de ces protocoles implique la définition de sous-ensembles homogènes de malades qui feront l'objet d'une randomisation entre les différentes attitudes thérapeutiques retenues.

En fait, la définition de sous-groupes homogènes est une démarche médicale classique comme l'atteste la remarquable nosographie établie à partir de la seule observation médicale. Il convient donc d'affiner cette nosographie en la complétant d'une classification pronostique.

L'élaboration d'une classification pronostique apparaît ainsi comme l'étape ultime d'une étude pronostique. La détermination du nombre de classes ainsi que la fréquence par classe constituent des difficultés pratiques dont l'approche est insystématisable, largement arbitraire. Un exemple en est donné par A. Auquier et coll. [10] dans la leucémie lymphoïde chronique.

Ainsi, une classification pronostique apparaît comme un outil de décision thérapeutique dont les protocoles ultérieurs doivent permettre l'évolution (introduction de nouveaux paramètres, réaménagement...)

2.2. Protocole expérimental

La nature et le nombre de questions posées concernant la seule adaptation thérapeutique sont tels que seul un protocole rigoureux pourra en apporter les réponses : certaines questions sont de nature thérapeutique (intérêt de l'adaptation, quantitative ou qualitative, du traitement), d'autres ont trait à la connaissance (validation de la classification et éventuelle amélioration).

Le protocole se compliquera davantage si l'on souhaite apprécier en plus l'intérêt de l'adjonction d'un nouvel agent thérapeutique (eg : apport d'une nouvelle drogue à une association chimiothérapeutique).

Les différentes questions retenues conduiront à planifier un essai thérapeutique caractérisé par ses objectifs nombreux et ses contraintes (éthiques, recrutement).

L'incidence du recrutement est importante : la classification permet la stratification du tirage au sort des différentes attitudes thérapeutiques retenues, mais chaque classe est autonome et requiert un nombre de sujets suffisant.

Cette contrainte peut conduire à limiter les objectifs du protocole, et, c'est d'ailleurs la situation dans laquelle nous allons désormais nous placer : on dispose d'une classification pronostique en 3 classes et on souhaite montrer l'intérêt de l'adaptation thérapeutique à la gravité : l'on dispose de 3 posologies ou 3 traitements d'aggressivité croissante.

Classes \ Traitements	1	2	3
1	X	X	X
2	X	X	X
3	X	X	X

a

Classes \ Traitements	1	2	3
1	X		
2		X	
3			X

b

Classes \ Traitements	1	2	3
1	X	X	
2	X	X	X
3		X	X

c

Classes \ Traitements	1	2	3
1	X		
2	X	X	X
3			X

b

Tableau I : Schémas de protocoles d'adaptation thérapeutique à la gravité.

Le tableau 1.a représente le schéma le plus complet qui permet de répondre à toutes les questions posées à condition de disposer pour chaque classe d'un recrutement suffisant. Mais ce protocle peut poser des problèmes éthiques : thérapeutique insuffisante pour des formes graves et thérapeutique trop aggressive pour des formes mineures.

Aussi, peut-on être tenté d'adopter le schéma illustré par le tableau 1.b : à chaque classe pronostique correspond un traitement. Ce protocole ne permet pas de répondre aux questions de nature thérapeutique. De plus, il ne permet pas d'étudier la classification, car chaque classe reçoit un traitement différent, donc il est impossible d'en évaluer le retentissement sur les paramètres pronostiques. Ce schéma anticipe la preuve de l'intérêt de l'adaptation thérapeutique qu'il ne peut en aucun cas fournir.

Il est donc indispensable de maintenir une variabilité thérapeutique. Les tableaux 1.c et 1.d représentent des schémas simplifiés, compromis entres les contraintes éthiques et les nécessités expérimentales qui assurent la progression thérapeutique et l'acquisition des connaissances.

Le schéma 1.c élimine pour les classes extrêmes la thérapeutique extrême : la réponse thérapeutique est complète pour la classe intermédiaire, mais n'est que partielle pour les autres : s'il s'agit d'une posologie, de meilleurs résultats avec la posologie intermédiaire conduiront dans la classe 1 à s'interroger sur les résultats de la posologie la plus forte, donc on pourra être amené à réaliser un nouvel essai pour cette classe comparant posologie intermédiaire et posologie forte. Quant à la validation de la classification, elle n'est complète que pour le traitement 2.

Quant au schéma 1.d, il permet de répondre à la seule question : faut-il adapter le traitement pour les classes extrêmes ? De plus ce schéma permet la validation de la classification pour l'attitude thérapeutique intermédiaire.

CONCLUSION

L'intérêt de l'adaptation thérapeutique à la gravité nous paraît suffisamment important pour justifier un effort de recherche méthodologique dans plusieurs domaines : explication de critères de jugement à issues multiples, procédures internes et externes de validation de résultats pronostiques. Une condition indispensable à cette démarche est l'existence de facteurs pronostiques importants et stables, fait relativement rare actuellement dans les maladies chroniques. Enfin, la nécessaire preuve de l'intérêt de cette stratégie thérapeutique implique la mise en place de protocoles expérimentaux comparant, à gravité homogène, tout ou partie des attitudes thérapeutiques envisageables. Ces protocoles requièrent l'introduction de grands nombres de malades et impliquent la mise en place de groupes coopératifs.

BIBLIOGRAPHIE

1 Kaplan EL, Meier P. Non-parametric estimation from incomplete observations. J Am Stat Assoc. 1958 ; 53 : 457-481.

2 Asselain B, Andrieu JM, Rioux P, Teillet F, Chastang Cl, Bayle-Weisgerber C, Lemercier N, Casassus P, Gremy F. Clinical consequences of multiple criteria right censored data analysis in Hodgkin's disease. MEDINFO 80, Lindberg, Kaihara Ed, NORTH-HOLLAND Publi. C°. 1980 ; 991-995.

3 Prentice RL, Kalbfleish JD, Peterson AV, Flournoy N, Farewell VT, Breslow NE. The analysis of failure time data in the presence of competing risks. Biometrics. 1978 ; 34 : 541-554.

4 Cox DR. Regression models and life-tables (with discussion) JR Statist Soc. 1972 ; B, 34 : 187-220.

5 Golmard JL, Guillard A, Chastang Cl. Application du modèle de Cox à l'établissement d'une classification pronostique de la détérioration intellectuelle dans la maladie de Parkinson. MIE 81. Proceedings Springer-Verlag. 1981.

6 Coronary Drug Project Research Group. Factors influencing long-term prognosis after recovery from myocardial infarction. Three years findings of the coronary drug project. J Chron Dis. 1974 ; 27 : 267-285.

7 Byar DP, Corle DK. Selecting optimal treatment in clinical trials using covariate information J Chron Dis. 1977 ; 30 : 445-459.

8 Mosteller F, Tukey JW. Data analysis and regression. Addison-Wesley, New-York. 1977 ; 133-163.

9 Miller RG. The jackknife : a review. Biometrika, 1974 ; 61 : 1-15.

10 Auquier A, Dighiero G, Chastang Cl, Binet JL. Elaboration d'une classification pronostique dans la leucémie lymphoïde chronique. MIE 81, Proccedings, Springer-Verlag. 1981.

A COMPUTER AIDED SYSTEM OF IMPROVING THERAPEUTIC MEASURES BY LONG TERM FOLLOW-UP

Lothar Horbach

Institute for Medical Statistics and Documentation

Erlangen, Germany

SUMMARY

A computer aided system of follow-up observations of defined diseases is implemented. Information about the individual pattern of findings at the onset of therapy and during the course of disease leading to good or poor results is documented. The system supports the communication of information to the different medical services involved. On the base of the documented data the parameters of multivariate models of prognosis are estimated. By the aid of these models the attribution of future patients to different prognostic groups is quantified and gives useful advice in therapeutic decisions.

1. INTRODUCTION

The problems of design, documentation and statistical evaluation of controlled clinical trials have been largely discussed in recent years and are of actual interest. But even if the application of certain types of drugs, operations or radiation is legitimated by clinical trials or by long experience there is always need of further improvement. Especially severe therapeutic measures such as cancer and cardiovascular surgery, treatment with special drugs, radiotherapy etc. applied in the early or acute phase of the disease do not lead to the entire functional and anatomic restitution. Further observation and, sometimes, care are necessary in the individual case. In this sense these patients can be regarded as patients in a chronic state of disease. Our computer aided system in Erlangen in a first step supports the combined activities of clinicians and general practitioners in follow-up observations and after-care by the storage and transfer of informations. A sufficiently big set of such observations of a defined therapeutic group gives a sound empirical base for the critical evaluation of the results by the applied therapeutic measures. The important question is put: How differ good and poor results by a certain therapy in the pattern of medical findings at the onset? The answer to this question can give us a key to better differential therapeutic decisions. Some ways of solution and some experience concerning the functions of our information system in this field of clinical investigation are presented in this paper.

2. FACTORS INFLUENCING EFFECTS OF THERAPY

The effects of therapeutic measures are more or less influenced by intervening factors.

- The individual pattern of the disease to be treated, e.g. stage and grade of cancer
- Common biological attributes, e.g. sex and age
- Genetic factors, e.g. those determining enzymatic defects
- Associated chronic diseases, e.g. diabetes, hypertension
- Social, sociological and environmental factors, e.g. family care

These factors influencing therapeutic results must be evaluated not only one by one, but also by their potential combinatory effects leading to a multivariate grouping of patients with good or poor results. For the patients with bad prognosis better alternative therapeutic measures are sometimes at hand or must be developed.

3. DESIGN OF FOLLOW-UP STUDIES WITH THE AIM OF GIVING ADVICE TO FUTURE THERAPEUTIC DECISIONS

In order to work out differential rules for therapeutic decisions which can be generalized first of all according to the rules of statistical inference the qualitative delimitation of the nosological population of patients to be involved has to be made. In practise the definition of the disease and/or the therapeutic indication is completed by listing exclusive criteria in the presence of which a patient has to be excluded from the follow-up study, e.g. patients exceeding a certain age.

Only a close collaboration between clinicians and specialists of statistics and informatics can lead to the right choice of relevant variables to be observed and documented. In every case identifying data of the patient, intervening variables and variables characterizing the course of the disease, and details of therapy (e.g. dose, compliance) have to be gathered following standardized schedules of observations. The spacing of observations in the course of follow-up must correspond to the dynamics of the pathological process.

4. DATA HANDLING

The application of multivariate models demands a complete and exact recording of the essential data entering into the calculations. Data acquisition is done during the stationary phase in hospital as well as during ambulatory controls of the discharged patients.Data are entered into the system by terminals with the aid of displays by a dialogue including controls of completeness, form and plausibility. The recruitment and calling in of patients for clinical reexamination at a certain date are completely supported by the computer with its central data bank.

The flow of clinical data is determined by the existing computersystem (Horbach, Überla (1), Meyer-Bender and others (2)). The configuration of this system is characterized by a subdivision into 3 levels:

- This first level is a multitude of mainly unintelligent terminals for data acquisition, retrieval and dialogue functions
- The second level consists of two communication processors also fulfilling certain real-time functions
- The third level is a general purpose computer with the functions of data base management, calculations etc.

This system enables to control data input, record linkage into patient files from different places and at different times, procedures of calling in patients to reexaminations, computational work and graphical representation of results. The development of the multitude of programs fulfilling the different functions of the system necessitates due regard to modern principles of software engineering.

5. MULTIVARIATE STATISTICAL MODELS OF PROGNOSIS AND THEIR APPLICATION

In a first approach to our problem the linear discriminant function was used to calculate vital risks for patients with myocardial infarction (HORBACH and others (3,4). This method was initiated by HUGHES and others (5) and by NORRIS and others (6). The findings observed at the onset of therapy figure as K variables in individual vectors

$$\mathfrak{x} = (X_1, X_2, \ldots, X_K)$$

of two groups of patients: those alive after a certain interval of time and those who died within this interval. Under the assumptions of multivariate normal distributions and equality of covariance matrices, the linear discriminant function

$$D\ (X) = a_1X_1+a_2X_2+\ldots a_KX_K$$

ascertains a maximal separation of the two groups. The individual values of the function D (X) of the two groups have generally overlapping but distinctly differring distributions. If the whole range of the two distributions is divided into classes of values D (X), groups of more or less different prognosis can be discerned.

CORNFIELD (7) has formulated a special model for the calculation of risk using the formula of BAYES. The conditional probability of an unfavorable result of a therapy M-an individual vector of variables X given - can be estimated by

$$\hat{P}\ (M\,|\,X) = \frac{1}{1+e^{-(a_0+D(X))}}$$

Under the assumption of an appropriate a_0, the estimation P (M|X) is calculated using again the linear discriminant function D (X). There is a rather good fit of the letalities estimated by the model to those observed.

The logistic model of Cornfield also can be calculated estimating the coefficients $a_0, a_1, \ldots, a_K$ by the method of maximum likelihood. Numerical procedures which can be used are those by NEWTON-RAPHSON or by WALKER and DUNCAN (8). The use of the maximum likelihood estimation leads to a still better fitting of expected to observed letalities than the linear discriminant function.

Applicating these models usually the distinction between early and late deaths, e.g. by myocardial infarction is made. This distinction points out the need of caculating prognostic indices as a function of time, e.g. expected individual survival curves under given circumstances of nosological pattern and therapy.

COX (9) has presented a model responding to these requirements. By this model all available informations of the follow-up of patients are taken into account. The estimating function of the survival time P(t) has the form

$$P(t) = e^{-e^{\beta_1X_1+\beta_2X_2+\ldots+\beta_nX_n}\,\Lambda(t)}$$

The unknown parameters $\beta_1, \beta_2, \ldots, \beta_n$ and the unknown cumulative hazard function Λ which characterizes the intensity of dying as a function of time are estimated on the base of the individual observation vectors at the onset of therapy and the documented survival time. Procedures of calculation have been presented by COX (9) and by KALBFLEISCH and PRENTICE (10). A special modification was worked out by GUNSELMANN (11). With the aid of the model life expectancy curves for future patients can be easily calculated.

AID FOR THERAPEUTIC DECISIONS BY QUANTIFIED PROGNOSIS

The special interest in the use of the outlined multivariate models differs from one type of therapeutic measure to the other one. The application of the linear discriminant function evaluating an international study of therapy in myocardial infarction (HORBACH and others (4)) provided very interesting results. The following variables entered into the observation vector: age, pulse rate, systolic blood pressure, blood flow in the limbs, signs of heart failure, arrhythmia, shock, localisation of the infarction in the septum, localisation in the apex, enlarged QRS-complex, atrial fibrillation, cerebral confusion. The distribution of D (X) of 994 patients who survived and of 264 patients who died within 6 weeks were overlapping but differred distinctly. The whole range of the two distributions was divided into classes of values D ($\mathfrak{X}$) with different prognosis. In the most favorable class comprising 400 patients, letality amounted to 3%, in a class of 58 patients with poorest prognosis the corresponding value was 83%. Further analysis showed that the drug which was to be tested - compared to the reference serie of controls - had a relatively better efficacy in patients with generally better than lower life expectancy; in the latter classes no beneficial effect could be detected.

An application of the COX model of big interest is going on in a follow-up study referring to the surgery of rectal cancer. There is a distinct zone of the localisation of rectal cancer in which two types of operation - extirpation with artificial anus or resection - can be taken into consideration. We have at our disposal documented follow-up observations of patients with comparable findings during operation, who were treated partly by extirpation, partly by resection. The data of these cases served to estimate the parameters of the COX model. For future cases the calculation of curves of individual expectancy of relapse of cancer and/or death as a function of time for both types of operation gives useful advice in deciding which type of operation has to be accomplished. The observation vector is chiefly supplied by the clinical pathologist intra operationem taking into account different variables characterizing stage, grading and the size of the tumor (HERMANEK (12)).

Further follow-up projects concerning the therapy of other cancer localisations and precancer, cardiovascular and other diseases are now implemented in our therapeutic information system.

BIBLIOGRAPHY

(1) Horbach L, Überla K. Rahmenplanung zum Einsatz der elektronischen Datenverarbeitung für die Medizinischen Fachbereiche der Bayerischen Universitäten. Erlangen 1977

(2) Meyer-Bender BA, Greiller R, Horbach L, Lange H-J, Seidel H, Überla K. Interfaces in a Computer Network for the Medical Schools in Bavaria. Lecture Notes in Medical Informatics Nr. 5, Proceedings of Medical Informatics, Berlin, Springer, p.763-773

(3) Horbach L, Gunselmann W, Just H. Schicketanz KU, Schmidt W. Verlaufsindizes bei Herzinfarkten.Bericht 19. Jahrestagung der Dtsch.Ges.f.Med.Dok. u. Statistik, Mainz 1974, Schattauer, Stuttgart

(4) Horbach L, Just H. Klinisch-therapeutische Studie: Trasylol bei Herzinfarkt. Intensivmedizin 1979; 16: 338-360

(5) Hughes WL, Kalbfleisch JM, Brandt EN, Costiloc JP. Myocardial infarction prognosis by discriminant analysis. Arch.Intern.Med. 1963; III: 338-360

(6) Norris RM, Brandt PWT, Caughey DE, Lee AJ, Scott PJ. A new coronary prognostic index. Lancet 1967: 274-278

(7) Cornfield J. Joint dependence of risk of coronary heart disease on serum cholesterol and systolic blood pressure: a discriminant function analysis. Fed.Proc. 1962; 21: 58-61

(8) Walker SH, Duncan DB. Estimation of the probability of an event as a function of several independant variables. Biometrika 1967; 54: 167-179

(9) Cox DR. Regression models and life tables (with discussion). J.R.Statist.Soc. 1972; B 34: 187-220

(10) Kalbfleisch JD, Prentie RL. Marginal likelihoods based on Cox's regression and life model. Biometrika 1973; 60: 267-278

(11) Gunselmann W. Multivariate Prognosemodelle in der Medizin. Habilitationsschrift 1979, Erlangen

(12) Hermanek P. "Grading" und "Staging". Bedeutung für die klinische Onkologie. Fortschr. der Medizin 1978; 96: 520-524.

ELABORATION D' UNE CLASSIFICATION PRONOSTIQUE DANS LA LEUCEMIE LYMPHOIDE CHRONIQUE

Ariane AUQUIER+, Guillaume DIGHIERO++, Claude CHASTANG+, Jacques-Louis BINET++

\+ Groupe INSERM U 88 : Méthodologie Informatique et Statistique en Médecine
CHU Pitié-Salpétrière - 91, Boulevard de l'Hôpital - 75634 PARIS Cedex 13

++ Service d'Hématologie
Hôpital Pitié-Salpétrière - 47 Boulevard de l'Hôpital - 75651 PARIS Cedex 13

Staging has achieved wide acceptance in many types of cancer as a basis for therapeutic decisions. The highly variable course of Chronic Lymphocytic Leukemia (CLL) justifies adaptating treatment to the severity of the disease provided the existence of a good prognostic classification. Therapeutic progress is demonstrated by randomized trials planned according to such a classification. The sizes of these trials must be large enough in each stage in order to achieve statistically powerful conclusions. The requirement of large numbers is in conflict with the relatively rare incidence of CLL. Therefore if a prognostic classification is to be used in randomized trials of CLL, it should not have too many stages. The existence of classifications in CLL with four or five stages led us to reconsider the staging problem in CLL. In this paper we present an analysis of survival data of two series totalizing 295 patients using the Cox model in order to identify important prognostic factors. This analysis led us to propose a new classification of CLL in three stages. We were able to confirm its prognostic value on four other series of patients. We discuss how this new classification was used in the planning of the new randomized trial of the CLL cooperative group of the French Society of Hematology.

La Leucémie Lymphoïde Chronique (LLC) est une maladie d'évolution très variable : certains malades meurent dans l'année suivant le diagnostic, d'autres vivent plus de dix ans. Les travaux récents de RAI et coll.[1], Binet et coll.[2], Rundles et coll.[3] et Montserrat et coll.[4] ont contribué à une meilleure connaissance pronostique de la LLC; ces auteurs, en s'appuyant sur l'étude de courbes de survie tracées pour différentes valeurs de variables cliniques et biologiques, ont proposé des classifications en quatre ou cinq stades. La multiplicité de ces classifications a abouti à une volonté générale d'adopter une classification unique afin de faciliter les échanges entre spécialistes de la maladie. La grande variabilité d'évolution des malades atteints de LLC justifie l'adaptation thérapeutique à la gravité. Les progrès dans le traitement de la maladie seront donc mis en évidence par des essais thérapeutiques planifiés selon une classification pronostique.

Comme le discutent Chastang et coll.[5], les effectifs de ces essais doivent être suffisamment importants à l'intérieur de chaque stade pour pouvoir mettre en évidence des différences entre traitements avec des risques de première et deuxième espèce suffisamment faibles. Or, pour réaliser de tels essais, nous devons également tenir compte de la faible incidence de la LLC. On estime en effet qu'il y a environ 1000 nouveaux cas de LLC en France actuellement chaque année. Des essais thérapeutiques ne pouvant s'étirer sur de trop nombreuses années, on ne peut classer les LLC en trop de stades, ce qui diminuerait d'autant le recrutement de chaque stade. Or, sans nier la valeur pronostique des classifications existantes, nous avons trouvé, à l'usage, qu'elles comportaient trop de stades pour permettre la mise en place d'essais thérapeutiques utiles. Nous avons donc reconsidéré le problème de classification dans la LLC, en tentant une recherche de facteurs pronostiques à l'aide du modèle de Cox, ce qui nous a conduit à proposer une classification en 3 stades. Nous avons pu en confirmer la valeur pronostique sur d'autres malades et enfin nous avons utilisé cette classification dans le protocole du nouvel essai randomisé du Groupe Coopérateur de la Société Française d'Hématologie pour le traitement de la LLC.

1. MATERIEL ET METHODES

1.1. Les malades

Cette étude a été réalisée à partir de deux échantillons de malades. Le premier (la série rétrospective) est constitué des malades à partir desquels Binet et coll.[2] ont établi leur classification en 1976. Cette série, mise à jour à l'occasion de notre étude, comportait 129 malades. Nous n'en avons retenu que 99 car une trentaine de malades présentait des valeurs manquantes pour l'une au moins des variables considérées dans l'analyse : ganglions cervicaux, axillaires, inguinaux, rate, foie, plaquettes, hémoglobine, âge, sexe, lymphocytose. Le recul maximal est de 193 mois.

La seconde série de malades, la série prospective, est issue du protocole randomisé LLC 76 activé en Mai 1976. Les 196 malades de cette série présentent un recul maximal de 41 mois. Les deux séries de malades ont été analysées séparément d'une part en raison du recul très différent, d'autre part en raison de la qualité des données bien supérieure lorsqu'il existe un protocole, ce qui implique un recueil prospectif.

1.2. Analyse statistique

Le critère étudié est la survie calculée à partir de la date de randomisation pour la série prospective. Pour la série rétrospective, nous avons choisi de calculer la survie à partir du début de l'observation clinique. Cette étude est réalisée alors que tous les malades ne sont pas encore décédés, donc les temps de survie se présentent sous la forme de données censurées : pour les seuls malades décédés la survie totale est connue, pour les autres on n'en connaît qu'une limite inférieure (laps de temps entre la date initiale d'observation et la date de dernière consultation) . L'analyse de ces données censurées est possible sans perte d'information grâce à des méthodes statistiques adaptées : celle de Kaplan et Meier [6] permet d'estimer des courbes de survie, et on peut chercher à expliquer la variabilité des temps de survie grâce, entre autres, au test du log-rank [7] et au modèle de Cox [8].

Dans le modèle de Cox on fait l'hypothèse que chaque malade (i) a un risque de décès instantané (ou probabilité de décès à un instant t sachant que le malade était vivant jusqu'alors), noté $r_i(t)$, qui dépend à la fois de l'instant t et d'un certain nombre de variables - celles dont on cherche à déterminer l'apport à la connaissance pronostique. Plus précisément, le logarithme de ce risque $r_i(t)$ se modélise dans le cas de 3 variables X, Y, Z par :

$$\log\left[\frac{r_i(t)}{r_o(t)}\right] = ax_i + by_i + cz_i \quad ;$$

$r_o(t)$ est une fonction du temps. Plus la valeur de la combinaison linéaire $(ax_i+by_i+cz_i)$ est élevée, plus le risque de décès instantané est élevé et donc plus est élevée la probabilité que le malade meure tôt. Ces paramètres (a, b, c) sont estimés à partir des données (X, Y, Z) et des temps de survie censurés et on peut en tester l'égalité à zéro.

Les variables retenues pour l'analyse ont été codées soit de façon binaire (tumeur palpable = 1, non palpable = 0; sexe masculin =1,féminin = 2), soit de façon continue (plaquettes, hémoglobine, âge divisés par leur valeur maximale; pour la lymphocytose on prend le logarithme divisé par 10 en raison de la distribution dissymétrique).

2. RESULTATS

La meilleure qualité des données nous a conduit à étudier en premier lieu la série prospective. Après avoir étudié l'incidence pronostique des variables retenues prises isolément, nous avons utilisé le modèle de Cox pas à pas sur ces 196 malades. La variable la plus explicative est la numération de plaquettes. Au deuxième pas la variable qui, associée aux plaquettes, permet de mieux expliquer la survie est l'hémoglobine. Puis associée aux plaquettes et à l'hémoglobine vient la palpation de la rate, dernière variable sélectionnée. Nous avions en effet décidé d'interrompre l'inclusion de variables dès que la vraisemblance maximale des paramètres (critère qui traduit la probabilité attachée à la valeur optimale de ces paramètres étant donné les valeurs des variables de base et des temps de survie censurées) n'augmenterait plus que de façon non significative. Le critère de sélection (-2 log - vraisemblance) est passé de 271.112 avec zéro variable dans le modèle à 238.760 avec les 3 variables retenues. Le modèle de Cox ainsi sélectionné s'écrit :

$$\text{Log}\left[\frac{r_i(t)}{r_o(t)}\right] = -3.70\ (\text{plaquettes}/450) - 4.70\ (\text{hémoglobine}/180) + 0.61\ (\text{rate})$$

Les tests statistiques qui permettent de juger de l'égalité à zéro de ces 3 paramètres ont respectivement les valeurs 2.70($p < 0.01$); 3.79($p < 0.01$); 1.33($p > 0.05$). Ce modèle indique l'effet péjoratif d'une thrombopénie et d'une anémie. Une splénomégalie semble aussi être un signe péjoratif, ceci de façon non significative. Ce modèle permet de calculer un score pour chaque malade, score d'autant plus élevé que la thrombopénie et l'anémie sont sévères et la rate présente. La Figure I visualise la valeur pronostique de ce score : les malades de la série prospective ont été répartis en 3 groupes (score < -5.2 ; $-5.2 \leqslant$ score < -3.4, score $\geqslant -3.4$) pour lesquels on a tracé les courbes de survie. On notera l'évolution particulièrement péjorative du troisième groupe. La valeur pronostique de ce score se trouve confirmée par la série rétrospective où l'on aboutit, avec les malades répartis en 3 groupes selon les mêmes bornes, à des courbes de survie significativement différentes (Fig. II). Le groupe de plus mauvais pronostic est bien évidemment caractérisé par une grande fréquence d'anémie ou de thrombopénie (73 % pour la série prospective, 82 % pourla série rétrospective).

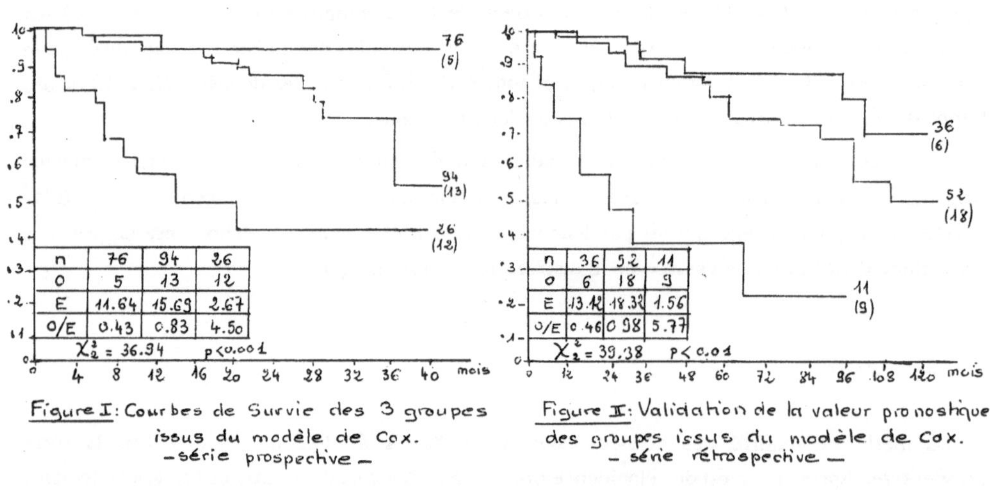

Figure I: Courbes de Survie des 3 groupes issus du modèle de Cox. – série prospective –

Figure II: Validation de la valeur pronostique des groupes issus du modèle de Cox. – série rétrospective –

Ainsi l'analyse de la série prospective et sa validation sur la série rétrospective retrouvent le caractère péjoratif de la thrombopénie et de l'anémie dont l'importance était dejà soulignée dans les autres classifications de la LLC : thrombopénie et anémie caractérisent en effet les groupes d'évolution la plus péjorative de ces classifications. La consistance de ce résultat à travers différentes séries nous a conduit à isoler les malades atteints d'anémie ou de thrombopénie (Hb $<$10g/l et/ou plaquettes $<100{,}000/mm^3$) - 27 dans la série prospective et 13 dans la série rétrospective - et d'en faire le groupe le plus péjoratif de notre classification.

Il aurait été possible de définir notre groupe le plus péjoratif par les scores les plus élevés issus du modèle de Cox plutôt que par des seuils d'anémie et de thrombopénie. Ceci ne nous a pas paru souhaitable en raison des complications supplémentaires qu'entraîne dans la pratique clinique courante le calcul d'un score pour chaque malade. D'autre part nous n'avions pas pour cette étude d'argument statistique solide pour préférer une méthode à l'autre étant donné les effectifs dont nous disposions. D'un point de vue statistique, nous rencontrons une difficulté analogue dans la définition d'un seuil : pourquoi choisir 10 g plutôt que 11 g comme seuil d'anémie ? C'est un choix essentiellement arbitraire pour lequel les arguments statistiques ne peuvent pas être décisifs en raison des faibles effectifs [9].

Nous avons poursuivi notre analyse en utilisant les sous-groupes de malades non thrombopéniques et non anémiques (169 malades dans la série prospective, 86 dans la série prospective), afin de rechercher des facteurs pronostiques qui auraient pu être masqués par le caractère très péjoratif de l'anémie et de la thrombopénie dans les groupes entiers. Le faible nombre de décès dans la série prospective (15 sur 169) nous a conduit à ne plus la privilégier dans notre analyse et à utiliser également la série rétrospective (24 décès sur 86 malades). A nouveau par une utilisation pas à pas du modèle de Cox, nous avons isolé comme facteurs les plus liés à la survie l'adénopathie inguinale et l'hépatomégalie pour les 86 malades rétrospectifs et, pour les 169 malades prospectifs, la splénomégalie et l'adénopathie axillaire. Ces résultats montrent l'importance de l'atteinte tumorale pour expliquer la survie des malades ni thrombopéniques ni anémiques. Le codage binaire des variables traduisant le syndrome tumoral nous a conduit à considérer le nombre d'aires tumorales palpables comme critère prédictif. Cet index peut varier de 0 à 5 puisque nous considérons 5 aires tumorales : les ganglions inguinaux, cervicaux et axillaires (que l'atteinte soit uni-ou bilatérale), la rate et le foie. L'étude de cet index sur les deux séries montre que globalement il détient une valeur pronostique non significativement différente de celle des scores calculés à partir de l'un ou l'autre des modèles de Cox (ceci est établi par comparaison de vraisemblances). La visualisation des courbes de survie tracées par nombre d'aires palpables nous a conduit à diviser les malades en deux groupes, selon qu'ils présentent plus ou moins de 3 aires palpables. Ces deux groupes associés au groupe des malades thrombopéniques et anémiques définissent la nouvelle classification que nous proposons (Fig. III).

Hb $\geqslant$ 10g/l et Plaquettes $\geqslant$ 100,000/mm^3	$<$ 3 aires palpables	Stade A
	$\geqslant$ 3 aires palpables	Stade B
Hb $<$ 10g/l et/ou Plaquettes $<$ 100,000/mm^3	quelque soit le nombre d'aires palpables	Stade C

Figure III : Nouvelle Classification de la LLC

Les Figures IV et V présentent les courbes de survie par stade des séries prospective et rétrospective : médianes de survie d'environ 2 ans pour le stade C, 7 ans pour le stade B et non encore atteinte pour le stade A.

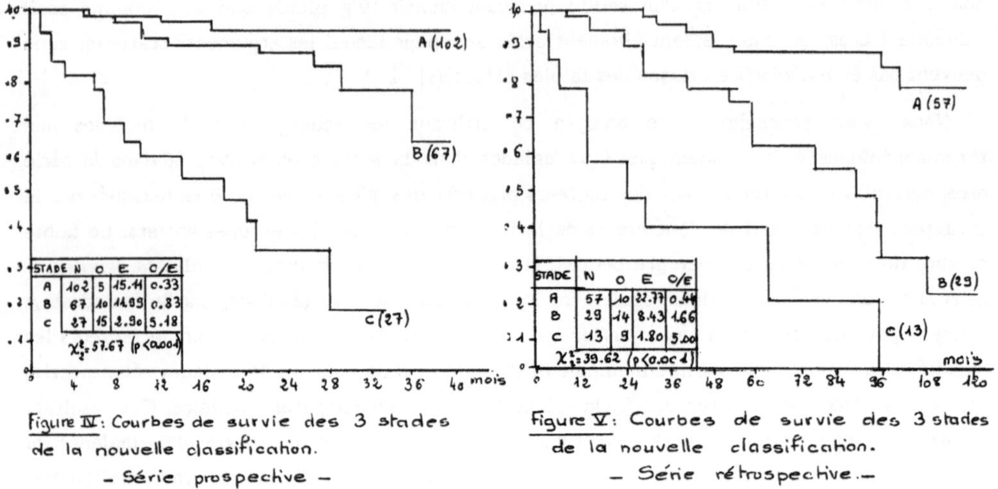

Figure IV : Courbes de survie des 3 stades de la nouvelle classification. – Série prospective –

Figure V : Courbes de survie des 3 stades de la nouvelle classification. – Série rétrospective. –

3. DISCUSSION

C'est une pratique courante dans le domaine de la cancérologie d'établir des classifications utilisées lors de la décision thérapeutique (Maladie de Hodgkin, cancer du sein,...). Bien que ces classifications aient un caractère arbitraire dû à l'aspect continu de la maladie au moment du diagnostic, elles sont néanmoins nécessaires si l'on veut adapter le traitement à la gravité.

L'étude présentée ici fournit un exemple d'élaboration d'une classification pronostique à partir d'une méthodologie statistique qui permet de prendre en compte simultanément plusieurs variables susceptibles de détenir une valeur pronostique. C'est ainsi que par des utilisations pas à pas du modèle de Cox, nous avons pu dégager l'importance de la thrombopénie et de l'anémie et, dans un second temps, celle du syndrome tumoral chez les malades non thrombopéniques et non anémiques. Ceci nous a conduit à proposer une classification en 3 stades basée sur ces variables (Fig. III).

Le but d'une telle démarche est d'une part d'améliorer la prédiction de l'évolution des malades et d'autre part d'utiliser la classification dans des essais thérapeutiques où l'on cherche à adapter le traitement au pronostic (voir à ce sujet l'article de Chastang et coll. [5]). Or on sait que des facteurs pronostiques mis en évidence dans une série de malades ne détiennent souvent pas une aussi bonne valeur pronostique dans une autre série de malades. Une étape essentielle dans l'élaboration d'une classification est donc de vérifier que sa valeur pronostique n'est pas due à un aspect particulier de l'échantillon à partir duquel elle a été établie. Une façon simple de valider la classification proposée est de la tester sur d'autres séries de malades. Lors d'une présentation de cette classification à l'occasion d'une réunion internationale sur la LLC (Paris, Novembre 1979), nous avons pu nous assurer la collaboration de 4 centres d'hématologie qui ont validé la nouvelle classification sur leurs données. Les différences entre les courbes de survie des stades A, B et C se sont retrouvées dans les 4 séries totalisant plus de 600 malades, comme en témoignent les tests du log-rank ($\chi^2_2 = 23.16$, $P < 0.001$; $\chi^2_2 = 30.15$, $p < 0.001$; $\chi^2_2 = 50.56$, $p < 0.001$; $\chi^2_2 = 27.42$, $p < 0.001$).

Le groupe coopérateur français d'étude de la LLC a adopté cette classification pour son nouveau protocole. Ce protocole vise à répondre à trois questions :

- pour le stade A, est-il nécessaire de traiter les malades par le chloraminophène, puisque leur évolution semble être bonne ?

- pour le stade B, où les malades ont une évolution intermédiaire, quelle est la valeur d'une polychimiothérapie (COP) par rapport au chloraminophène ?

- pour le stade C, où la médiane de survie se situe autour de 2 ans, est-il utile de traiter les malades par une polychimiothérapie plus aggressive (CHOP) ?

Le schéma de randomisation de la Figure VI est donc utilisé pour répondre à ces questions.

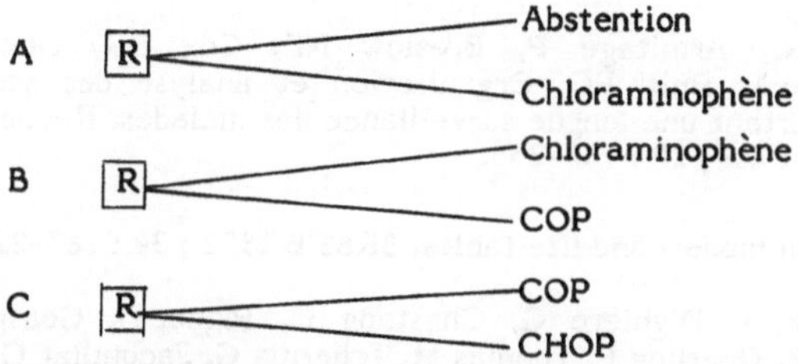

Figure VI : Schéma de randomisation du protocole LLC 80

Il s'agit donc de trois essais randomisés distincts, mais avec des traitements communs entre stades : la moitié des malades des stades A et B reçoivent du chloraminophène, la moitié des stades B et C du COP. Ces attitudes communes permettront, lors de l'analyse de ce protocole, de tester partiellement la classification chez des malades qui auront reçu un traitement homogène. Dans les séries utilisées soit pour l'élaboration soit pour la validation de la classification, il est en effet difficile de séparer l'incidence du traitement hétérogène de la valeur pronostique de la classification. Quelques comparaisons dans nos séries de malades nous laissent cependant penser que l'interaction entre traitement et classification, si elle existe, n'est que très faible.

Le protocole LLC 80 souligne l'importance d'une bonne connaissance pronostique lorsqu'on cherche à adapter le traitement à la gravité. Ces conséquences thérapeutiques justifient la réalisation d'études pronostiques planifiées et analysées à l'aide d'une méthodologie statistique adaptée.

REFERENCES

1 Rai KR, Sawitsky A, Cronkite EP, Chanana AD, Levy RN, Pasternack BS. Clinical staging of Chronic Lymphocytic Leukemia. Blood 1975 ; 46 : 219-234.

2 Binet JL, Leporrier M, Dighiero G, Charron D, D'Athis P, Vaugier G, Merle-Berat H, Natali JC, Raphael M, Nizet MG, Follezou JY. A clinical staging system for Chronic Lymphocytic Leukemia, Prognostic significance. Cancer 1977 ; 40 : 855-865.

3 Rundles RW, Moore JO. Chronic Lymphocytic Leukemia. Cancer 1978 ; 42 : 941-945.

4 Montserrat E, Rozman C. Sub-classification of stage II Chronic Lymphocytic Leukemia with prognostic implicatoins. Lancet 1979 ; 2 : 854.

5 Chastang C, Asselain B, Auquier A, Gremy F. Décision thérapeutique établie à partir de la connaissance pronostique. Problèmes méthodologiques. Proceedings MIE Toulouse, Mars 1981.

6 Kaplan E, Meier P. Non-parametric estimation from incomplete observations. J Am Stat Assoc. 1958 : 53 : 457-481.

7 Peto R, Pike MC, Armitage P, Breslow NE, Cox DR, Howard SV, Mantel N, McPherson K, Peto J, Smith PG. Organisation et analyse des essais thérapeutiques comparatifs comportant une longue surveillance des malades. Revue d'Epidémiologie et de Santé Publique, 1979 ; 27 : 167-255.

8 Cox DR. Regression models and life tables. JRSS B 1972 ; 34 : 187-220.

9 Binet JL, Auquier A, Dighiero G, Chastang C, Piguet H, Goasguen J, Vaugier G, Potron G, Colona P, Oberling F, Thomas M, Tchernia G, Jacquillat C, Boivin P, Lesty C, Duault MT, Grémy F. A new prognostic classification of Chronic Lymphocytic Leukemia derived from a multivariate survival analysis. To appear in Cancer (1981).

DIFFICULTES DANS L'ETABLISSEMENT D'UNE CLASSIFICATION PRONOSTIQUE A DES FINS DE DECISION THERAPEUTIQUE DANS LA LEUCEMIE AIGUE LYMPHOBLASTIQUE DE L'ENFANT

Cl. CHASTANG[1], M.F. AUCLERC[2], J.P. CHANTALOU[1], M. WEIL[2], Cl. JACQUILLAT[2], F. GREMY[1]

1 Groupe INSERM U 194 : Méthodologie Informatique et Statistique en Médecine, 91 bd de l'Hôpital, F-75634 Paris Cedex 13

2 Service d'Oncologie Médicale, Groupe Pitié-Salpétrière 47, bd de l'Hôpital, F-75651 Paris Cedex 13

In acute lymphoblastic leukemia, the present therapeutic progress is due to a better use of the known chemotherapy : drugs association, different ways of administration, adaptation to severity... The therapeutic adaptation is evidently based on the identification of efficient pronostic factors. Taking the remission duration as a response variable, we undertook a prognostic study of 1288 children with ALL divided into 4 groups, each receiving homogeneous treatments. The pronostic factors of the 08 LAL 74 protocol (third chronological group) are more numerous than those of the two first groups and the prognostic information is more important. The therapeutic adaptation and the modification in the nature of the first relapse could be taken as a possible explanation but this explanation cannot be proved in the absence of an experimental design. The 10 LAL 76 new protocol leads us to invalidate this hypothesis and gives moreover some results in contradiction with those of the 08 LAL 74 protocol for identical therapeutic subgroups. This fact has not yet been explained. So, the analysis of these 4 groups validates only the well-known pejorative prognostic value of a leucocytosis greater than 35000 and /or the existence of a tumoral syndrom. Therefore, the present study shows the real interest of a more rigorous methodological approach : validation of prognostic results, definition of protocols in order to show the interest of treatment adaptation to severity and inclusion of larger samples of patients.

De 1950 à 1970, la découverte de médicaments nouveaux a transformé l'évolution de la leucémie aigue lymphoblastique : alors que la mort intervenait en quelques semaines avant 1950, il est désormais possible d'obtenir, grâce à une chimiothérapie, une rémission (disparition des signes de la maladie) pour 90 % des enfants, et de prolonger cet état par l'association de différentes techniques thérapeutiques, puisque la médiane de survie atteint désormais 4 ans. En l'absence de nouvelles chimiothérapies, les hématologistes ont cherché depuis 1970, à améliorer les associations de médicaments (polychimiothérapies) et leurs modalités d'administration dans le temps.

Le groupe de chimiothérapie de la Société Française d'Hématologie a, dans cette perspective, développé des essais thérapeutiques randomisés où le traitement était adapté au pronostic. C'est ainsi que le protocole 08 LAL 74 activé en 1974 prévoyait une "agressivité" thérapeutique adaptée à un score pronostique défini à partir de l'étude de 650 malades, enfants et adultes, traités à l'Hôpital Saint-Louis de 1964 à 1973. Trois éléments prédictifs d'une évolution péjorative avaient été identifiés : âge supérieur à 15 ans, leucocytose supérieure à 35000 él./mm^3, existence d'un syndrome tumoral. La posologie de base est administrée aux malades présentant un seul critère de gravité ; en l'absence de signe de gravité, la posologie est diminuée d'un tiers ; deux ou trois critères de gravité conduisent à une posologie augmentée d'un tiers. Ce protocole ne permet donc pas de prouver l'intérêt de l'adaptation de la posologie à la gravité.

En 1980, nous avons repris l'étude pronostique de la leucémie aigue lymphoblastique de l'enfant afin de préciser la classification pronostique, outil de décision thérapeutique.

Ce papier ne vise pas à définir et à justifier une telle classification, mais présente les difficultés de cette démarche.

I. MATERIEL ET METHODES

Cette étude pronostique de la LAL concerne les enfants traités de 1964 à 1979 selon les protocoles de l'Unité de chimiothérapie de l'Hôpital Saint Louis. En effet, contrairement au travail réalisé en 1973, nous avons dissocié enfants et adultes : la LAL de l'adulte s'isole par sa symptomatologie, ses résultats thérapeutiques, ses éléments pronostiques et ses indications thérapeutiques qui en font pratiquement une maladie différente.

Schématiquement, on peut distinguer 3 groupes de malades :

Groupe I : 551 enfants inclus dans les protocoles de l'Hôpital Saint Louis de 1964 à mars 1974. Le traitement d'induction comprend prednisone et vincristine, associées éventuellement à d'autres chimiothérapies et est poursuivi par un traitement d'entretien et des réinductions. A partir de 1969, ces protocoles prévoient une prophylaxie méningée intensive (1).

Groupe II : 405 enfants du protocole coopératif 08 LAL 74 (activé d'avril 1974 à octobre 1976) qui vise à apprécier l'apport de l'endoxan à la polychimiothérapie prednisone, vincristine et daunorubicine. Ce protocole prévoit une adaptation de la posologie en fonction du score de gravité (2).

Groupe III : 332 enfants du protocole coopératif 10 LAL 76, activé de novembre 1976 à décembre 1979. Ce protocole prévoit aussi un ajustement thérapeutique à la gravité et teste l'intérêt de plusieurs associations.

L'analyse de ces données intervient nécessairement alors qu'une proportion variable de malades selon les protocoles sont vivants en rémission. Aussi, sont utilisées les méthodes adaptées à l'analyse de données tronquées : estimation de Kaplan-Meier (3), log-rank test (4) et modèle de Cox (5).

II. RESULTATS

II.1. Choix du critère de jugement

La fréquence des rechutes hématologiques et leur incidence sur le pronostic vital avaient fait choisir la rémission hématologique comme critère d'évaluation thérapeutique. Cependant, d'autres rechutes surviennent (méningée , testiculaire), aussi, nous avons décidé d'utiliser comme critère de jugement la rémission globale, délai entre la date de rémission et l'apparition de la première rechute, quelle que soit sa nature. Ce critère est utilisé sous la forme simplifiée de variable tronquée à deux modalités (rémission, rechute).

II.2. Incidence du traitement

Les malades du groupe I (1964-1974) peuvent être subdivisés en 2 sous-groupes selon l'existence d'une prophylaxie méningée, ce qui fut le cas à partir de 1969: avant 1969 le taux de rémission globale à 5 ans est de 13 %, après 1969, il est de 32 %. Par ailleurs, la nature de la première rechute (tableau II) justifie cette division.

Quant aux protocoles 08 LAL 74 et 10 LAL 76, leur analyse ne met pas en évidence de différence significative selon la nature du traitement reçu après randomisation. Aussi, l'effet thérapeutique des différents bras sera négligé.

Ainsi, cette étude pronostique envisage 4 groupes de malades : IA (1964-1968), IB (1969-1974), II (08 LAL 74), III (10 LAL 76).

II.3. Variables pronostiques

Le tableau I donne, pour chaque paramètre étudié, le degré de signification du test de log-rank et permet, de juger de la variabilité pronostique entre ces 4 échantillons : seule la leucocytose détient une valeur pronostique significative pour les 4 séries. On notera l'absence de valeur pronostique de l'atteinte médiastinale pour le protocole 08 LAL 74, résultat en contradiction avec les autres séries et avec les données de la littérature. Par ailleurs, l'étude pour les trois premiers échantillons des variables traduisant le syndrome tumoral hormis l'atteinte médiastinale (rate, foie, adénopathies, autres tumeurs) semble montrer une force pronostique croissante au cours du temps. Mais ce résultat n'est pas retrouvé dans l'analyse du protocole 10 LAL 76 dont le profil pronostique s'apparente davantage à celui du groupe IA (1964-1969).

La valeur pronostique constante du score, établi en 1973, n'est pas surprenante car traduit l'existence d'une leucocytose supérieure à 35000 et d'un syndrome tumoral, paramètres dont la valeur pronostique est constante.

	Nombre de classes	Groupe IA 1964-1969	Groupe IB 1969-1974	Groupe II Protocole 08LAL74	Groupe III Protocole 10LAL76
Nombre de malades		368	183	405	332
Malades mis en rémission		323	164	363	296
Effectif étudié		305	159	363	296
Age	5	0.05	0.50	0.12	0.14
Sexe	2	0.09	0.20	0.002	0.56
Globules blancs	5	$<10^{-4}$	$<10^{-4}$	0.04	0.02
Blastes sanguins	4	$<10^{-4}$	$<10^{-4}$	0.04	0.14
Blastes médullaires	4	0.36	0.55	0.50	0.79
Médiastin	2	$<10^{-3}$	$<10^{-3}$	0.13	$<10^{-4}$
Rate	4	0.40	0.003	0.04	0.06
Foie	4	0.10	0.03	$<10^{-3}$	0.33
Adénopathies	4	0.02	0.24	0.004	0.12
Autres tumeurs	2	0.99	0.13	0.002	0.80
Plaquettes	4	0.27	0.34	0.03	0.32
Score	3	$<10^{-3}$	$<10^{-4}$	0.002	0.007

Tableau I : Eléments pronostiques de la rémission globale : degré de signification du log-rank test (les variables quantitatives ont été polytomisées, eg globules blancs en 5 classes (1) <5000, (2) $\geq 5 < 15000$, (3) $\geq 15 < 35000$, (4) $\geq 35 < 100\ 000$, (5) $\geq 100\ 000$).

Situation en décembre 1979	Groupe IA 1964-1969		Groupe IB 1969-1974		Groupe II Protocole 08LAL74		Groupe III Protocole 10LAL76	
	♂ (183)	♀ (122)	♂ (82)	♀ (77)	♂ (211)	♀ (152)	♂ (179)	♀ (117)
Vivant en RC	11	18	23	26	73	75	112	73
Décédé en RC	19	11	3	6	15	14	5	4
Rechutes	153	93	56	45	123	63	62	40
1ère rechute hématol.	43%	45%	45%	69%	53%	82.5%	71%	82.5%
1ère rechute méningée	38%	51%	27%	24%	6.5%	9.5%	14%	15%
1ère rechute {testicul. / ovarienne	9%		10.5%		27%	1.5%	5%	
R. Hémato-méningée	6%	4%	10.5%	7%	3%	5%	5%	2.5%
R. testiculaire associée	4%		7%		10.5%	1.5%	5%	

Tableau II : Nature de la première rechute

2.4. Nature de la première rechute

La rémission globale étudie le délai de la rémission sans prendre en compte la nature de la première rechute. Or, comme le montre le tableau II, la première rechute diffère selon les protocoles. Ce tableau est simplificateur dans la mesure où n'intervient pas le délai de rechute : eg les rechutes testiculaires apparaissent plus tardivement que les rechutes hématologiques. L'introduction d'une prophylaxie méningée efficace à partir de 1969 a abouti à une réduction importante du risque méningé. Parallèlement, les rechutes testiculaires, isolées ou associées, augmentent en fréquence jusqu'au protocole 08 LAL 74, puis elles semblent diminuer dans le protocole 10 LAL 76 (3+3). Cet effectif n'est pas explicable par le faible recul actuel.

2.5. Modèle de Cox

	Groupe IA 1966-1969	Groupe IB 1971-1974	Groupe II 08LAL74	Groupe III 10LAL76
Effectif	305	159	339	253
p<0.05	Globules blancs Médiastin (SCORE) Ganglions	Globules blancs (SCORE) Médiastin Rate Foie	Foie (SCORE) rate Globules blancs Autre tumeur Sexe Blastes sanguins Plaquettes Ganglions	(SCORE) Médiastin Globules blancs Ganglions Rate
p>0.05	Sexe Age Foie Rate Autre tumeur	Ganglions Autre tumeur Sexe Age	Age Médiastin Blastes médull.	Age Blastes médull. Blastes sanguins Plaquettes Foie Autre tumeur Sexe
sous-ensemble "résumé"	Globules blancs Médiastin	Globules blancs Médiastin	Foie Autre tumeur Sexe Globules blancs	Médiastin Globules blancs Blastes médull.

Tableau III : Modèle de Cox et rémission globale

Afin d'appréhender simultanément l'information pronostique de ces variables, le modèle de Cox (5) a été appliqué à l'explication de la rémission globale. Le nombre important de valeurs manquantes a conduit à éliminer les blastes sanguins et médullaires et les plaquettes lors des analyses des protocoles 1964-1974.

Le tableau III donne donc pour chaque groupe la liste des paramètres ordonnés selon leur incidence pronostique (déduite de la vraisemblance observée avec un seul paramètre explicatif) et le sous-ensemble de paramètres résumant l'information pronostique globale (déterminé par la procédure de pas à pas ascendant). On constate l'absence de continuité pronostique au cours du temps (qui serait restituée si l'on "supprimait" soit le protocole 08 LAL 74, soit le protocole 10 LAL 76). Nous avons établi une classification pronostique en 3 groupes à partir du protocole 08 LAL 74 dont l'application aux autres protocoles aboutit à une différence significative (p=0.01) seulement pour le groupe IB (1969-1974).

A l'exception du protocole 08 LAL 74 pour lequel il est possible d'individualiser 3 groupes d'effectif équivalent, la même démarche utilisant le modèle de Cox permet seulement d'isoler un faible pourcentage de malades dont l'évolution est péjorative : leucocytose supérieure à 35000 et atteinte médiastinale (l'association de ces deux critères ou l'existence isolée d'une leucocytose supérieure à 100 000 renforce la gravité). Il s'agit de 91 malades du Groupe IA (305), 35 malades du Groupe IB (159) et 85 du protocole 10 LAL 76 (296).

Ce résultat - subdivision en 2 classes pronostiques - n'est pas contradictoire avec la valeur prédictive du score à 3 modalités : en effet, les scores 1 et 2 sont peu différents dans leur évolution et le score 3 est attribué aux sujets présentant une leucocytose supérieure à 35000 et/ou une atteinte médiastinale.

III. DISCUSSION

L'analyse pronostique de 4 groupes d'enfants présentant une leucémie aigue lymphoblastique conduit à des résultats contradictoires qui ne nous permettent pas d'isoler des facteurs pronostiques stables. D'autre part, ces analyses ne prennent pas en compte des éléments dont l'importance n'est probablement pas négligeable.

III.1. Résultats contradictoires

L'interprétation des résultats ne pose pas de difficultés jusqu'au protocole 08 LAL 74. En effet, les protocoles 1969-1974 assurent une amélioration de la durée de la rémission, probablement due à la prophylaxie méningée, et permettent l'apparition de nouveaux facteurs pronostiques.

Le protocole 08 LAL 74 améliore à nouveau la rémission globale, ce qu'on ne peut pas imputer de façon causale à l'adaptation de la posologie à la thérapeutique, en l'absence de randomisation entre dose standard et dose adaptée. La comparaison, à score constant, des protocoles IB (1969-1974) et du 08 LAL 74 montre des résultats identiques pour le score 1, un léger bénéfice au score 2, et une différence significative au score 3 (10 % et 32 % de rémission à 5 ans). Ainsi, on pourrait avancer l'interprétation suivante : l'adaptation de la posologie tend d'une part à annuler les éléments de pronostic péjoratif (leucocytose, atteinte médiastinale) et d'autre part, l'amélioration résultante permet à de nouveaux facteurs pronostiques d'émerger d'autant plus que la rémission s'achève sous des formes nouvelles (rechute testiculaire).

Cette hypothèse est appuyée par l'étude, chez les garçons du 08 LAL 74, des éléments pronostiques de la rechute hématologique et de la rechute testiculaire : aucun paramètre n'est pronostique de la rechute hématologique alors que globules blancs, blastes sanguins et plaquettes sont des éléments pronostiques de la 1ère rechute testiculaire.

Le protocole 10 LAL 76 est de conception voisine de celle du 08 LAL 74 (drogues, agressivité thérapeutique selon la gravité). Donc, on pouvait, a priori, s'attendre à observer des résultats analogues : durée de rémission, nature de la 1ère rechute et éléments pronostiques.

Si ces 2 protocoles ne sont pas différents quant à la durée de la rémission, la nature de la première rechute et ses éléments pronostiques les opposent. Cette discordance est soulignée par l'existence d'un bras commun : la moitié des malades du 08 LAL 74 et le quart de ceux du protocole 10 LAL 76 ont fait l'objet de la même attitude thérapeutique. Ces 2 groupes sont homogènes quant aux variables pronostiques. La nature de la première rechute apparaît différente : par exemple, 23 rechutes testiculaires sont dénombrées parmi 107 garçons du 08 LAL 74 alors qu'une seule est apparue dans le bras identique du 10 LAL 76 (44 garçons) ($p < 0.10$, log-rank test). Nous n'avons pas, pour l'instant, d'explication de ces modifications observées au cours du temps. Les premières hypothèses à vérifier concernent l'application effective des modalités thérapeutiques.

III.2. Eléments non pris en compte dans cette étude pronostique

III.2.1. L'analyse du critère de jugement utilisé - durée de rémission globale - ne prend pas en compte la nature de la rechute (6).

III.2.2. L'analyse des protocoles 08 LAL 74 et 10 LAL 76 ne fait pas intervenir l'adaptation de la posologie à la gravité. Or l'analyse des résultats du 08 LAL 74 et du 10 LAL 76 montre un "resserrement" des courbes relatives aux 3 scores, sans qu'il soit possible d'affirmer que cet aspect est lié à l'adaptation thérapeutique en l'absence d'un protocole rigoureux.

III.2.3. Cette analyse n'étudie pas, en raison du trop grand nombre de valeurs manquantes, des paramètres dont la valeur pronostique est affirmée par de nombreux auteurs : classification cytologique FAB, lymphocytes T.

CONCLUSION

Cette analyse pronostique de la rémission globale de la leucémie aigue lymphoblastique de l'enfant montre la fragilité des conclusions d'une étude pronostique: une même attitude thérapeutique conduit à des résultats variables dans le temps, et le traitement est susceptible d'interférer avec les éléments pronostiques. Pour pallier ces difficultés, il convient donc de planifier des protocoles parfaitement rigoureux, prévoyant des bras communs au fil des protocoles, permettant d'apporter la preuve de toute action grâce à une procédure expérimentale. Par ailleurs, ces protocoles doivent inclure un grand nombre de malades (plusieurs centaines) et ce d'autant plus qu'on cherche à adapter le traitement à la gravité.

REFERENCES

1 Jacquillat Cl, Weil M, Auclerc MF, Auclerc G, Chastang Cl, Flandrin G, Izrael V, Schaison G, Degos L, Boiron M, Bernard J. Prognosis and treatment of acute lymphoblastic leukemia. Study of 650 patients. Cancer Chemother Pharmacol. 1978, 1, 113-122.

2 Jacquillat Cl, Weil M, Auclerc MF, Schaison G, Chastang Cl, Harousseau JL, Bauters F, Olive D, Griscelli Cl, Bonnet M, Lamagnere JP, Bernard J. Applications de l'étude des facteurs pronostiques au traitement des leucémies aigues lymphoblastiques de l'enfant (< 20 ans). Le protocole 08 LAL 74. Actua Hématol. 1980, 14, 152-169.

3 Kaplan EL, Meier P. Non parametric estimation from incomplete observations. J Am Stat Assoc. 1958, 53, 457-481.

4 Peto R, Pike MC, Armitage P, Breslow NE, Cox DR, Howard SW, Mantel N, Mc Pherson K, Peto J, Smith PG. Design and analysis of randomized clinical trials requiring prolonged observation of each patient. I. Introduction and design. Br J Cancer, 1976, 34, 485-512. II. Analysis and examples, Br J Cancer, 1977, 35, 1-39.

5 Cox DR. Regression models and life-tables (with discussion). J R Statis Soc, 1972, B34, 187-220.

6 Prentice RL, Kalbfleisch JD, Peterson AV, Flournoy N, Farewell VT, Breslow NE. The analysis of failure time date in the presence of competing risks. Biometrics, 1978, 34, 541-554.

A HEURISTIC MEDICAL DECISION MAKING ALGORITHM AT A TROMBOSIS CENTRE

Hein C. Bisterbosch, Herman H. P. J. Lemkes, Ria J. Boekhout-Mussert and Albert M. Vossepoel

BAZIS, University Hospital,
Rijnsburgerweg 10 2333 AA Leiden
The Netherlands

ABSTRACT

An algorithm for computer assisted coagulation control is presented. An existing algorithm based on a pharmaco-kinetic model was insufficiently accepted by the physicians using it.
In close co-operation with the physicians a decision-tree approach was developed which gained an obvious high acceptance.
The resulting dosage proposals were divided into three output flows: "no", "experimental" and "good" proposals. The "good" proposals, 40 % of all cases, do not require inspection by the physician any more.

1.0 INTRODUCTION

The aim of oral anticoagulant therapy is to prevent thrombo-embolic phenomena by reducing a patient's blood clotting activity to within an individually assessed therapeutic range (between 5 and 10 % Thrombotest for most of the patients).

The response of a patient to anticoagulants strongly depends on:
- the individual patient's sensitivity to anticoagulants, which may change over a period of time
- other medications
- illness
- eating and drinking habits

Thus, the control of the patient's coagulation time is made difficult by external influences.

The long term character of therapy with oral anticoagulants is apparent from the fact that one third of all patients receive treatment with anticoagulants for one year or longer.

In the Netherlands, the anticoagulant therapy is often delegated to regional specialized Thrombosis Centres, such as the Leiden Thrombosis Centre (LTC), with:
- 5400 out-patients
- 88000 prescriptions yearly
- 12 staffing (2 physicians)
- 14 out-patients clinics

The centre services a region with 400.000 inhabitants.

1.1 METHODS

The anticoagulants used are phenprocoumon and acenocoumarol.
The assay method used for measuring the coagulation time is Thrombotest time according to Owren.

At LTC, the real time Information System for Thrombosis Centres (ISTC), is in full operational use since 1974 [1,2].
ISTC shares the facilities of the integrated Hospital Information System (HIS) of Leiden University Hospital [3].

The communication between ISTC and its users is strictly conversational, in contrast with current practice elsewhere [4,5,6].
Typical response times are in the order of 1 second, also at peak-load times, which is about 100 times faster than with a microcomputer approach [7].
Video display units are used to exchange information with physicians and nurses of LTC.

1.2 PREVIOUS EXPERIENCE WITH A CLINICAL DECISION MAKING MODEL

From 1974 up to November 1980 we have been working with a computer assisted anticoagulant control system based on a pharmaco-kinetic model.
In this model the patients anticoagulant history was condensed in 3 individual parameters; the anticoagulant level, the sensitivity to anticoagulant and the rate of change in this sensitivity.
The parameters in this system were tuned statistically.
A proposal consisted of a calculated dosage and a calculated appointment period.

In practice, the elaborate pharmaco-kinetic model did not perform as well as expected because:

- the physician could not understand why the computer made a specific proposal;
- the physician often judges a patient case in a rather empirical way. If he "feels" that a patients coagulation time is on its way to the target value in the therapeutic range, he continues with the former same dosage and appointment period.

The whole medical history with, where possible, a dosage and appointment period proposal, is printed at each visit of a patient. It is for use by the physician, who checks all proposals and gives a prescription to patients without a proposal.

The percentage of patient cases which got a prescription whitout physici intervention shows large variation over time as may be illustrated by the following table:

1975	1976	1977	1978	1979	until 1980-11-11	after 1980-11-11
41 %	55 %	63 %	56 %	40 %	41 %	57 %

Note that the figures up to 11-11-1980 relate to patients using phenprocoumon only, the figure after 11-11-1980 is related to patients using phenprocoumon as well as patients using acenocoumarol.

1.3 DEVELOPMENT OF THE DECISION TREE

To achieve a greater degree of acceptance of the proposals, we decided to develop a "decision tree" which should incorporate all the empirical rules the physicians are using.
Only for the calculation of dosage adjustments a simplified pharmaco-kinetic model is used.
The decision tree is a heuristic algorithm incorporating a sequential decision-making process in which the patient cases are divided into specific subclasses.

Our purposes were threefold:

- With regard to the individual patient:
  To give him such an optimal combination of dosage and appointment period, that the chance of the coagulation time going above or below the therapeutic range is minimal, and the length of the appointment period is maximal.
- With regard to the control system:
  To maximize the percentage of patient cases for which it is possible to give a proposal, and
  to increase the acceptance of the proposals up to an ideal 100 %.
  Also to limit the usage of the system to patients with a reasonable predictable behaviour.
- With regard to the physician:
  The proposals are given by the empirical algorithm according to strict rules that are defined together with the physicians.
  The algorithm is not subject to individual feelings as the physicians are. Because classes of proposals that turn out to be always 100 % accepted do not require inspection anymore, the physician can be partially replaced.
  The "good" proposals can be authorized automatically by the system.

Most of the patients have the following therapeutic range:

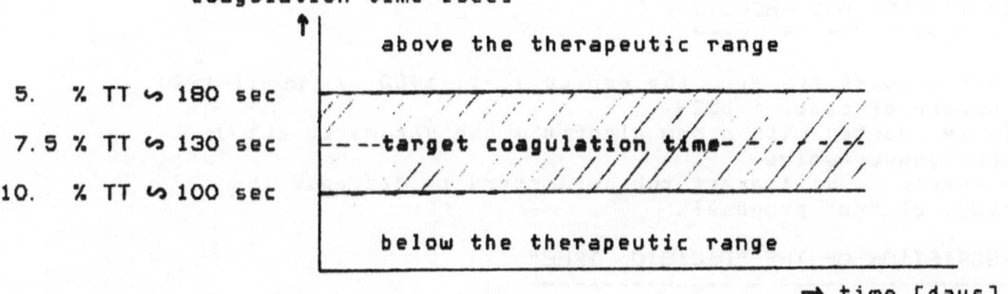

The aim of coagulation control is to keep the patients coagulation time (CP) within in therapeutic range in course of treatment.

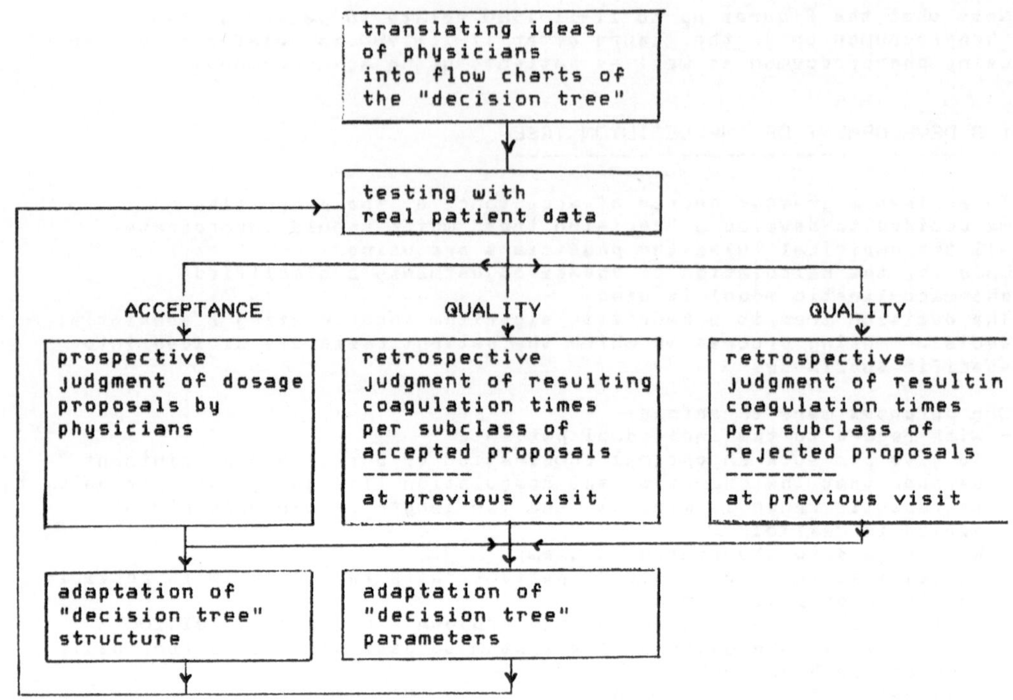

In this iterative process the structure of the "decision tree" was define(and a preliminary adjustment of the parameters was performed.
In this way we developed our heuristic medical decision making algorithm.
Although its structure is fixed in the computer program, all the algorithm's parameters can be altered on line.
We are continuously working on further optimization of the algorithm's parameters to increase the percentage of "good" proposals.

2.0 REALISATION AND RESULTS

The shown results are from the period 11-11-1980 / 28-11-1980
Total number of cases = 5329
Because we started with a new algorithm the parameter set-up is rather conservative.
In the future we will adapt the parameters to decrease the percentage of "no" proposals.

2.1 DESCRIPTION OF THE "DECISION TREE"

The heuristic algorithm has the following functions:
- judging the medical history, while taking into account:
    the number of previous appointments

. starting and stopping with medicines that interfere with the anticoagulant used
. remarks entered by nurse or physician during the last appointment period
. actual and previous coagulation time

- classifying the patient's case into one of the three main categories by a system of heuristic rules and boundary conditions.
  These 3 categories ,"no" proposal, "experimental" proposal or "good" proposal are printed in 3 separate flows.
  This is for the use of the physicians who authorize these proposals for each category separately.
  The main categories have, amongst others, the following different properties:
  . "no" proposal: the algorithm judges itself incapable of making a proposal for this case, e.g. patients using interfering medicines or having strongly varying coagulation times.
  . "experimental" proposal: the dosage proposed by the algorithm is changed compared with the patient's previous one.
    The "experimental"proposals are intended to be critically reviewed by the physicians.
  . "good" proposal: the dosage proposed by the algorithm is equal to the patient's previous dosage
    The "good" proposals are intended to be authorized automatically in the future, requiring a continuous acceptance of 100 %.
- assigning a specific subclassification number to the patients case in the heuristic decision-making algorithm.
  On the medical history is printed at each visit of the patient, an explanatory text according to the specific subclassification number.
- determining the appointment period.

The 3 flows can be described by the following diagram:

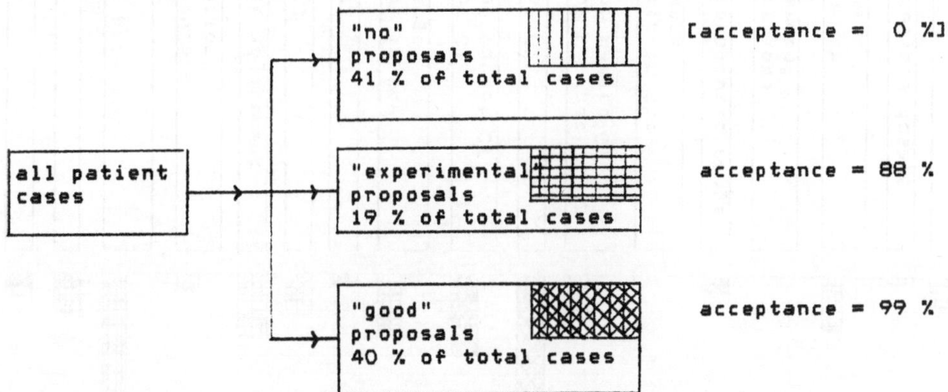

So in 57 % of all patient cases a prescription is made without physician intervention (cf. the table in section 1.2).

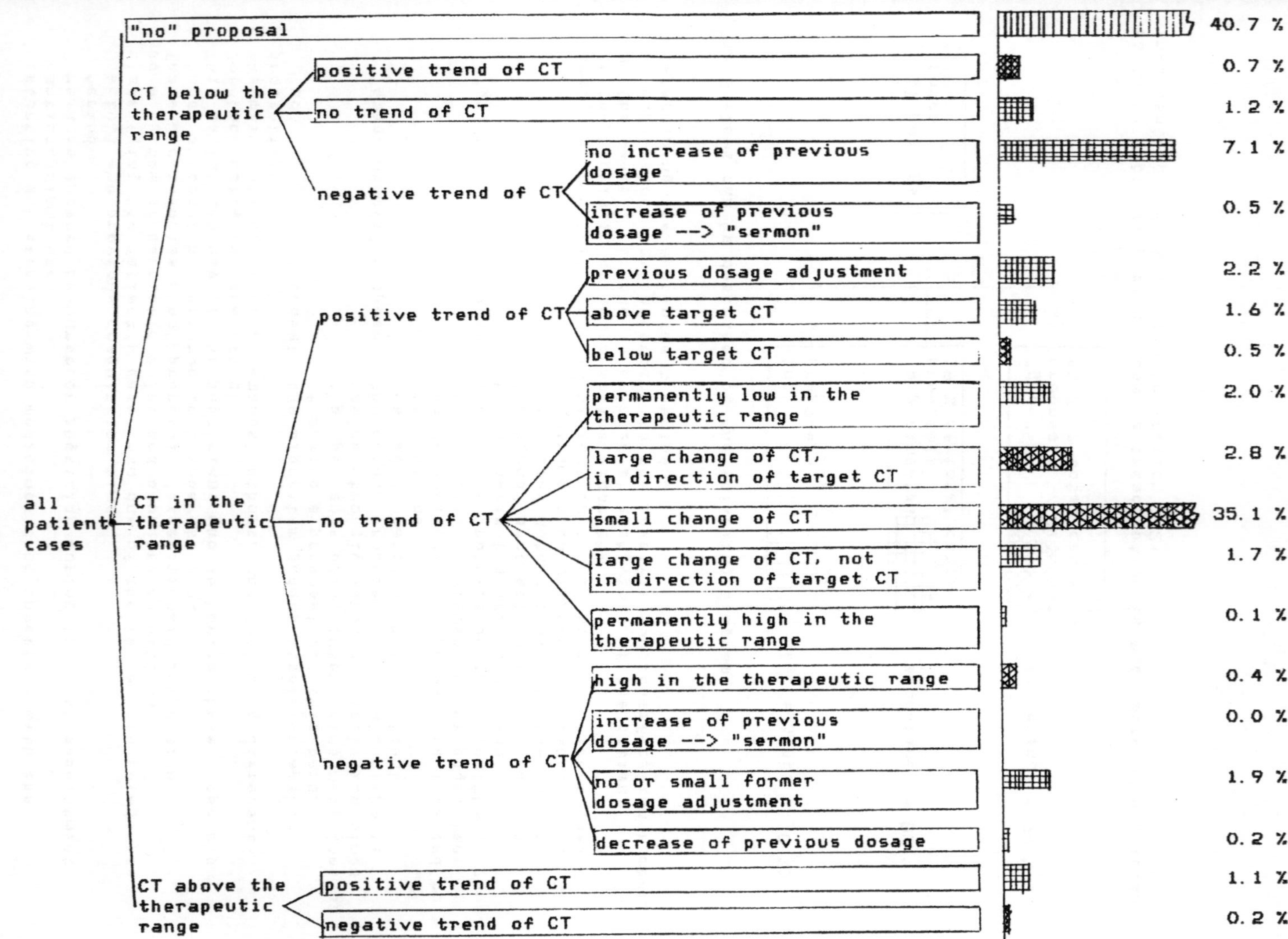
"no" proposal
CT below the therapeutic range
positive trend of CT
no trend of CT
no increase of previous dosage
negative trend of CT
increase of previous dosage --> "sermon"
previous dosage adjustment
positive trend of CT
above target CT
below target CT
permanently low in the therapeutic range
large change of CT, in direction of target CT
all patient cases
CT in the therapeutic range
no trend of CT
small change of CT
large change of CT, not in direction of target CT
permanently high in the therapeutic range
high in the therapeutic range
increase of previous dosage --> "sermon"
negative trend of CT
no or small former dosage adjustment
decrease of previous dosage
CT above the therapeutic range
positive trend of CT
negative trend of CT
40.7 %
0.7 %
1.2 %
7.1 %
0.5 %
2.2 %
1.6 %
0.5 %
2.0 %
2.8 %
35.1 %
1.7 %
0.1 %
0.4 %
0.0 %
1.9 %
0.2 %
1.1 %
0.2 %

2.2 CALCULATION OF DOSAGE ADJUSTMENT

When the algorithm decides that a dosage adjustment is necessary, it aims for the target coagulation time in the patients therapeutic range.

The heuristic algorithm does not use curve fitting of previous dosages.

$$\frac{\text{New dosage}}{\text{Old dosage}} = \left(\frac{\text{corrected target coagulation time}}{\text{corrected actual coagulation time}} \right)^{[\text{dose-effect ratio}]^{-1}}$$

The method of correction is determined by the assay method used to measure the coagulation time.

It is clear that the dose-effect ratio is the most important parameter in this formula.
Previous investigation [2] has shown that the calculated dose-effect ratio strongly varies from patient to patient.
However, for the individual patient this parameter is very hard to obtain with sufficient accuracy.

So we have to resort to choose one value for all patients.
In order to select this value we simulated the patient's response to a dosage adjustment for different values of the dose-effect ratio.
The physicians chose the value of 6, which for them, was most acceptable.

2.3 OPTIMIZATION OF THE CLASSIFICATION IN THE "DECISION TREE"

For each class in the decision tree we measure the stability of the classification.
I.e., we measure at the next visit of the patient whether the coagulation time is below, above or within the therapeutic range.

2.4 ACCEPTANCE

The acceptance of a class of proposals strongly depends on the individual physician.
Previous experience has taught us that the physicians use the system optimally if they only change the proposals they strongly disagree with [2].
Retrospective evaluation reveals whether changes in the proposals were essential or marginal.
Furthermore, this evaluation teaches us about the acceptability in each subclass, which may lead to adaptation in the characteristics of the subclass.

2.5 QUALITY

Evaluation of the resulting coagulation time, at the next appointment of the patient, is set up to improve quality of decision making by both ISTC and physician. In the case of accepted proposals it reveals for each subclass the quality of the ISTC and physician.
In the case of changed proposals the ISTC is able to predict a resulting coagulation time based on the dose-effect relation.
This predicted value can be compared with the actual value, at the next appointment of the patient, resulting from intervention by the physician.

3.0 CONCLUSIONS

The proposals of the formerly used purely pharmaco-kinetic model were hard to understand for the physicians.
So we developed in close co-operation with the physicians a decision-tree that splits up the individual patient cases into subclasses.
Only a dosage adjustment is calculated by a simplified pharmaco-kinetic model. This approach gained a high degree of acceptance among the physicians.

A practical result is that a separate output flow of "good" proposals can be split off. These proposals, having an acceptance of 100 % can be authorized automatically. In this way the physicians are partially replaced by the medical decision making algorithm.

With the subclassification approach we obtained the tools to measure and improve the quality and acceptance of each specific subclass separately.

REFERENCES

1. Wiegman, H. and A.M. Vossepoel(1977) A computer program for long-term anticoagulation control, Comp. Progr. Biomed. 7, 71-84
2. Vossepoel, A.M., and H. Wiegman(1977) Computer assisted medical practice in anticoagulation control: theory, practice and evaluation, in: Medical Computing, eds. M.Laudet et al. (Taylor & Trancis, London) pp. 375-389; also in: Med. Inform. 2, 125-140.
3. Bakker, A.R.(1977) Implementation approach and evaluation of the use of Leiden University Hospital Information System, in: Medinfo 77 eds. D.B. Shires and H. Wolf(North- Holland, Amsterdam) pp. 943-947
4. Sheiner, L.B.(1969) Computer-aided long-term anticoagulation therapy, Comput., Biomed. Res. 2, 507-518.
5. Hoffer, E.P., K.D. Marble, P.M. Yurchak, G.O.Barnett(1975) A computer-based information system for managing patients on long-term oral anticoagulants, Comput. Biomed. Res. 8, 573-579
6. Visser, J.(1976) Manual for automation of out-patient anticoagalation treatment, (in Dutch: Handleiding voor de automatisering van poliklinische antistolbehandeling), (Ziekenhuis de Weezenlanden, Zwolle)
7. Powers, W.F., P.H. Abbrecht and D.G. Covell Systems and Microcomputer Approach to Anticoagulant Therapy IEEE Trans. Biomed. Eng. 27(1980) 520-523

COLON AND RECTAL CARCINOMA, REGISTRATION OF A PROSPECTIVE TRIAL

T. Wiggers* and G.I.H. van Wandeloo**

* Surgical Department St. Annadal Hospital (head: Prof.Dr.J.M.Greep)

** Data processing Department (head: Drs.J.Jager)

State University Limburg, Maastricht, The Netherlands.

Introduction

Cancer of the large intestine is a disease with an increasing incidence in the Western countries. With the current surgical technics the survival figures have reached a steady level (1). With the question how to improve these results, two prospective trials were started in January 1979. In one trial different surgical technics are used. In the second trial pre-operative radiotherapy is used. A multi-institutional study was started in 7 hospitals in the Southern part of the Netherlands to become a sufficient number of patients for statistical analysis. At the first admission an inquiry form containing 80 different items have to be filled. Follow-up is organised during a period of five years using a fixed scedule (figure 1). All laboratory values and investigations have the intention to estimate the disease free interval. If the patient shows a recurrent disease then all these investigations are no longer necessary and the day of his death is recorded only.

follow-up

Maanden *	3	6	12	18	24	30	36	42	48	54	60
Lab.chemie (zie protocol)	X	X	X	X	X	X	X	X	X	X	X
CEA	X	X	X	X	X	X	X	X	X	X	X
X-thorax		X		X		X		X		X	
X-colon		X		X				X			
Scintigrafie		X		X		X		X		X	
Recto / coloscopie		X				X				X	

*) = months

figure 1

We needed a very good registration system to get reliable figures for analysis (2). The participants had to be motivated to keep their administration well organised and to produce their data in time. It quickly became evident that we needed computer facilities both for administration and statistical analysis.

Demands

Our demands can be summarised as follows:

1. to register the data of all patients;
2. to print listings and verify these data;
3. to have summary print-outs for the participating specialists which are suitable for their patient files;
4. to consult, to add to and to modify the obtained data;
5. to print periodically follow-up forms with only the necessary questions;
6. to check every month whether the completed follow-up forms are sent back;
7. to allow authorised persons only to enter to the data;
8. finally to make statistics possible.

System design

The system designed had the following characteristics:

1. it was developed on a VAX 11/780 and the input was done via a terminal;

2. the interactive procedures were developed in Datatrieve-11;
3. the batch programs were written in COBOL;
4. a statistical application was made for SPSS (Statistical Package for the Social Sciences).

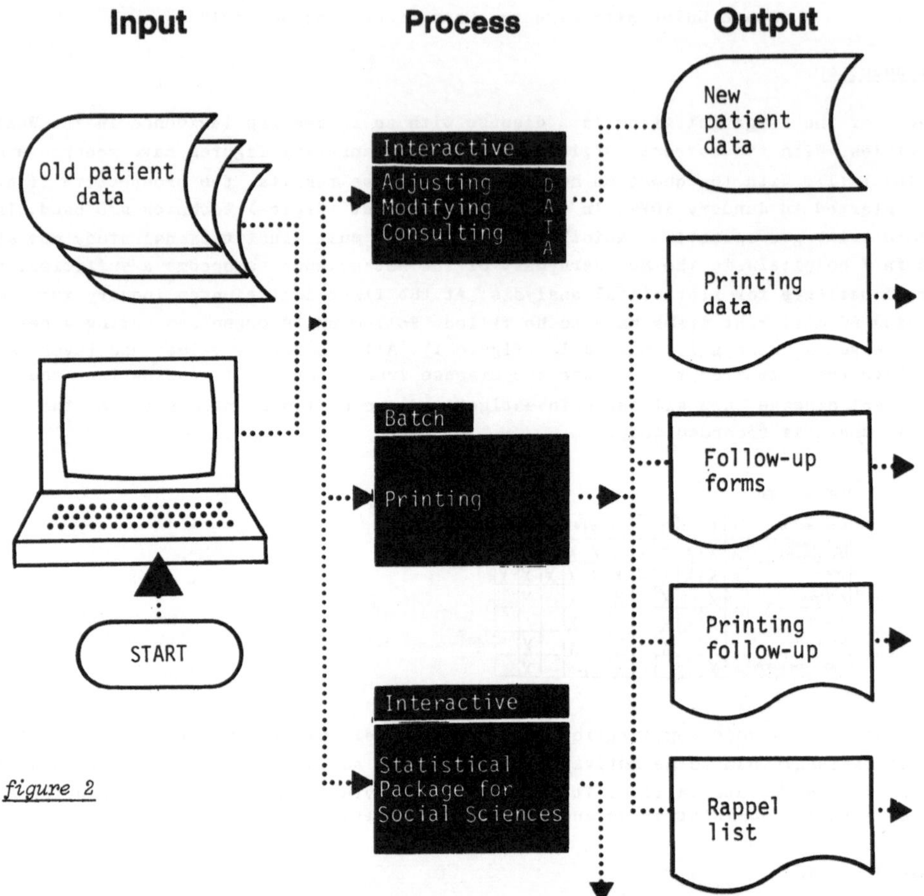

figure 2

In figure 2 you see the scedule with on the left the necessary input and on the right the output.

Results

100 Patients are entered yearly. 300 Pre-printed follow-up forms are sent out and entered after filling. To enter, modify and consult these data, a special procedure has been made (figure 3). By typing one of the commands a procedure is automatically started and shows sequentially all the required items and the number of the right question has to be typed only. The program screens for non logic errors during the run. The batch program is started by the command: print. This program has several procedures to print the right listings, follow-up forms, error-lists and rappel-lists. All these procedures are done automatically. F.e. if a patient has died in the post-operative phase you can enter the data as if he was still living. At the moment you type the date of his death the program stops producing follow-up forms and keeps the data for statisti-

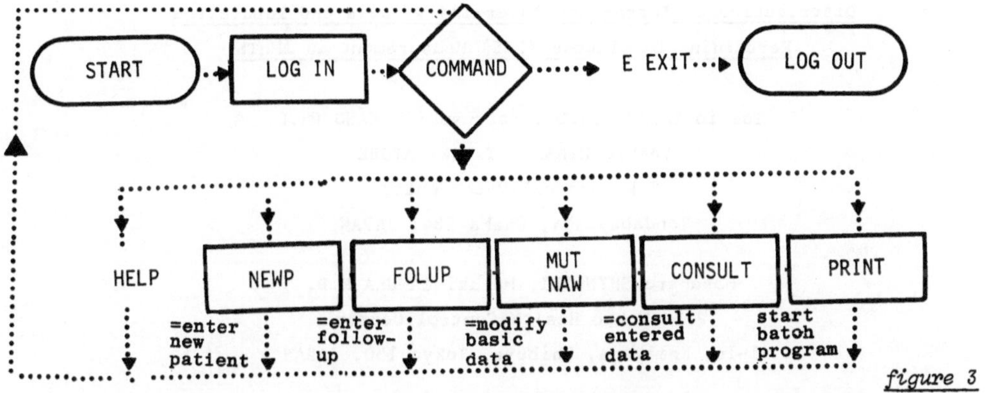

figure 3

cal analysis only. If during the follow-up definite signs of recurrent disease are detected the computer stops asking all the necessary questions which were necessary to detect these recurrence and in the next form only the day of his death and adjuvant therapy are asked for. A list of missing data is printed every month if completed follow-up forms are not entered in time.

Trialnr 223851980402

History dd 21-07-80

1.01 First symptom	: Bloodloss per anum
1.02 Current bowel habits	: Not changed
1.03 First symptom-admission	: Within 1 year
1.04 First symptom-G.P. visit	: Within 1 year
1.05 Previous bowel diseases	: None
1.06 Appendectomy	: No
1.07 Time previous bowel diseases	: Not applicable
1.08 Family history	: Negative

Laboratory investigation dd 25-07-80

figure 4

Here you see an example of a part of the summary of the input data. It is printed in a proper size and can be kept in the participating specialists' patients file. All these data can be used for statistical analysis. We have the possibility of using SPSS.

Conclusion

A system has been designed to help both administration and statistical analysis of this colon and rectal carcinoma trial. The system fullfils our demands and can be run in the hospital on a selfreliant base without specific knowledge of computers.

References

(1) Olson RM, Perencevick NP, Malcolm AW, Chaffey JT. Patterns of recurrence following curative resection of adenocarcinoma of the colon and rectum. Cancer 1980; 45: 2969-2974.

(2) Mzabi R, Himal HS, Demers R, Maclean LD. A multiparametric computer analysis of carcinoma of the colon. Surg, Gyn and Obst. 1976; 143: 959-964.

Distribution of Intra- and Inter-Individuals and Population Pertaining to Glucose (FBS) Measurement in AMHTS

Toshio YASAKA Ph.D., Katsuyuki NAKANO Ph.D.
Yoshio HIRAKI, Takaki ATOBE
P.L. Medical Data Center
Tondabayashi, Osaka 584, JAPAN

Masaharu SHINBORI, Masaki TAMURA M.D.
P.L. Tokyo Health Control Center
1-16, Kamiyama, Shibuya, Tokyo 150, JAPAN

An intensive study on the relationships among the intra-individual, the inter-individual and the population distributions has been performed in order to give further understanding to the 'normality' of test results. The test results of more than 15 regular visits by 737 patients to an automated multiphasic testing system are used to estimate the inter-individual distribution which would have been impossible to attempt otherwise. This paper concentrates on glucose results to clarify the situation.

1. INTRODUCTION

The P.L. (Perfect Liberty) Health Control System has accumulated, in it's ten year operation, the members' semi-annual test results at the P.L. Medical Data Center, equipped with an IBM 3031 system using D/B and D/C systems. These periodical test results, easily accessible due to the IDAM system (1) were investigated and reported on their clinical significance (2, 3) and the concept of 'subject specific physiological fluctuation ranges' or, the individual normal range, was developed. In order to cope with observing the individual fluctuations which is sometimes very small compared with the range of population, the long-term quality control, it was found, is a vital necessity and its errors are not admissible (4).

The delicate situation, required to deal with the small changes and the long term quality control error in measurements, necessitated us to look into the problem of distribution types, and some of experiences on this problem were reported already due to our advantages that there are 15 or measurements pertaining to each individual (5).

This paper, concentrating on the fasting blood sugar or glucose measurement, describes the method of identifying the intra- and inter-individual distribution, and some clinical significances of the resultant distributions.

2. MATERIALS AND METHODS

At their semi-annual check-up, blood was drawn from the P.L. Health Control members in a seated position between 9:00 am and 11:00 am after at least 10 hours of fasting after the previous day's evening meal. Members were socially active executives, professionals or factory owners etc., and their spouses.

The Technicon SMA 12/60 has been used throughout the time during which the blood samples used in the present study were analyzed for such factors as, CPK, calcium, total protein, cholesterol, glucose, uric acid, albumin, A/G, LDH, SGOT, alkaline phosphate, total bilubrin and BUN. Similarly, the Colter Model S was utilyzed for hematology measurements throughout this period.

The population demography, grouped by sex and age is given in Table 1, and the results from each individual are 15 or more.

Table 1. Subjects grouped according to sex and age

age group	20's	30's	40's	50's	60's	70's-	total
male	4	60	129	126	88	22	429
female	1	27	105	105	61	9	308
total	5	87	234	231	149	31	737

The individuals are grouped according to their age at the 8th examination which is located in the middle of the 15 examinations.

The population distribution in its ordinary sense (from whatever source the materials are obtained - a hospital outpatient department, an aerial survey, or anywhere else) is a distribution of a single sample from each individual which contains both the variation due to the individual's specificity and that due to within the individual's fluctuation.

Let us denote the single sample distribution by $f(x|\mu,\sigma^2)$ in terms of its density function, whatever the type of distribution; the distribution of means by $f_m(\bar{x}_{i\cdot}|\mu_m,\sigma_m^2)$; and the distributions of individuals by $f_i(x_{ij}|\mu_i,\sigma_i^2)$. Then it follows, that

$$\hat{\mu} = \bar{x} \text{ and } \hat{\sigma}^2 = s_x^2 \quad \text{from} \quad f(x|\mu,\sigma^2),$$

$$\text{that} \quad \hat{\mu}_i = \bar{x}_{i\cdot} \text{ and } \hat{\sigma}_i^2 = s_i^2 \quad \text{from} \quad f_i(x_{ij}|\mu_i,\sigma_i^2)$$

$$\text{and that} \quad \hat{\mu}_m = \bar{\hat{\mu}}_i \text{ and } \hat{\sigma}_m^2 = s_{\hat{\mu}_i^2} \quad \text{from} \quad f_m(x_{i\cdot}|\mu_m,\sigma_m^2)$$

whereas from the point of view of the joint distribution of the intra- and inter-individual distribution (Figure 1),

$$\text{(i)}\quad \hat{\mu} = \hat{\mu}_m = \bar{x}.. ,\ \hat{\sigma}^2 = s_G^2 + s_P^2$$

where $s_G^2 = \hat{\sigma}_m^2$ and $s_P^2 = \bar{\hat{\sigma}}_i^2$. Now,

$$\text{(ii)}\quad \hat{\sigma}_m^2 \doteqdot s_m^2 = s_G^2 + \frac{1}{n} s_P^2$$

since theoretically each μ_i has a variance of $\frac{1}{n}\cdot\sigma_i^2$, and when n is large $s_m^2 = s_G^2$ and thus $\hat{\sigma}_m^2 = s_G^2$ which is, for all practical purposes, $s_G^2 = s_{\hat{\mu}_i}^2$. In this study n = 15, therefore s_m^2 includes 6, 7% of the intra-individual variance. Therefore, it follows that

$$\text{(i')}\quad \hat{\sigma}^2 = s_{\hat{\mu}_i}^2 + \bar{\hat{\sigma}}_{i\cdot}^2$$

Figure 1 Concept for constructing the single sample distribution of the population from the distribution of sample means and sample distributions of individuals (for details, see text)

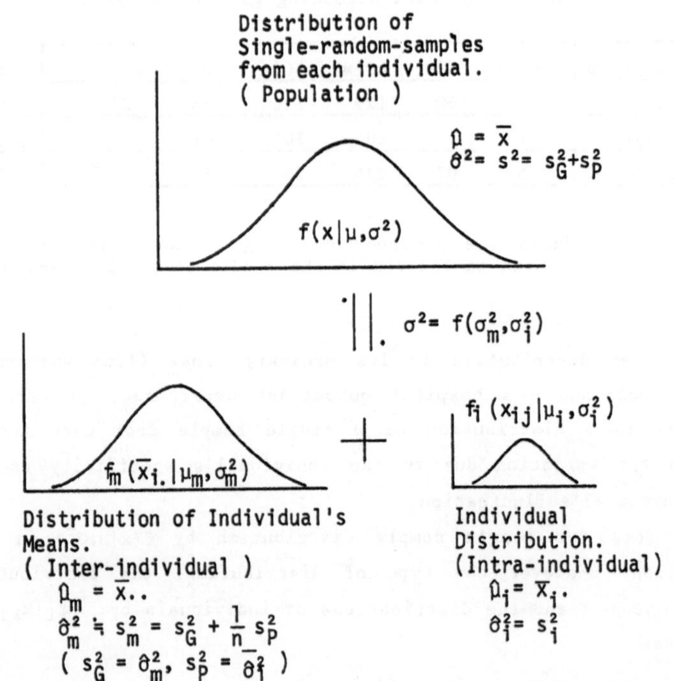

The distribution types are examined with respect to the three distributions: $f(x)$, $f_m(\bar{x}_i)$ and $f_i(x_{ij})$. Actually, a set of various types of transformations (including the transformations $y = x$, $\ln x$, $x^{1/2}$, $(\ln x)^{1/2}$, $(\ln x)^{1/3}$, x^2, $(\ln x)^2$, x^3, $(\ln x)^3$ and $\ln(\ln x)$) is applied to sample values and after the transformation the normality of these sample distributions is tested by the cummulant method (skewness $z_1 = |g_1| / \sigma_{g_1}$ and kurtosis $z_2 = |g_2| / \sigma_{g_2}$, where $g_1 = k_3/k_2^{3/2}$ and $g_2 = k_4/k_2^2$) for small samples, namely, for the intra-individual sample distributions where n = 15 and by the ordinary moment method for larger samples, namely, for the single sample distributions and the distributions of means (where n = 429 or the like, for both of the latter).

3. RESULTS

3.1. The Intra-individual Distribution

The normality hypothesis which we assumed throughout the previous studies, in respect to the cummulant method for small samples, cannot be denied either the 1% significance level or the 5% significance level with respect to individual distributions after application of Smirnov-Grubbs rejection test. This holds for almost all AMHTS test items including the serum glucose measurement under any of the transformations previously listed. Thus, it was natural to assume that the individual distribution is Gaussian normal without variable transformation.

The details, for serum glucose, of the percentage of patients showing normality, are shown in Table 2.

Table 2. The percentages of individuals' distributions that conformed with "normality" after the long-term quality control correction and the Smirnov-Grubbs rejection test are applied. (glucose, 737 males and females)

LTQC	S-G	X	Lnx	$X^{1/2}$	$X^{1/3}$	X^2	X^3	Ln(LnX) [1)]
–	-	86.43	86.02	85.89	86.02	86.02	85.21	85.48
	+	96.74	96.34	96.20	96.07	95.52	96.20	96.34
+	-	83.18	82.63	82.63	82.63	82.50	81.00	82.09
	+	95.52	96.34	95.93	96.07	94.98	94.30	95.93

1) $(\text{LnX})^n$, n= 2, 3, 1/2, 1/3 are omitted but including these there were no significant differences of the rate among all these transformations at the 5% significance level.

3.2. The Inter-individual Distribution

Unlike other AMHTS tests (the SGOT distribution excepted), the glucose distribution of both mean and single sample distributions does not conform, to any of the transformations listed above, under a test of normality with 5% significance level. Some of the observed skewnesses and kurtosises, are summarized in Table 3, and suggested that it may be far more convenient to regard the intra-individual distributions as normal under other types of variable transformations, e.g. lognormal, $X^{1/2}$, $X^{1/3}$, etc..

Actually, the means distributions and the single sample distributions of the two tests, glucose and SGOT, do not conform to normality under any type of variable transformation (Table 3). In order to exclude the excessively wide fluctuations,

Table 3. Observed skewness and kurtosises of the distribution of means and the single sample distribution with intra-individuals untransformed and with the long-term quality control correction.

			X			LnX			$X^{1/3}$		
a	b	dist.	G1	G2	n	G1	G2	n	G1	G2	n
-	-	mean	3.712	23.587	419	2.575	14.000	419	2.923	16.655	419
		random	3.615	24.416	429	2.155	12.692	429	2.594	15.800	429
	+	mean	0.783	4.017	405	0.660	3.832	407	0.747	4.028	407
		random	0.605	3.820	419	0.412	3.715	421	0.529	3.879	421
+	-	mean	3.733	24.063	429	2.577	14.211	429	2.930	16.940	429
		random	4.431	37.673	429	2.359	15.952	429	2.945	21.190	429
	+	mean	0.774	4.020	415	0.654	3.848	417	0.742	4.047	417
		random	0.682	4.397	419	0.516	4.416	422	0.580	4.424	421

a: + Smirnov-Grubbs test applied within individual distributions and
- not applied.

b: + Smirnov-Grubbs test appplied to individuals' means and
- not applied.

Table 4. Observed skewnesses and kurtosises, means and standard deviations of the distribution of means and the single sample distribution with intra-individual distributions transformed by $X^{1/3}$. (With LTQC correction and Smirnov-Grubbs test applied for intra-individual distributions and also the χ^2-test applied for large variances with 1% point)

		X					LnX				
S-G for inter-individual	dist.	G1	G2	n	mean†	s.d.†	G1	G2	n	mean†	s.d.†
-	mean	0.864	6.421	404	4.7481	0.10587	0.721	5.604	404	1.5575	0.022111
	random	0.555	4.867	404	4.7521	0.13130	0.415	4.467	404	1.5582	0.027460
+	mean	0.303	2.829	403	4.7464	0.10048	0.248	2.795*	403	1.5572	0.021112
	random	0.279	3.581*	403	4.7504	0.12706	0.180	3.479*	403	1.5579	0.026675

† : values are shown as are transformed.

* : conforms with normality at an 1% significance level.

which are possibly of multi-modulity, individuals with a variance greater than the 1% point of the χ^2 distribution of a degree of freedom 14, or 15, the number of samples from an individual, minus 1, are rejected. With this filtration, the distribution of means conformed well with normality under a lognormal transformation (Table 4).

Thus out of the population of 429 individuals, 25 were rejected due to their large variances and out of the remaining 404, one was rejected since in this case the mean value lay outside the distribution of the means after the lognormal transformation. The resulting distribution has as its mean and standard deviation, 1.5572 (106.87 on the original scale) and 0.021112 respectively, and the m + s.d. and m + 2s.d. being 113.86 and 121.30 respectively.

3.3. The Single Sample Distribution

The sample distributions obtained from the single samples from each individual are examined and the parameters are shown in Table 3 and Table 4 in parallel to those of the distributions of means. The results from the above distributions are similar. With the intra-individual distribution as it stands, there were no single sample distributions under any of the listed variable transformations which conformed with normality; but, with the intra-individual distribution transformed by $X^{1/3}$ and with individuals with variances greater than the 1% point in the distribution rejected, the single sample distribution conformed with the normality both with no transformation and with lognormal transformation.

Thus, after exploring all the listed transformations by applying them to the intra-individual distributions, the distributions of means and the single sample distributions, it was found that the only transformation under which the distribution of means and the single sample distributions conform with normality is the lognormal transformation with $X^{1/3}$ transformation for the intra-individual distribution and with Smirnov-Grubbs rejection test applied to both the intra- and inter-individual distributions and with the individuals having a large variance excluded. For convenience, let us denote this composite transformation, f, as $f = \ln(X^{1/3})$.

4. CLINICAL SIGNIFICANCE AND CONCLUSION

To the P.L. Tokyo Health Control Center (actually one of the AMHTS facilities affiliated with the P.L. Health Control System), a specific clinic is attached for mildly diabetic patients (6). Here, medical records of detailed examinations are maintained in addition to the regular health check-ups records. Against these medical records, the significance of the newly obtained parameters from the distribution of means is evaluated in comparison with those from the glucose distribution in an ordinary sense.

In Figure 2, with a glucose distribution model given at the top, a comparison of intervals based on the ordinary scale after the $Ln(X^{1/3})$ transformation specified as $m + \sigma < x \leqq m + 2\sigma$ and $m + 2\sigma < x$, and the findings given in the medical records are shown.

Figure 2 Comparison of the intervals specified as $m + \sigma < x \leqq m + 2\sigma$ and $m + 2\sigma < x$ in the glucose distribution (males) between the intervals as such from the ordinary scale and those given after the $Ln(x^{1/3})$ transformation.

DM : the diabetes mellitus type by 50g-0-GTT and/or diagnosed as such by physician
B : the border-line type by 50g-0-GTT and/or diabetes mellitus suspected
OX : the oxihyper type by 50g-0-GTT
U : renal diabetes diagnosed or suspected
N : normal in respect to diabetes and/or hyperglysemia
The individuals in the population concerned are sorted by their individual mean values and arranged with magnitude decreasing from right to left.

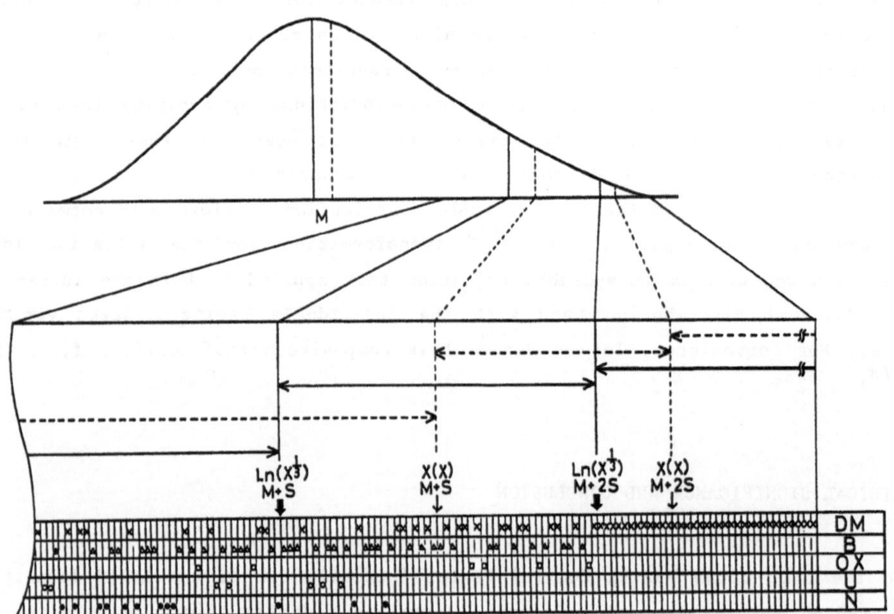

In the lower rectangular chart for findings, individuals' test results are sorted according to their mean values, with values decreasing from right to left. Among them, those marked X in the row DM are those that have been classified as the DM type on the 50g-O-GTT, those marked Δ in the row B are those that have been classified as the border-line type, those marked □ in the row OX are those classified as the oxihyper type, and those marked O in the row U are those found to be renal diabetics and those marked • are normal. The class DM includes those diagnosed diabetes mellitus cases in the more general sense, and class B includes those who are suspected diabetes mellitus cases.

This population has as its mean and standard deviation, 107.69 (mg/dl) and 9.28 (mg/dl) respectively after the Smirnov-Grubbs test has been applied to both the intra- and inter-individual distributions, accordingly the points of $m + \sigma$ and $m + 2\sigma$ are 116.97 and 126.25 and likewise, under $Ln(X^{1/3})$ transformation, when the scale is reverted to the usual, it has as its mean, $m + \sigma$ and $m + 2\sigma$, 106.87, 113.86 and 121.30 repectively.

What is remarkable is that the point $m + 2\sigma$, from the $ln(X^{1/3})$ transformation, so clearly divides the hyperglycemic interval into that which solely includes those diagnosed as diabetes mellitus cases and that which includes other types. This does not happen with the $m + 2\sigma$ point from the ordinary mean and standard deviation.

Parallelly, chronic hepatitis were well differentiated from other hepatic diseases such as hepatic insufficiency. When similar transformations were applied on the individuals' distributions (log x), and the distribution of means $(\log x)^{1/2}$ with the test of 1% point of χ^2 distribution.

This is the only fact that can be stated positively, but what is suggested is that the method applied may pave the way for the more precise and deep interpretation of the characteristics of measurement distributions of AMHTS tests (biochemistry, hematology and other physiological tests) and therefore the information obtained through these tests may be better organized especially in terms of 'normal ranges'.

REFERENCES

1) T. YASAKA, et al.: "Clinical Data Evaluation and the PL Health Control Information System", Computer Programs in Biomedicine, Vol(8) pp 51-70, 1980.
2) T. YASAKA: "Health Control Data-Base System and Subject-Specific Normal Range", MED. INFORM., Vol(1) pp 105-132, 1976.
3) T. YASAKA, et al.: "Normalized Q-sum Method for Clinical Data Evaluation (Homeostasis Dynamics)", Medical Computing, ed. M. Landet et al. Taylor and Francis, London, pp 311-328, 1977.
4) T. YASAKA, et al.: "The long-term quality control and clinical data evaluation of individuals in AMHTS", MED. INFORM., Vol(4) pp 173-185, 1979.
5) T. YASAKA, et al.: "Distribution Types: Population and Intra- and Inter-Individual Distributions", MEDINFO 80. eds Lindberg D.A.B. and Kaihara S. North Holland. pp 1269 - 1273, 1980 MEDINFO 80 Proceedings.
6) M. TAMURA, et al.: "Metabolic disease information system", Medical Computing, ed. Laudet, M., et al., Taylor and Francis Ltd., London, pp 281-291, 1977.

MODELES QUANTITATIFS DE GENETIQUE EPIDEMIOLOGIQUE

Alice GUEGUEN et Denise SALMON
INSERM U 88 - CHU Pitié-Salpétrière

Analysis of inheritance of simple mendelian traits, as blood groups markers and some rare diseases, were the only possible field in medical genetics a few years ago. Recent advances in computerized medical records and in computer based algorithms of computation open a new field of research : genetic epidemiology.

Three different methods are reviewed : the partition of variance, the path analysis and the mixed model. The partition of variance may be applied to any sort of pedigree, by summation of log likelihood and results into computation of genetic and environmental components. The path analysis was first described by Sewall Wright : a diagram expresses the relationships among the variables in the model by means of paths. It is attractive but unfortunately implies that more parameters be estimated than the number of observed correlations makes possible. A simplification of the model is often necessary. Finally, complex segregation analysis in the mixed model of Morton and Mc Lean incorporates the effects of segregation at a major locus, a polygenic effect and sibling environmental effect, this last one, however, confounded with polygenic dominance. This last method is very sensitive to transformation of the data, skewness simulating a major gene effect in some cases.

Jusqu'à ces dernières années, la génétique humaine se divisait en deux domaines distincts. Le premier voyait l'application sans failles de la ségrégation mendélienne classique de gènes allèles, codés par un même locus ; c'est le sort par exemple, du système ABO de groupe sanguin, de maladies rares à transmission dominante comme l'achondroplasie ou récessive comme la galactosémie. A l'opposé, d'autres pathologies semblaient frapper certains membres d'une même famille sans obéir clairement aux lois de Mendel. Il était courant d'émailler les publications de termes comme la pénétrance, rapport du nombre de cas observés au nombre de cas attendus selon un taux de ségrégation mendélien ($\frac{1}{4}$ ou $\frac{1}{2}$) ou comme l'expressivité, ce dernier mot traduisant le fait que deux sujets atteints dans une même famille n'expriment pas la maladie avec la même intensité. Pénétrance et expressivité ne sont en fait qu'une formulation commode pour masquer notre ignorance du mode de transmission exact du caractère étudié. Tant qu'à faire, la classique notion de "terrain" , chère aux cliniciens de l'école classique est tout aussi convenable pour exprimer le fait que, dans certaines familles, on est plus susceptible de développer une affection pathologique donnée.

Cependant, des modèles définissant cette génétique complexe peuvent être édifiés désormais et confrontés à des données réelles : la génétique épidémiologique devient à notre portée, puisque l'ordinateur nous permet d'une part la gestion de dossiers familiaux complexes, d'autre part l'introduction de modèles mathématiques comportant plusieurs paramètres dont la signification peut être testée.

On peut distinguer trois approches du problèmes : la partition de la variance observée, la méthode des chemins de Sewall Wright (6), l'analyse de la ségrégation dite complexe.

1. La partition de la variance repose sur un modèle additif et linéaire sans interaction entre le génotype et le milieu. La variance phénotypique est égale à la somme des termes $\sigma^2_a, \sigma^2_d, \sigma^2_e$ qui sont respectivement les variances : additive, due à la dominance et due à l'environnement. La méthode de Keneth Lange, Joan Westlake et Anne Spence (3) a été développée pour des arbres généalogiques de tailles et de structures variables. Pour un arbre généalogique de n sujets, on dispose de n mesures individuelles d'un caractère quantitatif $x' = (x_i, i=1..n)$. Etant donnés deux sujets i et j, on définit deux coefficients à partir de leurs liens de filiation à savoir ϕ_{ij}, probabilité qu'un gène pris au hasard pour un locus donné de i soit identique par descente à un gène pris au hasard pour le même locus de j et Δ_{ij}, probabilité que deux sujets i et j possèdent deux gènes identiques par descente pour un locus donné. Ω, la matrice de variance covariance de cet arbre généalogique a pour éléments :

$$\mathrm{cov}(x_i, x_j) = 2\sigma^2_a\phi_{ij} + \sigma^2_d\Delta_{ij} + \sigma^2_e \quad\quad i = 1 \dots n \quad j = 1 \dots n$$

Soit $u' = (u_i, i=1, n)$ l'espérance mathématique de $x' = (x_i, i=1,n)$ avec $u_i = u_m$ si l'individu i est de sexe masculin et $u_i = u_f$ s'il est de sexe féminin.

Si on suppose la multinormalité des mesures, le log de la vraisemblance s'écrit :

$$L = -\tfrac{1}{2}\log|\Omega| - \tfrac{1}{2}(x - u')\Omega^{-1}(x - u)$$

Le log de la vraisemblance de plusieurs arbres est maximisé par la méthode des scores de Fisher. On obtient ainsi des estimations des différents paramètres sur lesquels des tests d'hypothèses peuvent être effectués par des rapports de vraisemblance. Des modèles basés sur un décomposition plus fine de la variance peuvent être élaborés comme le montre l'exemple suivant dans lequel la variable étudiée est le nombre de crêtes digitales à partir d'un échantillon de 150 familles comprenant 590 individus (Anne Spence, J. Westlake et K. Lange (5)).

Les auteurs ont supposé l'existence d'une variance due à l'environnement commun σ^2_c (environnement intra-utérin). Après estimation des paramètres, trois hypothèses ont été testées : $\sigma^2_d = 0$, $\sigma^2_c = 0$, $\sigma^2_d = \sigma^2_c = 0$. Chacune de ces hypothèses a été rejetée au seuil de 1 %. La variance due à la dominance est peu importante mais significative, résultat qui n'avait pu être trouvé par des méthodes classiques.

2. La méthode de l'analyse des chemins repose sur l'élaboration d'un diagramme exprimant les relations entre plusieurs variables mesurées sur des individus apparentés ou non. Ces variables peuvent être observées (exemples : le phénotype, ou encore un index d'environne-

ment familial commun) ou rester non directement accessibles à l'observation (ex. : le génotype moyen du couple parental, ou encore l'environnement familial commun et l'environnement aléatoire). Des chemins fléchés affectés chacun d'un coefficient relient ces différentes variables. Si le chemin est unidirectionnel, il exprime une relation de cause à effet (ex. : l'action du génotype sur le phénotype). S'il est bidirectionnel, il exprime une corrélation entre deux variables (ex. : corrélation entre les génotypes des parents).

Les différents coefficients de corrélation (interclasses ou intraclasses) calculés sur des paires de variables mesurées (par exemple coefficient de corrélation entre les phénotypes de deux frères) se déduisent de la lecture du diagramme et sont égaux à des "sommes de chemins" ; ils sont donc fonction de paramètres à estimer.

En pratique, on estime les paramètres par la méthode du maximum de vraisemblance. Il faut toutefois remarquer que cette estimation n'est possible que si le nombre de paramètres est inférieur au nombre de coefficients de corrélation calculés (exemple : corrélation entre deux frères élevés ensemble par leurs parents, corrélation entre deux frères, l'un élevé par ses parents, l'autre élevé par des parents adoptifs, corrélation entre un enfant et son père adoptif, etc...).

On s'attache moins en fait, aux valeurs des estimations obtenues pour chaque paramètre défini dans le modèle qu'aux tests de sous hypothèses (tests de rapport de vraisemblance) qui permettent, en confrontant les deux vraisemblances obtenues sur un modèle complet à k paramètres et sur un modèle incomplet à k - m paramètres, de tester l'existence ou l'inconsistence des m paramètres absents du second modèle.

Dans Analysis of Family Resemblance, Rao, Morton et Yee (4) ont donné une description détaillée de la méthode et étudié des exemples, entre autres le poids à la naissance. A partir de différents coefficients de corrélation entre jumeaux de même sexe, ou de sexe différent, frères, demi frères paternels et demi frères maternels, les auteurs ont trouvé que l'héritabilité seule ne peut expliquer les données. L'environnement commun maternel explique une grande part de la variance phénotypique : 55 % en supposant qu'il n'y a pas d'héritabilité et 49 % si on l'introduit, celle-ci représentant alors 8 % de la variance totale.

Nous donnons ci-dessous pour illustrer la méthode un exemple simple d'analyse des chemins, à savoir la corrélation parent-enfant.

La diagramme présenté comporte certaines hypothèses : l'effet de l'environnement (E) et le génotype (Y) agissent sur le phénotype (Z) de manière additive et ne sont pas corrélés ; on suppose également qu'il n'existe pas d'interaction entre les gènes (épistasis).

D'autre part, on décompose (Y), valeur génotypique en une valeur linéaire (L) et une déviation due à la dominance (D), ces deux valeurs n'étant pas corrélées.

Enfin, on sait que la corrélation parent-enfant pour la variable L, valeur linéaire du génotype, est de $\frac{1}{2}$. Les index p et e font référence au parent et à l'enfant. h représente l'effet du génotype sur le phénotype, et e celui de l'environnement sur le phénotype, g celui de L valeur linéaire du génotype sur le génotype, et d celui de la déviation due à la dominance sur le génotype.

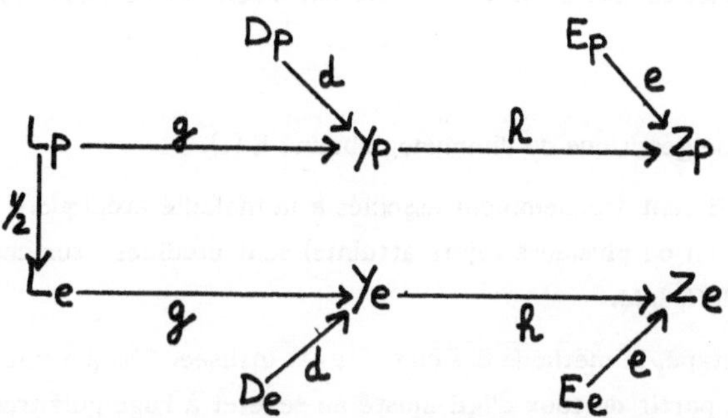

La variance phénotypique σ_z^2 est égale à la somme de la variance d'origine génétique σ_y^2 et de la variance due à l'environnement σ_e^2. h^2 et e^2 représentent respectivement les pourcentages de variance d'origine génétique et environnementale ; on a la relation $h^2 + e^2 = 1$.

Quant à la variance d'origine génétique σ_y^2, elle se décompose en deux termes : σ_l^2 variance génétique additive et σ_d^2 variance due à la dominance. De manière similaire, g^2 et d^2 représentent les proportions de variance additive et de variance due à la dominance avec la relation $g^2 + d^2 = 1$.

3. Les modèles complexes de ségrégation (Morton et Mac Lean) font intervenir sur un effet polygénique (dû à l'addition de plusieurs systèmes génétiques), a) la ségrégation d'un locus majeur de type mendélien de fréquence q, b) des effets aléatoires et c) l'effet du milieu commun aux membres d'une même fratrie. L'effet du locus majeur est défini par une distribution de moyenne M sur laquelle interviennent un déplacement t dû au génotype et un déplacement d dû à la dominance. L'effet polygénique suit par hypothèse, une distribution normale (0, $\sigma^2 g$) et peut être décomposé en une part b due au génotype parental moyen et une part y propre à chaque sujet. L'effet du milieu suit, par hypothèse également, une distribution normale et peut être décomposé en une part commune à tous les membres de la fratrie et une part aléatoire. Il en découle que le phénotype des enfants ne dépend du phénotype des parents que par l'intermédiaire du génotype.

Les tests de sous hypothèses, par les rapports de vraisemblance, permettent de tester l'hypothèse d'existence du gène majeur ($q \neq 0$, $t \neq 0$), d'effets polygéniques ($\sigma^2 g = 0$), d'effets du milieu.

Ce modèle extrêmement séduisant, n'est pas exempt de critiques : il est impossible d'y distinguer une corrélation entre frères/soeurs due au milieu d'un effet polygénique avec dominance. D'autre part, tout écart à la normalité dans la distribution du caractère étudié peut simuler un gène majeur. En effet, le test q = t = 0 est extrêmement sensible aux transformations de données.

Deux exemples d'études sur des familles permettront d'éclairer l'exposé des méthodes.

1er exemple

Gerrard, Rao, Morton : étude génétique de l'immunoglobuline E (1).

Des taux élevés d'IgE sont fréquemment associés à la maladie atopique. 173 familles (145 normales, 28 comportant un ou plusieurs sujets atteints) sont étudiées : sur chaque sujet, sont dosés les taux d'IgE, IgA, IgG, IgM.

Dans une première étape, la méthode des chemins est utilisée. Chaque sujet est défini par une variable P, calculée à partir du taux d'IgE ajusté au sexe et à l'âge puis transformé et par une variable index I calculée de façon analogue à partir de la corrélation entre le taux d'IgE et celui des autres Ig. 6 variables P_P I_P P_M I_M P_E I_E mesurées sur le père (P), la mère (M), l'enfant (E) fournissent 15 corrélations ; s'y ajoute une corrélation entre le phénotype de deux enfants. Les corrélations attendues selon le modèle sont définies à partir du diagramme. L'estimation des paramètres par le maximum de vraisemblance, et les tests de rapport de vraisemblance démontrent l'existence de facteurs génétiques et aussi des effets dus au milieu.

On décide alors de passer à une étude plus approfondie par l'analyse de la ségrégation, tout en sachant que ce deuxième modèle, parce qu'il ne suppose pas de corrélation due au milieu entre parents et enfants va conduire à une surestimation de l'héritabilité.

On standardise tout d'abord à l'intérieur de chaque génération, le taux d'IgE de chaque sujet puis on cherche par le maximum de vraisemblance, la transformation qui normalise au mieux les distributions de la variable standardisée, sous 3 hypothèses différentes : une seule distribution, un mélange de deux ou trois distributions ; le modèle à deux distributions est retenu parce que le mieux ajusté aux données. Ceci revient à dire qu'il existe un locus majeur d'effet complètement récessif ou complètement dominant sur la transmission du taux d'IgE.

L'analyse de "ségrégation complexe" est alors effectuée sur la variable transformée. Les tests de sous hypothèses (plus importants, rappelons-le, que les estimations proprement dites des paramètres) montrent qu'il existe un effet polygénique et un locus majeur régulateur d'effet complètement récessif : les sujets porteurs de deux gènes récessifs présentant des taux élevés d'IgE.

2ème exemple

Etude de l'hémochromatose héréditaire (Kravitz et al) (2)

Des sujets porteurs d'un fer sérique anormalement élevé sont susceptibles de développer une cirrhose. Un arbre généalogique important a pu être étudié en Utah. La variable quantitative retenue pour base de l'étude est la saturation de la transferrine. D'autre part, l'analyse sur chaque membre de cette famille des taux de fer sérique, de ferritine sérique, d'excrétion urinaire du fer provoquée par la déféroxamine, complétée éventuellement par une biopsie du foie, permet de trichotomiser cet échantillon en sujets à surcharge élevée de fer, en sujets à surcharge modérée de fer et en sujets normaux.

On est donc ici en présence d'une maladie à seuil : à partir d'un seuil donné de surcharge ferrique, la maladie métabolique se déclenche.

Le modèle retenu est celui du locus majeur à deux allèles. La "liabilité" ou susceptibilité d'un sujet à développer la maladie est définie par la somme de son taux de saturation de la transferrine et d'un effet du milieu, de distribution normale. Un échantillon de sujets normaux sur lequel est mesuré le taux de saturation de la transferrine est introduit dans le corpus de données. Par le maximum de vraisemblance, on peut dès lors estimer la variance de l'effet du milieu et le seuil du taux de saturation de la transferrine au delà duquel se déclenche une atteinte clinique.

De surcroit, l'analyse de la liaison génétique démontrée auparavant entre le système HLA, marqueur qualitatif, et le locus régulateur du taux d'IgE, marqueur quantitatif, apporte sur certains sujets des informations supplémentaires. Ce fait est important car le dépistage précoce des sujets à risque est ainsi amélioré et débouche sur une prévention efficace.

Toutes ces études sont idéalement achevées quand les méthodes de liaison génétique permettent de localiser un tel gène régulateur, ou encore quand les progrès de la biochimie débouchent sur la définition d'un modèle physiopathologique. Elles sont cependant extrêmement prometteuses à l'heure actuelle et devraient nous permettre de démonter le mécanisme de l'hérédité des maladies à risque, diabète, hyperlipidémies, athérosclérose.

REFERENCES

(1) Gerrard JW, Rao DC, and Morton NE. A genetic study of immunoglobulin E. Am J Hum Genet 1978 ; 30 : 46-58.

(2) Kravitz K, Skolnick M, Cannings C et al. Genetic linkage between hereditary hemochromatosis and HLA. Am J Hum Genet 1979 ; 31 : 601-619.

(3) Lange K, Westlake J and Spence MA. Extensions to pedigree analysis. III. Variance components by the scoring method. Ann Hum Genet Lond 1976 ; 39 : 485-491.

(4) Rao DC, Morton NE and Yee S. Analysis of family resemblance. II. A linear model for familial correlation. Am J Hum Genet 1974 ; 26 : 331-359.

(5) Spence MA, Westale J. and Lange K. Estimation of the variance components for dermal ridge count. Ann Hum Genet Lond 1977 ; 41 : 111-115.

(6) Wright S. Genetics 1921 ; 111-178.

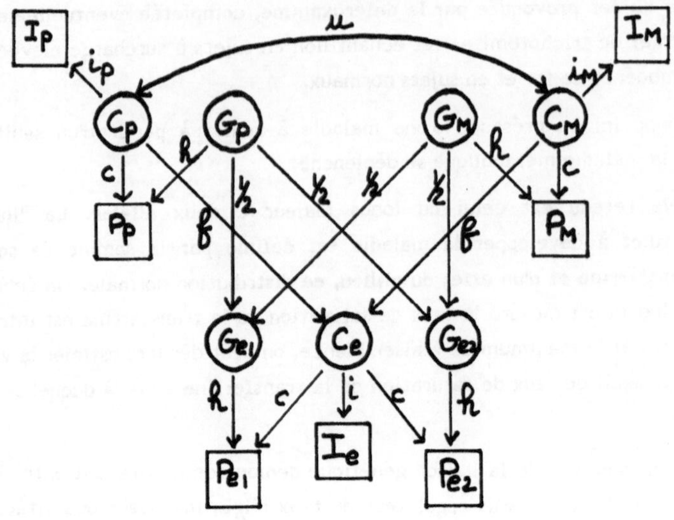

u : corrélation entre l'environnement du père et l'environnement de la mère

i_P : effet de l'environnement du père sur son index d'environnement

i_M : effet de l'environnement de la mère sur son index d'environnement

i : effet de l'environnement d'un enfant sur son index d'environnement

c : effet de l'environnement sur le phénotype

f : effet de l'environnement d'un parent (père ou mère) sur l'environnement de l'enfant

h : effet du génotype sur le phénotype

Les variables I (index d'environnement) et P (phénotype) sont observées

Les variables C (environnement) et G (génotype) ne sont pas observables

La corrélation entre le phénotype de la mère P_M et l'index d'environnement de l'enfant I_E est égale à : icf (1 + u).

A D.B.M.S. FOR AN EPIDEMIOLOGICAL RESEARCH ABOUT MENTAL DISEASES AND RELATIVE HOSPITALIZATION: INITIAL RESULTS AND DEDUCTONS OF A PRELIMINARY STUDY ON ABOUT TWO YEARS.

Vito MIRIZIO - Maurizio RAFANELLI - Fabrizio L.RICCI

Istituto per l'Analisi dei Sistemi e Informatica - C.N.R.
Via Buonarroti, 12 - 00184 ROMA - ITALY

SUMMARY.

In the recent years studies and research about mental health have been mainly concerned with the prevention of psichic disease and the programming of medical assistance. In this paper we are described: a) the purpose of this research; b) a data recording method, related to some characteristics of the patients; c) an admission form to use for epidemiological research; d) the characteristics of the D.B.M.S. that has been implemented and of the query language used; e) first results and some considerations about them .

PREVENTION OF MENTAL ILLNESS AND THE EPIDEMIOLOGICAL PROBLEM.

A "case-register" in the following definition of J.K.Wing is a collection of data on experiences of a population, living in a definite area, with particular medical or social services. The fundamental characteristics of such a case-register are: a) the continuous updating with data coming from all the hospitals, from which results the chronological development of admissions of subgroups of the population to the different hospitals; b) the preliminary knowledge of the main socio-demographic indexes of the area under inquiry. Our research is developed in the district of Rome, (that has a population of over 4 millions of people), where there are about 9,000 admissions in one year in about 30 public and private clinics. This research has not focused the attention on the desease itself and its causes, but: 1) on possibilities of correlating data on in-patients to socio-demographical data concerning the people who live in the area served by the psychiatric institution; 2) on some characteristics of in-patients (living area, civil status, ecc.) and on the most relevant conditions of in-patient admission; 3) on the individualization of groups of population under high risk of hospitalization.

METHODOLOGY AND CHOISE OF VARIABLES.

The computerized patient case-register for psychiatric epidemiology was developed in two different stage: a) the organizational stage (i.e. the planning of the psychiatric hospitalization form (P.H.F.) and its storage); b) the preparation of the management instruments (i.e. the data base and its query language).

The choice of significative variables has taken into consideration both the epidemiological aim of the inquiry and the tipical problems of computerized data management systems. The formalization and codification of P.H.F. items were performed with regard to: a) the formal aspect of data; b) semantic meaning (that is"not ambigu ty"); c) proper use of symbology; d) simple compilation of form and verification of correctness of the codification.

PRIVACY.

The preservation of "patient-privacy", as no individual subject can be identified from the data stored on the computer data base, was easily obtained by means of a code assigned to the patient, formed by 16 characters and manually compiled by sociologists and public health assistants that filled out the P.H.F.. This code is a simple elaboration of surname, Christian name, birth-date and sex, having a low probability of synonymy (See App.1).

THE MATHEMATICAL MODEL OF P.H.F.

The data set R related to one hospitalization is defined by means of a hierarchical type procedure in the following manner:

$$\begin{cases} R=(R_1)_1 U(R_2)_1 U \ldots U(R_n)_1 \\ (R_i)_1=(R_{1,i})_2 U(R_{2,i})_2 U \ldots U(R_{m,i})_2 \\ \ldots\ldots \\ (R_J)_{K-1}=(R_{1,J})_K U(R_{2,J})_K U \ldots U(R_{P,J})_K \end{cases} \qquad (1)$$

where $i = 1,2,\ldots,n$

j = index vector, whose dimension is k-1 and whose term to the bottom right of the brackets specifies the hierarchical level to which the set belongs.

For such a set the following properties are true:

$$(R_{\bar{i}})_J \cap (R_{\bar{h}})_J = \Phi \qquad (2)$$

$$(R_{\bar{i}})_J \cap (R_{\bar{h}})_e = (R_{\bar{h}})_e \qquad (3)$$

with $j > e$ and where:

$(R_{\bar{i}})_J$ and $(R_{\bar{h}})_J$ are the ith and the hth element of the jth level;

$(R_{\bar{h}})_e$ is the hth element of the eth level belonging to the branch of the tree whose root is the $(R_{\bar{i}})_J$ element.

THE P.H.F.: PRATICAL REALIZATION.

The P.H.F. that we created and the one presently used, consists of 27 items, subdivided in: administrative, private (of the patient and of head of family, if different, about occupation, work sector and position at work), admission and dismissal data (with notices about condition of admission, of presentation and of dismissal, about the place where the patient is going, etc.(See App.2).

THE DATA BASE.

The data base, organized on mass storage by means of a simple file, has possibility of access through 5 different research channels and a theoretically unfinite number of sub-channels (in this case they are 35). This system uses a query language that is extremely simple to learn and use. The system-package is a single segmented program, written in Assembler Univac 1100 and in Fortran V and implemented on the University of Rome computer Univac 1100/82.

This record is inserted into the data base, associating a "position descriptor" to it. Every channel is composed by extracting the descriptors related to that channels from the records. Then we associate to that descriptor the address set of only those records that contain that descriptor. The sequence of operations that carries out the research of the records, containing a certain descriptor, takes place in the following manner:

1) research on the table is done, through the system directory on the index directory table, in the central memory, and the desired channel segment (index block) is localized;

2) the desired index block is transferred from mass storage to central memory (first access to mass storage);

3) a new research on the table is done to localize the channel descriptor in the index block, so as to individualize in what channel block the above mentioned channel descriptor is memorized;

3) the channel block, found in step 3, is transferred from mass storage to central memory (second access to mass storage);

4) the last step on the table supplies the number of informations associated to the channel descriptor with the related addresses associated to this descriptor.

In Fig. 1 these phases are illustrated.

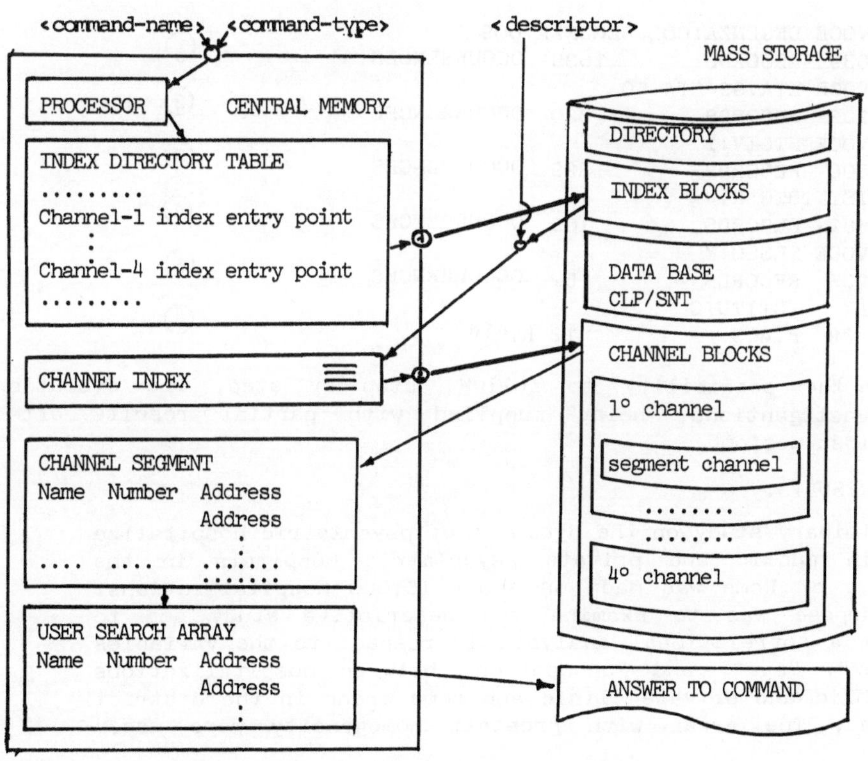

Fig. 1

A peculiar characteristic of this system is that only two accesses to mass storage, independent of the data base dimension, are needed to individualize the "number" of available records, for every "phase of research". Moreover the system can be utilized by different users at the same time. Finally the system, in addition to the above-mentioned merits, is structured in such a way that the part which resides in the central memory occupies no more that 22 K-words, independently of the dimension of the data base on which we are working.

THE QUERY LANGUAGE.

The fundamental characteristics of the query language are:

- its simplicity of use, even for non-specialized staff;
- the possibility to carry out phases of research by means of successive selections, declaring the various bonds with every new step and combining the bonds logically, in any way whatever;
- the possibility to utilize the system either in batch or in demand.

Let us give an example of a simple sequence of instruction (scanning with one research key); "we want to know the number of hospitalizations (6) related to patients of male sex (5), unmarried (3), between thirty and fifty years old (2), whose stay (1) in private clinics (4) lasted less than ten days (1)":

```
>LOOK VOCE DEGENZA:001=DEGENZA:009
     1639  RECORDS        1639  OCCURRENCES          (1)
>LOOK VOCE ETA:39=ETA:50
     3233  RECORDS         820  OCCURRENCES          (2)
>LOOK VOCE STCIV:1
     4506  RECORDS         329  OCCURRENCES          (3)
>LOOK ISTITUTO R.4*
     5582  RECORDS         108  OCCURRENCES          (4)
>LOOK VOCE SESSO:M
     6935  RECORDS          52  OCCURRENCES          (5)
>DISPLAY   ISTITUTO
       39  R.409            13 R.414                 (6)
```

We note the possibility to follow, step by step, the evolution of investigantions, being supplied with partial results after every instruction.

FIRST RESULTS.

A preliminary study on the dynamics of psychiatric hospitaliza tion in public and private psychiatric hospitals in the district of Rome was made on about 15,000 hospitalizations. Its purpose was to examine the descriptive study and to perform a correlational analysis in respect to the variables of "sex", "age", and "occupation" between hospitalizations in pubblic and private clinic and some areas in the district of Rome. The areas with greatest homogeneity were used, individualizing four types:

1) areas inhabited prevailingly by the upper middle class, in urban territory only;
2) areas inhabited prevailingly by the middle class, in urban territory and with extensive rural zones;
3) areas inhabited prevailingly by the working class, in urban territory and with some rural zones;
4) areas inhabited prevailingly by the working class, only in rural zones.

The analysis of the last type (four area) gave such a difference in the structure for age that it was not possible to formulate any deductions at this level.
Instead the examination of histograms, performed by our investigations and related to the first three types (see Tab.1,2 and 3), permit us to make these first affirmations:

a) type one area (see Tab.1) has a high percentage of elderly population, with old-age index variable between 130.23 and 132.60 (we define "old-age index" as the ratio between population older then 60 years and population from 0 to 15 years).
   The age-band that is principally present in the psychiatric hospitals is from "35-49 years" (indipendent of sex).
b) type two area (see Tab. 2): here the oldage index varies between 46.23 and 59.95; we have noticed that for men there is no particular age group that is more likely to have to undergo hospitalization.
   Instead there is a prevalence of women over 65 years of age in psychatric hospitals (and, in part, also from 35 to 49 years).
c) type three area (see Tab. 3): the old-age index varies between 31.62 and 32.60; for men the age-bands mainly present are from 35 to 49 years (and in part over 65 years) while for the women such age-bands are, also here, over 65 years of and in part from 35 to 49 years.

▨ PATIENTS MEN
▦ PATIENTS WOMEN
▭ POPULATION OF THE AREA

1 Age-band=20-34 years
2 " " =35-49 "
3 " " =50-64 "
4 " " =65 years and over

All the values are in per cent.

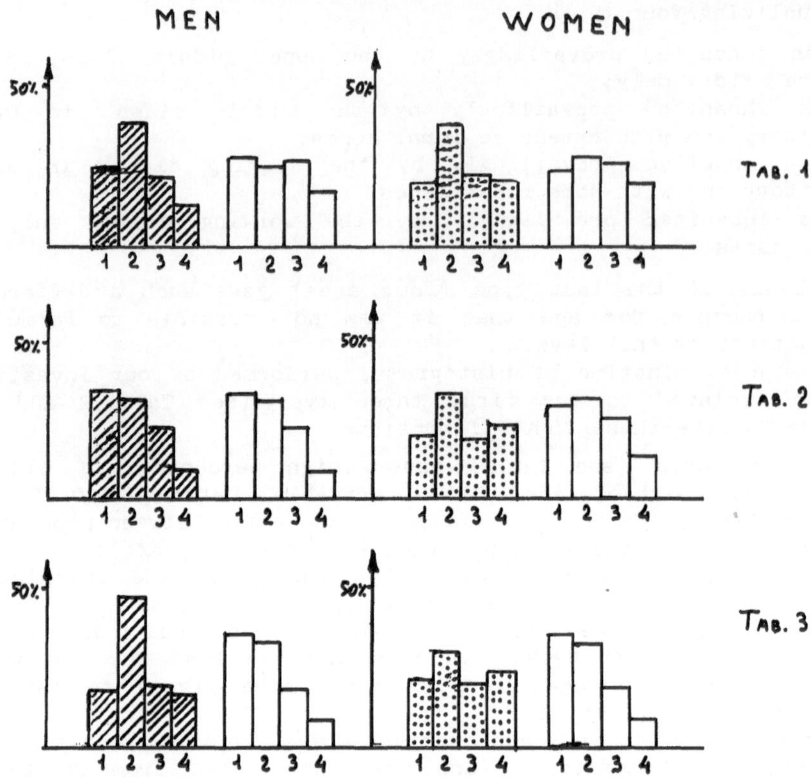

CONCLUSIONS.

The creation of a population-register can be justified only on the condition that the research project be combined with practical iniziatives: the data made available by this new survey instrument must therefore be ever increasingly inserted, in a dynamic and constant manner into vaster, more complete social and health programs.

With this D.B.M.S. it has been possible to follow the movement of patients through various hospitals (the "history" of the patient) and to organize and elaborate statisticly the data retrieval in the data base, in accordance to descriptive-correlational research, attempting to make out the differences between sub-group by means of comparisons.

The importance of these studies, still in course, is in the fact that have changed the aim of the investigation from one of an epidemiological character to a preventive one: that is, from the individuation of the causes of the mental illness, to the analysis of the institutional response given to psychic disturbances.

APPENDIX 1.

In Fig.2 is showed an example of code obtained by a surname, Christian-name, birth-date and sex.

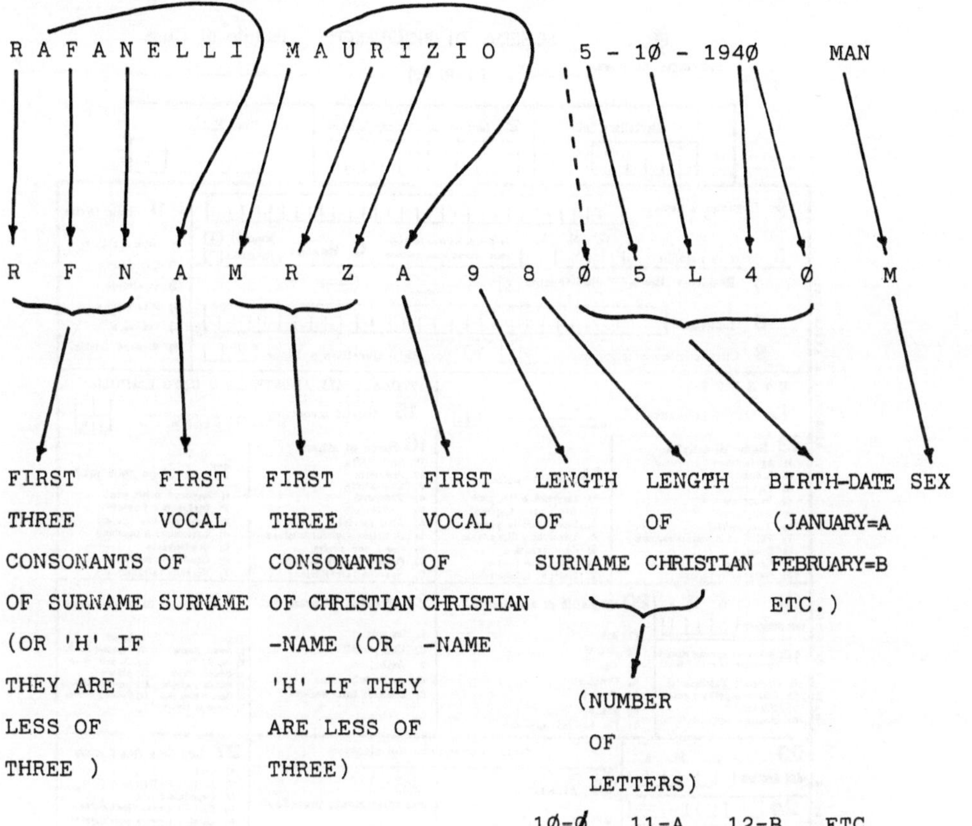

Fig. 2

APPENDIX 2.

In Fig. 3 the psychiatric hospitalization (P.H.F.) form is showed.

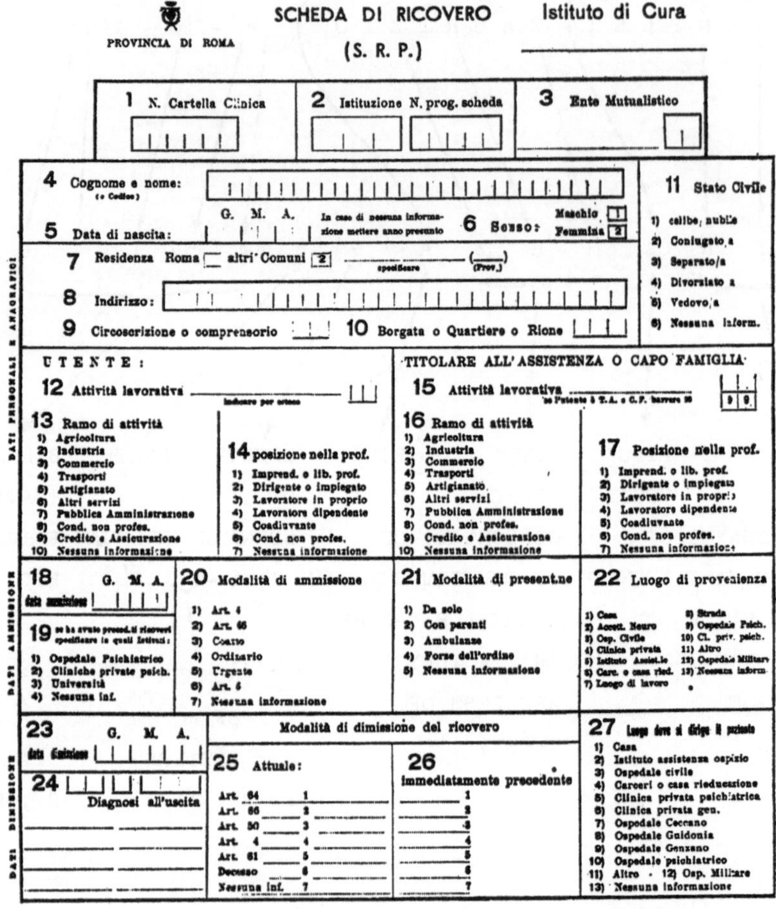

PROVINCIA DI ROMA

SCHEDA DI RICOVERO
(S. R. P.)

Istituto di Cura

1 N. Cartella Clinica

2 Istituzione N. prog. scheda

3 Ente Mutualistico

DATI PERSONALI E ANAGRAFICI

4 Cognome e nome: (o Codice)

5 Data di nascita: G. M. A.

In caso di nessuna informazione mettere anno presunto

6 Sesso: Maschio 1 Femmina 2

7 Residenza Roma altri Comuni 2 specificare (Prov.)

8 Indirizzo:

9 Circoscrizione o comprensorio

10 Borgata o Quartiere o Rione

11 Stato Civile
1) celibe, nubile
2) Coniugato/a
3) Separato/a
4) Divorziato/a
5) Vedovo/a
6) Nessuna inform.

UTENTE:

12 Attività lavorativa (indicare per esteso)

13 Ramo di attività
1) Agricoltura
2) Industria
3) Commercio
4) Trasporti
5) Artigianato
6) Altri servizi
7) Pubblica Amministrazione
8) Cond. non profes.
9) Credito e Assicurazione
10) Nessuna informazione

14 posizione nella prof.
1) Imprend. o lib. prof.
2) Dirigente o impiegato
3) Lavoratore in proprio
4) Lavoratore dipendente
5) Coadiuvante
6) Cond. non profes.
7) Nessuna informazione

TITOLARE ALL'ASSISTENZA O CAPO FAMIGLIA

15 Attività lavorativa (se l'utente è T.A. e C.F. barrare 99) 9 9

16 Ramo di attività
1) Agricoltura
2) Industria
3) Commercio
4) Trasporti
5) Artigianato
6) Altri servizi
7) Pubblica Amministrazione
8) Cond. non profes.
9) Credito e Assicurazione
10) Nessuna informazione

17 Posizione nella prof.
1) Imprend. o lib. prof.
2) Dirigente o impiegato
3) Lavoratore in proprio
4) Lavoratore dipendente
5) Coadiuvante
6) Cond. non profes.
7) Nessuna informazione

DATI AMMISSIONE

18 G. M. A. data ammissione

19 se ha avuto preced.ti ricoveri specificare in quali Istituti:
1) Ospedale Psichiatrico
2) Cliniche private psich.
3) Università
4) Nessuna inf.

20 Modalità di ammissione
1) Art. 4
2) Art. 66
3) Coatto
4) Ordinario
5) Urgente
6) Art. 6
7) Nessuna informazione

21 Modalità di present.ne
1) Da solo
2) Con parenti
3) Ambulanze
4) Forze dell'ordine
5) Nessuna informazione

22 Luogo di provenienza
1) Casa
2) Accett. Neuro
3) Osp. Civile
4) Clinica privata
5) Istituto Assist.le
6) Carc. o casa ried.
7) Luogo di lavoro
8) Strada
9) Ospedale Psich.
10) Cl. priv. psich.
11) Altro
12) Ospedale Militare
13) Nessuna inform.

DATI DIMISSIONE

23 G. M. A. data dimissione

24 Diagnosi all'uscita

Modalità di dimissione del ricovero

25 Attuale:
Art. 64 1
Art. 66 2
Art. 50 3
Art. 4 4
Art. 61 5
Decesso 6
Nessuna inf. 7

26 immediatamente precedente
1
2
3
4
5
6
7

27 Luogo dove si dirige il paziente
1) Casa
2) Istituto assistenza ospizio
3) Ospedale civile
4) Carceri o casa rieducazione
5) Clinica privata psichiatrica
6) Clinica privata gen.
7) Ospedale Ceccano
8) Ospedale Guidonia
9) Ospedale Genzano
10) Ospedale psichiatrico
11) Altro - 12) Osp. Militare
13) Nessuna informazione

Fig. 3

REFERENCES.

(1) Ammanniti M., Rafanelli M., et al., Indagine sull'ospedalizzazione psichiatrica nella Provincia di Roma; organizzazione di un registro di popolazione, Rivista di Psichiatria, vol.XIII, N.6,Nov.-Dic.1978.

(2) Anderson J., Forsythe J.M., Information processing of medical records, North Holland Ed.1970.

(3) Bachev S., Petkova E., A national computer-based epidemiological information system, Methods of information in medicine, N.15, 1976.

Berkeley C., Privacy and the patients' right to information, Medc.Res.Eng., Jan.-Feb. 1971.

Birtchnell J., The use of a psychiatric case register to study social and familiar aspects of mental illness, Soc.Scient.Med., N.7, Feb. 1973.

(6) Cassano G.B., Tansella M., et al., Tecniche di automazione in psichiatria, Il pensiero scientifico (Ed.), 1974.

(7) Dow J.T., Designing computer software for information systems in psychiatry, Computer and Biomedical Research, N.8, 1975.

(8) Kaplan R.W., Brunjes S., The enrollment file: a key module of a clinical data base, Methods of information in medicine, N.15, 1976.

(9) Krupinski J., The use of computerized patients' registers in psychiatric epidemiology, Medinfo 77, North Holland Ed., 1977.

(10) Maccacaro G.A., Problemi di medicina preventiva, Appl.Biomed. del Calc.El. N.2, 1971.

(11) Mc Mahon B., Pugh H., Epidemiology: principles and methods, Lit. Brown and Comp., 1971.

(12) Miles H.C., Gardner E.A., A psychiatric case register in planning community mental health services, Arch. Gener. Psych. N.14, 1966.

(13) Rafanelli M., Un sistema di gestione di una base di dati socio-sanitari per uno studio di tipo epidemiologico sui ricoveri nelle cliniche psichiatriche, Ist. Automatica, Univ. di Roma, R.78-07, Maggio 1978.

(14) Rafanelli M., Ricci F.L., CLP/SNT: un sistema per la gestione automatica di un archivio sanitario ad uso epidemiologico, Ist. Automatica, Univ. di Roma, RI.78-02, Dic. 1978.

(15) Torre E., Marinoni A., L'epidemiologia psichiatrica e la prevenzione delle malattie mentali, Appl.Biom. del Calc.El. N.2 1972.

(16) Wing J.K., Epidemiological methods and the clinical psychiatrist, In Sainsburg P., Kreitman Ed., 1975.

ETUDE DES FACTEURS DE RISQUE ALIMENTAIRE DANS LES CANCERS DU RECTO COLON

Geneviève MACQUART-MOULIN, Jean-Pierre DURBEC,
Jacqueline CORNEE et Patrice BERTHEZENE

Equipe de Mathématiques Informatique de
l'U.31 de l'I.N.S.E.R.M.
MARSEILLE - FRANCE

Ce travail a été mené en collaboration avec les Professeurs Pierre BRICOT, Georges MICHOTEY, Henri SARLES et les Docteurs Henri BRANDONNE, Alain DUBAU, Georges GASTAUD, Bernard SIGNOURET, Robert VILLANI.

SUMMARY

By means of a retrospective study, this work intends to examine the influence of dietary factors on the occurence of colorectal cancer.

The variables studied are concerning the daily mean alimentary consumptions of simple and complex glucides, saturated and non-saturated lipids, animal and vegetal protides, dietary fibres, vitamins, mineral constituents. The study convers 97 patients having an adenocarcinoma of colon or rectum, verified by anatomopathology. The control subjects came from Functional Rehabilitation Centres (surgical traumatisms consecutive to industrial, traffic accidents, etc...) and did not show any known digestive affection.

The appreciation of the alimentary consumption was carried out by means of a detailed individual questionnaire.

Results show a decrease in relative risk with high consumptions of complex glucides, total fibres, cereal fibres, vegetable fibres, E-vitamin and potassium with male subjects.

The risk equally decreases with female subjects for high consumptions of vegetables and fruits of current consumption, E-vitamin and potassium.

However, the risk increases with female subjects for high consumptions of animal protides.

1 - INTRODUCTION

Le cancer du recto-colon est actuellement le premier des cancers digestifs. Il représente 10,8 % de la mortalité par cancer chez l'homme et 16 % de la mortalité par cancer chez la femme.

Les travaux de Burkitt D.P., Cummings J.H. et Modan B. (1, 2, 3) ayant montré une relation possible entre le mode de nutrition et l'apparition de ce cancer, ce travail se propose, dans une étude rétrospective, d'étudier l'influence d'un certain nombre de facteurs alimentaires : glucides, protides, lipides, fibres alimentaires, vitamines, alcool et tabac.

2 - MATERIEL ET METHODES

2.1 - Echantillonnage :

L'étude porte sur :

- 97 malades atteints de cancer du colon ou du rectum, provenant de 8 Services de Gastro-Entérologie et de Chirurgie Digestive de Marseille. Les malades sont interrogés dès leur admission à l'hôpital. Ne sont retenus que les sujets ayant un adénocarcinome prouvé par l'anatomopathologie et dont le diagnostic de cancer remonte à moins d'un an (1ère hospitalisation).

- 97 sujets témoins provenant de Centres de Rééducation Fonctionnelle (traumatismes chirurgicaux consécutifs à des accidents de travail, de la route et autres ...) qui ne présentent aucune affection digestive et qui ne sont soumis à aucun régime alimentaire.

Les distributions des âges dans les deux échantillons ont été contrôlées et sont, par suite, identiques.

2.2 - Enquête alimentaire :

Une appréciation de la consommation alimentaire a été effectuée au moyen d'un interrogatoire individuel détaillé sur l'alimentation, les boissons et le tabac. Le questionnaire alimentaire proprement dit est inspiré de celui mis au point par la section de Nutrition de l'INSERM au Vésinet (4). L'interrogatoire porte sur la période précédant les premiers troubles afin d'éviter les modifications récentes que le malade peut de lui-même apporter à son alimentation.

La conversion des aliments en protides, lipides, glucides, vitamines, éléments minéraux, a été réalisée au moyen des tables de correspondance classiques. Pour les fibres, les résultats sont calculés d'après la table de correspondance de Southgate (5).

Pour faciliter la conversion des aliments en fibres alimentaires, les légumes ont été regroupés en cinq classes et les fruits en six : légumes catégories 1, 2, 3 suivant que leur teneur en fibres est en moyenne de 1 g %, 2.8 g % et 4.6 g % ; pommes de terre (2 g %) et légumes secs (16 g %) ; fruits catégories 1, 2, 3 selon que leur teneur en fibres est en moyenne 0.65 g %, 1.40 g %, 2,10 g % ; bananes (3.4 g %), fruits oléagineux (8.3 g %), fruits secs (15.4 g %).

Les variables étudiées sont au total : les glucides simples et complexes, les lipides saturés et insaturés, les fibres alimentaires, les protides animaux et végétaux, les éléments minéraux, l'alcool et le tabac.

2.3 - Méthodologie statistique :

Risque relatif :

Le risque de cancer du recto-colon, pour une consommation journalière moyenne de la classe k, peut se définir comme la probabilité d'observer un cancer chez un sujet ayant une consommation de fibres k, soit p (1/k).

On se propose d'étudier le risque relatif du cancer du recto-colon en fonction des différentes variables dont, en particulier, la consommation journalière moyenne en fibres.

Ceci peut se faire au moyen des modèles Log- linéaires pour les tables de fréquence. Les propriétés de ces modèles sont explicitées par Kullbak et Gokhale (6), Bishop et coll. (7).

Principe de la méthode :

Les données se présentent sous la forme de tables de fréquence à plusieurs critères de classification (par exemple : cancers-témoins, consommation moyenne de fibres, d'alcool, etc...).

L'analyse statistique de cette table de fréquence à l'aide de modèles Log-linéaires permet l'étude des relations entre les différents critères de classification étudiés.

En fait, on se propose de montrer comment la probabilité qu'une observation tombe dans une cellule donnée dépend des relations mutuelles entre les variables servant à la classification. Le risque relatif de cancer peut se définir, pour les mêmes classes de consommation de fibres, comme le rapport de la probabilité précédente à la probabilité p(1/1) d'observer un cancer chez un sujet dont les consommations sont les plus basses. Avec les notations utilisées, le risque relatif peut s'écrire :

$$r_k = \frac{p(1/k)}{p(1/1)}$$

En toute rigueur, le risque relatif se définit comme le rapport de l'incidence du cancer du recto-colon pour la classe k à l'incidence pour la classe de consommations les plus faibles. Les probabilités p(1/k) ne peuvent être estimées dans une enquête rétrospective. Les estimations de ces probabilités nécessiteraient une enquête prospective concernant un échantillon de grande taille dans la population générale.

Il conviendrait, de plus, de vérifier dans tous les cas la présence ou l'absence de cancer du recto-colon. Tous les sujets devraient donc être soumis à des examens médicaux approfondis, ce qui est évidemment impossible.

Dans les études rétrospectives malades-témoins, seul le risque relatif peut être approché. Les seules informations disponibles obtenues par échantillonnage sont relatives à la répartition des consommations journalières moyennes de fibres dans une population de cancer et une population de sujets témoins. Ces informations permettent d'estimer la probabilité pour qu'un sujet présentant un cancer i=1 ou témoin i=2 ait des consommations journalières moyennes correspondant à la classe k, soit : p(k/i) cette probabilité. Cependant, si on fait l'hypothèse que le cancer du recto-colon est une maladie rare dans la population générale, on peut montrer, par un calcul simple sur les probabilités, que la quantité :

$$\rho_{ik} = \frac{p\ (k/1)}{p(1/1)} \times \frac{p(1/2)}{p(k/2)}$$

peut être prise comme approximation du risque relatif du cancer étudié (r_k). Il faut noter que ρ_k s'exprime en fonction des probabilités qui peuvent être estimées dans une étude rétrospective malades-témoins.

Soit E_1 l'échantillon de N cancers et E_2 celui de N' témoins. n_{ik} désigne le nombre de sujets de l'échantillon i dont les consommations sont dans la classe k. Les données se présentent sous la forme de tables de fréquence à p critères de classification dont l'une correspond à la classification en cancers et témoins.

Des hypothèses sur les relations mutuelles entre les facteurs sont alors proposées (indépendance, indépendance conditionnelle) ; les fréquences observées n_{ik} doivent alors satisfaire des contraintes imposées par les hypothèses étudiées pour que celles-ci soient satisfaites. On peut montrer par exemple, à l'aide des propriétés des familles de distributions exponentielles, qu'il est possible de déterminer une table de fréquence qui satisfasse ces contraintes et qui soit la plus proche possible de la table de fréquence observée. Soit n_{ik} le terme générique : l'écart entre les tables observées et calculées peut être mesuré par la quantité :

$$I = 2\sum_k n_{ik} \ \mathrm{Ln} \frac{n_{ik}}{\widehat{n_{ik}}}$$

la sommation devant être effectuée sur toutes les cellules de la table de fréquence observée. Si les hypothèses de départ sont vérifiées, on trouve que I peut être comparé à une variable aléatoire suivant une loi du χ^2 à d degré de liberté ; d correspond au nombre total de cellules de la table moins le nombre minimum de relations indépendantes entre les fréquences impliquées par les hypothèses testées. En fonction de la valeur obtenue pour I et par comparaison à la quantité d'une variable aléatoire suivant une loi du χ^2 on pourra rejeter ou accepter les hypothèses proposées. La méthode précédente se ramène à une décomposition du logarithme des fréquences en une somme de termes correspondant à des effets ou interactions entre les variables. Cette décomposition fait apparaître de façon explicite l'approximation choisie pour le risque relatif comme un terme d'interaction entre les différentes variables et la classification cancers-témoins; Le risque relatif peut alors être explicité en fonction des paramètres du modèle.

3 - RESULTATS

Les risques relatifs observés ont été calculés pour l'ensemble des variables étudiées. Les facteurs alimentaires ont été considérés isolément et seul un petit nombre a été retenu. Pour les hommes ils figurent dans le Tableau I.

TABLEAU I - RISQUE RELATIF DE CANCER DU RECTO-COLON CHEZ LES HOMMES EN FONCTION DE L'ALIMENTATION

Consommation journalière	Cancers FO*		Témoins FO*		Risque relatif	Intervalle de confiance à 95%	χ^2 ***
Fibres totales (g/jour)							
< 19	14	(14.57)**	9	(8.43)	1		
19 - 22	10	(10.35)	9	(8.65)	0.71	0.21 - 2.44	5.55
23 - 28	11	(8.61)	8	(10.39)	0.88	0.03 - 0.26	(2 ddl)
≥ 29	8	(9.48)	18	(16.52)	0.29	0.09 - 0.93	
Fibres céréales (g/jour)							
< 11	35		27		1		4.26
≥ 11	8		17		0.36	0.14 - 0.97	(1 ddl)
Fibres des légumes totaux (g/jour)							
< 12	36		27		1		5.44
≥ 12	7		17		0.31	0.35 - 0.11	(1 ddl)
Vitamine E (UI/jour)							
< 8.5	16	(14.62)	5	(6.38)	1		
8.5 - 11.5	8	(10.78)	11	(8.22)	0.23	0.06 - 0.88	9.85
11.5 - 15	13	(11.58)	14	(15.42)	0.29	0.08 - 1.02	(2 ddl)
≥ 16	6	(6.02)	14	(13.98)	0.13	0.03 - 0.54	
Potassium (mg/jour)							
< 3 350	36		28		1		4.51
≥ 3 350	7		16		0.34	0.12 - 0.94	(1 ddl)

* FO : fréquences observées

** Entre parenthèses figurent les fréquences calculées sous l'hypothèse de variation linéaire du risque relatif

*** χ^2 : stastitique du rapport du maximum de vraisemblance (test d'homogénéité)

On peut remarquer que le risque relatif observé ne varie pas toujours de façon monotone, en particulier pour les fibres totales (χ^2 d'homogénéité = 5.55, 2 degrés de liberté (ddl), où on peut noter toutefois une diminution en fonction de la quantité consommée (test de linéarité $\chi^2 = 3.89$, ddl = 1). La vitamine E paraît être un facteur important (χ^2 d'homogénéité = 9.85, ddl = 2). Le risque relatif approché décroît linéairement en fonction de la consommation journalière en vitamine E (test de linéarité $\chi^2 = 7.458$, ddl = 1). L'effet des fibres provenant des légumes totaux sur le risque relatif de cancer du recto-colon paraît significatif (χ^2 d'homogénéité = 5.44, ddl = 1 ; il en est de même pour les fibres des céréales (χ^2 d'homogénéité = 4.26, ddl = 1). La quantité de potassium ingérée en moyenne par jour jouerait également un rôle dans la diminution du risque relatif (χ^2 d'homogénéité = 4.51 ; ddl = 1).

Pour les femmes (Tableau II), le risque relatif observé ne varie pas toujours de façon monotone, en particulier pour la consommation de fibres provenant des fruits de la catégorie 3 (χ^2 d'homogénéité = 5.74, ddl = 2) et la consommation en potassium (χ^2 d'homogénéité = 6.19, ddl = 2). On peut noter pour ces deux facteurs une diminution significative du risque en fonction de la quantité consommée (test de linéarité $\chi^2 = 5.63$, ddl = 1 pour les fruits catégorie 3, et $\chi^2 = 5.106$, ddl = 1 pour le potassium).

Par contre, le risque relatif augmente avec la consommation journalière en protides animaux (χ^2 d'homogénéité = 4.65, ddl = 1).

TABLEAU II - RISQUE RELATIF DE CANCER DU RECTO-COLON CHEZ LES FEMMES EN FONCTION DE L'ALIMENTATION

Consommation journalière	Cancers FO*		Témoins FO*		Risque relatif	Intervalle de confiance à 95%	χ^2
Protides animaux (g/jour)							
< 45	13		24		1		4.65
≥ 45	41		31		2.44	1.07 - 5.53	(1 ddl)
Fibres des fruits catégorie 3 (g/jour)							
< 3	21	(20.58)**	11	(11.42)	1		
3 - 5.9	21	(21.85)	23	(22.15)	0.48	0.19 - 1.22	5.74 (2 ddl)
≥ 6	12	(11.58)	21	(21.42)	0.30	0.11 - 0.83	
Potassium (mg/jour)							
< 2.000	16	(14.90)	6	(7.10)	1		
2.000 - 2.599	12	(14.20)	14	(11.80)	0.32	0.09 - 1.08	6.19 (2 ddl)
≥ 2.600	26	(24.90)	35	(36.10)	0.28	0.10 - 0.81	

* FO : fréquences observées

** Entre parenthèses figurent les fréquences calculées sous l'hypothèse de variation linéaire du risque relatif

Il faut noter que, chez les hommes, le risque relatif est plus bas pour des consommations élevées en glucides complexes (R.R. = 1 pour une consommation moyenne < à 130 g/jour et R.R. = 0.16 pour une consommation > 180 g/jour) et en fibres provenant de l'ensemble des fruits (R.R. = 1 pour une consommation moyenne < 7 g/jour, R.R. = 0.53 pour une consommation > 7 g/jour).

Pour les femmes, le risque relatif est plus bas pour des consommations élevées en fibres des légumes de la catégorie 2 (R.R. = 1 pour une consommation moyenne < 4g/jour, R.R. = 0.47 pour une consommation > 8 g/jour), et en fibres provenant de l'ensemble des légumes (R.R. = 1 pour une consommation moyenne < 15 g/jour, R.R. = 0.5 pour une consommation > 15 g/jour).

On doit noter que, ni la consommation d'alcool, ni la consommation de tabac n'ont d'effets apparents sur le risque relatif de cancer du recto-colon. Ceci est en désaccord avec certains résultats antérieurs qui ont mis en évidence la consommation de bière et de cigarettes comme facteur de risque (M.E. Breslow and James E. Enstrom (8)).

4 - DISCUSSION

Ce travail porte sur l'étude des facteurs de risque alimentaire dans les cancers du recto-colon. Les variables étudiées concernent les glucides, les lipides et les fibres, les vitamines, les éléments minéraux, l'alcool et le tabac. Une telle étude est difficile à aborder par le biais d'une enquête rétrospective portant sur les habitudes alimentaires. En effet, les hypothèses nécessaires pour une étude précise du risque relatif nécessitent :

1) que les malades et les témoins choisis soient issus de la même population et représentatifs de leurs sous-populations respectives ;

2) soit que la maladie considérée soit rare dans la population générale, ou comme l'a montré Miettinen (9) que la population soit stable au cours du temps.

En ce qui concerne nos échantillons, ils ne sont certainement pas représentatifs de la population générale et la maladie concernée ne peut être considérée comme rare. Toutefois, on peut admettre que la quantité utilisée pour estimer le risque relatif est, malgré tout, un indicateur valable de la corrélation entre la présence de la maladie et les facteurs considérés.

La méthode d'analyse choisie permet d'étudier une table de fréquence de façon complète et exhaustive en tenant compte des effets interactions entre les variables et elle offre le moyen de tester un certain nombre d'hypothèses vraisemblables sur les liaisons entre maladie et facteurs. Les résultats sont, en particulier, interprétables en terme de risque relatif contrairement à la méthode logistique.

Les résultats montrent que le risque relatif diminue pour une consommation élevée en glucides complexes chez les hommes. Il n'y aurait pas d'effet chez les femmes. Pour les lipides aucune variation significative n'a été mise en évidence dans aucun des deux sexes. Le risque relatif augmente significativement chez les femmes avec la consommation en protides animaux, mais rien de significatif n'a été noté chez les hommes. Les résultats sur les fibres sont particulièrement intéressants, puisque le risque est significativement diminué chez les hommes quand la quantité totale de fibres ingérées augmente (et particulièrement celles des céréales et des légumes).

Chez les femmes, le risque diminue pour des consommations élevées en légumes et en fruits (et plus particulièrement pour les légumes catégorie 2 et les fruits catégorie 3).

Pour de fortes consommations de vitamine E et de potassium, le risque relatif diminue aussi bien chez les hommes que chez les femmes.

Ces résultats peuvent être rattachés à un certain nombre d'hypothèses physiopathologiques. En effet, les fibres auraient un effet protecteur sur la muqueuse intestinale, en absorbant, en diluant ou en éliminant les acides biliaires insaturés qui jouent le rôle de carcinogènes ou de cocarcinogènes. De même, la vitamine E pourrait jouer un rôle indirect par ses propriétés d'antioxydants.

Il paraît donc utile de poursuivre de telles recherches épidémiologiques sur les relations entre nutrition et cancer, car il semble du plus haut intérêt de dépister les populations à risque sur lesquelles une surveillance particulière devrait être exercée.

REFERENCES

(1) BURKITT D.P. Epidemiology of cancer of the colon and rectum. Cancer. 1971 ; 28 : 3-13

(2) CUMMINGS J.H. Dietary factors in the aetiology of gastrointestinal cancer. J. Hum. Nutr. 1978 ; 32 (6) : 455-65

(3) MODAN Baruch, M.D. BARELL Vita B.A., LUBIN Flora, R.D. et al. Low fiber intake as an etiologic factor in cancer of the colon. J. Nat. Cancer Inst. 1975 ; 55, n° 1 : 15-17

(4) CUBEAU J., PEQUIGNOT G. Enquête méthodologique testant la validité d'un interrogatoire portant sur l'alimentation passée d'un groupe de sujets de sexe masculin. Rev. Epidémiol. Med. Soc. Santé Publique. 1976 ; 24 : 61-67

(5) Mc CANCE and WIDDOWSON, in "The composition of foods", A.A. PAUL and D.A.T. SOUTHGATE, H.M. Stationnary Office, London , 1978

(6) KULLBACK S., GOKHALE D.V. The information in contingency tables. Marcel Dekker Inc., New York, 1978

(7) BISHOP Y., FIENBERG S., HOLLAND P.N. Discrete multivariate analysis, theory and practice. MIT press. Cambridge, Massachussets, 1977

(8) BRESLOW N.E. and ENSTROM James E.. Geographic correlations between cancer mortality rates and alcohol tobacco consumption in the U.S.A. J. of the Nat. Cancer Inst. 1974 ; 53, n° 3

(9) LELLOUCH J. HEMOND D. L'estimation du risque relatif dans les enquêtes rétrospectives. Rev. Epidem. et Santé Publi., 1980 ; 28 : 127-129

Nous tenons à remercier Madame A. ROQUEPLO, diététicienne, qui a effectué les interrogatoires alimentaires.

Nous remercions également les Centres de Rééducation Fonctionnelle de Valmante, Rosemond,Chanteclerc, Mazargues, Les Feuillades, La Pointe-Rouge (Marseille) où les témoins ont été recueillis.

HOW TO MEASURE THE EFFECTIVENESS OF INTERVENTION TRIALS

F.H.BONJER, A.P.M.VAN DER LEE
Department of Cardiology
University Hospital Leiden
The Netherlands

A.H.JONKERS
Netherlands Institute
for Preventive Medicine
Leiden, The Netherlands

SUMMARY

A method for the quantitative assessment of intervention effects in the absence of a conventional control group is presented. It is based on the assumption that confounding influences can be estimated from the group below the level where intervention started. The statistical problems which still await solving are discussed.

INTRODUCTION

A committee for the detection and prevention of ischaemic heart disease in industrial populations started its activities in 1971 under the name COPIH. Between 1971 and 1975 some 21500 male workers were screened for the first time. Those who showed an elevated level on risk factors for coronary artery disease were given advice and guidance in order to reduce these levels. Reexamination of 15000 workers took place between 1975 and 1977.

The reasons for not appearing for a second visit are generally known. For the majority these were economic such as lay-offs and the like.

No control group was formed because at the time it was considered unethical to deprive an examinee of an adequate advice. Intervention consisted of advice and guidance about eating and smoking habits or physical activity, with or without medication.

THE MATERIAL AND THE PROBLEM

From the numerous data of the screening procedure a single parameter has been selected for this paper: the serum cholesterol level. This was measured throughout by the same method in laboratories which were centrally controlled. A high serum cholesterol is generally accepted as a risk indicator for coronary artery disease and is supposed to be susceptible to intervention methods.

The easiest way to judge the results of first and second examination and thereby a possible effect of intervention is the comparison of the mean values.

A better insight can be obtained from the comparison of the mean values at first and second examination of classes formed on the basis of the first examination results (figure 1).

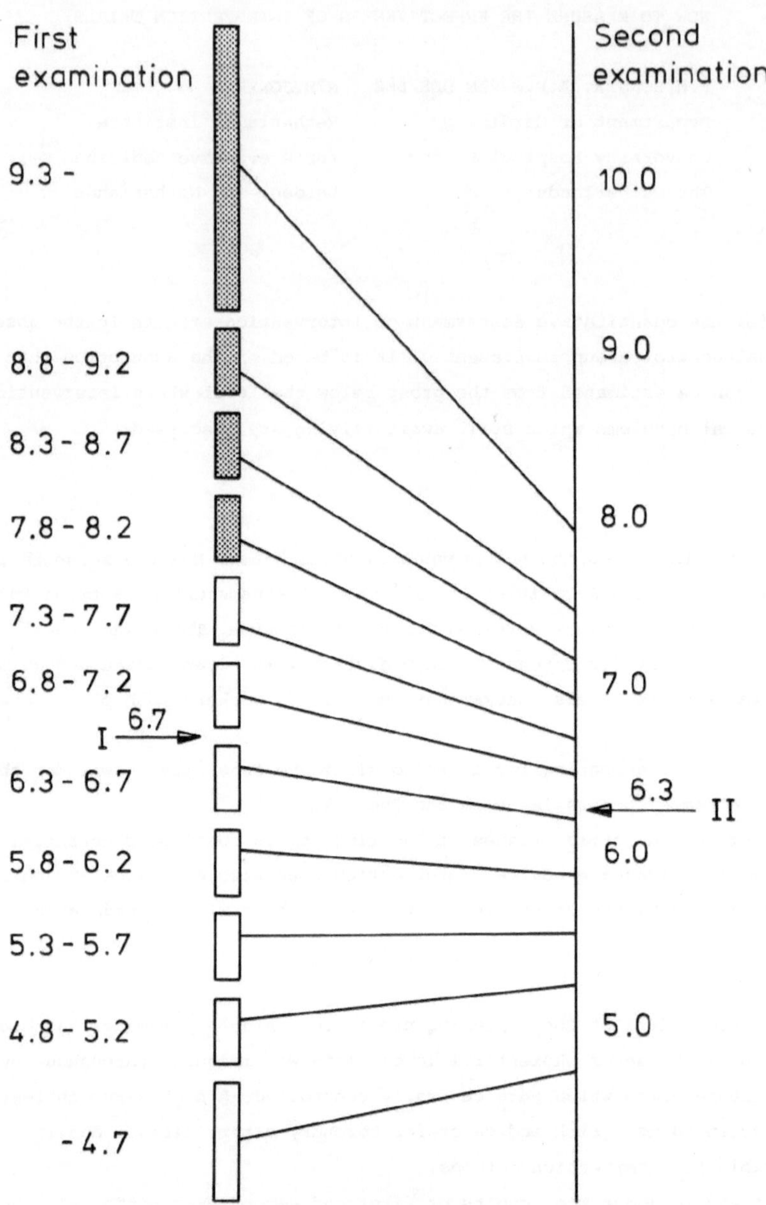

Figure 1 Serum cholesterol mean values of first and second examination in mmol/l. I and II indicate mean values. n = 15300

It is quite obvious that the groups which were initially high have values at second examination which are considerably reduced.

The statistical phenomenon of regression to the mean is clearly present. The crucial question is whether the drop of initially high values is in excess of this regression.

A number of factors has to be taken into account when considering this possible excess. Selection of the study population may have taken place because those who had an extreme initial value and stayed high have dropped out. This is a reasonable hypothesis in case of a biological parameter, that can be considered as a risk factor.

Ageing generally has but little effect on cholesterol levels.

But changes in the habitual nutritional pattern of the general population may well cause an overall lowering.

The problem is how to isolate the effect of intervention from the other factors mentioned.

The conventional approach to such a problem is based on comparison of data obtained from an intervention group and from an adequate control group. As has been stated in the introduction, such a control group is not available in the frame of the COPIH project. In the approach presented here the control group function is executed by those examinees who had initial values below the cut off point of 7.8 mmol/l and who, for that reason, were not exposed to intervention. As this group was subject to the same complex of other influences as the intervention group, it can be used as a predictor for the total effect this complex had on the intervention group. (Cook, Campbell 1979)

Figure 2 shows a scattergram of a 10 % sample of the individual values of first and second examination. The figure is divided at the level where intervention started. The left part represents the group without intervention and is supposed to show the result of all influences with exception of intervention. Differences between the right and the left part may then be ascribed to intervention, provided the assumption is justified.

In more general terms the problem can be stated as follows. Having two truncated distributions we want to test if they are parts of one distribution or not. As yet we do not know how to test this.

In figure 3 the data were reduced to regression lines for left and right part. The shift and rotation of the line to the right as compared with the line for the left part may be due to intervention.

Formulated in general terms again: we want to know whether these two regression lines are parts of the same line or are really different. Underlaying this formulation is of course the assumption that we are justified in computing regression lines for these two truncated distributions.

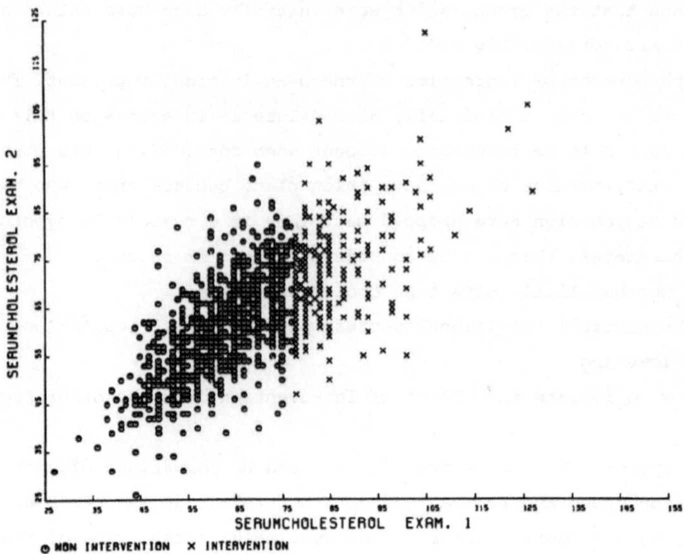

Figure 2 Serum cholesterol values of first and second examination. Intervention was applied whenever initial values of serum cholesterol were above 7.8 mmol/l. Each symbol represents at least one individual.

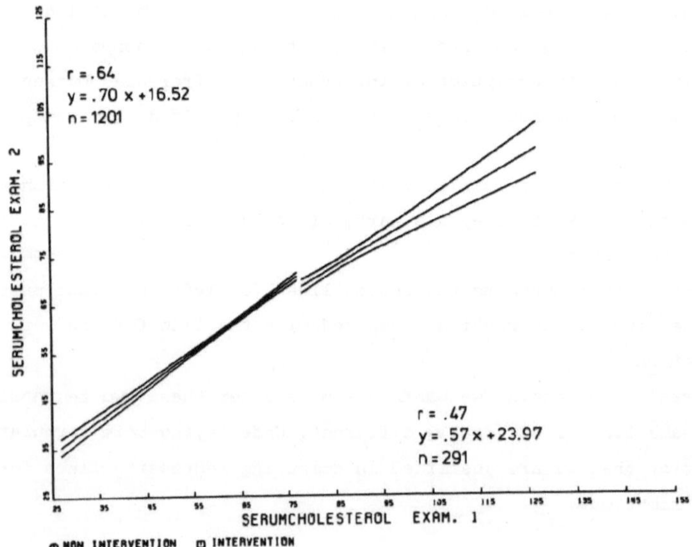

Figure 3 Regression lines for serum cholesterol values above and below an initial level of 7.8 mmol/l (95 % confidence limits).

DISCUSSION

The problem presented here is one which is common to many intervention schemes. These schemes were started with the aim to provide a service. Only later, when one tried to evaluate what was being done, arose the problem which we have put before you.
We really have come to ask your advice in solving it. Whether or not there is a real intervention effect in the COPIH data which were used as an example is, at this point, not relevant.
The first question is whether it is justified to use the results of the group below the intervention point, the group to the left in our figures, as a predictor for all kinds of confounding influences. We think we are justified to do so for two reasons. Firstly these influences should operate regardless of the level of cholesterol. Secondly, we looked at data from a study of 575 apparently healthy Dutch people, who did not receive intervention regardless the initial cholesterol level found. They were examined in 1970 and 1973 with three years between examinations. Figure 4 shows the scattergram of their individual values. There is no hint here of the two parts which we saw in the COPIH data of figure 2.

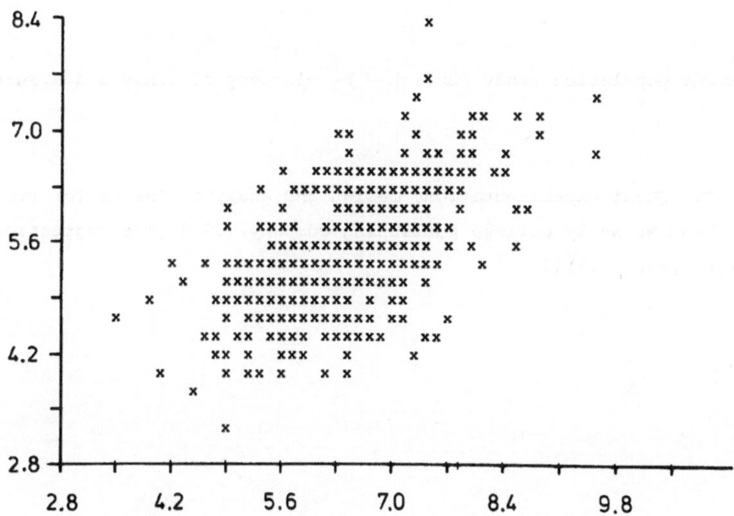

Figure 4 Serum cholesterol values of first and second examination (without examination) from the Vlagtwedde population study. Each symbol represents at least one individual. r = .61 n = 575

The second question relates to the computation of the regression lines for the two truncated distributions. Is the conventional method still aplicable in this situation? We do not really see why not, but we may be wrong in this.

The third question follows from the second. If regression lines can be computed, how can one test if the lines for the two truncated distributions are significantly different?

Finally one would like, of course, to quantify the intervention effect provided the foregoing problems can be solved. We think it would be reasonable to use for this the extrapolation of the regression line of the non intervention part. The difference between the expectation derived from this and the actual observations would be an expression of the magnitude of the intervention effect.

It would be extremely useful for many physicians working on intervention if these problems could be clarified.

CONCLUSION

Although not all statistical aspects of the approach presented here are completely understood, it seems to be possible to assess the effectiveness of intervention trials in the absence of a conventional control group.

ACKNOWLEDGEMENT

Data of the Vlagtwedde population study published by courtesy of J.May and J.Burema.

REFERENCE

Cook ThD, Campbell DT. Quasi-experimentation, design and analysis issues for field settings. Chicago. Rand Mc.Nally college publishing company. 1979. The regression-discontinuity design, page 137-142.

A Computer System for Occupational Health Epidemiology

by

Carl-Göran Anjou (1), Kjell Andersson (2), Olav Axelson (3)
Christer Edling (3), Per-Johan Samuelsson (1), Ove Wigertz (1)

Department of Medical Informatics, Linköping University, Linköping (1) and
Departments of Occupational Medicine, Regional Hospital, Örebro (2) and
University Hospital, Linköping (3), Sweden

ABSTRACT: To support the analysis of cohort data with comparison to the national averages of morbidity or mortality, a computer-based program system has been developed for the determination of expected numbers of cause-specific deaths as well as expected cases of cancer disease in a cohort. The features of the system refers to such operations as interactive data entry employing error-checking routines, data storing, fast and efficient data retrieval and permits various options with regard to exposure conditions and induction-latency periods. This paper describes the general principles of this program, and gives one example of a concrete application for which the system has been used.

This work was financially supported by the Swedish Work Environment Fund (Grant No 79/371 A).

1. INTRODUCTION

Various risk factors for disease have been identified through epidemiological research both in medicine at large and in occupational health in particular. During the last decade there has also been an increasing interest for epidemiological studies and considerable methodological development has taken place. Epidemiological projects tend to be laborious, however, and therefore it is desirable to utilize computer technique as far as possible, especially for the realization of a more or less routineous surveillance of various worker populations with exposure to known or suspected health hazards. Such surveillance would require databases for individual exposure, data on outcome in disease and epidemiological and statistical programs for data evaluation.

Information about disease is reasonably easy to achive in some countries, at least as far as cancer disorders and causes of death are concerned since available through the national health statistics. More difficult is to achieve exposure information, especially the more detailed one which goes beyond such crude indicators of exposure as occupational title, years in a particular job etc. However, the intent of this communication is not to discuss these general aspects but to present the principle and use of a computerized program for cohort or follow-up studies both with regard to open and closed cohorts and with some options regarding the induction-latency period aspect as particularly relevant in cancer studies but important also in the context of other disorders.

2. SYSTEM ORGANIZATION

The functional organization of the system is shown in figure 1. It consists of the occupational exposure database which basicly contains employee information regarding person identification, time of employment, types and levels of exposure and a medical record containing significant prior diagnosis and causes of death. All diagnosis are coded according to the International Classification of Disease, ICD, 1965 (WHO 1965). In order to provide mortality and incidence rates there is an additional database containing national age and sex specific rates for cancer disorders and causes of deaths. The system also supports such operations as interactive data entry, database management, selective retrieval, updating and editing support for all data. In order to ensure a high degree of data quality the system performs validity checks at data entry, e.g. if the first year of employment precedes the birth year an error message is displayed, etc.

A considerable amount of effort has been devoted to make the system easy to use for the unexperienced user. The dialogue used for interactions between the user and the system is a mix of a command language, i.e. the user controls the actions of the system by issuing different commands, and a guided dialogue where the user is promted for input. At all levels there are help information available where the user gets further explanations and comments.

The main objective of the system is to determine the expected numbers of cause-specific deaths or cancers. To achieve this a number of requirements on the system design has been considered. As many workers often encounter multiple exposures in their jobs, the need of registration of multiple exposure has emerged as an essential feature of the system.

Another requirement has been that the system should accommodate several periods of employment. To achieve this the program can take three periods of employment into consideration with the possibility to accumulate information of up to ten different types of occupational exposure.

3. PRINCIPLE OF THE PROGRAM

The computer program is based on the principle of observation of person-years at risk, i.e. during a particular calendar year a certain individual contributes with a person-year at observation in a specific category of age and sex. For a given cohort, the program provides the aggregate of age and sex specific person-years under observation during the study period, and, in a second step, multiplies the matrix of person-years with the matrix of national age and sex specific incidence rates for the respective calendar years and summarizes the resulting fractional contributions to obtain the expected numbers of cause-specific deaths or cancers (cf MacMahon and Pugh 1970, Axelson and Ulander 1975). In a third step a comparison is made with the observed numbers in terms of point estimates and selected confidence intervals for the rate-ratio along with p-values based on the Poisson distribution (Cutler, Schneiderman and Greenhouse 1954)

After executing the RUN-command a menu of all options available is displayed. From this level selection and execution of different tasks may be done. The first option, assigned to compute the expected numbers, sets up a list of instructions for the conditions to be entered for the process of selecting individuals. Data may be retrieved from the exposure database selected in accordance with the given conditions or retrieved by the SEARCH program. The latter method provides the facility of defining sub-cohorts, i.e. specifically selected groups of employees, to be entered to the evaluation program. Thus information might be obtained about the effects of particular exposure situations, either pure or selected aggregates.

The first step in the evaluation process is to compute the distribution of person-years that each individual at risk contributes during each calendar year of the study period. The criteria for selecting an individual to become a member of the cohort is given by the period of exposure, period of induction-latency, exposure category, i.e. the level of exposure, types of agents and smoking category (cf table 1). Other background variables than smoking might be considered as well.

In the second step the obtained person-year distribution will be multiplied with the national age and sex specific mortality or incidence rates to obtain the expected cause-specific deaths or cancers. Several disorders within the cohort may be studied and selection of the particular rate takes place through the ICD-code. Ranges of ICD-codes can be specified and entered to the program, e.g when studying the outcome of all types of tumors, the program aggregates all over the ICD-range 140-209 (according to ICD 1965); a result printout is shown in table 1.

3.1 The ageing problem

When a population of active and retired workers is followed for a number of years the magnitude of the risk or rates will usually increase in the older age categories. In order to control this ageing of the cohort the program provides three options. The first option enables the user to decide which age categories he wants to have excluded. This implies that the upper tail of the person-year distribution can be cut off from an arbitrary age category. An age category includes five years. The second and third option enables the the cohort to be handled according to two different approaches, namely letting the cohort be open or closed. When the evaluation is carried out for the closed cohort alternative an individual who has become a member of the cohort can only leave by cause of death. It should be noticed in this context that national cancer rates are based on the average population thus including person-years in the denominator also from individuals already suffering from cancer. In the open cohort alternative the condition for leaving the cohort is determined by the year of retirement or some other suitable criterion. That means, when a person has terminated his employment or the otherwise defined observation frame he is no longer contributing person-years at observation. This condition can be used in a rather flexible way, e.g. by an option providing the possibility to extend the leaving condition to comprise the last year of employment plus an arbitrary number of years, or one might use retirement as the rejection criterion. The fact that the cohort can be treated in different ways makes the program a powerful tool for the exploratory analysis of associations between occupational exposure and illness.

3.2 The induction-latency period and requirements of exposure.

An important parameter when studying health problems is the induction-latency period. The range of this period can be assumed to vary considerable from one disease to another and specific studies of this phenomenon are desirable. To the complexity of the relationships between the induction-latency period, exposure and illness contributes the fact that in cancer disorders the intensity of exposure seems to influence the length of the induction-latency period (Hueper and Conway 1964). To allowe for these aspects in the evaluation process, the program provides a number of options. When computing the expected numbers of deaths or cases of disease it is possible to chose any number of years for the induction-latency period. Since the length of the induction-latency period for some disorders at different exposure levels is not well known, a graph of the rate-ratio or rate-difference as a function of induction-latency for a certain disease can be displayed on the CRT. Similarly, the amount of exposure can be defined through a criterion for admission to the cohort, e.g. an exposure time of, say, one year might be required. Again, as with regard to induction-latency it is possible to obtaine the rate-ratio or rate-difference as a function of the exposure time.

4. PRACTICAL EXAMPLE

A practical example of using the computer system may be taken from a pilot study testing the hypothesis that exposure to diesel exhausts might increase the mortality from cardiovascular diseases and cancer as due to carbon monoxide and mutagenic effects from the exhausts. The study encompassed a closed cohort of all men employed in a bus company at any time during 1950-1959, some of these employees beeing exposed to rather high levels of exhausts in the context of service and repair work. The total cohort was divided into three categories, clerks (0), bus-drivers (1) and bus-garage workers (2). This latter group was supposed to be the most heavily exposed to diesel exhausts.

The study period was 1951-1978 and the outcome variable was taken as total deaths, deaths from malignant diseases (ICD 1965, 140-209) and deaths from cardiovascular diseases (ICD 1965, 390-458). There was no loss to follow-up in this cohort but a problem arose in the analysis of the data due to a suspicion of an increased fraction of smokers in the cohort as compared to the general population.

However, the smoking habits of the cohort itself could not be fully established but a questionnaire survey was made among the men who were employed in the bus company in 1979 and it was assumed that the obtained cross-sectional view of the smoking habits was reasonably representative also for the cohort.

The expected numbers of cause-specific deaths in the total cohort and in the different subcohorts were calculated by means of the computer program providing table 1, which was then further refined for presentation elsewhere (Edling et al 1980). A correction was undertaken for smoking in calculating the expected numbers of deaths for cardiovascular diseases according to a principle presented some years ago (Axelson 1978).

In conclusion the result of this pilot study was that during 1951-1959 there were 129 men employed contributing with 3161.5 person-years under observation. Without any conditions applied with regard to induction-latency period and exposure time, the total cohort showed a significant overmortality from cardiovascular diseases with 12 observed deaths compared to 6.36 expected. This overmortality was found to be referable to people who had worked in the garage (exposure category 2). As indicated above the program allowes for various requirements on the induction-latency time; requiring at least ten years of exposure and 15 years of induction-latency period, the total cohort was reduced to 79 men providing 1093.5 person-years at observation. With this option, there is still an overmortality among the bus-garage workers and under the conditions applied in the evaluation, this group showed a fourfold increase in risk of dying from cardiovascular diseases ($p < 0.05$).

5. DISCUSSION

The presented computer program for analyzing cohort data with reference to the national averages of morbidity or mortality is a first step in creating an interactive computer assistance for epidemiological data evaluation. Further development should allow also for comparison of two or several cohorts with regard to various levels of exposure, including a reference cohort. In comparison between observed numbers of cases in a specificly defined cohort and the expected numbers as calculated from national rates, there is usually no possibility to more explicitly deal with confounding factors other than age and sex as directly controlled in the program.

Should deviating smoking habits be associated with a particular occupational exposure there are usually no smoking-specific national rates to compare with but just adjustments are nevertheless possible as based on correction technique presented elsewhere (Axelson 1978). Corrections of this type was made in the study of garage personnel but is not yet available directly in the interactive computer program. In developing a variant of this program for handling of comparisons between various exposure-specific sub-cohorts, it will be possible to build in also a sub-routine for checking and adjusting for various exposure-related risk factors, i.e. confounding factors.

REFERENCES

1. AXELSON O., ULANDER A.: Epidemiologi, efter föreläsningar av O.S. Miettinen. Yrkesmedicinska kliniken, Regionsjukhuset i Örebro och Arbetarskyddsfonden, 1975

2. AXELSON O.: Aspects on confounding in occupational health epidemiology. Scand J Work, Environ Health 4: 98-102, 1978.

3. CUTLER S.J., SCHNEIDERMAN M.A., GREENHOUSE S.W.: Some statistical considerations in the study of cancer in industry. American Journal, publ hlth 444, 1159-1166, 1954.

4. EDLING C., KLING H., ANJOU C.G., AXELSON O.: Kohortstudie över dödlighet bland anställda i ett kommunalt bussbolag. 29. Nord. yrkeshyg. möte, Oslo, Nov 3-5, 1980. Yrkeshygienisk institutt HD842, Oslo 1980

5. HUEPER W.C., CONWAY W.D.: Chemical carcinogenesis and cancers. Springfield, Ill: Thomas 1964.

6. MACMAHON B., PUGH T.F.: Epidemiology, principles and methods. Boston: Little, Brown & Co, 1979.

7. WHO. Manual of the International Statistical Classification of Diseases, Injuries and Causes of Death. 1965 Revision, Geneva, World Health Organization 1967.

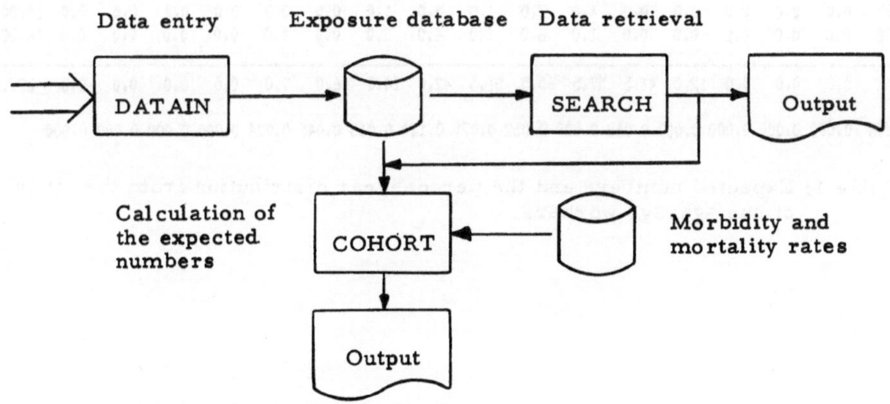

Fig 1: Blockdiagram of the system

THE EXPECTED NUMBERS OF DEATH IN ALL TYPES OF TUMORS (MALE)

STUDY:	GARAGE	POPULATION:	129	RISK-RATIO:	4.73
STUDY PERIOD:	1951 - 1978	COHORT MEMBERS:	20	CONF.INT.:	0.57 - 17.11
EXPOSURE TIME:	>10	REJECTED:	109		
LATENCY PERIOD:	15	PERSON-YEARS:	289.0		
EXPOSURE CATEGORY FOR DIESEL EXHAUSTS:	2	EXPECTED NUMBER:	0.4224		
SMOKING NOT CONSIDERED		OBSERVED NUMBER:	2		

CALCULATION TO AGE CATEGORY 90-
TYPE OF COHORT: CLOSED
DATE 24-NOV-80

YEAR	AGE CATEGORIES 15-19	20-24	25-29	30-34	35-39	40-44	45-49	50-54	55-59	60-64	65-69	70-74	75-79	80-84	85-89	90-	PER.YEAR	EXP.NUM
1951	0.0	0.0	0.0	0.0	0.0	1.0	1.5	0.0	0.0	0.0	0.0	0.0	0.0	0.0	0.0	0.0	2.50	0.00200
1952	0.0	0.0	0.0	0.0	0.0	0.0	2.0	1.0	0.0	0.0	0.0	0.0	0.0	0.0	0.0	0.0	3.00	0.00357
1953	0.0	0.0	0.0	0.0	0.0	0.0	2.0	1.0	0.0	0.0	0.0	0.0	0.0	0.0	0.0	0.0	3.00	0.00334
1954	0.0	0.0	0.0	0.0	0.5	0.0	2.0	1.0	0.0	0.0	0.0	0.0	0.0	0.0	0.0	0.0	3.50	0.00345
1955	0.0	0.0	0.0	0.0	1.0	0.0	2.0	1.0	0.0	0.0	0.0	0.0	0.0	0.0	0.0	0.0	4.00	0.00337
1936	0.0	0.0	0.0	0.0	0.0	1.0	1.0	2.0	0.0	0.0	0.0	0.0	0.0	0.0	0.0	0.0	4.00	0.00430
1957	0.0	0.0	0.0	0.0	0.0	1.0	0.0	2.0	1.0	0.0	0.0	0.0	0.0	0.0	0.0	0.0	4.00	0.00639
1958	0.0	0.0	0.0	0.0	0.0	1.0	0.0	2.0	1.0	0.0	0.0	0.0	0.0	0.0	0.0	0.0	4.00	0.00616
1959	0.0	0.0	0.0	0.5	0.0	1.0	0.0	2.0	1.0	0.0	0.0	0.0	0.0	0.0	0.0	0.0	4.50	0.00618
1960	0.0	0.0	0.0	0.5	1.0	1.0	0.0	2.0	1.0	0.0	0.0	0.0	0.0	0.0	0.0	0.0	5.50	0.00676
1961	0.0	0.0	0.0	0.5	2.0	1.5	1.0	1.0	2.0	0.0	0.0	0.0	0.0	0.0	0.0	0.0	8.00	0.00935
1962	0.0	0.0	0.0	1.0	2.0	3.0	1.0	0.0	2.0	1.0	0.0	0.0	0.0	0.0	0.0	0.0	10.00	0.01369
1963	0.0	0.0	0.0	1.5	2.0	3.0	1.0	0.5	2.0	1.0	0.0	0.0	0.0	0.0	0.0	0.0	11.00	0.01384
1964	0.0	0.0	0.0	1.0	3.0	1.0	3.0	1.0	2.0	1.0	0.0	0.0	0.0	0.0	0.0	0.0	12.00	0.01522
1965	0.0	0.0	0.0	0.5	3.0	2.0	3.0	1.0	1.5	1.0	0.0	0.0	0.0	0.0	0.0	0.0	12.00	0.01449
1966	0.0	0.0	0.0	2.0	2.0	2.5	3.5	1.0	2.0	1.0	0.0	0.0	0.0	0.0	0.0	0.0	14.00	0.01593
1967	0.0	0.0	0.0	3.5	2.0	2.0	5.0	1.0	1.0	1.0	1.0	0.0	0.0	0.0	0.0	0.0	16.50	0.02284
1968	0.0	0.0	0.0	1.0	5.0	2.0	4.0	2.0	0.5	1.0	1.0	0.0	0.0	0.0	0.0	0.0	16.50	0.02205
1969	0.0	0.0	0.0	0.0	5.0	3.0	2.0	4.0	0.0	1.0	0.5	0.0	0.0	0.0	0.0	0.0	15.50	0.01876
1970	0.0	0.0	0.0	0.0	4.0	3.0	3.0	4.0	0.0	1.0	0.0	0.0	0.0	0.0	0.0	0.0	15.00	0.01560
1971	0.0	0.0	0.0	0.0	4.0	2.0	3.0	4.0	1.0	1.0	0.0	0.5	0.0	0.0	0.0	0.0	15.50	0.02385
1972	0.0	0.0	0.0	0.0	4.0	2.5	2.0	5.0	1.0	0.0	1.0	1.0	0.0	0.0	0.0	0.0	16.50	0.03455
1973	0.0	0.0	0.0	0.0	1.0	6.0	2.0	4.0	2.0	0.0	1.0	0.5	0.0	0.0	0.0	0.0	16.50	0.03058
1974	0.0	0.0	0.0	0.0	0.0	6.0	2.5	2.0	4.0	0.0	1.0	0.0	0.0	0.0	0.0	0.0	15.50	0.02704
1975	0.0	0.0	0.0	0.0	0.0	5.0	2.0	3.0	4.0	0.0	0.5	0.0	0.0	0.0	0.0	0.0	14.50	0.02404
1976	0.0	0.0	0.0	0.0	0.0	4.0	3.0	2.0	4.0	1.0	0.0	0.0	0.0	0.0	0.0	0.0	14.00	0.02376
1977	0.0	0.0	0.0	0.0	0.0	4.0	3.0	1.0	5.0	1.0	0.0	0.0	0.0	0.0	0.0	0.0	14.00	0.02415
1978	0.0	0.0	0.0	0.0	0.0	1.0	6.0	1.0	4.0	2.0	0.0	0.0	0.0	0.0	0.0	0.0	14.00	0.02713
P.YEAR	0.0	0.0	0.0	12.0	41.5	59.5	60.5	51.5	42.0	14.0	6.0	2.0	0.0	0.0	0.0	0.0	289.00	
EXP.NUM	0.000	0.000	0.000	0.002	0.012	0.029	0.052	0.079	0.114	0.065	0.045	0.024	0.000	0.000	0.000	0.000		0.42240

Table 1: Expected numbers and the person-year distribution from the study of bus –garage workers.

THE DETECTION OF DISEASE CLUSTERING WITH LONG AND VARIABLE INCUBATION PERIODS

R. R. Harris
Department of Mathematical Statistics and Operational Research
University of Exeter
Exeter, England

1. INTRODUCTION

For diseases of unknown or uncertain aetiology, it is often of interest to test epidemiologically hypotheses concerning the possible existence of an infectious agent. Notably such studies concern Burkitt's Lymphoma (1), childhood leukaemia (2) and multiple sclerosis (3). Since Knox (4) originally formalised the concept of space-time interaction and formulated a statistical test for its existence, a number of other tests have been proposed and applied to various diseases and conditions. When contemplating an infectious agent, it is clearly of importance to consider case-to-case contact and hence to consider the incubation, or latent, period of the disease. Although most of these statistical tests are not conceptually adequate for use with diseases other than those with very short incubation periods - they only consider one place and one time for each patient - Pike and Smith (5) consider a susceptible-infective model which does appear to be logically applicable to such situations in that it allows the natural history of the disease to be specified in terms of a period of susceptibility (during which the patient would have contracted the disease) and a period of infectivity (during which the patient would have been able to infect other potential patients). The statistical test formulated by Pike and Smith considers, for all possible pairs of patients who are infective and/or susceptible within the area under study during the study period, whether or not one patient was in the right place at the right time to infect the other patient. The test statistic is the number of such concordant pairs. Under the null hypothesis of no space-time interaction, the approximate distribution of the test statistic is available for testing this null hypothesis against the hypothesis of space-time clustering of the form specified in the hypothesised natural history of the disease.

2. METHODOLOGY

In order to study the behaviour of infectious diseases, a simulation program has been developed at the University of Exeter and data output from this program may be used to investigate the performance of the

Pike-Smith test, in particular when the diseases have long and variable latent periods. Such studies have been briefly undertaken on the earlie and simpler tests using real data from diseases *known* to be infectious but obtaining the data required for the Pike-Smith test is time-consuming and expensive, so that it has only been carried out for diseases of unknown aetiology. Simulation provides an inexpensive alternative.

The program establishes a specified number of communities various distances apart and of varying population sizes and age structures. One person in a particular community is assumed to contract the disease and their infective period and date of onset are specified, together with the probability of actually infecting another person with whom they are assumed to have had contact, namely those in their own or surrounding communities which fall within their area of infectivity - assumed for simplicity to be a circle of given radius. Other cases are therefore generated and these then go on to possibly infect other members of their own or surrounding communities. The use of life-table data allows the structure of communities to be changed through time and a survival distribution is postulated for those who contract the disease. The program is sufficiently general to allow infective, susceptible and incubation periods to be distributed with various probability distributions and therefore provides a very general model for an infectious disease, in particular fulfilling the requirements of the Pike-Smith model.

3. RESULTS

In the chronic diseases that have been investigated for the existence of space-time interactions, features invariably present are the low but constant incidence rate and the postulation of a long and variable incubation period (IP). Sets of data of this form have been obtained from the simulation program for long (relative to the postulated IP) time periods and interest has been centred upon the performance of the Pike-Smith test for long and variable lengths of IP. The results reported in this work consider lengths of IP which arise from normal distributions with mean values from 10 to 25 years and with coefficients of variation up to 20%. In each case sets of data were generated for a period 10 times the length of the mean IP and the Pike-Smith test applied. Sartwell (1966) has exhibited that for short average lengths of IP a log-normal distribution provides a good fit for the distribution of IP but no such evidence exists for long mean lengths so in this study a normal distribution was considered more appropriate.

Full tabulation of the results obtained is expansive but a number of general features emerge. As would be expected with coefficient of variation zero, that is a fixed length IP, the Pike-Smith test reports significant clustering (conventionally using .05 significance level) but when the coefficient of variation was increased to 2% results became insignificant (that is, the test is not observing the space-time interaction known to be present) at the above quoted level for all mean lengths of IP tested.

4. DISCUSSION

The evaluation of any statistical test based on (simulated) data must have its limitations but it is clear (and theoretical arguments can easily be advanced though not quantified) that for diseases of long and variable IP the Pike-Smith test is generally not sensitive enough to exhibit the existence of space-time interactions. The obvious manoeuvre of reducing the significance level is clearly not available since in an actual application the test may then report space-time interactions due to non-causative agents, for example mobility of populations. However full tabulations of simulation results may give useful guidance as to when the test may be reliably used. The effect of other aspects of the natural history of the disease on the usefulness of the Pike-Smith test need to be, and are currently being, investigated.

5. REFERENCES

(1) Williams EH, Smith PG, Day NE, Goser A, Ellice J, Tukei P, Space-time clustering of Burkitt's Lymphoma in the West Nile District of Uganda. Br J Cancer. (1978) ; 37 : 109-122.

(2) Smith PG, Pike MC, Till MM, Hardisty RM, Epidemiology of childhood leukaemia in Greater London. Br J Cancer. (1976) ; 33 : 1-8.

(3) Neutel CI, Walter SD, Mousseau G, Clustering during childhood of multiple sclerosis patients. J Chron Dis. (1977) ; 30 : 217-224.

(4) Knox EG, The detection of space-time interactions. Applied Statistics. (1964) ; 13 : 25-29.

(5) Pike MC, Smith PG, Disease clustering : a generalization of Knox's approach to the detection of space-time interactions. Biometrics. (1968) ; 24 : 541-556.

(6) Sartwell PE, The incubation period and the dynamics of infectious disease. Am J Epid. (1966) ; 83 : 204-216.

ECONOMICAL IMPLICATIONS OF THE ADVANCED TECHNOGICAL APPLICATIONS TO THE CARE OF HANDICAPPED AND CRONICALLY ILL

N.GIANOTTI,A.ANDREANI

SOGESS-Sistemi Organizzazione e Gestione Servizi
Sociali e Sanitari
Via Turati, 29 20121 MILANO -ITALY-

Through the constant aid of reliable technology extramural instead of intramural care is possible for chronically ill and handicapped, costs might be saved and patients become more indipendent, self-reliant and co-subjects of the process.
If health economists confirm these conditions in analytical studies a better formulation of the law of economics of substitution among inputs of production function for health services might be:"Positive economic benefits can always be reached when in a care or cure process a patient -object is substituted by a patient -subject".

The aim of this paper is to consider some of the economic implications in applying bio- and electromedical technologies in health services.

The process of automation and the replacement of labour with capital

The first consideration is due to the fact that as often as not the technologist or, more in general, the person in charge of technological applications in welfare services tends to believe in the principle that it is always more economical to replace labour with capital, through automation.

Past analyses, based on so-called microeconomics, reveal that when applying the economic theory to industry the behaviour of the function of cost of total production and per unit produced, fluctuates in relation to the changes in its composition (fixed costs: machinery, plant, capital, etc., and variable costs: labour, consumption, maintenance, etc.) as a consequence of the continuous process of technological innovation and automation of production.

This kind of analysis concludes that, for given production intervals, this process brings about a continuous improvement in efficiency as the labour factor is progressively substituted by capital,represented by more and more automated equipments and capital goods.

The improved performance levels are measured on the basis of either a better quality product at equal production costs or higher productivity due to lower unitary costs for the same product. Where the two production factors, capital and labour, cannot be exchanged, for instance when the organic composition of a product cannot be altered, an increase in productivity is not feasible unless for higher levels of labor productivity.

But if this reasoning is true for industrial production processes for which automation was originally theorized and applied; it might be a mistake to reach the same conclusion in the case of services production, and in particular health services. In fact, in the latter, the structural and organization references of the "production process" are different and consequently the presupposition of automation is likewise different inasmuch as the "labour factor" (health operator) cannot be replaced to the same extent as occurs in the industrial production processes and in most cases it cannot be eliminated. This is the main reason, among many, as to why on an historical level, development of automation in health services would not always confirm the validity of cost-saving in the substitution mentioned. (1)
On the other hand if the introduction of automation could have brought significant cost-saving also in health services, attributing this to the law of substitution of labour by "capital" (technology) does not always seem convincing.

The real substitution process in health services

The second consideration is that this conclusion is a far too mechanistic interpretation of the real substitution process brought about the introduction of automation in health services.

The proposal to gradually automate all jobs done by a human being, end-owing the machine with all the necessary know-how, would inevitably fail in welfare services. Not only would it be nonsense to think of a complete and generalized replacement of health operators, but expropriating them of know-how and skill, through the use of technology, is conceptually wrong and would bring about the opposite results.

Should automation cause this effect then the qualitative/quantitative performance of the replacement would prove a failure, as success is strictly correlated with the availability of information capable of convincing the participants of "health production" (patients and medical staff alike) of its advantages.

The most important qualitative novelty of this technology is in fact that it should allow the patient to participate more directly in the control process.

In conclusion, the objective is to provoke a wider participation in the medical decision-making process, not only by the patient but also by the local community in general (2).

A few significant examples

The previous remarks most certainly apply to the technology used in dialysis, especially home-dialysis, or for partially assisted dialysis where the self-reliancy of the patient, involved in his own rehabilitation, is fundamental (3).

In this case technology has reached a level that guarantees sufficient reliability as far as instrumentation is concerned and a very satisfactory degree of automatic monitoring through built-in machine logic.

The patient is protected against mishaps and can confidently play the leading role, no longer an object of the therapeutic-rehabilitation process.

This has also made it possible to shift patients from intramural care to extramural care thus streamlining considerably organization and reducing administration costs.

In Italy it is estimated that with an adequate extramural semi-assisted dialysis program (10% of patients), home patients (30%) and hospital pa tients (60%), developed in parallel with kidney transplants, it would be possible to reduce total investment costs by 50% and annual costs by 10%. Excluding the cost of transplants yet further reductions could be achieved since the annual costs of semi-assisted dialysis are 20% lower than those of hospital treatment and as much as 30% lower than those of home treatment.

Another case in the rehabilitation of handicapped people is represented by electrostimulated neurolysis. This therapy, simpler than the previous one, can replace in continuation the onerous but more desultory assistance of specialized staff.

Backed up by an adequate and tinely rehabilitation program this technology contributes to a quicker recovery of motor handicapped people and an earlier return to extramural care (4).

The most important result is the possibility of handling one's own rehabilitation, enjoying a greater and in some cases, total autonomy. From an economic viewpoint the most evident result lies in a reduction of the period of time required to reach the break-even point between hospital costs, rehabilitation program cost and the saving in otherwise necessary nursing costs (5) (6).

Yet other examples can be found in dealing with handicapped people. Applications using sophisticated technologies and requiring interdisciplinary "engineering" of technologists, doctors, date processing specialists, etc., are today generalized for blind people, for the deaf and dumb (wrist communication devices, computer terminals enabling the dumb to communicate on the telephone).

Considerable progress has been made in the field of protheses, artificial organs and limbs and in human robotics. The field of examples is yet vaster and can be extended to diagnostics, monitoring and therapeutic sectors.

Similar positive evaluations can in fact be found following the application of the "full-proof" diagnostic technology and of computerized monitoring of blood pressure with wrist devices for the hypertensive (provided consumerism is curbed), 24 hours around the clock EEG measurements with portable devices for controlling epileptic children, remote monitoring during rehabilitation of heart ill and home treatment of haemophilia.

Recently the conclusions of a study lasting several years about home treatment of haemophilia, revealed that there is a decisive increase in self-reliancy in these patients and a corresponding reduction in costs of assistance (7).

<u>A trend in research for welfare economics</u>

In conclusion, the essential technological aim to be pursued is that technology must be reliable and able to give sufficient information to allow "lay" control of care and cure programs. Other conditions required and trends to be followed are: miniaturization of hardware, simple controls in device monitoring and interaction capability, simple and reduced maintenance, and so on.

From an organization viewpoint it must be possible to replace intramural with extramural care even for chronically ill and handicapped or temporarily handicapped people or at the most to transfer patients earlier from the first type of care to the second. More and more patients and voluntary people can be included in the drift of health care and cure processes.

Through the constant aid of technology, costs are saved, there is a corresponding reduction in medical staff and thus, patients become more independent, self-reliant and co-subjects of the process.

Rigorous economical researches are still to be carried out to assess condition for saving more than just inflated expenses.
If health economists confirm this condition in analytical studies regarding all or a large part of case studies (since in many situations the introduction of sophisticated intramural technologies has failed to reduce costs), then a better formulation of "the law of economics of substitution among inputs of production function" can be found for the health economics field. Thus, while the traditional "law of economics of substitution among inputs of production function" states that economic (but not only economic) benefits can be correlated with the ef -

fect of substituing labour by capital (automation), then a better definition of "a law of economics of substitution among inputs of production function" in health might be "Positive economic benefits can always be reached when in a care or cure process a patient-object is substituted by a patient-subject".

Is this conclusion true? A wide field of research is open to health economists.
Its challenge or its results might be to develop and plan interdisciplinary researches in new technologies, more capable than the traditional ones of changing impact on patients, on other subjects and on the organization of welfare services.

Bibliography

(1) Gianotti N.,Axerio G. Aspetti economici dell'applicazione della tecnologia nell'organizzazione dei servizi sociali e sanitari. Proceedings of "La tecnologia nella Pianificazione ed organizzazione dei servizi sociali e sanitari" Regione Autonoma Friuli-Venezia Giulia 1977.

(2) Tancredi TL and Barsky AJ Technology and Health Care Decision Making-Conceptanalizing the Process for Societal Informed Consent - Medical Care, 1974; 12: 250-261

(3) Blazy CR, Deley SM, Rosenquist BJ, Jensen WM, and Eschbach JW, The importance of patient training in home hemodialysis; Ann. Intern. Med. 1970; 73: 841.

(4) AA.VV.- Stroke: does rehabilitation effect outcome? Arch. Phys.Med. Rehabil. 1975; 56: 300-320

(5) Matsumoto N, Whisnant JP, Kurland LT and others Natural history of stroke in Rochester, Minnesota 1955 through 1969: extension of previous study, 1945-1954. Stroke, 1973; 4: 20-29

(6) Gianotti N, Della Corna L Considerazioni di natura economica sulla riabilitazione in Italia. Documenti Sanità 1976; 3: 215-19

(7) Kanfert JM Social and psychological responses to home treatment of haemophilia. J of Epid. and Com. Health 1980; 34: 194-200

LES INDICATEURS DE SANTE ADAPTES A L'ETUDE DES MALADIES CHRONIQUES INVALIDANTES

Jean-Claude HENRARD
Consultation de Gérontologie
CHU Paris Ouest
Paris, France

1. SUMMARY

Disablement is complex in nature being biomedical as well as social. Its study needs to identify separate concepts - WOOD has proposed three separate concepts, impairment, disability and handicap - which allow to develop disablemnt indicators. We have constructed selected indicators in order to assess the health status of the elderly and especially their disablement. The selected indicators are presented as well as some exemplary results of their application. They seems to give a sensitive view of the different factors and dimensions of disablement. This is an indispensable step before trying to consider ways in which the impact of disablement might be reduced.

2. INTRODUCTION

2.1 L'émergence des maladies chroniques dans les années 50 soulève le problème des limites du modèle Pastorien de la maladie (étiologie - lésion anatomique - signes et symptômes). Un tel modèle ne rend pas compte des conséquences de la maladie qui réduisent ou interdisent les activités quotidiennes. Une approche plus comportementale le permet mais impose de faire appel à de nouveaux concepts tels que l'invalidité. L'invalidité est souvent conçue en termes de limitation des performances dans une ou plusieurs activités essentielles de la vie quotidienne (1).

2.2 La mesure de l'invalidité a été effectuée par de nombreux auteurs selon deux approches (2). La première est l'évaluation chez des individus de leurs capacités à accomplir certaines fonctions physiques, mentales, comportementales ou activités de la vie quotidienne. La seconde est l'identification des groupes d'individus remplissant des critères d'incapacités prédéterminés (nombre de sujets ne pouvant manger seul, sortir de chez eux etc...). Ces divers travaux ont une vision simplificatrice de l'invalidité. Sa nature complexe à la fois biomédicale et sociale nécessite l'éclatement de ce concept.

2.3 Dans ce travail nous voudrions présenter : les concepts appropriés à l'étude de l'invalidité, les indicateurs élaborés pour sa mesure, des exemples de leur application lors d'une enquête de santé, en population.

3. LES CONCEPTS APPROPRIES.

3.1 La nature complexe de l'invalidité nécessite la distinction de concepts différents. WOOD dans le but d'améliorer les informations sur les conséquences des maladies chroniques a proposé trois concepts distincts : la déficience, l'incapacité, le handicap, liés en une séquence allant du biologique au social (3, 4).

3.2 La déficience se définit par une quelconque perturbation des structures ou fonctions anatomiques, physiologiques ou psychologiques de l'organisme. L'extériorisation des déficiences donne lieu à des limitations fonctionnelles. De telles limitations peuvent à leur tour donner lieu à des restrictions d'activités ou incapacités. L'état de santé physique et mental d'un individu correspond à l'existence ou non d'un ensemble de déficiences et d'incapacités.

3.3 En cas de mauvais état de santé, l'accomplissement de certains actes ou de certains comportements fondamentaux pour le maintien de la vie de chacun en tant qu'être social peuvent être socialement difficile ou impossible. La socialisation d'un problème de santé peut être définie par le concept de handicap. Le handicap est le désavantage social conféré par l'incapacité et la déficience mais aussi par un environnement défaillant. Le handicap résulte pour chaque individu des altérations de l'état de santé physique et mental et des conditions d'environnement personnel (relations sociales, logement, ressources économiques) et collectif (habitat, services sanitaires et sociaux existant). Il traduit une déviation par rapport aux normes habituelles pour l'âge et le sexe.

4.1 LES INDICATEURS MESURANT L'INVALIDITE.

4.1 A partir des concepts l'on peut construire des indicateurs qui soulèvent deux sortes de problèmes. Le premier est le choix des activités ou dimensions servant à mesurer déficiences, incapacités et handicaps. Le second est le choix du système de graduation pour chacun des indicateurs utilisés (5). Nous avons élaboré de tels indicateurs lors d'une enquête destinée à apprécier l'importance des problèmes de santé et les conditions de vie d'une population âgée de 65 ans et plus vivant à domicile dans un arrondissement de Paris (6).

4.2 La recherche de déficiences a porté sur l'existence ou non depuis au moins six mois de douleur et/ou limitation des articulations des membres et du tronc, de troubles cardio-respiratoires, sensoriels, neurologiques, de séquelles de traumatisme, de dépression et autres problèmes de santé.

4.3 La recherche d'incapacités a concerné les activités manuelles, celles dues à des mouvements des membres et du tronc, les activités de déambulation, les soins personnels et enfin les activités ménagères.

CHAMP D'ACTIVITE	NOMBRE D'ACTIVITES	EXEMPLE
A. MANUELLES	3	. ECRIRE
A. DUES AUX MOUVEMENTS	8	. ATTRAPER UN OBJET HAUT SITUE, SE PENCHER EN AVT
A. DE DEAMBULATION	4	. MARCHER, SE LEVER D'UN SIEGE
A. DE SOINS PERSONNELS	6	. SE COUPER LES ONGLES DE PIED
A. MENAGERES	2	. PREPARER LES REPAS

TABLEAU I : RESTRICTIONS D'ACTIVITES (INCAPACITES)

Pour chaque champ d'activité plusieurs gestes ou activités ont été étudiés. Une échelle de sévérité a été établie selon le degré de capacité pour chaque composant retenu.

4.4 Les handicaps ont été recherchés dans cinq dimensions : dépendance physique, déplacement, occupations, intégration sociale, suffisance économique (Tableau II).

DIMENSION DU HANDICAP	ELEMENTS RETENUS
DEPLACEMENT	ETENDUE DES DEPLACEMENTS
INDEPENDANCE PHYSIQUE	DEGRE DE DEPENDANCE DANS LES ACT. : . SOINS PERSONNELS . MENAGERES . DEAMBULATION
OCCUPATIONS	IMPORTANCE DES OCCUPATIONS : . PROFESSIONNELLES . SOCIALES . DE LOISIR
INTEGRATION SOCIALE	. FREQUENCE DES RELATIONS SOCIALES . IMPORTANCE DES OCCUPATIONS SOC. . SENSATION OU NON DE SOLITUDE
SUFFISANCE ECONOMIQUE	OUI OU NON

TABLEAU II : HANDICAPS

Un ou plusieurs éléments ont été analysés pour chacune des dimensions choisies. La graduation des handicaps s'est effectuée plus ou moins simplement selon les dimensions :

- Quatre catégories ont été retenues selon l'importance de la réduction des déplacements.
- Quatre catégories ont été distinguées à partir de l'intervalle de temps pouvant séparer deux interventions (7) destinées à répondre aux besoins créés par la dépendance physique.
- Deux catégories ont été distinguées pour la suffisance économique (oui ou non).
- Pour les occupations on a d'une part recensé les restrictions pour chacune des occupations analysées ; d'autre part élaboré une échelle à quatre niveaux selon l'importance de l'ensemble des occupations.
- Enfin en ce qui concerne l'intégration sociale on a d'une part

construit un indicateur de fréquence des contacts sociaux, d'autre part un indicateur synthétique à quatre niveaux obtenus par addition des différents scores attribués à chacun des éléments pris en compte.

5. APPLICATIONS DES INDICATEURS.

5.1 Dans certains cas il est utile d'identifier les éléments de chacun des trois niveaux de la séquence de l'invalidité pour lesquels une intervention modifierait dans un sens favorable le déroulement de la séquence. En ce qui concerne le déplacement par exemple il importe de ne pas méconnaitre les incapacités ou les déficiences d'amont. Ainsi, parmi les 54 personnes (sur un total de 204 interrogées) ayant dit avoir une réduction de leurs déplacements, 45 avaient une restriction ou une incapacité pour au moins une activité des membres inférieurs, du tronc ou de la déambulation. Parmi les 9 n'ayant pas de restriction d'activité de ce type, 7 avaient une déficience expliquant la réduction des déplacements (atteinte cardio-respiratoire, sensorielle, dépression, troubles de l'équilibre), les 2 restant avaient de mauvaises conditions sociales (ressources insuffisantes, étage élevé sans ascenseur). Tableau III.

		DEGRE DE CAPACITE		
	TOTAL	INCAPABLE	RESTREINT	NON RESTREINT
ETENDUE DU DEPLACEMENT	N	N	N	N
CONFINE A DOMICILE	23	13	9	3
CONFINE AU QUARTIER	27	13	11	3
DIFFICULTE DANS LES DEPLACEMENTS HORS QUARTIER	25	8	12	5
TOTAL	54	22	23	9

TABLEAU III : Relation entre l'étendue des déplacements et les restrictions d'activité dues aux mouvements et à la déambulation. (La fréquence des restrictions individuelles n'est pas exclusive, leur addition dépasse le total).

Dans l'ensemble les 54 sujets rapportaient 83 déficiences : 32 d'ordre rhumatismale, 21 de nature cardio-respiratoire, 15 sensorielle, 6 séquelles de traumatisme et 4 neurologiques.

5.2 Avant d'entreprendre une action visant à réduire tout handicap, il est particulièrement important de distinguer ce qui est dû au social et ce qui est dû au bio-médical. Par exemple, dans le cas d'une réduction des relations sociales qui n'est pas un handicap en soi mais le devient en cas de mauvais réseau social ou incapacités physiques, une action visant à pallier cet handicap ne peut être entreprise qu'après avoir fait la part des différents facteurs responsables. Ainsi, la réduction des contacts sociaux apparait plus fréquente chez des personnes ayant une limitation des déplacements vivant seul et encore plus nettement chez ceux n'ayant plus d'enfant vivant (Tableau IV).

	TOTAL	RESTRIC DEPL	VIV SEUL	SS ENFT
EFFECTIF	200	54	86	67
FREQUENCE DES RELATIONS	%	%	%	%
AU MOINS UNE FOIS/SEM.	76,5	63,0	67,4	49,3
AU MOINS UNE FOIS/MOIS	15,0	14,8	17,4	31,3
MOINS SOUVENT	8,5	22,2	15,1	19,4

TABLEAU IV : FREQUENCE DES RELATIONS SOCIALES CHEZ LES SUJETS AYANT UNE RESTRICTION DES DEPLACEMENTS, VIVANT SEUL, SANS ENFANTS.

5.3 Incapacités et défaillance de l'environnement peuvent cumuler chez un même individu. Il en était ainsi dans notre enquête pour de nombreuses femmes âgées de 75 ans et plus : elles étaient souvent seules (chez prés de 80%), avec des ressources économiques faibles (chez 40%), des difficultés pour les activités managères (chez 48%), pour celles des soins personnels (chez 25%) etc... Cet ensemble cumulatif des facteurs défavorables donne lieu à une rareté des contacts sociaux (inférieurs à une fois par semaine dans 65 p. cent des cas) une diminution des occupations (chez 55%) une réduction des déplacements (chez 50%) etc...

Ce groupe est à haut risque d'être placé définitivement en institution lorsque les services sociaux palliatifs sont insuffisants.

5.4 Les cinq dimensions retenues doivent être considérées comme un handicap potentiel tant que n'ont pas été prises en compte les données de l'environnement. Celles-ci peuvent corriger les désavantages conférés par la restriction d'activité qui reste alors une incapacité plus ou moins marquée sans conséquences sociales. Dans le cas contraire la restriction d'activité donne lieu à un handicap. Par exemple, 8 des 96 femmes de l'échantillon interrogé, étaient totalement dépendantes pour préparer les repas. Cet aide elles le recevaient toutes et n'avaient donc pas à proprement parler de handicap.

6. CONCLUSION.

L'utilisation d'indicateurs de déficience d'incapacités et de handicap permet d'avoir une vision probablement adéquate des différents problèmes de santé soulevés par les différentes dimensions de l'invalidité, d'identifier les groupes particulièrement défavorisés, de prendre en compte les données de l'environnement. Tout ceci est indispensable avant d'entreprendre des mesures destinées à combattre l'impact individuel et collectif de l'invalidité.

7. REFERENCES BIBLIOGRAPHIQUES.

(1) Garrad J. et Bennett A.E. A validated interwiev schedule for use in population surveys of chronic disease and disability. Brit. J. Prev. Soc. Med. 1971, 25 : 97-104

(2) Wood P.H.N. et Badley E.M. An epidemiological appraisal of disablement. In recent Advances in Community Medicine. Ed. Bennett A.E. Churchill Livingstone, Edinbourg, 1978.

(3) Wood P.H.N. Classification of impairments, and handicaps. (WHO/ICD 9/Rev. CONF/75.15) Genève - Organisation Mondiale de la Santé 1975.

(4) International classification of impairments, disabilities and handicaps - a manual of classification relating to the consequences of disease. Organisation Mondiale de la Santé 1980.

(5) Williams R.G.A., Johnston M., Willis A. et Bennett A.E. Disability

a model and measurement technique. Brit. J. Prev. Soc. Med., 1976, 30 : 71-78.

(6) Henrard J.C. Epidemiology of disablement in the elderly. Int. Rehab. Med. 1980, 2, sous presse.

(7) Isaacs B. et Neville Y. The needs of old people. The "interval" as a method of measurement. Brit. J. Prev. Soc. Med. 1976, 30 : 79-85.

RHUMATISME CHRONIQUE ET RESTRICTION D'ACTIVITE
RESULTATS D'UNE ENQUETE DE POPULATION

M. CHAVANCE[1], B. CASSOU[2], P. LAZAR[3], J.C. HENRARD[4]

1 INSERM U 194, 91, bd de l'Hôpital, F-75634 Paris Cedex 13
2 Centre de Rnumatologie, Hôpital Tenon, 4, rue de la Chine, F-75020 Paris
3 INSERM U 170 - Villejuif, France
4 Consultation de Gérontologie, Ste Perrine, Paris

A population survey was carried out to estimate the prevalence and consequences of rheumatic diseases. Notions of impairment, disability and handicap have been used, and indicators have been built up to get measurements of them. 19.5 % of the subjects were suffering from at least one chronic rhumatismal impairment. 77 % of them were presenting at least one functional limitation and 59 % an activity restriction in at least one of the 4 investigated dimensions. Nevertheless, these results are biased since the answer rate is only 52 %. The analysis of the relation between the answer rate and the impairment rate allows us to bring down the latter from 19.5 % to 13 %. As regards the nature of the indicators, deficiency and functional limitation are essentially biomedical ; activity restriction,taken as a handicap indicator, while depending on biomedical state, is largely function of social and professional environment.

1. INTRODUCTION

Les maladies rhumatismales sont parmi les plus fréquentes des maladies chroniques et invalidantes (1). Les données épidémiologiques sur l'invalidité rhumatismale sont très peu nombreuses. Jusqu'à présent en France, c'est de façon indirecte que l'on a tenté d'évaluer l'ampleur du problème, à partir de dossiers administratifs, des statistiques hospitalières ou de données étrangères. La seule enquête de population française a été conduite par un bureau d'étude, DELBARRE (2) rapporte que 22 % des 3,522 personnes interrogées se plaignaient de rhumatismes au moment de l'enquête ; appelés à noter de 0 à 10 la gêne provoquée par la maladie. 39 % d'entre eux (8.6 % de la population générale) se sont attribués une note supérieure ou égale à 8. A l'étranger les taux de prévalence rapportés s'échelonnent de 7 % au Japon, SCHISHIKAWA (3) à 23 % en Australie, NELSON et LANCASTER (4). Aux USA, l'enquête "Health Interview" effectuée en 1960-62 sur un échantillon représentatif a montré (5) que 21.6 % des sujets âgés de 45 à 64 ans se plaignaient de rhumatismes ; chez 3.4 % des sujets, il existait également une limitation d'activité et ce taux passait à 2.4 % si les rhumatismes étaient la première cause de cette limitation.

Au cours du 4ème trimestre 1978, nous avons mené une enquête de population afin d'évaluer la fréquence et les conséquences de la pathologie rhumatismale. Nous avons pour cela utilisé les concepts de déficience, d'incapacité et de handicap définis par WOOD (6) et exposés ici par HENRARD (7), pour la mesure desquels nous avons construit des indicateurs. Nous présentons une partie des résultats en nous efforçant d'évaluer l'importance du biais et de préciser si les indicateurs sont de nature différente.

2. MATERIEL ET METHODES

Trois arrondissements de Paris (IIIe, XIIIe, XVIIIe) ont été choisis ainsi qu'une ville moyenne de la banlieu sud (Arpajon). Dans chacun de ces secteurs, une zone a été délimitée, 168 immeubles ont été tirés au sort, 883 personnes de 30 ans et plus vivant dans 715 foyers ont été interrogées par les enquêteurs de formation non médicale. La proportion de portes ouvertes a été de 52 %.

Le questionnaire a été construit de la manière suivante :

1. Informations élémentaires sur la composition de chacun des foyers des immeubles tirés au sort.
2. Pour tous les sujets d'un foyer âgés de plus de 30 ans, le questionnaire individuel comporte une série de questions sur la présence pendant plus de 6 mois de douleurs et/ou de limitations lors des mouvements des différentes articulations du tronc ou des membres. L'existence d'une déficience rhumatismale a été définie par l'existence d'une réponse positive à l'une de ces questions.
3. Pour tous les sujets présentant une déficience rhumatismale, le questionnaire individuel se poursuit par
   a. une série de questions portant sur des gestes simples explorant la limitation fonctionnelle. Pour le membre supérieur, par exemple, trois gestes ont été retenus : attraper un objet haut situé, serrer un objet, ouvrir un robinet. Pour chaque geste, l'échelle suivante a été utilisée : geste possible sans difficulté : 0, possible avec difficulté : 1, impossible : 2. Les sujets ont été classés en 3 groupes en fonction du score total pour le membre considéré : 0 : pas de limitation ; 1 ou 2 : limitation modérée ; 3 ou plus: limitation sévère.
   b. Des questions explorant la restriction d'activité dans quatre domaines : soins corporels, déplacements, tâches ménagères, activités professionnelles.

L'influence de l'âge, du sexe et de la catégorie socio-professionnelle du chef de famille sur les 3 indicateurs de déficience, de limitation fonctionnelle et de restriction d'activité a été étudiée en utilisant le risque relatif (R.R.). Pour chacune des 3 variables socio-démographiques divisées en 2 classes (moins de 60 ans, contre 60 ans et plus ; masculin contre féminin ; ouvriers, employés ou petits commerçants contre cadres moyens, cadres supérieurs ou professions libérales). Le risque relatif est égal au rapport des taux de l'indicateur choisi dans chacune des classes, par exemple $\frac{\text{taux de déficience chez les femmes}}{\text{taux de déficience chez les hommes}}$. Le risque relatif mesure alors l'augmentation (R.R.$>$ 1) ou la diminution (R.R.$<$ 1) du risque de déficience pour les femmes par rapport aux hommes. L'âge intervenant de façon importante, les taux calculés par sexe et par groupe de CSP ont été standardisés par rapport à l'âge.

3. RESULTATS

3.1. Taux observés

172 sujets (19.5 %) présentaient au moins une déficience rhumatismale chronique ; 132 sujets (77 % des déficients présentaient au moins une limitation fonctionnelle dont 53 (31 % des déficients) une limitation sévère ; 101 sujets (59 % des déficients) présentaient une restriction d'activité dans l'une au moins des dimensions explorées (Tableau I).

Tableau I : Résultats bruts de l'enquête

Foyers	Réponses	sujets de 30 ans et plus	Déficients	Déficients présentant une limitation fonctionnelle	Déficients présentant une restriction d'activité
1360	715 52 %	882	172 19.5 %	132 77 % des déficients	101 59 % des déficients

3.2. Evaluation des biais

Ces résultats sont évidemment biaisés : les sujets interrogés ne peuvent qu'être différents, dans leur ensemble, de ceux qui n'ont pas été trouvés à leur domicile par les enquêteurs. On constate par exemple que la répartition des sujets de l'échantillon par âge et par sexe est différente de celle observée 3 ans plus tôt dans les mêmes zones lors du recensement général. Il est possible de redresser les chiffres obtenus en appliquant les taux spécifiques observés par âge et par sexe aux effectifs correspondant fournis par le recensement de 1975. Le taux de déficience rhumatismale est ainsi ramené de 19.5 % à 18.6 %. Ce chiffre est vraisemblablement plus près de la réalité, mais la démarche suivie permet de redresser (en partie) la composition de l'échantillon non de corriger les biais sur les taux spécifiques par âge et par sexe. Cela ne peut être fait qu'en considérant la source même du biais.Le procédé le plus classique consiste à réinterroger systématiquement un échantillon représentatif des sujets qui n'ont pas répondu à l'enquête initiale. Il est efficace si les conditions d'enquête permettent un taux de réponse de l'ordre de 100 % lors de cette deuxième phase ; pour des raisons financières, il était malheureusement impossible à mettre en eouvre ici. Une procédure alternative consiste, à partir d'une hypothèse sur la nature du facteur de biais, à effectuer une mesure pragmatique de la relation entre les intensités du facteur de biais et du biais résultant.

On observe une relation négative entre le taux de réponse et le taux de déficience rhumatismale. En effet, le coefficient de corrélation linéaire entre les transformées logistiques de ces deux taux mesurés sur les 114 immeubles parisiens ($r = -0.23$)

est significativement différent de zéro au seuil = 0.05 . Il est possible de préciser cette relation et d'obtenir la valeur du taux de déficience rhumatismale sous l'hypothèse d'un taux de réponse de 100 %. La figure 1 représente les immeubles parisiens en fonction du taux de réponse T_R et du taux de déficience T_D ainsi que le taux moyen de déficience rhumatismale pour les immeubles dont le taux de réponse est compris entre $\frac{k}{10}$ et $\frac{k+1}{10}$ (k variant de 1 à 9). On remarque que la courbe joignant ces points moyens est décroissante, un seul point est aberrant de ce point de vue. Il est donc raisonnable de prendre l'intersection de de cette courbe avec la droite d'abscisse T_R=1 comme estimation du taux de prévalence de la déficience dans la population générale. On obtient ainsi un taux de l'ordre de 13 %.

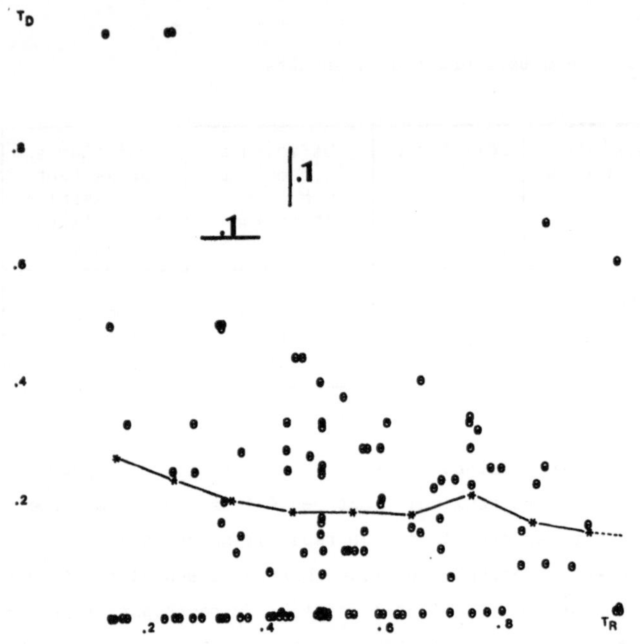

Figure 1 : Représentation des immeubles parisiens en fonction du taux de réponse T_R et du taux de déficience rhumatismale T_D

En ce qui concerne les taux de limitation fonctionnelle et de restriction d'activité parmi les rhumatisants, aucune relation significative avec le taux de réponse n'a été constatée. Il n'y a donc pas lieu de corriger sur ce point des résultats de l'enquête.

3.3. Relation de la restriction d'activité avec la déficience et la limitation fonctionnelle (Tableau II)

Du point de vue de la localisation des déficiences, c'est l'atteinte du membre inférieur qui entraîne le taux le plus élevé de restriction d'activité (67.5%) puis l'atteinte du rachis (44.8 %) et celle du membre supérieur (14.3 %). Pour les sujets présentant plusieurs déficiences de localisations différentes le taux de restriction d'activité est identique à celui des sujets dont la déficience ne concerne qu que les membres inférieurs.

Parmi les sujets présentant une limitation fonctionnelle on retrouve la même hiérarchie : membre inférieur (62.8 % de restriction d'activité),rachis (50 %), membre supérieur (25 %). Ce pourcentage est en général plus élevé que celui rencontré dans le groupe des sujets déficients. Ceci est particulièrement net dans les deux groupes présentant des limitations multiples (88.8 % et 84 % contre 65 % et 66.7 %).

La restriction d'activité augmente par ailleurs avec le nombre de localisations atteintes et l'intensité de la limitation fonctionnelle.

Localisation de la déficience ou de la limitation	Nombre de sujets déficients	dont sujets avec restrictions d'activité		Nombre de sujets limités	dont sujets avec restrictions d'activité	
membre supérieur uniquement	14	2	14 %	20	5	25 %
rachis uniquement	29	13	45 %	18	9	50 %
membre inférieur uniquement	40	27	68 %	35	22	63 %
membre supérieur et inférieur	20	13	65 %	9	8	89 %
diffuse	69	46	67 %	50	42	84 %

Tableau II : Nombre et pourcentage de sujets présentant une restriction d'activité selon la localisation de la déficience ou de la limitation fonctionnelle

3.4. Influence des variables socio-démographiques (Tableaux III et IV)

Le risque relatif (R.R.) de déficience pour les sujets de plus de 60 ans est égal à 2.3 ; autrement dit, ces sujets ont un taux de déficience (29.1 %) 2.3 fois plus élevé que celui des sujets de moins de 60 ans (12.9 %). Les femmes ont un taux de déficience standardisé par rapport à l'âge supérieur à celui des hommes (R.R. = 1.6). Par contre, il n'y a pas de liaison entre déficience et C.S.P. (R.R. = 1.1).

La limitation de fonction est au moins aussi liée que la déficience avec l'âge (R.R. = 2.9) et le sexe (R.R. = 1.7) et également non liée avec la C.S.P. (R.R. = 1.2).

La restriction d'activité appréciée globalement n'apparaît liée ni à l'âge (R.R. = 1.2) ni au sexe (R.R. = 1.0) ni à la C.S.P. (R.R.=1.3). Cependant le tableau IV, qui permet d'apprécier l'influence des 3 variables socio-démographiques sur la restriction d'activité dans chacun des 4 domaines étudiés, amène à corriger ces appréciations :

- soins personnels : la restriction d'activité est liée à l'âge (R.R. = 3.3) non liée au sexe (R.R. = 1.1) très liée à la CSP (R.R. = 7.8).
- déplacements : résultats analogues, mais les différences sont atténuées en particulier pour la C.S.P.
- tâches ménagères : elles n'ont été étudiées que chez les femmes (absence de réponses chez les hommes). Leur restriction est moins liée à l'âge (R.R. = 1.9) et à la C.S.P. (R.R. = 1.3).

- activités professionnelles : elles n'ont été étudiées que chez les hommes de moins de 60 ans car seule la CSP du chef de famille a été recueillie, et dans de nombreux cas un doute existe quant à l'activité professionnelle du conjoint. La restriction de ces activités est très liée à la CSP (R.R. = 6.9)

	Age $\geq$ 60 ans/$<$ 60 ans	Sexe+ Fem./masc.	C.S.P.+ manuel/non manuel
Déficience	$\frac{29.1}{12.9} = 2.3$	$\frac{23.2}{14.3} = 1.6$	$\frac{21.5}{19.1} = 1.2$
Limitation fonctionnelle	$\frac{24.4}{8.5} = 2.9$	$\frac{18.1}{10.4} = 1.7$	$\frac{15.1}{13.0} = 1.2$
Restriction d 'activité	$\frac{63.5}{51.4} = 1.2$	$\frac{58.7}{61.3} = 1.0$	$\frac{62.6}{49.3} = 1.3$

Tableau III : Risque relatif de déficience, de limitation fonctionnelle et de restriction d'activité en fonction de l'âge (prévalence parmi les sujets de 60 ans et plus sur prévalence parmi les sujets de moins de 60 ans), du sexe (prévalence parmi les femmes sur prévalence parmi les hommes) et de la CSP (prévalence parmi les travailleurs manuels sur prévalence parmi les non manuels)

+ taux standardisés en fonction de l'âge

Domaine d' activité	Age $\geq$60 ans/$<$60 ans	Sexe+ Fem./Masc.	C.S.P.+ manuel/non manuel
Soins personnels	$\frac{24}{7.3} = 3.3$	$\frac{17.6}{15.7} = 1.1$	$\frac{19.4}{2.5} = 7.8$
Déplacements	$\frac{45.2}{16.2} = 2.8$	$\frac{33.8}{36.6} = 0.9$	$\frac{35.9}{29.5} = 1.4$
tâches ménagères (taux calculés pour les femmes)	$\frac{26.7}{14.0} = 1.9$		$\frac{23.4}{17.7} = 1.3$
activités professionnelles (taux calculés pour les hommes de moins de 60 ans)			$\frac{62.5}{9.1} = 6.9$

Tableau IV : Risque relatif de restriction d'activité dans les quatre domaines étudiés en fonction de l'âge (prévalence parmi les sujets de 60 ans et plus sur prévalence parmi les sujets de moins de 60 ans), du sexe (prévalence parmi les femmes sur prévalence parmi les hommes) et de la CSP (prévalence parmi les manuels sur prévalence parmi les non manuels)

+ Taux standardisés en fonction de l'âge

4. DISCUSSION

Le taux de prévalence des déficiences permet de juger l'importance des rhumatismes chroniques dans la population étudiée. Le taux mesurée, 19.5 %, est surestimé car le taux de réponse n'a été que de 50 %, et ce sont en majorité les sujets les plus jeunes et sans déficience qui étaient absents lors de la visite de l'enquêteur. Une étude du biais ainsi introduit a permis de ramener à 13 % la prévalence des déficiences rhumatismales. Ce chiffre est compatible avec ceux rapportés dans d'autres études de population : 7 % au Japon (3), 13 % en Tchécoslovaquie (8), 19 % en Grande Bretagne (9), 22 % aux USA (5), 23 % en Australie (4). Il est important de de souligner que si les plus grands efforts doivent être déployés pour travailler dans des conditions de rigueur méthodologique aussi parfaites que possible, il n'est pas toujours possible d'éviter l'introduction d'un biais. Cependant, diverses techniques peuvent alors être mises en oeuvre pour le corriger.

En ce qui concerne la limitation fonctionnelle et la restriction d'activité, que nous avons pris comme indicateurs de l'incapacité et du handicap, nous avons constaté des taux de 77 % et 59 % parmi les déficients rhumatismaux, ce qui correspond à des taux de prévalence dans la population générale de 10 % et 7.7 % également compatibles avec les résultats déjà publiés, 8.6 % de "gêne importante" en France (2), 3.4 % de restriction d'activité aux USA (5). Il n'est pas apparu nécessaire de corriger les taux de limitation fonctionnelle et de restriction d'activité parmi les déficients.

En ce qui concerne la nature des indicateurs utilisés, on constate que la restriction d'activité est liée à la déficience et à la limitation fonctionnelle. Le plus grand pourcentage de restriction d'activité observé, pour une topographie donnée, parmi les 132 sujets limités que parmi les 172 déficients peut s'expliquer par une sévérité plus grande des atteintes dans le 1er groupe. La limitation apparaît ainsi comme l'expression de la sévérité des déficiences. Mais la restriction d'activité ne semble pas n'être que la simple conséquence de ces 2 variables bio-médicales. Déficience et limitation de fonction sont très liées à l'âge et au sexe mais peu liées à la CSP du chef de famille. Au contraire, la restriction d'activité étudiée globalement n'apparaît liée ni à l'âge, ni au sexe, ni à la CSP. Il est néanmoins surprenant que la restriction d'activité ne soit pas liée davantage avec l'âge. Il faut remarquer que les sujets de moins de 60 ans avaient plus de facilité que leurs aînés à exprimer une restriction d'activité professionnelle puisque ces derniers n'étaient interrogés que sur les conditions de leur départ à la retraite. En fait l'analyse de la restriction d'activité, en distinguant chacune des 4 dimensions étudiées met en évidence l'effet âge, en particulier pour les soins corporels et les déplacements, ainsi qu'un effet considérable de la CSP pour les soins personnels, les activités professionnels et, dans une moindre mesure les déplacements. Ainsi, il semble bien que ces indicateurs soient de nature différente. Déficience et limitation de fonction sont essentiellement bio-médicales, la restriction d'activité, qui est un indicateur de handicap est certes, fonction de l'atteinte bio-médicale mais dépend largement de l'environnement social et professionnel.

REFERENCES

1 Reynolds MD. Prevalence of rheumatic diseases as causes of disability and complaints in ambulatory patients. Arthritis Rheum. 1978, 21 : 377-382.

2 Delbarre F. Les rhumatismes en France. Journée de communication sur l'arthrose, Paris 8 mai 1977. Laboratoires Chibret-LaboratoiresMerck Sharp et Dohme.

3 Schichikawa K, Mayeda A, Komatsubara Y et al. Rheumatic complaints in urban and rural populations in Osaka. Ann Rheum Dis. 1966, 25 : 25-31.

4 Nelson SG, Lancaster HO. A morbidity survey of rheumatism ib Sydney. Med J Austral. 1959, 46 : 190-193.

5 NCHS. Chronic conditions and activity limitation, United States, July 1961, June 1963. Vital and Health Statistics, séries 10, n° 17, P.H.S., Washington, US Government Printing Office.

6 Wood PHN. Classification of impairments and handicaps. WHO/ICD9/REV.CONF/7515, Geneva, World Health Organization, 1975.

7 Henrard JC. Les indicateurs de santé adaptés à l'étude des maladies chroniques invalidantes. MIE 81, Toulouse, 9-13 mars 1981.

8 Sitaj, Straka L, Niepel G. The occurence of rheumatic diseases on the basis of an examination of the population as a whole. Bratislavske Lekarske Listy, 1954, 34 : 612-639.

9 Kelgren JH, Lawrence JC, Aitken-Swan J. Rheumatic complaints in an urban population. Ann Rheum Dis. 1953, 12 : 5-15.

INFORMATIQUE ET HANDICAPES :
ESSAI DE TYPOLOGIE DES METHODES D'ASSISTANCE

P. Demarne

IBM - FRANCE

PARIS

La question que peuvent se poser de nombreux spécialistes, mais aussi le grand public et bien entendu les handicapés, est la suivante : quel peut être aujourd'hui le contenu de l'intersection (déjà explorée ou bien à explorer) entre les possibilités de l'informatique et les besoins des handicapés ?

Il s'agit en fait d'une intersection probablement très riche, si l'on songe tant à l'arborescence complexe du handicap faisant lien entre physiologie, pathologie, psychologie et sociologie, qu'à celle des applications de l'informatique certainement accrue ces années dernières des conquêtes du microprocesseur, pour ce qui concerne surtout les opérations ponctuelles et locales,et des conquêtes du télétraitement en temps réel (plus récemment nommé télématique) à très vaste échelle.

Si nous essayons de clarifier les relations qui existent ou pourraient exister entre ces besoins humains et les productions de l'ordinateur - nommons "assistances" ces dernières - nous sommes conduits à examiner des schémas du type H(-) (difficultés humaines) et I(+) (assistances compensatrices de l'informatique) et tels que, dans une certaine mesure l'on puisse espérer que H + I tende vers l'annulation.

Bien entendu, et nous tenons à le souligner pour de fortes raisons, le secours matériel d'une machine si perfectionnée soit-elle, ne couvrira jamais totalement les besoins de l'être humain privé de certaines de ses capacités "normales" (ou théoriques) dans une physiologie et une société données.

Notons en passant que le handicap participe lui aussi d'une construction mentale. Il est souvent la description de l'idée que la société se fait d'une fonction physiologique "gommée".

C'est pourquoi le vécu apparaît souvent si loin du décrit, du stéréotypé, et pourquoi, les aides mécanistes participant de la même architecture sont fréquemment d'une pauvreté aussi consternante pour l'utilisateur que pour le concepteur (exemple de l'orthopédie "lourde" pour les paralysés).

A contrario, il serait très injuste d'oublier les progrès du rapprochement Homme-Machine dans la lutte contre les déficiences physiologiques. L'expression même de "poumon d'acier" par exemple en disait long voici une trentaine d'années encore sur ce rapprochement contre-nature certes, mais salvateur.

Les progrès de l'assistance respiratoire si décisifs en quelques décennies montrent parmi d'autres, qu'une adaptation sans cesse plus poussée de la machine à l'homme rend non seulement l'aide tout à fait tolérable mais contribue fortement à la faire oublier : scaphandriers d'hier, plongeurs autonomes d'aujourd'hui.

Pour en revenir à l'informatique que nous ne souhaitons pas magnifier outre mesure, il est clair que nous ne savons pas au juste comment la situer par rapport au handicap.

Une première idée fort simple apparaît ici. Pour explorer le sous-ensemble Handicap-Informatique nous pourrions tout d'abord établir un tableau donnant sur une dimension les principaux handicaps humains et sur une seconde dimension les applications de l'informatique permettant de compenser les handicaps considérés.

Approche un peu élémentaire certes, car, comme on le sait les handicaps, même très circonscrits sur le plan de la physiologie humaine, entraînent des conséquences souvent difficiles à évaluer sur d'autres plans ... psychologique, social, professionnel ...

Il s'agit donc là d'un point de départ, rien de plus, pouvant stimuler des recherches et, à terme,d'utiles applications.

Une réflexion un peu plus évoluée peut intervenir ici à partir du travail du Docteur Wood qui paraît faire autorité chez les spécialistes. Nous en retiendrons que pour lui le concept de HANDICAP résulte de la DEFICIENCE (perturbation des structures anatomiques, physiologiques, ou psychologiques de l'organisme) et de l'INCAPACITE (manifestation fonctionnelle de la déficience).

Le HANDICAP serait finalement la socialisation plus ou moins difficile selon l'environnement, des problèmes physiques et mentaux de l'individu atteint de déficience(s) entraînant incapacité(s).

Pour l'observateur moyen c'est évidemment l'incapacité qui est perceptible et assez directement intelligible. La déficience requiert pour sa définition précise des connaissances et des méthodes d'investigation généralement très élaborées et se situe bien loin du handicap. A titre d'exemple combien de beaux diagnostics neurologiques précoces sont-ils loin de donner un aperçu du handicap à moyen terme ou à long terme. De même le handicap dans ses résonances socio-économiques et socio-culturelles variées demeure-t-il très délicat à définir à partir du tableau de ou des incapacités.

Nous aurions donc tendance dans une approche large, à centrer les efforts communs des hommes de science, des médecins, des rééducateurs, des travailleurs sociaux, des handicapés eux-mêmes autour de la notion d'INCAPACITE. Ce qui n'empêcherait pas en aval de projeter cette incapacité dans l'espace social pour définir les handicaps au sens de Wood.

Si nous reprenons maintenant les grandes familles de difficultés invalidantes nous pouvons nous en tenir aux Incapacités Mentales, Incapacités Sensorielles, Incapacités Motrices, Incapacités Viscérales. Elles se subdivisent évidemment et il en est d'autres aussi selon le sens que l'on donne au concept de viscère.

Le problème devient alors en prenant des exemples pour fixer les idées : que peut apporter l'informatique à une incapacité mentale exprimée par un syndrome amnésique ? Que peut apporter l'informatique à une incapacité sensorielle aboutissant à la cécité ? Que peut apporter l'informatique à une incapacité motrice résultant d'un traumatisme médulaire ? Que peut apporter l'informatique à un diabétique ?

Quand on examine avec soin les réponses possibles à ces questions on s'aperçoit que notre désir serait de pouvoir pallier directement la déficience (aide directe) par exemple rendre la vue. En réalité dans bien des cas cela est actuellement impossible mais nous pouvons tourner certaines difficultés (aide indirecte) et faciliter la lecture pour le non-voyant par la traduction automatique du Braille.

Il est aisé de passer des incapacités aux handicaps quand on évoque les problèmes sociaux, professionnels, culturels auxquels ces incapacités conduisent.

Nous explorons en quelque sorte l'ensemble que nous nommions tout à l'heure H(-).

En face de cet ensemble se situent les grandes familles d'applications de l'informatique telles que nous les connaissons aujourd'hui et savons les maîtriser.

Dans la perspective qui nous importe nous devons incontestablement retenir :

- le <u>traitement du signal</u> (ex : prothèses automatisées ; frappe de caractères par reflet d'un mince rayon de lumière sur l'oeil du "dactylographe" paralysé...)
- le <u>traitement de l'information</u> (ex.déjà donné de la transposition d'un texte usuel en Braille et réciproquement)
- les <u>banques de données</u> (ex : documentation automatisée au service de la recherche ; de l'emploi ; des conditions de vie quotidienne...)
- les banques de données avec <u>interactivité</u> poussée (ex : enseignement assisté par ordinateur, passation de tests professionnels, aménagement de postes de travail à domicile, jeux culturels...).

Le premier et le dernier de ces domaines nous paraîssent devoir évoluer énormément dans les années qui viennent grâce aux progrès techniques des micro-processeurs et aux progrès sociaux permettant d'envisager la décentralisation de certains types de tâches (télé-travail) en même temps que la possibilité de relier par de vastes réseaux, mondiaux à la limite, tous ceux qui pourraient participer à une oeuvre commune (ex : information,de l'agence de presse au journal à domicile, éventuellement "sur mesures").

Cette évocation peut donc sans aucun doute nous permettre de progresser avec méthode dans l'examen des assistances possibles de l'informatique au handicap. Pour chaque incapacité il suffit de s'interroger systématiquement sur ce que pourrait apporter un traitement convenable du signal, un traitement de l'information, une ou plusieurs banques de données interactives.

Il serait je crois fastidieux de revenir sur bien des constatations encourageantes qui font que notre propos est tout le contraire d'un exercice scholastique.

Des enfants autistiques qui apprennent mieux au terminal qu'avec un maître vivant comme nous le disait il y a bien des années déjà le Professeur Jean Claude Pagès aux déficients moteurs, provisoires ou définitifs pour lesquels le terminal serait la solution de tant de problèmes graves, on peut imaginer la gamme des thèmes informatiques dérivant de l'examen de nos manques, de nos difficultés de nos gênes. majeures.

Le malheur, il faut l'avouer maintenant après quelques pas dans une problématique pleine de promesses, c'est que pour le moment, et pas seulement en Europe, le bilan des intersections Handicap - Informatique est extrêmement pauvre.

Après avoir interrogé nos correspondants en Europe, Afrique et Moyen-Orient, après avoir fait paraître dans une revue spécialisée une pressante demande d'information, après avoir consulté plusieurs spécialistes qualifiés, nous aboutissons aux trois conclusions suivantes :

- sauf pour les mal-voyants l'informatique est très peu utilisée en faveur des handicapés (expériences pour mal-voyants signalées en Suède, Belgique, Italie ; pour sourds-muets en France)
- un certain nombre d'expériences scientifiques possibles ne paraîssent pas avoir été amorcées
- il n'existe aucun centre de documentation spécifique pouvant permettre de situer les efforts nationaux, et internationaux dans ce domaine.

Il résulte de cette brève réflexion émanant de ce que nous pourrions nommer <u>l'informatique sociale</u> deux suggestions que nous croyons profondément utiles pour des millions d'enfants et d'adultes par le monde :

1) que le monde savant pourrait apporter son immense compétence à l'examen méthodique du tableau que nous avons esquissé, où les multiples possibilités de l'informatique seraient systématiquement expérimentées dans la large gamme des handicaps ramenés selon Wood aux insuffisances et incapacités.

2) que dans le même temps un Centre de Documentation sérieux, scientifique, puisse être créé, recueillant les résultats de telles recherches et permettant à tous ceux qui pensent détenir quelque résultat de les verser dans un réservoir commun, unique, central, à l'échelle du pays voire de l'Europe.

   Pour bien des raisons ce Centre de Documentation concernant l'Aide Informatique aux Handicapés, devrait à notre avis se sîtuer, au moins initialement, dans un cadre universitaire, un

C.H.U. par exemple. Cela pour permettre l'élaboration de travaux aussi objectifs que faire se peut en dehors des poussées contraires et bien naturelles, des groupements d'handicapés dont les constats mènent, c'est évident, à la revendication parfois très ou trop sommaire, et des Pouvoirs Publics évidemment plus soucieux d'efforts réglementaires et budgétaires que d'analyses techniques précises pourtant nécessaires avant toute décision globale.

Bref, Handicap et Informatique représentent à notre avis une immense espérance, mais c'est à la science qu'il faut en confier l'étude sérieuse, la pratique sociale permettant les ajustements nécessaires.

"HOME COMPUTERS AND THE HANDICAPPED"

J.C. Tabary, C. Tabary
F.R.A. 18 - INSERM
Hopital R. Poincaré F.92380-Garches

Certain severely handicapped people like spastics or tetrapegics, are totally unable to move or perform everyday tasks without assistance. Highly sophisticated electronic devices have been developed in an attempt to help these people. These devices have clearly benefitted from recent developments in electronics and the latest aids are very similar in conception to home computers.

In addition, computer miniaturization since 1978 has enabled "maid of all work" home computers to be put on the market at very competitive prices. Among other items, they provide opportunities of games, means of communication and teaching aids; thus the handicapped,always insufficiently integrated into our social life should be the first to take advantage of these computers.

This electronic evolution prompted us to develop the use of home computers by the physically handicapped, and we believe it is of interest to share the experience acquired in this field.

-:-:-:-:-

I-Problems involved in the use of computers by physically handicapped people.

The use of a home computer by a physically handicapped person involves several problems :

A-Financial difficulties

These are not very serious, as even a highly sophisticated computer is far cheaper than a specialized device for the handicapped, and a computer with enough basic functions will cost no more than an electric typewriter. Almost all the computers on the market can be gradually upgraded. Additional facilities expected in the near futur include a growing second hand market, lower prices and very simple devices which can be plugged into the family TV set. It is hoped that a complete home computer set, including a typewriter, will shortly be available for no more than 1000 or 2000 french francs, 250 or 500 US dollars.

B-Use of the computer

Using a computer is harder than using a device especially designed for handicapped people. In the latter type of machine, all circuits are permanently connected and immediately usable. A computer is based on many different circuits that must be logically connected before it can work. This provides much more flexibility but necessitates a different program for each use. Severely handicapped people who cannot manipulate an electric typewriter, cannot give instructions to a computer via a keyboard and cannot themselves load the pre-recorded programs.

C-Solving these problems.

The solutions are much easier than they seem. In most cases, a whole keyboard is not necessary for the use by a handicapped person. It is possible to implement programs which only require an answer of "yes or no", given by pressing a single key. By displaying groups of items of decreasing size on the computer's screen, the user can select one item from a very large number by two or three well-timed pressures on a single key. The circuits closed by this key are of very low voltage and involve no risk of electric shock. It is very simple to connect two wires corresponding to the two lugs of an electric key. As any kind of switch connected to the other end of those two wires will act as a key, different kinds of switches can be used for different categories of handicapped people, and computers can therefore be equipped with several such keys.

The loading into the computer of programs previously stored on magnetic tape can be easily learned by anyone in charge of helping handicapped people in their everyday life. Once the program is loaded, the computer is ready for use by the handicapped person.

Certain more complicated program loaders allowing the handicapped person to choose the program he desires from a program library are also available. This library can be indefinitely extended, as even if only one switch is used.

Consequently, the only remaining problem is the designing of special programs for the handicapped. We believe its solution does not require specialized programmers. It is true that some programming languages are complicated and hard to learn for non-specialists, but others can be learned and applied without difficulty. Most home computers use BASIC, a language for beginners. And once a program has been written, it is easily duplicated and can be used by people who know nothing about programming.

Moreover the firmware technique is expected to be on the market soon. Firmware is a solid-state program which can be plugged into the computer, making it the complete equivalent of a specialized device for the handicapped which requires no loading of pre-recorded programs.

In conclusion, all the above problems can be solved and should not hinder the use of home computers by handicapped people.

II-What can a computer offer a handicapped person ?

A distinction should be made between the severely handicapped and those able to use a normal or slightly modified key-board.

A-Severely handicapped.

Communication is one of the computer's obvious uses. It must provide a way of communicating in writing for the tetraplegic, who cannot write, and all the means of communication for the dyskinetic who can neither speak nor write. A computer also offers all kind of possibilities to people unable to grasp normal written language. For instance, a computer makes it possible to manipulate and translate into normal written characters a language that is symbolically easier to grasp, such as a pictographic language especially designed for the handicapped and easily programmed on a computer. It is also easy to add a voice synthetizer to the computer and turn it into a mean of active communication.

Another general use is environmental control. A multiple choice program can easily open or close any switch on any circuit. For example, tape and video-tape recorders often have switches which are hard to use for a handicapped person but can be replaced by relays opened or closed by the computer.

The computer can also be connected to a telephone. The handicapped person can select a phone number from a pre-recorded list and make his own calls.

B-Moderately handicapped people.

If a handicapped person is capable of using a keyboard, he can benefit from all the computer's advantages. These are well advertised by the programs already on the market : they includes all kinds of teaching aids, games for one or more players or against the computer and drawings.

In addition - and this is very important - a handicapped person interested in programming can soon learn to write his own programs and help others by his knowledge and experience.

III-Results of our own experience.

We did not encounter many technical difficulties. We chose the least expensive devices because they were intended for home use by handicapped people who could not afford expensive machines. Special switches were easy to build. With manufacturer's permission, two wires were soldered to the lugs of one key after removal of the keyboard lid. An ordinary switch soldered to the other end of the wire was quite sufficient to enable easy use of the computer, because a well designed program does not require precise contact with the switch.

All the programs we used had two specific routines :

- an input routine that breaks an idle loop whenever the single pre-selected key or one of several keys is pressed. This routine allows the execution of a program to be influenced by the choices which the user makes from several possibilities offered by the program itself.
- a bolting routine with a blank period immediately after a key is pressed. This blank means that the computer ignores any unintentional renewed pressure on the key for certain amount of time after the initial pressure. It allows the use of ordinary switch even by dyskinetic persons, since successive pressures during a specified period have the same effect as a single pressure.

The duration of the periods between choices and bolting times can naturally be specified in the program to suit each handicapped person. Periods can be chosen by a healthy assistant or by the handicapped person himself, depending on the nature of the program. For environmental control, special relays are used which command line voltage and computer circuitry, relay instruction is simple and only costs about 100 french francs per switch at most.

Having solved these technical problems, we were able to assess the advantages afforded by a computer to a physically handicapped person. It seems that in the communication field, they are not very great. We are not qualified to assess them in the sphere of environmental control, as we were only able to study this area superficially. On the other hand, the home computers advantages were obvious in the fields of teaching aids, occupationnal therapy and games. The use of the computer was also beneficial in psychological or neuro-medical exploration.

COMMUNICATIONS : It is fairly simple to design programs which only require the handicapped person to use a single key, when writing on the screen. The letters of the alphabet are grouped in lines on the screen and the different lines are successively underscored by a cursor. The key must be pressed when the line wanted is indicated by the cursor. The same process is renewed for the choice of a particular letter from the letters in the previously chosen line.

T H I S T E X T H A S B E E N T Y P E D W I T H A
S I N G L E K E Y . . . .

E	A	S	?	I	N
T	R	U	L	O	P
C	D	M	V	Q	F
G	B	H	J	X	Y
Z	K	W	1	2	3
4	5	6	7	8	9

Screen display during a simple writing program.

At the end of each operation, the letter chosen is printed at the top of the screen, after the letters chosen earlier.

The method is fairly slow, not because of delays caused by the computer but on account of the motor handicap of the user. We designed more sophisticated programs than those just described, in order to speed up writing, but the understanding of such programs demands greater intellectual ability from the user.

We do not believe it is possible to save more time by the other kinds of programs, which means that the low writing speed determines the limits of this method as a means of communication. Oral communication through yes-no answers between a healthy person used to handicapped people and a physically handicapped person unable to speak or write is easily sustained and by comparison, the advantages of computer communication are slight. Our writing programs are of much more help in teaching handicapped how to read and spell, and can be used as sub-routines for answering, in teaching or game programs. In these cases, it is also possible to offer a direct choice between different answers, by pressing a key when a possible answer is proposed.

We used pictograms as a means of communication. This is must easily done by drawing a series of pictograms on transparent paper. When placed against the screen, the paper adheres by static electricity. A program can provide a cursor which underlines the successive pictograms, and when this cursor reaches the one chosen by the user, he presses the key to select it. Even young children can very easily use those pictograms but they will probably not be able to articulate them so as to form a language. Nevertheless, it seems to us very important to have a practical way of testing a means of communication so widely publicized by the Bliss Method. Perhaps it will be easier to estimate more precisely what can be expected of this method when its pictograms are combined with a transistor and voice synthetizer enabling the Bliss pictograms to be directly expressed in everyday language. The home computer is obviously the ideal central unit for such a translation system.

PROGRAMMED TEACHING : Our computer appears to be a success in this field. Programs were designed to require short answers only, mostly of the yes or no ; alternatively, they require a simple choice between a few numbers. Grammar, arithmetic or general knowledge can easily be taught and tested under such conditions ; although computer teaching has been criticized, the brief question-and-answer method is increasingly used. Programmed teaching for the handicapped usually consists of a list of computerized questions and answers rather than a real course ; in this case, the computer offers the best type of dialogue possible between a teacher and a handicapped student.

DRAWING : We have designed drawing programs which only use a single key. Some of the programs on the market using several keys can be adapted to the handicapped. However, as in the communication field, this technique, ahead, slow and boring for a healthy person, becomes unbearably so for a severely handicapped one, and moreover, the less handicapped are usually very good at drawing.

Practically speaking, drawing is useful for rehabilitation when it forces the handicapped person to demonstrate a capacity for time-space representation. Again, it is efficient in teaching but not as a routine means of drawing.

EXERCICES IN TIME-SPACE REPRESENTATION : Here the computer is of great help ; it adds a notion of movement and controlled timing to ordinary exercices. Programs with single-key answers dissociate the physical task from the space representation tasks. The experience acquired with physically handicapped children shows that motricity and space representation are independent. The suppression of movement difficulties allows correct assessment of space representation efficiency and the invention of exercices specifically adapted to developing such efficiency. In our resarch, we used simple exercices, designed for example, to study eye movement in physically handicapped people. It is simple to obtain the random appearance of signs on a computer screen, and then to judge the handicapped person's ability to concentrate his gaze on one point, according to criteria of time and distance.

GAMES : Many games for computers are sold on the market. They can easily be modified to allow the use of a single key or a few keys. Consequently, finding suitable games for handicapped people is not a technical problem. The benefits of such programs are greater for the handicapped than for others. Card games become possible even when a physical handicap prevents holding of cards. However, the greatest advantage is that a handicapped person always has a partner to play with, which is especially important for a category of people whose social integration is difficult.

-:-:-:-

In conclusion, what we have described is only a beginning. Home computers have only been on the market in France for two years, so that our experience is still limited. Nevertheless, the beneficial results we have already obtained and the ease with which they can be propagated to a large number of people, give us reason to think that the home computer can become the everyday companion of the physically handicapped.

SUMMARY

Recent facilities in Electronics have given everyone a possible access to home computers able to fullfill many tasks, namely the tasks performed previously by very expensive electronic devices especially designed for helping severely handicapped people as means of communication and environment controls. In comparison, the home computer appears cheaper and more versatile. This paper reports a six-months experience with the use of home computers for physically handicapped people and gives the results obtained in the fields of communication, games, teaching aid and occupational therapy.

RESUME

Les progrès récents de l'Electronique ont mis à la disposition du grand public des petits ordinateurs capables d'effectuer de très nombreuses tâches, notamment les tâches effectuées antérieurement par de coûteux systèmes électroniques construits spécialement pour aider les grands handicapés sur le plan de la communication et du contrôle de l'environnement. En comparaison, l'ordinateur familial est beaucoup moins cher et beaucoup plus performant. Cet article relate une expérience de six mois portant sur l'usage d'ordinateurs familiaux auprès de grands handicapés moteurs et fait part des résultats acquis sur le plan de la communication, de l'aide à l'enseignement, des jeux et de la rééducation

APPLICATION OF INFORMATION TECHNOLOGIY IN REHABILITATION

Prof. Dr. W. Augsburger
Forschungszentrum für Rehabilitation und Prävention
Stiftung Rehabilitation Heidelberg
Postfach 10 14 09
69 Heidelberg - Federal Republic of Germany

- Abstract -

The Stiftung Rehabilitation Heidelberg belongs to those institutions responsible for providing existential means and social security in the Federal Republic of Germany. As supporting body of large facilities for the handicapped, research centres and institutes for rehabilitation and prevention, it has contributed since the Fifties toward expanding efforts aimed at smoothing the path of the severely disabled and especially the disadvantaged groups of disabled people leading them to an independent existence and complete integration into the community. The Stiftung is also concerned with educating the public with regard to the situation of the handicapped and the struggle to remove prejudice.

Taking the Stiftung Rehabilitation Heidelberg as an example, it is the intention to present here present and future usages of information technology aimed at realizing these tasks in vocational, medical and social rehabilitation, and to discuss future priorities and projects of information technology.

1 INFORMATION TECHNOLOGY IN REHABILITATION

1.1 Changes in rehabilitation

The change in industrialized countries from infectious diseases to the chronic ones caused by the affluent society, and, in medical care,
from the curative, remedial concepts to a holistic view of man as centrepoint of a vocational and social surroundings is confronting society with new tasks and types of services.
As a result of environmental damage, behavioral deficits of the individual and fateful occurrences, disease or accident, increasingly more handicapped persons, survived patients with multiple disabilities or invalids require the maintenance or restoration of their health as well as services which would enable them to use their individual residual functional abilities so as to obtain the most out of their life and work conditions.

In order to determine the number of disabled persons involved - it is estimated that there are about 4 - 5 million disabled in the Federal Republic of Germany and about 13 million in the European Community - and in order to be able to prepare optimal individualized rehabilitation plans, it is necessary to unify terms, criteria and procedures. As long as this premise is lacking, the disabled will suffer directly or indirectly the negative effects arising therefrom. Moreover, there are no adequate and regular statistics which could make an analysis of the situation and requirements of rehabilitation possible.

1.2 Stiftung Rehabilitation

The Stiftung Rehabilitation has faced up to these tasks and has set as its aim the social and vocational integration of the disabled with the intention of restoring the unlimited communication between the disabled person and his environment, and enabling him to participate fully to the social and economic life. In order to achieve this and in order to perform the tasks necessary thereto, the Stiftung Rehabilitation has set up facilities as well as developed instruments and methods in its research centre whose services and application for the ill and the disabled concentrate upon the following characteristics

- o cognitive and occupational skills
- o psychic and physical functions
- o social behavior

Due to the individual's increasing demand for different services outside these pre-set characteristics, it is essential to coordinate the various services such as medicine, psychology, education, sociology, engineering and administration in order to view from a holistic viewpoint strictly individual and non-independent characteristics and to prepare optimal treatment or rehabilitation plans.

Such holistic approaches are being implemented by integrated service systems in the model centres of the Stiftung Rehabilitation

- o the Heidelberg Vocational Retraining Centre (with 1700 training and residential places for disabled adults)
- o the Rehabilitation Institute for Vocational Assessment (approximately 200 places)
- o the Rehabilitation Hospital Heidelberg (approx. 110 beds)
- o the Rehabilitation Centre for Children and Adolescents in Neckargemünd
  (comprehensive school with 370 places
  vocational training facilities with 400 places
  inpatient treatment with 80 beds
  rehabilitation assessment with 60 places)
- o the Karlsbad Rehabilitation Hospital (approx. 675 beds)

Within this context, information technology has taken over important tasks in the service systems and in administration.

1.3 Emphasis of information technology

The application of information technology at the Stiftung Rehabilitation is concentrated on three main points:

- o removal of restricted communication and occupational possibilities of disabled persons with specific disabilities of various forms through compensation of effects of disability by means of technical aids for bridging reduced functions.
- o supporting rehabilitation services of the specialized fields of medicine, vocational training and school education, psychology, administration, social service, and other specialized units in the facilities of the Stiftung Rehabilitation.
- o developing instruments in the area of information and documentation in rehabilitation and for the purpose of analysing the causes of disability and rehabilitation processes.

In order to accomplish these tasks as well as development projects, the Stiftung makes use of a large-scale data processing system which is connected to over 350 data terminals in dialogue form. The various facilities of the Stiftung are provided with data processing services via remote data processing.

2 Examples of application of information technology

2.1 Compensation of effects caused by disability
- Model workplaces for the severely disabled -

In our opinion, however, vocational rehabilitation is not the final objective. It is rather the social rehabilitation that is at the forefront while the vocational rehabilitation represents an element or a prerequisite for social integration of the disabled.

This means that our interest should not be directed only toward vocational rehabilitation, but that we should think in terms of vocational and social integration which guarantees to the maximum extent secure, long-term jobs for the handicapped.

The jobs which can be secured on a long-term basis are, in our opinion, to be found in the field of information technology, this being particularly true for the severely disabled.

The following considerations form the basis of our project 'Development of Model Workplaces for the Severely Disabled':

- o In the foreseeable future, an increasing number of jobs in many areas of industrial life will be assigned to computerassisted information systems of enterprises.
- o Jobs with information processing characteristics offer favorable opportunities for severely disabled people.
- o The effects of disability can be compensated through disability-specific adaptations of the man-machine interface.
- o There are sufficient initiatives and prerequisites for the creation of jobs in and outside an enterprise within the field of application of information systems in enterprises.

Technological innovations not only make jobs redundant, they also produce new ones. For a large number of disabled in our society who are precluded from full social integration, because due to their limited motor skills they are unable to find a suitable job despite vocational rehabilitation and proper qualification, it is of existential importance that this disadvantage can be completely removed with the aid of technological devices already available today, and that these new jobs made accessible also to this group of disadvantaged persons.

There are already concrete signs for the development of such real job situations when one looks at some forms of homebound employment (text processing, book-keeping) and at occupations using increasingly computer-assisted company-own information systems at the level of administrative decisions. Particularly suitable in this respect are such jobs which obtain (nearly) all their work materials via computer processing.

With specific modifications of the man-machine interface these workplaces can be developed and adapted for disability groups with particular types of disabilities through the use of computerized working methods.

In order to secure with our research projects a wide spectrum of job opportunities and to create new jobs for a large number of disabled persons, thus reducing the unemployment level among the disabled, the development of new jobs must be based on hardware and software products which are already being widely used in practical work.

Such a software package has been implemented already on our data processing system.

2.2 Supporting rehabilitation services

- computer-assisted instruction -

First and foremost aim of the vocational retraining centre is the vocational rehabilitation of disabled persons. Since this process must be completed within a limited period of time and, in addition, medical, psychological or sociological obstacles often have to be overcome, efforts must be untertaken to ensure an efficient and humane form of rehabilitation.

Bearing the humane aspects in mind, these aims can be economically satisfied only through the massive intervention of technical media. The specific use of modern teaching and learning materials is indispensable if one is to achieve a successful rehabilitation. In this context, the computer holds a key position.

The computer usage includes application which aid or support the teacher/instructor the learner and the administration.

The CAI package is written in the interactive language APL (A Programming Language). Approx. 230 terminals are connected with this computer in a network that covers the German language region.

More than 600 teaching and learning programs are accessible to 4.000 registered rehabilitees who are undergoing professional training. In 1979 these programs have been used 130000 times.

These CAI programs are equivalent to approx. 500 hours of classroom teaching and mostly covering basic subjects that involve a great share of exercises. In addition to this, we offer simulation programs and didactic games in a great variety of areas.

At the present moment, all CAI programs conceived for typewriter terminals are being adapted for CRT display. This will make it easier to use CAI packages more widely in the Federal Republic of Germany.

We are in the process of transferring - within the framework of projekt KODA (cf. list of references) sponsored by the Federal Government - our CAI system from an IBM 3033-N onto a SIEMENS 7.521.

The costs of CAI are dependent upon numerous factors. According to our experience, one CAI dialogue hour incurs 3 to 4 DM of system costs, provided the CAI takes up 10 - 15 % of the entire data processing system.

2.3 Information, documentation and Data Analysis
- hospital information system -

The current form used at the Stiftung Rehabilitation for documenting rehabilitee and patient data fulfils only partly the demands placed upon it. Where a storage of rehabilitee data was at all undertaken, it was done for one specialized area alone and, in most cases, independently from the documentation of other specialized units.
The aim of the planned information system for the model centres of the Stiftung Rehabilitation is to prepare an overall concept for a patient-related data storage in a data base which corresponds to the situation and demands of practice and of new documentation application.
At the present moment the following partial projects are being carried out:

- o basis documentation at the Karlsbad Rehabilitation Hospital
- o social anamnesis at the Heidelberg Vocational Retraining Centre
- o vocational rehabilitation at the Karlsbad Rehabilitation Hospital
- o routine medical examinations of disabled persons at the Heidelberg Vocational Retraining Centre.

Logical data structure of the rehabilitation documentation

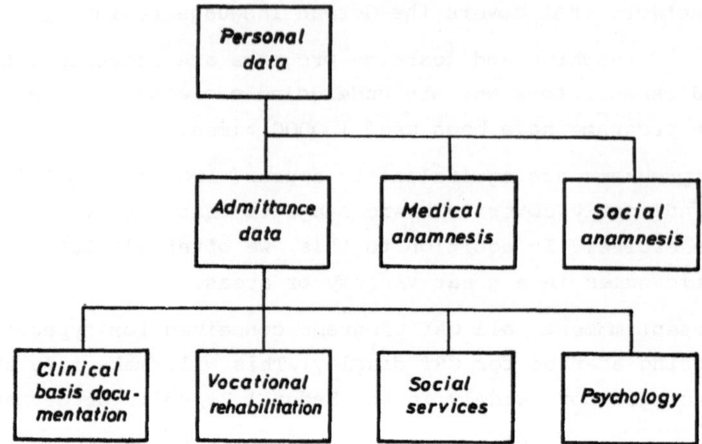

Compared to the personnel costs for the documentation in specialized departments, the data processing costs for the rehabilitation documentation system are negligible.

The rehabilitation documentation system is based on a concept applicable to different specialties; the clinical basis documentation represents simply an integral element of the rehabilitation documentation system. The clinical basis documentation, though, corresponds to the state-of-the-art.

3. Prospects

Possible undesired side effects of information technology developments and their impact on society and disadvantaged groups such as the disabled and elderly are increasingly gaining importance besides the more technically based problems. We consider this to be a challenge and believe that it is our task for the future to increase our efforts in this regard and work towards a situation which will enable us to identify such side effects early enough and take adequate countermeasures. It is our hope that our first functional experience with a more humane use of computers, as practiced in the field of rehabilitation, will find many followers and wide imitation. Another step forward towards this goal will be our project model workplaces for the severely disabled and the establishing of data bases of rehabilitation client characteristics.

Literature

1. BOLL, W.: Die Rehabilitation in der Bundesrepublik. In: Der Kompaß Heft 4, 1975

2. JOCHHEIM, K.-A. / WINDORFER, A. / u. a.: Zielsetzung der Rehabilitationsmöglichkeiten und Grenzen. Jochheim, K.-A./Scholz, F.J.(Hrsg.) Rehabilitation, Bd. I, S 14-24 Thieme Verlag, 1975

3. AUGSBURGER, W.: Informatik und Rehabilitation. In: Rehabilitation - Praxis und Forschung. Springer Verlag, Heidelberg 1977

4. AUGSBURGER, W.: Educational System. In: Lecture Notes in Computer Science, vol. 49, Springer Verlag, Berlin-Heidelberg-New York 1977

5. HAUNGS, LAMPL: Functions in APL to Assist the Programming and Servicing of CAI-Lessons. In: APL 76-Conference Proceedings. ACM, New York 1976

6. KOLLER, S. / WAGNER, G. (Hrsg.): Handbuch der medizinischen Dokumentation und Datenverarbeitung Schattauer Verlag 1975

7. EHLERS, C.Th. et al.: Datenverarbeitung im Klinikum der Georg-August-Universität Göttingen, Beschreibung des Gesamtsystems. Göttingen 1979

8. SAUTER, K. / REICHERTZ, P.L. / ZOWE, W. /WEINGARTEN, W. / FINKE, D. KLONK, J.: Datenbank-gestütztes Patienteninformationssystem für ein Universitätsklinikum 1977, GMDS-Jahrestagung Göttigen 1977

9. WEDEKIND, H.: Datenbanksystem I, II 1974 BI Wissenschaftsverlag Mannheim-Wien-Zürich

GERIATRIC MEDICINE - ITS DATA NEEDS AND INFORMATION USAGE

J. Anderson, Department of Medicine, King's College Hospital, Denmark Hill, London SE5.

M.S. Kataria, Department of Geriatric Medicine, St. Francis' Hospital, St. Francis' Road, London, SE22.

S.K. Das, Department of Geriatric Medicine, St. Helier Hospital, Carshalton, Surrey.

Summary

A system analytical view of the data involved in geriatric medicine has been made. It outlines the use of such tools as logical data flows, data dictionaries, feedback loops, data storage and output and privacy and confidentiality needs. The importance of such an analysis is stressed before system design.

Introduction

Society is now having to come to terms with longevity of an increasing number of its members and the quality of life of those who are past the age of retirement. This is particularly so as the number of people over 75 years old increases. There is no doubt that both in family practice and in hospitals the major part of medical consultation and advice is sought for by this age group of patients. The only other group creating heavy 'consultation' load is that of infants and children (1).

Thus we have identified a group of patients some of whom require continual management and 'chronic care', where information from many resources is both important and in some cases vital. There is a need to coordinate such data for the medical team to guide and control the care of these patients. Naturally data from multiple sources of expertise is needed for appropriate medical decision making and management. This may be from doctors, geriatricians and general practitioners, nurses, physiotherapists, occupational therapists, speech therapists, social workers (a multi-disciplinary medical team). In many cases there is reliable information from family and friends (2).

Thus we have been finalising the data requirements for improving medical decision making and relating such input data with the resulting outcome. These outcomes must relate not only to the medical but to the psychological needs of the patient and their social environment. Such information is of great use to guide the patient's management, sometimes over long periods of time when doctors, nurses, etc. will have to keep updating it to encompass current difficulties and events. This requires not only the efforts of a multi-disciplinary team but also a uniform, accurate and complete information system (3).

To practise satisfactory medical surveillance it is necessary to prevent events by anticipating them. For example, if we are informed that the stairs in the patient's house are difficult and dangerous and the patient is unsteady, then action has to be taken to inspect and install handrails, or if need be to try and change the environment such as changing the location of the bedroom.

Methods

To specify what users require is a major function of system analysis. There are several tools available for this purpose and we will illustrate their use.

a) Logical Data Flow

The Logical Data Flows proceed stepwise in design from an overall description and model of the data flows to the specification of detailed information flows at each stage.

Figure 1

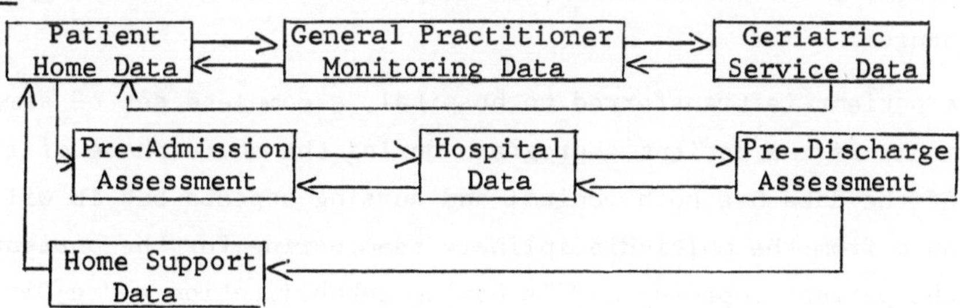

Figure 1: This gives an overall model of the basic data flows in geriatric care.

The detailed data flows developing from Figure 1 will be illustrated descriptively. The Patient Home Data set which includes the name, address and telephone number of the patient, the age, family membership and support of the family and friends with an overall physical, psychological and social assessment is the key data considered by the General Practitioner Monitoring (GPM) procedure. It not only has the Patient Home Data but checks and updates this data as necessary. If the patient is over the age of 75 years the general practitioner receives a special fee for this service so it has other attributes. When there is a deterioration in the Patient Home Data, the General Practitioner Monitoring data changes and a consultation for hospital care may be arranged with the local geriatrician. He will check to see if there is data about this patient in his Geriatric Service Data. If not, he will update it according to the data provided by the general practitioner.

Arrangements are made by the geriatrician for the multi-disciplinary team, including a nurse, occupational therapist and social worker to visit the patients home and complete a Pre-Admission Assessment. The data deals with all aspects of the patient's state including the environment. As well as including medical data there will be data about physical performance of the patient, whether he can get out of bed, dress himself and be continent during the day and night. There will be psychological data about the mental state of the patient and his emotional state. Social data will reflect his competence and the support that has been given by the family, friends, voluntary and other agencies. An environmental assessment will take into account the patient's disabilities and what support can be given by appropriate changes.

If the patient is transferred to hospital, a complete set of similar data monitors the patient's progress during the acute phase of illness. Most of the data has both medical and nursing aspects but it will also have data from the multi-disciplinary team caring for the patient. When the patient improves and is having rehabilitation a Pre-Discharge Assessment is made of a similar nature to the Pre-Admission Assessment.

The appropriate physical, social and environmental support are considered and the Home Support Data provided as a basis to support the patient on his return home. This recognises both family, voluntary and other supporting services including 'meals on wheels' and a 'home help' service.

b) Feedback Loops

The first feedback loop is the General Practitioner Monitoring data which keeps the data about the patients state and updates it regularly and brings key issues to the notice of the general practitioner. The next loop is between the Geriatric Service Data and the Patient Home Data where the patient may receive support from geriatric services such as the Day Centre and the Day Hospital. Here patients can be observed as well as encouraging social interaction and support. The third feedback loop is between the Pre-Admission and Pre-Discharge Assessment so that the improvement of the patient's medical, physical, psychological, social and environmental state can be ascertained.

This data will also interact with the home support data of the patient on his return home and it will be monitored to see that the supports provided are appropriate and useful. This area involves conditional decisions based on data.

c) Data Dictionary and Data Elements

Such a project needs a detailed data dictionary and the appropriate specification of data elements which will be used at each stage and their values must be agreed by the users. There may be general overall meaningful descriptive categories such as old people, old people frail, and/or elderly and/or sick. Each discipline involved in the multi-disciplinary care team needs an appropriate vocabulary. We have adopted the Systematic Nomenclature of Medicine (SNOMED) as our basic medical document not only because of its comprehensiveness and post-coordinated attributes, but also because it is possible to develop micro-glossaries to cover the specific vocabulary related to geriatric care.

d) Data Output

Data is output at each major step of the caring process to update other areas and also used to provide appropriate feedback loops and to trigger appropriate medical actions. It is also used by the geriatrician to coordinate the efforts of the multi-disciplinary team both in and out of hospital, especially in relation to the Pre-Admission and Pre-Discharge Assessments.

Information is also required to coordinate hospital services with community services on discharge. It is important that both hospital and community services be coordinated effectively to provide the maximum help to the patient. Thus the patient data reflects itself in data output, so that it is ensured that if appropriate data is input then the desired output can be computed. This is a re-iterative process during the analysis.

e) Data Storage

In the analysis we have avoided specification of the specific means of data storage leaving this as a design task during system implementation. What is essential is that the appropriate data requirements be revealed by the reiterative process of analysis and both flow and content specified at each stage. Different data storage procedures can then be considered in relation to the frequency of response times.

f) Privacy and Confidentiality

No one person in the multi-disciplinary team can deny responsibility for privacy and confidentiality and it is the doctors role to ensure that appropriate actions are taken. All members of the care team must be able to access all data but others may only require certain specific data appropriate to their needs or are given information by the doctor when necessary. Certainly there is a need to consider carefully the availability of information and its dissemination including statistical management information.

Discussion

The use of some of the major tools in this system analysis of geriatric care have shown that they lead to positive results which clarify the roles of the necessary data. Further information has to be provided about who is responsible for its collection. At present we have decided that it will be the responsibility of the different members of the team to enter the data appropriate to them. This may be done by completing forms and questionnaires as backup or entering data through visual display units or other devices. Monitoring procedures will use visual display units.

Doctors and other members of the multi-disciplinary team must not only be able to use set programs for specified output but also must be able to formulate their own queries and scan the appropriate data to get such queries answered. The essential part of the system analysis exercise is that it reveals to the users of the system the kind of information system which has been implicitly accepted but which has to be made explicit to work automatically.

Often in the iterative processes of analysis new insights are gained into the usefulness of data. It does emphasise that data takes time and resources to collect and it is not worth collecting if this is just an academic exercise but must be used to provide useful and necessary output. Thus the whole emphasis of care records changes as the necessary relationship to effectiveness receives more emphasis. It also provides a necessary model which can be updated to meet changing conditions.

References

(1) Bodenham, K.E. and Wellman, F. A Report for the Scottish Home and Health Department for a Health Service Information System. Nuffield Provincial Hospital Trust, Oxford University Press, 1972.

(2) Das, S.K., Anderson, J. and Kataria, M.S. Computer orientated basic research programming in geriatric medicine and geriatric case taking. Age and Ageing (1975) 4: 63.

(3) Das, S.K., Anderson, J. and Kataria, M.S. Geriatric Case Taking. Abstracts, Proc. 10th International Congress of Gerontology (1979) 11: 57.

L'EVALUATION DES BESOINS DES PERSONNES AGEES DANS LA PERSPECTIVE DE LA GESTION DU SYSTEME DE SOINS ET SERVICES PROLONGES

C. Tilquin, C. Sicotte

Equipe de recherche opérationnelle en santé (EROS), Département d'administration de la santé, Université de Montréal, C.P. 6128 Montréal, H3C 3J7, Canada

ABSTRACT

A three stage need assessment system has been developed. First social/mental/physical needs are assessed by a nurse or a social worker. Second, services needs (nursing, physiotherapy, occupational therapy, medical services, social services, support services) are assessed by a multidisciplinary team on the basis of the first assessment. Third, the type of program requested by the elderly is decided on the basis of the second assessment by a management committee.

The presentation will focus on the description of the instruments supporting the assessment process and on their validity and reliability. One will then discuss the way this instrument is used in Quebec for deciding on the placement of elderly people in domiciliary or institutional programs, and for the planning of regional health and social services networks.

INTRODUCTION

En 1977, a été entrepris le développement du système CTMSP 77 d'information pour la gestion du réseau de programmes de soins et services prolongés aux personnes âgées. Par programme, nous entendons toute organisation de soins et/ou services aux personnes âgées: aide familiale, soins à domicile, centre de jour, hôpital de jour, centre d'accueil, hôpital de soins prolongés, ...etc. Par réseau, nous entendons l'articulation de tous les programmes visant une même population, pour en faire un ensemble intégré, où les ressources se complètent et sont conçues en fonction des besoins de la population à desservir.

Le système CTMSP 77 a été conçu pour permettre l'identification, l'évaluation et la mesure des besoins de la personne âgée qu'elle vive à domicile ou en établissement. Il a été développé et validé selon le schéma suivant:

MODULE D'IDENTIFICATION ET D'EVALUATION DES BESOINS

La première composante de ce module est un <u>formulaire d'évaluation de l'autonomie</u> physique, psychique et sociale de l'individu. Ce formulaire est rempli lors d'une

		SERVICES REQUIS				
		Fréquence hebdo.	Durée prob.		TOTAL	
			- 3 ms	+ 3 ms	- 3 ms	+ 3 ms
ASPECT INTELLECTUEL	☐ Fonctionnement intellectuel........................... 3					
	☐ Fonctionnement intellectuel........................... 6					
ASPECT PSYCHO-AFFECTIF	☐ Fonctionnement psycho-affectif........................ 6					
	☐ Fonctionnement psycho-affectif........................10					
ASPECT PHYSIQUE	☐ Fonctionnement perceptuel, sensoriel, sensitif......... 4					
	☐ Fonctionnement perceptuel, sensoriel, sensitif......... 8					
	☐ Fonctionnement physique............................... 3					
	☐ Fonctionnement physique............................... 6					
	☐ Fonctionnement physique............................... 9					
	<u>Fauteuil roulant</u>					
	☐ Transferts.. 6					
	☐ Déplacements.. 6					
	☐ Recommandations.......................................12					
	<u>Entraînement aux A.V.Q.</u>					
	☐ Hygiène et confort.................................... 4					
	☐ Hygiène et confort.................................... 9					
	<u>Entraînement aux A.V.Q.</u>					
	☐ Entretien et cuisine.................................. 4					
	☐ Entretien et cuisine.................................. 9					
	☐ Enseignement de nouvelles méthodes de travail.......... 6					
	☐ Orthèse: ajust. et réentraînement (2 séances consée.).. 4					
	☐ Prothèse: ajust. & réentraînement (2 séances consée.).. 4					
	<u>Barrières architecturales:</u>					
	☐ Recommandations.......................................12					
	☐ Enseignement à l'entourage immédiat.................. 4					
		TOTAL				
	☐ Programmes d'activités (non-professionnel)............ 6					
	☐ Programmes d'activités (non-professionnel)............12					

☐ Une évaluation plus poussée est requise

Pourquoi?____________________ Type d'évaluation____________________

<u>CE BENEFICIAIRE RECOIT ACTUELLEMENT DES TRAITEMENTS EN ERGOTHERAPIE</u> ☐ Oui ☐ Non

NO. DOSSIER____________________

NOM____________________

Figure 1

Module de mesure -

Formule pour l'ergothérapie (milieu institutionel)

entrevue avec la personne âgée (et avec le soignant, en institution). L'entrevue est faite soit par une infirmière, soit par un travailleur social. Un espace est prévu dans le formulaire pour l'inscription des impressions, commentaires et suggestions de l'interviewer.

La seconde composante du module d'identification et d'évaluation des besoins est un formulaire d'évaluation médicale. Il est rempli par le médecin du client à domicile et équivaut à un examen complet majeur. Pour le client en établissement hospitalier ou d'hébergement, le formulaire peut être rempli soit par le médecin, soit par l'infirmière sur la base du contenu du dossier médical.

La validité de contenu de ce module a été testée en posant la question de savoir s'il était possible, sur la base de l'information receuillie par ce module, pour un comité multidisciplinaire de décider des besoins de services de l'individu (voir module suivant). On a ainsi conduit diverses expériences où l'information à la disposition du comité variait et où les supports d'information utilisés changeaient.

MODULE DE MESURE

Le module de mesure est un ensemble de formules de mesure du niveau des soins et services requis par la personne:

- une formule pour les soins infirmiers qui est la formule de mesure du niveau PRN 76 (voir autre communication)
- une formule pour le service social
- une formule pour la physiothérapie
- une formule pour l'ergothérapie (figure 1)
- une formule pour les soins médicaux
- une formule pour les services de soutien (figure 2)

Ces formules sont remplies par un comité multidisciplinaire (un travailleur social, une infirmière, un médecin, une ergothérapeute et une physiothérapeute) sur la base de l'information contenue dans les formulaires d'évaluation d'autonomie et d'évaluation médicale.

Toutes ces formules sont du même type que la formule PRN 76 de mesure du niveau. Chacune est constituée d'un ensemble de critères ou facteurs qui sont tous des actes

ORGANISATION MATERIELLE		SERVICES REQUIS				
		Fréquence	Durée probable		Total hebdo.	
			- 1 ms	+ 1 ms	- 1 ms	+ 1 ms
	☐ Préparation des repas	21/sem.				
		TOTAL				
		Fréquence	Durée probable		Total annuel	
			- 1 ms	+ 1 ms	- 1 ms	+ 1 ms
	☐ Emplettes	2/mois				
	☐ Entretien ménager	2/mois				
	☐ Travaux lourds - planchers	6/an				
	☐ Travaux lourds - grand ménage	2/an				
		TOTAL				
	Au besoin / Transport avec accompagnement					
	- véhicules normaux	☐				
	- véhicules spécialisés	☐				

PRESENCE		Fréquence hebdo.	Durée probable		Total hebdo.	
			- 1 ms	+ 1 ms	- 1 ms	+ 1 ms
	☐ Présence 20 heures sur 24 ....(20 hres)................					
	☐ Présence 24 heures sur 24 ....(24 hres)................					
		TOTAL				

VIE SOCIALE		Fréquence hebdo.	Durée probable		Total hebdo.	
			- 1 ms	+ 1 ms	- 1 ms	+ 1 ms
	☐ Contacts d'amitié (téléphones)..........(15 min.)................					
	☐ Contacts d'amitié (visites)............(45 min.)................					
	☐ Repas communautaires....................(60 min.)................					
	☐ Services récréatifs.....................(30 min.)................					
	☐ Services récréatifs.....................(60 min.)................					
	☐ Services récréatifs.....................(120 min.)................					
	☐ Programme d'activités...................(60 min.)................					
	☐ Programme d'activités...................(120 min.)................					
		TOTAL				

REFERENCES

☐ Nutrition
☐ Podiâtrie
☐ Optométrie
☐ Psychologie
☐ Soins dentaires
☐ Denturologie
☐ Pastorale
☐ Autre(s) ________________
☐ Programme d'activités physiques

☐ Une évaluation plus poussée est requise

Pourquoi? ________________ Type d'évaluation ________________

EROS - CTMSP 77 ©

NOM ________________

NO. DOSSIER ________________

Figure 2

Module de mesure -

Formule pour les services de soutien (milieu institutionel)

ou interventions de soins et/ou de services et qui sont pondérés en terme du nombre de minutes requis pour leur exécution par jour ou par semaine. Ces formules ont toutes été développées par des comités d'experts de chacune des disciplines concernées sur la base de données recueillies dans le milieu.

L'ensemble du module de mesure du système CTMSP 77 a été validé sur son contenu par sa méthode même de construction. Une étude de fiabilité a été effectuée et s'est avérée concluante. D'autres études de fiabilité et de validité sont actuellement en cours.

MODULE D'AIDE A LA DECISION ET AU CONTROLE

Le module d'aide à la décision et au contrôle à court terme est en cours de développement en même temps qu'il est testé dans la réalité puisqu'il est implanté au niveau d'un territoire de département de santé communautaire. Le genre de décision et de contrôle dont il est question ici est la certification et la recertification du placement des personnes âgées dans le réseau. Il s'agit donc de s'assurer que ceux-ci reçoivent et continuent à recevoir les services du programme du réseau de soins et services prolongés qui est le mieux à même (donner juste ce qu'il faut, ni trop, ni trop peu) de répondre à leurs besoins.

Le module d'aide à la décision et au contrôle à court terme est constitué d'un ensemble de mécanismes et procédures visant à aider les gestionnaires du réseau à assurer et maintenir un placement "approprié" des clients.

L'information de base nécessaire pour prendre de telles décisions et assurer un tel contrôle est fournie par le module de mesure du système, plus précisément par le dossier des formules de mesure du niveau des soins et services requis par le client. Une fois que ce dossier a été rempli par le comité multidisciplinaire, l'information qu'il contient est résumée sur une formule synthèse (figure 3) qui rend compte essentiellement du niveau de chacun des types de soins et services requis par le client, de la fréquence et du terme de ces soins et services.

Par ailleurs, des mécanismes ont été mis au point pour amener les gestionnaires du réseau à définir chacun des programmes de celui-ci en terme des niveaux de chacun des types de soins et services qu'il offre au client type qu'il admet.

Un comité d'admission a la charge de certifier et recertifier le placement des clients dans tous les programmes du réseau. Il prend ses décisions sur la base des deux ensembles d'informations quantitatives et objectives mentionnées ci-dessus; à savoir le portrait du client en terme de niveaux et le portrait de chaque programme en terme des niveaux de soins et services offerts à son client moyen.

	Unités de mesure	SERVICES REQUIS TOTAL Court terme	Long terme
Préparation des repas	fois/semaine		
Organisation matérielle	fois/année		
Présence	heures/semaine		
Vie sociale	heures/semaine		
Soins infirmiers - infirmières	heures/semaine		
Soins infirmiers - autres	heures/semaine		
Services médicaux - généralistes	visites/année		
Services médicaux - spécialistes	visites/année		
Service social	heures/mois		
Physiothérapie - A	heures/semaine		
Physiothérapie - B - milieu spécialisé	heures/semaine		
Ergothérapie	heures/semaine		
transport - véhicules normaux			
- véhicules spécialisés			

Services de soutien/références: 1-______ 2-______ 3-______

Services médicaux/consultation: 1-______ 2-______ 3-______

Services médicaux/références: 1-______ 2-______ 3-______

Sercices requis une seule fois

Services soutien: ______ Service social: ______

Soins infirmiers: ______ Physiothérapie: ______

Services médicaux: ______ Ergothérapie: ______

DECISION: ______

Nom du bénéficiaire: ______ No. dossier ______

Figure 3

Module d'aide à la décision et au contrôle - Formule synthèse (milieu institutionel)

Le module d'aide à la décision et au contrôle à long terme utilise l'information produite par le module de mesure et le module d'aide à la décision et au contrôle à court terme pour aider les gestionnaires du réseau dans leur tâche de planification du réseau en fonction des besoins de la population âgée.

En effet, l'utilisation systématique du module de mesure du système pour évaluer les besoins des clients permet de constituer petit à petit un portrait complet des besoins de soins et services de la population et les mécanismes de recertification assurent la constante mise à jour de ce portrait. De plus les décisions de placement et de revision de placement lorsque confrontées avec les besoins des individus placés, laissent apparaître les écarts qui peuvent exister entre les types de programmes disponibles et le nombre de places disponibles dans ces programmes d'une part, et les besoins de la population âgée d'autre part. Sur la base de ces informations sur les besoins de la population et son évolution, sur les programmes disponibles et sur la façon dont les besoins sont satisfaits, les gestionnaires peuvent planifier le réseau de soins et services prolongés pour qu'il soit toujours adapté aux besoins de la population âgée.

L'ACCESSION A LA QUALITE DE LA VIE REVENDIQUEE PAR LES HANDICAPES

S.PANNIER*

SUMMARY

Four thousand participants met at the World Rehabilitation Congress in Winnipeg (23rd - 27th, 6 , 1980), 10% of them were severely handicapped persons with motor and sensory involvement and representing 101 countries.

The leitmotiv of this Congress was their complete integration in society. They refuse being considered as assisted, claim their right as a minority among others, the right of working, of sharing responsibilities in the community and not only survival but quality of life as well.

The World Disabled Association has been created. It is meant to use its influence with authorities so as to change the state of mind of people and find the necessary solutions. At the very beginning of the Handicapped Persons' World Year, a number of considerations with regard to the participation of the French-speaking in this powerful international mouvement.

INTRODUCTION

Est considérée comme handicapée toute personne qui, pour des causes motrices, sensorielles, viscérales ou intellectuelles, ne dispose pas, à titre provisoire ou définitif, de l'intégrité des capacités de l'homme normal.

* Pr.S.PANNIER, Hôpital Raymond Poincaré, 92380 GARCHES, F.

Le handicap constitue une gêne dans le vécu quotidien du sujet qui en est atteint. L'objectif de la médecine -et tout spécialement de la médecine de rééducation-est de faire le bilan de cette gêne, compte tenu de l'être humain auquel elle a à faire et de sa situation dans la société. De pallier, ensuite, au mieux, les conséquences personnelles et sociales du handicap.

Que représentent,numériquement,ces handicapés dans notre population ? Il est très difficile, à ce sujet, d'avoir des chiffres précis, étant donné l'absence -paradoxale- dans notre pays de statistiques officielles. On peut néanmoins se baser sur un travail effectué en 1966 par GROSSIORD qui, procédant par recoupements successifs, concluait qu'une fois regroupées les catégories motrices, sensorielles et viscérales (les handicapés intellectuels étant exclus) un peu plus d'un français sur 50 serait un handicapé.
Les implications de ces notions de base sont, à l'évidence, nombreuses et complexes. Elles sont, au premier chef, d'ordre médical. Les handicaps relèvent de causes extrêmement variées. C'est ainsi qu'en prenant par exemple le domaine exclusivement moteur ils peuvent être d'ordre traumatologique, rhumatologique ou neurologique, atteignant un être humain à n'importe quel âge de sa vie, parfois dès sa naissance.

De nombreux autres champs que celui de la médecine, au sens classique du terme sont concernés : ceux, en citant pêle-même, de l'appareillage, de la psychologie, de la sociologie, de l'économie, de la politique également.
Des choix de société doivent, en effet, obligatoirement être faits vis à vis de ces handicapés -dont,il convient d'y insister, l'espérance de vie est actuellement, dans la plupart des cas, du même ordre de grandeur que celle de la population moyenne. Ces choix concernent bien entendu, non seulement les soins mais aussi, de façon logique, la réintégration des handicapés dans la société.
Cette dernière suppose tout un ensemble de mesure très diverses parmi lesquelles nous citerons la suppression des barrières architecturales (de façon à régler les problèmes d'accessibilité des locaux, y compris pour les personnes circulant en fauteuil roulant), la remise au travail.
En fait, ce qui est déterminant en la matière c'est qu'existe l'état d'esprit -la volonté- de la part de la société pour que cette réintégration soit effective. Du côté des handicapés on verra que le retour dans une vie aussi proche que possible de la normale -une vie de qualité- est revendiquée de façon de plus en plus nette. C'est ce qui est apparu très nettement au Congrès de Winnipeg.

Le Congrès mondial de REHABILITATION INTERNATIONAL a eu lieu du 23 au 27.6.1980 à Winnipeg (CANADA). Nous allons tenter de rendre compte de quelques uns des principaux aspects de cette importante rencontre. Celle-ci avait été longuement préparée à l'avance par des réunions tenues à l'échelon national dans les divers pays participants. Elle était destinée à avoir une grande diffusion, à l'orée de l'année mondiale des handicapés. Cette diffusion sera, sans aucun doute, assurée par diverses voies et, déjà, par la promulgation de certains textes par l'U.N.E.S.C.O.

Nous citerons, dans un premier temps, les points qui nous ont paru être les plus importants dans ce Congrès, les uns après les autres, sans chercher à établir une classification particulière.

Dans un deuxième temps, nous nous livrerons brièvement à quelques réflexions que nous avons été amené à faire à ce sujet.

1 - PRINCIPAUX ASPECTS DU CONGRES DE WINNIPEG.

1 - 1 - L'importance de la participation était, à l'évidence, impressionnante. 4000 personnes, représentant 101 pays, ont été présentes pendant 5 jours, avec assiduité.
Il s'agissait d'une majorité anglo-saxonne, mais la communauté francophone n'était pas absente; nous y reviendrons.

Les pays en question étaient de ceux que l'on dit développés (Amérique du Nord, Europe de l'Ouest, Japon) mais aussi de ceux qui sont considérés comme étant en voie de développement (Inde, Indonésie, Afrique par exemple)

10% des participants environ étaient eux-mêmes des handicapés : handicapés moteurs sévères dont beaucoup étaient en fauteuil roulant (souvent électriques, certains modèles nouveaux paraissant peu encombrants, très maniables, très " performants "). Mais des handicapés sensoriels, aveugles, sourds étaient également présents. Un tel pourcentage de non valides nous a semblé assez inhabituel par rapport à ce que nous observons habituellement dans les Congrès auxquels nous avons pu participer : qu'ils soient nationaux ou internationaux, médicaux ou médico-sociaux. Il a incontestablement apporté un poids supplémentaire à cette assemblée, dans le sens du pragmatisme et de l'authenticité de sa réflexion.

Les autres membres présents appartenaient à diverses instances des pays sus mentionnés préoccupés par le sort des handicapés; représentants, à un haut niveau des pouvoirs publics, d'associations nationales et internationales de handicapés, des équipes soignantes (médecins, para médicaux, travailleurs sociaux), sociologues, économistes, chefs d'entreprise etc...

1 - 2 - La diversité des sujets abordés -médicaux,sociaux,économiques- durant ces 5 jours, au cours de séances multiples, a permis de faire un tour très complet des problèmes posés, dans beaucoup de pays du monde, aux handicapés en eux mêmes et dans leurs relations réciproques avec la société à laquelle ils appartiennent.

1 - 3 - L'unicité des points de vue exposés à propos de ces thèmes divers par les orateurs quels qu'ils soient -handicapés ou non- était frappante. Le dénominateur commun, l'objectif constamment visé: étaient l'intégration, l'assimilation des handicapés dans la société.

1 - 3 - 1) Celles-ci impliquent des solutions pratiques. Des témoignages personnels de handicapés, des relations d'expériences concluantes filmées ou non, ont été présentées à ce sujet en grand nombre.

Il en ressort que les handicapés refusent désormais de subir passivement les hospitalisations prolongées -sauf en cas de nécessité médicale, bien sûr- la ségrégation en centres dits spécialisés, -sauf évidemment passage en vue d'une formation professionnelle réaliste -et, à fortiori la relégation en hospices- même s'ils sont dits " humanisés ".
Ils veulent rentrer dans leur foyer ou bien en constituer un. Ils y vivront éventuellement seuls et de jeunes handicapés sévèrement atteints, des tétraplégiques par exemple, ont fait état sur ce plan, avec humour, d'expériences personnelles réussies à force de courage. Sinon, ils vivront en petits groupes, (6 à 8 en général) réunissant des handicaps lourds mais divers, constitués de personnes qui se sont choisies par affinités.

De toute façon, la médicalisation est limitée au minimum logique, selon les normes générales, en cas de besoin, (appel au médecin traitant ou au spécialiste). La conception, vis à vis des tierces personnes est identique.
Cela suppose que l'autonomie maxima soit assurée par des aides techniques, des aménagements intérieurs et du matériel de contrôle de l'environnement. Dans cette perspective, la " machine à saisir à distance " ou " téléthèse ", qu'elle soit allemande (HEIDELBERG), américaine (STANFORD, U.C.L.A.) ou française (SPARTACUS), pourra rendre au maximum les services que l'on attend d'elle; cela d'autant plus qu'il n'est pas déraisonnable de penser qu'au prix de certains aménagements des commandes, une même machine pourra servir à plusieurs handicapés.

Cela suppose également que les barrières architecturales (escaliers, dénivellations de trottoirs, difficultés de parking etc...) soient abolies afin que le handicapé puisse sortir de son logement et circuler aussi librement que possible en ville. Il en est ainsi, déjà, souvent dans de nombreuses cités anglo-saxonnes et aussi dans quelques villes françaises : Lorient par exemple.

1 - 3 - 2) L'intégration du handicapé dans la société implique en second lieu un certain état d'esprit :

De la part des handicapés qui refusent un statut " d'assistés ". Ils réclament au contraire, le plein droit au travail, la pleine participation aux responsabilités de la communauté. Ils veulent, dans l'ensemble, non seulement obtenir la survie que leur donne actuellement la médecine mais également accéder à une certaine qualité de la vie.

De la part de la société qui doit changer son état d'esprit vis à vis des handicapés devant être considérés comme une minorité à part entière parmi d'autres -afin de les intégrer en son sein.

Deux remarques s'imposent à ce sujet :

- La première est que cette attitude des handicapés, outre qu'elle est parfaitement logique sur le plan humain, paraît bien répondre aux difficultés de la situation économique actuelle. Elle correspond, d'autre part, à l'esprit qui a toujours été celui du médecin de rééducation. Plutôt que d'être placé à vie (une vie dont l'espérance de durée peut être proche de la normale, à condition que les complications cutanées et urinaires bien connues soient évitées) dans des hospices, même plus ou moins aménagés mais habituellement sous équipés en personnel, il est hautement souhaitable que les handicapés, même " lourds ", retrouvent un maximum d'autonomie; qu'ils rentrent dans une vie aussi normale et d'aussi bonne qualité que possible; qu'ils travaillent à nouveau, autant que faire se peut, ce qui les " motive " et les rend productifs sur le plan de la collectivité. Des recherches sont effectuées actuellement dans certains pays, les Etats-Unis notamment, qui montrent que certains travaux, éventuellement délicats, peuvent être effectués -dans l'industrie électronique par exemple- par de très grands handicapés qui n'étaient pas auparavant des intellectuels ; ces derniers peuvent se reclasser, en principe, on le sait, sans difficulté insurmontable. Et, même dans la conjoncture actuelle, avec les problèmes posés par le marché du travail, on ne voit pas pourquoi les handicapés n'auraient pas, pour trouver un emploi, des chances égales aux valides. Il s'agit là d'un état d'esprit à instaurer dans la communauté comme nous le disions ci-dessus et, finalement, d'un choix de société.

- La deuxième remarque est que le problème, rejoignant celui des personnes âgées,restera très difficile pour les handicapés vieillissants. Il faudra encore trouver des solutions adaptées, satisfaisantes sur le plan humain.

1 - 4 - Un puissant courant s'est manifesté au cours de ce Congrès,aboutissant, on l'a dit, d'une préparation préalable de plusieurs années. Difficilement réversible, semble t-il, il a engendré :

1 - 4 - 1) La création d'une association mondiale des handicapés (World Disabled Association = W.D.A.).
Celle-ci, fait notable, se définit comme une union apolitique de consommateurs -et l'on sait le poids croissant que prennent de telles associations dans la société économique actuelle. Le principe de base de cette structure est que l'on envisage de plus en plus couramment le handicap en termes de coûts -sous entendu à la charge de la communauté. Cette estimation nécessiterait d'ailleurs des études socio-économiques approfondies faisant intervenir, entre autres, des comparaisons sérieusesavec d'autres types de coûts,à charge pour la société. Quoiqu'il en soit, les handicapés,acceptant le principe d'être des consommateurs -de soins par exemple- réclament en contre partie certains droits concernant leurs besoins : soins de bonne qualité, suppression des barrières architecturales (qui ne sont d'ailleurs paut-être que maintenues artificiellement par une société qui veut les ignorer) et surtout, satisfaction de ces revendications fondamentales qui sont l'accession à une certaine qualité de la vie et à la pleine participation aux responsabilités de celle-ci.

1 - 4 - 2) La Charte des handicapés, approuvée solennellement par les congressistes réunis à Winnipeg, est un volumineux document dans lequel sont consignés les divers problèmes médicaux, sociaux, économiques etc... posés par le handicap, tels qu'ils ont pu être définis par de nombreuses commissions ayant travaillé dans les divers pays participants ainsi que les solutions préconisées pour y remédier. Avec les amendements apportés par les délégations présentes au Congrès, il est le reflet de cet état d'esprit actuel des handicapés que nous avons essayé de rapporter ainsi que de leur volonté d'une structuration en un groupement déstiné à peser efficacement, dans les années à venir, sur les décisions des pouvoirs publics concernés. Publié à l'occasion du Congrès, ce document est destiné à une grande diffusion; il sera notamment promulgué prochainement par l'U.N.E.S.C.O.

2 - LES REFLEXIONS QUE NOUS AVONS PU FAIRE AU RETOUR DE CE CONGRES, BRIEVEMENT RESUMEES, concernent les points suivants :

2 - 1 - Faiblesse de la participation francophone :

Venant du Canada français, de Suisse, du Liban, de Centre Afrique, de France, les participants francophones, à une estimation grossière, ne représentaient que environ 1% de la population présente à ce Congrès mondial (4000 personnes, rappelons-le).

Ces personnes n'étaient nullement préparées à constituer une délégation homogène -à la différence de la plupart des délégations anglo-saxonnes (Japon compris). Ainsi s'est posé,une fois de plus,le problème de la place de la francophonie dans le monde anglo-saxon.

2 - 2 - L'état d'esprit latin face au handicap :

Il nous a paru, à l'évidence, à notre retour, une fois de plus, bien différent de celui des anglo-saxons. Même dans les milieux médicaux spécialisés, un certain manque d'intérêt, voire une certaine méfiance, continuent à se manifester pour ce qui se passe en dehors de nos frontières, quelqu'en soit l'importance.

Non moins grave est l'ignorance dans laquelle est tenu et se tient le public français vis à vis de la question posée par le handicap ; si cette dernière est posée de façon théorique, les réponses individuelles comme celles de la collectivité, continuent à être bien souvent celles du rejet.

Bien différent paraît, sur ce plan, le pragmatisme anglo-saxon.

2 - 3 - Nous espérons que l'année mondiale des handicapés changera quelque chose à cet état de fait. Mais il faudrait, pour cela, une meilleure circulation de l'information. Il faudrait surtout que soit fait nettement et avec une volonté sincère, tenace d'efficacité, le choix de société nécessaire pour trouver des solutions aux problèmes posés par le handicap dans une civilisation qui se dit évoluée. C'est ainsi, nous semble t-il, que pourra se modifier de façon réellement positive l'état d'esprit concernant ce sujet dans notre pays, dans le sens annoncé, rappelons-le, par la loi française du 30.06.1975 en faveur des personnes handicapées.

ADVANCES IN ASSISTIVE SYSTEMS FOR LOCOMOTION DEFFICIENCIES

Rajko Tomović
Faculty of Electrical Engineering
Belgrade, Yugoslavia

SUMMARY:

Trends in the design of externally powered ortheses for locomotion defficiences are reviewed. Two advanced approaches in this field are described. A new technology of self-fitting modular orthosis with soft interface has been tested on patients with locomotion defficiencies. In addition, the application of non-numerical control for the knee-locking function in the case of above-knee amputation is presented. The above-knee prosthesis has been designed as autonomous unit including the microprocessor controller and the power supply.

INTRODUCTION

The era of externally controlled assistive devices for rehabilitation purposes has started with upper extremity prostheses. For many years to come this trend persisted in rehabilitation engineering. As a matter of fact, the same development pattern applies to industrial robotics where the design of manipulators was given priority. A systemic concern for locomotion robots and corresponding rehabilitation applications followed with a delay the research efforts in upper extremity control.

It would be certainly interesting to analyse the reasons for the above course of development. Speaking of industrial robotics, there is no doubt that feasible applications of locomotion machines are much more restricted than the scope of tasks performed by manipulators. However, the same thinking cannot be extended to medical robotics. As known, patients having locomotion defficiencies are not a negligible group of the total handicapped population. Nonetheless, active assistive devices for lower extremities are practically nonexistent in terms of field applications. Next, we shall try to produce some explanations for such a state of affairs.

DESIGN PROBLEMS

Although control problems involved in locomotion activity are simpler than control tasks met in upper extremity activities, the over-all man-machine interaction in rehabilitation of locomotion functions is technologically challenging. In the first place, the power supply needed to support autonomous locomotion activity is considerable. At the current stage of external power supply technology, autonomous locomotion activity on level ground is limited to a 1-2 hours, not to speak of more power consuming tasks like stair climbing and similar. On the other hand, the magnitudes of transmitted static and dynamic forces in external control of locomotion are much higher than in most manipulation tasks. At least, they cannot be reduced below certain limits given the body weight and anatomy of the patient.

In normal environmental conditions locomotion, as known, consists of repetitive cycles involving joints with smaller number degrees of freedom than the hand and arm skeleton. Due to all above facts passive prosthetic and orthotic devices for lower extremities have a better chance to compete with corresponding active systems. Shortly, the dividing line of passive versus active assistive devices for lower extremities favours much more the passive solutions in comparison to the same case of upper limbs.This may explain to some extent the delayed appearance of active assistive devices for locomotion defficiencies.

RESEARCH TRENDS

Locomotion activity has been extensively studied as part of general research in neurophysiology and biomechanics. However, modern control enginnering's interest in locomotion machines is of relatively recent date. The first attempts to relate automata theory and animal locomotion go back to the paper presented by Tomović /1/. In a subsequent paper, the theoretical background was laid down for the use of finite state approach in the design of orthotic and prosthetic devices for lower extremities /2/.

Practical applications of computer controlled orthotic devices for locomotion defficiencies are related to active exoskeleton /3/. Although this research in rehabilitation engineering proved to be of considerable theoretical and general interest, the use of machines of such a commpexity does not seem to be feasible in field conditions.

Another interesting trend in the design of advanced assistive devices for lower extremities has been given the name "soft suit" orthosis. However, the first models of soft suit orthosis had, as known, several serious drawbacks not to mention the highly simplified on-off control using compressed air. A more advanced technology of soft suit orthoses for lower extremities based on modular design has been proposed by a group of French -Yugoslav scientists /4 /.

At this moment, above research is still of exploratory nature. There is no intention to enter here into the detailed assessment of what has been accomplished so far in this respect. However, the great value of above mentioned research lays in the fact that many essential aspects of man-machine interaction in the design of assistive locomotion systems have been clearly brought out into the foreground. In order to overcome existing constraints preventing successful application of advanced assistive devices for locomotion defficiencies, new approaches have been recently proposed of which we shall speak below.

THE SELF-FITTING ORTHOSIS

The basic idea of self-fitting technology of assistive devices relies on following principles,

1. Modular Design. The term modular in this context refers to joint modularity. For instance, the assistive device can be applied to the knee joint and extended, if needed, to the hip joint without the need to modify the existing structure. In other words, modules are additive and any combination of assisted joints on both legs is possible with the available elements.

2. Prefacricated Parts. The self-fitting orthosis consists of prefabricated parts which are supplied in standard sizes.

3. Adaptivity. Orthosis length is adaptive to patient´ s anatomy due to the use of telescopic arrangement. The same arrangement takes care of the adaptivity of the external joint to the patient´ s knee motion so that precise alignment of the orthosis is not necessary. Consequently, the requirement for the strict fitting of the orthosis must not be observed. Thus, the procedure to put the orthosis on is highly simplified and the time needed to perform this activity greatly reduced.

4. Soft Interface. The basic idea of soft interface has been retained. However, the soft interface consists in this case of just normal tight trousers of commercially available staff. The trousers are equipped with pockets into which the prefabricated parts are inserted and joined

together by the patient himself without the aid of any tools.

5. Self-fitting. Once the trousers are taken on, the orthosis is assembled on the patient from the kit containing the prefabricated parts. This is, thus, the first on-line fitting assistive system since all existing solutions are designed as off-line fitting devices. In addition, no mechanical or other workshop assistance is needed to fit this orthosis to the patient. Just the help of a tailor is required to prepare the trousers.

6. Functional additivity. The self-fitting orthosis has been designed from the very beginning as a multipurpose assistive system. Since knee joint can be locked passively as well as by voluntary action, the device may be used as a long brace. At the same time, an active, fully autonomous, microprocessor controlled, module is under development which can be attached to the desired joint transforming thus the device into externally powered orthosis. Having in mind adaptive features of this orthosis and the soft interface used to transfer the forces, a special control philosophy was developed which generates joint motions independently of fixed coordinate system. More of this will be said in the next part of the text.

Fig. 1 shows the set of prefabricated parts needed for the assembly of the orthosis.

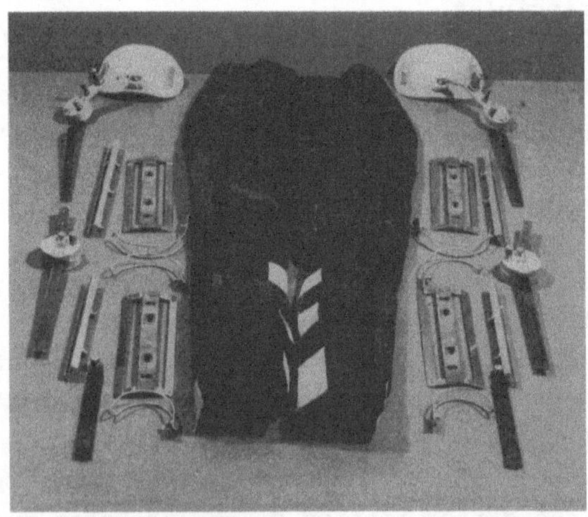

Fig. 1. Parts of the self-fitting orthosis

In Fig. 2 a standing patient using the orthosis as a long brace is shown while in Fig.3 the sitting position is displayed.

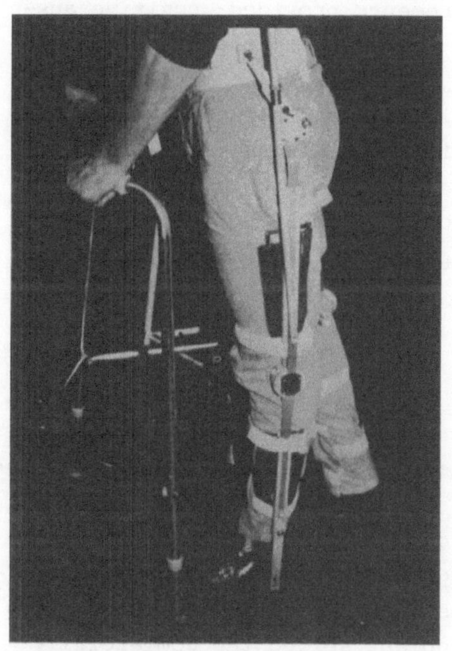

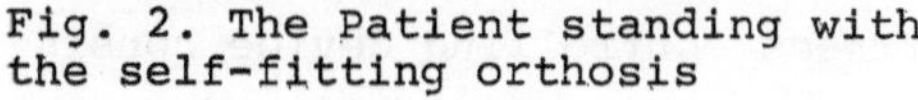

Fig. 2. The Patient standing with the self-fitting orthosis

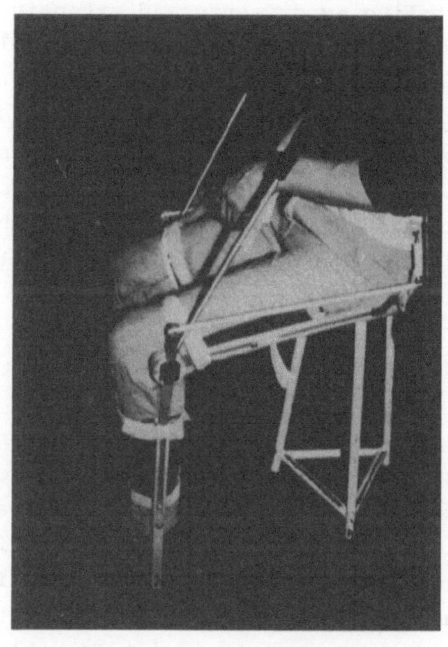

Fig. 3. The Patient sitting with the self-fitting orthosis.

The development of the self-fitting orthosis opened several new fundamental problems in rehabilitation engineering. Namely, the orthosis as such, in off-body position, is a mechanically undermined structure as is the human skeleton when left by itself. The assistive device will become a mechanically determined structure only when attached to the human body. Here we have an example of man-machine interaction which can be studied as a structure only in its integrated biomechanical form. Mathematical models for such structures have been proposed by D.Popović /5/.

Evidently, to use trousers made of commercially available staff is an attractive idea. However, in order to prove the feasibility of this approach two important questions had to be answered. Namely, can the "ski"-type or "blue-jeans" -type trousers stand the static and dynamic forces appearing in standing-up, sitting down and locomotion of the orthosis -patient system? The second question is related to the force transfer. As known, the interface of any assistive system has to be such that no damage to patient´s skin and other life functions is caused. Interesting experiments and extensive measurements provided positive answers to both questions so that clinical tests with patients carrying self-fitting orthosis were undertaken.

So far preliminary tests to derive indications about the feasibility of self-fitting orthosis to assist different kinds of patients with impaired locomotion functions are carried out in Yugoslavia, Japan, the Netherlands. In principle, the orthosis is intended for patients with locomotion defficiencies but with preserved upper body functions.

KNEE-LOCKING CONTROL

Several Rehabilitation Engineering Centres in the world have suggested that, instead of complex locomotion machines, rather simple active control should be added to the available lower limb prostheses in order to assist the knee-locking function. Such a control system has been developed by the Faculty of Electrical Engineering, Belgrade, for the needs of the Veterans Administration Hospital, New York.

As a starting point for this development served the commercially available skeletal prothesis with passive knee-locking mechanism. In our case, the knee-locking and the stiffness controlling device consists of the hydraulic cylinder equipped with an electrical micromotor which acts upon the fluid flow, Fig. 4. The hydraulic on-off actuator is under the microprocessor control. However, the control philosophy used for the knee-locking is new and remains valid for locomotion control in general.

The control approach applied here is of a non-numerical nature. The basic idea is to equip the prosthesis with artificial reflex loops. This is accomplished by using:

a: artificial proprioceptive and exteroceptive sensors,

b: tactile rather than visual pattern recognition.

For the knee-locking reflex loop following artificial sensory information is required;

- on-off touch sensors to detect which part of the foot is in contact with the ground,
- knee-angle measurement,
- vertical line detection.

All the sensors are located at the appropriate places of the skeletal prosthesis.

On the basis of sensory feedback, the microcomputer takes the decision to lock or unlock the knee joint of the prosthesis. The control algorithm is derived from observations of the normal gait and control theoretical considerations. Namely, it has been pointed out that the continuous locomotion control can be replaced by finite state algorithms and logical (boolean) expressions using sensory feedback as input /1,2./ For instance, to detect the intention to initiate the walking cycle, following logical condition must be satisfied,

(no foot contact with the ground and extended knee of the left (right) leg) and (foot contact with the ground and knee extended for the right (left) leg). A detailed description of the non-numerical algorithm for knee-control is found in the reference /6/.

Two important advantages of the logical locomotion control must be

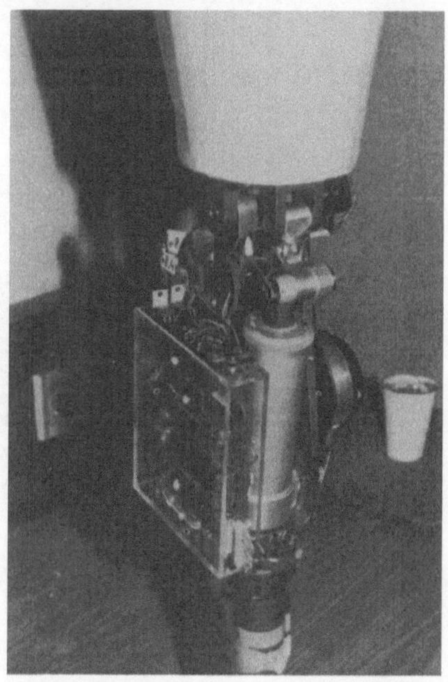

Fig. 4. The electrohydraulic actuator

emphasized. In the first place, logical control is, like the biological motion, independent of the fixed coordinate system except for the vertical line. Consequently, it is highly insensitive to trajectory perturbations and modifications of the body position. Besides, logical control is to a large extent modular so that, for example, the knee-locking algorithm operates without inputs from other joints.

Several models of the prosthesis have been built for clinical tests. The control system, including the power supply, is added as a module to the passive skeletal prosthesis. The weight of such a self-contained module is 1.2 kg. The control unit allows for two hours of autonomous walking on level ground at this stage of technology development. A patient equipped with such a prosthesis is shown in Fig. 5.

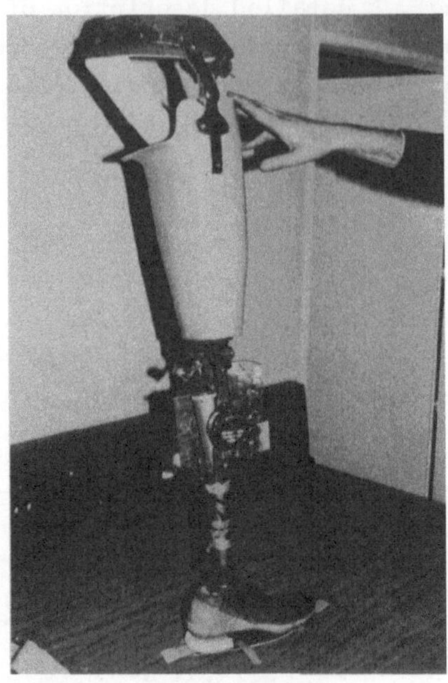

Fig. 5. Patient fitted with active above-knee prosthesis.

KNEE-MOTION CONTROL

While clinical tests with the knee-locking control are under way, a more advanced control module is being developed. Namely, instead of just active locking function, the full extension-flexion knee cycle can be externally controlled. For this purpose, evidently, conventional trajectory control could be used. The disadvantage of this approach in rehabilitation engineering is obvious. It is too expensive in terms of the power supply. Consequently, above approach has been rejected.

The proposed knee-motion control unit is based on the principle of <u>partial</u> external power supply. The motor unit is designed as a four-state device:

1. Rigid state-locked knee.
2. Free state-loose knee.
3. Forward motion - knee extension.
4. Rearward motion - knee flexion..

The unit is under logical control with the above mentioned sensory inputs. In this way, the external power consumption is minimized since the available biological power source is used at maximum. The motor unit is self-contained, of modular design and interchangeable with the knee-locking unit. Such an approach permits multipurpose use of the prosthesis,

a. The conventional passive knee-locking mode.
b. The active knee-locking mode.
c. The active knee-motion mode.

The motor unit can be attached to the self-fitting orthosis as well. Thus, the passive orthotic device is transformed into an active assistive system having knee-motion control. As seen, we are aiming at a self-fitting orthotic technology which is both structurally and functionally modular. Detailed description of the motor unit will be presented at the International Symposium on External Control of Human Extremities, Dubrovnik, 1981.

CONCLUSION

Main intention of this contribution was to draw attention to new approaches in the field of lower limb assitive devices. After a dominant trend to use control engineering for rather complex locomotion machines, a renewed interest to improve assistive devices by superimposing some simple active control is also evident. In addition, advances in soft-interface technology and modular design can be observed.

REFERENCES

1. R.Tomović, "A General Theoretical Model of Creeping Displacement", Cybernetica, Vol IV, No.2, pp. 98-1o8, 1961.
2. R.Tomović, R. McGhee, "A Finite State Approach to the Synthesis of Bioengineering Control Systems", IEEE Trans., Vol. HFE-7, No.2, pp. 65-69, June 1966.
3. M.Vukobratović, D. Hristić, Z. Stoiljković, "Development of Active Antropomorphic Exoskeletons" Medical and Biological Engineering, pp. 64-80, 1974.
4. P.Rabishong, R.Tomović et al, "AMOLL Project", Proc.V Intern.Symposium on External Control of Human Extremities, Dubrovnik, pp.33-43, 1975.
5. D.Popović, "The Biomechanics of the Self-Fitting Orthosis", Proc. Rehabilitation Eng. Intern.Seminar, pp.25-40, Tokyo, July 1980,

published by Society of Biomechanics, Waseda University, Ookubo, Shinjuku-ku, Tokyo 160, Japan.
6. R.Tomović, "Remarks on Non-Numerical Nature of Locomotion Control", Proc. Rehabilitation. Eng. Intern.Seminar, pp. 14-24, Tokyo, July 1980.

SUBSTITUTING OF UPPER HUMAN EXTREMITIES FUNCTIONS- - WHERE WE ARE GOING? *)

A.Morecki and H. Borowski
Technical University of Warsaw

J.Kiwerski and R.Paśniczek
Metropolitan Rehabilitation Center

J.Ober
Institute of Biocybernetic and Biomedical Engng., Polish Academy of Sciences, Warsaw, POLAND

Summary

The paper presents some medical, technical and methodological aspects of the problem of supporting lost motorial functions of upper human extremities.

Some results obtained in application of hybrid system for supporting the grasp movements - alive manipulators - are described.

1. REASONS OF MOTOR DYSFUNCTION

Motor dysfunction can be caused either by a trauma or past as well as current sickness (like poliomyelitis, brain stroke, polineuropatia and myopathia). Another reason, which practically eliminates use of technical means in restoring of the motor functions, is muscular spasticity. The latter occurs in high level damage to the motion control system, in other words the damage to the central nervous system.

All these reasons have one feature in common: regardless of the level of the primary damage they cause total disintegration of motor functions and lead to various disturbances and constraints imposed on the functions of the inflicted motor organ. The primary changes are followed by secondary ones which deteriorate the passive properties of the extremity (influence for example, the extremity neutral position, change its range of motion etc.).

2. ANALYSIS OF RETAINED MOTOR FUNCTIONS

In a case of extremity paralysis, the patient's motor organ has to be analysed in order to reveal all activities and motions which can be used in compensation for the lost functions, or in control of an external supporting apparatus. Another reason for the analysis is to evaluate the extent of functional deficiency and to determine

*) This work was sponsored at Technical University of Warsaw by the National Science Foundation under Grant J-F7F0661-P.

the effectiveness of the retained biokinetic chain (its kinematic properties and strength capacity). These factors have to be considered later while choosing an adequate supporting device, though it should be used only if other means have failed.

Anticipated improvement in a chosen function, in prehension for example, obtained after a supporting apparatus has been mounted, should be weighed against the remining functions of the considered upper extremity. The analysis should include determination of retained positioning of the extremity, its transporting possibilities and dexterity. The latter reflects the patient's ability to perform short-range, multi--directional motions of high precision, as in writting. An example of wrong procedure is a case in which a high level amputee (amputation in shoulder joint) is fitted with an artificial arm with the self-adapting gripper.

In spite of bioelectric control engaging the muscles of the shoulder gridle, the utility of the device from patient's view is next to none, due to lack of positioning and manipulation of the gripper. More drastic examples can be found when the supporting apparata are mounted on the entire and inert extremity.

The deficite of the motor function cannot be considered apart from the extremity's sensory function. Existing sensory function (such as tactile feeling in the hand) calls for application of technical equipment in restoring prehension. Lack of this function creates very unfavourable conditions for application of any equipment, since the parts of the device exert a definite pressure on the patient's flesh and may irritate the skin and cause its mechanical damage.

Another important factor to be considered in patient's rehabilitation is functions compensation, which consists in taking advantage of other parts of the motor organ.

This unilateral deficit in manipulation with the full efficiency of the alternate extremity creates unfavourable situation from the technical point of view, because the healthy extremity soon begins to take over (compensate), at least partly,the functions of the deficient one. The situation is similar to that in which a man loses sight in one of his eyes. In such case, generally, no active prosthesis is used.

In complete paralysis of an extremity or in a case of bilateral amputation - - manipulators seem to be the only reasonable solution.

To conclude: fitting of a patient with an upper extremity prosthesis of a medical manipulator should be proceeded by a thorough analysis. Before a supporting device is applied the following tasks should be completed:

- possibly wide recognition of patient's motions and control sites,
- determination of real needs of a patient,adequate to his retained possibilities,
- determination of patient's emotional and psychic states and his predisposition to work with the apparatus,
- consideration of possibilities of patient's resuming his professional life with relation to his health, profession, family status, financial situation and the like.

3. METHODS OF SUPPORTING OF EXTREMITY FUNCTIONS

In this paragraph we shall present chosen methods employed in the process of supporting of, lost functions.

3.1. Methods using the external sources of energy

In these methods mainly external actuators and sources of energy are used to power the determined joints of the extremity. The procedure is explained in Figure 1.

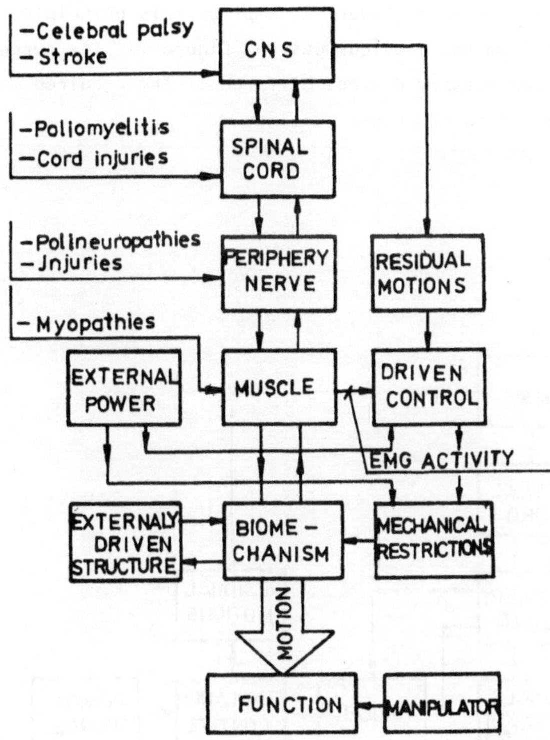

Figure 1

One should realize that in such case the structure is doubled which means that the external mechanical system (an orthostesis or a manipulator) is mounted on the biokinematic chain of the extremity. In an orthosteis, the external actuators are used to drive portions of the double chain |1|. In case of a manipulator mounted separatly from the extremity, whose activity is nil, the functions are realized exclusively by the technical device.

This is our belief that this way of restoring of the lost functions, without motor training of a patient has many drawbacks.

Apart from the presented motor factors, all possible control sites on the patient's body should be considered. Certain signals or motions (like that of a head) can be very useful in control of the equipment |2|.

3.2. Method using own and external sources of energy

In this method the links of the extremity are driven by the retained muscles powered from their own biochemical sources of energy. Low-energy external sources of electric energy used in this method play only the role of control switches for the system |3|.

A stimulation orthostesis, shown in Figure 2, employs this principle. The external orthostesis is different from the previous design (Figure 1). Its purpose is to shape the hand to block the unnecessary degrees of freedom. The required motion of the arm is performed by stimulation of proper muscles.

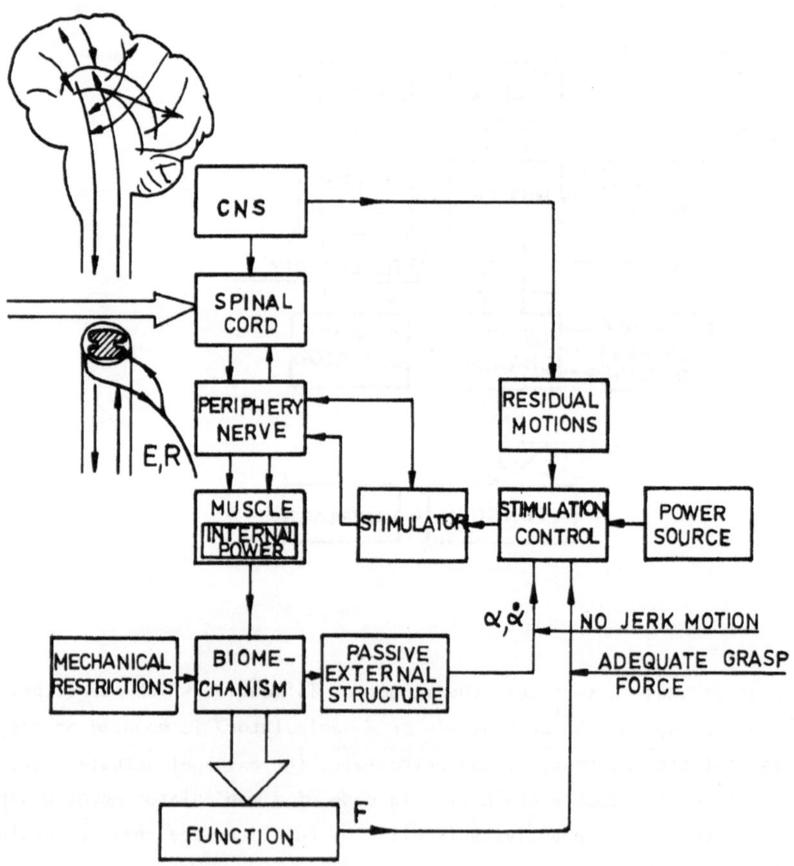

Figure 2

4. HYBRID METHOD FOR PREHENSION SUPPORTING - ALIVE MANIPULATORS

Damage to the spinal cord, regardless of the lesion level, results in vast changes in motor activity of the organism. The lesion site becomes a temporary or permanent breaking point of ascending and descending signal ways.

In such case the brain is isolated from information being sent from below-the--lesion part of the body served by the spinal cord and nerves. This lack of information makes the brain unable to form an adequate answer to what is really happening at the peripheral zone. On the other hand the commands sent by the brain do not reach the peripheral zone because the descending ways of information are blocked by the lesion.

In such situation all that happens at the peripheral zone cannot be controlled by the brain, and may be caused by that part of the spinal cord which extends below the lesion. Such activity can be manifested by spasticity which is uncontrolled, aimless and undirected muscular response to various stimuli coming from the peripheral zone. The patients with such damage are indifferent to such environmental stimuli as high and low temperature, pain and touch. They are also unable to perform a purposeful motion since the flow of necessary brain impulses through the spinal cord and peripheral nerves to the muscles is stopped.

Figure 2 shows in a simplified way the nature of the damage. Receptor (R) and effector (E) are intact. Neverthless, the centripetal stimuli received by the receptors reach only the spinal cord below the lesion, and cannot be transmitted higher to the brain. The effector, also intact, cannot fulfil its task becasue of the lack of the stimuli from the brain, controlling its activity.

In a case of C4 - C6 lesion the functions may be controlled directly either by stimulation of involved muscles, or by stimulation of their nerves. The latter methods is more effective due to a smaller amount of energy spent to achieve muscular contraction and the minimum number of used stimulators. Simple prehension can be controlled merely by two stimulators effecting the extension and flexion of the fingers.

In our studies concerning the stimulation of paralysed upper extremities (tetraplegy), we concentrated our efforts mainly on prehension control done by means of implant stimulators. In case of damage occuring on higher than C6 level it is impossible to use any auxiliary apparatus supporting prehension, because not only flexors, extensors of fingers and smaller muscles of the hand, but also the extensors of the wrist are paralysed. The investigations being carried on now are concentrated mainly on patient's smooth controlling of closing and opening motion of fingers in prehension.

Under physiological conditions the smooth motion of the extremity and exerting of the required force is associated with switching in a necessary amount of motor units excited from the central nervous system. In stimulation of nerves by means of a stimulator, the whole stem or undetermined part of the stem is excited. Therefore, the extension and flexion of the fingers are performed very rapidly. The functions are realized inaccurately and so is useless for the patient. Similar results were obtained in a group of several tetraplegics in years 1970-1975 |4,5,6|. In prehension process the fingers very often slide off an object or shift its position making it tumble over. This also happens when the grip is being loosend.

The studies on smooth, stimulated prehension, carried out in 1976-1980, included various methods of nerve excitation, both in open and feed-back control system, the controlled quantity being the angular velocty of the fingers.

The preliminary investigations were made for the system in which the grip force was controlled by change in voltage amplitude of stimulation impulses, duration and frequency of which were set to 0.2 ms and 50 kHz respectively. The record of fingers closing angle versus time (Figures 3a and 3b) shows that the motion is performed in a very short time and is independent from the rate of change of the voltage. The feed-back loop has small, if any, effect. The reason lies in a large inertia of muscles and time delay of signal transmition in neuromuscular system.

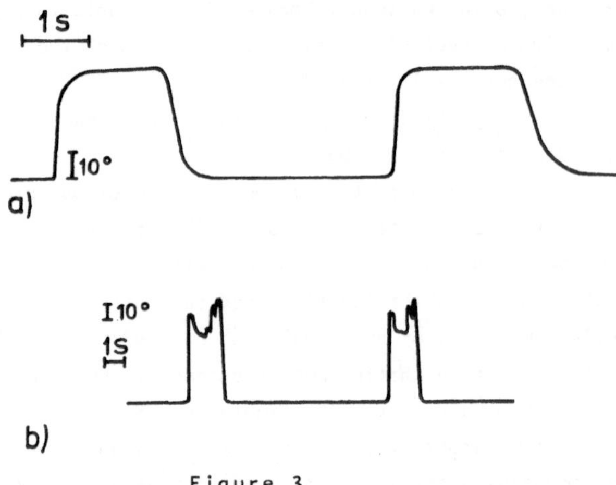

Figure 3

The further investigations showed that it is the first impulse of duration of about 50 μs, which causes almost the full closing of the fingers (more that 80% of the entire motion range). The estimated time delay is about 80 ms.

Another concept investigated was that, in which the controlled fingers flexion was coupled with stimulation of fingers extensors in order to slow down the motion after the predetermined angular velocity of fingers was exceeded.

The stimulation of the extensors was switched on command from the feed-back control system, and the amplitude of the impulses transmitted to the flexors increased in a linear way. The response of this control system turned out to be better than of the previous one. However, the time record of the fingers closing angle, shown in Figure 4, shown the considerable oscillations in comparison with the ideal case. Both,

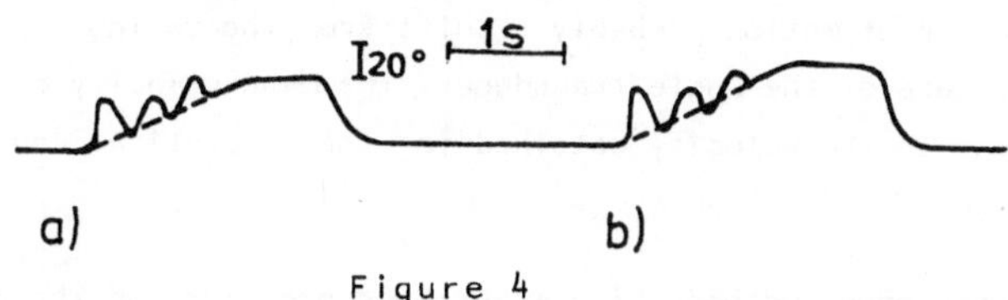

Figure 4

the closing time and the voltage build-up system of control comprises in a small sensitivity to resisting force. The time of motion measured from full extension to full gripping is independent from the resistance. The increase in the gain of the feedback leads to drop in stability of the fingers. For large values of the gain any disturbance, like brushing with fingers against an object or a roughness of the base, results in oscillating motion of the fingers.

Further, the properties of another method of fingers flexion control were investigated. In this method the impuls time, associated with the state of muscular excitation, was used to control flexion of the fingers. The amplitude of voltage was set so that 50 μs impulses caused no motion. The impuls time could be changed to 220 μs (the control done by change of applied voltage). Using this method in an open control system a record of fingers closing angle versus time was made, shown in Figure 5.

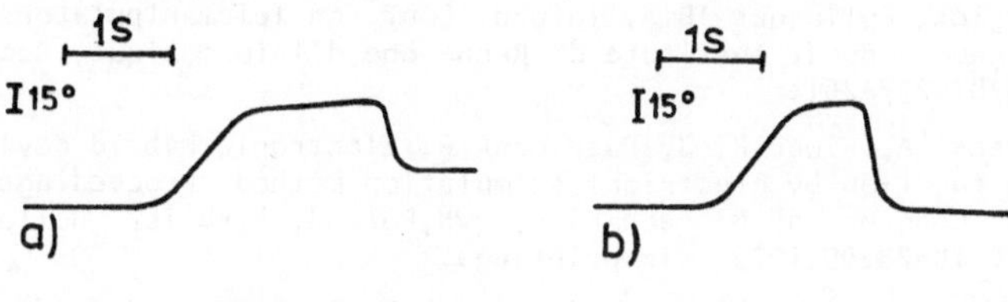

Figure 5

It is evident from the graph that the motion is performed without abrupt changes in acceleration. The deflections of the real graph from the theoretical relationship represented by a straight line are less than ±10%.

Figure 6 shows the record of the closing angle versus time made for the system fitted with a feed-back loop. In this case the performed motion is fairly smooth.

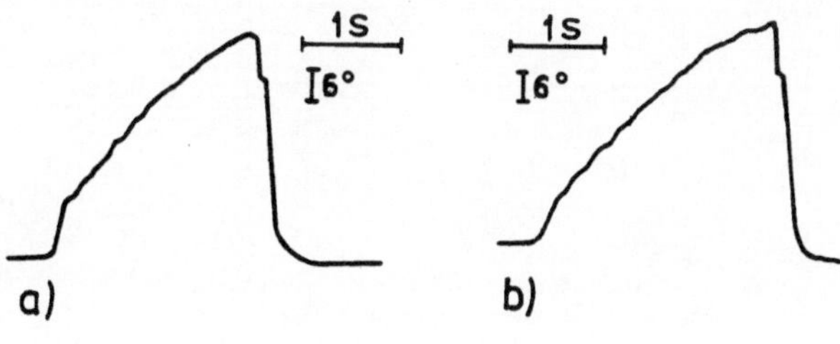

Figure 6

The step-wise character of motion probably results from the variable resistance of the mechanical structure of the angle transducer. The mean velocity of the motion is constant and close to the velocity obtained for the theoretical course.

5. CONCLUSION

Presented in this paper methods of prehension supporting and the results obtained in the years 1970-1980 show that the proposed hybrid method is very promising.

Possibility of performing smooth motion of the fingers (hand opening and closing) creates for the patients means of performing useful and functional motions.

6. REFERENCES

|1| Morecki A et al. Manipulators for supporting and substituting lost functions of human extremities. Proceedings, On Theory and Practice of Robots and Manipulators, Vol.I, Udine, 1974: 214-230.

|2| Ober JK, Leonhard J, Ogórkiewicz A. On the head manipulator for bilateral shoulder disarticulated children. Proceedings, Theory and Practice of Robots and Manipulators, PWN-Elsevier, 1977: 206-210.

|3| Paśniczek R, Kiwerski J, Wirski J and Borowski H. Some problems of implant stimulation applied to grasp movements. Proceedings of the IVth Intern. Symp. "Advances in External Control of Human Extremities", Belgrade, 1977: 584-602.

|4| Morecki A, Borowski H, Gasztold H, Kiwerski J and Paśniczek R. On two systems for tetraplegics. Colloques IRIA, Intern. Conf. on Telemanipulators for the Physically Handicapped. Institute de Recherche d'Informatique, Rocquencourt, Sept. 4-6,1978: 237-251.

|5| Weiss M, Morecki A, Kiwerski J, Paśniczek R. Electronic hybrid device for control of hand function by electrical stimulation method. Proceedings of the VIIth Intern. Congress of Biomechanics, PWN,Poland, Elsevier, Holland, Vol.A, Warsaw, Sept. 18-23.09.1979 (in printing).

|6| Morecki A, Weiss M, Kiwerski J and Paśniczek R. A new method for forcing lost grasping functions of extremities by use of an orthotic manipulator combined with implanted stimulators of nerves. Intern. Conf. on Medical Devices and Sports Equipment, August 18-20.08.1980, SF, Century 2, Emerging Technology Conferences, August 10-21,1980.

LE MAT$_1$*: TELETHESE POUR GRANDS HANDICAPES DES MEMBRES SUPERIEURS

PANNIER S.[1] VERTUT J.[2] GUITTET J.[2] KWEE H.H.[3]

ABSTRACT

The French SPARTACUS telethesis (MAT$_1$) developped for the severely handicapped having lost the use of bi-lateral prehension will be presented at this Congress. It will be compared with a certain number of similar foreign models.

The authors of this conference beleive that this machine, in spite of its high price, would enable the severely handicapped to lead a life as normal as possible, to save a good deal of hospital expenses and some hours of an aid as well (it is obvious that this aid will not be withdrawn for human reason.

INTRODUCTION

L'I.R.I.A.** a lancé en 1975 un projet pilote sous le nom de SPARTACUS, concernant une " machine à prendre à distance " ou téléthèse (il ne s'agit en effet ni d'une orthèse ni d'une prothèse). Cet appareil utilisant les ressources de la technologie moderne -notamment informatique- est destiné aux handicapés ayant perdu l'usage de la préhension manuelle bilatérale. Dans de tels cas, lorsque les solutions apportées par les petits appareillages ingénieux et peu coûteux, provenant essentiellement des ressources de l'ergothérapie, sont insuffisantes, de même que celles qui visent le contrôle de l'environnement,des machines plus sophistiquées doivent être mises à la disposition des grands handicapés. Ceux-ci manifestent, en effet, de plus en plus, le désir d'une plus grande autonomie allant dans le sens d'une réinsertion à part entière dans la société.

* Manipulateur automatisé pour tétraplégiques.
** Institut de recherche en informatique et en automatique. Voluceau - Rocquencourt , 78150 LE CHESNAY

1 - Pr.S.PANNIER , Hôpital Raymond Poincaré, 92380 GARCHES.
2 - VERTUT J. , GUITTET J. , C.E.A. Saclay , BP2, 91190 GIF SUR YVETTE.
3 - KWEE H.H. , Laboratoire SPARTACUS, I.U.T. Université Paris XII, 91000 EVRY.

1 - LES CHOIX AYANT PRESIDE A L'ELABORATION DE LA TELETHESE SPARTACUS.

Nous ne reprendrons ici que certains d'entre eux, définis lors de la concèption du projet (2).

- L'appareil est extérieur au patient, non anthopormophique. Cette solution a été jugée préférable dans un double but de simplification : en cherchant d'une part, à éviter le plus possible pour le handicapé les liaisons homme-machine assujétissantes; en limitant, d'autre part, les difficultés de fabrication -coûteuses- d'un exosquelette.

- Il est indépendant du fauteuil roulant (si celui-ci est nécessaire au handicapé) de façon qu'il soit le plus performant possible. Mais il peut être rendu automoteur.

- Son champ de balayage est aussi vaste que possible, aussi bien sur les plans de travail horizontal que vertical -un objet doit pouvoir être saisi en hauteur ou ramassé au sol. Il est ainsi plus " universel ", l'environnement n'étant modifié que dans les limites raisonnables. La charge maxima pouvant être soulevée contre pesanteur a été fixée à 3 kgs.

- La commande est réalisée par divers capteurs enregistrant au maximum les possibilités restantes du sujet (mouvements de la tête,des épaules,de la main si possible). Un laryngophone, un appareil de type Glottomat peuvent être utilisés -de préférence aux dispositifs de reconnaissance de la parole dont le coût est encore élevé.

- La machine est équipée de certains automatismes pour l'approche rapide, la saisie, la tenue, le toucher. Le " retour d'information " est assuré, certes, par la vision mais aussi par un retour sensoriel suppléant le tact et renseignant le handicapé sur les interactions entre la pince et l'environnement par présentation synthétique visuelle ou par stimulation cutanée convenablement localisée.

- Les normes de sécurité ont, bien entendu, été étudiées de façon très approfondie. C'est dans ce but que la vitesse de déplacement de la pince a été limitée à 0,5m/sec. Un débrayage automatique du système en cas d'incident, de phénomène parasite ou simplement de fatigue du patient est prévu.

Trois objectifs ont constamment influé sur la mise au point de cette téléthèse : ce sont la recherche de :

- Sa " transparence ", visant à ce qu'elle soit peu encombrante, suffisamment esthétique -compte tenu de son efficacité- et que sa commande soit logique et simple, nécessitant un minimum de contraintes.

- Sa " fiabilité ", sa maintenance devant absolument être assurée en permanence. En fait, les premières expérimentations ont montré que les chances de pannes étaient faibles ; elles proviennent surtout des systèmes de cablage électrique.

- Son " économie ". Le coût prévisible, élevé, de la machine sera influencé par plusieurs facteurs : la baisse du prix de l'informatique, même si ceux du domaine mécanique restent élevés ; l'importance des " retombées " industrielles (tâches répétitives en milieu hostile) étudiées parallèlement dans le projet SPARTACUS ; l'importance de la population -nationale, voire internationale- de handicapés concernés, compte tenu des services rendus dans leur réinsertion -l'aspect économique de celle-ci ainsi que sa qualité étant considérés dans cet optique comme des facteurs primordiaux.

2 - LA " POPULATION " DE HANDICAPES CONCERNES.

Une enquête a été faite (1) à partir d'un questionnaire adressé à 30 centres de rééducation français avec l'aide de l'I.R.I.A. et du bureau des statistiques du ministère de la Santé. Elle concernait les actes de la vie quotidienne : nourriture, lecture, écriture, distractions.

Centrée sur les tétraplégiques, elle a mon montré que ceux-ci seraient, en France, 3 à 4000 dont 2500 à 3000 traumatiques avec un chiffre prévisible de 150 à 200 nouveaux cas par an. Il faut tenir compte dans ces chiffres, à côté des tétraplégies traumatiques, d'autres séquelles neurologiques (P.A.A. ayant échappé à la vaccination, affections dégénératives relativement peu évolutives), d'affections rhumatologiques (certaines polyarthrites rhumatoïdes), d'amputations congénitales ou acquises bilatérales des membres supérieurs, de polytraumatismes ; dans ces derniers l'appareillage peut jouer un rôle éventuellement provisoire.

Les grands handicapés moteurs manifestent un désir toujours plus grand d'autonomie, de réinsertion professionnelle,sociale, de participation à la vie de la communauté. Dans ce sens, la présence auprès d'eux d'aides humaines (tierce personne) a des avantages indiscutables : soins, relations interhumaines qui ne peuvent être remis en question. Mais elle a aussi des inconvénients : dépendance, coûts ; ces derniers sont chiffrables : un travail récent indiquait qu'en cas d'économies en présence de temps de 50% d'une tierce personne, un télémanipulateur du type SPARTACUS serait amorti en 5 ans.

3 - RESULTATS INITIAUX : EXPERIMENTATION A PARTIR DU M.A.$_{23}$.

Depuis 1978, 4 adultes conservant des séquelles sensitivo motrices graves de tétraplégies hautes ne leur laissant, en pratique, que la commande volontaire des mouvements de la tête et des épaules, ont expérimenté le télémanipulateur M.A.$_{23}$. Celui-ci, construit pour l'industrie atomique par J.VERTUT et coll. a été adapté à la commande des handicapés par J.GUITTET et coll. Un protocole a été suivi : il comportait une série d'exercices concernant des assemblages de pièces, des suivis de trajectoires, des exercices correspondant aux gestes de la vie quotidienne : se nourrir, boire, écrire avec un scripteur,à la machine, téléphoner. L'insertion d'objets divers dans des surfaces évidées de formes correspondantes s'est montré comme étant, à l'usage, un excellent test de précisions. La durée d'apprentissage a été variable d'un patient à l'autre, ce qui peut s'expliquer par les données de leurs examens cliniques. La coopération a toujours été très fructueuse et source de progrès réciproques entre " chercheurs " et " expérimentateurs ".

4 - SITUATION ACTUELLE : REALISATION ET EXPERIMENTATION DU MAT$_1$. (3 - 4)

Les équipes sus mentionnées collaborent à la mise au point de la téléthèse MAT$_1$ destinée aux handicapés. Celle-ci devrait être mise à leur disposition dans certains services ou centres de rééducation dans le courant de l'année 1981. Signalons à ce sujet qu'un protocole expérimental commun est en cours d'élaboration entre l'équipe du projet SPARTACUS et certaines équipes étrangères, en particuliers américaines (STANFORD - U.C.L.A.) afin de comparer les performances des télémanipulateurs à partir de batteries de tests, tels que ceux que nous avons cités.

5 - AMORCE DE COMPARAISON DU PROTOTYPE FRANCAIS AVEC QUELQUES AUTRES PROJETS DE TELEMANIPULATEURS ETRANGERS.

Parmi les projets de ce type -dont le nombre ne dépasserait pas dans le monde une dizaine- nous ne citerons que trois d'entre eux que nous avons pu connaître précisément, voire expérimenter.

HEIDELBERG :

Il s'agit là d'une étude entreprise il y a plusieurs années déjà. Elle comporte un télémanipulateur (efficace mais volumineux et complexe) desservant un volume dans lequel l'aménagement de l'environnement a été très poussé. La commande est analytique (axe par axe) par action du menton sur des petits leviers. La formule retenue est donc mixte alors qu'en ce qui concerne la téléthèse française ainsi que les deux projets américains mentionnés ci-dessous les performances des appareils visent (dans la limite du raisonnable bien entendu) à une relative indépendance par rapport à l'aménagement de l'environnement. Il semble, qu'à notre connaissance du moins et sans que nous en sachions pour autant toutes les raisons, ce programme ait été peu développé.

STANFORD :

Les chercheurs de cette Université utilisent un manipulateur fabriqué dans le commerce (Unimate), donc relativement bon marché. Ses performances mécaniques sont actuellement inférieures à celles du prototype SPARTACUS; en particulier son rayon d'action efficace est faible : il ne va ni au sol ni en hauteur. Sa commande -essentiellement par la voix- fait l'objet d'études très poussées. Cette commande a, pour l'instant, l'inconvénient d'être lente et complexe. Le manipulateur sera prochainement monté sur un fauteuil roulant électrique, lui-même très " performant ". Une commande céphalique par l'intermédiaire d'ultra-sons est à l'étude. Elle sera plus confortable que la commande par des capteurs céphaliques directs.

U.C.L.A. :

A l'Université de Los Angeles est étudié un manipulateur comportant un bras télescopique qui semble très fonctionnel et peut aller au sol ainsi qu'en hauteur. Néanmoins, ses qualités mécaniques paraissent, là aussi, inférieures à celle de la téléthèse SPARTACUS. La charge soulevée est apparemment plus faible également. Une commande par la direction des yeux est en cours d'étude pour ce manipulateur. Cette commande est rapide et efficace mais, dans l'état actuel des choses, elle a l'inconvénient de nécessiter des réglages avant chaque séance d'utilisation.
Surtout, le principe actuel est tel que, dans certaines positions du " bras ", le regard directeur doit se détourner de la cible visée, ce qui constitue une gêne majeure pour l'utilisateur. Des solutions d'améliorations techniques sont en cours d'étude sur ce point précis. Cet appareil est d'ores et déjà monté sur le même fauteuil roulant électrique que celui qui sera utilisé à Stanford.

Il convient de noter que la téléthèse française dispose d'une avance par rapport aux projets américains sus cités du fait de l'expérimentation entreprise par des patients depuis 2 ans ; celle-ci a fourni déjà nombre d'appré-

ciations sur la question essentielle qui est celle de l' "interface" homme (handicapé) - machine (téléthèse).

CONCLUSIONS

La téléthèse " SPARTACUS " (MAT_1) s'inscrit dans un programme de réalisation de matériels d'assistance aux grands handicapés, destiné à augmenter leur autonomie et à faciliter leur réinsertion sociale. Même coûteuse, il est vraisemblable, comme tendent à le prouver des travaux en cours (5) qu'elle permettra à ces handicapés de parvenir à une réinsertion sociale de qualité tout en permettant certaines économies : raccourcissement des séjours en services et centres de rééducation, suppression des " placements de chroniques " désastreux et coûteux, économie et utilisation plus rationnelle du temps de présence des tierces personnes -qu'il n'est pas question, pour autant, de suplanter totalement tant leur rôle humain est important.

BIBLIOGRAPHIE succincte

1 DURAND J. , BOURLIOUX-GAVARDIN M. et PANNIER S.
Résultats préliminaires d'une enquête nationale sur les tétraplégiques.
Ann. Méd. Phys. 1978, 21, 3 , 312 - 325.

2 GUITTET J. , KWEE H.H. , QUETIN N. , YCLON J. , GROSSIORD A. , DURAND J. , PANNIER S.
A Telemanipulator for the Physically Handicaped : Manipulator Control Studies.
IRMA III, Bâle - Suisse , Juillet 1978.

3 VERTUT J. et GUITTET J.
Le système SPARTACUS : Conception du MAT_1
Conférence Internationale sur les Télémanipulateurs pour handicapés physiques. I.R.I.A. , Septembre 1978.

4 KWEE H.H. , GUITTET J. , QUETIN N. et YCLON J.
Manipulator Control Studies.
Automne 1979. Bulletin of Prosthetics Research, Veterans Administration, New-York.

5 TREMBLAY M.
Contribution à l'étude des aspects économiques liés à l'utilisation de la téléthèse SPARTACUS par des tétraplégiques.
Mémoire pour le C.E.S. de Rééducation et Réadaptation fonctionnelles. Paris 1980 , 56 p. dactyl.

Docteur E. MICHAUT - Monsieur F. PELISSE
C E R A V A L
2, rue du Parc - 94460 Valenton, France

CHAINE DE MESURE ET D'ANALYSE DE LA MARCHE GEREE PAR ORDINATEUR

SUMMARY - Until recently, gait analysis has been only possible by clinical observation, which does not give the details of the main causes of any anomaly.

These clinical observations do not give any concrete measurement or comparison with the same patient or with others patients.

With the use of automatic gait measurement system, which include forces plate transducers, and a small computer allows an objective study by measurement and recordings of the forces with the ground while walking. The computer calculates the data and automatically returns the final results in graphic pictures. In this way clinical observation is completed by a mecanical analysis of the phenomenon.

This method is used for the reeducation and limb-fitting of lower limb amputees.

INTRODUCTION - L'étude des forces exercées entre le pied et le sol au cours de la marche permet de connaitre les sollicitations reçues par le membre en appui. La connaissance de ces sollicitations est d'un intérêt capital pour la fabrication, le réglage et l'adaptation des prothèses des membres inférieurs.

Jusqu'à ces dernières années, la technique consistait à faire marcher le sujet à examiner sur un plateau de forces relié à un enregistreur graphique puis à dépouiller et à interpréter les courbes ainsi obtenues.

L'importance du travail et le délai qu'il imposait entre la prise des mesures et les résultats rendaient cette technique inutilisable en dehors du laboratoire de recherche. La précision des résultats était également médiocre car les points relevés sur les courbes ne peuvent pas être très nombreux et leur lecture introduit une erreur importante.

L'utilisation de l'ordinateur a donné à cette technique depuis 10 ans environ, le complément qui en fait le meilleur instrument de mesure pour l'évaluation de la qualité de l'appareillage des amputés des membres inférieurs.

PRINCIPE, MATERIEL ET METHODE - La figure (1) reproduit la piste de marche avec ses dimensions. Au centre de cette piste, deux plateaux de forces identiques de 170 cm de long et de 30 cm de large permettent le recueil successif de plusieurs posés de pieds droit et gauche. Cette disposition présente plusieurs avantages :

- la longueur de la piste est suffisamment grande pour qu'au moment du passage sur les plateaux de forces, le sujet ait une marche en régime établi, c'est-à-dire qu'il ne soit pas en phase d'accélération ou de freinage
- toutes les mesures nécessaires, une mesure sur le pied droit et une sur le pied gauche, sont recueillies en un seul passage.

L'utilisation d'un plateau de forces unique et de faibles dimensions nécessite au moins deux passages pour enregistrer les posés droit et gauche. Mais, étant donné les faibles dimensions du plateau, il est fréquent que le pied se pose à cheval sur le plateau et sur la piste de marche, ce qui rend la mesure inutilisable. C'est pourquoi le nombre de passages est, en général, supérieur à deux

- les mesures relevées sur chaque pied ont lieu au cours des posés successifs, la vitesse de la marche est donc rigoureusement la même pour les enregistrements du côté droit et du côté gauche
- le temps écoulé entre les deux appuis successifs est mesuré, la durée de la phase pendulaire est ainsi connue
- la période dite de double appui pendant laquelle s'effectue le transfert de l'appui d'un pied sur l'autre peut être étudiée également
- la durée du cycle de la marche qui est égale à la somme d'un appui et d'une phase pendulaire est connue
- la longueur des pas peut être calculée et, à l'aide de la durée du cycle, la vitesse de la marche est également déterminée.

L'ensemble de ces informations permet l'étude mécanique de chaque appui séparé comme il est fait avec un plateau simple de faibles dimensions mais, en plus, la reconstitution de la succession des phases et des cycles de la marche est possible.

Les plateaux de forces reposent, à chacun de leurs angles, sur un système mécanique muni de jauges de contraintes. La figure (2) reproduit le dessin côté des capteurs. Le pied (5) solidaire de la platine du plateau de forces (1) repose sur le levier (4) par un contact ponctuel, le levier (4) est fixé par la pièce (6) aux tubes soudés qui constituent le bâti (3) des plateaux de forces.

Les deux jauges de contraintes fixées sur le levier (4) sont reliées pour constituer un demi pont de Wheatstone, le capteur ainsi constitué est sensible aux seuls efforts verticaux imposés à la platine. De la même façon, les quatre jauges fixées sur le pied (5) sont reliées deux à deux pour constituer des capteurs à même de mesurer les composantes horizontales Rx et Ry de la résultante des forces imposées à la platine.

Chaque jauge est associée à un circuit imprimé comprenant une alimentation réglable et un amplificateur de mesure. Le gain des amplificateurs est tel qu'une force de 1 daN donne une différence de potentiel de 0.2 volts.

Le convertisseur A/D utilisé a une résolution de 12 bits pour des tensions comprises entre + et - 10 volts par rapport à la masse.

Configuration informatique : NOVA 3 de DATA GENERAL

- Unité centrale : 64 K octets
- Imprimante : 30 c/s
- Ecran
- Table traçante : BENSON 1130
- Unité de disque : 2 x 5 millions d'octets.

Chaque capteur est scrupté toutes les 100e de seconde. Le temps accordé pour franchir les 1.70 m des plateaux de forces est de 3 secondes, ce qui correspond à une vitesse de marche de 2 kilomètres par heure environ.

Le début et l'arrêt des mesures sont déclenchés automatiquement par le programme mis en mémoire machine lorsque les capteurs ne sont plus excités.

RESULTATS - La figure (3) reproduit l'ensemble des graphes tracés à la suite d'un seul passage sur les plateaux de forces.

Les courbes 1, 2, 8, 9, 10, 11 correspondent à la variation, au cours du temps, des composantes $\vec{Rx}$, $\vec{Ry}$, $\vec{Rz}$ de la résultante $\vec{R}$ des forces exercées entre le pied et le sol.

Les axes sont choisis de façon à ce que le trièdre (0/$\vec{Rx}$, $\vec{Ry}$, $\vec{Rz}$) soit de sens direct avec :

- $\vec{Rx}$ horizontale, dirigée dans le sens du déplacement
- $\vec{Ry}$ horizontale latérale
- $\vec{Rz}$ verticale.

Sur les mêmes axes que les courbes 1 et 2, la ligne horizontale d'ordonnée POI correspond au poids du sujet. Les courbes de repère 3 et 3' représentent le déplacement du point d'application de la force $\vec{Rz}$ le long du pied au cours de l'appui. Les schémas de pieds placés à droite des courbes fournissent l'échelle des ordonnées aux graphes 3 et 3', qui admettent en abscisse l'axe des temps communs respectivement aux courbes 1 et 2.

La courbe 12 représente les variations de $\vec{Rz}$ dans une succession de cycles de la marche, la première courbe complète est toujours un appui gauche.

La courbe 13 est obtenue en faisant la somme des courbes représentées en 12, elle représente donc la variation de toutes les forces verticales exercées entre les appuis et le sol.

Les courbes4, 5, 6 et 7 représentent schématiquement un pied de profil sur lequel est tracée, sous forme d'histogramme, la répartition des quantités d'appui exercées en chaque point du pied (courbes 4 et 5) et le vecteur résultant dans le plan sagittal des forces exercées entre le pied et le sol en différents temps de l'appui (courbes 6 et 7).

Simultanément, les valeurs remarquables (position et niveau des maximums, passage à zéro, durées d'accidents particuliers, etc...) sont transcrites par l'imprimante (figure 4). Une analyse comparative de chaque courbe des côtés droit et gauche est programmée ; le résultat de cette analyse est imprimé en clair à la suite des valeurs numériques. De cette façon, les principaux défauts concernant la prothèse ou la marche sont annoncés. La valeur globale de la qualité du résultat de l'appareillage est donnée par une note chiffrée.

L'ensemble de ces résultats est complété par des informations caractérisant le blessé (nom, âge, niveau et côté d'amputation, etc...) qui sont demandées à l'opérateur au cours du déroulement du programme.

DISCUSSION - La totalité des courbes, graphiques, textes et valeurs numériques est obtenue en 6 minutes.

Chaque courbe correspond à une représentation graphique de la marche projetée dans un plan, chaque phase du pas est divisée ainsi en plusieurs parties. Si l'observation de ce phénomène d'habitude trop rapide pour être appréciée est transformée en une lecture aisée, les anomalies par rapport à un cadre connu s'en détachent facilement. La correspondance des courbes avec la marche permet d'en apprécier de façon quantitative les défauts et les qualités, la sanction thérapeutique peut y être recherchée et de toute façon ce dossier conserve sa valeur dans le temps puisqu'il peut être un élément de comparaison ou de constatation d'évolution.

L'usage régulier de cette installation depuis plusieurs années au CRA pour l'appareillage des amputés des membres inférieurs nous a prouvé son efficacité. La présence de l'ordinateur rend quasi automatique le déroulement de toutes les opérations depuis la prise des mesures jusqu'à la sortie des informations, libérant ainsi l'opérateur de toutes les charges qu'exigent la surveillance et le maniement d'appareils de mesure. Ce dernier peut alors consacrer son attention sur le sujet examiné et veiller à ce que les mesures soient prises à un moment où aucun évènement extérieur ne perturbe le déplacement du blessé.

CONCLUSION - L'analyse faite actuellement sur la marche des amputés n'est pas définitive, les programmes sont modifiés régulièrement pour tenir compte des observations faites à l'usage.

D'autres mesures peuvent être associées à celles qui viennent d'être exposées sur les plateaux de forces, par exemple la marche avec soutiens (cannes et cannes béquilles) munis de capteurs permet d'étudier ces modes de déplacement et fournit un bilan des différents appuis au cours du déplacement. Des capteurs placés sur prothèse des membres inférieurs sont également utilisés pour compléter les informations nécessaires à la compréhension de certains défauts de marche des amputés.

L'extension de la méthode à d'autres marches pathologiques d'origines diverses (neurologique, orthopédique, etc...) nécessiterait seulement la modification des programmes pour adapter l'analyse des mesures enregistrées au handicap étudié.

Le fàible coût, la rapidité et surtout l'absolue innocuité de cet examen permettent de le recommander pour le suivi des divers déficits de l'appareil locomoteur.

BIBLIOGRAPHIE

(1) CAVANAGH P.R., MICHIYOSHI AE. A technique for the display of pressure distributions beneath the foot. Journal of Biomechanics 1980 ; 13 : 69-75.

(2) COOK TM, COZZENS BA, KENOSIAN H. A technique for force-line visualization. Rehabilitation Engineering Center, Moss Rehabilitation Hospital, Philadelphia, PA 19141. March 1979.

(3) GOLA MM. Mechnical design, constructional details and calibration of a new force plate. Journal of Biomechanics 1980 ; 13 : 113-128.

(4) LAMOREUX LW. Kinematic measurements in the study of human walking. Bulletin of Prosthetics Research. Spring 1971 ; BPR 10-15 :

(5) LORD G, GENTAZ R, GANDOLFI R. La marche normale et ses altérations après arthroplastie totale au membre inférieur. Revue de Chirurgie Orthopédique. 1977 ; 63 : 221.236.

(6) MICHAUT E, PELISSE F. Utilisation de l'ordinateur pour la mesure et l'analyse des principaux paramètres de la marche à l'aide d'une chaîne de mesures comportant des plateaux de forces. Acta Orthopaedica Belg. 1978 ; 44 : 809-823.

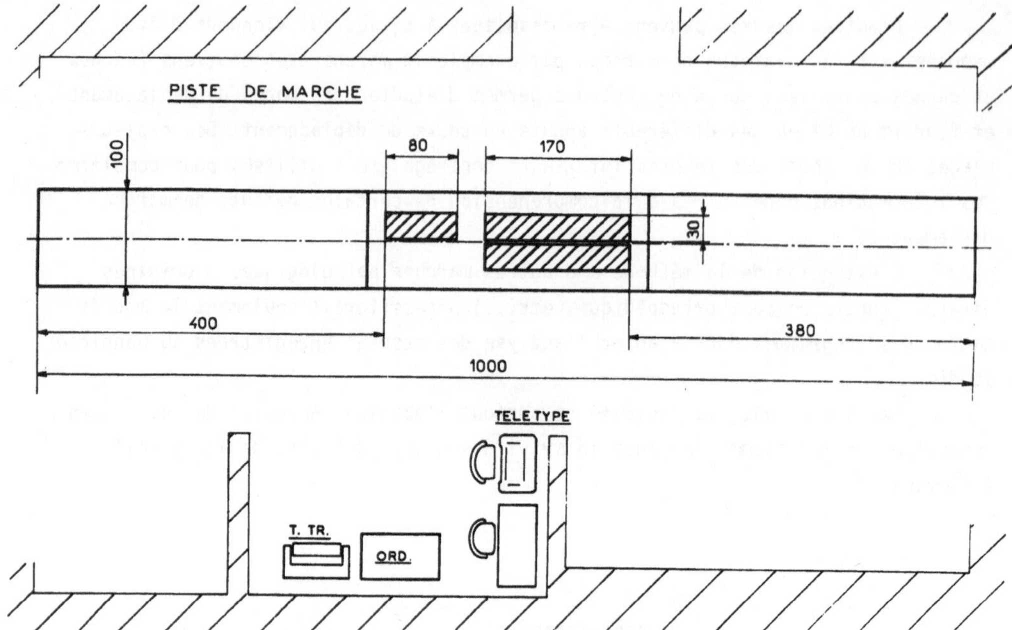

Figure 1 - Plan de la piste de marche. Les plateaux de forces sont inclus dans la piste et, en réalité, très peu visibles par le sujet examiné. L'installation comporte un plateau simple de 80 x 30 cm et un plateau double composé de deux plateaux de 170 x 30 cm.

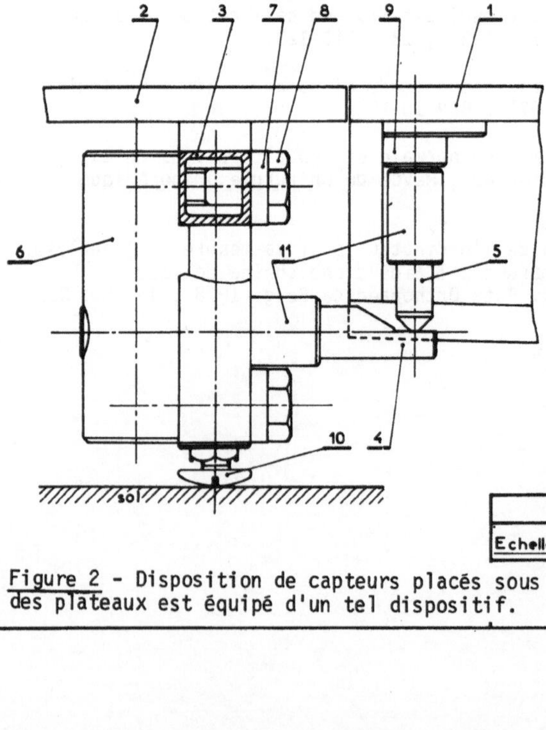

REP	NB	DESIGNATION	MATIERE
11	16	Capots de protection	A_U4G
10	4	Pieds reglables	
9	8	Support Cpt. Rx Ry	A-U4G
8	16	Vis H, M10_40	E 26
7	16	Rondelles carrées	Etiré
6	16	Support pour Cpt. Rz	A 56
5	8	Capteurs Rx et Ry	A_U4G
4	8	Capteurs Rz	XC 65 f
3	1	Bati (tube carré)	
2	1	Piste de marche	Bois
1	2	Plateau	Bois

C_E_R_A_V_A_L

Echelle : 1

Figure 2 - Disposition de capteurs placés sous les plateaux de forces. Chaque angle des plateaux est équipé d'un tel dispositif.

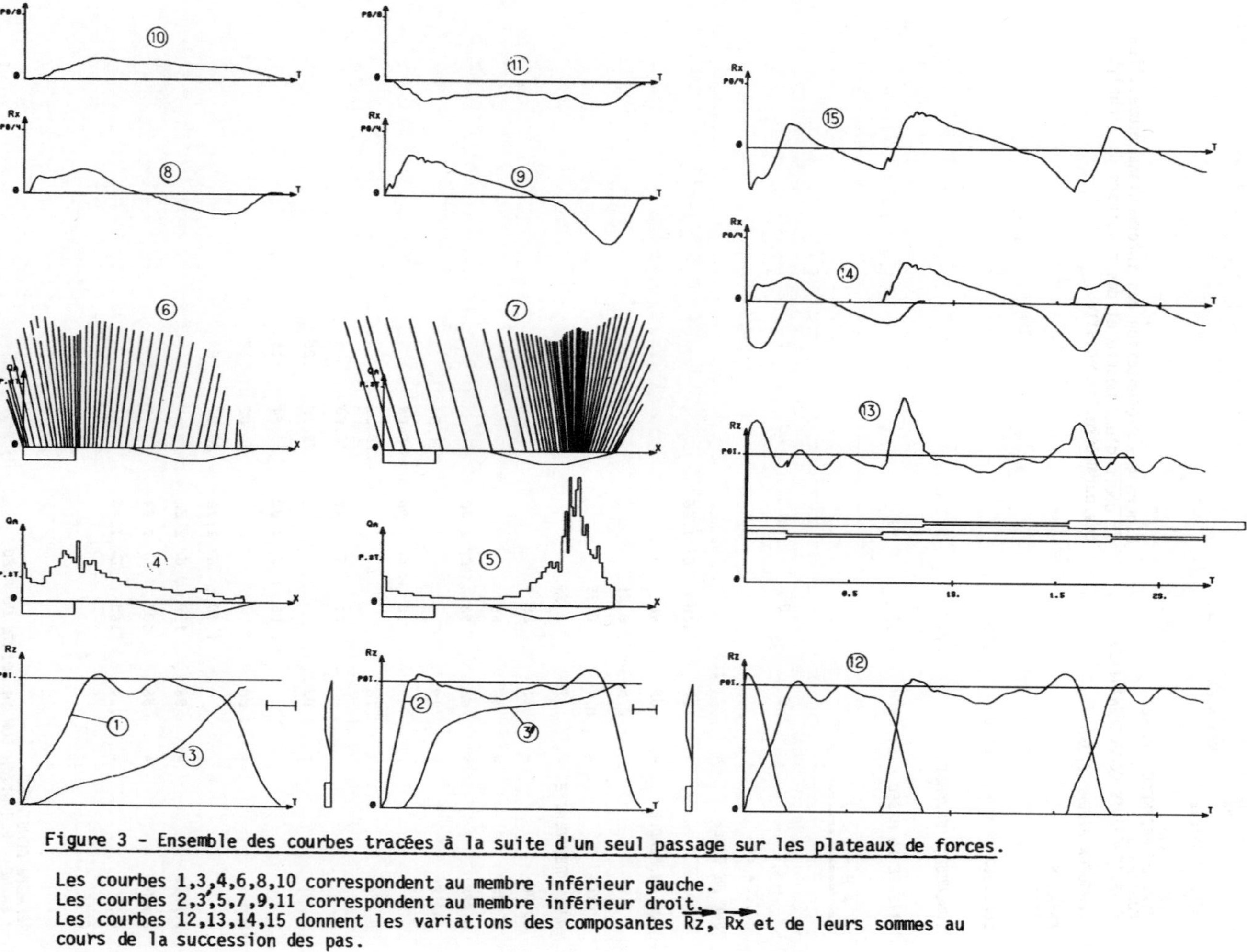

Figure 3 - Ensemble des courbes tracées à la suite d'un seul passage sur les plateaux de forces.

Les courbes 1,3,4,6,8,10 correspondent au membre inférieur gauche.
Les courbes 2,3',5,7,9,11 correspondent au membre inférieur droit.
Les courbes 12,13,14,15 donnent les variations des composantes $\vec{Rz}$, $\vec{Rx}$ et de leurs sommes au cours de la succession des pas.

11 - 6 - 80
9 / 58 / 7
NOM:ALEX A
NIVEAU:CUISSE
COTE:G
AGE:34 ANS
TYPE DE PROTHESE:CONTACT
SOUTIEN:0
RENSEIGNEMENTS COMPLEMENTAIRES:

LONGUEUR PIED= 275MM

ESPACES :

LONGUEUR D'UN PAS EN CM : 129

LONGUEUR D'ENJAMBE : 74 424

VITESSE EN M/SEC. ET KM/H : 0.83 2.98

APPUIS
================

		G	D	R	%C	T
POIDS= 64						
DUR DE CYCLE	=	156.				
T.APP	=	87	110	G/ 1.26		
DUR.PH.PENDUL	=	69	46			
A/CYC	=	0.56	0.71			
P/CYC	=	0.44	0.29			
APPUI/PENDULAIRE	=	1.26	2.39			
GD-DG	=	21	20			
A.SIMP	=	46	69			
Q.APP	=	62	93	D/ 1.50		
0-0,8P	=	19			21.84	
			10	G/ 1.90	9.09	
0,8P-0	=	16			18.39	
			11	G/ 1.45	10.00	
1.MAX.	=	1.03			29.89	26
			1.06	G/ 1.02	13.64	15
2.MAX.	=	1.00			54.02	47
			1.10	G/ 1.10	80.91	89
Q.RX>0.	=	53	139	G/ 2.62		
Q.RX<0.	=	58	107	G/ 1.84		
Q.RY	=	114	165	G/ 1.45		
COTE	=	5				

DEFAUTS CONSTATES
J.SAINE : ELEVATION SUR LA POINTE DU PIED
PROTHESE : DEFAUT D'APPUI

Figure 4 - Présentation des informations recueillies au cours d'une mesure et des résultats de l'analyse des paramètres enregistrés.

ROLE OF GRAPHIC SUPPORT IN STANDARDIZATION OF COMMUNICATION AIDS FOR THE MOTOR HANDICAPPED

P. Morasso, V. Tagliasco, R. Zaccaria
Istituto di Elettrotecnica, Università di Genova
Genoa, Italy

ABSTRACT

Tailoring a communication device to a motor disabled child requires the availability, in the rehabilitation environment, of modularized systems which are based on several levels of standardization (mechanical, electrical, software). On this purpose, it is convenient to distinguish between 'Institutional Devices' and 'Personalized Devices', which are obtained from the former in the tailoring process by choosing and configuring the appropriate modules.
In particular, a graphic package is a very important module for an effective man/machine interaction. An implementation is described which is embedded in the BASIC interpreter of the LSI 11 microcomputer and which uses a low cost graphic terminal, such as the Matrox MLS 512.

1. INTRODUCTION

The experience acquired during the design and evaluation of the first prototype of the project LOGOS /1/ has made evident that the process of tailoring a communication device to a motor disabled child is far from a trivial task, because it imples an intimate knowledge and estimation capability of the sensory-motor integration mechanisms, which is mostly lacking.

It is then necessary to provide the rehabilitator, during the phase of tailoring, with a certain experimental capability which allows him to evaluate the effect of adjusting some parameters of the interactive child/device system at the psycho-physical, psycho-motor, logic, cognitive levels.

Furthermore, such experimental capability must be linked to the possibility of transferring the results from the experimental phase to the operative phase, during which the child uses a specifically configured device in his study/work environment.

The previous requirements can be satisfied (at the level of design criteria and architectures) by planning two levels of communication devices:

i) Institutional Device,
ii) Personalized Device.

The Institutional Device must be easily programmable, for the purpose of easily varying the interactive techniques (scanning, delays, codes, etc.), the graphic characteristics, the input transducers, the output actuators, the operative functions (e.g. simple writing, word processing, environment control, etc.).

The personalized Devices are particular configurations of the previous system adapted to the particular needs of individual subjects.

2. ROLE OF STANDARDIZATION

The achievement of the above mentioned goal imples that the designer/rehabilitator has the availability of modularized systems in which commercially available equipments are used as much as possible and which are based on several levels of standardization, from mechanical/electrical specifications (bottom) to "abstract object" definitions (top), such as software packages (Fig. 1).

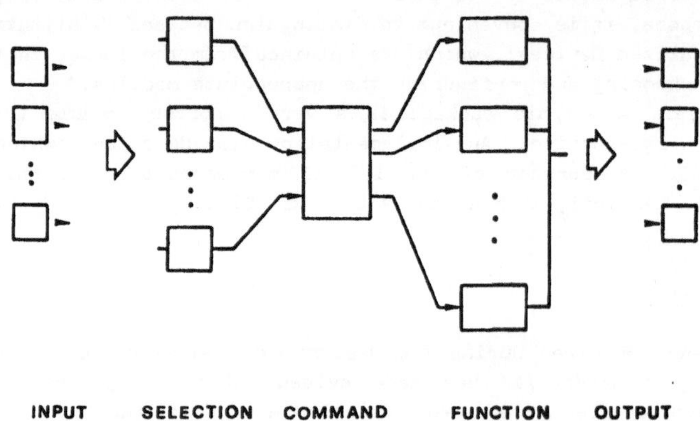

Fig. 1 Main modules of a flexible communication device for motor disabled subjects.

Some standardization proposals were impled in all LOGOS stages (e.g. size and resolution of displays, statistic functions, sensors, etc.); nevertheless, we deem important to analyze this problem with more detail.

All Items of the following (open) list are both suggestions of the past LOGOS experience and its underlying phylosophy for the future.

Input/Output

A mechanical and electrical standard should be defined for all peripheral interfacing (possibly, a well spread communication standard, such as bit-serial RS 232 or byte-serial IEEE 488).

Peripherals

Low cost, "usual" devices (homogeneous with respect to the I/O standard) may include: digital audio cassette, mini floppy disc, printer, commercial TV set interface, music generator, etc.. Devices with a little amount of autonomous computing capability ('intelligent' peripherals) could be very useful in environment control tasks such as, for example, automatic phone dialling.

Software

Since a language is to be proposed, BASIC is a very good candidate for allowing flexibility, ease of use in the rehabilitation environment and ease of configuring personalized systems; furthermore, BASIC can be easily extended to include the required Real Time Functions (such as I/O driving, clock management, etc;).

Software Packages

An institutional device should be provided with some high level procedures, with access by means of simple instructions of the language (e.g. "CALL" in BASIC). Let us point out the following:

i) statistical information on the language spoken by the subject;

ii) graphic generator, as discussed later, with high resolution for alphanumeric or quasi-alphanumeric symbols;

iii) visual schemes (linear, matrix-like, circular, morse-like, etc.);

iv) analog sensor filtering;

v) sound generation (which is relevant for training children).

However, such a work of standardization needs to be not only "open minded", but also aware of the parallel growth of communication media for "normal people", with refernce to the large area of "consumer electronics".
For example, we may quote the following relevant phenomena:

i) a spread of common TV-based generalized data networks, like "Teletext" and "Viewdata";

ii) a circulation of written texts (books, journals, etc.) on digital supports like floppies or cassettes or also via phone network;

iii) an increasing use of telemonitoring, even only for alarm signalling in case of danger or damege (e.g. for the elderly living alone).

3. <u>GRAPHIC SUPPORT</u>

In a previous paper /2/ some aspects of standardization were investigated, but the role of graphic support was not clearly evidentiated.

In effect, even if the experimentation of the LOGOS prototype in a rehabilitative environment is not yet terminated, it is already possible to point out the importance of a factor which was understimated in a preliminary design phase: motor disabilities are almost invariably associated with sensory-perceptual malfunctions, particularly of visual type.

A direct consequence of this fact is that common character generators (5x7 or 7x9 pixels) are inadequate. Such a low resolution indeed is compatible with the characteristics of the visual system only if characters are "small" (i.e. about one degree of visual angle).

If these characters are enlarged, to overcome defects of visual acuity or irregularities of the visual field, the result is what we may call "Lincoln effect" (*), which even worsens the recognition of graphic signs.

In addition, a set of quasi-alphabetic signs (e.g. symbols, small objects, pets) would be desirable in most cases.

It is then necessary to develope a generator system of graphic signs (characters or other) with a much higher resolution, without resorting, however, to the direct storage of all the pixels, which is practical only for low resolution signs because it requires a storage proportional to n*n.

The graphic unit which was chosen for representing high resolution graphic signs is the horizontal segment (the "filling segment"), associated with a segment scanning generation technique, which requires a storage proportional to n.

High resolution, on the other hand, requires another representation level, in which are defined larger aggregation sttuctures, but in a small number, from which the graphic signs can be composed.

In other words, the graphic sign generator acquires the characteristics of a data base.

The graphic support which was developed consists of a program for the creation of the binary data file on a PDP11 minicomputer, with the use of the Tesak VD501 image acquisition/processing system.

The data file can then be used for generating graphic signs on a graphic video terminal which has a refresh memory of 512x512x1 pixels (e.g. a low cost system such as Matrox MLS 512).

Each graphic sign stored in the data file is built starting with a complete pictoric image which first is digitized and then is coded.

An acquisition program allows the operator to extract a nxn square, where n is the basic resolution of the graphic sign. A particular useful value for n is 60, because it allows easily to obtain reduction factors of 1/2, 1/3, 1/4, 1/5, 1/6 in the display phase (Fig. 2, 3).

During the acquisition of graphic signs it is possible to modify interactively incorrect details, pixels by pixels, as shown in Fig. 4.

In the coding phase, the nxn square is examined line by line, looking for edges which identify filling segments. Each couples of edges so found represents a "stroke" of the graphic sign. With four strokes it is possible to represent a large variety of signs and this value was assumed in the implementation. Each graphic sign is then coded as a list of, at most, four strokes and the whole graphic sign file, which can be used subsequently for sign generation, is structured as follows:

(*) This effect is related to the famous photograph of the american president, digitized with a low resolution. The face can be better recognized far away (i.e. with a low enlargement) than with a close look (i.e. with a big enlargement). This effect has to do with the low-pass filtering characteristics of the human visual channel.

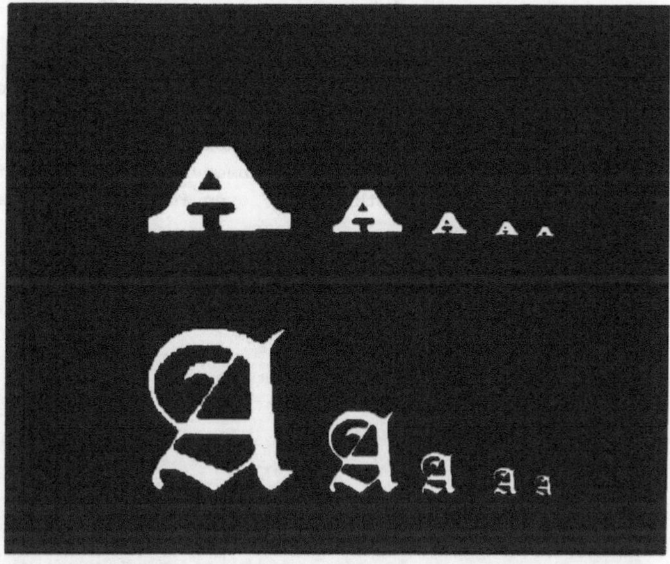

Fig. 2. Display of two graphic signs with different amplification factors. The basic graphic sign, stored in the data file, is the second from the left, for both fonts. The other signs were obtained using a magnification factor of 2/1, 1/2, 1/3, 1/4, respectively.

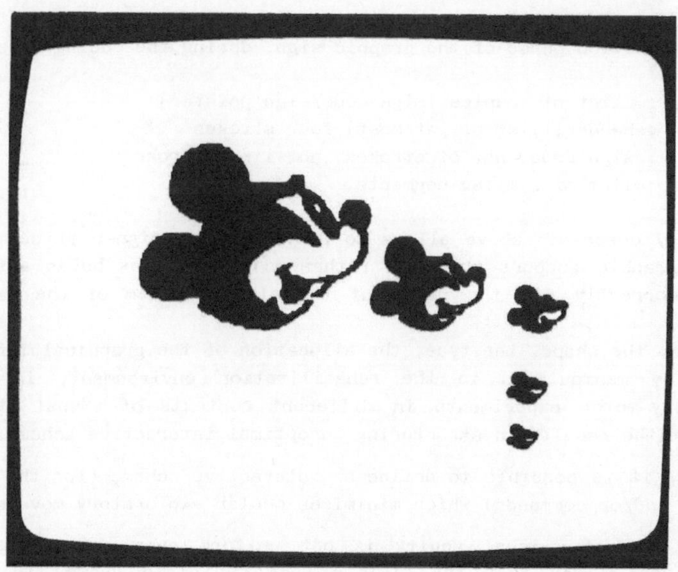

Fig. 3. Display of a non alphabetical sign with different magnification factors. The basic graphic sign, stored in the data file, is the second from the left. This picture makes evident a peculiarity of the coding algorithm, on the basis of which the graphic sign file is built. This algorithm extracts form the image, for each raster line, couples of edges, no more than four of them. It is possible to observe that such limit eliminates only a detail of the mouth, even in a complex graphic sign as the "mickey mouse".

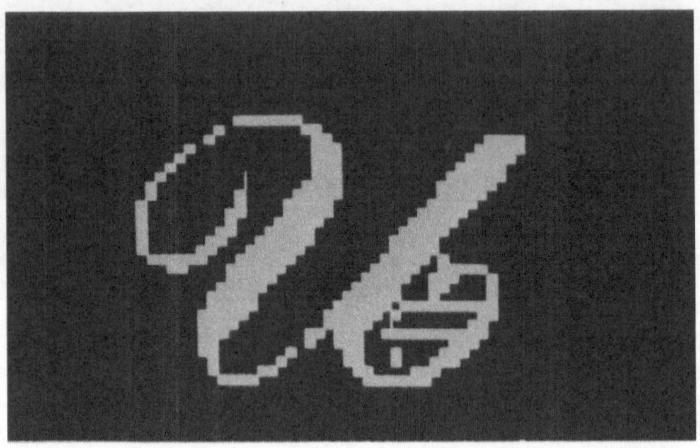

Fig. 4. Interactive correction of incorrect details, during the acquisition phase of the graphic sign, during the coding phase.

```
sign directory := list of couples (sign code/sign pointer)
sign           :=header, list of (at most) four strokes
header         :=sign code, no. of strokes, no. lines/stroke
stroke         :=list of filling segments.
```

The methodology described above allows to provide the designer of communication aids with a graphic support which is rather little complex but is sufficiently powerful to correctly fit the needs of the visual system of the handicapped person.
In other words, the shape, the type, the allocation of the graphical information must be easily manipulated in the rehabilitation environment, in order to perform sensory-motor experiments in different contexts of visual stimulation and to exploit the results in structuring an optimal interactive scheme.

In particular, it is possible to define an interactive scheme (for the selection of characters and/or commands) which minimizes ocular exploratory movements.

As a matter of fact, visual acuity is not uniform over the retina, but it varies, in such a way that the minimum resolved angle grows linearly with excentricity.

As a consequence, the graphic support described above allows to arrange in a circle the characters (as in Fig. 5) and this allocation guarantees that approximately all the characters are perceived with the same resolution, when the fixation point coincides with the center of the figure.

The effectiveness of this type of presentation, with respect to the traditional matrix-like or list-like arrangement, is under experimental evaluation.

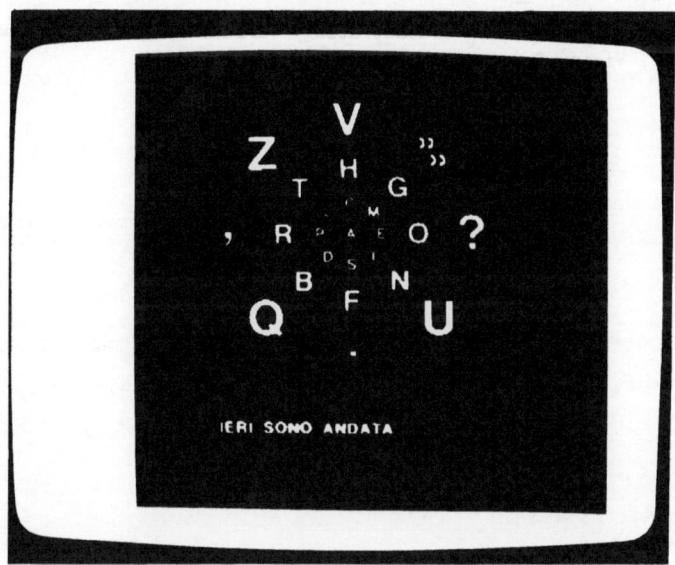

Fig. 5.. In this interactive scheme, a cursor (not shown in the figure) scans the characters according to a spiral path. When the cursor points to the desired character, the child activates the selection key.

Work supported by the Italian Research Council, Special Project on Biomedical Engineering.

Presented at the 3rd Medical Informatics Europe - Tolouse, March 9-13, 1981

REFERENCES

/1/ Morasso, P., Sandini, G., Tagliasco, V., Vernazza, T., Zaccaria, R.:"LOGOS: a microprocessor based device as a writing aid for the motor handicapped", Med.& Biol. Eng.& Comp., 16, 309, 316, 1978

/2/ Morasso, P., Penso, M., Suetta, G., Tagliasco, V.:"Towards standardization of communication and control systems for motor impaired people", Med.& Biol. Eng.& Comp., 17, 481-488, 1979

/3/ Austis, M., "A chart demonstrating variations in acuity with retinal position", Vision Res., 14, 589-592, 1974

MICRO INFORMATIQUE, TELEMATIQUE ET REINSERTION SOCIO-PROFESSIONNELLE DES GRANDS HANDICAPES MOTEURS. UN EXEMPLE PRATIQUE.

P. GERIN[+], M. EYSSETTE[x], M.A. GONON[+], D. BOISSON[x], G. BAILLY[+].

+ C.E.M.I. INSERM, 16, Avenue du Doyen Lépine, 69500 BRON FRANCE, TéL. (7)854.65.78)

x Service de Rééducation Fonctionnelle. Hôpital Neurologique, 59 Boulevard Pinel, 69003 LYON, Tél. (7) 853.81.81).

SUMMARY

SCRIBE is a microprocessor based multipurpose aid for the severely motor handicapped. A two-channel input uses signals from microswitches activated by short range mouth movements. Self adaptating to individual speed of users, SCRIBE thus writes on a video screen. An editor allows for correcting this text before printing. SCRIBE controls several external devices (telephone, tape recorder, ...) and an internal permanent data file.

Connected to a terminal of videotex system, as Teletel, it gives the handicapped an opportunity to use its possibilities for an effective socio-professional rehabilitation.

Les progrès de la réanimation médicale ou chirurgicale sauvent certes aujourd'hui des malades auparavant perdus, mais au prix parfois de handicaps moteurs irréversibles majeurs.

La rééducation de ces patients a bénéficié elle-même de travaux considérables, et assure leur stabilisation. Par contre, beaucoup moins de résultats ont pu être obtenus jusqu'ici pour l'étape ultime de cet effort thérapeutique, à savoir la réinsertion socio-professionnelle.

Nous voulons montrer ici comment deux pôles de l'informatique actuelle -la micro-informatique et la télématique- peuvent s'associer pour apporter à ce niveau des possibilités susceptibles de transformer cette situation. Et celà à propos d'un appareillage, réalisé dans notre laboratoire (le C.EM.I.) et testé depuis plusieurs années "au lit du malade" : le système SCRIBE (1).

Précisons que nous avons en vue ici des patients présentant de très gros handicaps moteurs, tétrapléqiques ou équivalents, mais avec conservation des fonctions intellectuelles.

Il peut s'agir de séquelles de lésions traumatiques, virales, vasculaires, dégénératives, anoxiques.

I - Les fonctions à remplir :

L'activité professionnelle envisagée est du type conseil-information. Elle rompt l'isolement du sujet, met à profit la qualification spécifique qu'il avait ou qu'il acquiert et ne demande que l'exécution d'un minimum de tâches mécaniques, assez facilement automatisables.

Les fonctions dont l'exécution est nécessaire pour effectuer un tel travail sont :

- L'utilisation du téléphone, pour répondre ou pour appeler, avec dans ce dernier cas la possibilité de recourir à une liste pré-établie de correspondants habituels ;
- La prise de notes, soit orales, sur enregistreur magnétique, soit écrites ;
- La rédaction de textes, avec toutes possibilités pour leur mise au point avant leur frappe définitive ;
- L'utilisation de fichiers, à deux niveaux différents : soit un petit fichier personnel (avec diverses fonctions : élaboration, modifications, consultation), soit un vaste fichier public (avec surtout la fonction de consultation).

II - Les commandes :

Toutes ces fonctions doivent pouvoir être accomplies par le sujet lui-même, donc à partir de commandes motrices résiduelles très restreintes (par exemple, de simples mouvements de mâchoire).

Elles doivent aussi respecter diverses exigences :

Transparence : le capteur doit être aussi peu visible que possible, et en tout cas ne pas gêner l'utilisateur, que ce soit par lui-même ou par son mode d'utilisation.

Ainsi doit être éliminé, à notre avis, tout dispositif reposant sur la détection de mouvements oculaires ou de contractions musculaires faciales ; mais aussi les appareils nécessitant l'observation permanente d'un panneau d'indications (caractères alpha-numériques ou ordres divers), comme les matériels de Carba (2) ; ou à fortiori ceux réclamant des mouvements permanents de la tête pour assurer le balayage d'une matrice par un contacteur mécanique (3) ou optique (4).

Il faut choisir au contraire, dans toute la mesure du possible une commande motrice dont l'usage ne comporte pas de gêne et de fatigue. Un mouvement résiduel au niveau d'un membre sera préféré à un mouvement de la mâchoire, celui-ci à un mouvement de la tête (5-6).

Adaptation : le capteur doit être adapté mécaniquement à l'utilisateur, mais ceci à partir de quelques versions de base peu nombreuses, pour ne pas en élever le coût. Surtout, le dispositif doit pouvoir s'adapter, dans son rythme d'utilisation, aux possibilités de chaque sujet, et à leurs variations dans le temps, et ceci de préférence de manière automatique, ce qui n'est pas le cas dans les appareils proposés jusqu'ici.

Apprentissage : le mode d'utilisation du capteur doit être aussi simple que possible et le dispositif doit comprendre des modes de fonctionnement facilitant l'apprentissage, et aidant à l'utilisation, pour réduire les risques d'erreur et la fatigue.

Ainsi, nous avons refusé la simplicité technique de l'utilisation d'un codage ASCII, pourtant proposé (7) mais uniquement à des handicapés informaticiens, ce qui limite par trop le domaine d'application.

L'informatique actuelle permet de répondre à ces divers besoins d'une manière efficace, sur le plan technique et sur le plan économique. Le microprocesseur assure, au niveau de l'utilisateur, l'interface spécifique ; la télématique ouvre des domaines d'application pour lesquels une haute qualification professionnelle n'est pas nécessaire.

III - Solution technique réalisée :

Nous avons réalisé, et fait évoluer au cours d'essais cliniques au long cours, un dispositif micro-informatisé satisfaisant aux exigences ci-dessus. Orienté vers la communication écrite, il a été baptisé "SCRIBE".

Il met en oeuvre un microprocesseur 8080 de INTEL (8). Un logiciel de base de 6 K ROM (8 bits) assure le décodage des signaux envoyés par l'utilisateur, à partir d'un code dérivé du Morse. Il s'adapte automatiquement au rythme de l'utilisateur, quel qu'il soit. Il informe ce dernier des ordres qu'il vient de recevoir, de ce qu'il propose d'effectuer, et lui rappelle éventuellement les commandes à utiliser : tout ceci facilite beaucoup l'apprentissage, pour lequel il faut cependant compter 8-10 jours, à raison d'une séance de 1-2 H/jour. A ce stade, quelques clefs sur le panneau avant permettent une assistance temporaire par un aide extérieur, pour l'exécution de certaines fonctions. Des logiciels spécifiques (jusqu'à 16 K ROM, 8 bits) peuvent y être associés.

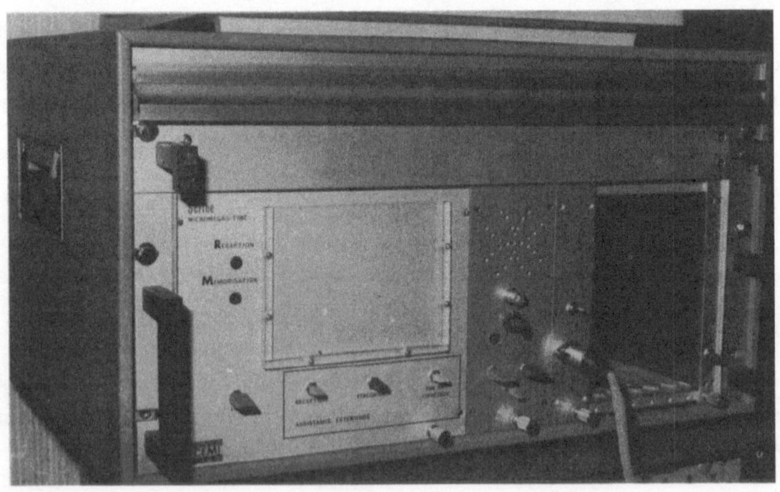

Les caractères alpha-numériques sont visualisés sur un écran vidéo (16 lignes de 32 caractères), dont la ligne inférieure est consacrée aux indications fournies par SCRIBE. Ces caractères peuvent servir soit à rédiger des "instructions" définissant des commandes (par exemple, pour l'utilisation du téléphone ou d'un magnétophone : 7 relais de puissance sont disponibles), soit à mettre au point et imprimer des textes, avec un éditeur adapté. La liaison avec l'imprimante est du type à boucle de courant.

Un "calepin de notes" est constitué par 1 K de mémoire vive alimentée sur batterie, avec une autonomie de plusieurs mois ; l'utilisateur peut le remplir, modifier, imprimer son contenu, à volonté.

Diverses formes de capteur ont été réalisées, comportant deux contacts. Une version miniaturisée est incorporée à un moulage en résine de la voute palatine, sa mise en oeuvre étant effectuée par des mouvements de la mâchoire. Nous avons adopté à ce niveau le principe d'un contact de proximité (par champ magnétique) pour éliminer la fatique entraînée par un capteur de pression (9).

Par fil, ou par un boîtier à ultra-sons, le capteur est connecté à un module d'entrée assurant la protection contre tout risque d'électrocution et éventuellement la détection et l'élimination de fausses commandes (mouvements involontaires mal dirigés ou répétitifs).

Ceci permet de résoudre de manière efficace le problème posé (cf. 10-11) pour permettre l'utilisation par des sujets présentant des séquelles d'encéphalopathie cérébrale infantile avec incoordination motrice ("infirmes moteurs cérébraux"). On utilise alors trois contacts au lieu de deux, et on abandonne le codage temporel.

En ce qui concerne sa connexion à un réseau télématique, SCRIBE ne doit pas remplacer le terminal de télématique. En effet, il faut que son écran propre puisse continuer à jouer son rôle de bloc-notes, même pendant l'utilisation du réseau. Bien que cela aboutisse à la présence de deux écrans, leur spécificité justifie cet investissement. Par ailleurs, incorporer à SCRIBE le logiciel lui permettant de dialoguer avec le réseau serait lourd en mémoire morte. La solution la meilleure est donc le remplacment par SCRIBE du seul clavier du terminal télématique, ce qui suppose seulement l'adjonction d'une carte interface et d'un logiciel limité.

Ainsi, SCRIBE est adaptable à l'utilisation du système Vidéotex, pour services Teletel et annuaire électronique.

Ce dispositif a été utilisé par des malades très divers, avec des mouvements résiduels d'un doigt, ou de la mâchoire, ou même seulement de la tête.

IV - Utilisation professionnelle :

A) SCRIBE peut permettre par lui-même une activité professionnelle, quand y suffisent l'utilisation du téléphone (12), la prise de notes, la rédaction de courrier ou de documents divers.

Ceci suppose cependant un niveau de qualification assez élevé : possibilité, par exemple, d'assurer un enseignement par correspondance, un conseil en gestion.

De ce fait, ceci ne peut concerner qu'un nombre restreint de ces grands handicapés moteurs. Il serait donc très intéressant d'échapper à cette limitation.

Or, c'est la possibilité offerte récemment par le développement de la télématique.

B) On peut escompter en effet que le nombre d'abonnés de ce réseaux ne se développera que progressivement. Dans un immeuble ou groupe d'immeuble, un handicapé pourra alors remplir, pour leurs habitants, de multiples fonctions d'information, de réservation, d'exploitation de banques de données, etc... Et cela sans que soit nécessaire alors une longue formation professionnelle. Une activité rémunérable, effectuée à domicile mais en contact avec de très nombreuses personnes, devient parfaitement possible dans ces conditions.

C) A un degré de plus, des activités de documentaliste spécialisé vont certainement être nécessaires, pour établir et exploiter les banques de données des réseaux ; par exemple, les données bibliographiques scientifiques.

D) Enfin, on peut escompter un développement ultérieur de la télématique dans le sens télé-enseignement (utilisation de bibliothèques enregistrées ; enseignement programmé). Ceci pourrait transformer la formation professionnelle de handicapés, en permettant notamment de les maintenir dans leur environnement habituel. Une des branches ouvertes ainsi est constituée par l'informatique elle-même.

SCRIBE est particulièrement bien adapté à cet usage, parce qu'il assure aussi l'usage du téléphone, parce qu'il comprend un véritable éditeur de texte au lieu de n'être qu'une machine à écrire, parce qu'il a un propre fichier interne conservable, parce qu'il permet de commander des dispositifs annexes tels qu'un magnétophone. Son rythme d'écriture est du même ordre que ceux des divers systèmes proposés, soit de l'ordre de 60 caractères par minute, bien assez pour utiliser efficacement de tels systèmes, d'autant plus que le texte conversationnel peut être préparé par avance, avant l'appel du système Vidéotex.

Bien que certains aient proposé de connecter leur dispositif d'assistance à des ordinateurs (cf. 3-13), le branchement sur un système télématique n'a pas, à notre connaissance, été encore perçu dans tout son intérêt potentiel au niveau de la réadaptation des grands handicapés moteurs.

V - Aspect économique :

Un élément pratique essentiel, dans la description d'un appareillage d'assistance pour handicapés, est constitué évidemment par son prix de revient.

Il est intéressant de préciser que le prix des composants entrant dans la fabrication d'un prototype de SCRIBE est de quelque 14 000 F (plus l'imprimante). Une production industrielle bénéficiant, du fait de la série, d'un prix de revient (composants) nettement moindre. Ceci peut être comparé aux 10 000 F de Logos (10) moins performant.

Ceci doit être complété par le prix de la connexion avec un réseau de télématique, qui est fonction de ce dernier.

On reste donc dans une enveloppe de coût qui, comparée au prix de journée des formations professionnelles en milieu spécialisé, et au prix des soins à domicile, apparaît suffisamment modeste pour présenter également un réel intérêt au point de vue économie de la santé.

Si en outre la possibilité d'utilisation des systèmes télématiques par de tels handicapés est prévue dès la conception ou la mise en place de ces systèmes, le coût de leur adaptation s'en trouvera sans doute allégé.

VI Conclusion :

En combinant les intérêts de la micro-informatique et de la télématique, le système SCRIBE permet de modifier profondément les possibilités de réinsertion socio-professionnelle des grands handicapés moteurs.

Il constitue en effet un appareillage satisfaisant sur les divers plans des performances techniques, de la transparence et du coût.

1 - GONON M.A., MORENVAL F., GERIN P., PERNIER J., BAILLY G., RUBEL P., RAGUSIN P., BEZ M. : Scribe : un système d'aide aux grands handicapés à base de micro-processeur. Med. Biol. Eng. and Comput. 1980, 18, 206-212.

2 - BAUMANN U., HAUBER B., SCHIAN H.M. : Rapport sur l'utilisation d'un appareil de communication et de maîtrise de l'environnement à l'école et à l'hôpital. Carba. Edit. 1977, 132 pp.

3 - VASA J.J., LYWOOD D.W. : High speed communication aid for quadriplegic, Med. Biol. Eng. 1976, 14, 445-450.

4 - SOEDE M., STASSEN H.G. : Lightspot operated typewriter for severely disabled patients. Med. Biol. Eng. 1973, 11, 641-644.

5 - ROESLER H., PARSLACK V. : Medical manipulators. General considerations on the design criteria of manipulative technical aids for quadriplegics. 1st CISM-IFTOMM Symp. on Theory and Practice of robots and Manipulators. Udine 5-8/9/73.

6 - AGZARIAN J., READ J.H. : A multiaccess interface for the disabled. Med. J. Aust. 1973 (1), 300-302.

7 - LYWOOD D.W., VASA J.J. : Computer terminal operating and communication aid for severely handicapped. Med. Biol. Eng. 1974, 12, 693-697.

8 - RUBEL P., BAILLY G., GIARD M.H., Microprocessor based biomedical instrumentation A modular approach. 11th Internat. Conf. Med. Biol. Eng. Ottawa, 1976.

9 - BONTRAGER E.G., NICKEL V.L., SCOTT I. : Intra-oral telemetry control for orthotic power systems. Proc. Int. Telemetering. Los Angeles. 1972.

10 - MORASSO P., SANDINI G., SUETTA G., TAGLIASCO V., VERNAZZA T., ZACCARIA R. : Logos : a microprocessor based device as a writing aid for the motor handicapped. Med. Biol. Eng. and Comput. 1978, 16, 309-315.

11 - ILES G.H. : A scanning communication aid for severely handicapped children. 11th Internat. Conf. Med. Biol. Eng. Ottawa, 1976, P. 414-415.

12 - LE NOUVEL P., BOULANGER Y., MORIN G., BELLIARD H., BESSON R., Téléphone et handicap physique. Annales Med. Physique, 1979, 22, 309-319.

13 - VIDAL J.J. : Adaptive computer communication prosthetics for persons with severe motor handicap. 30th ACEMB. 5-9 Nov. 1977.

René DISSOUBRAY
Institut National de Jeunes Sourds
Paris, France

AUTO CONTROLE DE CERTAINS PARAMETRES DE LA PAROLE CHEZ LES SOURDS. UN PROTOTYPE D'AIDE VISUELLE

The acquisition of speech requires the interactive development of articulatory skills and perceptuals skills. It can be expressed so : one can articulate as one can hear, and one can hear as one can articulate.
The primary effect of deafness on the acquisition of speech is the removal of the facility for acoustic monitoring of articulation.
Visual aids palliate, in a certain part, the lack of acoustic perceptions.

Analogic ones were known for many years but they are not very useful , each one being able to indicate only one parameter.
We have used a data processing aid which provides the same functions as the analogic ones , but on a screen only. It also has a lot of other possibilities like games, drawings, etc. It offers alternatives and variety in training strategies. The main drawback is that this kind of apparatus is not wearable and so, it cannot replace the acoustic feedback, always present in the speech auto-training of hearing children.

The prototype was of a good help for correcting some articulatory errors, deficiency in rythm and pitch but the defects were often coming back when the deaf was not before the screen. We think that the best results we can obtain will be during the first childhood of our deaf children.

1. LE PROBLEME DE LA COMMUNICATION.

Les sourds entre eux se comprennent fort bien à l'aide de la langue des signes. Ce type de communication s'étend souvent à la famille, parfois au proche entourage, mais il ne convient pas aux relations socio-professionnelles avec les entendants qui ne connaissent pas cette langue.
La communication avec les entendants passe donc par divers apprentissages :

perception du langage oral, par l'entraînement auditif et la lecture labiale.
du langage écrit, par la lecture.

émission de parole, à l'aide d'auto contrôles auditifs, visuels et tactiles.

2. LA PERCEPTION AUDITIVE.

C'est la qualité des informations acoustiques perçues qui détermine, pour la plus grande part, la qualité de l'articulation. Madison & Fucci (1) ont noté, sur 100 enfants âgés de 6 ans 4 mois à 7 ans 6 mois, une corrélation significative entre la qualité de leur articulation et leur possibilité de discrimination phonémique.

Ils notent également que, selon divers auteurs, c'est entre 7 et 9 ans que ces possibilités articulatoires et de discrimination arrivent à maturation.

Les récents progrès dans le domaine de la qualité des prothèses auditives (contours d'oreilles) et surtout le nombre croissant d'enfants appareillés et pris en charge avant l'âge de 2 ans, ces nouvelles données ont beaucoup modifié le tableau des conséquences habituelles de la surdité, même importante.
Ces enfants conservent une voix claire et sont généralement capables d'acquérir une articulation et un rythme d'élocution satisfaisants. L'utilisation efficace qu'ils peuvent faire de leurs restes auditifs, associée aux informations que procure la lecture labiale, leur permet de percevoir un minimum d'informations phonétiques et prosodiques susceptibles de les aider à l'imitation de la parole et à l'auto contrôle de leur émission.

Pendant cette période d'apprentissage, l'intervention de l'orthophoniste reste toujours nécessaire et primordiale. Les automatismes s'installent progressivement, à partir d'auto contrôles kinesthésiques, et deviennent plus tard de solides habitudes

3. PERCEPTION TACTILE ET VISUELLE.

De nombreux enfants sourds ayant une perte auditive trop importante ou ayant été appareillés trop tardivement, ne peuvent pas utiliser efficacement leurs perceptions auditives, même associées à la lecture labiale. Pour eux, l'apprentissage de la parole doit utiliser d'autres voies sensorielles, tactiles et visuelles.
Un tel apprentissage nécessite la présence du spécialiste et le concours d'appareils ; il ne pourra pas s'effectuer en situation de communication naturelle et restera très artificiel. Les résultats seront donc insuffisants, et il faudra pratiquer de nombreuses corrections tout au long de la scolarité.

3. 1 INFORMATIONS TACTILES.

Nous noterons seulement (puisque notre sujet est limité aux aides visuelles), que les informations recueillies par la main ont longtemps suffi à apprendre la parole aux sourds, au temps où l'on ne connaissait pas l'électronique. En effet, certains caractères phonétiques et prosodiques de la parole sont perçus facilement et efficacement par le toucher du larynx et de différentes parties du visage qui transmettent plus ou moins les vibrations laryngées. La qualité du souffle, sa direction, sa température, apportent également de précieuses indications.

3. 2 INFORMATIONS VISUELLES.

Il s'agit essentiellement, pendant la période d'apprentissage de la parole, de la connaissance de la position des organes phonateurs visibles et de la lecture labiale. Le décodage du message oral sera assuré par la lecture labiale également, complétée par les expressions et attitudes, des gestes naturels et, dans un autre domaine, l'utilisation des restes auditifs.

4. LES AIDES VISUELLES, DE CONCEPTION ANALOGIQUE.

Les unes représentent l'évolution de l'intensité ou de la mélodie, en fonction du temps.

Les autres apportent des indications au niveau du phonème :

Indicateurs de S , de nasalité, de voisement

Spectrographes

Oscilloscope

Certains paramètres sont parfois représentés sur la même courbe : intensité et mélodie, cette dernière étant témoin du voisement.

4. 1 L'OPINION DES UTILISATEURS.

Si l'oscilloscope a encore de nombreux partisans (il est utilisé par les orthophonistes sous le nom de "Phonaudioscope"), c'est sans doute parce qu'il permet, à l'aide d'un seul appareil, diverses représentations de la parole : la durée, l'intensité, le nombre d'émissions vocales, le voisement qui produit un signal périodique et le bruit des consonnes sourdes dont le signal est aléatoire.
Dans l'ensemble, ces aides visuelles de conception analogique sont peu utilisées. Il leur est reproché de ne pas fournir une représentation de la parole qui soit en rapport avec les mécanismes articulatoires, de ne fournir d'indication, pour la plupart d'entre elles, que sur un seul paramètre, ce qui nécessite l'utilisation de plusieurs appareils, encombrants et coûteux. Par ailleurs, ce type d'appareil n'est pas évolutif, et ses images, toujours les mêmes, ne suscitent pas longtemps l'intérêt des enfants.

Enfin, si l'on excepte l'indication de la mélodie de la phrase, pratiquement incontrôlable par les perceptions tactiles, les autres indications que procurent les aides visuelles traditionnelles ne permettent pas d'obtenir de meilleurs résultats que les anciennes techniques de démutisation lorsqu'elles sont pratiquées par un rééducateur qui connaît bien son métier.

4. 2 L'INTERET DE CES APPAREILS.

Il faut néanmoins souligner certains aspects positifs :

- la précision de la représentation et sa fixité sur un tube à mémoire permet à l'enfant de prendre conscience de certains défauts difficiles à repérer par les voies sensorielles.
- les auto contrôles perceptifs n'aboutiraient qu'à une réalisation approximative de nombreux phonèmes s'ils n'étaient précisés par les indications de l'orthophoniste. Les indicateurs de S , de CH , les spectroscopes, permettent l'auto contrôle de certains phonèmes.
- enfin, il est important que l'enfant puisse juger lui-même de la qualité de ses réalisations, sans dépendre en permanence de l'avis de l'adulte.

5. APPORTS DE L'INFORMATIQUE A LA CONCEPTION DES AIDES VISUELLES.

5. 1 LES CONDITIONS D'UTILISATION SONT TRES DIFFERENTES.

Un seul appareillage suffit à de multiples représentations : un écran, un mini-ordinateur et un clavier de commande.

Le sujet se trouve enfin en face d'une tâche attrayante et qu'il peut varier , ce qui maintient sa motivation : sur l'écran, il peut faire apparaître des dessins sur lesquels il peut agir ; il peut même construire des figures, répondre à des sollicitations ; il est récompensé de ses réussites par l'inscription de son score ou d'une figurine enjouée.

Voici, à titre d'exemple, une réalisation de Nickerson, Kalikow & Stevens (2) :

La présence d'une "bulle" indique si S ou Z sont émis.
La présence de la pomme d'Adam indique le voisement.
L'intensité est représentée par la grandeur de la bouche
La hauteur de la pomme d'Adam dépend de la hauteur du fondamental.

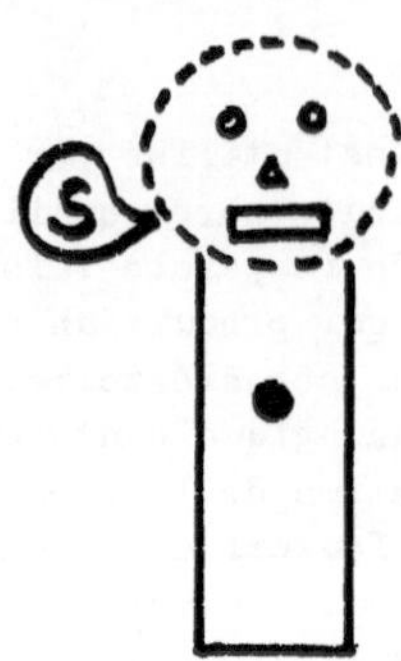

5. 2 DE NOUVELLES POSSIBILITES DE RECONNAISSANCE .

M.C. Haton utilise un système automatique de reconnaissance de mots (3) où des erreurs minimes d'articulation ne sont pas détectées tandis que de grandes variafions de durée et de rythme ne sont pas admises.

Cornett, Beadles et Wilson (4) travaillent sur un projet de transcription de certains éléments phonétiques de la parole reçue ou émise, en temps réel, dans un code visuel dont les indications complètent celles apportées par la lecture labiale. L'appareil est portatif et ses indications pouvant être utilisées en permanence, il constituera une véritable aide à la communication. Les prototypes actuellement expérimentés n'apportent que 60% de réponses exactes et doivent donc être encore perfectionnés.

Une recherche ayant pour objectif la réalisation d'une aide à la communication en français est également entreprise par le Centre Scientifique de IBM France, avec la collaboration de l'INJS de Paris.

6. LE PROTOTYPE IBM-INJS, SES POSSIBILITES.

La description de l'appareil faisant l'objet d'une autre communication, nous nous bornerons à décrire son utilisation.

6. 1. LA REPRESENTATION DE L'INTENSITE.

6. 1. 1. A L'AIDE DE COURBES.

Une courbe modèle étant mise en mémoire dans la partie supérieure de l'écran, le sujet essaie de l'imiter dans la partie inférieure.
Les variations d'intensité provoquent le déplacement vertical du spot pendant que le balayage horizontal s'effectue d'une manière continue ou sur commande manuelle.

6. 1. 2. A L'AIDE DE JEUX PROGRAMMES.

Le balayage lent et automatique de l'écran ne se produit que lorsque le sujet émet de la voix, ce qui produit le déplacement vertical du dessin mobile, selon les variations de l'intensité.

Pour les 5 jeux actuellement programmés, le mobile revêt différentes formes :

- une croix ou une flèche, qui doit suivre différents types de couloirs, sans en toucher les bords. Le score affiché au départ diminue d'un point chaque fois que le mobile quitte son couloir.
- un chameau, qui doit se déplacer sur un écran parsemé se palmiers, sans les heurter, mais qui doit boire trois mares. Chaque palmier heurté ôte un point, et chaque mare bue en ajoute deux.
- un canard, qui doit manger 18 vers répartis sur l'écran, sans se faire attraper par trois loups, ce qui coûterait 5 points à chaque fois.

Il est assez difficile d'obtenir un score maximum pour la plupart de ces jeux, et les enfants se passionnent pour améliorer leurs performances.

Deux exemples des jeux proposés :

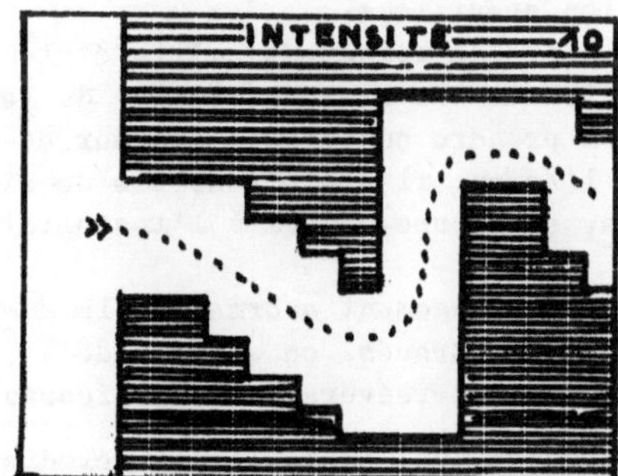

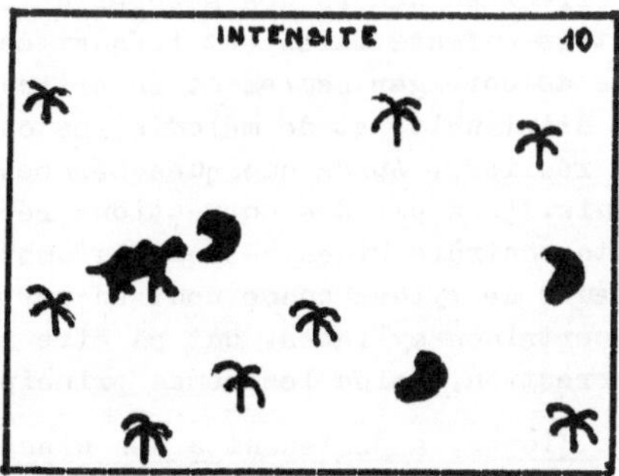

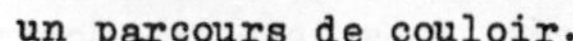

un parcours de couloir. Le jeu du chameau parmi les palmiers.

6. 2 LA REPRESENTATION DE LA MELODIE.

Les courbes (à départ déclenché ou à balayage continu) ainsi que les 5 jeux, sont les mêmes que les représentations utilisées pour l'intensité. Toutefois, on dispose de 4 échelles de fréquences, correspondant aux voix d'enfants, de femmes et d'hommes. La quatrième échelle utilise des fréquences plus étendues, pouvant servir indifféremment aux trois catégories de voix.

7. EXPERIMENTATION.

L'appareil est installé dans une cabine d'orthophonie de l'Institut National de Jeunes Sourds de Paris. On lui a adjoint un amplificateur et un casque afin que l'enfant puisse contrôler sa voix en même temps qu'il en voit une représentation.

Ce proto-type a été conçu dans le cadre d'une recherche jointe : IBM - INJS de Paris, afin d'extraire un certain nombre de paramètres de la parole, première étape d'un travail beaucoup plus vaste sélectionnant des informations qui, com-

plétées par la lecture labiale, permettraient une intelligibilité suffisante de la parole. Cette première étape réalisée, nous avons voulu éprouver la fiabilité de la détection de ces paramètres et,parallèlement, expérimenter l'utilisation de leur représentation visuelle avec des enfants déficients auditifs.
L'aide visuelle qui a résulté de ce double objectif ne convient pas à l'apprentissage des premières réalisations vocales. C'est donc avec des enfants plus âgés que nous avons expérimenté, plutôt pour corriger des erreurs que pour enseigner.

7. 1 LES RESULTATS.

Le professeur et les élèves d'une même classe ont utilisé l'appareil pendant un semestre de l'année scolaire dernière, pour la correction de défauts d'articulation ou de rythme. La moyenne d'âge des enfants était de 10 ans. Ils ont eu, selon les cas, de 5 à 15 séances chacun.
L'un d'eux avait une voix de tête et ne parvenait pas à la modifier en contrôlant la perception des vibrations à la poitrine et au larynx, selon les procédés classiques. Moins de 10 séances lui ont suffi pour corriger ce défaut, définitivement semble-t-il, grâce à la surveillance attentive de son professeur qui reprenait chaque erreur en dehors des séances de rééducation spécifique.
Deux autres enfants faisaient fréquemment des erreurs de voisement qu'ils étaient capables de corriger seulement en articulant lentement. La mise en mémoire de leurs courbes d'intensité et de mélodie les ont aidés à prendre conscience des corrections à réaliser. Après quelques séances devant l'écran, il a été possible de fixer ces acquisitions par des corrections répétitives, en classe, jusqu'à l'installation d'un auto contrôle kinesthésique automatique.
Des défauts de rythme concernant en particulier un allongement anormal de la durée de certaines syllabes, ont pu être repérés sur les tracés, ce qui a aidé à leur correction, selon les mêmes principes, grâce à la persévérance du professeur.

4 autres élèves, appartenant à des classes différentes, ont travaillé la mélodie.
Les séances de rééducation n'étaient pas pratiquées par les professeurs des enfants, ce qui explique sans doute l'infériorité des résultats obtenus, par rapport à ceux des enfants qui sont suivis par la même personne, en cabine comme en classe.
Christophe, 15 ans, sourd profond, a une voix de tête. Il a renoncé à porter sa prothèse depuis plusieurs années. Au cours des quatre premières séances, un fondamental plus grave n'a pu être obtenu que par hasard, par tâtonnements et sans pouvoir répéter les réussites. A la 10ème séance, il était capable, toujours après quelques tâtonnements, de conserver un fondamental normal. La correction aurait certainement été définitive si elle avait été poursuivie systématiquement quelque temps encore, en classe comme à la maison.
Frédéric, 11 ans, sourd sévère appareillé, est notre plus brillant sujet. Il a commencé sans pouvoir moduler la mélodie de sa voix. Maintenant, après 19 séances, il réussit le jeu du chameau parmi les palmiers sans une seule erreur. Cependant, les automatismes ne sont pas encore acquis, puisque ce garçon ne peut pas encore moduler la hauteur de sa voix lorsqu'il ne dispose pas du contrôle visuel.
Ahmed et Ali, 7 et 8 ans, sourds profonds appareillés mais n'ayant que 2 ans de scolarité, ont eu beaucoup plus de difficultés. Leur premier problème a été de tenir constante l'intensité de leur voix pendant quelques secondes. Une fois ce

premier pas franchi, il n'a pas été possible, après 8 séances d'obtenir des modifications contrôlées de la valeur de leur fondamental. L'un comme l'autre ne réussissent à émettre une voix plus aiguë que par à-coups, en augmentant brutalement l'intensité, presque comme un cri.

7. 2 CONCLUSION.

L'appareil que nous avons utilisé s'est montré parfaitement fiable et capable d'extraction des paramètres choisis : durée, intensité, mélodie, quel que soit le locuteur, voisement et énergie.
Il a été d'une grande efficacité pour montrer des défauts d'articulation et de rythme chez des sujets dont la vitesse de l'articulation ne permettait pas de déceler ces erreurs à l'aide du contrôle tactile.
Par contre, on a pu vérifier que, la période normale d'apprentissage une fois dépassée, les mauvaises habitudes sont très difficiles à combattre et ne peuvent disparaître qu'au prix d'un travail long et persévérant, à condition que le sujet soit motivé suffisamment.
Devant ces difficultés, nous avons décidé d'étudier de nouvelles présentations de jeux et un système de commandes simplifiées afin de réaliser un appareil qui puisse être utilisé avec succès par les tout petits, pendant la période favorable aux apprentissages.
Quoi qu'il en soit, le problème de l'extraction des paramètres est à présent résolu. Cela représentait une première étape -de beaucoup la plus simple- vers le second objectif : l'aide à la lecture labiale, qui présente un intérêt sans aucune mesure avec ces premières réalisations.

REFERENCES

1 Madison C L , Fucci D J,Perceptual and motor skills 1971 ; 33 :831-838.
2 Nickerson R S, Stevens K N, Teaching speech to the deaf : can a computer help . Proc nat conv ACM August 1972 : 240-250.
3 Haton M C, Haton J P,Le système SIRENE ;Rev Générale ens déf audit 1979 : 103-8.
4Cornett R O,Beadles R,Wilson B, Automatic cued speech ; 1977 Conf on speech analyzing aids for the deaf, Gallaudet College, Washington DC.

VERS UN ENSEIGNEMENT DE LA PAROLE ASSISTE PAR ORDINATEUR ?

S. BARTH, G. ADDA, G. ROINSOL

Institut National de Jeunes Sourds de CHAMBERY B.P. 15
73160 COGNIN - FRANCE

SUMMARY : After a short description of the state of the art in the domain of visual speech training aids for the deaf, we shall present the programs we have used for two years with children of the pre-school department of the National Institute for the deaf at CHAMBERY.

I LES DIVERS TYPES D'AIDES VISUELLES CLASSIQUES

La question que se posèrent, en 1972, R.S. NICKERSON et K.N. STEVENS : "Teaching speech to the deaf : can computer help" n'a probablement pas reçu de réponse définitive à cette heure. Proposons-nous, tout d'abord, d'en cerner les raisons.

Plusieurs décades de chercheurs ont produit un nombre étonnant de systèmes susceptibles de faciliter l'apprentissage de la parole par les enfants déficients auditifs. Nous n'en dresserons ici qu'un catalogue sommaire. Le lecteur intéressé pourra trouver une bibliographie plus complète dans S. BARTH (2).

On distingue en général :

- les jouets animés par la voix,
- les indicateurs de phonèmes (logoscope, visible speech, détecteurs de fricatives et de nasales...)
- les vocoders visuels,
- les indicateurs d'accent et de mélodie.

Le mode de fonctionnement de ces appareils est presque entièrement analogique.

I - 1) Exploitation et critique pédagogique

Les jouets commandés par la voix introduisent, d'une manière flagrante, une démarche ludique soumise à des impératifs : "je parle et l'auto roule" ; "je me tais et l'auto s'arrête". L'enfant émettra de la voix non pour faire plaisir à l'adulte, mais pour obtenir un résultat (ici le mouvement de l'auto) qui ne peut apparaître par aucun autre moyen, et découvrira parallèlement le pouvoir de la parole.

Les concepts de jeu et de règle nous semblent capitaux en matière d'aide visuelle. Le premier pour la motivation qu'il renforce, le second pour les limites qu'il impose.

Il faut malheureusement reconnaître que l'expérimentation pédagogique de certains de ces systèmes (il en existe aussi qui n'ont jamais été évalués...!) n'a guère permis de dégager une réelle méthodologie de l'apprentissage de la parole par leur intermédiaire. Deux raisons peuvent être principalement évoquées:

- inadaptation du jeu : les appareils amusent l'enfant, lui plaisent, mais ne l'aident pas à progresser autant qu'il le serait souhaitable.

- inadaptation des règles : la représentation visuelle de la parole est d'une trop grande complexité au niveau :
  - des patterns engendrés,
  - de la comparaison de faits locutoires différents.

Celle-ci entraîne naturellement pour l'enfant une difficulté d'apprentissage, voire l'incapacité à associer les schémas moteurs de la parole aux éléments du code visuel engendré par l'appareil.

Ajoutons que les variabilités inter et intra-locuteur des réalisations acoustiques des phonèmes, des mots, des phrases contribuent à rendre difficile les tâches d'imitation de modèles (courbes mélodiques, spectogrammes...). Il semble que la grande finesse d'analyse de certains systèmes, joue paradoxalement contre l'efficacité pédagogique (que devient la notion de sécurisation liée à celle de repère ?). Toutefois, nous n'abonderons pas dans le sens de la nécessité d'une précision sommaire des paramètres extraits car les effets en seraient aussi catastrophiques au niveau de l'utilisateur !

Enfin, n'oublions pas qu'un bon nombre d'aides visuelles d'utilisation trop complexe ont fini prématurément la brillante carrière à laquelle on les destinait.

I - 2) <u>Les systèmes informatisés</u>

L'appareil de NICKERSON et STEVENS (13) a été le premier système d'enseignement de la parole assisté par ordinateur. En France, il faut citer :

- un programme développé en 1974 au Laboratoire d'Informatique pour la Mécanique et les Sciences de l'Ingénieur (S. BARTH, J.S. LIENARD) susceptible de permettre la correction du rythme et des transitions phonétiques (2).

- le projet SIRENE du Centre de Recherche en Informatique de Nancy (12).

- le système I.B.M. expérimenté à l'Institut National de Jeunes-Sourds de Paris.

- le système de l'I.N.J.S. de Chambéry.

II DESCRIPTION DES MODULES UTILISES

En nous fondant sur les constatations faites précédemment, nous avons entrepris la conception d'un système modulaire d'aide visuelle à l'apprentissage de la parole. La modularité concernant d'une part les paramètres acoustiques, d'autre part la complexité de la tâche demandée à l'élève.

Nous ne décrirons, dans la suite de cet article, que quatre modules dont l'utilisation est réelle au sein du service d'Education Précoce et des classes maternelles de notre établissement. Trois concernent le niveau sonore, et un la pause de la voix. Leur évolution vers une forme opérationnelle a été le fruit d'une expérimentation pédagogique dont les résultats ont toujours dicté les modifications effectuées.

1) Les moyens techniques

Notre laboratoire possède un mini-ordinateur PDP 11/20 avec 24 K mots de mémoire muni d'un tiroir Time-Data XO et d'une console de deux disques DEC RK 05 augmentant la capacité de 2,4 Mmots de 16 bits.

Afin d'utiliser ce système pour l'enseignement, nous avons adopté la configuration simplifiée suivante (fig. I).

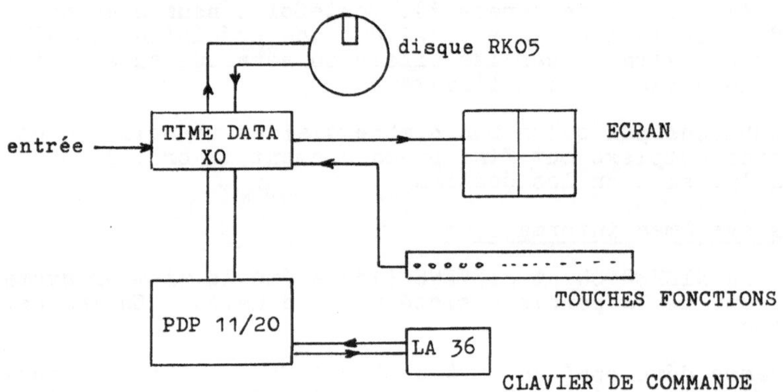

Fig. 1. Configuration du système modulaire d'aide visuelle de l'I.N.J.S. de Chambéry.

Son principal avantage est la souplesse de mise en œuvre tant du point de vue de la programmation S. BARTH (2), que de l'utilisation S. BARTH (2).

2) Acquisition et traitement du signal

Les signaux de la parole sont pré-traités par un intégrateur (constante de temps : 10 ms) ou par un extracteur de mélodie (modèle Institut de Phonétique de Grenoble), échantillonés (Fe = 100 Hz) et numérisés sur 10 bits.

L'acquisition se fait par blocs, suivant la technique du "double buffer" par l'intermédiaire de programmes appartenant à la bibliothèque du T.S.L. (Time Series Language). Le traitement (lissage, comparaison à des seuils...) est effectué par des programmes écrits en assembleur (MACRO 11 du RT 11 VØ3 de Digital Equipment).

Le pré-traitement nous a paru indispensable pour obtenir une visualisation "temps réel" compatible avec un travail de rééducation.

3) Chargement et exécution des programmes

L'ensemble des programmes correspondant à chaque module est stocké sur disque. Le chargement et l'exécution de l'un d'entre eux est effectué par l'intermédiaire des touches fonctions et d'instructions cataloguées. Chaque module possède une procédure de sortie qui réactive les touches pour une nouvelle sélection.

4) Programmes de visualisation

Chaque programme de dessin est écrit en assembleur. La visualisation se fait sur une unité TEKTRONIX 6Ø3 dont on n'utilise pas le mode de mémoire. Aucun scintillement n'est observable.

5) Prise de conscience des émissions vocales

Nous visualisons un "bonhomme" (fig. 2) dont la taille est proportionnelle au niveau d'émission. La figure obtenue peut être réduite à un point ou déborder des limites de l'écran, les comparaisons intermédiaires étant possibles. La variation de la taille se fait en synchronisme avec celle du niveau sonore.

Fig. 2.

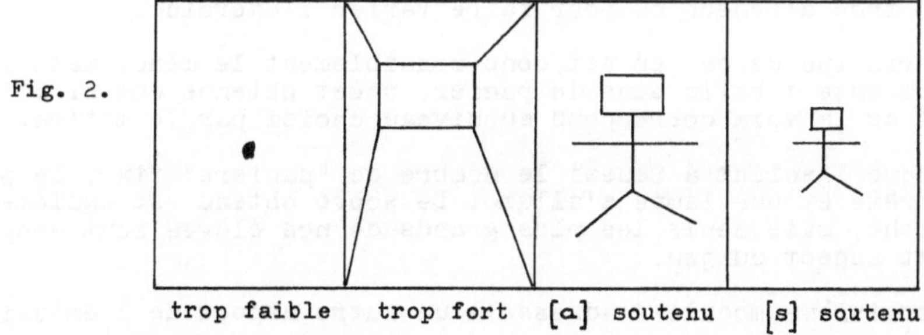

Ce jeu est le premier présenté à des enfants soit aphones, soit n'ayant que des émissions de voix involontaires ou incontrôlées.

Après une période de mutisme généralement observée, l'enfant est rapidement tenté d'obtenir lui aussi ce dessin lumineux et se rend vite compte que le seul moyen de réussir est d'émettre de la voix.

Dès qu'il a compris qu'il peut aussi agir sur la taille de la figure, il ne se lasse pas de passer du grand au petit "homme" en faisant varier l'intensité de son émission vocale.

Le but et les limites de ce jeu étant atteints, nous passons alors au second module.

6) <u>Placement du niveau sonore entre deux limites</u>

L'enseignant fixe au départ le nombre de réussites qu'il impose à l'élève et celui des essais infructueux qu'il permet. Une émission vocale provoque le départ de la balle sur une trajectoire parabolique dont le paramètre de commande est le niveau sonore (fig. 3). Celui-ci est moyenné sur 100 ms.

Fig. 3.

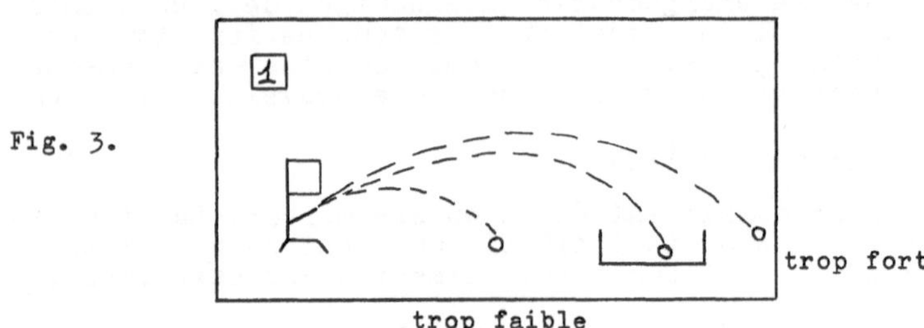

Le jeu s'arrête lorsque le score obtenu est égal au nombre de réussites fixé ou lorsque le nombre d'échecs a été atteint.

Le professeur peut alors modifier le facteur d'amplification et les deux paramètres de départ pour encourager l'élève qui aurait subi trop d'échecs ou pour faire varier l'exercice.

Le principe de ce jeu est donc sensiblement le même, mais la récompense : balle dans le panier, n'est obtenue que si l'intensité de la voix correspond au niveau choisi par le maître.

Lorsque l'enfant a réussi le nombre de "paniers" fixé, le jeu s'arrête et une lampe s'allume. Le score obtenu est également affiché, mais seuls les plus grands de nos élèves sont sensibles à cet aspect du jeu.

La troisième module s'adresse à un autre aspect de l'émission vocale.

7) Tenue de la voix

Le jeu consiste à faire monter la barre horizontale en maintenant une émission sonore à un niveau constant pendant un temps facilement programmable par l'enseignant (fig. 4).

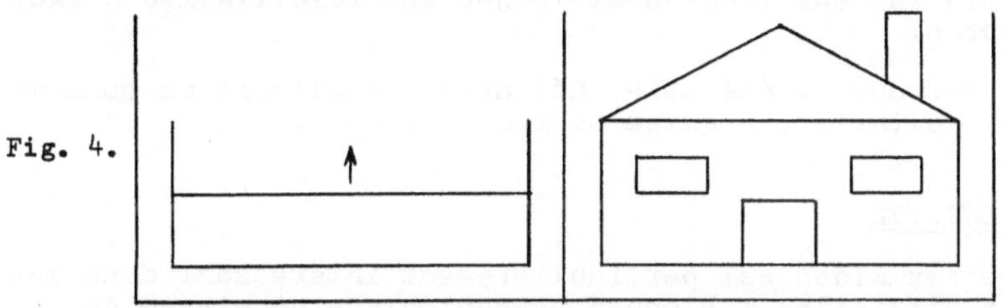

Fig. 4.

Lorsque la tenue n'est pas constante, la barre oscille de bas en haut. Si la tenue a duré le temps prévu, le rectangle se ferme et une maison est dessinée (Fig. 4). Le rééducateur peut alors modifier le temps de montée de la barre pour moduler le travail de l'élève.

Ce dernier jeu est celui qui plaît le plus aux enfants. C'est aussi celui qui nous paraît le plus pédagogique, car il aide l'enfant à acquérir un des mécanismes le plus important pour la compréhension ultérieure de sa parole : la maîtrise du souffle et de la tension musculaire.

8) Pose de la voix

La pose de la voix consiste à faire acquérir à l'enfant sourd un registre compatible avec celui des entendants du même âge.

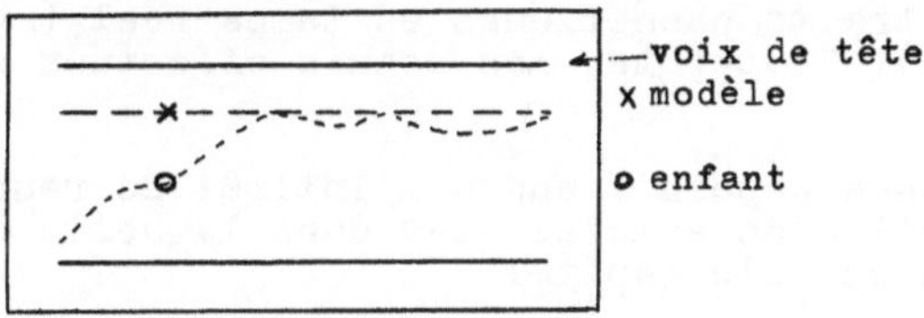

Au début du jeu, le professeur donne :

- la hauteur du fondamental qui servira de modèle,
- une valeur limite, à ne pas dépasser, correspondant à la voix de tête,
- la durée du balayage.

Les deux premières valeurs sont tirées de graphiques représentant des moyennes en fonction de l'âge publiées par KENT (10).

Le travail consiste à suivre la trajectoire du modèle pendant un temps fixé par la durée du balayage sans interrompre l'émission laryngée ni prendre une voix de tête.

Dès que l'enfant émet un son, le modèle et sa réalisation apparaissent sur l'écran. Ils se déplacent tant que les deux conditions ci-dessus sont réalisées. En cas d'échec, seules les deux barres persistent sur l'écran et le jeu est réinitialisé à gauche de l'écran.

Lorsque le parcours a été effectué, nous visualisons un bonhomme dont la taille varie (en guise de renforcement).

III PERSPECTIVES

L'apport de ces aides est particulièrement intéressant dans les cas réputés difficiles : blocage psychologique au niveau de l'émission de la parole, voix de tête persistante (utilisation des modules mélodie). Pour les cas normaux, ils offrent des exercices attrayants par enrichissement de l'environnement scolaire.

Pour répondre au troisième critère, à savoir la simplicité d'utilisation, nous avons commencé l'étude, en liaison avec l'Université scientifique et médicale de Grenoble, de l'implantation de ces aides visuelles sur un système à micro-processeurs.

Cette solution devrait permettre une utilisation courante dans le cadre d'une classe. Elle est financée par un contrat de recherche libre de l'I.N.S.E.R.M.(*).

D'autres programmes sont en cours d'expérimentation. Ceux-ci sont destinés au rythme, à l'acquisition des voyelles et des fricatives,et à la syllabation. Pour ces derniers, en dehors des difficultés que pose la définition d'une visualisation pédagogiquement pertinente, surgit le problème de la reconnaissance automatique de traits phonétiques en temps réel (reconnaissance quasi immédiate). Toutefois, les essais effectués semblent prometteurs.

L'expérience ainsi menée depuis 2 ans a l'intérêt de réunir une équipe pluridisciplinaire de spécialistes dans laquelle l'utilisateur potentiel joue un rôle capital.

(*) contrat n° 808002 : "conception et expérimentation d'une aide visuelle à l'apprentissage de la parole pour les déficients auditifs".

BIBLIOGRAPHIE

1) G. ADDA, S. BARTH : la découverte du pouvoir de la parole sur l'enfant sourd. Colloque International "pré-langage" - Besançon - 1979.

2) S. BARTH : application des procédés de reconnaissance automatique de la parole à l'aide aux déficients auditifs profonds. Thèse, Ecole Nationale de la Santé Publique, Paris, 1975. Prix Philips décerné par l'A.F.E.R.L.A. 1976.

3) S. BARTH, R. CHULLIAT : étude sur les anamorphoses fréquentielles des formants vocaliques en fonction de l'âge. Colloque International d'Audiophonologie, Paris, 1977.

4) S. BARTH, R. CHULLIAT : étude sur la variabilité et la normalisation des structures phonétiques en vue de l'amélioration du langage oral chez les déficients auditifs. Bulletin d'Audiophonologie n° 5, Besançon, 1977.

5) S. BARTH, R. CHULLIAT : modifications inter-locuteurs de l'échelle formantique. 9e Journées d'Etudes sur la Parole du Groupe de la communication parlée du G.A.L.F., Lannion, 1979.

6) S. BARTH, R. CHULLIAT : étude comparative de la trajectoire du F2 dans la parole des déficients auditifs et dans celle des entendants. XIe J.E.P. du Groupe de la Communication Parlée, Strasbourg, 1980.

7) M.L. COHEN : the A.D.L. sustained phoneme analyser.Am. Ann. Deaf n° 113, 1978.

8) R.G. CRICHTON, F. FALLSIDE : the development of a deaf speech training aid using linear prediction analysis. Speech Communication Seminar, Stockholm, 1974.

9) C.J. GUEGUEN, A.H. MAISSIS : un système d'aide aux sourds profonds. 10e Assises de la Prothèse Auditive, Paris, 1972.

10) R.D. KENT : anatomical and neuromuscular maturation of speech mechanism : evidence from acoustic studies. J. of Speech and hearing research, sep. 1976, vol 19 n° 34.

11) C. LEGROS : reconnaissance des voyelles et application à la rééducation de la parole. Revue Acoust. n° 44, 1978.

12) J.P. HATON, M.C. HATON, M. LAMOTTE : Sirène : un projet de système interactif pour la rééducation vocale des enfants non-entendants, 6e J.E.P. du G.A.L.F., Toulouse 1975.

13) R.S. NICKERSON, K.N. STEVENS : teaching speech to the deaf : can computer help? Proc. Nat. Conv. A.C.M. August 1972.

AN OPTICAL CHARACTER RECOGNIZER

A. DA RONCH, R. SPINABELLI, C. PAGURA
Istituto per Ricerche di Dinamica dei Sistemi
e di Bioingegneria del CNR (LADSEB)
Corso Stati Uniti 4, 35100 Padova

SUMMARY

An optical character recognizer for the blind is described, based on the following elements: an image digitizer using an array of solid state photosensors; a microprocessor controller which implements the recognition algorithms; an output terminal. The algorithms perform the following main functions: thinning, by which 'skeletons' of images are obtained; segmentations, i.e. subdivision of the written text into lines and of each line into single characters; normalization of the images in size; extraction of topological features of the skeletons from their graph representation, and selection of some metrical data; pre-selection and recognition by comparison with stored models. The device is intended for personal use.

1. INTRODUCTION

A printed character recognizer for the blind is being developed at LADSEB. The project started with a preliminary investigation among the potential users on the main facilities that such a device should provide, and then the design specifications were outlined. It was first pointed out that the recognizer should be oriented to individual users, and therefore be portable and inexpensive in order to make the handicapped user independent of other persons or social services in accessing printed information; in addition, reading speed should be comprised between 10 and 20 characters per second; finally, the use of the device should require as little manual intervention from the user as possible.
The above requirements are fulfilled firstly by optimizing the image transformation algorithm, so that execution time and memory occupation can be kept low, without exceeding an error rate of 5% (i.e., 5 unidentified characters out of 100). The implementation of such algorithms on a dedicated microprocessor network can further improve processing speed. As for the input device, it must be based on automatic scanning of the image, to improve speed and to ensure minimum handling problems on the user's side.

2. DESCRIPTION

The conversion from printed text to a form acceptable by the blind is shown in the block diagram of figure 1. The functions performed by each block are described in the following.

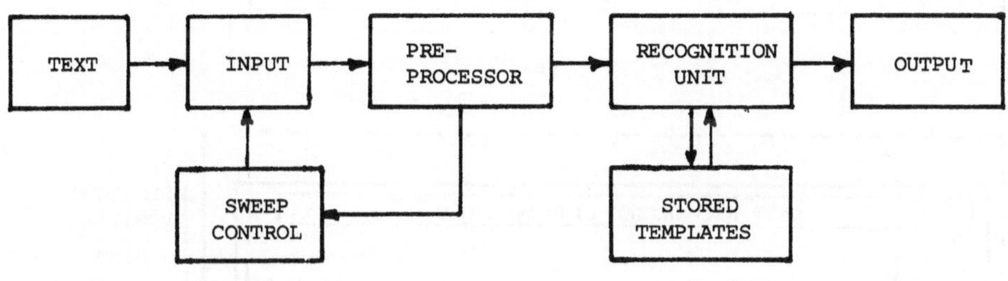

Figure 1. Block diagram.

2.1. Input block

It is an optoelectronic scanner, formed by a single array of 256 photodiodes, which scans the image automatically through two types of motions (figure 2). The first motion (a) is perpendicular to the array and scans a band of printed lines from left to right. This motion has a constant speed, related to the output rate of the signal produced by the optoelectronic device, and allows fitting a square grid to the image.

The optoelectronic device generates an analog output signal whose amplitude is proportional to the average gray level in each square element of the grid. The signal is processed by a contrast correcting circuit and then quantized to a sequence of binary values obtained through comparison with an adaptive threshold calculated from the extreme gray levels (i.e., white and black) of the text. We assume "0" to represent white and "1" to represent black. The bit string obtained in this way is then transmitted syncronously to the preprocessor block and stored in a representation matrix.

The second type of scanning motion (b) is controlled by the processor and allows scanning the subsequent set of lines, after acquisition and recognition of the previous set.

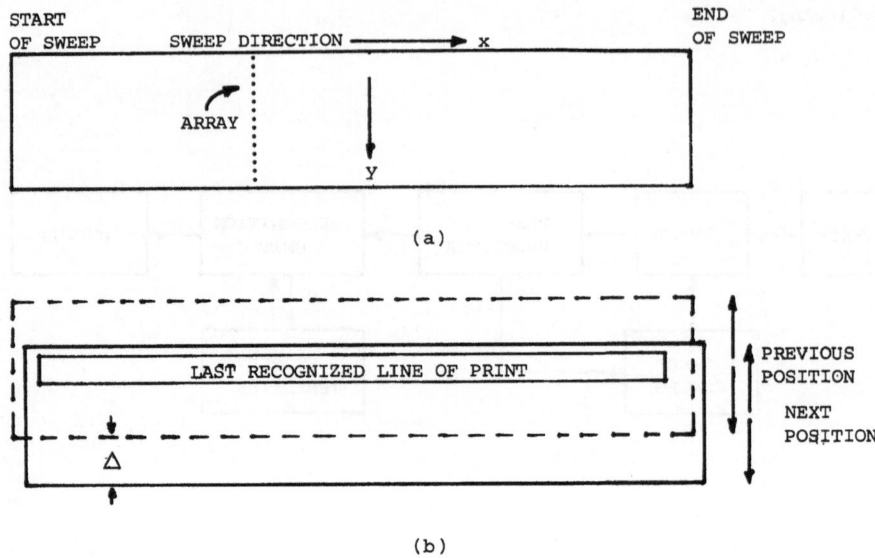

Figure 2. The two mechanical scanning motions and their relationship with the image: (a) constant speed motion, parallel to lines; (b) step by step forward motion (Δ = amplitude of step).

2.2. Preprocessor block

This block allows transforming and recoding the image, and segmenting it into lines; each line is then segmented into characters. Such operations can be grouped as follows:

Thinning. It is performed over sets of black elements ("dots") to obtain the so-called "skeletons" of the original sets, preserving connectivity and form. This operation is performed by a dedicated hardware device (Da Ronch and Spinabelli (1)) which receives the digital signal produced by the Input block. It consists mainly of shift registers interlaced with logic units, which allow analysing the digitized image in real time and erasing the dots not belonging to any skeleton. The processing system receives the data output by the thinning device, and stores them in the aforementioned representation matrix.

Sweep alignment. The detection of the angles between the x_r axis of the printed lines and the scanning direction is performed by a trial-and-error algorithm which searches for the direction along which the maximum number of 1's (dots) is measured in the matrix. This angle has two thresholds of tolerance: ± 8° and ± 20°. Below the lower threshold the image is accepted for further processing, while between the two thresholds the scanning system readjusts its x axis. Above the upper threshold the text must be repositioned by the user, and this is signalled by the device. In the last two cases the acquisition must be repeated.

Detection of the printed lines. It is assumed that the straight lines enclosing each printed line be oriented as described in the preceeding paragraph and be positioned at the minima of amplitude in the dot density histogram, calculated along the orientation direction.

Image recoding. The binary matrix description of the skeletons is transformed into a Freeman code description (Freeman (2)); the skeletons are subdivided into connected sets, with the addition of the matric data required for an exact reconstruction of the original image. The connected sets are detected and stored sequentially, according to the acquisition order.

Segmentation. The segmentation of printed lines into characters corresponds to associating connected sets and single characters; in general for printed characters there must be a one to one correspondence. This operation is carried out through two types of tests, and therefore it implies two types of decisions. In the first type of test (characters formed by several sets) the mutual position of the rectangles enclosing consecutive sets is checked, and we can extract information about the spacing between consecutive words and punctuation. The second type of test (several characters forming a single connected set) compares the enclosing rectangle with the statistics of the available sets.
Confidence thresholds are established for the decisions on the associations; in case of uncertainty between various choices these are passed over to the recognition system, which makes a decision according to its own specific criteria.

2.3. Recognition unit

This block examines one character at a time and attributes it a semantic value through comparison with the templates constructed during the learning phase. The result is stored in a memory area that can be accessed by the Output block.
Among the available algorithms, two groups have been selected and coded into independent procedures, in order to cover a wide range of fonts compatibly with a reasonable saving in computer space. The two procedures run in parallel processing the same image and their results are fed into a decision making stage. They are both divided into three steps: 1) feature extraction; 2) preselection; 3) comparison with the templates.
One of the procedures is based on the recognition of the topologic features of the image and it is called "Topology" (Beghi et al (3)). The other is based on a dot by dot comparison between the image and a number of masks, and is called "Mask".

Topology. The structure of the image is detected and coded in terms of a graph, i.e. a set of nodes and arcs (figure 3). The nodes are further classified according to the number of arcs they belong to, as "ends" and "crossings". Metric data are also required to discriminate between images having the same structure but sufficiently different shapes. Therefore, the length and two angles were associated to each arc: the first angle is measured between the chord and one cartesian axis, the second between the arc's midpoint and the nodes. The sign of the angles is based on the convention introduced by the Freeman code.

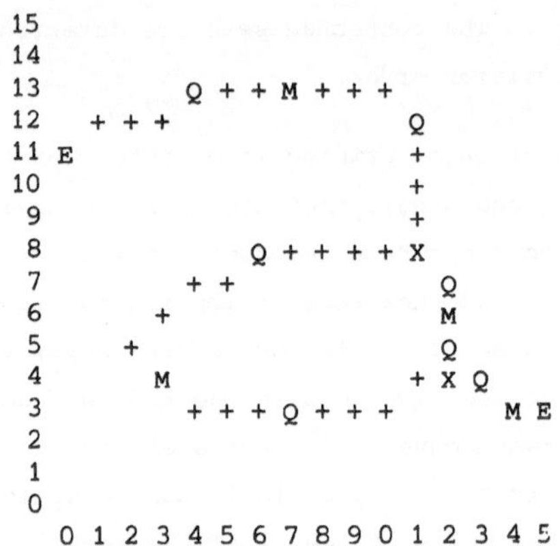

x = crossing node

E = end node

M = midpoint of each arc

Q = quarter-distance point

Figure 3. An example of skeleton.

Preselection is based on parameters related to the numerosity of elements in the image; the templates are ordered using such parameters as keys. Each key denotes the group of templates to be selected.
The actual comparison is performed by matching the structures of the given image with the templates, and by checking that metric differences are within bounds.

<u>Mask</u>. The original image is normalized through a linear transformation of the axes, in order to allow its matching with the resident masks, contained in 16 x 16 square matrices (figures 4, 5). The transformation parameters are calculated so that a fraction of the original dots fall within a pre-fixed rectangle inside the square matrix.

15							1	2	1							
14					2	9	13	14	14	10	6	1				
13			2	8	13	13	8	6	6	11	12	9	1			
12		8	8	10	8						4	10	7	1		
11	1	2	4	4	1						3	7	9	2	1	
10				2			1	1	1	1	4	8	6	6	2	
9						1	3	4	5	9	10	14	13	7		
8				1	8	10	13	13	15	11	10	9	12	8		
7			1	7	7	8	4	2				3	8	11		
6			3	14	7	2					1	2	8	11		
5			13	8	2						1	4	8	11		
4		7	15	10	2				1	2	8	12	16	13	2	2
3			1	14	18	19	20	19	19	18	14	7	6	10	17	16
2				1	2	3	2	1							1	1
1																
0																
	0	1	2	3	4	5	6	7	8	9	0	1	2	3	4	5

Figure 4. Mask templates: histogram of the occurrence of dots over 22 samples.

15																
14						+	+	+	+	+	+					
13				+	+	+	+	+	+	+	+	+				
12		+	+	+	+						+	+	+			
11			+	+								+	+			
10											+	+	+	+		
9								+	+	+	+	+	+	+		
8					+	+	+	+	+	+	+	+	+	+		
7				+	+	+	+							+		
6				+	+								+	+		
5			+	+								+	+	+		
4		+	+	+							+	+	+	+		
3				+	+	+	+	+	+	+	+	+	+	+	+	+
2																
1																
0																
	0	1	2	3	4	5	6	7	8	9	0	1	2	3	4	5

Figure 5. The result of thresholding the histogram of figure 4 at 1/6 of the number of samples.

The data required for preselection are related to the numerosity of dots and absolute values of Freeman vectors in the normalized image. These too are used as ordering keys denoting groups of templates: this method is less time-consuming than a sequential comparison of the values of parameters with the corresponding confidence intervals of templates.
Direct comparison with a mask requires counting the number of coincidences between points of the given image and points of the mask. The scores obtained for preselected masks are made statistically comparable by subtracting from each one the "expected score" of each mask (defined as the average score of the samples used to form the mask itself).

2.4. Decision block

It is in charge of solving possible ambiguities arising from either uncertainties in segmenting a line into characters, or from disagreements between the two recognition algorithms. It calculates which, among normal alternative subdivisions, has the highest global score; to solve the second type of ambiguity it can either use some weighting coefficients that allow classifying the answers, or it can introduce a contextual analysis in terms of probability of groups of characters.

2.5. Output block

Two output methods are envisaged: speech synthesis performed by a dedicated processor, and Braille code output in a volatile form through a board containing several pin matrices. The pins can be made to stick out of the board, thus allowing tactile recognition. Both solutions will adopt commercial devices.

3. DISCUSSION

At the present stage of the project the following parts have been implemented: the scanning system, the preprocessing hardware; the algorithms are being installed on a minicomputer; the construction of templates and validation of procedures has begun recently.

A microprocessor in a "system development" configuration is used to evaluate memory and time occupation of the various processing stages, in order to design a dedicated prototype with a multi-microprocessor architecture. Such a system will contain also the facilities for user interaction.

Acknowledgements

The authors are deeply indebted to G.P. Toffano of the Electronic Laboratory who painfully assembled the prototype.

REFERENCES

1. Da Ronch A., and Spinabelli R., 1977, "Assottigliamento di immagini in tempo reale", Simposio AEI, Trieste, Italy.
2. Freeman H., 1961, "On the encoding of arbitrary geometric configurations", IRE Trans. Electronic Computers, EC-10(2), 260.
3. Beghi L., Da Ronch A., Segato E., Spinabelli R., 1978, "Un riconoscitore di caratteri per non vedenti", 15^ Convegno Internazionale BIAS, Milano.

MAN-MACHINE COMMUNICATION
(Overwiew of automatic aid systems for the blind)

Jaime LOPEZ KRAHE
Departement ISSV - Laboratoire Image - ENST -
46 rue Barrault 75634 PARIS cédex 13

1. SUMMARY

The modern information processing capabilities offer a new approache to blind's problems. Mobility and recording are studied in relation to modern technology. Our aim is to present a survey of the relevant works and to propose a synthesis of the corresponding studies, along with some prospects for the future.

2. INTRODUCTION

Information-processing systems offer notable possibilities of improving the way of life and the social integration of the blind. There are indeed approximately 16 million in the world with two major problems :

Mobility : Up to now, the problem of self governing transportation has been "solved" by canes or trained dogs.

Reading:For the blind, it is a very important problem to have acces to the common written information systems which still constitute the essence of a memory communication net work. The Braille system (1) was invented 150 years ago. It makes use of a binary code with 6 bits per character, translating an alphabet of 64 characters.From a psychophysiological point of view, this system is well adapted to the sense of touch. Consequently it allows appreciable reading speeds.
Magnetic recording is another approach. It constitutes a quite easy means to obtain "spoken-books", but the serial reading is not very satisfying ; furthermore magnetic recording requires a human operator and can hardly be automated.

3. MOBILITY AIDS

These systems deliver information about environment, in order to make mobility easier. We have mentionned only the traditionnal systems such as canes, guide dogs... or some collective equipments (suppression of architectural barriers, guiding grooves on the pavements, acoustical signals, ...).

The main difficulty with electronical systems is that they should translate complex tridimensionnal information into some perceivable stimulus. In fact, they usually only detect obstacles such as walls, barriers, steps, holes, etc. The corresponding research follows two main tracks.

The "bionic cane" (2) represents, originally, the first one. In this system, a laser beam is used in order to localize the neighbouring objects by their reflexion. The cane must be moved angularly. Then, a triangulation process delivers tactile informations, related to obstacles.

Ultra-sound sonar systems are more wide-spread. The "binaural environmental sensor" (3) is the most developped one.

This system consists of spectacles with ultra-sound transmitter-receiver. The echo is mixed with the reference signal, and the corresponding differential frequencies generate audible signals. Those are transmitted to the ear, through mechanical contact with the bone. In this manner, the blind are able to receive additionnal acoustical information from environment which is important . The resulting amplitude and frequency informations depend on the reflexion characteristics of objects, their distance, the sweeping, etc. Unfortunately this system does not detect holes, so it only complements the cane.

4 - READING

In our opinion, two important classes of methods should be distinguished, among the machine-aid written systems :

- The "off-line" methods, for which a "translation system" is put in between the written informations and the blind. This is the case of the very important recording and editing systems.

- The "real-time" methods, for which a prosthesis is offering a direct signal transduction interface.

4.1. Off-line methods : the recording systems

In the past few years, the magnetic recording methods have performed important evolutions. Concerning analog recording, notable improvements have been proposed such as variable re-reading velocity systems (real-time resampling method), pointer devices for labelling, high storage capabilities etc. On the other hand major improvements result from the recent digital Braille recording machines (Digicassette, versabraille ...). In these machines, the Braille text is stored on a digital cassette (6 Braille tomes on a C 90). The usual input/output devices consist in a Braille keybord and a tactile Braille matrix, which offer very adapted reading/writting capabilities. These systems can also be connected either to classical writting-machines — which gives interesting possibilities of interconnection between Braille and normal printing — or to teleprocessing networks. Some efficient numerical set-up can be added, such as microprocessors, text-editors, etc. Therefore, these implements must be considered as very relevant solutions for our specific man-machine communication problems.

4.2. Off-line methods : the editing systems

At present time, the paper editing systems still play a major role. But the total available number of Braille documents is severely limited. Indeed, a specialized transcriber cannot copy more than 4000 words a day.

Clearly, computer sciences offer new approaches in this field. An instance, new algorithms are now implemented to edit music. One can easily imagine how the music edition was an intricate problem, before the introduction of automatic programming...

As far as the general editing problem is concerned (see figure 1) we shall follow the classical division : input, processing, output.

The input : The main idea is the following one. It is possible to use the digital records delivered by the classical editing processors (such as photocomposer of Optical Character Recognition) as automatic inputs for a Braille editor (4). In fact, besides the corresponding legal and administrative problems, several technical difficulties arrise (the recording materials and the input codes are very diversified, the graphics need a human operation..)

The information processing : It essentially consists in automatic code-translation problems. There exist 2 distinct Braille codes : integral Braille (Grade I) and stenographic Braille (Grade II). The former problem is simpler than the latter, which is closely dependant on linguistic conditions. Such grade II programs do exist for English (5), French (6)...
It must be fointed out that such information processing algorithms can be thought as a constitutive element of a general data-bank system (7).

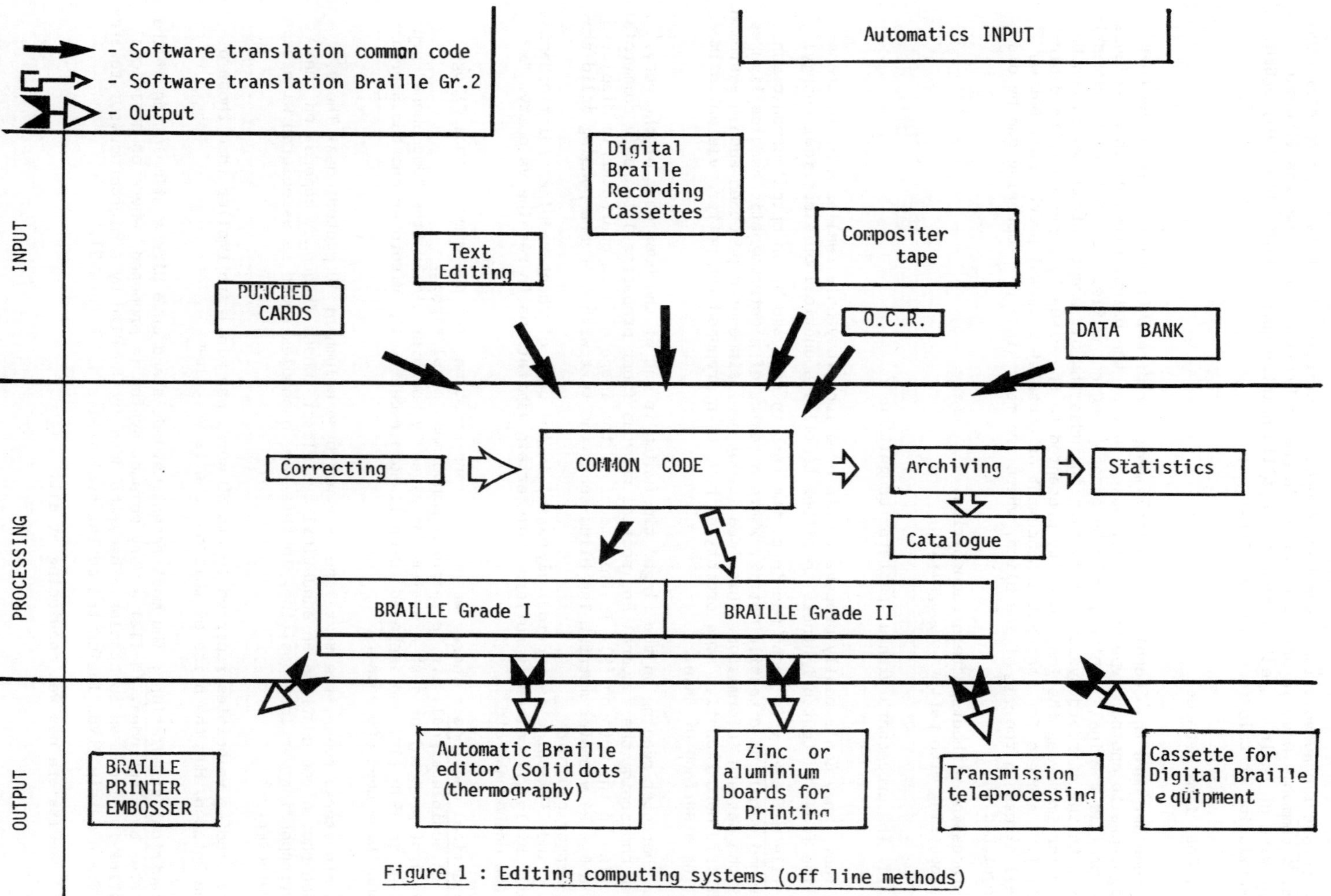

Figure 1 : Editing computing systems (off line methods)

The output : Many solutions have been proposed : Braille cassettes, Zinc or Aluminium boards commonly used in printing-works, Automatic Braille edited records (thermic engraving or resin projection methods, Braille printer output (IBM, TEM-8 BR, SAGEM...) Transmission or teleprocessing network...

4.3. Real time methods

We consider here the technical aids implements for direct translation from the text brightness to another type of energy, detectable by the blind. First of this includes the Braille terminals, which should be adapted and normalized in order to be compatible with the standard systems. This also includes the different methods which can be used for improving the image quality presented to the visually impaired (closed circuit T.V. systems for contrast enhancement or contrast reversal processes). But we shall stress in the case of the blind, where two main kinds of processing can be distinguished :

- processing without pattern-recognition,
- processing with pattern recognition.

4.3.1. The processors without pattern-recognition

In fact, they don't really process the information. They only realise a plain translation from the text brightness to either tactile, acoustical or electrical energy)

Tactile machines : In these machines, the text is analysed by an optoelectronic sensor and output on a tactile matrix, where a series of electromagnetic needles figures out the pattern information. This idea is not new, since Grim proposed such a system in 1880 (8). More recently, some prototypes have been proposed for pattern vision, stimulating a surface of skin.

For character reading on the finger tip (which is one of the best part of the body, when concerning the temporal and spatial nervous fiber properties) the only commercial machine is the Optacon (9). In this machine, the image of each character is displayed on a 6 x 24 vibrator matrix. The blind scans the text with a corresponding solid-state sensor camera.
The kind of machine is particularly useful in the case of short readings (dictionnaries mail, bills...), since it suffers from certain limitations in reading velocity, fatigue phenomena, etc...

Acoustical machines : There, we need a transformation from a bidimensionnal "image" to an audible signal, i.e. a temporal monodimensionnal signal.
The 1rst proposal of such a system was given by Fournier D'Albe (the "Optophone" proposed in 1910 (10) and improved later). More recently the Visotoner and the Stereotoner have been presented.

In the stereo toner, the text-line is swept by a column of 10 photodiodes. There, each photodiode controls an acoustical oscillator, whose frequency depends on the corresponding vertical position. In this way, a complex sound is associated with each character.

The reading velocities reported (up to 60 words per min.) are smaller than those of the Optacon. But the price of this machine is very low.

Electrical stimulation : The most recent methods stand on a direct stimulation of the cortex by electrodes. In (12) a very compact system is proposed, where an artificial retina is placed on spectacles. Then, the data are handled by a microprocessor towards a 8 x 8 matrix fixed inside the cortex occipital side (Figure 2).

The results are not yet convincing at all.

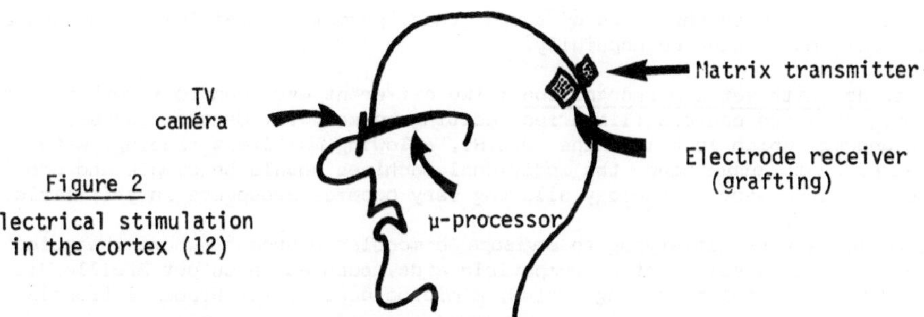

Figure 2

Electrical stimulation in the cortex (12)

4.3.2. The processors with pattern recognition : reading machines for the blind

We now describe complex information processors, where the characters are automatically recognized. Due to this feature extraction stage, the quantity of information received by the user is very optimized. So, the reading step becomes easier and faster (Braille codes, sound, synthetic voice, etc.).

The recognition step is the most difficult one. It has already been studied for the Optical Character Reading systems (O.C.R.). But for our purpose, the performances needed are quite different. The reading machines for the blind must be multifont but they can suffer a relatively high level of error-rate. Instead of such figures as 1/100 000 for O.C.R., we can admit only 1 to 5% since the human operator is able to correct errors, through context information and language redundancy . Furthermore the errors seem to be very systematic in this case, and we can avoid the need of a reject class.

Several systems have been proposed up to now. The author himself realized a prototype, in the Image laboratory of ENST (e.r. 1 to 4%, 150words per mn (13)). The more sophisticated system in this domain has been developped by Kurzweil (14) and includes a voice synthetisor.

5. PROSPECTS FOR THE FUTURE

After this survey of the various approaches, let us now clear out some ideas for the future :

Mobility aids : More compact systems are predictable, where microprocessors will recognize obstacles and set warnings. As far as the warning signals are concerned, they should not disturb the ear, which helps on mobility too.

Off-line methods : Braille edition. A particular effort must be made, in order to improve the inter connexion between the special purpose software and the general methods used in modern editing systems. This must allow a faster production of Braille documents.

Off-line methods : digital recording systems. Systems with transient output are very ecological. They do not use paper. The development of these digital recording machines should result in versatile man-machine interfaces. For them too, normalization efforts are needed (for storage on cassettes, for interfacing with teleprocessing terminals etc.).

Real-time methods, without pattern recognition. The Optacon can be considered as a finite product, compact and reliable. But it seems that this machine has reached the margin of psychophysiological limits. Nevertheless, since the brain is a very good pattern recognition machine, these simple methods are perhaps not to be doomed. It is not impossible that some evolution happens in acoustical machines, resulting from the actual research in sound synthesis and pattern recognition invariants. Such systems should be economical and well-suited to the congenital blind. If we suppose that the ear adapts itself easily to the space of sound, then, premature training of the congenital blind should be considered hopefully.

Real-time methods, with pattern recognition : Two different ways can be foreseen, for these systems. For large centers (libraries, editing houses...). General purpose machines are needed, which look like the O.C.R., allowing multifont reading, with low error-rates. On the other hand the individual machines should be simple and economical, the microprocessor technology allowing very hopeful prospects in this field.

In fact, it would be very satisfying to envisage a modular approach, where the blind would have at their disposal a lot of compatible aids, such as an output Braille display connected to a digital recording system, a microprocessor for Grade II translation, etc...
One of the final objective whould be to implement a whole man-machine communication system. With the actual hopes in computer and teleprocessing technology, we can expect that, in the future, the blind and the non-blind will be considered equivalently as fa as communication is concerned. The development of digital recording machines with transient output displays constitute a significant example of the new generation of man-machine communication services. When considering industry, it is not impossible to dream to such an evolutive process...

6. CONCLUSION

Today, science and technology offer hopeful possibilities to the blind, and to the handicapped in general. However, some very important conditions must be stated, as follows.

These technical aids cannot be considered as usual products. Indeed, the handicapped have the right to be informed, the right to work. These rights cannot be measured by the classical commercial criteria such as the short term economic efficiency, for instance. Furthermore, it is notable that they are high-technology products, with hopefully very few potential users...

We think that the two following principles should be admitted :

- that the corresponding research be supplied by administrative organisations, according to more general criteria, taking care of the remarks above mentionned.
- that they be subsidized as aids by the Social Security systems.

In fact, this leads us to social, or even, political problems...

7. BIBLIOGRAPHIE

(1) UNESCO. L'écriture Braille dans le monde; Unesco publication Paris 1953

(2) HOOVER. "Foot travel without sight : foot travel at valley Forge" Outlook for the blind - Vol. 40. pp. 246-251 - N.Y. 1946

(3) KAY L. "Ultrasonic spectacles for the blind" Proc. Int. Conf. on sensory devices for the blind . R. Dufton, Ed. London 1967n pp. 275-292

(4) Int. Conf. Computerised Braille Production - London June 1979

(5) FORTHIER, P.A. KEETING, D. "Data processing in the service of the blind" Convention Informatica 1977 - Paris, 20-23 Sept. 1977

(6) TRUQUET M. Braille Grade II translator Program - NCC - N.Y. Juin 1976

(7) PUIG de la BELLACASA R., LOPEZ KRAHE J. - Applicationes de las telecomunicaciones y de la informatica a la rehabilitacion, educacion y asistencia de ciegos, ciegos-sordos y dedicientes visuales - Fundesco n°54 - Madrid Julio 1979

(8) GALLOIS - Anaculoscope de C. Grim - Bulletin "Le Valentin Haüy" - Paris octobre 1883

(9) BLISS J. - A reading Machine with Tactil Display - Visual Prosthesis Ac. Press 1971

(10) FOURNIER D'ALBE E.E. - "The OPTOPHONE : An Instrument for reading by ear" Nature Vol. 105 - London May 1920 - pp. 295-296

(11) SMITH G.C. - The steteotoner Reading Aid for the Blind. A progress report Proc. of Carnahan Conference on Electronic Prosthesis - Lexington, 19-21 sept. 1973 pp. 74-76

(12) BRINDLEY G.S., LEWIN V.S. - "The visual sensations produced by electrical stimulation of the medical occipital cortex"- J. Physial n°196, London 1968

(13) LOPEZ KRAHE J. -"An Optical Reading Machine for the Blind"Optica Hoy y mañana - Proc. of ICO-11 - Madrid - Sept. 1978

(14) KURZWEIL R.C., KLEINER A. -"A description of the Kurzweil Reading - Machine and a status Report on its testing and Dissemination"- Bull. of Prosthesis Research Spring 1977.

L'ORDINATEUR ET L'APHASIQUE

Evelyne ANDREEWSKY et Gérard DELOCHE
INSERM U.84
Hôpital de la Salpêtrière
47, Bd de l'Hôpital
75634 Paris Cedex 13/France

Summary

(The computer and the aphasic)

Both the computer and the aphasic have problems in handling natural language.

A cognitive approach of language-handling mechanisms is carried out, starting from the acknowledgment of these problems, on one hand (Artificial Intelligence concepts and applications -i.e., respectively "procedures" or "speech synthesis"- given its theoretical framework, and neuropsycholinguistic facts - its experimental data).

The relevance of computers in neuropsycholinguistic experiments is illustrated, on the other hand, with an example (a "lexical decision" task) where the presentation of stimuli and the analysis of subjects answers are both under the control of a micro-computer.

We derived such specific applications from this research as computer-aided learning and rehabilitation of written language.

1. INTRODUCTION

L'ordinateur et l'aphasique ont au moins ceci en commun : les difficultés qu'ils éprouvent à utiliser la langue (naturelle).

-Rappelons, en ce qui concerne l'ordinateur, que les travaux d'Intelligence Artificielle, dans la mesure où ils impliquent des traitements linguistiques élaborés (en traduction automatique, dialogue homme-machine, reconnaissance de la parole, etc..) n'ont guère dépassé le stade du laboratoire.

-En ce qui concerne les aphasiques, rappelons que leurs troubles du langage ne se traduisent pas par une baisse concernant, de manière uniforme, les performances du malade. Celui-ci peut présenter, au contraire, des déficits linguistiques spécifiques. Ces déficits, d'origine organique, reflètent l'absence de certains traitements psycholinguistiques, dans la mesure où on conceptualise les relations entre "neuro" et "psycho" en terme d'une dualité de type "matériel-logiciel". Dans ces conditions, l'éventail des déficits aphasiques reflète celui des diverses composantes constituant le système neuro-psycholinguistique normal.

On conçoit alors que l'ordinateur, permettant de simuler les composantes de ce système, soit associé à l'aphasique, dont les déficits en reflètent des propriétés spécifiques.

Nous allons d'abord donner un exemple associant Intelligence Artificielle et Neuropsychologie en une démarche théorique de psychologie cognitive; nous présenterons ensuite un exemple de l'aide que peut apporter la micro-informatique dans l'expérimentation en psycho-linguistique. Nous présenterons enfin des applications de ces recherches à la rééducation de certains troubles du langage des aphasiques.

2. INTELLIGENCE ARTIFICIELLE ET PROCEDURES NEURO-PSYCHO-LINGUISTIQUES

Les modèles psycholinguistiques développés en Intelligence Artificielle, et simulés sur ordinateur, explicitent certains traitements inhérents au langage. La neuro-psycholinguistique permet de valider expérimentalement ces modèles.

Exemple : Une première difficulté à laquelle se heurtent les traitements automatiques de la langue, est la détermination de la classe grammaticale des mots. Par exemple, un "synthétiseur de la parole" (1) (système permettant de faire énoncer par un ordinateur mots ou textes fournis sous forme écrite), dépourvu d'analyseur syntaxique, ne peut fonctionner correctement. Il ne pourra notament pas énoncer correctement les homographes non homophones comme dans :

les poules du couvent couvent;

ou il est un as; tu as du vent d'est, etc..

si les classes grammaticales des mots soulignés n'ont pas été déterminées:

D'une manière générale, le problème des ambiguités syntaxiques s'est révélé crucial pour toutes les applications qui (cf. liste du § 1) impliquent de près ou de loin la compréhension. La désambiguation syntaxique apparaît ainsi comme une composante nécessaire à tout système de compréhension du langage, même le plus rudimentaire.

"Rudimentaire" est sans doute un qualificatif qui s'applique à la compréhension linguistique de certains aphasiques. C'est ainsi que les aphasiques "agrammatiques", (dont les énoncés sont dépourvus de marque syntaxique : seuls y figurent substantifs et verbes sans flexion) ne comprennent le langage que partiellement : en effet, ils ignorent en réception (comme dans leurs énoncés) tout ce qu'indiquent : relations syntaxiques, temps et forme des verbes, etc..

Ces malades ont-ils "perdu" la syntaxe (comme l'affirme la littérature neuropsychologique)? Si tel était le cas, aussi partielle que soit leur compréhension, elle s'inscrirait alors en faux quant à la nécessité (cf. ci-dessus) d'une désambiguation syntaxique, dans tout système, même élémentaire, de compréhension.

Une expérience très simple permet de montrer que chez ces malades, la composante de "désambiguation syntaxique" fonctionne toujours : en effet, si on leur fait lire à haute voix des phrases comportant notamment des homographes tels que "car" ou "or", (substantifs ou conjonction), on constate que ces mots, toujours énoncés quand ils figurent dans une phrase en fonction de substantif, ne le sont jamais s'ils sont en position de conjonction : on a là la preuve expérimentale de l'action (implicite) d'une désambiguation syntaxique.

C'est ainsi que, à travers l'agrammatisme, la composante "désambiguation syntaxique" est isolée des autres mécanismes syntaxiques (qui, eux, ne fonctionnent plus); certaines propriétés spécifiques de cette composante - postulée théoriquement en Intelligence Artificielle, ont ainsi pu être expérimentalement étudiées (2), en faisant lire à haute voix à ces malades du matériel linguistique approprié.

3. EXPERIENCES NEURO-PSYCHO-LINGUISTIQUES CONTROLEES PAR MICRO-ORDINATEUR

Les micro-ordinateurs sont bien adaptés aux expérimentations psycholinguistiques; en effet, leurs écrans affichent (par construction) des textes alphanumériques (ou des images video) : les stimuli des expériences; leurs claviers peuvent servir à recevoir, pour les enregistrer, les réponses des sujets -des plus simples (oui/non) aux plus élaborées-. D'autre part, si cela est nécessaire, les conditions expérimentales peuvent être modifiées et adaptées automatiquement à chaque sujet, au fur et à mesure des réponses fournies; enfin, le prix modique de ces appareils, la simplicité de leur utilisation et leur encombrement réduit sont des atouts qui manquaient aux terminaux d'ordinateurs.

3.1. Compréhension lexicale en lecture

Certains phénomènes observés dans la lecture à haute voix des aphasiques (cf. § précédent) amènent à remettre en question les modèles classiques des mécanismes de lecture ("conversion" de l'écrit en oral) et à postuler que la lecture à haute voix est médiatisée par la compréhension. On conçoit alors que des expériences de lecture de mots puissent valider des hypothèses quant aux modalités de leur compréhension.

3.2. Conditions expérimentales

Mots ou séquences de lettres ne constituant pas un mot (ex: mirpe) sont affichés un à un sur l'écran du micro-ordinateur. On teste les facteurs linguistiques (ex: classe grammaticale) qui influent sur le taux d'erreur et de temps de réaction des sujets à la question : "est-ce un mot de la langue"? (cette expérience est dite de "décision lexicale"). Il faut que le temps d'affichage soit adapté à chaque sujet si on veut utiliser les taux d'erreurs produits: si le temps d'affichage est trop long, on n'observera pas d'erreur - s'il est trop court, les réponses seront souvent données au hasard. Un temps de 20 à 100 ms convient en général. Un algorithme modifiant ce temps permet de l'ajuster pour chaque sujet, en fonction des réponses de celui-ci à un pré-test.

- Réponses des sujets

Les sujets répondent "oui" ou "non" par l'intermédiaire de deux boutons poussoirs; chaque réponse est enregistrée ainsi que l'intervalle de temps qui la sépare de l'affichage du stimulus ("temps de réaction" du sujet).

- Analyse des réponses

Les taux d'erreurs et les temps de réaction sont calculés pour chaque classe d'items lexicaux (par exemple : classe des fonctionnels, d'une part, et substantifs, de l'autre), pour chaque sujet et pour l'ensemble des sujets. Ces analyses, comme l'ensemble de la mise en oeuvre des expériences de "décisions lexicales" sont, bien entendu, automatisées.

3.3. Résultats

Un des résultats (3) de ce type d'expérience sur les sujets adultes normaux, est que les substantifs sont reconnus de manière sensible à leur fréquence dans la langue, alors que ce n'est pas le cas pour les fonctionnels: les procédures correspondant à ces traitements sont donc différents. Cette même expérience réalisée sur des alexiques ("dyslexiques profonds") (4) permet d'affirmer l'indépendance de ces procédures de reconnaissance : celle traitant des substantifs étant, pour ces malades, la seule qui soit conservée. C'est ainsi que ces expériences de "décision lexicale" amènent à valider des modules du système de la lecture.

4. REEDUCATION DU LANGAGE DES APHASIQUES

Une première technique de rééducation concerne un type d'apprentissage du langage écrit, irréalisable sans le secours d'un ordinateur : il s'agit d'apprentissage sans visualisation des erreurs. Cette technique a été éprouvée et testée avec la rééducation de sujets aphasiques (5). Des exercices appliqués à la syntaxe de la langue et à la signification des mots ont été dérivés de cette technique.

4.1. Apprentissage de l'orthographe sans visualisation des erreurs

L'apprentissage habituel de l'orthographe consiste en dictées, permettant de contrôler les performances de l'élève. On lui signale ses fautes, mais celles-ci sont restées auparavant suffisamment longtemps sous ses yeux pour avoir de grandes chances d'interférer avec la mémorisation souhaitée : celle de l'orthographe correcte des mots.

Pour éviter la visualisation des mots à l'orthographe erronée, on adopte la technique suivante : on introduit un micro-ordinateur pour filtrer les erreurs en visualisant seulement ce qui, tapé sur le clavier, est correctement orthographié : (en cas d'erreur, un signal sonore retentit (la signalant ainsi immédiatement) et la lettre erronée n'est pas affichée; l'élève ne peut continuer sans l'avoir corrigée).

Les résultats de ce type d'apprentissage se sont révélés très positifs pour les enfants dysorthographiques (6), et une aide à la rééducation des aphasiques utilisant cette même technique a fait l'objet d'un mémoire d'orthophoniste (7). Un prototype spécialisé a été développé en vue de cette application (8).

4.2. Aide à la thérapie mélodique et rythmée du langage

Une technique récente, qui fait preuve d'efficacité dans la rééducation du langage des aphasiques, est la "thérapie mélodique et rythmée". Celle-ci consiste à associer aux phrases une mélodie bien marquée. Cette association diminue beaucoup les difficultés de verbalisation de certains malades (9).

L'introduction d'un micro-ordinateur permet de matérialiser les rythmes à suivre, à la fois visuellement (au moyen de traits verticaux sur l'écran, espacés proportionellement aux temps), et par des "bip" sonores; la tâche du patient est d'appuyer sur une touche à chaque "bip". Ses performances sont visualisées sur l'écran, et il peut ainsi comparer ses réponses avec le rythme de référence, en un "feed back" visuel.

4.3. Aide à la rééducation de la lecture

L'apprentissage de la lecture, comme la rééducation, est en règle générale controlée par l'enseignant au moyen des énoncés de l'élève : on fait lire celui-ci à haute voix.

Bien que de nombreux travaux (10) montrent que convertir graphemes en phonèmes (b, a ⟶ /ba/) n'aide pas l'élève à accroitre ni la qualité ni la rapidité de sa compréhension, mais celle de cette conversion, la lecture à haute voix reste l'exercice privilégié auquel recourent les enseignants. Il existe cependant des méthodes, destinées aux enfants, qui favorisent spécifiquement la compréhension de l'écrit, plutôt que sa conversion en oral. Les progrès de l'élève sont contrôlés, dans ces méthodes de "lecture silencieuse", au moyen de batteries de questions portant sur le sens des phrases et des textes écrits.

L'adaptation de ces méthodes à la rééducation des alexiques nous a semblé pouvoir être accompagnée utilement des techniques micro-informatiques : on affiche un texte sur l'écran du micro-ordinateur; des questions concernant son sens apparaissent sur l'écran et le malade y répond par l'intermédiaire du clavier. Le temps mis pour lire le texte, le pourcentage de bonnes réponses aux questions et l'évolution de ces paramètres sont calculés et affichés à la fin de chaque exercice : c'est ainsi que le micro-ordinateur "dialogue" avec le patient; ce dialogue permet à l'alexique d'agir sur le déroulement de sa propre rééducation (en choisissant textes et vitesse de présentation) et d'avoir l'évaluation chiffrée de ses performances, que la machine fournit au fur et à mesure.

Ce type de rééducation de l'alexie est en cours d'essai; des essais analogues sont également en cours dans un Institut parisien spécialisé, pour l'apprentissage de la lecture par des enfants sourds-muets.

5. CONCLUSION

Théories cognitives et pratique de l'ordinateur dans nos recherches nous ont conduits à proposer des méthodes d'apprentissage (et/ou de rééducation) du langage, aidées par micro-ordinateur, matérialisant les applications pratiques de ces recherches théoriques.

Comme ces applications amènent à réfléchir sur les mécanismes du langage, on peut affirmer que l'ordinateur et l'aphasique auront encore bien des choses à se dire - et à nous dire !

REFERENCES

(1) Liénard JS. Le processus de la communication parlée. Introduction à l'analyse et à la synthèse de la parole. Masson, Paris, 1977.

(2) Andreewsky E, Seron X. Implicit processing of grammatical rules in a classical case of agrammation. Cortex. 1975 ; Vol XI, 379-390.

(3) Dési M. Effets de fréquence en "décision lexicale" : influence de la classe grammaticale des mots. Diplôme de maitrise de psychologie.

(4) Patterson KE. What is right with "Deep" dyslexic patients ? Brain & Language. 1979 ; 8 : 111-129.

(5) Seron X, Deloche G, Moulard G, Rousselle M. A computer-based therapy for the treatment of aphasic subjects with writing disorders. Journal of Speech and Hearing Disorders. 1980 ; 45 (1) : 45-58.

(6) Deloche G, Seron X, Saillant B, Moulard G, Chassin G. "Rééducation programmée d'un cas d'agraphie". Acta Neurologica Belgica. 1976 ; 76 : 201-211.

(7) Drai S. Perspective d'utilisation d'un ordinateur dans la rééducation de l'orthographe. Mémoire d'orthophonie, Université Paris VI. 1977.

(8) Jutier P, Andreewsky E, Deloche G, Nicolas P. Micro-processor based system using a commercial tape recorder both as a digital and audio device. MECO : Advances in Measurement and Control, Vol. 3. 1978 ; 796-799.

(9) Van Eeckhout P. Apport de la mélodie et du rythme dans les rééducations sévères. Rééducation orthophonique. 1979.

(10) Foucambert J. "Quelques pré-supposés théoriques de l'enseignement habituel de la lecture". Psychologie et Education, "Les processus psychologiques de la lecture". 1978 ; 21-26.

"Expert Systems": Their Nature and Potential.

H.R.A. TOWNSEND

An "expert system" is a large and complex program that aims to model, more or less explicitly, the way in which a human "expert" is able to solve problems in a particular domain. Medical diagnosis and management (in specialised areas) is an obvious application, but experience in solving social or engineering problems can be captured in a similar way.

The computer system consists of two principal parts, a database of knowledge (the "knowledge base") and a control program (the "inference mechanism") which interprets the "particular facts", which are the input to the program, in the light of the knowledge base in order to arrive at the "advice" which is the end result or output of the program.

The inference mechanism employs a form of deduction and treats the problem as that of proving a theorem in a modified first order predicate logic. The knowledge base consists of a collection of simple logical relations, expressed in symbolic form which can be printed out in an easily understood format as follows:-

If A then B

where A is a logical formula consisting of "facts" (or "predicates"), linked by the logical connectives "AND" and "OR", while B indicates some action to be carried out if the logical formula is evaluated as true. For example:

<u>If</u> one of the patients symptoms is brief losses of consciousness
<u>and</u> the patient's age is close to 10 years
<u>then</u> a likely diagnosis is petit mal epilepsy.

These logical relations are generally called rules and the action part may be viewed "passively" as a "consequence" or actively as a desired "goal".

A "fact" is conveniently modelled as an "object-attribute-value" triple. In this case a patient (the object) has many attributes, one of which is "age" and the value of this attribute in a particular patient may be 10 (years). Similarly the patient has a number of "symptom" attributes, one of which may have the value "brief losses of consciousness".

Of course, in medical diagnosis (and in most other fields as well) nothing is ever certain and strict logical deduction is therefore rarely, if ever, applicable.

Consequently a good deal of effort in the development of expert systems has gone into exploring techniques of "judgemental reasoning", i.e. combining evidence which is more or less certain in order to arrive at a suitable measure of belief or disbelief in the logically implied conclusion.

In the example given, we may either assume that "brief losses of consciousness" is an indisputable fact or we may allow the physician (or possibly even the patient who might be filling in a symptom questionnaire or even operating a simple computer terminal) the option of stating some approximately quantitative degree of confidence in the statement; e.g. in this case perhaps 0.5, meaning that mother thinks the child is having brief losses of consciousness when asked directly but isn't really sure. "Close to 10 years", however, should be susceptible of more precise definition (assuming that the child's age is accurately known) and is really shorthand for a whole set of rules associating different ages with different degrees of credibility of the suggested diagnosis.

This raises an interesting point concerning the representation of knowledge. There are two possible representations:

1) extensive or tabular
2) intensive or algorithmic.

Each has its own advantages and disadvantages. The algorithmic form can often be made very compact but on the other hand certain relations, particularly those which are non-linear, discontinuous, or very complex, may be difficult or impossible to express as a suitable algorithm, while certain other algorithms although expressed economically may take a very long time to compute, or in extreme cases the computation may never halt. Tabular representation is much more suitable for complex and ad-hoc mappings but tends to take up impracticably large amounts of memory.

The art of artificial intelligence lies largely in choosing representations which can work in practice with finite resources of both space and time.

Although the object-attribute-value relation is widely used and is very general it may turn out as a somewhat procrustean mould into which to force a real world model. An alternative, which is being actively explored, is the frame or prototype. The underlying notion is one of "jumping to conclusions" - when we go into a room we expect four walls, a floor and a ceiling. We expect a carpet, linoleum or matting on the floors, doors and windows in the walls, perhaps pictures, and a plain ceiling perhaps with light fittings. Any given room may violate these expectations but most of them don't.

Similarly if we observe a doctor interviewing a patient, after a few routine questions it becomes obvious that the doctor has selected a "prototype" diagnosis and subsequent questions are directed to testing whether the selected prototype (syndrome - diagnostic category or what you will) is a good fit to the particular individual. If it proves not to be so - if the effort is too procrustean - then the prototype is discarded and a new one selected. Thus a prototype or frame is a constellation of attribute-value ranges which collectively represent a concept (such as a diagnosis). The difficulties are mainly those of selecting a suitable prototype in the first place, and later of knowing when to abandon a poorly fitting prototype and try another.

To go back to the more strictly logical inference mechanisms one of the simplest and easiest to understand is the so-called "modus ponens" reasoning. Consider the simple set of rules below in which letters from the alphabet have been substituted for "facts".

1) A & B → F
2) C & D → G
3) E → H
4) B & G → J
5) F & H → X
6) G & E → K
7) J & K → X

The arrow "→" implies "THEN", thus the first rule reads
If A is true AND B is true THEN F is true.

Suppose that in a particular case we discover by observation that "facts" B, C, D, and E are "untrue", and we wish to discover if X is therefore true.

The computer will consider those rules which could be used to infer the truth of X, i.e. those rules (5,7) which have an X on the right hand side of the arrow. Each such rule is tested to see if each of the facts on the left hand side are known to be true, any unknown fact being treated in the same way as the original fact X - a technique known as "recursion".

Thus:-

X may be deducted from Rule 5 or Rule 7.
1) Starting with Rule 5, are F & H true?
2) F can be shown to be true if A & B are both true (Rule 1).
3) A is not known to be true, so this attempt fails.
4) Continuing with Rule 7, are J & K true?
5) J can be shown to be true if B & G are both true (Rule 4).
6) B is known to be true "a priori".
7) G can be shown to be true if C & D are both true (Rule 2)
8) C is known to be true "a priori".
9) D is known to be true "a priori".
10) Therefore G is true.
11) Therefore J is true.
12) K can be shown to be true if G & E are both true (Rule 6).
13) G is already known to be true (step 10).
14) Therefore K is true.
15) Therefore X is true.
Q.E.D.

The great advantage of this technique is that an explanation can be quite easily generated simply by recapitulating the rules involved in the successful reasoning chain as shown by lines 5 to 16 above.

This capacity to "explain itself" is one of the most important characteristics of an "expert system".

There are successful diagnostic systems based simply on Bayes' rule which are supplied with a list of symptoms and signs from which a calculation is made, taking account of prior probabilities, to give the posterior probabilities of a list of selected differential diagnoses. Such systems can play an important part in improving the performance of young doctors, particularly by encouraging methodical habits and also by providing a rapid feedback of correct assessments, but they are quite unable to provide any kind of explanation because the techniques employed to arrive at the answer are totally foreign to the way a human mind naturally approaches the problem.

Expert systems on the other hand, because they explicitly model at least some characteristics (hopefully the rational characteristics) of human thought can explain by simply laying bare the relevant bits of their internal processing.

Example:-

12) Do you consider R.E. James to be a compromised host in the sense that s/he has increased susceptibility to infection (Alcoholic, diabetic, uremic or immunosuppressed)? ** Why

(1.E.) Why is it important to determine whether organism-1 is a contaminant. It has already been establised that

(1.1.) This bone culture was taken from a sterile source therefore, if

(1.2.) R.E. James is a compromised host then there is suggestive evidence (6) that the Peptostreptococcus is not a contaminant. (Rule 106).

(Excerpt from a session with Mycin by the author)

Furthermore the same techniques can be used to model the likely (or desirable?) thought processes of a human learner so that a student who is stuck for the next question to ask (observation to make or test to perform) can request the computer for assistance.

Example:-

**TOPIC

We are discussing the degree of reversibility of airways obstruction of PATIENT-7.

Hypotheses you should be considering are: none, insignificant, slight, good and significant.

**WHAT IS THE CHANGE IN FORCED EXPIRATORY VOLUME?

The change in Forced-Expiratory-Volume (1sec.) after bronchodilation of M. Smith is 31.

**WHAT IS THE CHANGE IN RESISTANCE?

The change in Resistance after bronchodilation of M. Smith is 28.

We have substantially completed our discussion of the degree of reversibility of airway obstruction of M. Smith.

Would you like to make a hypothesis now (as opposed to gathering more information)?

**NO

We will now consider evidence that leads to a conclusion about the degree of reversibility of airway obstruction of M. Smith.

Here is a conclusion that you may not have considered ....

The fact that the change in Forced-Expiratory-Volume (1sec.) after bronchodilation of M. Smith and the change in Resistance after bronchodilation are known is evidence that there are bronchodilation test results (RULE Ø28)

Given the post bronchodilation test results, does this tell you that the degree of reversibility of airway obstruction is slight?

**YES

No, given this fact, we can conclude that the degree of reversibility of airway obstruction of M. Smith is significant (RULE Ø2Ø)

The degree of reversibility of airway obstruction would be slight when the change in Forced-Expiratory-Volume (1sec.) after bronchodilation of the patient is between 1 and 5.

Fig.8. Excerpt from PUFF Tutorial.
(From W.J. Clancey et al. Computer applications in Medical Care, October, 1979.)

But again there are many problems for which this kind of careful logical deductive reasoning is not appropriate.

For example it is difficult to use a strictly logical approach to the problem of reconstructing a jigsaw puzzle. A better method is to spread all the pieces out on a large table and identify groups which probably belong together, for example, the sky in the upper part of the picture, fields or trees in the lower part and figures in the foreground. As soon as any two pieces which fit together are identified, assembly can begin and the completed picture grows from several of these small "foci" as more and more pieces are found which fit with those already assembled until finally the growing regions coalesce and all that remains is to fill in the gaps.

This sort of strategy can be modelled by a number of knowledge systems which share a common database and act in parallel, each searching the database for particular patterns of facts from which deductions and new assertions can be made. The whole procedure is rather like a group of children who get together on a rainy afternoon to assemble a large jigsaw puzzle as a joint exercise. A formidable scheduling problem of course arises - in the case of children, to keep them from quarrelling, but in the case of computer processors, which are more patient, to prevent them from becoming locked in a "deadly embrace" in which each process is waiting for another to finish before it can proceed with its own task. A related and even more difficult problem to be faced by these parallel systems is that of being able to backtrack. If two pieces of the jigsaw happen to fit together but do not really belong together, then in order for the picture to be completed they must at some stage be taken apart again. This operation of discarding an unsuccessful hypothesis and trying again can be fairly simply implemented for a single process, but the difficulties are compounded for numbers of co-operating processes. Furthermore in anything like a complex problem, backtracking needs to be guided by an efficient strategy for selecting the next hypothesis (frame or prototype etc.) if the deductive system is to have any hope of making progress.

The problems can be ameliorated by adopting an hierarchical organization with low level processes combining primitive observations and passing the results upwards to processes operating at successively higher levels of abstraction.

There is another way in which this notion of a conceptual hierarchy can be applied:- We can reason about the way in which we approach the problem. Referring back to the simple example given earlier, there was a choice between using Rule 5 or Rule 7 in order to deduce the truth of X. The attempt to perform the deduction using Rule 5 failed. If we had started with Rule 7 on the other hand we would have been able to go directly to the solution. Could we devise rules to advise us which rules to try first? These can be called 'meta rules' - rules about rules - in the example we might have had a rule:-

<u>If</u> there are rules with J in the premise
<u>then</u> try these rules preferentially.

The advantages of using the rule formalism to guide the evaluation process are similar to those which can be adduced for using rules in the first place. "Knowledge expressed in rules comes in modular chunks which are easy to understand and easy to change."

You may by this time be wondering if there is really any practical use for what seems to be a rather "ivory tower" approach to abstract problem solving by large complex computer programs which attempt to model human thought.

At the Pacific Medical Centre in San Francisco there is a pulmonary function laboratory where just such a system (appropriately called 'PUFF') is in daily use. Patients coming into the laboratory submit to a number of routine tests of pulmonary capacity, air-flow, lung compliance and blood gas estimations. These are all summed up in half a page of numbers giving the values of all the various estimates. This mass of numbers however, requires a good deal of expertise to interpret and is quite useless as a report to be sent out to the refering clinician. The 'PUFF' program receives this batch of numbers and applies logical rules to determine the best explanation, finally producing a written report, giving in comprehensible English, the indicated conclusion e.g. "The patient is suffering from obstructive airways disease" together with a list of the most important findings providing evidence for this conclusion as well as standard recommendations for therapy etc.

Example:-
Smoking probably exacerbates the severity of the patient's airway obstruction, discontinuation of smoking should help to ease the symptoms, good response to bronchodilators is consistent with an asthmatic condition and their continued use is indicated, the high diffusing capacity is consistent with asthma.
Pulmonary function diagnosis: Severe obstructive airways disease, asthmatic type.

(From Jan S. Aikins, HPP-79-10)

The reports are of course checked by the consulting physician before they are sent out. On the afternoon when I was there only two, out of a batch of some two dozen, required a hand written annotation - in both cases to take account of prior examinations, the results of which were 'unknown' to PUFF.

The program was initially developed using a system EMYCIN which consists of the inference mechanisms developed for MYCIN, a program which is able to provide expert diagnostic assistance to a physician treating patients with septicaemia and meningitis. After the PUFF rules (some 40 in all) had been developed and proven the Emycin environment (Emycin runs on a large PDP 10 at the SUMEX facility at Stanford University, California), the entire system was coded by hand in BASIC to run in batch mode on a moderate sized PDP 11 at the Pacific Medical Centre.

Puff is in a sense unusual because the "human interface" is all at the output. Assembling descriptive phrases to produce a report which reads in a reasonably natural and connected manner is not too difficult in a restricted domain, it becomes much harder as the domain of discourse becomes more complicated. As users become more accustomed to intelligible computer output, there is likely to be an increasing demand for fluency as the surprise that a computer can produce anything other than simple numbers wears off.

The human interface for input data is however an even more difficult problem. We often hear it said that no ordinary user can be expected to manipulate a typewriter keyboard. Suggested alternatives vary from the exotic - voice or hand written input - to the simplest - YES/NO/? buttons.

Most of the expert systems in current use rely on conventional VDU terminals and use YES/NO or menu selection techniques wherever practical, reverting to straightforward input, backed by automatic spelling correction and extensive immediate validation checks, for more complex questions. This is probably the sensible technical "state of the art" solution, but a great deal of care is still needed to phrase questions comprehensibly and to ask questions in an intuitively "reasonable" sequence. Internal representational devices such as meta-rules and prototypes are of great help here.

I have previously emphasised the importance of the ability of expert systems to explain their actions. Most existing systems are still a little clumsy in this respect, but the needed improvements are more cosmetic than fundamental because the systems are at least deliberately designed to use computational mechanisms, like logical deduction, which can be understood in human terms.

The outstanding problem today is how to create, modify, update, improve and debug the knowledge base. The use of production systems consisting of modular, largely independent rules has been a great step forward. Techniques for organising rules - meta rules and prototype structures - help by keeping the knowledge explicit and correspondingly more comprehensible, but the knowledge still has to come from somewhere in the first place.

There are two possible sources, on the one hand we may question a human expert - or panel of experts - on the other hand we may try to devise computer programs, which formulate new rules by a process of induction.

Expressing knowledge as rules which can be used in a production system is not easy. It is an art, just as writing conventional sequential, algorithmic computer programs is also an art and both require considerable but different skills. A high level computer language such as ALGOL, PASCAL or ADA provides a framework for expressing algorithms and supplies useful control structures such as "For..step..until..do.." Furthermore such languages continually check that references to objects, whether data objects or program objects, are fully and consistently specified. In a similar vein, programs are being developed for constructing expert systems, these could well be languages in the same sense as Algol etc., but because AI workers commonly use the environment provided by interactive LISP, expert systems are usually created interactively by a sort of bootstrapping operation involving an expert system whose expertise lies in constructing expert systems!

```
Example:-
You need to specify:  Rule  evaluator,Knowledge  sources,Control
You may modify:  Hypothesis  structure
(AGE keeps track of what has and has not been specified)
What do you want to do next?
:: kn
What is the name of the KS you want to create or add rules to?
```

```
:: wholesentencerules
(New knowledge source)
What events invoke this knowledge source?
:: always (Always means any event can be a precondition to this knowledge source)
Between which Hypothesis levels does this KS make inferences?
From?
:: letter
To?
:: alphaletter
From?
:: none
Which links are used to record inferences made by this KS?
:: possiblevalue (Possiblevalue links will connect elements from the letter
                  level to possible values in the alphaletter level)
Inverse link?
:: possiblevalue/of
Link?
:: assignedvalue (Assignedvalue links will connect positively assigned values
                  from the alphaletters to the crypt letters on the letter level)
Inverse link?
:: assigned/to
Link?
:: none
Do you want to use multiple or single hit strategy for this KS?
You can specify Onceonly with Single or Multiple.
:: single onceonly (Single to fire only one rule and Onceonly to mark that rule
                    so that it won't be fired again)
Local variables can be defined as (variable value) or (variable).
Define a local variable.
:: (wordnodes ($value 'cryptogram part))
(Store the node names for the word nodes in WORDNODES. The function $VALUE
retrieves those names by following the "part" link from the CRYPTOGRAM node)
Define a local variable
:: (word)
Define a local variable.
:: (irs)
Define a local variable.
:: done
                        (From H. Penny Nii and Nelleke Aiello. HPP-79-4)
```

Some systems of this kind, attempt to classify new rules as they are being created and to assist the "Rule provider more or less actively".

```
Example:-
    (The expert is in the middle of a normal rule acquisition sequence, when he
    mentions an organism name that the system has never encountered before.)
The new rule will be called RULE384
  If 1 - THE SITE OF THE CULTURE IS BLOOD
     2 - THE PORTAL OF ENTRY OF THE ORGANISM IS THE URINARY TRACT
     3 - THE PATIENT HAS NOT HAD A GENITO-URINARY MANIPULATIVE PROCEDURE
     4 - CYSTITIS IS NOT A PROBLEM FOR WHICH THE PATIENT HAS BEEN TREATED
  Then
     1 - THE ORGANISM IS LIKELY (.4) TO BE AN E.COLI
```

```
Sorry, but I don't understand  THE ORGANISM IS LIKELY (.4) TO BE AN E.COLI
because these words are unknown:  E.COLI
(TEIRESIAS finds it cannot generate any interpretations of the text, so it reprints
the original line, and specifies where the trouble is.  This makes it possible for
the expert to figure out what it is that is new to the system.)
Would you care to try rephrasing that?
++**Y
(Please use *'s to mark what you think might be a new clinical parameter or a new
value of a clinical parameter)
     1 - THE ORGANISM IS LIKELY (.4) TO BE AN *E.COLI*
(While the language in this example is very simple, there are more complex cases
where it would be quite hard to decide from the context what sort of new item the
expert had in mind.  To avoid the necessity for more sophisticated natural language
handling, he is asked to mark off the new word or phrase with asterisks.)
It looks as though  E.COLI
refers to a new value of a clinical parameter, correct?
++**Y
  ....is it a new value of the identity of an organism?
++**Y
(...and with the new item clearly marked, the system can then do some very simple
 pattern matching to decide what's going on.)
                                                   (From Randal Davis.  AIM-283.)
```

The attempt simply to capture existing human knowledge is inevitably limited, if for no other reason, by the number of cooperative humanexperts available. It is tempting to try and devise techniques for exposing computers directly to the facts and letting them divine rules for themselves. A fairly simple technique described by Quinlan is as follows:- Suppose that we have a large collection of fixed-length records with fields as shown,

Sex (M/F)
Age (in years)
Social class (I,II,III,IV)
Cigarette smoker (YES/NO)
Area of residence (London, Southern England, Midland, Wales, Northern England, Scotland)
Lung cancer (YES/NO)

and say that we wish to predict the incidence of lung cancer from the other data. There are well known statistical techniques for tackling such problems, but as I have already pointed out statistical formulations are not susceptible to easily understood exposition.

Instead we take a random sample of, say 100, records and select the attribute which best divides the sample. This allows us to formulate a simple rule:- <u>If</u> an individual is a cigarette smoker
<u>then</u> lung cancer is likely to be recorded.

The simple rule can perhaps be elaborated:-

<u>If</u> an individual is a cigarette smoker
<u>then</u> conclude "Member of Subject Risk (SR) group".
<u>If</u> an individual is SR
<u>and</u> social class IV
<u>then</u> conclude "Member of High Risk (HR) group".

The most economical expression of all such rules is a "decision tree" which successively partitions the sample on each attribute

```
If cigarette smoker
  then if social class = IV
       then if age = 40 to 50
            then if area of residence = Midlands
                 then diagnosis lung cancer          (25)
                 if area of residence = Scotland
                 then diagnosis lung cancer          (10)
                 else diagnosis not lung cancer      (30)
            else      diagnosis not lung cancer      (20)
       else           diagnosis not lung cancer      ( 4)
  else if sex = M
       then           diagnosis lung cancer          ( 1)
       else           diagnosis not lung cancer      (10)
```

Next the decision tree procedure is tested on more cases randomly selected from the data and any "exceptions" (i.e. misclassified examples) are retained and added to the original sample. When - say - 10 such exceptions have been gathered the entire procedure is carried out again on the expanded sample to derive a new (revised) set of rules, or decision tree. This iteration is carried out again and again until no exceptions are found, or until exceptions are sufficiently rare for the rules to be considered practical and useful.

Ross Quinlan has studied the properties of such a procedure in the context of predicting the outcome of a chess endgame. I have also obtained promising results from applying the procedure to predict diagnoses from records of descriptions of Electroencephalograms.

An alternative but related technique involves the use of a teacher to present a carefully planned sequence of examples and counter-examples. In this latter case the emphasis is on the ability of the program to define attributes (or concepts) to enable it to distinguish between positive and negative examples, whereas the iterative procedure takes the attributes as given and concentrates on the problem of economical decision, using a fixed set of attributes and considering the resulting rule (or decision tree) as a "concept".

In whatever way an expert system is constructed, whether by deriving rules in consultation with human experts or by some automatic learning procedure, the result, when a working system has been achieved, is a codified, tested body of knowledge which represents the essence of expertise in the domain. Provided that it is not too complex, it can be reprinted in human language as a rule book or code of practice which may be quite simply used by ordinary humans in every day life. This phenomenon has been termed "knowledge refining" and is perhaps the most unexpected aspect of the use of computers as an aid to thought.

Summary

Expert systems provide a developing corpus of techniques for storing human knowledge in the context of automatic retrieval. The techniques of symbolic logic are used to improve the quality of the data and provide useful and manageable recall. The result is comprehensible not only as to factual content but also may be placed in context. Techniques are being developed which will allow Expert Systems to acquire new knowledge either from a teacher or by surveying large numbers of data records.

H. R. A. TOWNSEND 1981

AIDE A L'EDUCATION DE LA PAROLE DES ENFANTS SOURDS

Francis DESTOMBES (x) et René DISSOUBRAY (xx)

(x) IBM France, 36 avenue R. Poincaré, 75116 Paris
(xx) INJS, 254 rue Saint-Jacques, 75005 Paris

1. RECHERCHE JOINTE INJS-IBM FRANCE

Le prototype présenté est un système expérimental d'aide à la rééducation de la parole pour les enfants sourds, qui a été conçu et développé par le Centre Scientifique IBM France dans le cadre d'une recherche jointe avec l'Institut National de Jeunes Sourds de Paris (INJS). Il permet d'analyser la voix d'un enfant ou de son professeur, et d'afficher en temps réel sur un écran une représentation de paramètres vocaux. Le but est de fournir un moyen de contrôle visuel à l'enfant, afin de pallier la déficience de son contrôle auditif, et d'aider le professeur dans une séance de rééducation de la parole.

Une première version a été installée à l'INJS, qui procède à son évaluation dans le cadre réel de l'éducation de la parole, et peut ainsi identifier au fur et à mesure les modifications fonctionnelles qui peuvent améliorer l'utilité ou la facilité d'emploi du système. Afin de faciliter l'évolution du prototype pour prendre en compte ces améliorations, la conception a été faite en cherchant à réaliser les fonctions par logiciel plutôt que par des dispositifs matériels, chaque fois que cela était techniquement possible.

2. MATERIEL

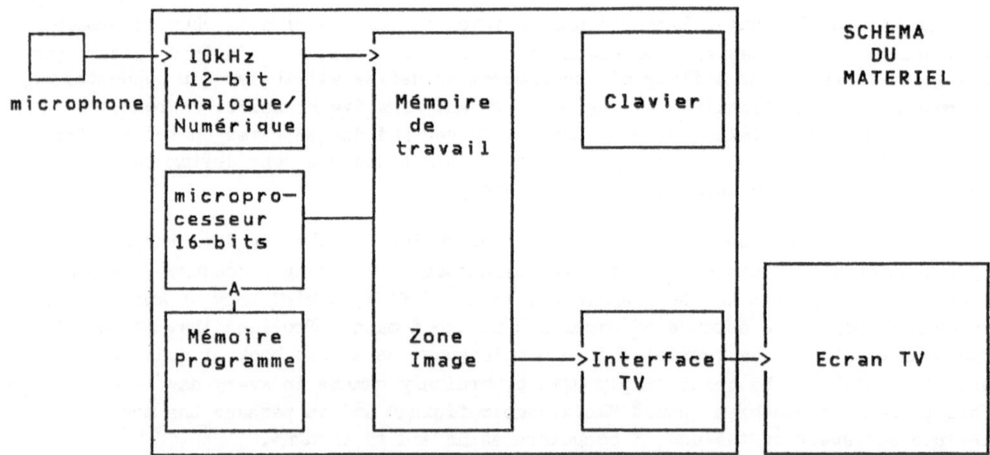

Les fonctions réalisées par le matériel se limitent à:

- Filtrage analogique à 5 kHz et échantillonnage à 10 kHz.
- Conversion des échantillons d'analogique en numérique (12 bits).
- Affichage d'une image sur l'écran de télévision connecté. Cette image (256 lignes de 256 points) est régénérée 50 fois par seconde à partir d'une matrice de 256x256 bits contenue dans la mémoire du système. La réalisation des différents graphismes affichés (caractères, courbes, dessins animés) est donc entièrement sous le contrôle du logiciel.

3. LOGICIEL

Comme il a été indiqué, les fonctions essentielles du système sont réalisées par le logiciel contenu dans la mémoire morte, en particulier:

- Calcul de l'intensité et de la fréquence fondamentale à partir du signal vocal échantillonné à 10 kHz.
- Affichage des résultats de calcul sous forme de courbes en fonction du temps. Possibilité de séparer l'écran en deux parties pour comparer les résultats de l'enfant à ceux du professeur.
- Affichage de résultats sous forme de jeux animés par la voix.
- Défilement vertical de l'image (flot continu d'informations) grâce à un processeur programmable d'entrées/sorties contenu dans l'interface d'affichage. Cette possibilité a été définie afin d'utiliser le système pour des recherches sur l'assistance à la lecture labiale. Elle pourrait peut-être s'avérer utile également pour l'éducation de la parole, en affichant simultanément de multiples paramètres vocaux, et non seulement l'intensité et la fréquence fondamentale.

4. CONCLUSION

L'informatique a renouvelé l'intérêt pour la recherche sur les aides technologiques pour l'éducation de la parole (voir bibliographie). Le prototype présenté illustre deux aspects importants de l'apport potentiel des microprocesseurs dans ce domaine. D'une part, la rapidité des calculs permet d'effectuer des traitements informatiques complexes en temps réel sur les données d'origine (ici, le signal vocal échantillonné), qui restent donc disponibles pour une évolution ultérieure des fonctions du système. D'autre part, la souplesse du logiciel offre une grande variété de présentations visuelles des résultats de calcul, afin de les rendre plus exploitables ou plus attrayants.

Néanmoins, une utilisation effective des techniques informatiques suppose la prise en compte des facteurs humains, qui sont particulièrement importants dans une telle application. C'est pourquoi ce prototype doit être considéré comme un outil d'assistance aux professeurs, éducateurs spécialisés ou orthophonistes, dont le rôle est essentiel pour évaluer son utilité, et pour définir les améliorations fonctionnelles qu'il est souhaitable de lui apporter.

5. BIBLIOGRAPHIE

(1) S. Barth : Application des procédés de reconnaissance automatique de la parole à l'aide aux déficients auditifs profonds; Thèse INJS, 1975.

(2) F. Destombes : Utilisation d'APL dans la construction d'un système microprocesseur; Etude F.006 Centre Scientifique IBM France, janvier 1980

(3) F. Destombes, H. Reine : raster scan TV interface; IBM Technical Disclosure Bulletin, Vol. 22, No. 11, 11 avril 1980

(4) F. Destombes, G. Baudry, M.D. Di Benedetto, H. Reine, J.P. Tubach : Un système microprocesseur d'aide à l'éducation de la parole; Congrès AFCET Informatique, 24 Novembre 1980.

(5) J.P. Haton, M.C. Haton : SIRENE : un projet de Système Interactif pour la Rééducation vocale des Enfants Non-Entendants Rev. Gén Ens. Déf. Auditifs, 4ème trimestre 1975, pages 203-9.

(6) A. Risberg : Visual aids for speech correction; Amer. Ann. Deaf, 113, 1968, pages 178-94

(7) J. Martony : On the correction of the voice pitch level for severely hard of hearing subjects; Amer. Ann. Deaf, 113, 1968, pages 195-202.

(8) J. Martony : Visual aids for speech correction : summary of three years' experience; In G. Fant (ed.), Speech communication ability and profound deafness Washington, 1970, pages 345-9.

(9) R.A. Nickerson, K.M. Stevens : Teaching speech to the deaf: can a computer help?; IEEE trans. Audio Electroacoust., 21, Oct 1973, pages 445-55.

MICROINFORMATIQUE ET REEDUCATION DU LANGAGE

Gérard DELOCHE,* Philippe VAN EECKHOUT,†
Evelyne ANDREEWSKY,* Xavier SERON▲ et Pierre JUTIER.**

1. INTRODUCTION

Les méthodes traditionnelles de rééducation (ou d'apprentissage) du langage se heurtent aux problèmes que posent les erreurs de l'élève. Il s'agit là d'un problème important car, d'une part, les méthodes "sans erreurs" rendent l'apprentissage plus efficace et, d'autre part, les corrections délivrées n'assurent pas leur non renouvellement. Ainsi, dans l'écriture manuscrite sous dictée, le sujet peut fort bien retenir l'orthographe erronée au lieu de la forme correcte des mots. Pour supprimer les effets négatifs de l'apparition des erreurs sur les performances des sujets, quatre conditions doivent être requises :

a) toute erreur doit être signalée sans délai;

b) elle ne doit pas être visualisée par le sujet;

c) la suite de l'exercice est conditionnée par la correction de l'erreur;

d) la difficulté des exercices doit être adaptée aux capacités du sujet; des procédures de facilitation visent à la prévention des erreurs.

Ne pouvant satisfaire à la condition b dans le cadre des exercices habituellement pratiqués dans un centre de rééducation du langage, nous avons utilisé des systèmes informatiques où le contrôle instantané de l'activité du sujet permet un traitement différenciel des erreurs. Nous présentons ici deux applications de cette démarche expérimentale : l'aide à la rééducation de certaines dysorthographies et l'aide à la thérapie mélodique et rythmée du langage.

---

* INSERM U.84, 47 Bd. de l'Hôpital, 75013 Paris,
† Service du Pr. F. Lhermitte, 47 Bd. de l'Hôpital, 75013 Paris.
▲ Service de Neuropsychologie, Université de Louvain, Belgique.
** INSERM U.88, 91 Bd. de l'Hôpital, 75013 Paris.

2. REEDUCATION DES TROUBLES DE L'ORTHOGRAPHE

2.1. Méthode

Le système se compose d'un clavier de machine à écrire et d'un écran TV reliés à un miniordinateur. Le thérapeute dicte une série de mots choisis en fonction du trouble particulier à rééduquer. La liste de mots ayant été préalablement enregistrée, le programme dispose ainsi de l'orthographe correcte de ceux-ci. Aussi longtemps que le sujet ne se trompe pas en sélectionnant les touches du clavier, les lettres correspondantes apparaissent sur l'écran. En cas d'erreur, un bref signal sonore retentit, avertissant ainsi immédiatement le sujet qu'il vient de faire une erreur (condition a); la lettre correspondante n'est pas affichée (condition b réalisée par suppression du "feedback" visuel en cas d'erreur); l'affichage des lettres est bloqué tant que l'erreur n'est pas corrigée (condition c). La condition d est satisfaite au moyen d'information visuelle sur le nombre de lettres qui constituent le mot (à l'aide de petits cadres) et par une progression des difficultés des exercices liée à un taux de réussite élevé (90%). Enfin, les listes de mots ont été constituées à l'issue d'une recherche des règles de passage du code oral au code écrit portant sur les 5000 mots les plus fréquents du français. Les exercices portent ainsi sur un échantillon illustrant les règles les plus usitées et leurs principales exceptions.

2.2. Résultats

Notre objectif thérapeutique étant la récupération de l'orthographe en écriture manuscrite, cette méthode de rééducation ne se justifie que dans la mesure où il y a (partiellement au moins) transfert de l'apprentissage réalisé dans cette situation (machine à écrire) à la situation habituelle (écriture cursive). Une amélioration significative des performances en écriture manuscrite a été mise en évidence à l'issue des rééducations expérimentales entreprises, aussi bien avec des adultes aphasiques (1) qu'avec des enfants dysorthographiques (2).

3. THERAPIE MELODIQUE ET RYTHMEE

Cette thérapie, dérivée de la technique MIT (3) est utilisée avec succès chez des sujets aphasiques pour le déblocage des mutismes et la suppression des stéréotypies (4).

Toutefois, certains aphasiques, qui ne peuvent reproduire des rythmes ou des mélodies simples ne peuvent bénéficier de cette thérapie. Certains exercices, portant sur la reconnaissance, la reproduction et la création de rythmes et de mélodies sonores permettent cependant d'amener ces malades au niveau où la thérapie mélodique et rythmée pourra être entreprise. L'appareillage utilisé se compose d'un micro-ordinateur, d'un écran TV, d'un clavier et d'un haut parleur. Les rythmes sonores sont visualisés sur l'écran; le sujet intervient en programmant ses propres rythmes et mélodies grâce aux touches du clavier.

4. CONCLUSION - PERSPECTIVES

L'efficacité de ce type de technique tient, selon nous, à la véritable interaction qui s'établit entre le sujet et le programme d'apprentissage (traitement différentiel des réponses, déclenchement de procédures de facilitation) ainsi qu'à l'aspect ludique des exercices (jouer avec un clavier de machine à écrire et un récepteur TV). Enfin, les progrès rapides de la technologie des micro-processeurs permettront bientôt de rendre largement accessible (faible coût, souplesse d'utilisation) des systèmes autonomes (5).

5. REFERENCES

(1) Seron X, Deloche G, Moulard G, Rousselle M. A computer-based therapy for the treatment of aphasic subjects with writing disorders. Journal of Speech and Hearing Disorders, 1980 ; 45 : 45-58.

(2) Deloche G, Rousselle M, Moulard G, Seron X. Rééducation assistée par ordinateur dans certaines dysorthographies. Rééducation Orthophonique, 1978 ; 16 (99) : 9-24.

(3) Sparks R, Helm N, Albert M. Aphasia rehabilitation resulting from melodic intonation therapy. Cortex, 1974 ; 10 : 303-316.

(4) Van Eeckhout P, Allichon J. Rééducation par la mélodie des sujets atteints d'aphasie. Rééducation Orthophonique, 1978 ; 16 (99) : 25-32.

(5) Jutier P, Andreewsky E, Deloche G, Nicolas P. Microprocessor-based system using a commercial tape-recorder both as a digital and audio device. In Proceedings of Measurement and Control Symposium, Athens, 1978; Vol.3 : 796-799.

ON THE DESIGN OF AN AUTOMATIC HOSPITAL

KRISHNA KANT

APPROPRIATE AUTOMATION PROMOTION LABORATORY

ELECTRONICS COMMISSION

E-WING, PUSHPA BHAVAN

NEW DELHI - 110062

SUMMARY

The paper discusses the application of computer aided diagnosis approach to provide the cheap, efficient and easily approachable medical facility. A centralized computer communication network (with a central computer and intelligent terminals) system with medical and patients data bases and diagnosis software system on the central computer has been discussed. This system acts as a automatic hospital/ health care centre.

1. INTRODUCTION

Computer aided diagnosis has been a subject of research since more than twenty years. The approaches developed to design the computer algorithm to diagnose a disease, based on a set of symptoms can be categorised as statistical or logical. The statistical models are based on the Bayes' theorem (1,2) of conditional probability, linear discriminant functions (3,4) and matching procedures (1). The logical algorithm uses decision tree model using sequential questioning methods (4,5,6). In both the approaches a data base structure has to be developed to store, update, insert, delete and retrieve the information regarding diseases, symptoms and the relation among them. A typical configuration (7) of a computer aided diagnostic system for development, test and use is shown in Fig. 1.

The present paper describes an on-line computer communication network for automatic diagnosis and treatment prescription.

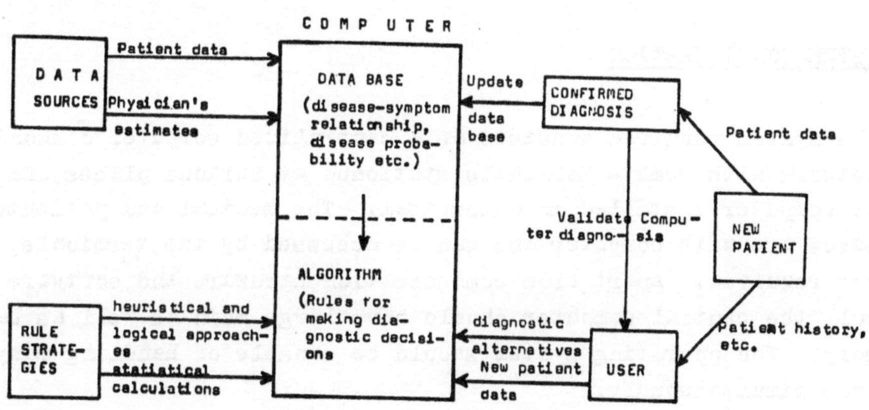

Fig.1: Computer Aided Diagnostic System - development, test and use

2. MEDICAL FACILITIES AND PROBLEMS

The objective of providing an efficient, fast and cheap medical facility to each individual cannot be achieved with the existing number of physicians and medical facilities. Moreover, because of that the physician in various hospitals and health care centres are heavily loaded and patients have to wait for a long time for their turn to see a physician. This not only deteriorates the performance of physicians but also has adverse effects on patients. There are also places (for example - heavy snowfall areas during winter) where regular medical facility cannot be provided. In Japan (Tohoku district and areas facing sea) remote health care stations are opened and examination sheet/ patient's history are communicated to a centralized hospital (TSUGAWA - Cho in Japan) using facsimile. On receiving the transmitted sheets the physicians write indications for treatments which are sent back using facsimile units. In this system the problem of transportation has been solved by computer communication. But the patients have to wait longer and physicians are equally loaded.

Thus there is a need of the application of automatic diagnosis to solve this problem.

3. SYSTEM CONFIGURATION

The system required consists of a centralized computer communication network with remote terminals stationed at various places and central computer installed in a hospital. The medical and patients data bases are with computer and can be accessed by the terminals, whenever required. Apart from communication hardware and software protocol, the central computer should have large main as well as back up memory. The operating system should be capable of handling many terminals simultaneously.

4. MEDICAL AND PATIENTS DATA BASES

Following factors should be considered while constructing a medical data base:-

- source of information
- diseases included
- number and types of indicants to be used

Medical text books, physicians' and experts' opinions and estimates hospital and emergency room medical records, etc., form the possible sources of information, to be stored in data base.

It is not necessary to include all the classes of diseases. There are total 17 major disease classes in ICDA. The data base should include only those classes/subclasses which do not need any emergency treatment or expert opinions (e.g. category V, VI and XVII). For other types of diseases the software should recommend suitable expert physicians.

Indicants are defined to include the features of patients' conditions like patient history, symptoms, examination results, etc. The number and type of indicants in the data base effects the diagnostic accuracy. The more powerful are the indicants, the more accurate the diagnosis (8). But clearly the data base in this application cannot include the indicants like lab. test, etc.

Thus following information will be stored in the medical data base:-

- symptoms
- diseases
- treatments
- expert physicians for all the types of diseases.

Moreover a data base of patients particulars, symptoms, disease diagnosed and treatment prescribed should also be maintained.

5. DIAGNOSIS SOFTWARE SYSTEM

The diagnosis software is the heart of the system. For this application, the diagnosis should be based on the logical approach. The system should be interactive i.e. it should ask as many questions as possible. While feeding the answers, the patients should be required to input minimum possible. As an example - A typical software system DOCTOR developed asks questions and a patient is required to input only either Y (for Yes) or N (for No) in response to these (See APPENDIX).

As soon as a patient accesses the system it should bring into main memory the complete history of the patient from data base. The further diagnosis and prescription should be based on the information stored in patients database. If the patient's condition is serious the system by itself should be able to send a call for ambulance at that particular terminal. If the patient is not serious and the system is not able to diagnose then it should suggest the patient to go to a particular physician based on the type of disease. The system can also to produce the case history of patients at the computer so that it can reach the particular physician prior to the patient. This will help physician during examination of the patient.

6. DOCTOR

This software system has been developed by using language TICOL on SILENT-700 (Texas Instruments Inc.) Intelligent Terminal. It is fully interactive and diagnoses the simple diseases like malaria on the basis of answers received from patients. If it is not able to diagnose it recommends a doctor suitable to patient. A typical output of system is placed at APPENDIX.

7. CONCLUSIONS

The concept of automatic hospital, though easy to conceive, is very difficult to implement in practice. The implementation requires a major development of the software systems, along with the logical algorithms for various classes of diseases. The system developed should be tested by simulating with real life data, from hospital records, to successfully demonstrate acceptability to and compatibility with users.

REFERENCES

1. Approach to a reliable program for computer aided medical diagnosis; Birk R.E, ENDRES L., McDonald J.C. Proctor L.D., Rinaldo J.A. and Rube C.E., Aerosp. Med. 45 (1974).

2. Computer assisted diagnosis of abdominal using estimates provided by clinicians, Leaper D.J., Horrocks J.C., Stainland J.R. and DE Dombal F.T., Br. Med. Jr. 4(1974).

3. The use of multiple measurements in taxonomic problems, Fisher R.A. Ann. Engen. 7(1972).

4. Mathematical methods in medical diagnosis, Croft D.J. and Machol R.E., Ann. Bomed. Eng. 2(1974).

5. Is computerized diagnosis possible? Croft D.J., Comput. Bio-Med. Res. 5(1972).

6. Rules for sequential diagnosis; Rector A.L. and Ackerman E, Comput. Biomed. Res 8(1975).

7. Computer aided medical diagnosis, Rogers, W., Ryack B. and Moller G. Inter. Jr. Biomed. Comput. 4(1979).

8. A comparison of methods for automated diagnosis of thyroid dysfunction, Nordyke R.A., Kulikowski C.A., and Kulikowski C.W., Comput. Biomed. Res. 4(1971).

APPENDIX

```
+++++++++++++++++++++++++++++++++++++++++++++++
YOU ARE WITH AN EFFICIENT AND FRANK DOCTOR

PLEASE BE FRANK IN CONVAYING YOUR TROUBLE

ATTN. LADIES! I AM NEUTRAL .SO BE FRANK.
+++++++++++++++++++++++++++++++++++++++++++++++


++++  ARE YOU A LADY?Y


++++ COULD YOU LIKE TO GO TO A LADY
     DOCTOR IN CASE I AM NOT ABLE TO
     DIAGNOSE?Y


++++ ARE YOU HAVING FEVER?Y


++++  ARE YOU HAVING PAIN?N


++++ ARE YOU FEELING COLD?Y


++++  ANY THING ELSE?N
+++++++++++++++++++++++++++++++++++++++++++++++

  YOU ARE SUFFERING FROM MALRIA .GET

  YOUR BLOOD TESTED.TAKE A DOSE OF

  CHLOROQUINE SUITABLE TO YOUR AGE.


+++++++++++++++++++++++++++++++++++++++++++++

GOOD LUCK

+++++++++++++++++++++++++++++++++++++++++++
```

```
◆◆◆◆◆◆◆◆◆◆◆◆◆◆◆◆◆◆◆◆◆◆◆◆◆◆◆◆◆◆◆◆◆◆◆◆◆◆◆◆◆◆◆◆◆
YOU ARE WITH AN EFFICIENT AND FRANK DOCTOR

PLEASE BE FRANK IN CONVAYING YOUR TROUBLE

ATTN. LADIES! I AM NEUTRAL .SO BE FRANK.
◆◆◆◆◆◆◆◆◆◆◆◆◆◆◆◆◆◆◆◆◆◆◆◆◆◆◆◆◆◆◆◆◆◆◆◆◆◆◆◆◆◆◆◆◆



◆◆◆◆  ARE YOU A LADY?N



◆◆◆◆ ARE YOU HAVING FEVER?Y



◆◆◆◆  ARE YOU HAVING PAIN?Y



◆◆◆◆ ARE YOU FEELING COLD?N



◆◆◆◆  ANY THING ELSE?N



◆◆◆◆◆◆◆◆◆◆◆◆◆◆◆◆◆◆◆◆◆◆◆◆◆◆◆◆◆◆◆◆◆◆◆◆◆◆◆◆◆◆

  TAKE ANALGINE AND RELAX.



◆◆◆◆◆◆◆◆◆◆◆◆◆◆◆◆◆◆◆◆◆◆◆◆◆◆◆◆◆◆◆◆◆◆◆◆◆◆◆◆
GOOD LUCK

◆◆◆◆◆◆◆◆◆◆◆◆◆◆◆◆◆◆◆◆◆◆◆◆◆◆◆◆◆◆◆◆◆◆◆◆◆◆◆


  MORE?N
```

THE EVOLUTION OF A DATA COMMUNICATIONS NETWORK IN AN UNIVERSITY HOSPITAL

Rita M James and Richard O Viale
Hospital University of Pennsylvania
Philadelphia, Pennsylvania 19104

Summary. The Hospital University of Pennsylvania has designed and completed the first of three phases of a data communications network. The network has a star topology, and its message protocol is based on message broadcasting. The central node, governing the network, is currently linked to five peripheral systems: Laboratory, Radiology, Financial, Admissions, and Patient Management. Technically the network has presented no problems. Its modularity parallels the Hospital's organization and catalyzes indepth departmental analysis and system design. Aspects of physical planning for the network were not unusual. In our hands, the methods for training large numbers of users needs more investigation. Most importantly, the network is cost beneficial.

1.0 Introduction. The Hospital University of Pennsylvania (HUP), in Philadelphia, is currently in the beginning of the second of three phases of the implementation of a data communications system. Briefly the three phases are

- -Develop and install a star network consisting of the already existing Laboratory, Radiology, and Financial systems and the newly designed Admissions and Patient Management systems (1,2)
- -Design, develop, and install a Medical Records system and an Out-Patient Registration system, both as new nodes in the network
- -Extend the Patient Management functionality to include all Nursing Station data communication activities and expand the network to encompass all ancillary services.

The star network concept has given HUP a degree of flexibility not usually found in hospital information systems. This flexibility arises from the independent nature of each network node; the design of each nodal system is limited only by the message protocol for communicating with the central node. In this concept, system management and control remain at the departmental level, but at the same time interdepartmental cooperation is enhanced.

The focus, herein, is on the flexibility, as already exhibited in the first phase, of the star network concept. Our experiences in design, policy, procedures, training, physical planning, and costs are discussed. Since no system is ideal, disadvantages of this approach are also noted.

2.0 First Phase Network. The first phase of the HUP data communications system involved the existing Radiology, Financial, data base, and Laboratory systems and the newly designed Admissions and Patient Management systems. The Radiology and the Laboratory systems each use DEC PDP 11/70's. The Financial and data base management systems are Shared Medical Systems' (SMS) products and are resident off-site at the SMS disaster-proof data center on a complex of large-scale IBM computers. The Admissions and the Patient Management systems, although designed to be independent of one another, share one PDP 11/70 and, as such, share some master files; however if the need arises, they can be separated.

Each of the four computers is linked to a centralized PDP 11/34. The task of this "communicator" is to receive messages (reports, results, transactions) from the peripheral nodes and to broadcast them to the nodes designated by Hospital management to receive the messages. In the event that a node is not operational, the "communicator" spools that node's messages for later transmission. If the "communicator" is not operational, the peripheral systems, all of which were originally designed as stand-alone systems, queue their respective transmissions until the "communicator" returns on-line.

The whole network is now supporting 197 terminals and printers, located throughout the Hospital. These devices are distributed by system as follows:

System	Terminals/Printers
Laboratory	30
Radiology	30
Financial	12
Admissions	31
Patient Management	94

Information currently flowing on the network is limited to admission, discharge, and transfer transactions; laboratory results; radiology reports; patient status and condition; and patient insurance and billing data. The Admissions, Medical Records, Business Office, Information Service, Housekeeping, Pathology, and Radiology departments as well as the Nursing Stations use and contribute to the network.

2.1 Technical Critique of the Star Network. The star network concept, which uses broadcasting (and not distributed data bases) and which was designed by one of us (ROV), required a prolonged vendor search because only a few exhibited the expertise and willingness to develop the design; Shared Medical Systems was ultimately selected for the network project because, of the hospital system vendors at the time, only they had done significant research in this area. The SMS implementation has presented no technical difficulties.

In the operations sphere the star network concept requires a greater degree of coordination and computer operator responsibility in Data Processing than is needed in other configurations. Master file maintenance for the several systems requires exacting coordination. Preventative maintenance must be precisely scheduled since different systems have different periods of low activity; although this may be a scheduling problem for Data Processing, it minimizes disruptions from the user point of view. The variety of operating systems lengthens the computer operators' training period and, ideally, always requires two operators to monitor the systems.

The network's modularity provides two important technical advantages. Since each system can operate by itself if necessary, computer equipment failures are significantly less pervasive than for other configurations. The second advantage is only now being tested; the Laboratory system is being replaced and, to-date, no function of the other modules has been degraded. If this advantage is realized, then the star network concept with message broadcasting has a flexibility, which is important in this era of rapidly changing hardware, not found in other configurations.

3.0 Systems Design. Several practical design advantages were discovered during the first phase of the project. As part of the systems design process, an analysis of policies and procedures for each network department is performed; from this analysis emerges a framework for system development consistent with the department's policies. The modularity permitted internal departmental analysis to be performed in a step distinct from the analysis of data needs outside the department. Thus the analyses have been able to be done in much greater depth with the given resources than if the Hospital were analyzed as a whole. Besides serving the systems' design, including backup procedures, the indepth analyses gave the Administration an opportunity to update policies and procedures and to have them in force before the introduction of the respective systems.

3.1 System Users' Manual. In each vendor's contract, the Hospital has successfully negotiated clauses which specify development of a Users' Manual jointly prepared by the Hospital and the vendor. The Users' Manual defines in great detail the system which will be implemented and is the document from which the vendor's programmers will work. The joint preparation assures the Hospital that its specifications are incorporated into the system and defines for the vendor all standards which it must meet. If the Hospital and vendor agree on its contents, then the Manual is appended to the contract, but if either party deems the contents unsatisfactory, the contract may be terminated.

3.2 User Participation in Design. The departmental approach permitted by the network's modularity, the development of the Users' Manual, and the departmental management demanded participation by the users from the earliest stages of system introduction. Departmental management must declare and justify the need for a system. Since supervisory personnel may not be able to provide the detailed steps of all the department's functions, all levels of personnel must participate in the system analysis. Departmental management and supervisory personnel form part of the Users' Manual preparation committee. After the department's internal needs are defined, other Hospital entities participate in defining their respective informational needs from the departmental system. Thus this approach relies heavily on the users' recommendations for design of the departmental system.

4.0 System Implementation. With the completion of the nodal system's design, efforts are shifted to implementation activities. These focus upon planning for the physical and environmental aspects of the installation and monitoring the status of the project.

4.1 Physical Planning. The Hospital is contractually responsible for meeting the physical and environmental specifications provided by the vendor. This responsibility includes the following tasks:

- The various work stations must be prepared for the equipment.
- Cable routes, junction boxes, terminations, and cable acquisition must be planned. The laying of cable in HUP's case was not a minor undertaking. The eleven building complex used more than 15,000 meters of 3-pair, 6-pair, 19-pair, and 27-pair cable to link the network's first phase terminals to the Data Processing machine room's computers; twenty-one junction boxes were strategically located in order to accommodate growth to more than 500 terminals.
- Expansion and upgrade of the machine must be planned, insuring ample electrical capacity, air conditioning, fire extinguishing equipment, and alarm detection.

These plans were made and carried out to accommodate all three phases of the data communications project.

4.2 Project Monitoring. The chief tasks of monitoring center on the physical plant preparation, hardware installation and testing, and, most importantly, software installation and testing. The first two tasks are primarily ones of coordinating contractors, Hospital personnel, and vendors.

The monitoring of software involves three steps, which must be performed for each software entity, including the operating system. First, the software must be checked against the Users' Manual. Second, it is loaded into a "shadow" or training system and tested for competence vis-a-vis the existing software. The software is left in the training system until the specific users are familiar with its function. Third, the software is moved onto the production system, where monitoring is in the form of responding to users' comments. Failure at any one of these steps results in starting the steps again after the software has been corrected and redocumented.

4.3 Project Implementation Organization. At HUP a project team was organized to coordinate and expedite all implementation activities. This team is directed by one of us (RMJ) and includes representatives from the engineering and planning departments as well as the vendor firms. The rennovation project added to the committee a professional construction manager, who directed the activities of the subcontractors. In this ongoing project persons are temporarily added to the committee as their expertise is needed.

5.0 Training. The user training task was the most time-consuming activity undertaken during the first phase network installation. Since the Hospital does not have a department dedicated to personnel training, the responsibility for staff training was assigned to Data Processing. After examining the approaches of several hospitals to computer user training, these basics emerged:

- A training area, away from patient care areas, was set up in order to allow the trainees to concentrate on the instruction.
- Each system's software specifications included a "shadow" or training system, allowing users to have actual computer experience before the system's introduction.
- A Users' Guide was developed for reference to the system's functions. These documents explain the departmental system in simple, non-technical terms and are organized in a step by step procedural format.

5.1 Training Methods. Two distinct training methods were applied during the training programs. For the Admissions module Data Processing trained all users and evaluated their performances; follow-up sessions were scheduled as needed. For the Patient Management module Data Processing trained key people from the Nursing Station; these individuals in turn trained the remaining staff in their areas. The first approach was used because the numbers were small and the tasks highly specialized. The second method evolved because of the large number of Nursing Station personnel (about 2,000 physicians, nurses, and clerks) who needed training for the Patient Management module; this training was somewhat simplified because their first phase functions are primarily queries.

5.2 Training Results. Neither of the two approaches proved more effective than the other. In the one-on-one training, sessions were often slowed by digressions into procedural areas, indicating the need to broaden the scope of this kind of training. While the second method was the only one possible, given Data Processing's resources, it resulted in poor to excellent secondary training, as one might expect. Ultimately, Data Processing had to supplant the training of the worst cases.

Unless a hospital can absorb the costs of a staff education department and the employees' training time, training will be adequate at best. Without such a department the most effective training is experience, trial and error. The benefits of the methods tried at HUP probably do not justify their costs.

6.0 System Costs. Ultimately the measure of any production system is its costs as compared to its benefits. The whole network is currently costing $5.92/patient-day. The second phase is expected to add one-half dollar/patient-day to this total. The projected cost of all three phases is $7.50/patient-day in inflated 1983 dollars; the Data Processing budget including personnel is expected to remain slightly below two percent of the Hospital budget throughout the project. Since the previously existing Laboratory, Radiology, and Financial systems, costing $5.07/patient-day, were already cost-justified as part of their respective implementations, only the incremental cost of the first phase network need be analyzed for benefits; this cost is 85 cents/patient-day.

6.1 System Benefits. Since the data communications first phase has not been operational for a whole fiscal year, the benefits of creating the network can only be projected from three months of financial reports. Benefits have accrued from a one day decrease in outstanding accounts receivable days ($40,000), from a decrease in uncaptured daily room charges ($400,000), and from a decrease in unbillable ancillary services ($600,000); these projected yearly benefits total $4.62/patient-day. Thus the benefits of adding the Admissions and the Patient Management systems and of creating the network exceed their costs by roughly a factor of four.

Bibliography.

(1) Levin M, Morganer R, Packer B. Laboratory Data Management: A Distributed Data Processing Solution. Proc. Fourth Annual Symp. on Computer Applications in Medical Care (IEEE Cat. No. 80CH1570-1); 1980 : 502-4.

(2) Arenson RL, Gitlin JM, London JW. An Operational Management System for Radiology: Innovative Techniques. Proc. Fourth Annual Symp. on Computer Applications in Medical Care (IEEE Cat. No. 80CH1570-1); 1980 : 142-8.

Title: THE VENEREAL B.E.D.E.

Author: Peter A Wigodsky, B.Sc., M.Sc., M.B.C.S., M.I.D.P., F.R.S.S.

Interviews for B.E.D.E. began in August 1979 and the following results are for the first 531 patients. Both male and female patients were interviewed over a range of more than 40 questions in a maximum 5 minutes session. The sample was somewhat selective in that it was only possible to visit the Department regularly on Mondays and Wednesdays, with random visits on alternative days throughout the period.

Initially a pilot questionnaire was employed for some 60 patients and in the light of its applications and results, amendments were made and the master questionnaire introduced. The questionnaire is efficiently structured so as to reduce both coding errors, respondent error and computational errors.

For some 61% of the patients interviews, this visit was part of their first series of visits to the department; thus there is a 39% return level to the same department - this was substantially more than originally thought.

The patient is asked of the time interval between symptoms arising, or being requested to visit the D.G.M., or deciding themselves to come along and actually arriving at the department. Three alternative time spans are presented to the patients and the results are listed below.

TIME INTERVAL	FREQUENCY	PERCENTAGE
Less than 1 week	390	73.3
2 - 4 weeks	69	13.0
More than 4 weeks	69	13.0
Not answered	3	0.7
		100

This first map shows the percentage distribution of the population by place of residence, as given by the respondent. The key, as indicated, is in three main fields with the boroughs in purple having (1)%, orange (1-3)%, and yellow (3-5)%. There are though, three boroughs which have higher individual percentages. These are the City of London (5.3%), Islington (14.8%), and Hackney (7.3%). Discussions with the receptionist within the Department of Genital Medicine, who must complete a standardised form for D.H.S.S. records, confirmed my suspicions that this inflated City rate is caused by patients using the address of their place of work as a means of obtaining further anonymity. The same may apply to some of their claims to live in Hackney. The Boroughs of Islington and Hackney are both easily accessible to the city, where St. Bartholomew's Hospital is situated.

The somewhat low rate for the City of Westminster is quite likely due to the fact that there are three other clinics in the West End area. Those named areas in the right hand corner follow a similar key for the 'dormitory commuter belts' who have employment in the City.

This second map illustrates the percentage distribution of the sample population by geographical area of employment. Not too surprisingly, the areas of the City, and Islington were most prominent with 45%, and 6.7% respectively.

This demographic pyramid and the proceeding one show the percentage distribution of diagnoses by sex of the total patients from each gender. This D series follows the diagnosis coding at St. Bartholomew's:-

D01 : Other Trepenomal Diseases
D02 : Other Conditions
D03 : No V.D.
D04 : Conditions referred elsewhere
D16 : Other conditions requiring treatment
D26 : L.S.& A.(or B.X.O.) Lichen Scelerosis and Atrophicus (or Balanitus Xerotica Obliterans)

The most interesting aspect of this graph is the percentage differences between males and females in the D03 category. Almost one quarter of those male patients interviewed were clear as compared with only 10% of female patients.

Both these tables contain cumulative frequency percentage distributions for patients with up to five diagnoses from patients records. The DHSS coding is as follows:-

A02 : Secondary Syph.
A03 : Latent Syph.
B01 : Post-Pubertal Gon.
C04 : N.S.U.
C07 : Candida
C09 : Pubic Lice
C11 : Warts

The two most prominent features on the C-series are the male patients with C04 diagnoses and female patients with C07. Between all series diagnoses, more categories of male patients are qualified as compared with females.

This pie chart shows the distribution of the sample population by marital status. Unlike the quarterly return forms for the DHSS, status here could be classified from one of single, married, cohabiting, divorced, separated, widowed or unmarried mothers. (By cohabiting is meant where two people are sharing a flat or house and are having regular sexual liasons with one another). 19% of the population were cohabiting (at the time of the interview). Not too surprisingly, half the population were single.

The next series of questions enquired of the age when the patient left school, and whether or not they went on to any further or higher education. Not too surprisingly the distribution was bimodal, with 30% leaving at 16 years of age and 29.5% at 18 years of age.

A staggering 63% said they went on to some form of further or higher education and for this group, their distribution amongst academic sites are listed below. Those listed as other include police cadet school, maritime colleges, etc.

The patients were asked how they knew of the DGM at St. Bartholomew's Hospital. The range of responses was very interesting indeed. Responses recorded as 'common sense' included the patient looking in a telephone directory under "V.D." and also an intuitive guess that a hospital the size of St. Bartholomew's would have such a department.

CATEGORY RESPONSE	FREQUENCY	PERCENTAGE
Already knew	16	3.0
Doctor (G.P.)	137	25.8
Contact	51	9.6
Friend	94	17.7
Family	6	1.2
Common Sense	213	40.1
Samaritans	3	0.6
Others	11	2.0
	531	100

If the patient was in the second series of visits, that knowledge of the department would be recorded from the first instance of having to visit the department.

Several questions relating to alcoholic drinking habits were asked. Using one unit of alcohol as one half pint of beer, or 1 measure of spirits or 1 glass of wine, the average was about 30 units per head per week. Some 61% of patients said that they would drink alcohol on a regular basis (i.e. more than twice a week).

These patients had an average alcoholic rate of 40.6 units per week, and an average time interval of some 54 months at their respective rates. Correlation coefficients using S.P.S.S. were used to identify positive relationships and Cramer's V proved the most reliable.

This table shows the value of V for drinking habits and the first diagnosis as recorded from the patients notes. Unlike other medical statistical tables, the number of persons applicable in each relevant category is indicated. The clearest conclusion is that for the most frequent diagnosis there is a strong relationship with the patients alcoholic habits.

Questions were asked concerning the number of partners in the last one month, three months, and six months (at the time of the interview).

Some patients had difficulty in even estimating the number of partners in the past six months, and these were mainly promiscuous homosexuals.

This slide shows the correlation coefficients dichotemised between clear diagnoses and all other diagnoses. Although a couple of the coefficients are low, the under lying trend overall, is that the patients who were clear have a greater rate of promiscuity than those patients who had a positive clinical diagnosis. Further analysis showed that if a patient was clear at one period, the patient did not decrease the sex frequency or partner frequencies until such a positive diagnosis occurred.

Crosstabulation of Diagnosis (1) By Alcoholic Drinking Habits - Amount and Length of Time

MALE PATIENTS			FEMALE PATIENTS		
Diagnosis	No. Patients	Cramer's V	Diagnosis	No. Patients	Cramer's V
B01	36	0.94648	B01	12	1.00000
C04	119	0.63072	C04	32	0.93541
			C06	7	1.00000
C07	15	1.00000	C07	23	1.00000
C09	8	1.00000			
C11	27	0.91287	C11	10	0.78174
D02	39	0.91287	D02	5	1.00000
D03	95	0.65245	D03	12	1.00000

N.B. Cramer's V is a suitable measure of association, i.e. a measure of strength of relationship. V takes the value of 0 when no relationship exists, and the value of +1 when the variables are perfectly related.

A series of questions were given only to those patients who were male homosexuals. In total there were 93 such persons, who volunteered that they had had homosexual relationships or when asked, admitted so. All the values for mean, median and mode, gave a value of 19 years of first homosexual involvement (as active, passive or mutual masturbation partner) with a range of 31 years (7 - 38 years old). Of these 93 patients, 33 (35.5%) had had heterosexual relationships at some point in their lives, and an average age of 18 years was given as the age of such a relationship. Of course, within the 33 patients, a number of practising bisexuals are counted, and thus when asked how many heterosexual relationships (resulting in sexual liasons) they had had, an average of 12 was found.

Various questions to determine a range of sociological indicators are posed. In the first instance the distribution to the question of property status of home is given.

STATUS	FREQUENCY	PERCENTAGE
Owner	169	31.8
Rental	266	50.1
Parental	92	17.3
N/A	4	0.8
	531	100

In the second instance, a question on Car ownership was asked. If the patient had use of a company car, then this was recorded as a NO response, as this car is not owned by him personally.

CAR OWNER	FREQUENCY	PERCENTAGE
Yes	240	45.2
No	286	53.9
N/A	5	0.9
	531	100

In the third case, the number of meals eaten in a restaurant per month is enquired. This may initially seem rather an obscure question; in a draft paper at another London S.T.D. Clinic, the only positive cross tabulations occurred between both syphilus and gonorrhoea and frequency of eating out. I have made a clear dichotomy requesting ONLY those meals eaten out in an evening or weekend. This was necessary as I am quite sure that the reason for the above positive observation is almost entirely due to the high lunch time frequency of eating out. As the other hospital in question is in the West End (commercial section) of London, the vast majority of their out-patients would eat lunch out, thus giving a rather exaggerated frequency. Thus the table given is for meals not including weekday lunches.

NOS. MEALS PER MONTH (excluding lunches)	FREQUENCY	PERCENTAGE	CUMULATIVE PERCENTAGE
0	101	19.0	19.0
1	68	12.8	31.8
2	74	13.9	45.7
3	37	7.0	52.7
4	73	13.7	66.4
5	16	3.0	69.4
6	21	4.0	73.4
7	7	1.3	74.7
8	31	5.8	80.5
9	6	1.1	81.6
10	30	5.6	87.2
11 - 15	36	6.8	94.0
16 - 20	18	3.4	97.4
21 - 25	6	1.1	98.5
26 +	7	1.5	100.0
	531	100	

A series of questions enquiring of the present number of children the patient has, and whether or not any may want any more children in the future, and also how many more they would want.

NO. OF CHILDREN (present)	FREQUENCY	PERCENTAGE	CUMULATIVE PERCENTAGE
0	412	77.6	77.6
1	42	7.9	85.5
2	54	10.2	95.7
3	17	3.2	98.9
4	4	0.7	99.6
5	1	0.2	99.8
6	1	0.2	100.0
	531	100	

Some 53% of the patients interviewed said that they would want some or further children in the future. Bearing in mind that almost half the patients had single marital status, this was not too surprising.

This study is related to two previous lines of investigation.

a) The only other similar study which was performed was conducted by Drs. Alexander, Samways, Poole and Dale, and the departmental Physician-in-charge at the time was Dr. C Nicol at the Lydia Clinic of St. Thomas' Hospital, from January to March 1972. The conclusions of the paper include that there exists a significant relationship between incidence of S.T.D. and geographical location in the case of four Wandsworth and three Lambeth electoral wards (the two boroughs which the Lydia Clinic covers). These relationships are of importance due to the social and physical environmental effects of the determining influences upon the sexual activity of the people. The kinds of personal characteristics considered include age, sex, race or ethnic group, marital status, social class and economic status.

Disappointment was expressed to the fact that figures on patients were collected for three monthly attendance only, and it was felt that a further study of this nature is necessary. In a letter received by the author in late 1978 from Dr. J Barrow, the present Physician-in-charge at the Lydia Clinic, it was discovered that the study was an isolated one which has not yet been furthered or elaborated upon.

b) The most recent paper discovered concerning the socio-demographic aspects of the S.T.D. was in November 1978 when proofs of papers were received by the Editor of the B.J.V.D.; these papers were written by Drs. Fulford, Catterall, Dane, Hornville, Lim, Eysenck and Wilson.

The results of the socio-demographic factors were quite surprising.

"No consistent evidence was found to implement age, nationality or marital status as determinants of S.T.D. risk. Equally, occupation, examined both by the Registrar General, classification and for specific occupational sub-groups, showed no overall association with S.T.D. Among non-sexual social activities only one positive association was found - between eating out and gonorrhoea. It is concluded that social and demographic factors contribute little to the distribution of S.T.D."

SUMMARY : THE VENEREAL B.E.D.E.

The results from interviews of 531 patients from the Department of Genital Medicine, St. Bartholomew's Hospital, are discussed. The data was collected for six months commencing August 1979, and was processed within the Computer Unit of the Polytechnic of North London, using the hardware facilities of the DEC-10, and S.P.S.S. software during the summer of 1980.

Of the subjects, data was recorded in a structured interview lasting a maximum of five minutes and enquiries are made of the clinical history (related to any previous diagnoses at St. Bartholomew's), sexual history, demographic history, alcoholic drinking habits and several indicators of a socio-sexual nature. Of the samples discussed, 22% are female, 78% male of which 21.5% were homosexuals.

The most prominant features of the Study include the fact that some 63% of the sample went to follow some form of further or higher education, suggesting that the sample is well educated and aware of the implication of sexually transmitted diseases. Furthermore, the drinking habits of the regular drinkers was almost double that of the regular drinkers of the control group. The Study has established that some 19% of the sample are presently cohabiting, a marital status previously ignored in similar studies.

Concerning analysis of the sexual activity of the sample, the conclusion can be made that the sample is highly active, taking several sexual partners over a given period (maximum of six months) and that this rate continues until the patient is required to visit the department due to the fact that they have some symptoms, or as the result of being contacted by a previous partner who has some symptoms. There is thus reason to believe that the individual will take numerous partners over time until the need arises to visit the department.

The above study will eventually present results of approximately 1,000 interviews and the Study itself is part of a larger project that is currently being undertaken; this is dichotomised into retrospective as well as prospective sections.

The capture and processing of routine clinical data in a cardiology department.

Keith N. Williams and Michael M. Webb-Peploe
Cardiac Department
St. Thomas' Hospital
Lambeth Palace Road
London SE1 7EH
England

Summary Three optical mark reader (OMR) forms are used to store and process clinical and haemodynamic data. One OMR form records details of the cardiac catheterisation in summary form and is processed to produce an audit of catheter laboratory performance and an extract by which all cases having the same criteria can be identified for clinical research. A second OMR form records the symptoms, certain important points in the history, the physical signs and the chest x-ray, electrocardiographic (ECG) and echocardiographic findings. A third OMR form records the results of special investigations aimed at identifying cardiovascular and respiratory pathology. From these last two OMR forms the computer generates a clinical report for distribution to colleagues and the case notes. This report has given a significant saving of secretarial and medical time compared to previous methods and is acceptable to those who receive it.

1. INTRODUCTION

As part of the DHSS experimental medical computing program, St. Thomas' Hospital has developed a number of applications on a medium scale time-sharing computer capable of supporting some 30 terminals with concurrent batch processing. One major application is a microbiology result recording system (Williams et al, 1978)[1] which uses OMR techniques and a reading device in the laboratory. Many of the programs and software routines used by the application are table driven and their details have already been presented (Davidson et al 1979)[2].

2. THE SYSTEM

The cardiac application comprises two major parts; one OMR form recording details of cardiac catheterisation and two OMR forms recording the results of the clinical examination and special investigations for both inpatients and outpatients.

2.1 The catheter OMR form

This form, which will not be described in detail, records a summary of the catheters used and procedures employed at cardiac catheterisation, any complications, the haemodynamic and diagnostic findings. The data thus captured are used to produce management statistics and for retrospective research.

2.2 The patient examination OMR form

This document records the findings at a clinical consultation with particular emphasis on the physical examination. The top of the form records identifying information such as hospital number, age, sex, etc. Next comes a list of important events in the past history followed by the symptoms experienced by the patients. Then come details of the physical signs, the chest x-ray, ECG and echocardiogram. The doctor adds extra manuscript information on a separate sheet and this normally includes the past medical history, family history, and current drug therapy.

2.3 The investigations OMR form

Some patients require more extensive investigation and the results of the more common investigations associated with heart disease are included on this document. This OMR form has recently been implemented and allows for:-

- lung function tests including spirometry and gas exchange measurements together with blood gases
- 24 hr ECG monitoring giving the basic rhythm and identifying any rate disorders
- exercise testing specifying the peak load achieved and the reason for stopping the test together with details of ECG changes and symptoms, both during the test and in the recovery phase
- venous occlusion plethysmography identifying changes in peripheral blood flow
- myocardial perfusion scans giving the location and type of perfusion defect
- pyrophosphate ("hot spot") scanning
- first pass perfusion studies detecting intra-cardiac shunts and measuring ejection fraction
- gated blood pool measurements recording the location of abnormal myocardial movement together with an estimate of ejection fraction
- lung scans giving details of ventilation or perfusion defects and a diagnostic interpretation of the scan.

This OMR form is filled in as results become available and entered into the computer when all outstanding investigations have been reported.

2.4 Procedure

As convenient, the secretary takes all outstanding OMR forms to the microbiology laboratory and feeds them through the mark reader. She then returns to the cardiac department to "process" the form; this involves validation and reporting of errors by the computer and, if error free, keying in extra information. This extra information will normally be the free text written by the doctor, but may also include extra identifying information and diagnoses not covered by the OMR forms (noncardiac diagnoses are amongst those which are keyed in uncoded).

2.5 Output

The computer output from the patient examination and investigations OMR forms takes the form of a typed clinical report. All outstanding report are printed on the cardiac laboratory terminal and the secretary then adds by hand laboratory results such as haematology, biochemistry and serology. She then photocopies the completed report and distributes it to the patient's local doctor, the referring clinician, our surgical colleagues if appropriate, department files and hospital case notes.

2.6 Analysis facilities

The system can produce a variety of analyses to help the department perform more efficiently. In practice these are most often derived from the diagnostic information entered via the catheter OMR form, although there is no conceptual reason why that from the other OMR forms should not also be included. The analyses involved are:

2.6.1 An annual audit which monitors materials and techniques used and the associated complications of each. This information is used to prepare the annual catheter laboratory report and to review the effect of changes of technique on the complication rates.

2.6.2 A costing facility whereby each catheter, angiogram, and procedure is individually costed and accumulated automatically against the patient and by time and by source of referral.

2.6.3 An extract facility which enables the rapid identification of all records sharing any specified criteria. The researcher defines the characteristics of those records in which he is interested, enters these criteria into the computer and ends up with a list of those records which meet his requirements.

He would normally then use this list to access the case notes and proceed with his research by manual means. An investigator usually wishes to pull out all cases with a specified diagnosis and this can be done with a single pass of the data held on the system; however it is possible to make several passes, merging them together with BOOLEAN operators, to meet quite sophisticated logical requirements.

2.6.4 A variety of other analyses are available including listings of diagnosis frequency, of referral source loads, and of sequential changes in any selected variable to allow for longitudinal studies.

3. RESULTS

Some 9 months of computer analyst and programmer effort were required to implement and enhance the system over a six year period since 1974. A further 3 weeks were contributed by clinical staff in the cardiac department to help design the OMR forms and to assess the results.

3.1 Running costs

The routine operation of the system was readily absorbed into the daily work of all staff involved. In particular the marking and processing of the catheter OMR form proved to involve so little effort that it was unnecessary to time it. The patient examination OMR form together with its manuscript history sheet takes approximately 10 minutes to complete, as did the job of dictation which it replaced. Our secretarial staff take 40 minutes to enter some 40 examination OMR forms each week, but 30 of these minutes are spent commuting to and from the Microbiology laboratory. Annotating the records takes 2½ hours per week, nearly all of which are spent typing in free text data. (The investigations OMR form has just been implemented and will reduce this figure to an estimated 1¼ hours per week at equivalent throughput). Each report takes 2 minutes to print at 30 characters per second but no additional secretarial time is involved by the unattended operation of the terminal. Addition of laboratory results, photocopying and distribution are all tasks unchanged from the previous system. The total secretarial time of 3 hours 10 minutes spent operating the computer system compares very favourably with 25 hours previously spent in typing the dictated reports. From the operational saving must be deducted the cost of the OMR documents (15p) and the amortised cost of the typewriter terminal (c.£300 p.a.). The savings effected by the various analyses and listings produced by the computer are harder to quantify. The annual report used to take a doctor 10 days to prepare, this is now reduced to 1 day. The costing figures proved extremely useful not only in itemising departmental expenditure but in convincing the administration that the department cares about cost. The extract facility was and, with increasing frequen is used to identify categories of patients for research and teaching purposes. To identify these patients by manual means would be a prohibitively time consuming and boring task; with the aid of the computer it takes minutes rather than weeks to scan through a file containing some 3800 catheter records going back to 1973 and 1400 examination records since August 1976.

3.2 Computer characteristics

The programs were written in FORTRAN IV using assembler language subroutines for input/output and data manipulation. These sub-routines, together with a number of utilities and table pre-processors form an extensive package capable of handling data of variable length and format. Each OMR form takes an average of 5.7 CPU seconds and 308 disk accesses to process and the application uses 8.9 million bytes of random access storage.

By extrapolating our experience transferring other applications (William et al, 1975)[(3)], we can estimate that transfer of the cardiac applicatio to a suitable configuration would take approximately 6 man weeks. In addition the software mentioned above would need transcription and this is a far larger task involving perhaps an additional 10 man months. Once transcribed, however, the software would be available for any other OMR based application.

4. DISCUSSION

Two important factors in the successful implementation of the system and its acceptance by medical and technical staff were, first the use of OMR forms which made it unnecessary for them to acquire typing skills, and second the careful avoidance of parallel running which actually increases the total volume of work. A third factor was the speed and ease with which the computer was programmed to accept and analyse cardiac information and, perhaps more importantly, rapidly to effect changes.

The most important aspect of the catheter OMR form is that it enables any records with defined characteristics rapidly to be extracted from the dat file thus providing a powerful tool for research workers. Auditing laboratory performance is, we believe, an indispensable pre-requisite if standards of investigation and safety are to be maintained or improved Very few busy laboratories are, however, able to spare the time to carry out an effective audit by manual means. The costing facility has an obvious application in a private health care system, but in the National Health Service it has made all staff more aware of cost and provided useful facts and figures for discussions with administrative staff.

The patient examination OMR form is particularly important demonstrating, as it does, that it is possible quickly and easily to record the necessary information for a computer automatically to generate a report embodying history and physical signs together with the chest x-ray, ECG and echocardiographic findings. Furthermore, this clinical report is sufficiently readable, comprehensive and flexible to gain general acceptance by a large number of clinicians. We know of no other applications of OMR techniques to the recording of routine clinical in cardiology, although the anaesthetic department at Charing Cross Hospital in London uses an OMR form for recording the pre-, per- and post-operative assessment of the anaesthetic history. Many other clinical data recording systems exist and all have to some extent overcome the major problem of formalising clinical data to the point where it may usefully be stored on a computer. Most suffer, however, by either requiring the doctor to type in his information directly, a task he neither likes nor does well, or having him write it down for subsequent entry by a secretary, with inevitable delays and errors. With our system the doctor still uses pencil and paper to record his observations, but the paper is itself a computer input medium.

The operational drawbacks of our system stem mainly from our having to share an OMR reader with another department. A further deficiency centres on the need manually to transcribe laboratory results onto the finished reports. Since the St. Thomas' system now holds most of these blood results, this job will, we hope, soon be done for us automatically. Finally, in order to produce a complete clinical report, it is necessary to type in certain sections verbatim. These sections involve mainly the history and, in our experience, it is unlikely that this could be sufficiently well structured to use OMR techniques.

Discussions of cost are often clouded by the difficulty of accounting for the capital and revenue costs of shared hardware and software facilities. (The cardiac department shares a great many common facilities which enable it, and the hospital as a whole, to function; for example buildings, heating, lighting and administrative facilities including the computer.) We are fortunate in that, apart from disk storage, our machine utilisation is trivial and on this basis, therefore, our costs are around £600 p.a. whilst saving half a secretary.

Medical computing in England has been criticised in the past on a number of counts (Committee of Public Accounts, 1976[4], British Medical Journal

1977[5]) and progress in the field of clinical medicine somewhat slower than, for example, in the more peripheral areas such as laboratory (Goodwin and Smith, 1976)[6], administrative and nursing applications. Whilst not entirely applicable to other specialties, we feel that our OMR form is sufficiently broad-based to act as a model from which other physicians and surgeons could develop similar recording systems to suit their needs. We have demonstrated that it is possible easily to record the major part of the clinical consultation for a computer, and to make secretarial savings by doing so. Unless medical computing can be shown to work in a clinical environment there is a danger that computer professionals will increasingly regard it as difficult and unrewarding and that medical staff will continue to look upon all computer systems with suspicion, as time-consuming, expensive and unproductive gimmicks.

REFERENCES

(1) Williams KN, Davidson JMF, Phillips I, Rice E, Lynn E. A computer system for clinical microbiology. J Clin Path 1978. 1978 : 31 : 1193-1201.

(2) Davidson JMF, Williams KN, Robertson VS. Table driven and Optical Mark Reading systems for clinical and laboratory applications. Proceedings, Medical Informatics Berlin 1979 : 5 : 414-426 (Springer-Verlag).

(3) Williams KN, Davidson JMF, Ingram GIC. A computer programme for the analysis of parallel line bioassays of clotting factors. Br J Haem. 1975 : 31 : 13-23.

(4) Committee of Public Accounts, Sixth Report, 1965-1976 Session. London HMSO 1976.

(5) Br Med J Leading Article - Experience with Computers and our money. 1977 : 1 : 404.

(6) Goodwin CS, Smith BC. Computer printing and filing of microbiology reports. 1. Description of the system. J Clin Path. 1976 : 29 : 543-552.

THE PLACE OF THE COMPUTER IN CONTINUING MEDICAL EDUCATION

Phil R. Manning, M.D.
University of Southern California School of Medicine
Postgraduate Division
Los Angeles, California

Continuing education for the practicing physician should be centered around three approaches: Assistance in acquiring information, fellowship based on academic activities, and linkage of education to practice. Computer science research should facilitate linking of continuing education to practice in three categories: Indexing office records for educational needs assessment, providing information when and where it is needed, providing guidance to the physician at the time diagnostic and therapeutic plans are being made.

The need for lifelong learning in medicine is uncontested, but the methods by which it is best accomplished remain in dispute. The problem begins with the traditional medical school program, which emphasizes transfer of information more than techniques for organizing medical practice to facilitate continuing education. Most schools do not teach students how to determine their own educational needs, nor do most medical school faculty members practice in an environment which is organized to enhance education. Formal CME is usually viewed as a classroom activity based on vague goals and engaged in by passive learners. In addition, the time pressures of practice, active community service, and family responsibilities make it difficult for physicians and other professionals to pursue lifelong medical learning. I believe that the practicing physician can be better served than at present by the academic community, and that proper CME will inevitably improve patient care.

A program that would facilitate learning should have three components: (1) assistance in acquiring information, (2) fellowship based on academic activities, and (3) linkage of education with practice.

Information

Information transmission in CME allows for a wide variety of learning strategies, including classroom activities, print media, and audiovisual information-transfer. We have been studying the techniques physicians use to gain new knowledge beyond their formal training. In one study we found that the professional journal was most frequently the first source of learning about echocardiography, understanding its principles, and updating knowledge (1). Meetings and conferences were another major source. In another study we found that physicians learned about cimetidine primarily from medical journals and meetings (2). In the case of cimetidine, conversations with peers also provided a significant learning source.

In addition to the knowledge explosion we also have a knowledge delivery-system explosion. Technologic advances allow classroom activities to be brought to the physician's office, home, or automobile by way of the telephone, radio, television, and audio and video tapes (3). Audiovisual methods will undoubtedly become even more sophisticated with the application of videodisc systems and computer managed learning systems. Rapid access to motion and still pictures will permit problem-solving encounters. Future technologic developments and applications offer virtually unlimited potential for both information transfer and simulated problem solving. The danger is that physicians will be so inundated by uncoordinated audiovisual teaching opportunities that most of the material will go unused. Major efforts to provide more computer methods for simulation are probably not a priority. The marketplace will undoubtedly determine the final outcome.

Sociability

Even in an exciting, rapidly developing profession like medicine, boredom may creep into patient care when certain procedures become routine. For this reason, peer reinforcement and interaction are important in the pursuit of further knowledge. Affective group participation can be used not only to improve learning, but also to stimulate excitement about activities that may otherwise be viewed as routine.

Practice-Linked Continuing Medical Education

In addition to general information transfer and arousal of enthusiasm for practice, effective continuing education should be linked to actual events in practice. Promoting such a linkage will probably be the computer's most significant contribution to continuing medical education. It is here that research and development should be strengthened, since every physician's office will probably soon contain a computer terminal. The computer may help the physician continue education based on real events in practice in at least 3 ways: (1) indexing office records for educational needs assessment, (2) providing information when and where needed, and (3) providing guidance in decision making.

I will give examples of several existing computer projects, not to introduce them to you as you undoubtedly already know of them, but to emphasize the educational potential of the systems:

Indexing Office Records for Educational Needs Assessment

At the turn of the century, Sir William Osler suggested that Physicians file cases in 3 categories: clear cases, doubtful cases, and mistakes.

> "It is only by getting your cases grouped in this way," said Osler, "that you can make any real progress with your post-collegiate education. Only in this way can you gain wisdom with experience. It is a common error to think the more a physician sees, the greater his experience and the more he knows." (4)

Unfortunately, few American physicians follow this advice but, instead, file charts by patients' name only. Manually crossfiling by patients' problems is, of course, more difficult, but the ability to review and profit from one's experience would be a valuable dividend. Computer technology can certainly facilitate organization of data with use of a multiple cross-filing system. Brownstein from South Carolina has described a system that readily permits the crossfiling of patient data according to (1) the problems that a physician is seeing in his practice, (2) social and demographic characteristics of patients, (3) medications, (4) laboratory studies, and (5) vital signs (5). This method allows physicians to anlyze many aspects of their practice and to direct their study accordingly.

Providing Information When and Where Needed

Instead of supplying information in a postgraduate course or through random reading weeks or months before it is needed, computer technology permits rapid, direct access to information when the physician is developing diagnostic and therapeutic plans. Such a system is being developed at the Lister Hill National Center (6). This system, however, does not directly guide decision-making, since the physician must still apply the computer information appropriately in the management of the patient's problem.

Providing Guidance

Completion of the requirements of an effective continuing education program requires providing the physician with guidance in decision-making. The system "Internist" being developed at the University of Pittsburgh offers guidance by mimicking the diagnostic behavior of the "excellent clinican" (7). Another system developed by Dr. Lawrence Weed and co-workers at the University of Vermont is organized around the problem-oriented record, which consists of 4 major parts: The data base (patient history, physical examination, and laboratory studies); a list of the patient's problems as they are understood; diagnostic and therapeutic plans; and progress notes organized around individual problems (8). Information related to a problem is contained on more than 45,000 frames or displays. Appropriate medical knowledge relating to a specific problem may be displayed within milliseconds. In addition, when a physician is puzzled about a diagnosis, he may obtain a list of diagnostic possibilities as well as information about procedures to confirm or exclude certain options? Possible side effects, dosages, and cost of drugs can be displayed, as can normal values, indications, contra-indications, and costs of laboratory tests.

Determining Educational Needs

Continuing medical education (CME) is hampered by the primitive state of methods for determining the specific educational needs of individual physicians. The objectives of most educational programs are usually based either on needs perceived by faculty members or those stated by the participiating physicians. In some cases, educational needs are inferred from the results of a paper and pencil test and in recent years, medical record audits have become useful for identifying needs of groups of physicians in hospital practice.

Identifying educational needs in office practice represents a more difficult task than the identification of needs in hospital practice. Office records are usually not standardized and there are major time constraints on both physician and staff. External audits of medical records are expensive and are not feasible on a large scale.

The following precepts and constraints must be addressed by any approach designed to recognize individual needs in ambulatory care:

1. The educational needs should be identified from the physician's daily work with patients.
2. The program must be acceptable to physicians and should not disrupt office routine.
3. The atmosphere should encourage openness by rewarding nondefensiveness on the part of the physician.
4. Confidentiality should be maintained for both physician and patient.
5. The method for identifying educational needs should recognize important problems that lead to educational recommendations.

We are attempting to identify educational needs of individual physicians automatically by ongoing review of the products of practice: prescriptions, laboratory order forms, etc. This strategy enables us to gather information about the physician's practice without going to the office, reviewing patient records, or significantly altering office routine. Our current efforts involve analysis of prescription copies by a review committee consisting of an internist and 2 clinical pharmacists. Participating physicians use a specially developed NCR form which produces a duplicate of every prescription written in the office supplemented by additional information, including patient data, the condition prompting the prescription, and other significant medical problems and medications associated with the patient. The informtaion is used to develop individual instructional packets directed to prescribing problems noted in the committee's review.

Data from 44 physicians in primary care have been reviewed (9). The analysis shows wide differences in the way certain drugs are used and in the frequency with which common drugs are prescribed. The types of educational needs determined by this simple method include: (1) inappropriate indications for a drug, (2) high frequency of prescriptions for certain drugs, (3) inappropriate prescription of drugs with abuse potential, (4) inadequate instruction, (5) excessive dose, (6) inappropriate dosage intervals, (7) prescription of ineffective drugs, (8) potential drug interactions. The method has identified some type of educational need for nearly all physicians in the study. We believe that this relatively simple method provides more information about educational needs of individual physicians in prescribing practices than surveys, chart audits, or the perception of educational planners.

I am describing these early experiences with an almost automatic method of identifying educational needs from the products of practice to encourage individuals in computer research to suggest ways that computer science can streamline the acquisition and review of physicians' practice data. Since physicians will soon have ready access to computer terminals in their offices, it seems natural that this resource would be invaluable for data collection and retrieval for educational needs assessment. Even though using duplicate prescriptions takes little physician time, the time needed to supply the background information needed to adequately evaluate the prescription is estimated to be about 40 seconds per prescription. The prescription review is also lengthy and it seems reasonable that the computer could be a significant aid in processing the prescription data and in actually carrying out portions of the assessment automatically.

Conclusions

All professionals subscribe to lifelong learning, but time constraints necessitate aid for some in implementing this concept. To date, most CME has consisted of information transfer by the printed page, classroom activities, or audiovisual media. These methods are usually related to general problems rather than those specifically confronting the physician at a given moment. Current computer technology makes it possible to relate education to actual events in practice when the physician must devise diagnostic and therapeutic plans. Such continuing education should place less reliance on strict memory and should enhance professional growth from experience. Efforts to further develop, perfect, and field-test the linking of computerized continuing medical education to real events in practice should take precedence over simulation techniques and simple transfer of information.

References

(1) Manning, P.R. and Denson, T.A., How cardiologists learn about echocardiography: a reminder for medical educators and legislators, Ann Int Med 91 (1979) 469-471.

(2) Manning, P.R. and Denson, T.A., How internists learned about cimetidine, Ann Int Med, in press.

(3) Manning, P.R. and Millard, W.L., Technology for continuing medical education. HSRC/HCPC Health Care Technology Compendium Series, University of Missouri, Columbia, Missouri, September 1979.

(4) Cushing, H., The life of Sir William Osler (Oxford University Press, New York, 1940) p.328.

(5) Braunstein, M., The computer-based medical record in family practice in Medalie, J.H., Family Medicine, Baltimore. The Williams and Wilkins Company, 1978.

(6) Schoolman, H.M. and Bernstein, L.M., Computer use in diagnosis, prognosis and therapy, Science 22 (1978) 926-931.

(7) Pople, H.E., Meyers, J.D. and Miller, R.A., In proceedings of the Fourth International Joint Conference on Artificial Intelligence, USSR, Tablishi, 1975.

(8) Weed, L.L., Your health care and how to manage it. Vermont: Essex Publishing Co., Inc., 1978.

(9) Manning, P.R., Lee, P.V., Denson, T.A. and Gilman, N.J., Determining educational needs in the physician's office, JAMA 244 (1980) 1112-1115.

Education in Medical Informatics: A course Structure and a Curriculum

Barbara Kostrewski,
Centre for Information Science,
City University,
London E.C.1. U.K.

Abstract

A curriculum in Biomedical Information Science is presented. The course aims to prepare students for employment in health-care, the pharmaceutical industry and the information industry. The training was developed within the framework of a postgraduate course in information science.

1. Introduction

Education in medical information and documentation is a new field. Traditionally medical documentation, in the bibliographic and documentation sense, has been the province of librarianship and this aspect of medical documentation has a strong tradition in the UK. Medical informatics has attained an independent framework in Germany (1) and curricula have been developed in the USA (2,3,4,5); while Germany's professional institution, the Gesellschaft fur Medizinische Dokimentation Informatick und Statistik, grants distinctions (6). Furthermore professional acceptance is reflected in the curriculum of the 5 year degree in medical informatics (6,7). This rigorous approach to education for medical informatics is unique. It is characterized by an all embracing approach to medical documentation and information, conceptually supported by the tradition of Institutes of Documentation, Information & Statistics alongside research institutions. This contributes to a well defined professional and educational structure.

2. Objectives

At the City University, London, a postgraduate curriculum has been operational since 1975. The diversity of medical informatics demands several levels and directions of training. Also a distinction has to be made between the training of medical personnel in the use and appreciation of systems and the training of information personnel for systems development in health-care. The work described here relates to the latter.

3. Factors contributing to the Development of the Curriculum in Biomedical Information Processing

A framework for the curriculum was derived through discussions with present and potential employers. The programme, an option within the framework of a postgraduate Masters degree in Information Science (8), was started as a result of the congruence of several factors reflecting the multifaceted nature of health-care. The emphasis on the information processing within the pharmaceutical industry is strong. The major factor conttributing to this has been the fact that the pharmaceutical industry is the largest single employer of our graduates, (Figure 1.) However, the increased complexity of other domains to the practice of medicine has emphasized the importance of information storage and retrieval at all levels of medical application.

	MSc Full-time	Diploma Part-time
Industry	61	40
Pharmaceuticals	26	16
Chemicals	7	2
Oil	5	0
Other Manufacturing	11	9
Information Industry	12	15

FIGURE 1.

Employment of Diploma and Masters degree graduates, 1976 - 1979

Subject	MSc Full-time	Diploma Part-time
Mathematics (2)	4	0
Physics	17	10
Chemistry	18	18
Physiology/Biochemistry	22	13
Pharmacology	7	1
Pharmacy	7	6
Medicine	3	0
Botany	4	4
Zoology	22	7
Biology/Microbiology	26	22
Agriculture/Agricultural Biology	4	2
Ecology/Environmental Science	2	3
Metallurgy	1	2
Engineering	0	2
Geology	7	2
Geography	11	4
Economics	6	5
Law	1	1
Psychology	3	1
Library Science	1	5
Miscellaneous Sciences	4	5
Other	4	23
Ph.D.s	10	3

FIGURE 2.

The City University:

Subject Background of Students, 1975 - 1979

The strong biomedical bias of The City University course is emphasized by the high proportion of natural science graduates which the course attracts; their subject distribution is shown in Figure 2. The pharmaceutical industry is heavily information dependant, requiring specialized information processing techniques. Moreover, the 1968 Medicines Act precipitated a new and more rigorous approach to the handling of information relating to pharmaceutical compounds. Consequently the pharmaceutical industry has to gather and collate more information than had been hitherto necessary, and this resulted in the introduction of a new profession, that of the registration officers and their counterparts in the Medicines Commission. Indeed, the awareness of the complexity of the therapeutic process has emphasized the need for computerized support systems which aim to capture all known pharmaceutical parameters and the complex network of interrelationships relating to drug therapy. Thus the curriculum aims to provide foundations for employment in information processing in the biomedical and in the broadest sense. The tasks carried out by our graduates range from systems design and implementation to systems support and documentation.

The application fo computing within the medical domain broke new ground. Traditionally computing has been the servant of commerce with well defined groups of concepts and data structures. The hospital environment however, presents a diversity of data, both qualitiative and quantitiative, with a strong element of language dependence. Thus management information, stock control, patient data, clinical investigations and bibliographic support have to be recorded and monitored. These requirements are reflected in the curriculum.

The important role of information within hospital pharmacy departments has been stressed by the introduction of a new function, that of the information pharmacits, whose main concern is the design and use of information systems in their specific environment. Such systems aim to provide heuristic support by providing total information in relation to drug therapy taking all parameters into account. Several Pharmacists who completed this course are now involved in the implemenation of hospital drug information systems.

It can be seen therefore,that this interpretation of education for medical informatics represents a three horned approach, that is, the needs of industry, the needs of medicine and health-care and also those of commercial information suppliers, both systems-design houses and database vendors.

4. Course Organization

There are two parallel courses: A full-time calendar year M.Sc. course leading to a Masters degree in Information Science and a two year day release Diploma course supported by appropriate employment leading to a Diploma in Information Science. The Health Service, the Medical Research Council and the Pharmaceutical Industry have sponsored students on both courses. Both courses run parallel for the taught part of the course and supervised practicals.

The Academic year comprises of three 10 week terms followed by four months for an evaluative study and dissertation. The three ten-week terms are occupied largely by taught sessions and practicals.

The course content is dependant upon the foundations laid in the core modules which are taken by all students.

Students receiving a Diploma may qualify for an M.Sc. by submission of a dissertation.

Entrance Requirements

A prerequisite for both the M.Sc. and Diploma courses in Information Science is a first or upper-second class degree in a scientific discipline. These high entrance requirements may in exceptional cases be mitigated by relevant previous experience and a good employment record. Of the part-time students taking the Biomedical Option, a major proportion are employed in the pharmaceutical industry, relevant research institutions e.g. Medical Research Council, specialized information centres eg poisons units, hospitals and government departments. An analysis of first employment has shown that the organizations relating to the health-care in the broadest sense are the largest single employer of our graduates. (8)

Student Intake

The total annual student intake is about 35 full-time and 35 part-time students out of about 200 applicants. Approximately one third of each group choose to take the Biomedical Option. Therefore, there are about 24 students taking the Biomedical Option each year. Since 1975 about 100 students have attended the option.

5. The curriculum

The core modules cover the fundamental concepts of information processing encompassing, data processing, systems analysis, computing, systems design, management, research methods and the requirements of specialist groups.

5.1 The Application of Electronic Technology in Systems Implementation within the Biomedical Environment

This forms an extension of the Information Systems, Computing and Systems Analysis core modules, but relates specifically to the medical environment and specific tasks that ar to be performed. The use of Viewdata within this context is also considered.

5.2 Specialized Information Systems

(a) The structure and nature of data banks;
(b) The selection, preparation and input of specialized information eg chemicals;
(c) The design of specialized data banks eg Toxicology, Antibiotics;
(d) The role and organization of Specialized Information Centres e.g. Poisons Centres, Health Hazards.

5.3 Information Systems for Drug Development

The understanding of the process involved in the development and information support of a drug. These systems demand a knowledge of the following:

(a) Basic reference sources;
(b) The maintenance of laboratory reports;
(c) Recording of all synthesized compounds and tests;
(d) Screening: the analysis of results and their recording;
(e) Linear notations of chemical structures, e.g. Wisswesser Line Notation;

(f) Computer handling of chemical structures;
(g) Internal information systems for the handling of internal data and relevant external information;
(h) Adverse reaction monitoring including both
    Legislation and
    Procedures and systems design.
(i) The dissemination of information about products including the work of Medical Information Departments and preparation of promotional literature.
(j) Collation and preparation of drug data for registration.

5.4 Medical Information Systems

The diversity of this field is analysed and the variety and levels of provisions of information are stressed. The following aspects are considered:

(a) The structure of the Health Service and the Medical Profession;
(b) Dissemination of Information to Practitioners;
(c) Patient Scheduling Systems;
(d) The design of Patient Record Systems;
(e) Screening Systems;
(f) The development of information systems in the Hospital Pharmacy, consideration of the criteria for computerization;
(g) Systems for clinical investigation eg pathology, radiology, clinical chemistry;
(h) Signal analysis, physiological data and their interpretation eg E.C.G., E.E.G.;
(i) Provision of information within the Health Service;
(j) Information as a decision support, in therapy management and diagnosis of disease;
(k) Information as administrative support:
(l) Computers in the collection of data for epidemiological work;
(m) Computers in the understanding of physiological processes;

and finally have an understanding of the interdependence of these systems and procedures.

5.5 Bibliographic Information

The importance of the provision of bibliographic information cannot be underestimated both in the clinical and research environments. The provision of bibliographic support particularly in the context of database design and utilization is an important part of the course. The following aspects are considered: -

(a) The use of the principal bibliographic sources and database;
(b) Computerization of bibliographic holdings;
(c) Medical classifications and structured reference languages;
(d) The structure of the major databases, eg hierarchical, relational;
(e) The provision of bibliographic support to research teams,
(f) The use of commercial bibliographic databases: practical on-line search formulation and analysis of search statements and formulation for the appropriate systems.

5.6 Practical Work

The implementation of the principles taught on the course is illustrated by a range of practical exercises and projects involving systems analysis and design within the bio-medical domain. This is further emphasized by visits, to hospitals, specialist centres and industry.

Detailed investigations and research are frequently extended by work carried out during the three month dissertations; which cover a wide range of topics eg the semantic analysis of reference languages, an evaluation of medical databases, pharmaceutical information in hospitals. Many dissertations are carried out in collaboration with outside institutions and thus contribute to information systems development in a practical way.

6. Discussion

Information Science graduates, with training in biomedical applications, are in demand; thus the need for further development of education in medical informatics is indicated. The application of information and documentation techniques within the biomedical domain are taught at The City University as part of a postgraduate course in Information Science. The three levels of expertise in Medical Information and Documentation (ie, the Medical Documentation Assistant, The Medical Informatician and the Holder of the Certificate) which have become established in Germany, have not been implemented in the UK. The main reasons are the differences in the structure of the professional institutions and the education framework. At present there tends to be a reliance upon "on the job" training and knowledge acquired through experience particularly at lower levels of responsibility (eg assistants) or within specialist environments. However, a new qualified element is emerging the doctor interested and committed to information processing. At present, courses in Systems Analysis and Data Processing at both undergraduate and postgraduate levels, are not generally applications defined. Although specialist training, through individual projects, may be intergrated. Moreover, training tends to be related to fundamentals which may be transposed to most organizations and environments.

It can be deduced from the subject distribution of applicants (Figure 2.) that students with a Degree in the life sciences, medicine, pharmacy, pharmaology are attracted to the Information Science course at The City University because training relating to the disciplines of the health sciences is given.

A detailed analysis of tasks performed by those completing the biomedical option and and taking relevant employment is being carried out. This investigation will contribute to further course development. However, education is a projection into the future and the paradox is that this thrust can only be based on experiences gained from the past. With this in mind, the major objective of training is to teach our students to be aware of possibilities and to cope with changes, both in approach and technology, and to be flexible; moreover, they must be conscious of the enormous contribution made by biomedical information processing.

REFERENCES

(1) KOEPPE, P. The development of medical informatics in the Federal Republic of Germany. Methods of Information in Medicine. 1977 ; 16(3) : 160-167.

(2) BLOIS, M.S., WASSERMAN A. A Graduate Academic Programme in Medical Information Science. Medinfo '74. 1977 ; 217-223.

(3) ELLIS B.M., GATEWOOD L.C. A training programme in Health Computer Sciences. Proceedings NECC (National Educational Computing Conference) University of Iowa. 1979.

(4) Computer Applications in the Health Sciences. Prospectus, Case Western Reserve University. 1979.

(5) Pre and Post Doctoral Training Program in Medical Information Science (Director Dr. A.B. Lindberg) University of Missouri. 1979.

(6) MÖHR, J.R. Certifikat Medizinischer Informatiker. 1978 ; F.K. Schattauer Verlag, Stuttgart - New York.

(7) MÖHR, J.R., HOFFMAN, J. and LEVEN, F.J. A Specialized Curriculum for Medical Informatics - a review after 6 years of experience. Proceedings, MIB '79. 1979 ; 61-72.

(8) BOTTLE, R.T. Training of Information Specialists in the U.K. Paper presented at conference on: Training of Information Specialists. Pretoria 6-7 May, 1980.

AN EXAMPLE OF THE USE OF COMPUTER IN SURGICAL PEDIATRIC WORKGROUND

B. Falcidieno', C. Gambaro'', G. Romagnoli'''

'Ist.Mat. Applicata C.N.R.,Via L.B. Alberti,Genova,Italy

''Ist. Mat., Univ. Genova, Via L.B. Alberti, Genova, Italy

'''Div. Chir. Ped., E. O. Ospedali Galliera, Genova , Italy

1. INTRODUCTION

The decline in infant mortality, which began in the 1970's, was a result of the development of intensive therapy which, with always more sophisticated methods of biochemical, biophysical and clinical monitoring, permitted on the one hand a more attentive control of the patient, and on the other hand, a more complete knowledge of the events surrounding the patient, thereby reducing the work time. With this in mind, in the mid 1970's, together with other pediatric centers, we decided to construct, on various work levels (pre-operative, operative and post-operative) a control system for surgical pediatric patients (1). This system would refer to a certain computer which could be continually re-programmed, based on the most up-to-date biomedical knowledge and on the work habits of the team. In addition to hardware problems, which were overcome according to the principles of biomedical engineering, we found the biggest problem to be the construction of the oriented software. Such software had to be efficient; it could not be subject to the tendency towards obsolescence which often affects a closed system. Our most important aim has been to transform the biomedical concepts into mathematical terms, which can then be evaluated so as to enable the construction of programs which, by controlling biological equilibrium (considering even individual variations), can therapeutically counterregulate the events. The advantage of having a system like this is that it conforms to the characteristics a monitor for pediatric surgery demands. These needs can be delineated as follows: it must guarantee that the principal vital data is constantly measured, using, however, only the most non-invasive sensors; it must establish minimum and maximum normality estimates for a certain patient in terms of his/her physiology which is determined by his/her age, as well as for the pathology of his/her organs; it must signal and give time projections not only of any possible exceeding of vital parameters, but also of the tendency towards abnormality, which, in correlation with other data, could express a precise vital function (respiratory, renal, hepatic); it must develop a control system which in typical situations can counter-regulate the events always in the same way, as determined by the pre-established operating protocols, thus avoiding personal interpretations which do not have a precise value; it must memorize any event so as to enable a future critical evaluation. All of this must come about in the simplest way possible, taking into consideration the person who will use the system, the environment in which the system is installed and the often dramatic moments in which it will be used (2) (3).

2. THE USE OF THE COMPUTER

The computer, interactively used for clinical data processing, proved to be a very efficient support. The most important balances we have taken into consideration are: cardio-circulatory, respiratory, renal, hematological, coagulative, hydric and acid-base balances. In particular, while for the first four, we used the computer only for synthesizing, for the last two, we needed a long clinical research in order to carry out a practical therapeutic thesis. In addition we made a graphics system (4) to display data and in order to be able to help users to make a rapid synthesis of the clinical proceeding, thus saving time and pointing out the cases on which they must operate. This particular way of elaborating clinical data and handling user interface increases the number of cases which can be controlled by a single operator and makes potential users' training easier.

3. DATA ACQUISITION

Biophysical data of heart-rate, respiratory rate, central venous pressure and arterial pressure are inserted on-line by means of monitors. The average selection is made out of five data with variable times which can be selected by the operator. Biochemical, biophysical and hematological data, given by the available devices of automatic analysis, are inserted off-line. Even extemporaneous data of the patient's clinical evaluation are put in off-line.

4. RESULTS

The most important aim was to control the hydric-electrolytic-caloric balance from birth to fourteen years of age. For its solution we needed four years of clinical research, based on an analysis of all the literature available. We succeed in producing a physiopatological program which is adaptable to metabolic needs of surgical pediatric patients, to medical operator's requirements and to the possibility of reaching blood vessels. The clinical hardware application has been succesfully used on about 120 patients in three years . We also developed a program which calculates the acid-base balance by using blood microsamples. This program enables us to indirectly deduce hematochemical data, deductions which would otherwise require bigger quantities of blood. Using this program, we can even state a precise feedback in a determinate time. The system is actually used at the Surgical Pediatric Division of "E O Ospedali Galliera".

5. CONCLUSION

We are convinced that a computerized system which is dedicated to the clinical control of intensive therapy must be directed towards a physiopathological analysis of the events, rather than towards the simple archiving and memorizing of the data. The experience acquired in these years has strengthened this working philosophy, thus convincing us of the need to investigate, in a clinical sense, the use of the computer despite the inevitable difficulties brought about, and attention demanded by this procedure.

6. REFERENCES

(1) Falcidieno B, Gambaro C, Romagnoli G. A system design of clinical information processing to increase refined diagnostic and therapeutic methods in surgical pediatric work. Proceedings of the International Congress on Applied Systems and Cybernetics. Acapulco. 1980.

(2) Romagnoli G and others.L'impiego dell'elaboratore elettronico in chirurgia pediatrica. Ipotesi preliminare di lavoro. Minerva Pediatrica. 1978; 30.

(3) Ray C. Medical Engineering. Year Book Medical Publishers Inc. 1974.

(4) Newmann W, Sproull J. Principles of interactive computer graphics. 2nd ed.Mc Graw Hill, New York. 1979.

SIAM-DOCEO : ANAMNESE ET ENSEIGNEMENT MEDICAL ASSISTES PAR ORDINATEUR

M.-O. Houziaux*, M. Bartholomé*, P. Bartsch[¤], Ph. Bovy[¤],
M. de la Brassinne[¤], P. Lefèbvre[¤]
Université de Liège
* Faculté des Sciences appliquées, Laboratoire DOCEO, SMATI, B19, B - 4000 Liège
¤ Faculté de Médecine, Hôpital de Bavière, B - 4020 Liège

1. BREF HISTORIQUE

Le projet présenté ici se situe dans le prolongement de recherches engagées depuis près de deux décennies. Les premiers travaux du Laboratoire devaient aboutir en 1965 à la mise au point d'un système d'enseignement assisté par ordinateur (EAO) appelé DOCEO I (1). A partir de 1967, était expérimenté, sur une version modifiée de DOCEO I, un programme d'anamnèse assistée par ordinateur (AAO); il concernait les patients atteints de diabète sucré (2). L'analyse des résultats permit une riche moisson de données et suscita une réflexion de type pluridisciplinaire sur le contenu et la structure du dialogue patient-médecin. En 1971, le projet *"Anamnèse et enseignement médical assistés par ordinateur"* bénéficiait du patronage conjoint de l'Université de Liège et du Fonds de la Recherche Scientifique Médicale (FRSM). SIAM (Système Informatique d'Anamnèse Multilingue) - DOCEO II est entré dans sa phase opérationnelle en 1972, à la Policlinique médicale de l'Hôpital universitaire de Bavière (3).

2. OBJECTIF : SIAM-DOCEO II, DEUX SYSTEMES EN UN

2.1. Quoique différents par leur objet, l'anamnèse et l'enseignement offrent des similitudes fondamentales. Dans l'un et l'autre cas, le propos est de confier à un ordinateur pourvu de terminaux appropriés la tâche de simuler l'activité humaine dans un processus conversationnel. Ici et là, il s'agit de recueillir d'un interlocuteur (patient ou élève) des informations qu'il faut constamment confronter, par un traitement en temps réel, pour décider de la suite du dialogue. Enfin, en médecine comme en pédagogie, la considération du facteur humain constitue le premier et l'ultime point de référence : malades et étudiants doivent être traités dans le respect de leurs différences individuelles. C'est pourquoi SIAM-DOCEO II a été doté d'une souplesse maximale, son rôle, au demeurant, se limitant à fournir une aide au praticien dans l'exécution de tâches à caractère répétitif ou d'opérations logico-mathématiques parfois complexes.

2.2. L'adaptativité requise a pu être atteinte grâce à la mise au point d'un logiciel original, et notamment d'un Langage de programmation de Processus Conversationnels (LPC) accessible au non-informaticien, dont les diverses instructions ont été définies en fonction des besoins propres à la conduite d'un dialogue - didactique ou anamnestique - où se conjuguent les possibilités de l'informatique et de l'audiovisuel. En ce qui concerne le matériel, le système comprend un mini-ordinateur et un ensemble de terminaux audiovisuels conçus et réalisés au Laboratoire DOCEO (vidéo, projecteur et magnétocassette à accès aléatoire). En fin de séance, une imprimante délivre un protocole détaillé, de présentation normalisée, destiné au médecin ou au professeur, parfois aussi à l'élève.

3. APPLICATIONS

3.1. Anamnèse (SIAM)

On compte actuellement une dizaine de disciplines médicales pour lesquelles des programmes ont été élaborés. Nous en mentionnerons cinq, représentatifs de la diversité du projet AAO.

Le questionnaire de *diabétologie* vise avant tout à une collecte systématique de données anamnestiques auprès de diabétiques avérés qui se présentent pour la première fois à la consultation spécialisée de la Policlinique médicale. En *dermatologie*, un programme permet d'interroger les patients souffrant de psoriasis; il suggère en outre une classification des thérapeutiques les plus adéquates en fonction du cas clinique et offre la possibilité de procéder à des anamnèses complémentaires ultérieures(4). Le questionnaire destiné au bilan quadrimestriel des patients soumis à l'*hémodialyse* (rein artificiel) aborde les statuts clinique et social et explore tous les systèmes physiologiques (cardiovasculaire, respiratoire, nerveux etc.) puis fournit des propositions motivées de diagnostic différentiel et assure le suivi périodique de chaque patient (5). En *pneumologie*, le test de dépistage de la bronchite chronique, déjà utilisé sur des milliers de sujets de la région liégeoise, constitue l'instrument de base d'une vaste enquête épidémiologique, en cours depuis 1978 (6). Citons enfin le programme assurant la constitution en mode conversationnel du *dossier diététique*; grâce à la vitesse opératoire de l'ordinateur, il fournit, deux ou trois minutes après la fin de la collecte des données, outre un compte rendu détaillé des habitudes alimentaires du patient, un bilan nutritionnel extrêmement complet, qui exigerait deux ou trois heures de calculs à une diététicienne expérimentée.

Sauf pour le test de dépistage de la bronchite chronique - questionnaire simple et court-, c'est une auxiliaire médicale et non le malade qui effectue à la console les opérations de lecture des questions et de transmission des réponses : techniquement et psychologiquement, un intermédiaire humain paraît indispensable. Notons encore que, grâce à sa console audiovisuelle, le système SIAM permet un interrogatoire de patients non francophones.

3.2. Enseignement (DOCEO)

Sans parler de diverses applications qui ne relèvent pas du domaine médical, le projet DOCEO concerne différentes populations : patients, personnel paramédical, étudiants et médecins.

Ainsi, une série de leçons ont été élaborées pour l'*éducation des diabétiques insulinodépendants* (7). Elles ont trait à des matières qui relèvent essentiellement du domaine cognitif. Les exposés théoriques y sont toujours accompagnés de questions de contrôle et d'exercices qui sollicitent la déduction voire l'induction, plus que la mémorisation pure et simple. On prépare également des leçons destinées aux *patients soumis à l'hémodialyse à domicile*. Au niveau de l'enseignement supérieur paramédical, mentionnons la prochaine mise en oeuvre d'un cours multimédia où DOCEO interviendra dans l'*entraînement à la manipulation de l'appareil respiratoire d'Engström*. Enfin, un algorithme a été mis au point pour la conduite programmée de *travaux pratiques sur l'hyperglycémie provoquée par voie orale* : 24 cas ont été définis à partir de dossiers réels; le rôle de l'étudiant consiste à se prononcer sur les résultats de l'épreuve après avoir sollicité du système, avec un maximum de pertinence, des informations complémentaires relatives à l'anamnèse, l'examen clinique et les analyses biomédicales.

4. RESULTATS ET DISCUSSION

4.1. En AAO, chaque questionnaire porte sur un domaine défini et relativement limité : cette solution a permis d'éviter l'écueil d'une investigation superficielle et de moduler les méthodologies selon les besoins. Corollaire de cette option initiale : l'évidence de la responsabilité du médecin dans la synthèse d'une situation pathologique. Le mode conversationnel et programmé de collecte de données s'est révélé bénéfique à maints égards : fiabilité et homogénéité des informations recueillies, rigueur logique de l'interrogatoire, motivation des patients.

4.2. Pour des raisons d'ordre pratique et conjoncturel, l'exploitation du système DOCEO dans le domaine médical a été affectée d'un certain retard. Quoi qu'il en soit, les résultats acquis rejoignent les tendances qui se dégagent généralement des expériences d'EAO : gain cognitif important et forte réduction de la dispersion des résultats, motivation des sujets.

4.3. La mise au point des programmes s'est révélée des plus bénéfiques : en requérant des médecins et des enseignants une définition précise des objectifs et des concepts, elle les a amenés à cerner et à structurer un certain nombre de démarches traditionnellement attribuées à des processus exclusivement intuitifs.

5. CONCLUSIONS

SIAM-DOCEO II est un outil qui libère le praticien de tâches répétitives (parfois très complexes) et favorise ainsi la relation interpersonnelle. Les protocoles informatisés fournissent une grande quantité de données lisibles, fiables, homogènes, facilement exploitables pour des études séméiologiques et épidémiologiques. Méthodologiquement, l'expérience s'est révélée des plus fructueuses.

6. REFERENCES

(1) Houziaux MO. Les fonctions didactiques de DOCEO. XIIe Coll. Ass. Int. Péd. Exp. de Langue Française. Université de Caen. 1965 : 47 - 71.

(2) Lefèbvre P, Houziaux MO. Anamnèse assistée par ordinateur en diabétologie. Rev. Méd. de Liège. 1969; XXIV, 22 : 803 - 809.

(3) Houziaux MO. Le système d'anamnèse assistée par ordinateur de l'Université de Liège. Rev. Méd. de Liège. 1975;XXX, 16 : 528 -540.

(4) de la Brassinne M, Houziaux MO, Bartholomé M, Bianchi AR. Conversational Computer - Assisted Anamnesis for Classification and Treatment of Psoriasis. IIId Int. Symp. on Psoriasis, Stanford University. 1980. (Accepted for publication.)

(5) Bovy Ph, Houziaux MO, Mawet N, Rorive G. Computer-Assisted Anamnesis in Dialysed Patients. XVIIth Congress of the European Dialysis and Transplant Ass., Prague. 1980. Abstracts : 13.

(6) Bartsch P, Bartholomé M, Houziaux MO. Application du système d'anamnèse assistée par ordinateur "SIAM" au dépistage de la bronchite chronique. Rev. Méd. de Liège. 1978; XXXIII, 3: 91 - 98.

(7) Houziaux MO, Godart C, Scheen-Lavigne M, Bartholomé M, Luyckx A, Lefèbvre P. Une expérience d'enseignement assisté par ordinateur chez des patients diabétiques insulinodépendants. Scientia Paedagogica Experimentalis. 1978; XV, 2 : 215 - 250.

USE OF VIDEOTAPED RECORDINGS OF CONSULTATIONS IN TEACHING

Professor R. Harvard Davis, Department of General Practice, Welsh National School of Medicine, Cardiff, U.K.

Introduction

The clinical consultation is the central part of clinical method but it is difficult to teach the skills of the consultation. Traditional teaching of history taking tells the student what data should be collected but not how best to obtain it. The interviewing skills of experienced doctors in a number of specialties are defective and this results in consultations going wrong. Audiovisual recordings provide a unique means of studying the consultation process and can be used for teaching undergraduates the skills involved (1). This communication reports the results of studies which demonstrate that the technique can also be used in teaching young and experienced doctors in the field of primary care.

Method

Recordings of actual clinical consultations were made (2). A rating scale (the General Practitioner Interview Rating Scale) was devised to measure the interviewing skills displayed by doctors in the consultation (3). Inter-rater reliability (+0.87) and intra-rater reliability (+ 0.80) were obtained (Pearson Produce Moment Correlation Coefficient). The recordings were rated blind. 5 experienced General Practitioners and 9 young doctors in training for general practice had consultations recorded before and after receiving instruction in interviewing skills. Their scores on the rating scale were compared with those of a control group of 12 experienced general practitioners and 8 trainees.

Results

The experimental group of experienced general practitioners achieved significantly higher total scores on their final recordings (figure 1) and had higher scores than the control group on each of the variables in the rating scale. For six items the difference was significant. The experimental group of trainee general practitioners did not achieve the higher overall score within the control group after teaching, but separating the two groups into those in their first six months and those in their second six months of training showed a trend towards improvement in the latter (figure 2). They achieved higher scores on 16 out of 17 variables compared with the control group. The deterioration in both control and experimental groups in the first six months could be due to the traumatic effect of moving from hospital to primary care.

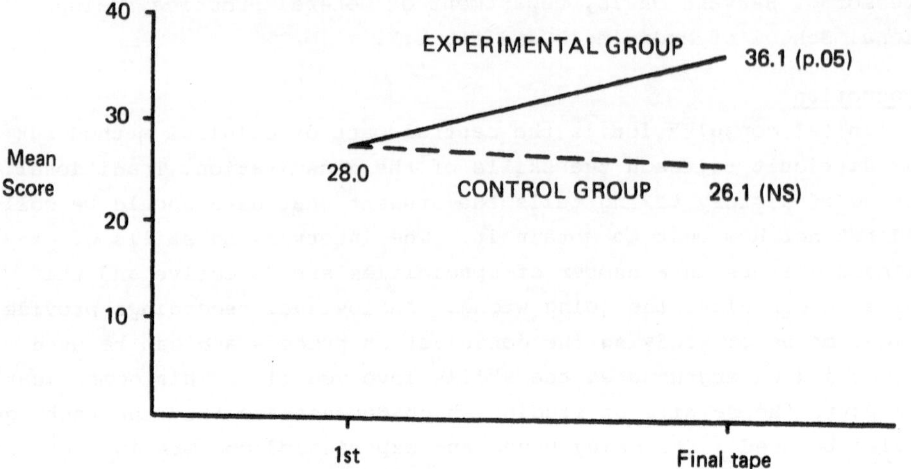

Figure 1. Experienced general practitioners. Mean scores of experimental and control groups before and after instruction.

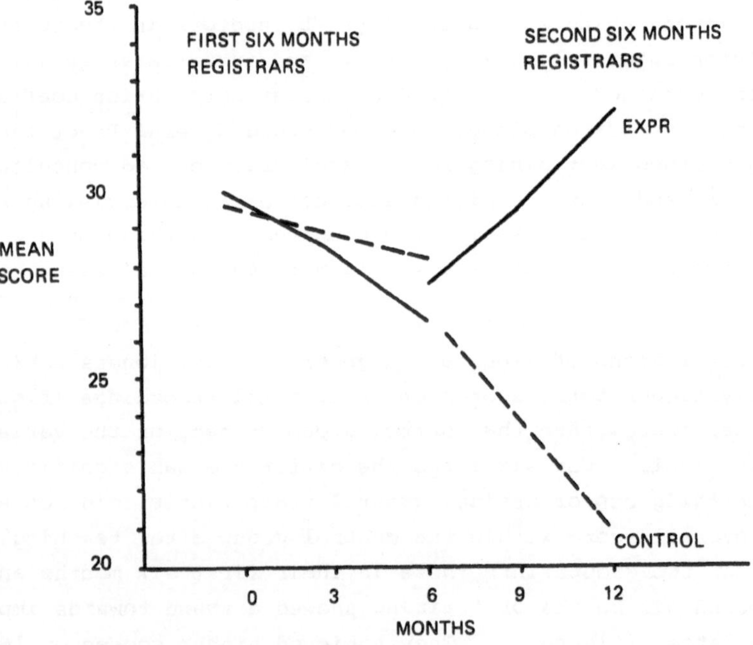

Figure 2. Trainee General Practitioners. A comparison of the mean scores during training.

Conclusions

The use of videotaped recordings of consultations is a valuable method of teaching interviewing skills in primary care. The use of this new teaching method has potential dangers which can be minimised by adherence to the following rules (4).

1. Newcomers to the technique should view their own tapes alone before being exposed to comment from others.
2. Any teacher using the technique must have had experience of having his own consultations recorded and reviewed by others.

Both these rules encourage acceptance of, and sensitise doctors to,the experience and encourage a positive supportive attitude.

3. Concentrate upon what is present in the recording, not upon what appears to be omitted.
4. The doctor whose tape is being recorded should initiate discussion because they readily identify their own faults and can often explain why.
5. Different groups have different needs. Stable groups meeting regularly are supportive, constructive and need less leadership. Ad hoc groups are less supportive, over-critical and over-defensive and need a leader to define aims and maintain control.

References

1. Maguire,G.P., Roc, P. Goldberg,D.P., Jones, S., Hyde, C.,O'Dowd,T., 'The value of feedback in teaching interviewing skills to medical students.' Psychological Medicine 1978, 8. 695-700.
2. Verby, J., Davis, R.H., Marshall, R.J., 'Television in General Practice'. J. Audiovis. Media in Med. 2. 56-58.
3. Verby, J., Holden, P., Davis, R.H., 1979. 'Peer review of consultations in Primary Care'. Brit. Med. J. 1979. 1. 1686-1688.
4. Davis, R.H., Jenkins, M., Smail, S.A., Stott, N.C.H., Verby, J., Wallace, B.B.,'Teaching with Audiovisual Recordings of Consultations' J. Roy. Coll. Gen. Practit. 1980. 30 333-336.

A COMPUTERIZED DATA ACQUISITION SYSTEM FOR MEDICAL GAMMA AND BETA SPECTROMETRY

H. Zeintl, R. Schosser, J. Seifert and K. Messmer

Institute for Surgical Research, University of Munich/FRG

INTRODUCTION

Gamma and beta spectrometry are frequently used in clinical chemistry (e.g. radioimmunoassays) and medical research (radionuclide tracer studies, microspheres etc.). The output data of a gamma or beta spectrometer is usually printed on a teletype or punched on paper tape. The analysis, however, is often performed on a computer. Therefore, the data has to be entered via a terminal keyboard or a paper tape reader. These manual activities are circumstantial, time consuming and error-prone, especially in case of several spectrometers. Therefore, a computerized system has been developed. It simultaneously records the output data of several spectrometers, evaluates the stored data and prints or plots the results.

METHODS

The automatic data acquisition system SANDRA consists of a PDP 11/03 microcomputer with two 0.5 MB floppy disk drives, a VT 100 console and a LA 36 printer with plot option. The SANDRA software package runs under the RT 11 V03B operating system. It is highly structured and subdivided into independent modules:

- dialog modules
- data recording modules
- evaluation modules.

The following types and numbers of spectrometers are currently connected to SANDRA:

- two multichannel gamma spectrometers (model 5921/5986, Packard Instrument Company, Inc.)
- one 3-channel gamma spectrometers (model 5375, Packard Instrument Company, Inc.)
- two 2-channel beta spectrometers (model 3255, Packard Instrument Company, Inc.)

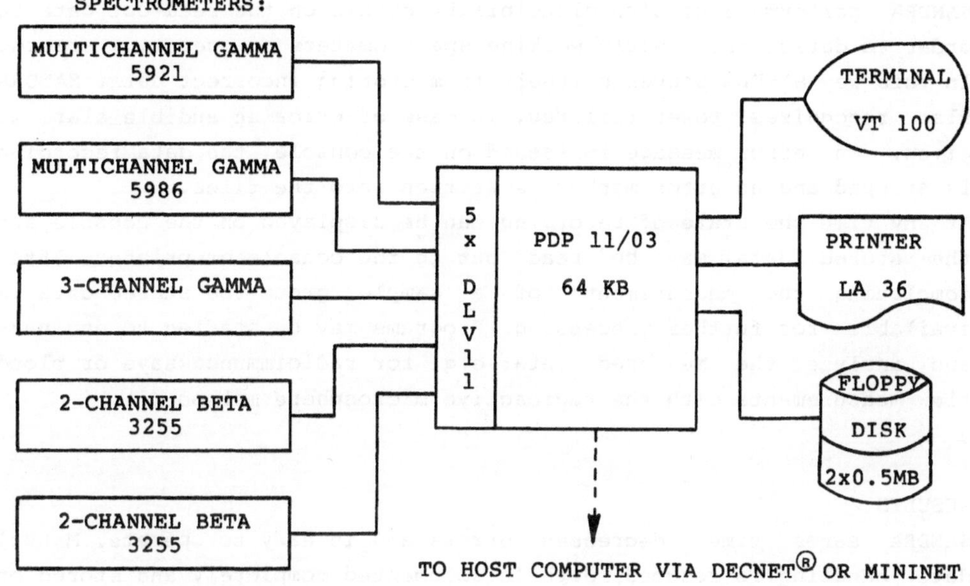

Figure 1 : Hardware configuration

After loading a spectrometer with a group of samples the operating modes and counting parameters are selected on the spectrometer and entered to the computer using a simple menu-oriented dialog on the console. In addition, comments on the measurement may be entered. After this opening dialog, SANDRA is ready to accept read-out data from the spectrometer and to store the data in a file on the floppy disk. Starting time and date of the measurement, entered comments and counting parameters are also stored in this file for documentation.

The content and format of the read-out data depend on the type of the spectrometer. The read-out data is generally composed of sample number, gross counts of each channel, net counts per minute, integral counts of each region of interest, energy of channels etc.. A data reduction is performed by SANDRA and normally only the counts per minute are stored in the file for further evaluation.

The background activity is measured and is automatically subtracted. Moreover a decay correction is done by SANDRA in case of radionuclides with a short half-life period (e.g. Iodine-131).

SANDRA performs extensive plausibility checks on the read-out data in order to detect incorrectly working spectrometers or operating errors. In this way SANDRA prevents itself from storing incorrect data. SANDRA also recognizes power failures. In case of error an audible alarm is given, an error message is issued on the console, the data recording is stopped and an error marker is written into the files.

At any time the state of recording can be displayed on the console and the stored data may be read out to the console or printer. After completing the measurements of a sample group the stored data is available for further processing. Programs may be started to evaluate and analyze the measured data: e.g. for radioimmunoassays or blood flow measurements with the radioactive microsphere method (1).

RESULTS

SANDRA saves time, decreases errors and is easy to operate. Manual data handling is reduced, data is documented completely and stored on a low cost floppy disk. With the data on the floppy disk, there are several possibilities for further processing by the computer. Due to the modular construction of the software package, SANDRA can be easily adapted to any spectrometer with a serial RS-232-C-Interface. In this case only the read-in module has to be changed.

CONCLUSIONS

The above described system SANDRA improves data acquisition, evaluation and documentation in medical gamma and beta spectrometry. The software is implemented in FORTRAN IV and uses about 45 KB memory. The hardware (PDP 11/03, floppy disk system, video terminal and printer) costs about $ 26000. SANDRA can be connected to a host computer via a serial link using commercial available software (DECNET® or MININET). Thus the data can be stored on the hosts data base and may be processed by larger evaluation programs.

REFERENCES

(1) Schosser, R., K.-E. Arfors and K. Messmer:
MIC-II - A program for the determination of cardiac output, arterio-venous shunt and regional blood flow using the radioactive microsphere method.
Comput. Programs Biomed. 9 (1979) 19-38.

A NOT LINEAR DISCRIMINATING METHOD GIVING BY A STUDY OF SERUM PROTEINS AN OBJECTIVE SUPPORT TO MEDICAL DIAGNOSTICS

G. SANDOR
Institut Pasteur
25, Rue du Docteur Roux
75015 PARIS

Y. LECHEVALLIER
I N R I A
Domaine de Voluceau
78150 LE CHESNAY

In order to obtain an informatic technic simple enough to give diagnosis in current clinical examination, we studied 5 serum proteins only, those having the maximal informative values, and discriminating increments of finite value were taken into account.

The following serum proteins where studied : albumin, orosomucoid, IgG, IgM, IgA.

A reproducible simple radial immunodiffusion technique was elaborated. The reference population composed by about 20. 000 university students had, itself, an internal variance of less than 0,1 %. A constant reference line allowed the calculation of concentrations in unknown samples thanks to an absolute dilution law (8)(5). Data concerning about 5 000 patients made access to statistical calculations for all common diseases of our countries.

The computer program was obtained by a two step mathematical evaluation : a) calculation of the most discriminating increments for the 5 variables taken individually ; b) calculation of the most discriminating combinations between the 5 variables by consideration of the concentration's domains established in the first step (2)(4).

The most discriminating increments were established by an adaptation to our problem of a method primitively proposed by Fisher (1). The computer program allows to find out the best cutting in domains when maximal Khi 2 values are obtained. Albumin and orosomucoid were cutted in 4 domains, IgM in 5, IgG and IgA in 6 (table 1).

DISCRIMINATING DOMAINS

	code number	symbols	albumin	orosomucoid	IgG	IgM	IgA
Strongly decreased	1	↓↓	<55,5		<44		<0,5
Moderately decreased	2	↓	55,5-73	<60	44-59	<42	0,5-55
Normal	3	→	>73	60-131	59-107	42-157	55-145
Moderately increased	4	↑		131-193	107-135	157-259	145-205
Strongly increased	5	↑↑		>193	135-208	259-525	205-530
Very strongly increased	6	↑↑↑			>208	>525	>530

Values in relative concentration percent.

For the calculation of the most discriminating combinations between the 5 variables, we begin by establishing a hierarchy amoung our 5 proteins according to their informative content. The proteins were arranged in order of decreasing informative content as follows ; albumin, orosomucoid, IgG, IgM, IgA. The following computer program allowed to range the patients' profiles in a matrice : Beginning with domain 1 for all 5 variables, we increased, at first, the domain numbers of IgA only. In the second step we increased also IgM domain numbers by associating to all 5 domains of IgM, taken in an increasing order, all 6 domains of IgA, taken as well in an increasing order. The same calculations were extended therefore to IgG, lastly to orosomucoid. Once albumin reached, we started again with isolated IgA increases, but all values were associeted now to albumin domain 2. The same process was repeated with domain 3 and lastly with domain 4 of albumin.

Similar profiles were now gathered together on the matrice and in order to obtain our informative groups, they were separated one from another by manual screening :

Groups	Albumin	Oroso-mucoid	IgG	IgM	IgA	Medical diagnosis
1	→	→	→ to ↑	→ to ↑	→ to ↑	Healthy persons atopic diseases benignant dermatoses
2	→ to ↓↓	→ to ↑↑	→ to ↑	→ to ↑	→ to ↑	Inflammatory processes without liver lesion nor immune attack (going from urticaria to generalized peritonitis.
3	↓ to ↓↓	→	→ to ↑	→ to ↑	→ to ↑	Isolated albumin decrease due either to an affected general status, or to an increase of protein catabolism (degenerative central nervous system diseases thyrotoxicosis).
4	→ to ↓↓	→ to ↑↑	↑↑ to ↑↑↑	→ to ↑↑	→ to ↑↑	Prevailing immune processes (collagenoses, extended suppurations).
5	↓↓	↓ to ↑	↑ to ↑↑↑	→ to ↑↑↑	→ to ↑↑↑	Chronical liver diseases.
6	→ to ↓	→ to ↓	→ to ↑↑	↑↑ to ↑↑↑	→ to ↑	Viral hepatitis
7	→ to ↓↓	→ to ↑↑	↑ to ↑↑	↑↑↑	→ to ↑	Polyclonal macroglobulinemia: tropical splenomegaly sleeping sickness.

Groups	Alb.	Oro.	IgG	IgM	IgA	
8	→ to ↓	↓ to ↑↑	↓ to ↓↓	↓ to ↓↓	↓ to ↓↓	Deficiency of immunoglobulin synthesis (agammaglobulinemia, chronical lymphocity leukemia)
9	↓↓	↓ to ↑↑	↓↓	→ to ↑↑	↓ to →	Extravascular loss of serum proteins (lipoid nephrosis exsudative enterites)
10	→ to ↓↓	→ to ↑↑	→ to ↑↑	→ to ↑↑	↓↓	Isolated IgA decrease. Ataxia telangiectasia; sporadic essential cases with recurrent infections for some of them
11_A	→ to ↓↓	→ to ↑↑	↑↑ to ↑↑↑	↓ to ↓↓	↓ to ↓↓	Monoclonal dysglobulinemias: IgG myeloma
11_B	→ to ↓↓	→ to ↑↑	↓ to ↓↓	↓ to ↓↓	↑↑ to ↑↑↑	Monoclonal dysglobulinemias : IgA myeloma
11_C	→ to ↓↓	→ to ↑↑	↓ to ↓↓	↑↑↑	↓ to ↓↓	Monoclonal dysglobulinemias : Waldenstroem's macroglobulinemia

For medical diagnosis purposes we may distinguish among several eventualities. Our serum protein study may have a pronostical meaning. The group 1, for instance, may help in a general health screening. Our study may evidence patho-physiological processes. Group 2, for instance, is characteristic for inflammatory lesions. Important and protracted immune processes are revealed further by group 4. Impairement of a given organ may be disclosed. This is the case for group 5 gathering together chronical liver diseases. Lastly a precise diagnosis also may be established. Group 6, for instance, is characteristic for viral hepatitis. Monoclonal dysglobulinemias as well present pathognomonic features (Group 11).

(1) W.D. FISHER : On grouping for maximum homogeneity. J. Amer. Statistical Assoc. 1958. 53. 789-798.

(2) Y. LECHEVALLIER : Classification automatique optimale sous contrainte d'ordre total. Rapport Laboria N° 200. 1977.

(3) G. SANDOR : Sémiologie biologique des protéines sériques. Edit. : Maloine, Paris, 1975.

(4) G. SANDOR, Y. LECHEVALLIER : Définition d'une grille de diagnostic tirée de l'étude des protéines sériques. Colloque IRIA. Analyse des Données. Versailles 1978.

(5) G. SANDOR, D. LODS, R. KERDILES; A. MAUROIS : Proposition d'un sérum de référence pour le dosage immunochimiques des protéines sériques. C.R.A.S. 1975, 281 D. 329-331.

Author Index